P9-DUU-323
02489270

k

Managed Care

NANDA Nursing Diagnoses and NIC Interventions

Practice Standards

Sexuality

Substance Abuse

Violence and Human Abuse

COMPREHENSIVE COMMUNITY HEALTH NURSING

Family, Aggregate, & Community Practice

RT

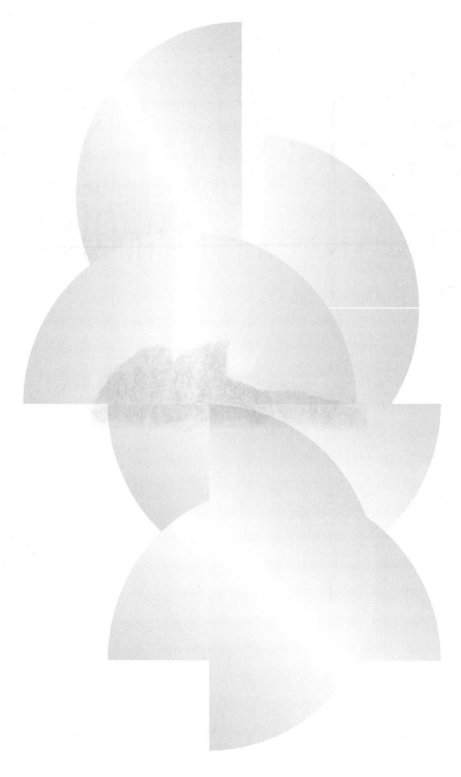

The logo for the book, interconnecting systems and subsystems, emphasizes a major focus in community health nursing practice—helping clients bring together in a meaningful way all the forces in their environment that influence their health and quality of life. Clients served by community health nurses, including individuals, families, aggregates at risk, and communities, often encounter environmental forces that impede growth. Community health nurses are uniquely positioned to help clients understand these forces and to mobilize coping strategies aimed at developing healthy, nurturing environments.

OKANAGAN UNIVERSITY COLLEGE
LIBRARY
BRITISH COLUMBIA

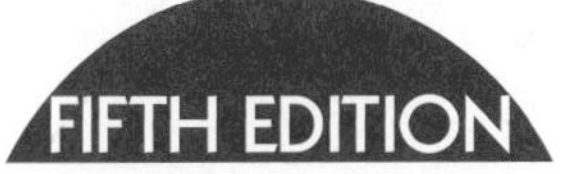

COMPREHENSIVE COMMUNITY HEALTH NURSING

Family, Aggregate, & Community Practice

Susan Clemen-Stone, RN, MPH
Associate Professor
Community Health Nursing
Division of Health Promotion
and Risk Reduction Programs
School of Nursing
University of Michigan
Ann Arbor, Michigan

Sandra L. McGuire, RN, EdD
Associate Professor
College of Nursing
University of Tennesee-Knoxville
Knoxville, Tennesee

Diane Gerber Eigsti, RN, MS
Assistant Professor
Department of Nursing
Miami University
Oxford, Ohio

with contributions by **Ella M. Brooks,** RN, PhD
Health Care Consultant
Brookings, South Dakota

with 177 illustrations

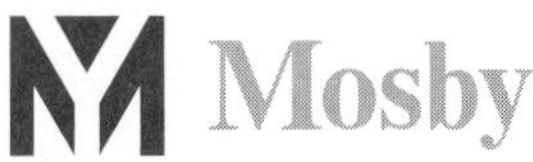

St. Louis Baltimore Boston Carlsbad Chicago Naples New York Philadelphia Portland
London Madrid Mexico City Singapore Sydney Tokyo Toronto Wiesbaden

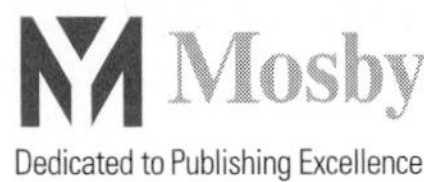

A Times Mirror Company

Publisher Nancy L. Coon
Editor Loren S. Wilson
Develomental Editor Brian Dennison
Project Manager Dana Peick
Project Specialist Catherine Albright
Designer Amy Buxton
Manufacturing Supervisor Karen Boehme
Cover Elizabeth Rohne Rudder

FIFTH EDITION
Copyright © 1998 by Mosby, Inc.
Previous editions copyrighted 1995, 1991, 1987, 1981

All rights reserved. No part of this publication may be reproduced, stored in a retrieval system, or transmitted, in any form or by any means, electronic, mechanical, photocopying, recording, or otherwise, without written permission of the publisher.

Permission to photocopy or reproduce solely for internal or personal use is permitted for libraries or other users registered with the Copyright Clearance Center, provided that the base fee of $4.00 per chapter plus $.10 per page is paid directly to the Copyright Clearance Center, 222 Rosewood Drive, Danvers, MA, 01923. This consent does not extend to other kinds of copying, such as copying for general distribution, for advertising or promotional purposes, for creating new collected works, or for resale.

Printed in the United States of America
Composition by Graphic World
Printing/binding by World Color

Mosby-Year Book, Inc.
11830 Westline Industrial Drive
St. Louis, Missouri 63146

Library of Congress Cataloging-in-Publication Data

Clemen–Stone, Susan.
Comprehensive community health nursing
p. cm.
Includes bibliographical references and index.
ISBN 0–8151–1324–2 (alk. paper)
1. Community health nursing. 2. Family—Health and hygiene.
3. Community health nursing—United States. I. McGuire, Sandra L.
II. Eigsti, Diane Gerber.
[DNLM: 1. Community Health Nursing. 2. Family Health. WY 106
C6255c 1998]
RT98.C56 1998
362.1'73—dc21
DNLM/DLC
for Library of Congress 97–35023
CIP

97 98 99 00 01/9 8 7 6 5 4 3 2 1

To Our Significant Others

Verna and Al J. Clemen, for their special love that promoted growth and family cohesiveness, and for encouraging and supporting independent thinking even when this was not the norm.

John and Sharon Clemen and **Sara and Henry Parks,** for their caring, friendship, and encouragement.

Denver Stone, for his love, unfailing support, and knowing just the right time to assist.

Teresa and Rick Stone, for their patience and understanding.

Holly Marie Huling, for bringing the joys of childhood into our life and for her loving ways.

To the memory of **Ike.**

Heiki-Lara Eigsti Nyce and Inge-Marie Eigsti, along with **Mark** and **Jim,** for their patience and loving.

John E. Gerber, for the joy he has brought.

Joseph, Kelly, and Kerry McGuire, and **Matthew Currin,** for their love, support, and encouragement.

Donald and Mary Lue Johnson, for their pride in this publication, their continued encouragement, and their love and interest.

Arthur and Sally Johnson, for the belief they instilled in the value of education, the role modeling they provided, and their constant love.

Judy Simpson, for her continued faith in and support of the nursing profession.

Alma Weale, for recognizing the importance of this publication and her unfailing encouragement.

Preface

The first edition of *Comprehensive Community Health Nursing: Family, Aggregate, and Community Practice* was published in 1981 to generate excitement about population and community-focused nursing practice as well as individual- and family-oriented care. It was obvious at that time that multiple societal and health care trends would significantly increase the opportunities and challenges for nurses in the community setting. The 1980s and 1990s were indeed characterized by major changes that have reshaped and expanded community health nursing practice. Clearly, health care delivery is shifting from the acute care setting to the community. Unprecedented needs in the community setting will require the development of new and innovative interventions for promoting health and preventing disease. Community health nursing's rich heritage in the community setting places this nursing specialty at a competitive advantage for stimulating innovation in practice.

As we approach the year 2000, community health nurses are uniquely poised to provide dynamic leadership in a health care system characterized by continuous and overlapping change. The emphasis in health care during the 1990s has moved from a national, holistic focus on health care reform to an era of rapidly evolving integrated managed care systems competing for public and private monies. These systems are designed to provide cost-effective, quality care for individuals and families. The future challenge for community health professionals will be to mobilize the resources necessary to meet the needs of populations at risk as well as individuals and families. Community health nurses have a strong background for mobilizing community resources and using them to address the needs of diverse client groups. They are also well grounded in their understanding of how to help clients move effectively across the health care continuum.

The mission in the future will be to build healthy, healing communities that provide access to health care for all. To assist practitioners to achieve this vision, the fifth edition of this text continues to provide a comprehensive foundation for community health nursing practice, including evolving approaches for addressing contemporary health issues. The educational preparation that makes community health nursing unique is its emphasis on community-oriented, population-focused practice from an interdisciplinary perspective.

THE FIFTH EDITION

Although the fifth edition of this book adheres to the original purposes of previous editions, a careful attempt has been made in the current edition to reflect the significant changes that have occurred within the field during the 1990s. As originally designed, this text was presented to help students and practitioners gain an understanding of the distinguishing features of community health nursing practice and the challenging nature of a specialty field committed to meeting the needs of vulnerable populations. The fifth edition speaks to the increasing challenges community health professionals will face as they strive to achieve health for all in the twenty-first century. It addresses the need to maintain a strong public health infrastructure to ensure access to care during a time of dwindling health care resources. Expanded discussion of the core public health functions of assessment, assurance, and policy development has been included. The advantages of broad-based coalitions at all levels of government that work in partnership with communities are highlighted.

Extensive revision in the book enriches its usefulness for students and practitioners. The role managed care plays in promoting the public's health is carefully explored. The opportunities as well as the challenges for the community health nurse in a managed care environment are identified. Expanded discussion on care management will help strengthen students' understanding of the pivotal role community health nurses play in helping populations in need access essential health care services. A creative partnership between a public health agency and a managed care organization, designed to address health care access disparities, is shared.

The profession is faced with unprecedented societal and health care changes that are significantly influencing client need and community health nursing practice. A new chapter, 12, Aggregate-Focused Contemporary Community Health Issues, has been added to present a more thoroughly developed discussion of aggregate-focused, contemporary community health issues. This chapter addresses the health disparities among minority populations; health risks associated with poverty, homelessness, and substance abuse; sexually transmitted diseases, HIV/AIDS; and violent and abusive behavior. Neglected public health mandates are highlighted throughout the text. Expanded content on infectious disease prevention and control in Chapter 11, Concepts of Epidemiology: Infectious and Chronic Conditions, and disaster management in Chapter 6, Environmental Health and Disaster Nursing, will help students gain an increased understanding of the multiple determinants of health and contemporary environmental health issues.

Nurses share with all health care professionals the need to examine carefully the delivery of their services in light of changing societal demands. Health care providers will face several critical challenges during the twenty-first century as they strive to maintain quality in health care delivery. They will need to become more accountable to those who purchase and use health services and more focused on demonstrating that they can provide cost-effective care that is measurable. Expanded content on nursing interventions and an increased focus on outcome assessment throughout the text will help students identify and evaluate appropriate community health nursing outcomes.

It is envisioned that a much stronger emphasis will be placed on providing preventive health services in the coming century. Several new tables have been added, most notably in Chapter 12 and Chapter 17, Health Promotion Concerns of Adult Men and Women, to help students identify relevant primary, secondary, and tertiary preventive interventions for combating contemporary health issues. It is also envisioned that the need for home health care and long-term care will significantly increase in the future. Discussion related to this need has been strengthened throughout, particularly in Chapter 21, Clients with Long-Term Care Needs: Home Health, Hospice, and Other Services. Trends are well documented by current literature throughout the text. Extensive information about where community health nurses can obtain up-to-date statistical data related to the health needs of at-risk aggregates, with resources that assist them in meeting community health needs, has been significantly updated.

Organization

The overall acceptance of the past four editions of this book have challenged us to preserve the basic framework of the original text while extensively revising the content to reflect the dynamic changes in health care service delivery. The framework for this text stems from the philosophy of community and public health nursing practice delineated in the definitions of the American Nurses Association and the American Public Health Association. These philosophies articulate the need for community health nurses to understand the environment in which they are functioning. They also address the unique orientation that community health nurses bring to any health care team: a holistic approach to promoting and protecting the health of individuals, families, and populations at risk from a community perspective. The two major parts of this book explore the unique role of the community health nurse from this perspective.

Part One presents a philosophical foundation for nursing practice in the community. It analyzes the origin, scope, and changing nature of community health nursing practice and examines community dynamics and societal and health care trends that influence the delivery of health, welfare, and environmental services. The emphasis is on the direct service functions of the community health nurse within the context of change and diversity. In Part One the reader is helped to analyze the concept of client from four perspectives—individual, family, populations at risk, and community—with a focus on providing culturally competent care. Special attention is placed on analyzing how the community health nurse uses the family-focused nursing process in collaboration with clients to implement and evaluate client-centered interventions.

Part Two stresses the value of working with aggregates at risk in the community. The needs of population groups across the life span are examined, and interventions for addressing these needs are presented. The importance of using the *Healthy People 2000* objectives to guide community assessment processes is articulated. The epidemiological process is presented as a tool for studying the determinants of health and disease frequencies in populations and for analyzing contemporary health issues. The emphasis is on using a partnership approach to health planning to build healthy, nurturing communities. In Part Two the reader is helped to gain an understanding of the role of the community health nurse in a variety of community settings such as schools, nursing centers, parishes, clinics, and work sites and how these settings provide important vehicles for reaching specific population groups. An increasing number of driving forces, including altered demographics, an emerging global and knowledge economy, technological innovation, growing consumer expectations, and emerging threats to to the health of our society, are influencing the competencies needed by practitioners to provide population-based care in the twenty-first century. The implications of these driving forces for nursing and skills needed by future health care providers are highlighted in Part Two. There is no question about the need for future practitioners to have strong critical thinking skills, effective communication capabilities, cultural skills, political competencies, business management and leadership skills, and lifelong learning skills. There is also no question about the increasing need to consider the ethical dimensions of practice and the importance of documenting the effectiveness of nursing interventions. Part Two reflects a strong future perspective.

Pedagogical Features

Comprehensive Community Health Nursing: Family, Aggregate, and Community Practice provides a foundation for discussion, dialogue, debate, and action both in the classroom and clinical setting. It was built on the belief that learning is a dynamic, collaborative process where students, faculty, and practitioners learn together. This book is designed to serve as a stimulus for bringing together the resources needed to address current and future health issues. It is envisioned that the classroom setting will serve as an environment where students can critically think about real-life client situations and clinical practice issues in the community setting. Several teaching/learning features of this text will prepare students for this type of classroom experience. *Objectives* are included at the beginning of each chapter to focus students' attention on the critical concepts needed to formulate guidelines for effective family- and population-based nursing interventions. Color illustrations and boxes throughout the text help students to quickly identify significant concepts, content, and nursing interventions. Careful attention was given to defining key concepts to facilitate students' understanding of them.

Six features of the book will help students obtain a *realistic perspective* of nursing care in the community setting. *A View from the Field* boxes enable the reader to understand community health nursing practice from the perspective of an experienced practitioner or client. These boxes help the student to examine the scope and exciting nature of nursing practice in the community setting, workload management issues, and client perceptions of health care delivery. Numerous *Case Scenarios* developed from clinical situations assist students to examine client needs and to apply theoretical concepts. *An Exercise in Critical Thinking* at the end of each chapter help students to think critically about client situations or the concepts covered in the text. These exercises reflect current issues encountered in the practice setting and encourage discussion and debate. The *Teaching Tips* boxes in Part Two help students to identify client learning needs and provide resources for facilitating the teaching process. The *Appendixes* provide valuable assessment tools and data that enhance students' abilities to use the nursing process with diverse client groups. Both the extensive *References* and *Selected Bibliography* provide historic and future information that aids students to gain a practical view of community health nursing practice. Several of these references encourage the student to challenge "what is" and dream about "what can be." These references can be used to promote lively debate in the classroom setting. The teaching/learning features of this text were designed to foster an *interactive approach* between faculty and students.

Revisions to the *Instructor's Resource Manual* will also assist educators to promote an interactive style of learning. The *Manual* highlights key concepts covered in each chapter and provides learning activities that promote critical thinking. Teaching aids for faculty are shared in the manual, including Class Preparation Resources, Learning Activities, Transparency Masters, and a Test Bank of approximately 800 questions.

ACKNOWLEDGMENTS

The authors are greatly indebted to family, friends, colleagues, students, and former faculty and associates for their support, guidance, and assistance as we revised this book. Special appreciation is extended to the following individuals:

- Beverly Smith, our administrative secretary and a special friend, whose painstaking efforts, patience, and dedication to our project made it a reality. This book could never have been published without her help.
- Bill Smith, whose "it only takes a little more to do it right" encouragement, as we began this process almost twenty years ago, provided the impetus to move forward. His willingness to share his wife's time will never be forgottten.
- Ella Brooks, who contributed two chapters to the fifth edition and who freely shared of her time to research the literature and critique the book.
- Roberta Asplund, Elizabeth Beach, Shu-Chen Chang, Marilyn Franecki, and Mo Qu, for their invaluable assistance with resesarch of the literature.
- Henry Parks, for helping us with our artwork and photography.
- Denver Stone, who willingly devoted considerable time to the tedious aspects of the manuscript preparation process. His commitment to quality was an inspiration to all of us.
- The reviewers of the book, who provided significant direction for the fifth edition revision.
- Colleagues from the service setting who have shared with us materials their staffs developed to facilitate the delivery of quality client services.
- Publishers and authors who graciously granted us permission to use information from their writings.
- The Mosby staff, especially Loren Wilson, Brian Dennison, Dana Peick, Catherine Albright, Cindy Deichmann, and Amy Buxton for their support, understanding, and concrete assistance.
- All our friends and family members who "understood" and allowed us to postpone events and activities.

Susan Clemen-Stone
Sandra L. McGuire
Diane Gerber Eigsti

A Note to the Student

Managed care. Health promotion. Populations at risk. These are words you hear quite frequently as you discuss the future of health care in courses throughout your nursing curriculum. Health care is changing. An increasing number of individuals, families, and groups will be treated in community settings as opposed to acute care settings.

What does this mean for you, the student nurse?

How can you prepare to meet the needs of clients in a changing health care environment?

How will you make a positive difference in the lives of people?

Are you ready?

Comprehensive Community Health Nursing: Family, Aggregate, and Community Practice is designed to equip you with a complete foundation for community health nursing practice and strategies for approaching contemporary community health nursing issues such as homelessness, teen pregnancy, substance abuse, and sexually transmitted diseases.

In this new fifth edition, we have included several features designed specifically to help you master the content more quickly and enjoyably.

Objectives are included at the beginning of each chapter and are designed to focus your attention on critical concepts.

A View from the Field boxes provide you with first-hand insight on chapter content from practicing community health nurses and their clients.

Case Scenarios clearly illustrate concepts with realistic examples.

An Exercise in Critical Thinking at the end of the chapter will encourage you to give deeper thought to concepts covered in the chapter.

Teaching Tips provide you with resources you need to direct clients toward healthy behaviors.

Appendixes provide you with assessment tools used by practitioners and important resource information.

References and **Selected Bibliography** for each chapter will provide you with additional reading opportunities and a starting point for further research.

Our hope is that this text will serve as a useful resource as you face the health care challenges that lie ahead, and that it opens the door to many career opportunities in the community setting. Best of luck in your chosen profession!

Susan Clemen-Stone
Sandra L. McGuire
Diane Gerber Eigsti

Brief Contents

UNIT SIX

Management of Professional Commitments

Appendixes

Contents

Appendixes

COMPREHENSIVE COMMUNITY HEALTH NURSING

Family, Aggregate, & Community Practice

PART ONE

A Foundation for Community Health Nursing Practice

Public health nurses have been leaders in improving the quality of health care for people since the late 1800s. They have been the vanguard of change for both the nursing profession and society as a whole, stressing the importance of establishing standards for nursing practice and education and of social reform to improve the quality of life for all individuals. Culturally sensitive, community-focused practice with an emphasis on addressing the needs of aggregates at risk and family-centered nursing care emerged as key principles in the specialty field of community health.

Our early leaders were role models for effective change. They dealt with community dynamics and worked to influence legislative processes that shape the direction of health, welfare, and environmental systems at all levels of government. Using multiple intervention strategies, they worked with communities as partners to promote health and prevent disease.

Our heritage involves over a century of caring—caring for communities, aggregates, and families. To continue the progress made by their early leaders, community health nurses must understand where and how their specialty began, the nature of current community health nursing practice, and how community forces contribute to or distract from the health of families and aggregates at risk. Part One presents the theoretical concepts essential for understanding these aspects of community health nursing practice. The *Healthy People 2000* mandate guides analysis of current health issues in the United States as well as needed health care reform. The organization of our evolving health, welfare, and environmental systems is discussed within the context of needed health care reform. The challenges are great. The opportunities to promote the health of communities are endless.

1

Historical Perspectives on Community Health Nursing

Objectives

Upon completion of this chapter, the reader should be able to:

1. Discuss the development of public health nursing in the United States.
2. Discuss how historical events have shaped the development of public health, nursing, public health nursing, and community health nursing.
3. Analyze the contributions of Florence Nightingale, Lillian Wald, and Mary Breckinridge to public health nursing.
4. Summarize historical events that influenced beliefs about educational preparation for community health nursing practice.
5. Analyze the development of a consciousness for the public's health.

Histories make [wo]men wise.

FRANCIS BACON

In 1993 public health nurses across the United States celebrated "A Century of Caring" (Division of Nursing, 1992). That year nurses and the American public celebrated public health nursing's first century of service and recognized the accomplishments of early public health nurses and their leaders, among them Lillian Wald, a brilliant political and social activist and the founder of public health nursing; Mary Breckinridge, a staunch advocate for children's health and founder of the Frontier Nursing Service; Mary Sewall Gardner, author of the first public health nursing textbook; and Lavinia Lloyd Dock, who devoted herself to helping women gain the right to vote. Today's nurses should be proud of such early public health nursing leaders! They are heroines and role models for persons committed to nursing, health care, and humanity. From the origins of public health nursing with Lillian Wald in 1893 to today, its practice represents a strong tradition of caring for communities, aggregates, and families! Public health nursing in the United States has a strong and proud history (see the box on the following page).

Historically, public health nurses have held a basic belief in human dignity, extended nursing care beyond the physical concerns of patients, recognized that illness could be prevented with health teaching, and realized that family and community contributed to a patient's illness and recovery. Community health nursing today is a culmination of the work that extraordinary women and men accomplished over a great many years. To better understand the development and evolution of contemporary community health nursing it is important to examine significant historical events. Examining history helps us to understand how public health nursing evolved and responded to societal needs.

IN THE BEGINNING

Nursing began when humanity began.

> The word nurse is a reduced form of the Middle English *nurice*, which was derived, through the old French *norrice*, from the Latin *nutricius* (nourishing). In Roman mythology, the Goddess Fortuna, in addition to her usual function as goddess of fate, was also worshipped as Jupiter's nurse (Fortuna Praeneste) and prayed to for hygiene in the public baths (Fortuna Balnearis). The earliest evidence in the prehistoric record shows that people sought to acquire a knowledge of pain-relieving remedies and to discover additional means of preventing disease. Nursing roles also developed in the desire to alleviate human suffering (Kalisch, Kalisch, 1995, p. 1).

Visiting nursing, or the care of ill people at home by a specialized group, has existed through the ages. Early deaconesses of the church were motivated by love and charity to care and comfort the sick poor. The New Testament is replete with stories of how the sick were visited. The Apostle Paul wrote of Phoebe in Rom. 16:1-2, "I commend to you our sister Phoebe, a deaconess of the church at

A Century of Caring (1893-1993) and Beyond: Select Events

1893 Lillian Wald founds the Henry Street Settlement in New York City
1895 Ada Mayo Stewart becomes the first industrial nurse
1898 Nurses' Settlement established in San Francisco
1900 Nurses' Settlement established in Richmond, Virginia
1902 Lina Rogers, working with the Henry Street Settlement, becomes the first school nurse
1909 Metropolitan Life hires public health nurses
1910 Public Health Nursing program at Teacher's College, Columbia University is started
1912 National Organization for Public Health Nursing (NOPHN) is established
Red Cross Rural Nursing Service is established
Children's Bureau is established
1916 Mary Sewall Gardner writes *Public Health Nursing*
1925 Mary Breckinridge founds the Frontier Nursing Service in Kentucky
1933 Pearl McIver appointed to USPHS as a public health nursing analyst
1942 American Association of Industrial Nurses established (later becomes American Association of Occupational Health Nurses)
1952 NOPHN becomes the National League for Nursing
1953 The journal *Nursing Outlook* begins publication (journal has a community health nursing focus)
1963 Public health nursing content required as part of baccalaureate nursing programs
1973 American Nurses Association (ANA) publishes *Standards of Community Health Nursing Practice*
1980 ANA and APHA develop definitions for practice in community health/public health nursing
1984 National Consensus Conference On the Essentials of Public Health Nursing Practice and Education was held
1986 National Center for Nursing Research established
ANA revises *Standards of Community Health Nursing Practice* and develops *Standards for Home Health Nursing Practice*
1988 Institute of Medicine publishes *The Future of Public Health*
1989 National Consensus Conference On the Educational Preparation of Home Care Administrators was held
1990 Association of Community Health Nursing Educators (ACHNE) publishes *Essentials of Baccalaureate Nursing Education for Entry Level Community Health Nursing Practice*
1991 ACHNE publishes *Essentials of Master's Level Nursing Education for Advanced Community Health Nursing Practice*
1992 ACHNE publishes *Essentials of Research Priorities for Community Health Nursing*
1993 National Center for Nursing Research becomes the National Institute for Nursing Research. Community-based practice is part of the nursing research agenda.
ACHNE publishes *Essentials of Differentiated Practice in Community Health*
1995 ACHNE publishes *Essentials of Community/Public Health Advanced Practice Nurse (C/PHAPN) Position Statement*
1996 APHA Public Health Nursing Section adopts a revised position statement on the *Definition and Role of Public Health Nursing*

Cenchreae . . . help her in whatever she may require from you, for she has been a helper of many and of myself as well." Phoebe is probably the first visiting nurse we know by name. The true ancestors of the modern nurse were noble deaconesses and early Christian women who were trying to do for their day what the nurse of today is doing for hers (Gardner, 1916, p. 3).

During the Middle Ages (500-1500 AD) epidemics of infectious diseases such as syphilis, scarlet fever, smallpox, influenza, and leprosy periodically swept civilization. The bubonic plague, or "Black Death," epidemic of 540 AD had an estimated death toll of 100 million, and some 800 years later it would claim a death toll of more than 60 million people (Kalisch, Kalisch, 1995, p. 12). Numerous factors added to the problem of infectious disease morbidity and mortality. Refuse was allowed to accumulate in streets and dwellings, human waste was dumped into public water supplies, and foods were often improperly stored and prepared. Personal hygiene was often neglected, and "to take a bath was to confess oneself ill" (Brainard, 1922, p. 29). There was practically no organized care of the sick in their homes (Brainard, p. 18). Superstition and folk medicine dominated health practices.

Throughout the Middle Ages monasteries and convents were erected in all parts of the world, and hospitals were often connected with them (Brainard, 1922, p. 16). Some religious orders existed primarily to provide nursing care to the sick. These early nurses included men who were drawn into military nursing orders, such as the Knights Hospitallers and Knights Templars. In such religious orders "the high born and rich and those of lowly birth alike gave their services to the care of the sick" (Gardner, 1916, p. 5).

The Renaissance (about 1500-1700 AD) brought about great political, social, and economic expansion and a revival of learning. Two important names from this period are St. Vincent de Paul and Mademoiselle Le Gras. In her book *Public Health Nursing*, Mary Sewall Gardner says of de Paul that "there is perhaps no more prominent figure in the history of public health nursing" (Gardner, 1916, p. 6).

In 1633 de Paul organized the Sisters of Charity (Kalisch, Kalisch, 1995, p. 28). The Sisters went from home to home, visiting the sick. As the movement spread and its numbers increased, problems with supervision arose. St. Vincent reorganized the group and appointed Mademoiselle Le Gras as supervisor. Together they made great contributions to the development of public health nursing, including providing education for those helping the poor and the sick, recognizing the need for professional supervision of caregivers, and helping people to help themselves. De Paul and Le Gras believed that one must determine the needs of the poor and disadvantaged, investigate the causes, and help supply solutions. Taken for granted by people today, these were entirely new concepts of charity for this time (Maynard, 1939).

For centuries, monasteries, convents, and religious orders stood for what was the best in nursing (Gardner, 1916, pp. 4-5). It is difficult to imagine how nursing could have sunk to the low levels it did between the end of the seventeenth century to the middle of the nineteenth century.

The Era of Sairy Gamp

> Nursing, like so many other things the history of which may be studied from century to century, has had its ups and downs, its bright periods of inspired effort, and its black periods of temporary degradation. It is not to the Sairy Gamps . . . that the ancestry of the modern nurse is to be traced. Sairy was but an unhappy incident in the history of nursing (Gardner, 1916, p. 3).

The change from nursing care given by devoted deaconesses to nursing care given by drunks and prostitutes is baffling. In *Martin Chuzzlewit*, published in 1844, Charles Dickens immortalized the prototype of the nurse of this era by describing a drunken, untrained servant, Sairy Gamp, as a nurse. In order to appreciate the great accomplishments of Florence Nightingale and early nursing leaders in raising the status of nursing, the conditions that were in existence when they began their efforts to establish nursing as a profession should be known.

At this time assistance programs for the poor and disadvantaged did not exist as we know them today, and social classes were rigidly stratified. Many people were starving, child labor was routinely practiced, housing was frequently inadequate, and personal hygiene and matters of public health were often ignored. Life expectancy was short and mortality rates were high. Medicine was at a low level, largely because the scientific basis for it was unknown, and health care was based on folklore and superstition. The huge slums of cities bred disease.

Nursing care in the western world had degenerated from care being given by deaconesses, sisters, and Christian women to care being given by beggars and vagrants. This change in the way care was provided began during the time of the Reformation (around 1500-1600 AD), when many church organizations were overthrown. After the Reformation the lack of nursing sisterhoods was deeply felt (Brainard, 1922, p. 70). Without the protection and acceptance lent it by the church, nursing lost much of its social standing. "Even during this dark period good and devoted women were giving their lives to the relief of suffering, but it was only individual effort, and as a rule in every country the great body of the sick poor were being cared for by overworked, ignorant, and unprincipled women, while the sick rich fared but little better" (Gardner, 1916, p. 8).

Nursing now existed in a low and dismal state, without organization or social standing; and no one who could possibly earn a living in some other way performed this service (Deloughery, 1977, p. 24). Those who sought nursing as a profession "lost caste thereby, for as one is judged partly by the company one keeps, a woman who began to practice nursing was almost certain to become corrupted if she were not so already" (Deloughery, p. 24).

With this background in mind, the contributions of Florence Nightingale to nursing, to public health, and to women are inestimable. Indeed, when Florence Nightingale began her career, it was a very dreadful thing to be a nurse.

FLORENCE NIGHTINGALE'S LEGACY

Florence Nightingale was the second child of William and Frances Nightingale. She was born on May 12, 1820 in Florence, Italy; her older sister Parthenope had been born the previous year in Naples. Her family was well-traveled, wealthy, and influential. Unlike other English girls of the day, Florence and her sister were well educated. As a young girl Florence mastered the fundamentals of Greek and Latin; studied history, mathematics, and philosophy; and wrote essays (Kalisch, Kalisch, 1995, p. 30). To her family's chagrin, Florence remained unmarried and expressed a longing to be a nurse. At age 25, her request to train as a nurse in an English hospital was rejected by her parents (Kalisch, Kalisch, p. 31). After a delay of many years, largely in deference to her family's wishes, she entered nurses' training in 1851 with Pastor Fliedner at Kaiserswerth on the Rhine, Germany.

Kaiserswerth

Theodor Fliedner was pastor in the town of Kaiserswerth. He and his young wife, Frederika, had started a Woman's Society for visiting and nursing the sick poor in their homes (Brainard, 1922, p. 74). In 1836 he started a hospital and a training school for deaconesses that is considered to be the first modern order of nursing deaconesses (Kalisch, Kalisch, 1995, p. 28). It was this training school that young Florence became determined to attend.

In the winter of 1849 Florence was touring Egypt with family and friends and spent time in Alexandria with the Sisters of Charity of St. Vincent de Paul (Kalisch, Kalisch, 1995, p. 31). The following spring she set out unaccompanied for Kaiserswerth, stayed there for 2 weeks, and left determined to return to train as a nurse (Kalisch, Kalisch, p. 31). The following year, with her ailing sister about to journey to the mineral springs of Carlsbad, Nightingale insisted on going to Kaiserswerth for nurses' training. Permission was granted on the condition that no one outside the family learn of her destination. Upon finishing training and returning home she entered the profession of nursing.

The Crimea

Shortly after her return to England, the Crimean War would offer Nightingale an opportunity and challenge as "Superintendent of the Female Nursing Establishment of the English General Hospitals in Turkey" (Kalisch, Kalisch, 1995, p. 32). The story of Miss Nightingale in the Crimea is legendary. Her work at Scutari has been chronicled by many, among them Longfellow, in his "Santa Filomena." It was there that she demonstrated that thousands of lives could be saved by intelligent nursing care and that capable nurses were needed in hospitals. She accomplished this in the face of overwhelming obstacles. Although the hospital at Scutari was designed to accommodate 1700 patients, when Nightingale arrived in 1854 there were 3000 to 4000 wounded men in it (Kalisch, Kalisch, p. 32). Many of these men lay naked, with no bed or blanket and no eating or laundry facilities. Within days of her appearance at Scutari she had a food kitchen operating, as well as a laundry. When Nightingale arrived at the Barrack Hospital, its mortality rate stood at 60%; when she left it was at 1% (Kalisch, Kalisch, p. 35). When the war ended in 1856 she returned to England and was determined to establish a school for nurses.

The First Modern Training School for Nurses

Upon returning to London, Nightingale established the first modern training school for nurses at St. Thomas Hospital in 1860. Interestingly, when the training school began most London physicians opposed the project; of the 100 physicians asked, only 4 favored the school (Kalisch, Kalisch, 1995, p. 36).

The opening of the St. Thomas school offered a new beginning for nursing. Nursing was viewed as a "calling" to a high duty, demanding the age-old characteristics of love, kindness, patience, and self-sacrifice; but now added to that was training (Brainard, 1922, p. 84). The principle that training was necessary to make a competent nurse was accepted; however, the knowledge of what that training should be was vague, and it was left to Florence Nightingale to show the way (Brainard, p. 84). Nightingale's training school set an example for other schools, including the one at Bellevue Hospital in New York City in 1873. The movement that would lead to University Schools of Nursing at Western Reserve and Yale had been set in place (Winslow, 1946, p. 331).

Originator of the Nursing Process and Nursing Research

Nightingale was the originator of the concept of the nursing process. The role of the trained professional nurse included assessment, intervention, and evaluation. In her famous *Notes on Nursing* she defined nursing as that care that puts a person in the best possible condition for nature to either restore or preserve health, to prevent or cure disease or injury (Nightingale, 1859).

From the very beginning of her career, Nightingale focused on the use of a scientific process to guide practice. "Nightingale (1885) encouraged nurses to be clear thinkers, and independent in their judgments" (Reed, Zurakowski, 1996, p. 47): She visualized the nurse as not merely an attendant for the sick but also a teacher of hygiene. She described the nurse as a "health missioner," a guide and teacher of health to the individual in the home. She recognized that "from the very nature of the case, compulsion can under no conditions work the changes we want to see wrought by the obedience of consent" (Winslow, 1946, p. 331). This was a very early affirmation of the principle that individuals are responsible for their own health and the role of the nurse is to promote the client's self-care capabilities.

Florence Nightingale is considered by many to be the first nurse researcher. She emphasized the importance of systematic observation, data collection, and statistical analysis in relation to nursing care. Her statistical research in British military hospitals in the Crimea showed that nursing interventions could make a difference in the morbidity and mortality rates of the soldiers. Her research report, *Notes on Matters Affecting the Health, Efficiency and Hospital Administration of the British Army,* led to both attitudinal and organizational changes in health care practices.

> Nightingale's theoretical ideas initiated a research tradition for nursing that provided a conceptual perspective and methodology for studying nursing phenomena. Her model was a highly significant landmark—signifying the birth of nursing science . . . Nightingale's research tradition thrives today regardless of the void of empirical nursing data that preceded and followed Nightingale. (Reed, Zurakowski, 1996, pp. 42, 48)

After Nightingale's work nursing research lay dormant for almost a century.

THE ESTABLISHMENT OF VISITING NURSING

Visiting nursing was greatly influenced by the modern public health movement and social awareness that occurred during the first half of the nineteenth century. The title given to this period in public health history is "The Great Awakening," and the person whose name is associated with it is an Englishman, Edwin Chadwick. In 1832 the Chadwick Report created a public awareness of the unsanitary, "unhealthy" conditions in which many English people lived, including the lack of proper refuse and sewage disposal, contaminated water supplies, improperly stored foods, and overcrowded dwellings. His report helped to bring about the passage of the English Public Health Act of 1848 and development of programs for the sick poor, and laid the groundwork for public support of visiting nursing. In 1850 an American public health pioneer, Lemuel Shattuck, wrote the Shattuck Report. It outlined many conditions similar to the ones mentioned by Chadwick and proposed public health solutions (see Chapter 4).

The modern concept of a nurse who provides care to families in the home was visualized and established in 1859 by William Rathbone of Liverpool, England. "It is to Mr. Rathbone that we owe the first definitely formulated district nursing association and in that sense he may be called the father of the present movement" (Gardner, 1916, p. 10). Rathbone was a wealthy businessman and philanthropist. His wife died after a long illness, and he had been impressed and comforted by the skilled home nursing care given to her in the months before she died. Rathbone had long been interested in helping the many poor people of Liverpool. If nursing care could help his wife, who had everything that money could buy, how much more might it do for people whose physical illnesses were made increasingly burdensome by their poverty. To test his idea, he employed Mrs. Mary Robinson, the nurse who had cared for his wife, to visit the "sick poor" in their homes. She was to instruct both the patient and the family in the care of the sick, give care, and teach hygienic practices. The experiment was so successful that Rathbone decided to establish a permanent system of district or visiting nursing in Liverpool (McNeil, 1967, p. 1).

A major problem in advancing district nursing for the poor was the fact that there were no nurses educated and prepared to do such work. In 1859, with the help and advice of Florence Nightingale, Rathbone founded a school for the training of visiting nurses on the grounds of the Liverpool Royal Infirmary. Within 4 years 18 nurses had graduated and were working in the city. These visiting nurses not only cared for the sick but also advocated health care and social reform.

The visiting nurse movement in England spread rapidly. In 1887 the Queen lent her support by establishing the Queen Victoria's Jubilee Institute for Nurses. Institute nurses received rigorous training and education. "A Queen's nurse was in every instance a graduate of a hospital giving a three years' course, and in addition she receives a six months post-graduate training in one of the homes of the Institute" (Gardner, 1916, p. 15).

VISITING NURSING IN THE UNITED STATES

> During all these years in which nursing in the Old World had been making such rapid and marvelous progress both in hospitals and in the care of the sick poor in their homes, nothing towards its development had taken place in the new world. When sickness entered the home of the colonist, therefore, the care of the patient devolved entirely upon the wife or the mother of the household, and upon her skill and experience depended the kind of nursing given, whether good or bad. The only outside assistance available was that of a friendly neighbor . . . (Brainard, 1922, pp. 180-181).

In 1839 Theodor Fliedner had accompanied two of his deaconesses to Pittsburgh in an endeavor to start visiting nursing in that city, but the undertaking did not prosper (Brainard, 1922, p. 194). A few other efforts were made to establish nursing sisterhoods and to introduce the Sisters of Charity into the homes of America's sick poor, but these efforts did not arouse the support of the public and were unsuccessful (Brainard, p. 194). Churches frequently provided some form of care for the sick, often in the form of home visiting and material relief. In the mid-1800s religious orders provided exemplary nursing service in American hospitals.

By the late 1800s large numbers of Americans were concerned with the poverty and misery experienced by so many people. Poverty was beginning to be seen as the result of social problems and conditions. People rallied around causes such as working to improve maternal and child health, abolish child labor, provide decent housing, and procure women's right to vote.

With the exception of the Ladies' Benevolent Society of Charleston and the Nurse Society of Philadelphia, no record exists of any system of home care for the sick poor in America up to the year 1877, when the Woman's Board of the New York City Mission hired a nurse, Miss Frances Root, to visit the sick poor (Brainard, 1922, p. 194). Miss Root was a graduate of the first class of the first training school for nurses in the United States, the Bellevue Training School for nurses in New York City. She was hired as a "missionary nurse" and was expected to use every opportunity to introduce religious counsel and words of Christian comfort (Brainard, p. 196). Her work was successful, and other such nurses were hired. The following year the New York Society for Ethical Culture hired missionary nurses. In 1889 the city health department in Los Angeles employed a nurse to provide home nursing care to the sick poor, one of the first recorded hirings of a nurse by an official, tax-supported agency (Rosen, 1958, p. 380).

The growth of our nation's cities, as well as the waves of immigrants to America, were two underlying reasons for the development of visiting nursing. Although every city had its rich people, the poor greatly outnumbered them. New York had the largest settlement of immigrants and thus faced the most problems concerning them (Figure 1-1). Dismal tenement houses were built for this huge influx of people, and living conditions were horrible. Very young children were expected to work 12 to 14 hours a day in dark, airless factories.

Visiting Nurse Associations

Visiting nursing in the United States, just as in England, was begun by groups of people who were greatly distressed by the conditions in which many poor people lived. American cities were growing fast, had large immigrant populations, large slum areas, and high rates of disease. These overcrowded cities posed many serious health problems. As visiting nurse associations arose they were often in these large cities and situated in low-income areas.

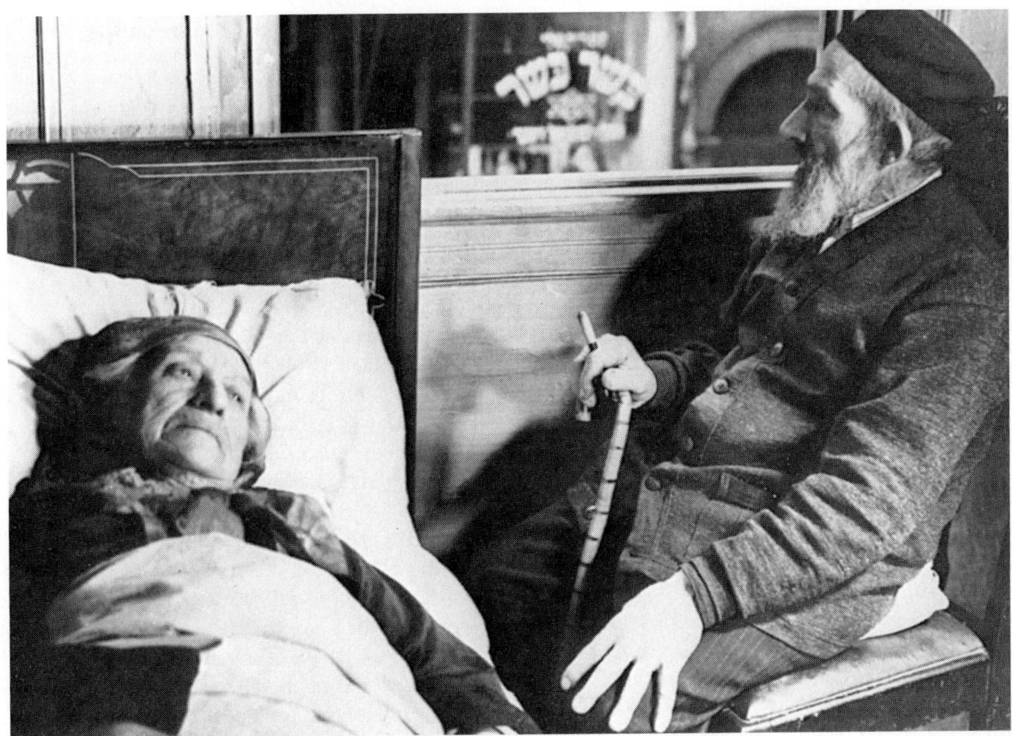

Figure 1-1 It was the year of the great blizzard, 1888, when this Russian blacksmith and his bride emigrated to the New World to build a life. Fifty years later, in sickness and in health, they were still together—thanks to a visiting nurse. *(Courtesy Visiting Nurse Service of New York City.)*

The first nursing association in America for the sole purpose of providing skilled care for the sick poor in their homes was the District Nursing Association in Boston in 1886. The association was heavily involved in teaching, as well as care of the sick, and soon changed its name to the Instructive District Nursing Association. Its original purposes and some nursing rules are given in the box at right. The Visiting Nurse Society of Philadelphia was founded later in 1886. The Philadelphia society had as its stated purpose "to furnish visiting nurses to those otherwise unable to secure skilled attendance in time of sickness, to teach cleanliness and the proper care of the sick" (Brainard, 1922, p. 219). Service was also given to people of moderate means who could afford to pay some for the care given, and this became one of the earliest known fee-for-service programs.

More visiting nurse associations were founded in Chicago (1889), Buffalo (1891), Kansas City (1892), Detroit (1894), and Baltimore (1896). Visiting nursing was now well established in the United States. However, it did not follow the English system established by Rathbone (Gardner, 1919, p. 29). In England Queen Victoria's Jubilee Institute for Nurses had set standards for the preparation of visiting nurses as well as for the care given by them. By 1890 21 separate organizations were engaged in visiting nursing in the United States. These organizations had no connection with one another and also had no common standards

Instructive District Nursing Association of Boston: 1886

ORIGINAL PURPOSES

1. To provide and support thoroughly trained nurses, who, acting under the immediate direction of the outpatient physicians of the Boston Dispensary, shall care for the sick poor in their own homes instead of in hospitals.
2. By precept and example to give such instruction to the families which they are called upon to visit as shall enable them henceforth to take better care of themselves and their neighbors by observing the rules of wholesome living and by practicing the simple arts of domestic nursing.

SOME NURSING RULES

1. Each nurse shall work for eight hours daily, employment on Sunday and holidays shall be exceptional, also night duty.
2. Nurses must be examples of neatness, cleanliness, and sobriety.
3. Nurses attending to contagious diseases shall be subject to special limitation in their attendance on other patients.
4. Nurses shall not interfere with the religious or political opinion of the patient.
5. Nurses shall not receive presents from patients, nor give money nor its equivalent.

From Brainard AM: *The evolution of public health nursing,* Philadelphia, 1922, Saunders, pp. 207, 210-211.

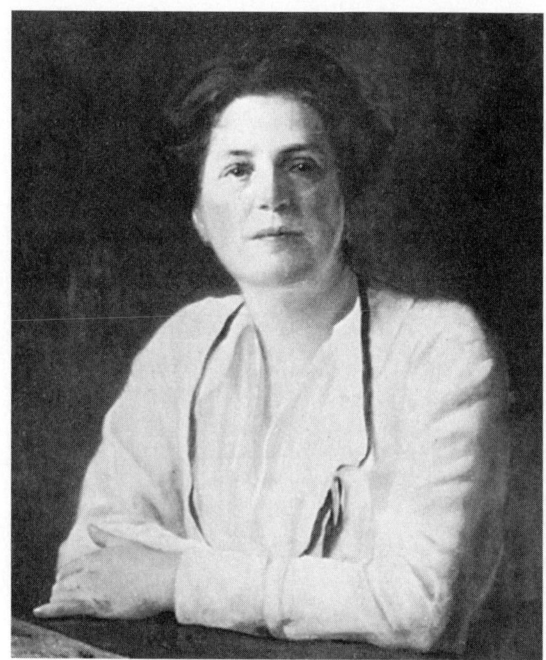

Figure 1-2 Lillian Wald, the nurse leader who was the "predecessor of modern public health nursing," was far ahead of her time. She promoted health and social reform at a time when it was not the norm for women to engage in such activity. Her accomplishments truly reflect the mark of a professional nurse. *(Courtesy Visiting Nurse Service of New York City.)*

of educational preparation for the caregivers. Cities and towns established their own visiting nurse services, and there was great diversity in the quality of organization and care given.

In 1896 the Nurses' Associated Alumni (now the American Nurses Association) was formed and helped to organize the nurses of the country into a professional group. This organization was the beginning of "group consciousness" among the visiting nurses of the United States.

ENTER LILLIAN WALD

Lillian Wald coined the expression *public health nursing* and is considered the founder of public health nursing in this country (Figure 1-2). Nightingale had originated the idea of "health nursing"; it was Wald who placed the word *public* in front of it so that all people would know that this type of service was available to them (Haupt, 1953, p. 81). *The House on Henry Street* is her story of the work she did as director of the Henry Street Settlement House.

Lillian Wald was born in 1867 and grew up in Rochester, New York. Though her family was not wealthy, her father, an optical goods dealer, provided a comfortable living for them. She studied at a private school and was an excellent student. Wald chanced to meet a graduate of the Bellevue Hospital Training School for Nurses who had assisted her sister during pregnancy. It was in this manner that she became interested in nursing. She graduated from training at New York Hospital in 1891 and supplemented her nursing instruction with a period of study at a medical college. During this medical college experience, she was asked to give classes in home nursing and bedside care to a group of women in the Lower East Side tenement district. This would become a turning point in Wald's career, and the point at which the concept of public health nursing was born:

> From the schoolroom where I had been giving a lesson in bed-making, a little girl led me one drizzling March morning. She had told me of her sick mother, and gathering from her incoherent account that a child had been born, I caught up the paraphernalia of the bed-making lesson and carried it with me.
>
> The child led me over broken roadways,—there was no asphalt, although its use was well established in other parts of the city,—over dirty mattresses and heaps of refuse,—it was before Colonel Waring had shown the possibility of clean streets even in that quarter,—between tall, reeking houses whose laden fire escapes, useless for their appointed purpose, bulged with household goods of every description. The rain added to the dismal appearance of the streets and to the discomfort of the crowds which thronged them, intensifying the odors which assailed me from every side. Through Hester and Division Streets we went to the end of Ludlow; past odorous fish-stands, for the streets were a marketplace, unregulated, unsupervised, unclean; past evil-smelling, uncovered garbage-cans; and—perhaps worst of all, where so many little children played—past the trucks brought down from more fastidious quarters and stalled on these already over-crowded streets, lending themselves inevitably to many forms of indecency.
>
> The child led me on through a tenement hallway, across a court where open and unscreened closets were promiscuously used by men and women, up into a rear tenement, by slimy steps whose accumulated dirt was augmented that day by the mud of the streets, and finally into the sickroom.
>
> All of the maladjustments of our social and economic relations seemed epitomized in this brief journey and what was found at the end of it. The family to which the child led me was neither criminal nor vicious. Although the husband was a cripple, one of those who stand on street corners exhibiting deformities to enlist compassion, and masking the begging of alms by a pretense at selling; although the family of seven shared their two rooms with boarders,—who were literally boarders, since a piece of timber was placed over the floor for them to sleep on,—and although the sick woman lay on a wretched, unclean bed, soiled with a hemorrhage two days old, they were not degraded human beings, judged by any measure of moral values.
>
> In fact, it was very plain that they were sensitive to their condition, and when, at the end of my ministrations, they kissed my hands (those who have undergone similar experiences will, I am sure, understand), it would have been some solace if by any conviction of the moral unworthiness of the family I could have defended myself as a part of a society which permitted such conditions to exist. Indeed, my subsequent acquaintance with them revealed the fact that, miserable as their state was, they were not without ideals for the family life, and for society, of which they were so unloved and unlovely a part.
>
> That morning's experience was a baptism of fire. Deserted were the laboratory and the academic work of the college—I never

returned to them. On my way from the sickroom to my comfortable student quarters my mind was intent on my own responsibility. To my inexperience, it seemed certain that conditions such as these were allowed because people did not know, and for me there was a challenge to know and to tell. When early morning found me still awake, my naive conviction remained that, if people knew things,—and "things" meant everything implied in the condition of this family,—such horrors would cease to exist, and I rejoiced that I had a training in the care of the sick that in itself would give me an organic relationship to the neighborhood in which this awakening had come. (Wald, 1915, pp. 4-8)

This "baptism by fire" changed the life of Lillian Wald.

The Henry Street Settlement House

Wald had an exceptional ability to inform and convince people about the need for health care and social change (Backer, 1993, p. 122). In 1893 she and Mary Brewster, her friend and classmate, were able to obtain funds from wealthy people to establish a Nurses' Settlement House in a slum section of the lower East Side of New York where the nurses would serve the sick poor and live among them. "By the end of the first month, Wald had begun to mobilize a vast array of the city's disjointed private relief and medical establishments to remedy her neighbors' ills" (Buhler-Wilkerson, 1991, p. 316).

The settlement house was nonsecretarian, as Wald believed that a nurse could be most effective if she were independent of any religious agency. She also insisted that nurses should be available to anyone who needed them, without the intervention of a doctor, establishing early in the history of nursing that the profession should be an independent one; families could refer themselves to the service without a physician referral. "Wald and Brewster quickly established the concept of the nurse ready to give her services in the home to all who needed them, making no distinction between those who could pay and those who could not, allied with no religious group, seeking to educate as well as to heal" (Kalisch, Kalisch, 1995, p. 175). Wald firmly believed in the dignity and independence of the people she served and thought that nurses should live in the neighborhood where they practiced so that they could better identify with the needs of the families served.

In 1895 the settlement house moved to Henry Street, where it still exists today. Lillian Wald was its head resident—the nurse in charge. By 1905 its staff of nurses was making almost 44,000 nursing visits a year (Kalisch, Kalisch, 1995, p. 176). Nursing service from the Settlement was available 24 hours a day (Fitzpatrick, 1990, p. 94). Those who could pay were charged 10 cents to 25 cents a visit to detach the stigma of charity or missionary work (Coss, 1989). Wald became an integral part of the community in which she lived. Her vision was to provide comprehensive health care from the client's point of view and encourage personal and public responsibility for health. The Henry Street Settlement house became known as an innovative force for health and human betterment in New York City and a model for other nursing agencies (Erickson, 1987, p. 18).

Lillian Wald has been honored for her social reform activities as well as her nursing achievements (see the accompanying box). Chapters in her book *The House on Henry Street* show some of this social zeal and include information on the nurse and the community, education and the child, the handicapped child, children who work, the nation's children, social forces, and "new Americans." Wald was a true humanist, committed to helping people improve the quality of their lives. She is a role model for public health nurses today and the predecessor of modern public health nursing. You can still visit the original Henry Street Settlement House. This settlement house provides a wide range of nursing, welfare, and social services. The Visiting Nurse Service of New York City evolved from the original Henry

A Look at Some Accomplishments of Lillian Wald

Lillian Wald's accomplishments are legendary and involve numerous "firsts" in nursing. She was an amazing woman whose ideas and programs were well ahead of her time. Wald transformed her nursing care into health and social policies. Her accomplishments are even more remarkable considering that she achieved them in a time when women did not even have the right to vote. The following is a list of some of these accomplishments

- Founded the Henry Street Settlement House and "public health nursing"
- Originated the idea of family-focused nursing
- Stressed the importance of health teaching in preventing disease and promoting health
- Established school nursing in the United States
- Was instrumental in establishing the Red Cross Town and Country Nursing Service to provide rural nursing
- Originated the idea of, and helped to establish, the U.S. Children's Bureau
- Established "milk stations" in New York City, where safe milk for infants and children could be obtained
- Was instrumental in securing changes in national child labor laws
- Was instrumental in securing better housing conditions in tenement districts and city recreation centers, parks, and playgrounds for children in New York City. (She even put playgrounds in the backyards of the nursing settlement houses)
- Provided summer camp experiences for poor inner city children
- Helped to establish graded classes for mentally handicapped children
- Provided humanistic care for immigrants to the United States
- Encouraged and taught courses in public health nursing
- Founder and first president of the National Organization for Public Health Nursing

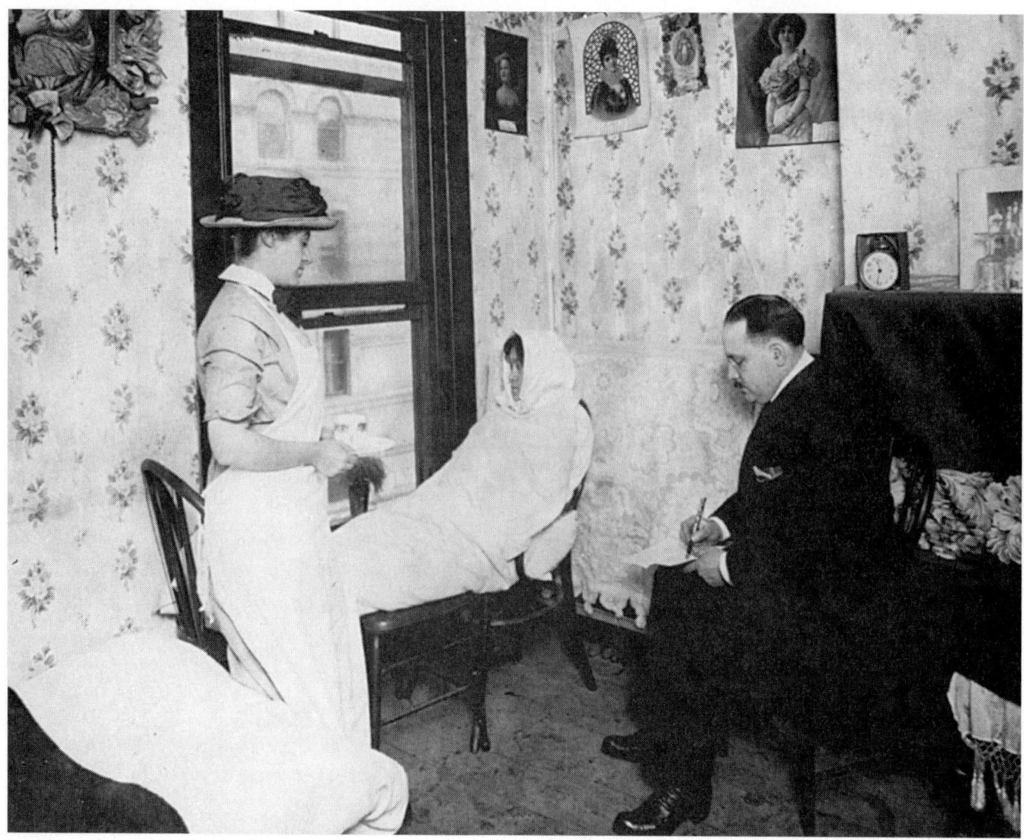

Figure 1-3 Convalescing from typhoid fever, New York City, 1912. *(Courtesy The Metropolitan Life Insurance Company of New York.)*

Street Settlement and provides an extensive range of nursing and home care services.

Other Nursing Settlements

The Henry Street Settlement was not the only nursing settlement in the United States. It is uncertain just how many settlements were established along the model of Henry Street, but it is known that some existed. Possibly the nurse's settlement whose work was most comparable to that done at Henry Street is the Nurse's Settlement of Richmond, Virginia (Brainard, 1922, p. 254). This settlement was started in 1900 by the entire graduating class of Richmond's Old Dominion Hospital. Unlike the Henry Street Settlement, no fees were charged. Other differences included that the Richmond nurses had other jobs, "volunteered" work at the settlement in their off-duty hours, and agreed to pay $5 every month for rent plus board for the days actually spent there (Erickson, 1987, pp. 17, 20). Within a short time the Richmond settlement reorganized, and three paid nurses were employed.

A Look at the Difference: Visiting Nursing and Public Health Nursing

Visiting nurse associations of the time primarily existed to nurse the sick poor in their homes—Lillian Wald's public health nurse expanded on that role. Not only did her nurses care for the sick poor at home, but they also practiced family-focused nursing, nursed the "whole" person, worked to improve social conditions, and provided health education, classes, and services in other settings such as clinics and schools (see A View from the Field). This early public health nursing role would later be reframed into its more contemporary role, which focuses on health education and primary prevention activities, providing care across socioeconomic groups, and nursing the community. The focus on the health of the community is reflected in the more contemporary use of the term *community health nurse*.

By 1912 public health nurses were supported by both private and public funds. The need for the skills and knowledge of this kind of professional was generally well recognized. They could be found in many kinds of agencies, as well as in both rural and urban settings (Figures 1-3 and 1-4). Table 1-1, compiled by public health nurse pioneer Mary Sewall Gardner, illustrates this distribution.

School Nursing Develops

A significant role for public health nurses in the early 1900s was school nursing. School nursing in the United States was begun by Lillian Wald. In 1902 health conditions of school

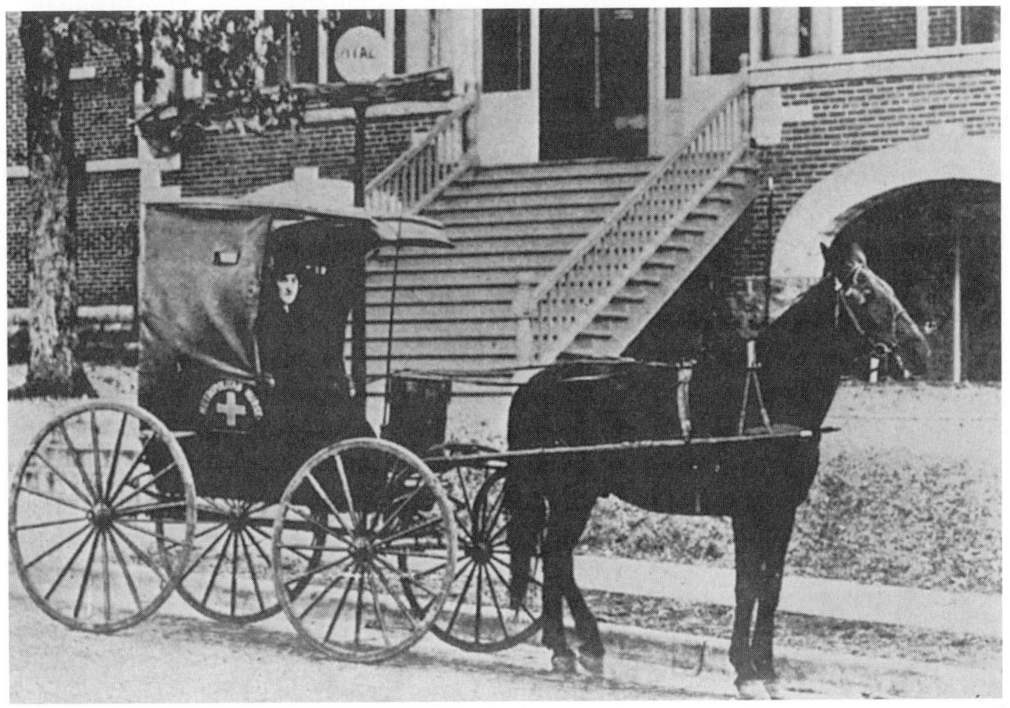

Figure **1-4** Public health nurse using horse and buggy before the advent of the automobile. *(Courtesy The Metropolitan Life Insurance Company of New York.)*

table 1-1 Distribution of Public Health Nurses in 1912

Visiting nurse associations	205
City and state boards of health and education	156
Private clubs and societies	108
Tuberculosis leagues	107
Hospitals and dispensaries	87
Business concerns	38
Settlements and day nurses	35
Churches	28
Charity organizations	27
Other organizations	19

NOTE: This list, used by the author in 1912, as secretary of a joint committee of the American Nurses Association and the Society of Superintendents of Training Schools, to circulate names of the agencies then known to be engaged in public health nursing, probably gives a reasonably true picture of the general distribution of nursing work among the different types of agencies. There were 78 letters sent to nurses working in that number of counties in Pennsylvania and 204 to nurses independently employed by the Metropolitan Life Insurance Company. From Gardner MS: *Public health nursing,* ed 3, New York, 1936, Macmillan, p. 40.

children in New York City were appalling. Thousands of students were sent home from school with diseases such as trachoma (an infectious eye disease), pediculosis, ringworm, scabies, and impetigo. They then played outside with the children from whom they had previously been excluded in the classroom (Wald, 1915, p. 51). Wald offered to show school officials in New York that with the assistance of a well-prepared nurse, fewer children would lose valuable school time and that it was possible to bring under treatment those who needed it.

Wald loaned a nurse to the New York City Health Department to accomplish these goals. The experiment was to be paid for with public funds. One month's trial with Lina Rogers, a nurse from Henry Street, proved to be immensely successful. Miss Rogers stated, "I selected four schools in the most crowded part of the city, which I visited daily, spending about one hour in each, after which visits were made to the homes. First of all, crude dispensaries were improvised in each school, and these were equipped each day with supplies donated by the Settlement" (Brainard, 1922, p. 269). The experiment was so successful that the New York Board of Health appointed twelve other nurses to assist in carrying on the work (Brainard, p. 270). The sum of $30,000 was approved for the employment of these nurses—the first municipalized school nurses in the world (Wald, 1915, p. 53), and the first use of trained nurses in any large number in health departments. School nursing remains an integral part of community health nursing today.

Tuberculosis Nursing

Surveillance for infectious disease control was a major function of early public health nurses. Throughout the nine-

A View from the Field — District Nursing in 1923

Historical Reprint In 1923 when this article first appeared in the February issue of THE PUBLIC HEALTH NURSE it was fairly common for board members to go with a public health nurse on her rounds for a day. Many agencies today would welcome the same opportunity but unfortunately the volunteer board member has less time available for this inside look into an agency. We may smile at the datedness of some of the descriptions but we will be quickly reminded that much of what was practiced then is practiced today. Read and enjoy!

The author of this piece was a member of the nursing committee, Public Health Nursing Department, The United Workers of Norwich, Connecticut.

Ruth N. Knollmueller
Historical Editor

A uniform of sober gray, relieved only by collar and cuffs of immaculate white linen, an armband bearing the letters P.H.N.—all of us know this uniform, most of us know the meaning of the letters, but how many stop to think of the deeper significance of the Public Health Nurse in terms of her community-wide service? Perhaps if the nurse tells us a bit about her daily travels it may help us to understand.

"How many calls have I made today? Twelve, no—thirteen in all. First I went to see a dear little girl, two years old, who has been so ill with empyema that for days we feared that we might lose her. A month ago she was operated on, and then a week later the doctor said that a second operation must be performed or the child would die. The Polish parents, almost frantic with anxiety, at first objected strongly, but finally consented to the second operation, and now the little girl is well on the road to recovery. Today I found her temperature normal for the first time in many weeks.

"My next patient was a young Greek woman who has a very interesting history. She had been an olive picker in her own country, but her eyes were turned toward the golden promise of America. The weary journey took three months, she tells me, and at the end was Ellis Island, with all that means of filth and disease. Small wonder that she caught an infectious skin trouble! I've been dressing the eruption every day for two weeks, but this is my last call, for the places are practically healed.

"In the near neighborhood there lives another Greek family. The children have been brought to our clinic and so I ran in for a friendly visit, before I went on to my case. We call in the homes of all our clinic babies, you know, to see if we can give help or advice or instruction.

"From babyhood to old age, from the cradle to the grave, indeed! My next patient was an old lady, and she died in my arms. But at least I had made her last days comfortable and she did so enjoy the attention. In all her long lifetime she had never known ill-health, had never had a nurse, and so my coming was a great event for her.

"The last call this morning I made on the three weeks' old baby of a young Russian woman. The mother had no doctor when her child was born, and her condition afterwards became so serious that a doctor had to be called. The doctor sent for me to assist in giving the necessary treatment, but all too soon it became evident that an operation must be performed. So the young mother was taken to the hospital and the wee baby was left in the care of a kind neighbor. I've been making friendly calls on the mother in the hospital, as well as keeping an eye on the new baby.

"After lunch I went to dress a bad case of leg-ulcers. My patient is a dear old lady, who has been suffering for forty years, hobbling about as best she could on crutches. At last the sores became so troublesome that she sent for a doctor, and he, realizing the necessity for constant attention, asked our department to send in a nurse. For five months I've been going there to do the dressings, and you simply can't imagine what improvement my patient has made. Already the crutches are discarded, and I have

From Young EE: A quiet day: a peep at some of the varied homes visited by a district nurse in the course of one "quiet day," *Public Health Nurs* 6:43-44, 1989.

teenth century tuberculosis was a leading killer among infectious diseases in the United States. The isolation of the tuberculosis bacillus in 1882 by Robert Koch showed that the disease was transmissible. Tuberculosis was a dreaded disease, and by 1915 there were more than fifteen hundred antituberculosis associations in the United States, including 35 state organizations (Gardner, 1916, p. 222). Tuberculosis patients were generally bedridden, and nursing care was often provided for them at home. Henry Street Settlement nurses regularly instructed patients and families about preventing and treating the disease (Wald, 1915, p. 54). In 1903, spearheaded by Lillian Wald, the New York City Health Department appointed three nurses (annual salary $900 each) to visit tuberculosis patients at home and teach the patients about sputum disposal and other aspects of care. The program was successful, and in 1905 the number of nurses was increased to 14. At the same time, agencies across the country were beginning to hire tuberculosis nurses. When Mary Sewall Gardner first wrote *Public Health Nursing* (1916), an entire chapter was dedicated to tuberculosis nursing.

Metropolitan Employs PHNs

A unique partnership between a private enterprise and an existing public health nursing organization greatly ex-

A View from the Field — District Nursing in 1923—cont'd

hopes that before long the ulcers will have disappeared. Think what that will mean to her, after all these long years of suffering. Do you wonder that I find a warm welcome in that home?

"Next I called on a young woman who had just come home from the hospital after an operation. The wound is not yet entirely healed, and so I have to dress it, but more than all that I try to cheer her up, because the period of convalescence seems endless to her and she gets so discouraged.

"After I left that little woman I stopped to see a young tuberculosis patient who has insisted upon coming home from the sanatorium, much against all advice. I do hope he is using the knowledge he gained in the sanatorium for his own progress and the protection of his family. I called upon him because he came to the tuberculosis clinic, and we try to keep in touch with all our clinic cases through friendly calling.

"The next case was an hourly nursing call—a case of grippe, needing baths to reduce temperature, and after I had finished making the patient more comfortable I made several short visits in the homes of clinic babies nearby.

"My last patient for the day was an old colored woman, who was once a slave. She's ninety-five and bedridden, needing daily care, but the house is spotlessly clean and she's such a cheerful old soul that it is a pleasure to do for her.

"It hasn't been a very exciting day, you see; there was nothing new or unusual, just a quiet day."

A quiet day! The work she does is as quiet and inconspicuous as the gray gown she wears, and yet it's so inclusive that today or tomorrow, directly or indirectly, it finds us all within the limits of its service.

panded public health nursing services in the early 1900s. Lillian Wald and Lee Frankel, founder of the Metropolitan Life Insurance Company Welfare Division, convinced the board of directors at Metropolitan that healthy policyholders would live longer, healthier lives and ultimately save the company money. In 1909 Metropolitan initiated the first public health nursing program for policyholders of an insurance company (Haupt, 1953, p. 81). Rather than employing their own nurses, the company used existing public health nursing services from the Henry Street Settlement, and services were available to all policyholders, with "sliding-scale" fees based on the ability to pay.

The Metropolitan project remained in place for 44 years. There were numerous contributions to public health nursing as a result of this project (Haupt, 1953). Among them are the following:

- The extension of bedside nursing care on a fee-for-service basis.
- The establishment of a cost-accounting system for visiting nurses that is used to this day.
- The reduction of mortality rates from infectious diseases. Mortality rates were reduced by half among the Metropolitan Life Insurance policyholders.
- The demonstration of how nursing and a business can work together to promote health.

Public Health Nursing in Rural Areas

While public health nursing in cities and towns was developing at a rapid rate at the beginning of the century, nursing service in rural areas was progressing slowly. No organized health service was provided in rural areas. Lillian Wald took action to correct this situation.

Lillian Wald was a member of the American Red Cross and expressed strong dissatisfaction at seeing the organization limited to the uncertainty and irregularity of service in war or calamity; she felt it wasteful to have a national organization inactive. She believed that the Red Cross was a logical facility to employ in promoting public health nursing in rural areas and scattered towns on a national scale (Dock, Pickett, Noyes et al, 1922, p. 1212). In 1912, the same year the Children's Bureau was formed, Lillian Wald asked her wealthy friend Jacob Shiff to donate money to the Red Cross so that a system of rural nursing could be developed. And so it happened that the Red Cross began a new department, the Town and Country Nursing Service, later named the Bureau of Public Health Nursing. The purpose of the department was to supply rural areas and small towns with trained public health nurses and to supervise their work. The Red Cross, however, did not assume the local financial responsibility for this work. Voluntary and charitable organizations, as well as fees for service, financed the nursing care given.

A Great American

Lillian Wald's work was widely recognized both in this country and abroad. In 1971 a bronze bust of Wald was placed in the Hall of Fame for Great Americans. An editorial about this event stated:

> The kind of health care Lillian Wald began preaching and practicing in 1893 is the kind the people of this country are still crying for. She demonstrated with no need to rest on formal research that

nursing could serve as the entry point—not only for health care, but for dealing with many other social ills of which sickness is only a part. She felt that nurses should go to the sick, instead of expecting the sick to come to them (and waiting for physicians to refer them); that care of persons in the home, especially of children, was far more effective and much less expensive except perhaps for those needing, to use her own word, "intensive" care. (A Prophet Honored, 1971, p. 53)

MARY BRECKINRIDGE

A remarkable leader in providing nursing services in rural areas was Mary Breckinridge. She founded the Frontier Nursing Service to provide public health nursing care to people in rural Kentucky. Like Wald, this remarkable woman dedicated her life to improving the health of the poor and underserved.

Almost from birth Breckinridge held a fondness and affinity for the people of Kentucky. Her father had been born and raised in Lexington, Kentucky. Her Grandmother Lees, a Kentuckian by birth, was a wealthy and charitable woman who spent a large part of her fortune on the education of Kentucky children. Mary said of her grandmother, "I doubt if she ever refused to help any Kentucky mountain child whose need she knew" (Breckinridge, 1952, p. 4). Young Mary would sit at her grandmother's feet and listen to the letters she read from the children she was helping. Later in life Mary would state, "Nearly a lifetime later, when I was living on money that came from my Grandmother Lees, it seemed altogether right to use this money to start the Frontier Nursing Service in the Kentucky mountains" (Breckinridge, p. 4).

Mary's family was well-to-do and travelled extensively. Although it was not deemed "proper" for her to receive a college education, Mary and her sister were educated by governesses and learned to speak both German and French. Mary loved her family and enjoyed her life but said, "I chafed at the complete lack of purpose in the things I was allowed to do. Several times I suggested to my mother that it would be nice to do something useful, but I never got anywhere with such an idea" (Breckinridge, 1952, p. 45). Later in life Mary would remedy that situation.

As a girl Mary frequently visited her uncle's plantation, and it was there that she learned to ride a horse—a skill that was a great asset to her in the Frontier Nursing Service. She would say of these times, "The happiest hours of my girlhood were spent on Oasis plantation in Mississippi and I loved it more than any place in the world. . . . We rode constantly when I was young, not only for fun but often because it was the easiest way to get about" (Breckinridge, 1952, p. 36).

Her life was marred by the early death of her first husband. Following his death she enrolled in nursing school at St. Luke's Hospital in New York City (Wilkie, Moseley, 1969, p. 27). She remarried after graduation, but this marriage ended after the death of her two children, an infant daughter and, soon after, her 4-year-old son. Her children gone and her marriage over, she began to devote herself to the work that would consume the rest of her life. She cherished the memories of her lost children and always had a special affinity for children, saying "My life was dedicated to the service of children" (Breckinridge, 1952, p. 111).

The Frontier Nursing Service

The Frontier Nursing Service was established in 1925. By 1930 six outpost nursing centers covered an area of 700 square miles and were serving nearly 10,000 people in southeastern Kentucky (Browne, 1966, p. 55). The service provided visiting nursing services; built a hospital; established medical, surgical, and dental clinics; and provided its famous nurse midwifery services. All nurses in the service were required to have nurse midwifery education in addition to their nursing and public health training.

The midwifery services were very successful and greatly reduced maternal and infant mortality. In looking at the first 1000 midwifery cases of the Frontier Nursing Service, it was noted that there were one third fewer stillbirths and one third fewer deaths among babies in the first year of life than among the general population of Kentucky, and that if such a service were available to all U.S. women there would be a savings of 10,000 mothers' lives a year, 30,000 fewer stillbirths, and 30,000 more infants alive at the end of the first month of life (Kalisch, Kalisch, 1995, pp. 279-280). The Frontier Nursing Service was an effort of love and caring and a great success! The Frontier Nursing Service in Hyden, Kentucky is still in operation today, and many agencies have modeled their programs after the work of Mary Breckinridge and the Frontier Nursing Service.

PROVIDING EARLY PUBLIC HEALTH NURSING SERVICES

Through the efforts of people such as Lillian Wald and Mary Breckinridge, public health nursing had emerged in the United States. Concepts of disease prevention and health promotion, personal responsibility for health and self-care, and use of community resources to promote health were all part of the practice of the public health nurse.

As is the practice today, often several different organizations in one city or county were carrying out home care. There were visiting nurses largely from philanthropic charity organizations caring for the ill and teaching families, and public health nurses (often from local health departments or employed by schools) teaching disease prevention and health promotion. To better define nursing roles and avoid duplication of services, a committee of representatives from numerous agencies interested in public health nursing in 1946 published guidelines on which public health nursing should be organized (Desirable Organization, 1946, p. 387).

The guidelines adopted by the committee agreed that a population of 50,000 was needed to support an adequate health program and that there should be one public health nurse for every 2000 people. Other principles included the following:

- That each public health nurse should combine the functions of health teaching, control of disease, and care of the sick
- That the community should adopt one of three patterns of organization that would best serve that community:
  1. All public health nursing service, including care of the sick at home, administered by the local health department
  2. Preventive services carried on by the health department with one voluntary agency, in close coordination with the health department, carrying responsibility for bedside nursing care
  3. A combination service jointly administered and financed by official and voluntary agencies, with all service given by a single group of public health nurses

It was agreed that it was important for public health nurses to be represented by a professional organization, have standards of practice, and be organized.

ORGANIZING PUBLIC HEALTH NURSES

Leaders among public health nurses, including Lillian Wald, Mary Sewall Gardner, Ellen Phillips Crandall, and Jane Delano, recognized the need to develop a professional organization and professional standards of practice. These same leaders clearly felt that only a new organization "whose sole object should be public health nursing would adequately meet the need" (Gardner, 1919, p. 41).

National Organization for Public Health Nursing

June 7, 1912 was a momentous day in the history of American public health nursing: at the annual meeting of the American Nurses Association and the Society of Superintendents of Training Schools, the National Organization for Public Health Nursing (now the National League for Nursing) was voted into existence with Lillian Wald as president. The two purposes of the National Organization for Public Health Nursing (NOPHN) were the stimulation and standardization of public health nursing and the furthering of relationships among all people interested in the public's health. It was the first national nursing organization to have a headquarters and paid staff. For a long period in the development of nursing it grew in power, set standards for practice, and influenced education by requiring certain curriculum content as a basis for employment (Fagin, 1978, p. 752). One of the unique features of the NOPHN was that membership was open to public health nursing agencies and other interested people as well as to nurses. Collaborative relationships among health and social agencies has always been a strength among those who work in public health nursing. The NOPHN became the National League for Nursing in 1952.

STANDARDS OF PRACTICE

Standards of practice are a hallmark of a profession, and it was long recognized that standards of practice needed to be developed for the profession. Although individual agencies provide conscientious and quality services, overall professional standards are needed. The first comprehensive statement of public health nursing objectives and functions was prepared by the NOPHN in 1931 (McIver, 1949, p. 65).

Standards of practice provide guidance in achieving excellence in care. They reflect current knowledge in the field and represent agreed upon levels of practice (ANA, 1986, p. 1). *Standards of Community Health Nursing Practice* were first written by the ANA in 1973. These standards were revised in 1986 and are presently being revised again. Currently both the American Nurses Association (ANA) and the American Public Health Association (APHA) are preparing documents that address excellence in public health/community health nursing practice. Chapter 2 discusses ANA's and APHA's beliefs about the scope of practice and standards of care for community health nurses.

EDUCATION FOR PUBLIC HEALTH NURSES

The education of public health nurses historically presented special problems because, traditionally, all nurses were prepared in apprentice-type programs in hospitals. Their curriculum was determined by the needs of the hospital and was controlled by the physicians. The education was illness- and individual-oriented and did not adequately prepare nurses to work in the community.

At the time of Lillian Wald, nurses going into public health nursing had to receive additional education following their basic nursing education. The first course in public health nursing was offered by the Boston Instructive Nursing Association in 1906 (McNeil, 1967, p. 4). However, considering the broad scope of a public health nurse's work, it soon became apparent that education for these nurses needed to be broad in scope. Because of the nurse's concern with social and educational problems, many early public health nursing programs were in teacher's colleges or university departments of sociology or social work.

In 1919, under the auspices of the Rockefeller Foundation and at the urging of concerned nursing leaders, the Committee for the Study of Public Health Nursing Education, with C-E.A. Winslow as chairman, began a 2-year investigation. Josephine Goldmark was secretary of the committee, and the study was later to bear her name.

The Goldmark Report

The purposes of the Committee were to study public health nursing education, to look at typical examples of public health nursing education and service, and to study the education afforded by hospital training schools, graduate courses for public health nurses, and special schools of a nonnursing type (Committee for the Study of Nursing Education, 1923, p. 2). The study was expanded the following year to look at the entire field of nursing education. Ten conclusions were reached that have profoundly affected the course of public health nursing, as well as of all nursing

Conclusions of the Committee for the Study of Nursing Education, 1923

Conclusion 1. That, since constructive health work and health teaching in families is best done by persons:

(a) capable of giving general health instruction, as distinguished from instruction in any one specialty; and

(b) capable of rendering bedside care at need; the agent responsible for such constructive health work and health teaching in families should have completed the nurses' training. There will, of course, be need for the employment, in addition to the public health nurse, of other types of experts such as nutrition workers, social workers, occupational therapists, and the like.

That as soon as may be practicable all agencies, public or private, employing public health nurses, should require as a prerequisite for employment the basic hospital training, followed by a postgraduate course, including both class work and field work, in public health nursing.

Conclusion 2. That the career open to young women of high capacity, in public health nursing or in hospital supervision and nursing education, is one of the most attractive fields now open, in its promise of professional success and of rewarding public service; and that every effort should be made to attract such women into this field.

Conclusion 3. That for the care of persons suffering from serious and acute disease, the safety of the patient, and the responsibility of the medical and nursing professions, demand the maintenance of the standards of educational attainment now generally accepted by the best sentiment of both professions and embodied in the legislation of the more progressive states; and that any attempt to lower these standards would be fraught with real danger to the public.

Conclusion 4. That steps should be taken through state legislation for the definition and licensure of a subsidiary grade of nursing service, the subsidiary type of worker to serve under practicing physicians in the care of mild and chronic illness and convalescence, and possibly to assist under the direction of the trained nurse in certain phases of hospital and visiting nursing.

Conclusion 5. That, while training schools for nurses have made remarkable progress, and while the best schools of today in many respects reach a high level of educational attainment, the average hospital training school is not organized on such a basis as to conform to the standards accepted in other educational fields; that the instruction in such schools is frequently casual and uncorrelated; that the educational needs and the health and strength of students are frequently sacrificed to practical hospital exigencies; that such shortcomings are primarily due to the lack of independent endowments for nursing education; that existing educational facilities are on the whole, in the majority of schools, inadequate for the preparation of the high grade of nurses required for the care of serious illness, and for service in the fields of public health nursing and nursing education; and that one of the chief reasons for the lack of sufficient recruits, of a high type, to meet such needs lies precisely in the fact that the average hospital training school does not offer a sufficiently attractive avenue of entrance to this field.

Conclusion 6. That, with the necessary financial support and under a separate board or training school committee, organized primarily for educational purposes, it is possible, with completion of a high school course or its equivalent as a prerequisite, to reduce the fundamental period of hospital training to 28 months, and at the same time, by eliminating unessential, noneducational routine, and adopting the principles laid down in Miss Goldmark's report, to organize the course along intensive and coordinated lines with such modifications as may be necessary for practical application; and that courses of this standard would be reasonably certain to attract students of high quality in increasing numbers.

Conclusion 7. Superintendents, supervisors, instructors, and public health nurses should in all cases receive special additional training beyond the basic nursing course.

Conclusion 8. That the development and strengthening of University Schools of Nursing of a high grade for the training of leaders is of fundamental importance in the furtherance of nursing education.

Conclusion 9. That when the licensure of a subsidiary grade of nursing service is provided for, the establishment of training courses in preparation for such service is highly desirable; that such courses should be conducted in special hospitals, in small unaffiliated general hospitals, or in separate sections of hospitals where nurses are also trained; and that the course should be of 8 or 9 months' duration; provided the standards of such schools be approved by the same educational board which governs nursing training schools.

Conclusion 10. That the development of nursing service adequate for the care of the sick and for the conduct of the modern public health campaign demands as an absolute prerequisite the securing of funds for the endowment of nursing education of all types; and that it is of primary importance, in this connection, to provide reasonably generous endowment for university schools of nursing.

From Committee for the Study of Nursing Education: *Nursing and nursing education in the United States*, New York, 1923, Macmillan.

(Committee for the Study of Nursing Education). These conclusions are in the accompanying box. As a result of this study, poor quality nursing schools were closed, qualified faculty members were hired, and the money allotted to education programs began to increase.

By 1921 public health nursing courses that met standards developed by the NOPHN were offered by 15 colleges and universities. These courses taught "preventive medicine," covering topics such as how to examine a class of children, how to find those who were developing measles, and how to visit in a home and evaluate tuberculosis contacts (Jensen, 1959, p. 236).

In 1944 the first basic collegiate program in nursing was accredited as including adequate preparation for public health nursing so that graduates did not need additional study to practice public health nursing after graduation from the basic nursing program (National Organization for Public Health Nursing, 1944, p. 371).

After 1963 no baccalaureate nursing program was accredited unless it prepared its graduates for public health nursing. This community health education has continued to be a major difference between the educational programs of baccalaureate nurses and diploma and associate degree programs.

During the 1980s a national consensus conference was held (USDHHS, 1985) and national studies were conducted (Blank, McElmurry, 1988; Jones, Davis, Davis, 1987) to examine the educational preparation needed to practice as a generalist (bacccalaureate prepared) and specialist (master's prepared) in public health nursing. A national consensus conference was also held to address education preparation for a specialist in home care (Cary, 1989). During this conference participants believed that a home care specialist needed strong preparation in public health nursing. Currently several documents address the essential concepts needed to function effectively in public health nursing (ACHNE, 1990, 1991, 1993, 1995; APHA, 1996; Blank, McElmurry, 1988; Jones, Davis, Davis, 1987; USDHHS, 1985). These concepts will be addressed throughout the text.

Professional Books and Journals

Books and journals are an important part of any educational program. It is through books and journals that the nurse can learn about the field, stay current, and find out about the progress in research and clinical practice.

In 1916 Mary Sewall Gardner wrote the first public health nursing text, aptly titled *Public Health Nursing*. On the very day that the NOPHN was formed, the Cleveland Visiting Nurses' Association presented its magazine, *The Quarterly*, to the group as a gift. *The Quarterly* later became *Public Health Nursing* and, still later, *Nursing Outlook*. It was an essential element to the development and dissemination of the public health nursing movement in the United States. Today numerous books and journals specifically address the practice of community health nursing.

THE EFFECTS OF WORLD WAR I ON PUBLIC HEALTH NURSING

By 1915 the role of the public health nurse was well established. However, with the advent of World War I in 1917 and the involvement of thousands of nurses in military service, public health nursing services were threatened. The American Red Cross investigated methods to deal with the situation (Roberts, 1954, p. 131). The efficient use of the limited supply of public health nurses was ensured by the Red Cross, which set up a roster of nurses who could be called upon to coordinate and supplement health resources. Emphasis was placed upon educational programs for the community as well as the control of communicable diseases. During World War I a nurse was loaned to the U.S. Public Health Service from the National Organization of Public Health Nursing to develop a public health nursing program for military outposts. This was the first public health nursing service to be established within the federal government (Gardner, 1916).

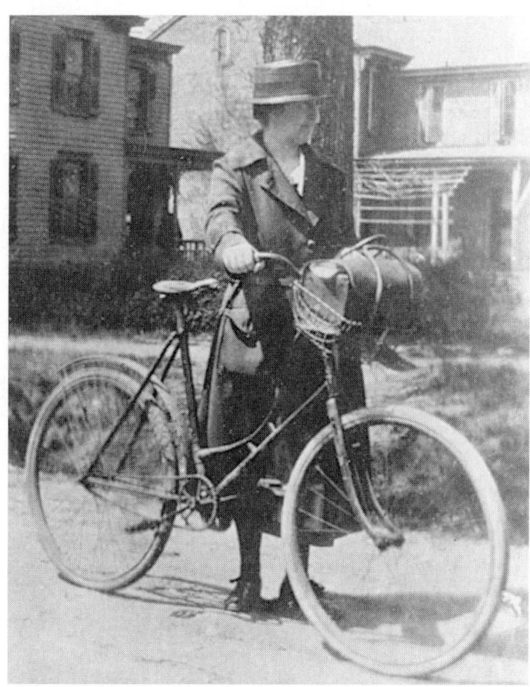

Figure 1-5 Public health nurse using a bicycle before the advent of the automobile. *(Courtesy The Metropolitan Life Insurance Company of New York.)*

The Vassar Training Camp for Nurses

A unique experience in the annals of nursing education was the Vassar Camp School of Nursing. Begun in 1918 and supported by the American Red Cross and the Council of National Defense, the program was based on the principle that the 3-year nursing course could be shortened to 2 years for students who had graduated from college majoring in other subjects. The purpose was to more rapidly fill the desperate need for nurses in wartime. Applicants to the program chose a college and were admitted into selected nursing schools across the country. Graduates of this program numbered 435; the program ended with the Armistice.

AFTER WORLD WAR I

Rapid changes came with peace. Economic prosperity, reaction to Prohibition, and the increasing use of the automobile created radical changes in the way people lived. These changes brought subsequent changes in public health nursing. The use of the automobile, for instance, permitted nurses to have easy access to rural areas and made once-closed areas accessible. The previous use of walking, bicycles, and horse and buggies made it difficult to reach many underserved populations (Figures 1-4, 1-5, and 1-6).

The poor physical condition of the nation's men, made evident in wartime, shocked the nation. About 29% of

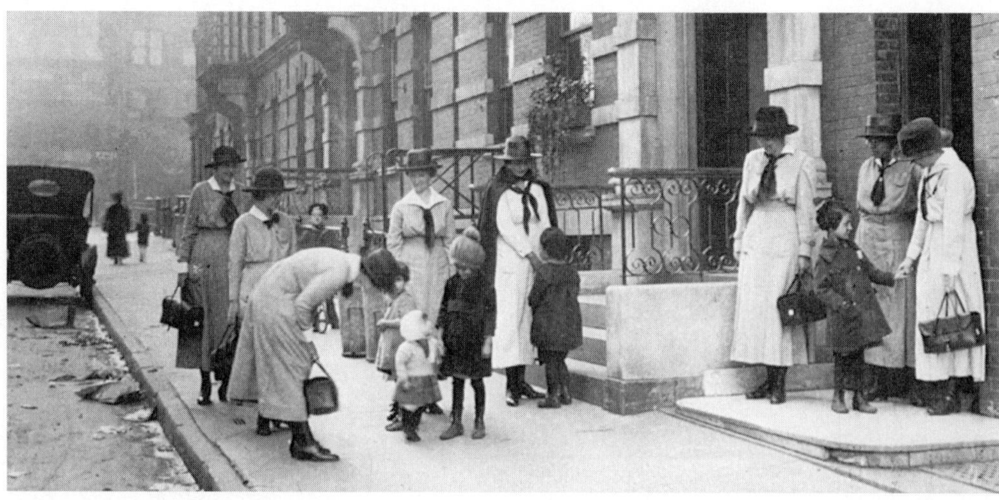

Figure 1-6 To these nurses of the 1930s, the city's streets were hospital corridors and family bedrooms their wards. Each carried cakes of soap to protect herself from germs and a whistle to guard herself from danger. *(Courtesy Visiting Nurse Service of New York City.)*

those called for service were unfit for military duty because of problems that in many cases were preventable (Roberts, 1954, p. 164). Health programs of both official and nonofficial private agencies grew as a result.

Before the war public health was a community affair administered under local self-government with slight state government supervision. In 1920 only 28 states had a statewide public health nursing program, and only five had divisions of public health nursing within state health departments (Roberts, 1954, p. 168). After the war there was an extraordinary phenomenon of the "nationalization of the public health," and public health become a subject of nationwide interest and concern (Smillie, 1952, p. 10).

During this time voluntary (non–tax-supported) agencies were very active in public health nursing activities. Two of these organizations were the American Red Cross and the National Tuberculosis Association (forerunner of today's American Lung Association). The Red Cross supplemented the work of health agencies and supported the idea that public health nursing should be the responsibility of municipalities, counties, and states. Public health nursing supervisors in some state health departments were also Red Cross supervisors. The National Tuberculosis Association provided public health nursing services to tuberculosis patients in many states (Fox, 1920, p. 180) (Figure 1-7).

The passage of the Shepherd-Towner Act of 1921 was a historic milestone in the evolution of public health and public health nursing. Studies by the Children's Bureau at the federal level showed that the United States had a higher maternal death rate than most other developed countries. This act, administered by the Children's Bureau, gave grants to states to develop programs that provided care to mothers, infants, and children.

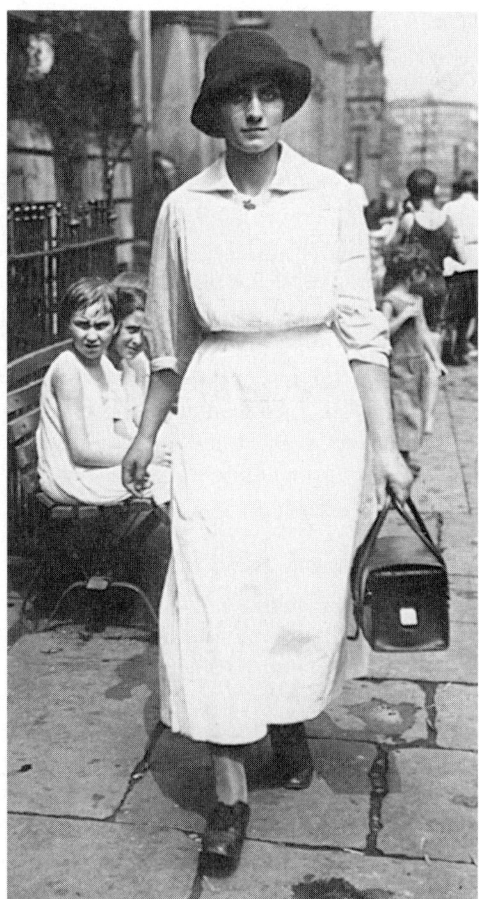

Figure 1-7 From the turn of the century on, the visiting nurse served as the first line of defense in the fight against diphtheria, tuberculosis, and other "killer" contagions of the era. *(Courtesy Visiting Nurse Service of New York City.)*

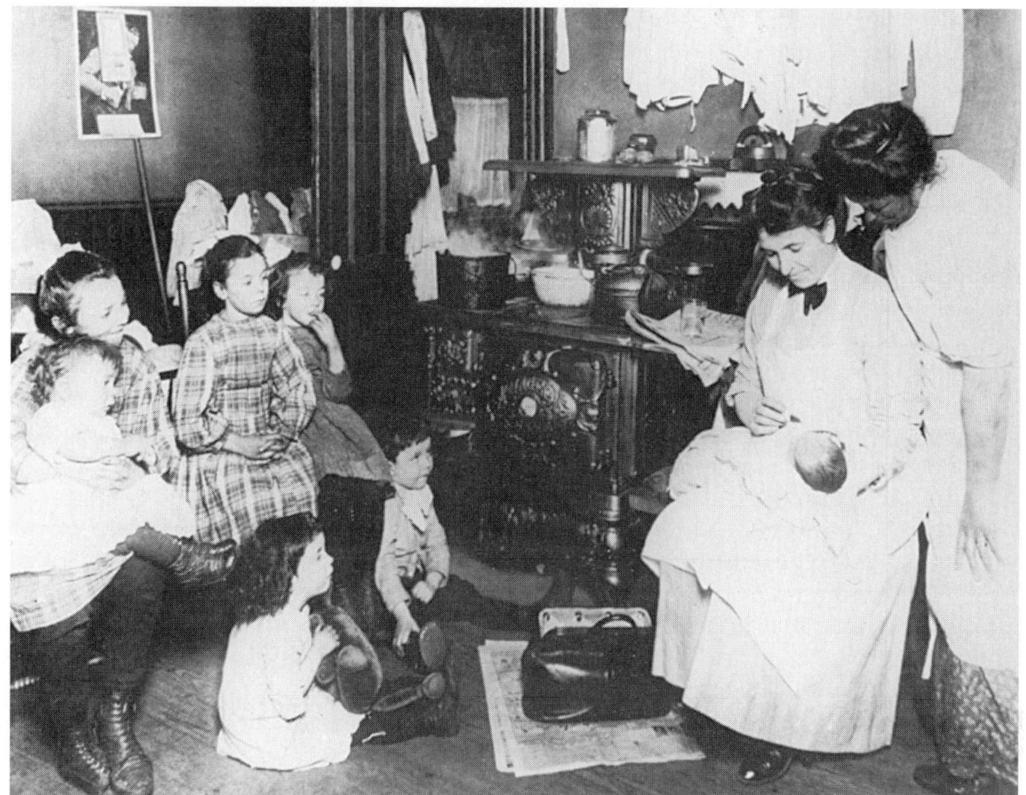

Figure **1-8** Involving the family in baby care, Boston, 1912. *(Courtesy The Metropolitan Life Insurance Company of New York.)*

Marie Phelan was appointed in 1923 as the first nurse consultant to the federal government in peacetime. At the request of state health departments she helped to develop programs that promoted the health of mothers and children (Figure 1-8). Her work had the effect of creating a demand for nurses to work with official health agencies to begin demonstration programs with mothers and infants and was instrumental in lowering the national maternal death rate.

The Great Depression and the Social Security Act

The Depression of 1929 forced many hospitals and schools of nursing to close, and the supply of nurses far exceeded the demand. In an effort to deal with many of the problems brought on by the Depression, the Social Security Act of 1935 introduced many government health and welfare programs and provided monies that aided in the expansion of public health nursing services (see Chapter 4).

Before 1935 only one third of the states had a public health nursing section within the state health department, and only 7% of the public health nurses employed had taken an accredited course in public health nursing. During 1936, the first year that money became available through the Social Security Act, over 1000 nurses received money to study public health nursing. By 1940 3000 nurses had received public health training in accredited schools, and 970 counties had developed full-time public health services (Williams, 1951, p. 156).

The Social Security Act and Public Health

Title VI of the Social Security Act focused on public health programs; its overall purpose was to elicit a public health program that would protect and promote the nation's health. Title VI was directly responsible for expanding and developing public health nursing programs and provided money for nurses to study public health. As a result of this legislation the public health nurse became an integral part of local health departments; the maternal and child health programs of the Social Security Act made the nurse's work with families essential.

Maternal-Child Health Expands

Historically, maternal-child health has been a major focus of community health nursing. Lillian Wald and Mary Breckinridge both were advocates for children's rights and supported programs that promoted maternal-infant health. In 1912, with the help of leaders like Lillian Wald, the Children's Bureau was created to help meet the needs of children. Title V of the Social Security Act greatly strengthened the public health nurse's ability to provide maternal and child health care to high risk families and expanded available services.

Funds from the Title V grant program were designed to improve the health of mothers and children who did not have access to adequate health care, particularly those from low-income families (see Chapters 4 and 15).

THE EFFECTS OF WORLD WAR II ON PUBLIC HEALTH NURSING

After World War II began in 1941, the nurse shortage became acute. The National Nursing Council, composed of six national nursing organizations, along with the aid of the U.S. Department of Education, requested $1 million to enlarge facilities for nursing education. Funding programs for nurses' training included Training for Nurses for National Defense, the GI bill, the Nurse Training Act of 1943, and Public Health and Professional Nurse traineeships.

The Public Health Service Act of 1944 consolidated existing federal public health legislation and provided for many public health programs (see Chapter 4).

Overall, World War II had a major impact on public health nursing. Specifically, the war influenced the following trends:

1. The importance of public health nursing service was recognized when public health nurses were declared essential for civilian work, although many of them entered military service
2. Maximum utilization of personnel was essential; official tax-supported public health nursing agencies combined with voluntary, non–tax-supported agencies to avoid duplication
3. Practical nurses were accepted as an important resource for nursing service
4. The establishment of priorities for health care became an important topic for discussion
5. Additional funds for nursing education became available and the fear of governmental control of education decreased. After the war, enrollment of nurses who were veterans or widows of veterans strained the resources of universities and agencies providing field experience.

When the war was over in 1945, President Harry Truman presented to Congress his recommendation for a comprehensive, national health care program in which nursing would have played an important role (Kalisch, Kalisch, 1995, p. 364). Truman recommended the following:

1. Federal grants for construction of hospitals and related facilities
2. Expansion of public health, maternity, and child health services
3. Federal grants for medical education, nursing education, and research
4. Establishment of a national social insurance program for the prepayment of medical costs
5. Expansion of present social insurance systems to furnish protection against loss of wages from sickness and disability

Charges of socialism from the American Medical Association ended the quest for national health insurance in 1949 and 1950 (Kalisch, Kalisch, 1995, p. 366). Today the United States still does not have a national health insurance program. The American Nurses Association strongly supported President Clinton's Health Reform Act in 1993; however, that act did not pass.

The Federal Government Provides Funding for Nursing Education

Right after World War II the nation recognized that a serious undersupply of nurses created critical situations in hospitals and health centers.

The government became involved in preparing new nurses with the passage of the Health Amendments Act of 1956, which authorized monies to aid registered nurses in the full-time study of administration, supervision, or teaching.

However, in 1963 the Surgeon General's Consultant Group on Nursing reported that there were still too few nursing schools and not enough nurses (U.S. Public Health Service, 1963). Based on these conclusions, the Nurse Training Act of 1964 was passed to provide money for nursing school construction and student nursing loans and scholarships.

THE BIRTH OF NURSING RESEARCH

Sigma Theta Tau, the international honor society in nursing, awarded the first known grant for nursing research in the United States in 1936 (Hudgings, Hogan, Stevenson, 1990, p. i). However, very little nursing research was being done at this time.

The decade of the 1950s is considered by many to be the birth of modern nursing research. In this decade the American Nurses Association (ANA) and the National League for Nursing (NLN) became actively involved in promoting nursing research. In 1954 ANA formed a Committee on Research and Studies, and in 1959 NLN established a Research and Studies Service. In 1952 the first nursing research journal, aptly named *Nursing Research,* was published.

By the 1960s ANA and NLN were at the forefront of nursing research activities. In 1962 ANA established nursing research priorities and published "Blueprint for Research in Nursing" in the *American Journal of Nursing.* In the 1960s new journals with a nursing research focus emerged, such as *International Journal of Nursing Studies* and *IMAGE.* In 1965 ANA held the first nursing research conference. These conferences were held yearly from 1965 to 1973 and were funded by grants from the Division of Nursing in the U.S. Public Health Service. In 1969 the first Center for Nursing Research in a college of nursing was established at Wayne State University College of Nursing in Detroit, Michigan (Werley, Shea, 1973, p. 217). H. Harriet Werley was the director of this program. Many early studies from the Center focused on community health nursing issues.

THE DECADES OF THE 1960s AND 1970s

Dating from the 1960s the federal government more aggressively took on the role of guardian of the nation's health. President Kennedy's inaugural address in 1961 is remembered for the words, "Ask not what your country can do for you—ask what you can do for your country." A new social consciousness swept the nation. The Constitution of the World Health Organization defined health as "complete physical, mental and social well-being and not just the absence of disease." This definition reflected inclusion of the mental and social aspects of health, as well as its physical aspects.

In the 1970s health care resources and services proliferated rapidly. Many Americans were insured under comprehensive health care insurance plans and began to see health as a right rather than a privilege. The ability to provide these health services led to numerous attempts to provide a national health insurance, though none were successful.

In 1972 Nurses for Political Action was organized, with headquarters in Washington, D.C. It became affiliated with the American Nurses Association and later changed its name to N-CAP, Nurses' Coalition for Action in Politics. Its purpose as a nonpartisan, nonprofit association was to obtain support for nursing from legislators, government officials, and the general public. The present health care system was fragmented and dominated by the medical profession, and nurses sought a place where they could help plan a system that comprehensively met the nation's health care needs.

In the 1970s all areas of nursing, including parent and child nursing, psychiatric nursing, and medical and surgical nursing, began discovering the community. These areas also began to emphasize the importance of the family to the patient, and the clear lines of distinction for what constituted public health nursing started to blur. However, it must be reemphasized that public health nursing was seen as a specialized area of practice with a broad comprehensive focus. Efforts were made to specifically define the nature, standards, and scope of public health nursing practice, and in 1973 standards of practice for community health nursing were developed by the American Nurses Association.

During the 1970s more non–health and allied health professionals began to work in the community. Social workers, physical therapists, occupational therapists, physicians' assistants, and home health aides were seen in public health settings. This increased the nurse's responsibility for coordinating care among the variety of health care providers. This responsibility continues to expand as the number of private agencies and health facilities involved in community-based practice multiplies. Health maintenance organizations, neighborhood health centers, free clinics, and numerous home health care programs represent some of the many facilities that sprang up in the community. The rapid development of health services and specialties created some confusion for people who found the existing health care system difficult to negotiate. People desperately needed someone to help them, and community health nurses offered hope.

The decade of the 1970s saw the more common usage of the term *community health nurse* instead of the historical term *public health nurse*. The term *community health nurse* was seen by many as "broadening" and better reflecting the holistic scope of practice and caring for the community. The term *community health nurse* was used in the standards of practice first published by the American Nurses Association in 1973.

The Expanding Role of the Nurse

By the 1960s the nursing profession began to look at new methods of meeting the health care needs of people, using advanced nursing practice, and extending the nursing role to take over some medical functions. The term *nurse practitioner* was first used at the University of Colorado in 1965 in a program that prepared nurses to provide comprehensive well-child care in ambulatory settings. The number of educational programs for advanced practice has risen rapidly, and the acceptance of advanced practice nurses (APNs) by the general public has been extremely positive. Today APNs provide primary care in many health care settings. Certification for these nurses is supported by major professional nursing organizations.

COMMUNITY HEALTH NURSING IN THE 1980s

The 1980s brought opportunities and threats to the health care setting. Consumers became more involved in pressing for healthcare reform and in examining methods to reduce their own risks for disease and disability (Roberts, Heinrich, 1985). Numerous health care delivery issues such as quality, accountability, and access came to the forefront, as did an increasingly well-educated and sophisticated consumer of health care. Renewed interest in home care services emerged, as did a greater focus on health promotion and disease prevention. There was intense interest about skyrocketing health care costs, cost containment, and quality assessment, and cost-containment measures were enacted at the federal and state level.

In the 1980s our nation's health status data reflected a dismal state of affairs. "Every key measure of maternal and child health in the United States worsened, failed to improve, or improved at a slower rate than in previous years. As a result the United States has fallen behind other countries with fewer resources on important health indicators such as infant mortality and low birthweight" (Children's Defense Fund, 1992, p. 1). The Institute of Medicine, in its classic report *The Future of Public Health,* addressed the fact that health care professionals and consumers were having to deal with immediate, enduring, and growing health care challenges (e.g., AIDS, health and welfare access issues for the poor and near-poor, an aging population, increasing poverty, and homelessness) with increasingly fewer resources (Institute of Medicine, 1988).

The 1980s were a time for reflection for consumer groups, health care professionals, and political leaders. Recognizing the serious state of affairs, all of these groups pushed for health care reform. Recognition grew that nurses are valuable resources in the health care system and can provide cost-effective preventive services.

The Healthy People Initiative

Probably one of the most significant occurrences in the 1980s was the beginning of the "Healthy People Initiative" with the publication of *Healthy People* in 1979 by the federal government. This document outlined health care needs in America and ways for addressing these needs. The following year, *Promoting Health, Preventing Disease: Objectives for the Nation* (USDHHS, 1980) outlined specific health priority areas and objectives that would guide the nation in its quest for health in the decade of 1980 to 1990. Chapter 4 discusses this initiative in more detail. This was the first time that the federal government had set national health priority areas and objectives and attempted to chart a course for the public health of the nation.

Nursing Research

The National Center for Nursing Research (NCNR) was authorized under the Health Research Extension Act of 1985 (Public Law 99-158) and was established on April 18, 1986 as part of the National Institutes of Health (NIH) in the USPHS. Its major purpose was to conduct a program of grants and funding to support nursing research and research training, expand the knowledge base in nursing, and promote health across the life span. Through the efforts of ANA and NLN and the support of nurses across the nation, the Center is the first and only national center for nursing research in the world.

With the establishment of NCNR, nursing research studies increased by leaps and bounds. NCNR became a major funding mechanism for nursing research. The accompanying box identifies national nursing research priorities. Other funding for nursing research includes the NIH's Institute of the Alcohol, Drug Abuse and Mental Health Administration, as well as many private funding resources (ANA, 1989).

On June 10, 1993 the NCNR became the National Institute of Nursing Research (NINR), the first and only one of its kind in the world. Nursing research in the United States is helping to shape nursing practice worldwide; American nurses can be very proud of their research heritage.

PRIORITIES RESULTING FROM SECOND CONFERENCE ON RESEARCH PRIORITIES IN NURSING PRACTICE

1—COMMUNITY-BASED NURSING MODELS (1995)
Develop and test community-based nursing models designed to promote access to, utilization of, and quality of health services by rural and other underserved populations.

2—HEALTH-PROMOTING BEHAVIOR AND HIV/AIDS (1996)
Assess the effectiveness of bio-behavioral nursing interventions to foster health-promoting behaviors of individuals of different cultural backgrounds—especially women—who are at high risk for HIV/AIDS, incorporating bio-behavioral markers.

3—COGNITIVE IMPAIRMENT (1997)
Develop and test bio-behavioral and environmental approaches to remediating cognitive impairment.

4—LIVING WITH CHRONIC ILLNESS (1998)
Test interventions to strengthen individuals' personal resources in dealing with their chronic illness.

5—BIO-BEHAVIORAL FACTORS RELATED TO IMMUNOCOMPETENCE (1999)
Identify bio-behavioral factors and test interventions to promote immunocompetence.

From National Center for Nursing Research: *Priorities resulting from second conference on research priorities in nursing practice*, Bethesda, Md., February 1993, NCNR.

THE CYCLICAL NATURE OF ISSUES IN COMMUNITY HEALTH NURSING

The issues that face community health nurses (CHNs) relating to common practices and education today are amazingly like those faced by Lillian Wald and her contemporaries. Impoverished families, lack of prenatal care, lack of elder care, malnutrition, lack of health care, babies born to destitute parents, communicable disease, and sexually transmitted diseases are problems that cross centuries. Human needs do not change or diminish—only our methods of dealing with them.

Recent cost-containment measures have affected the provision of health care services. State and local health departments need to critically examine each program that they offer, including community health nursing. Often programs lack adequate documentation of the effectiveness of community health nursing intervention. Preventive efforts and those that are long-term in nature are difficult to evaluate; thus CHNs must make such research a priority.

THE DECADE OF THE 1990s

As the decade of the 1990s comes to an end it is evident that the acute-care model of care delivery and disease-focused care and payment systems do not promote health, that many Americans remain uninsured and underinsured, that as America is aging many of the health care needs of the elderly go unmet, that managed care is not the answer to everyone's health care needs, and that vulnerable groups such as people who are handicapped, disabled, elderly, and minorities often have difficulty accessing appropriate health care. Although "Health Care for All" is a goal being promoted worldwide, it is not a reality for many Americans. As previously mentioned, the role of the advanced practice nurse is rapidly increasing to address unmet needs.

Health care planners, researchers, and practitioners note that we need to know more about the costs, effectiveness, quality, and safety of methods of health care. Methods to link health care management decisions to systematic information about outcomes of practice are necessary to improve the effectiveness of care and provide a firm basis for economic decision making. Alternatives to the health care system that we now have in place need to be explored. Nurses need to support their professional organizations in their efforts to provide quality, affordable, accessible health care for all Americans.

Healthy People 2000

Healthy People 2000 (USDHHS, 1990) continued the Healthy People Initiative for the decade of 1990-2000 and is referred to throughout this text. It built on the progress made with the *Healthy People* goals and objectives, added new priority areas, and set the course for America's health for the next decade. Nursing organizations were instrumental in the writing of the document, and nurses are playing a major role in accomplishing many of its objectives.

CHALLENGES FOR THE FUTURE

A key issue that will continue to challenge the profession throughout the next decade is the spiraling cost of health care. Medical costs are the fastest growing item in the federal government's budget. At the current rate of growth, spending for health care in the next 10 years will be in the trillions of dollars. If current rates of health care spending are maintained, problems with growing poverty, drug and alcohol abuse, teenage pregnancy, family violence, and the AIDS epidemic will have limited attention. There is no doubt that the current trend of managed health care will continue to expand. A significant challenge for nurses is to ensure quality care while delivering cost-effective care.

"Helping families to help themselves" was a creed of the earliest nurses who visited families in their homes. That creed is even more important for the contemporary community health nurse who cannot deal individually with the critical problems in our society. "In a free society public activities ultimately rest on public understanding and support, not on the technical judgment of experts. Expertise is made effective only when it is combined with sufficient public support, a connection acted upon effectively by the early leaders of public health" (Institute of Medicine, 1988). To be able to use the wealth of knowledge known about diseases and their prevention, we need to know more about how to communicate this to the public to mobilize their support. This is one of the major challenges for public health researchers and practitioners.

The challenges that need to be addressed in the twenty-first century are not insurmountable. Early public health nurse pioneers set the standards for the development of the nursing profession and for reform in health care delivery. They were on the cutting edge of the suffragette movement, the birth control movement, and the social reform movement that brought health care and civil rights to women, children, immigrants, prisoners, and the mentally ill. Their names are seen in the books that tell the story of our nation's history. Appendix 1-1 presents an overview of early nurse leaders whose lives we can celebrate today. They are models for our own professional and personal growth. Nursing leaders continue to have a strong voice in the public health concerns of our nation.

Individual nurses, as well as professional organizations, will be challenged to provide quality health care. We can be proud of the work our professional organizations have done to date to provide comprehensive health care to all, protect the rights of high-risk groups, and support the nursing profession. Nurses are at the cutting edge of research, education, and practice on the local, state, and national level.

SUMMARY

The beginnings of nursing can be traced to the beginnings of humankind, for there has always been a need for reducing pain with comfort measures. The early Christian church's contributions to nursing were significant, as were the organizational contributions of St. Vincent de Paul and Mademoiselle Le Gras to public health nursing. Florence Nightingale's legacy to professional nursing and to public health, along with the contributions of William Rathbone, the founder of public health nursing in England, provided the basis for public health nursing in the United States. Events in society at large have shaped nursing as a whole and the development of public health nursing. Public health nursing can be proud of its strong early leaders, such as Lillian Wald, Mary Breckinridge, and Mary Sewall Gardner.

Public health nurses used advances in the public health sciences to deal with the problems they encountered. The title of community health nurse came into being to emphasize that this field was for the community, not just people who were poor enough to use public assistance programs. How community health nurses organized themselves, along with methods of education for this area of nursing, shaped not only the development of this specialty area but also the entire field of nursing. Emphases in community health nursing, as well as nursing in general, are changing; the health scene is chaotic because there is no overall health plan. Community health nursing, with its focus on the health of aggregates, can involve nurses in health planning and in the necessary task of bringing order out of chaos.

CRITICAL *Thinking Exercise*

"Nursing has reached a point at which it is ready to use its history. Nursing can better evaluate its values and goals and chart its course to fulfill them if nurses have a fuller understanding of who they are and what they do, wish to be, and need to know.

If nursing is to continue to grow as a profession, knowledge of what has been done in the past and what factors influenced its growth are vitally important. It is in looking at nursing's history that safeguards can be established to ensure that the profession profits by its errors and recognizes its successes. If nursing does not study its history, its educational advances, its research, and its publications, it is doomed to repeat the same mistakes" (Hezel, Linebach, 1991, p. 272).

Examining nursing history and using it to analyze current trends and issues will help to ensure that community health nurses profit by errors and recognize successes. After reading this chapter and considering the state of our current health care system, complete one of the following exercises:

1. Select a current societal issue such as environmental pollution and examine the progress or lack of progress made in addressing the problem since early recorded history. Note the writings on the environment of Edwin Chadwick, Florence Nightingale, and Lillian Wald in this chapter.
2. Examine the characteristics of the current immigrants to the United States and consider how they are similar to and different from the immigrants in the early part of the century. How can community health nurses assist recent immigrants with their health needs?
3. Think about some of the achievements of early nursing leaders such as Lillian Wald and Mary Breckinridge and identify factors that facilitated and hindered their ability to accomplish goals. How would you personally deal with these inhibiting factors today?

REFERENCES

American Nurses Association (ANA): *Standards of community health nursing practice,* Kansas City, Mo., 1986, The Association.

American Nurses Association (ANA): *Education for participation in nursing research,* Kansas City, Mo., 1989, The Association.

American Public Health Association (APHA): *The definition and role of public health nursing: a statement of APHA public health nursing section,* Washington, D.C., 1996, APHA.

A prophet honored, *Am J Nurs* 17:53, 1971 (editorial).

Association of Community Health Nursing Educators (ACHNE): *Essentials for entry level community health nursing practice,* Louisville, Ky., 1990, ACHNE.

Association of Community Health Nursing Educators (ACHNE): *Essentials of master's level nursing education for advanced community health nursing practice,* Lexington, Ky., 1991, ACHNE.

Association of Community Health Nursing Educators (ACHNE): *Differentiated nursing practice in community health,* Lexington, Ky., 1993, ACHNE.

Association of Community Health Nursing Educators (ACHNE): *Community/public health advanced practice nurse (C/PHAPN) position statement,* Skokie, Il., 1995, ACHNE.

Backer BA: Lillian Wald: connecting caring with action, *Nurs Health Care* 14(3):122-129, 1993.

Blank JJ, McElmurry BJ: A paradigm for baccalaureate public health nursing education, *Public Health Nurs* 5:183-189, 1988.

Brainard AM: *The evolution of public health nursing,* Philadelphia, 1922, Saunders.

Breckinridge M: *Wide neighborhoods: a story of the Frontier Nursing Service,* New York, 1952, Harper & Brothers.

Browne HE: A tribute to Mary Breckinridge, *Nurs Outlook* 14(5):54-55, 1966.

Buhler-Wilkerson K: Lillian Wald: public health pioneer, *Nurs Res* 40(5):316-317, 1991.

Cary A: *Strategies for a collaborative future: the consensus report for the National Consensus Conference on the Educational Preparation of Home Care Administrators,* Washington, D.C., 1989, Catholic University of America School of Nursing.

Children's Defense Fund: *The state of America's children 1992,* Washington, D.C., 1992, The Fund.

Committee for the Study of Nursing Education: *Nursing and nursing education in the United States,* New York, 1923, Macmillan.

Coss C: Lillian D. Wald: progressive activist, *Public Health Nurs* 10(2):134-138, 1989.

Deloughery GL: *History and trends of professional nursing,* ed 8, St. Louis, 1977, Mosby.

Desirable organization of public health nursing for family service, *Public Health Nurs* 38:387-389, 1946.

Division of Nursing: *A century of caring: a celebration of public health nursing in the United States: 1893-1993,* Washington, D.C., 1992, American Public Health Association.

Dock L, Pickett SE, Noyes CD, et al: *History of American Red Cross nursing,* New York, 1922, Macmillan.

Erickson G: Southern initiative in public health nursing: the founding of the Nurses' Settlement and Instructive Visiting Nurse Association of Richmond, Virginia, 1900-1910, *J Nurs History* 3(1):17-22, 1987.

Fagin CM: Primary care as an academic discipline, *Nurs Outlook* 26:750-753, 1978.

Fitzpatrick ML: Lillian Wald: prototype of an involved nurse, *Imprint* April/May:92-95, 1990.

Fox EG, ed: Red Cross public health nursing, *Public Health Nurs* 12:175-181, 1920.

Gardner MS: *Public health nursing,* New York, 1916, Macmillan.

Gardner MS: *Public health nursing,* ed 1, revised, New York, 1919, Macmillan.

Gardner MS: *Public health nursing,* ed 3, New York, 1936, Macmillan.

Haupt AC: Forty years of teamwork in public health nursing, *Am J Nurs* 53:81-84, 1953.

Hezel LF, Linebach LM: The development of a regional nursing history collection: its relevance to practice, education, and research, *Nurs Outlook* 39(5):268-272, 1991.

Hudgings C, Hogan R, Stevenson JS, eds: *1990 directory of nurse researchers,* ed 3, Indianapolis, 1990, Sigma Theta Tau International.

Institute of Medicine, Committee for the study of the future of public health: *The future of public health,* Washington, D.C., 1988, National Academy Press.

Jensen DM: *History and trends of professional nursing,* ed 4, St. Louis, 1959, Mosby.

Jones DC, Davis JA, Davis MC: *Public health nursing education and practice,* Rockville, Md., 1987, Division of Nursing, USDHHS.

Kalisch P, Kalisch BJ: *The advance of American nursing,* ed 3, Boston, 1995, Little, Brown.

Kaufman M, Hawkins JW, Higgins LP, Friedman AH, eds: *Dictionary of American nursing biography,* Wesport, Ct., 1988, Greenwood Press.

Maynard T: *The apostle of charity: the life of St. Vincent de Paul,* New York, 1939, Dial Books.

McIver P: Public health nursing responsibilities, *Public Health Nurs* 41:65-66, 1949.

McNeil EE: *Transition in public health nursing,* John Sundwall Lecture, Ann Arbor, 1967, University of Michigan.

National Center for Nursing Research: *Priorities resulting from second conference on research priorities in nursing practice,* Bethesda, Md., February 1993, NCNR.

National Organization for Public Health Nursing: Approval of Skidmore College of Nursing as preparing students for public health nursing, *Public Health Nurs* 36:371, 1944.

Nightingale F: *Notes on nursing*, London, England 1859, Harris and Sons.

Nightingale F: Nurses, training of. In Quain R, ed: *A dictionary of medicine*, ed 9, New York, 1885, Appleton, pp. 1038-1043.

Reed PG, Zurakowski TL: Nightingale: foundations of nursing. In Fitzpatrick JJ and Whall AL: *Conceptual models of nursing: analysis and application*, ed 3, Stamford, Ct., 1996, Appleton and Lange, pp. 27-54.

Roberts MM: *American nursing, history and interpretation*, New York, 1954, Macmillan.

Roberts DE, Heinrich J: Public health nursing comes of age, *Am J Public Health* 75:1162-1172, 1985.

Rosen G: *A history of public health*, New York, 1958, MD Publications.

Shea FP, Werley HH: Research conducted at Wayne State University College of Nursing, *Nurs Res* 22:3, 268-270, 1973.

Smillie WG: *Preventive medicine and public health*, ed 2, New York, 1952, Macmillan.

U.S. Department of Health, Education and Welfare: *Healthy people*, Washington, D.C., 1980, U.S. Government Printing Office.

U.S. Department of Health and Human Services (USDHHS): *Promoting health preventing disease: objectives for the nation*, Washington, D.C., 1980, U.S. Government Printing Office.

U.S. Department of Health and Human Services (USDHHS): *Healthy people 2000: objectives for the nation*, Washington, D.C., 1990, U.S. Government Printing Office.

U.S. Department of Health and Human Services (USDHHS): Consensus conference on the essentials of public health nursing practice and education, Rockville, Md., 1985, Division of Nursing, USDHHS.

U.S. Public Health Service: *Toward quality in nursing: needs and goals. Report of the Surgeon General's consultant group on nursing*, Washington D.C., 1963, U.S. Government Printing Office.

Wald L: *The house on Henry Street*, New York, 1915, Holt.

Werley HH, Shea FP: The first center for research in nursing: its development, accomplishments, and problems, *Nurs Res* 22(3):217-231, 1973.

Wilkie KE, Moseley ER: *Frontier nurse: Mary Breckinridge*, New York, 1969, Julian Messner.

Williams R: *The United States public health service*, Bethesda, Md., 1951; Commissioned Officers Association of the U.S. Public Health Service.

Winslow, C-EA: *The conquest of epidemic disease: a chapter in the history of ideas*, Madison, Wi., 1943, University of Wisconsin Press.

Winslow C-EA: Florence Nightingale and public health nursing, *Public Health Nurs* 2:330-332, 1946.

Young EE: A quiet day: a peep at some of the varied homes visited by a district nurse in the course of one "quiet day," *Public Health Nurs* 6:43-44, 1989.

SELECTED BIBLIOGRAPHY

Allen CE: Holistic concepts and the professionalization of public health nursing, *Public Health Nurs* 8(2):74-80, 1991.

Bigbee JL, Crowder ELM: The Red Cross Rural Nursing Service: an innovative model of public health nursing delivery, *Public Health Nurs* 2:109-121, 1985.

Buhler-Wilkerson K: Bringing care to the people: Lillian Wald's legacy to public health nursing, *Am J Public Health* 83(12):1778-1786, 1993.

Buhler-Wilkerson K: Home care the American way: an historical analysis, *Home Health Care Serv Q* 12(3):5-17, 1991.

Carr AM: Development of public health nursing literature, *Public Health Nurs* 5:81-85, 1988.

Christy TE: Portrait of a leader: Lavinia Lloyd Dock, *Nurs Outlook* 17:72-75, 1969.

Christy TE: Portrait of a leader: Lillian Wald, *Nurs Outlook* 18:50-54, 1970.

Daniels DG: *Always a sister: the feminism of Lillian D. Wald*, New York, 1995, Feminist Press.

Dock LL and Stewart IM: *A short history of nursing*, New York, 1931, Putnam.

Dolan JA: *Nursing in society: a historical perspective*, Philadelphia, 1978, Saunders.

Fee E: The origins and development of public health in the United States. In Holland WW, Detels R, Knox G, eds: *Oxford textbook of public health*, ed 2, Oxford, 1991, Oxford University Press, pp. 3-22.

Fiedler LA: *Images of the nurse in fiction and popular culture, literature and medicine*, Albany, N.Y., 1983, Albany State University of New York Press.

Frachel RR: A new profession: the evolution of public health nursing, *Public Health Nurs* 5:86-90, 1988.

Gardner MS: The National Organization for Public Health Nursing, *Visiting Nurse Q* 4:13-18, 1912.

Hamilton D: Clinical excellence, but too high a cost: the Metropolitan Life Insurance Company Visiting Nurse Service (1909-1953), *Public Health Nurs* 5:235-240, 1988.

Mereness DA: From there to here in fifty years, *Nurs Outlook* 39(5):222-225, 1991.

Rathbone W: *History and progress of district nursing*, New York, 1890, Macmillan.

Robinson KR: The role of nursing in the influenza epidemic of 1918-1919, *Nurs Forum* 25(2):19-26, 1990.

Wald L: The treatment of families in which there is sickness, *Am J Nurs* 17(6):427-431, 515-519, 602-606, 1917.

2

Defining Community Health Nursing

Objectives

Upon completion of this chapter, the reader should be able to:

1. Articulate the distinguishing characteristics of community health nursing practice.
2. Formulate a personal definition of community health nursing practice, incorporating key concepts delineated by professional organizations.
3. Discuss the key concepts inherent in community health nursing practice.
4. Describe the mission of public health and how the concept of "Health for All" relates to this mission.
5. Understand the concept of client from the community health nursing perspective.
6. Identify the roles community health nurses assume in the practice setting and settings in which these nurses work.

The dogmas of the quiet past are inadequate for the stormy present and future. As our circumstances are new, we must think anew, and act anew.

ABRAHAM LINCOLN

As community health nurses approach the twenty-first century, daunting challenges and exciting opportunities are emerging. With the community becoming the focal point for health care, community health nurses are in a unique position to provide leadership in evolving managed care and integrated health systems. Their past heritage has provided them with the knowledge and skill to assist clients in moving across the health care continuum. However, with the health system changing so rapidly, the past can no longer be the only indicator for providing direction in practice. Circumstances are new and, accordingly, community health nurses must think anew and act anew!

The managed care movement has provided a stimulus for developing innovative approaches for addressing client needs in a more efficient manner. As these new approaches evolve, it is essential for community health nurses to establish mechanisms for monitoring client outcomes and for ensuring that the needs of all clients, regardless of their socioeconomic status, are met. "Managed care is not a magic bullet for solving all access and cost concerns and no amount of managed care can substitute for adequately financed programs that are well understood by beneficiaries, providers, and health plans alike" (Gold, Sparer, Chu, 1996, p. 153).

Although change is occurring in every aspect of the nursing profession, the basic values of community health nursing remain the same. Meeting the needs of disadvantaged individuals and groups has been a long standing obligation of community health organizations (Beery, Greenwald, Nudelman, 1996). The emphasis in community health nursing practice is on achieving community-wide health improvement (Salmon, 1995).

PERSPECTIVES ON COMMUNITY HEALTH NURSING PRACTICE

When public health nursing began in the early 1900s, it was a simple matter to define it as a specialty area within nursing. Public health nursing took place outside the hospital setting. It was "nursing without walls," nursing that was community-focused and family- and group-oriented. Early public health nurses functioned relatively independently and worked to maintain and improve the health of the entire community. Public health nursing was *"nursing for the public health"* (Brainard, 1921, p. 5).

Today, as the focus of health care continues to move outside the hospital setting and as more and more nurses assume expanded roles, defining community health nursing as a specialty area is less easily done. The definition becomes sharper and clearer, however, when one understands that the *nature of the practice*, not the *setting*, defines community health nursing as a specialty area. Nursing outside walls is not necessarily community health nursing. For example, pediatric nurses who do assessments of newborns in physicians' offices and nurses who counsel clients in mental

table 2-1 Practice Models of Community-Based Nursing and Community Health Nursing Compared

Model Component	Community-Based Nursing	Community Health Nursing
Goals	Manage acute or chronic conditions Promote self-care	Preserve/protect health Promote self-care
Client	Individual and family	Community
Underlying philosophy	Human ecological model	Primary health care
Autonomy	Individual and family autonomy	Community autonomy Individual rights may be sacrificed for good of community
Client character	Across the life span	Across the life span with emphasis on high-risk aggregates
Cultural diversity	Culturally appropriate care of individual and families	Collaboration with and mobilization of diverse groups and communities
Type of service	Direct	Direct and indirect
Home visiting	Home visitor	Home visitor
Service focus	Local community	Local, state, federal, and international

Modified from Zotti ME, Brown P, Stotts RC: Community-based nursing versus community health nursing: what does it all mean? *Nurs Outlook* 44:211-217, 1996, p. 212.

health centers are probably functioning as specialty-focused nurse *practitioners* with advanced physical assessment skills and preparation to exercise independent and collaborative judgment in the health care management of clients. The holistic *community* focus characteristic of community health nursing practice is not a major emphasis of nurse practitioners in many ambulatory care and other community-based health care settings. These practitioners place emphasis on managing acute or chronic conditions from an individual and family perspective. They are not necessarily oriented to the community (Goeppinger, 1984; Zotti, Brown, Stotts, 1996).

Several distinguishing characteristics differentiate community health nursing from community-based practice focused at the individual and family level of care (Table 2-1). Community health nursing is "nursing for the community's health." Its uniqueness lies in its emphasis on the health of the population as a whole. Because their focus is on the community, community health nurses provide care to individuals, families, and groups within the context and framework of the community (ACHNE, 1990, p. 1). This implies that community health nurses use information obtained from assessment and evaluation at individual and family levels to identify health needs and concerns at the community level (Conley, 1995). For example, it is not unusual for community health nurses to aggregate data from their family caseloads and to use these data to raise community awareness about major community health problems such as domestic violence or lack of access to primary health care services.

"Interventions at the individual and family levels are critical to the population-based role of public (community) health nursing, because they provide the linkage necessary to effectively interact with the community" (Conley, 1995, p. 4). Community health nurses address both the personal and the environmental aspects of health and deal with community factors that either inhibit or facilitate healthy living. Personal health involves the biopsychosocial and spiritual aspects of individual, family, and group functioning, whereas environmental health deals with people's surroundings—settings such as homes, schools, workplaces, or recreational facilities—and factors within these settings that influence health behavior. In community health nursing, nurses enter the environment in which people live and practice within that environment, in sharp contrast to the situation where the client enters the nurse's environment in a hospital or clinic. However, in addition to the one-to-one or single-family approach to health care, the community health nurse thinks in terms of populations within caseloads, districts, census tracts, cities, and group settings. Aggregates at risk within these populations, including families at risk, are identified so that preventive measures and resources can be targeted for them. This kind of community focus involves educating individuals and groups and changing the social and physical environments that cue and reinforce the choices people make. Environmental factors that generate patterns of disease and social problems in populations must be addressed to resolve many of our contemporary health concerns such as AIDS, teenage pregnancy, and toxic waste contamination (Institute of Medicine, 1988; Koopman, 1996).

The emphasis in community health nursing practice is on promoting health and preventing disease. Intervention strategies focus on providing health promotion services in group settings such as schools, work sites, or churches and in family environments. They also involve screening programs that are community based; environmental changes through persuasion, as illustrated by the public's use of seat belts; and regulation and the use of mass media (Shea, 1992, p. 787). The fact that smoking is now considered a health hazard and is no longer chic is a superb illustration of education at the community level through the mass media.

An example can best illustrate how the community health nurse expands community-based nursing by focusing on aggregates at risk and the community:

CASE *Scenario*

Julie Cherry, a community health nurse working for an official health department, was assigned a census tract as her population to be served. This census tract was located in a decaying area of town with substandard housing and no transportation, playgrounds, or parks. A large industrial complex lay in the census tract, and consequently large numbers of young laborers and their families lived there. There was no hospital located in the area and only one physician. The community health nurse received numerous referrals from the physician and outlying hospitals to visit young mothers who needed support with parenting their newborn children. The nurse assessed the need for a parenting group by talking with the families whom she served as well as with her supervisors. She and the families she visited planned a weekly sharing and support group that met in a neighborhood church. The group was well attended and generated community interest in developing a coalition designed to address the needs of young families with children. In addition to maintaining the support group, this coalition helped families in the neighborhood to address other areas of concern. For example, churches in the community obtained volunteers to transport families in need to medical appointments and established recreational activities for school-age children.

The nurse in this case scenario demonstrated critical elements in community health nursing: providing care to the unit of service—the family—and concurrently planning preventive health measures for an aggregate at risk—young families needing parenting and other family support services. This is a step beyond providing primary health care to families who need that level of nursing intervention, and is different from the one-to-one focus of care to a sick person in the hospital or ambulatory care setting. Another case scenario helps to clarify how community nursing concepts are applied in the practice setting when nurses work with families that have an ill family member.

CASE *Scenario*

Jack Webster is a community health nurse employed by a hospital-based home health agency. His caseload typically has a large percentage of people over 65 years of age with diagnoses such as congestive heart failure, diabetes, pneumonia, and hypertension. A common concern that Jack encounters with his clients is their inability to shop for food since they often cannot drive or walk to shop. It is difficult to rely on neighbors, and families frequently live long distances away from the inner-city neighborhood served by Jack. Jack worked with a local church to develop an organized cadre of volunteers who grocery shop for those clients who need this service. These volunteers also provide respite services that help to prevent caregiver role strain. Many primary caregivers in Jack's caseload are elderly and have major health concerns.

As was the situation with Julie Cherry, Jack Webster demonstrated how delivering one-on-one care to ill clients provided a window of opportunity for identifying population-focused needs within the community. Jack also worked collaboratively with a significant community system to meet crucial client needs and to provide a long-term solution to a community health problem.

The unique aspects of community health nursing practice do not negate direct individual client care or community-based nursing. One-to-one clinical practice, illustrated by pediatric nurse practitioners and geriatric nurse specialists, certainly has a place in community health nursing when it is performed for the explicit purpose of improving the level of health in a community. Nurses in these roles can have the expertise needed to plan for aggregates at risk and are also very valuable consultants for other community health nurses.

Although community-based practice and managed care are clearly emerging as major health care delivery strategies, community health nurses will continue to play a significant role in ensuring that the needs of vulnerable populations are met. They will work in partnership with clients and other health care providers in monitoring access to care and in identifying unmet needs among underserved groups. Financing a managed care program for low-income populations does not by itself resolve access problems created by diverse barriers to care. Nor does it necessarily provide a safety net for those near poor populations that are uninsured (Gold, Sparer, Chu, 1996). Public health agencies and managed care organizations have already recognized the need to establish mutually beneficial collaborative models for maintaining and improving the health of populations (Beery, Greenwald, Nudelman, 1996).

Beery, Greenwald, and Nudelman (1996) propose that a National Network be founded to advance the building of coalitions between managed care and public health that will address population-focused needs. They describe a managed care and public health youth initiative partnership that has created innovative intervention strategies for addressing the needs of young people in the community. This initiative supports a school-based health center and neighborhood programs aimed at reducing violence, teen pregnancy, drug abuse, and sexually transmitted diseases. It also addresses the medical needs of homeless adolescents and works to enhance educational and employment opportunities for young people. Creative partnerships such as the one described by Beery, Greenwald, and Nudelman are mutually beneficial for managed care and the public's health. The partnership model is increasingly being used to guide family and population-focused practice in the community setting (Courtney, Ballard, Fauver et al, 1996). This model is discussed in Chapter 14.

EVOLUTION OF TITLE OVER TIME

Historically, varying titles have been used to describe the type of nursing provided in the community setting, including district nursing, health nursing, visiting nursing, public health nursing, and community health nursing (McNeil, 1967). *District nursing,* which was the origin of our present concept of public health–community health nursing, was the title used by Rathbone when he hired nurses in England to care for the sick poor in their homes (see Chapter 1). When home nursing services were started in the United States, the term *visiting nursing* was used to identify the specialty area of practice that emphasized home-based nursing care. *Public health nursing* has its historical roots in Florence Nightingale's *health nurse* and Lillian Wald's *public health nurse*. Wald thought the word *public* denoted a service that was available to *all* people and, thus, coined the term *public health nursing* when she was director of the Henry Street Settlement in New York City. She hoped that by doing so the public would realize that the nursing services provided by the Henry Street Settlement were available to all individuals in the community. However, as federal, state, and local governments increased their involvement in the delivery of health services, the term *public health nursing* became associated with "public," or official, agencies and in turn with the care of poor people.

Home health nursing and *home care* were other titles that emerged with the development of the home health care industry. Government policy changes beginning in the 1970s, including Medicare's prospective payment system and the progressive use of third-party payments for noninstitutionalized care, fostered a rapid growth in home health care. The emphasis in home health care is on the delivery of health care services to families who are dealing with an ill family member in the home. Home health care nurses also address population-focused needs of at-risk home care groups.

The phrase *community health nursing* emerged out of an interest in reaffirming the original thrust of public health nursing practice: nursing for the health of the entire public/community versus nursing only for the public who are poor. Some people use the terms *community health nursing* and *public health nursing* interchangeably. It must be remembered, however, that not every nurse who works in the community setting is a public health–community health nurse. Public, or community, health nurses have a definitive philosophy of practice that is described in the next section of this chapter.

In this text, the terms *community health nurse* and *community health nursing* will be used to emphasize the major focus of the nurse's work—the community—as well as the underlying philosophy of population-focused practice. Community health nursing is viewed as a specialty area in nursing, oriented to promoting and protecting the health of populations. The reader will find that a variety of titles (e.g., home health nursing, visiting nursing, and community–public health nursing) are used in practice to identify nurses who work with populations as well as individuals and families. For example, it is common for official agencies such as health departments or departments of health and human services to use the term *public health nursing* to describe the population-focused practice of nurses employed by these agencies.

DEFINING COMMUNITY HEALTH NURSING: PURPOSES AND GOALS

Community health nurses have consistently examined the nature of their practice within the context of societal needs and have focused attention on developing standards for practice to guide quality improvement efforts. The National Organization for Public Health Nursing (NOPHN), founded in 1912, grew out of a concern for the rights and safety of clients. At that time, community health nursing professionals were finding that as their specialty-based practice was rapidly expanding to meet the needs of vulnerable populations nationwide, "there were no generally accepted standards for anything" (Gardner, 1975, p. 17). They "realized a body of poorly prepared and unsupervised nurses, some of whom might be without an ethical background for this work, were a dangerous element to let loose in the homes of the people and might easily jeopardize, in a short time, all the confidence we had been building throughout the country" (Gardner, p. 17).

One of the major purposes of the NOPHN was to promote standardization of community health nursing practice. "It was believed that the general public, as well as those involved in public health nursing affairs, had to be made aware of the importance of nursing standards" (Fitzpatrick, 1975, p. 38). Ella Crandall, the executive secretary of NOPHN, traveled over 32,000 miles in 1915 to carry out this mission. She spoke to countless lay and professional groups to inform the public about community health nursing and to promote standard setting within the profession (Fitzpatrick).

In recent times, the American Nurses Association (ANA) and the American Public Health Association (APHA), the two professional organizations that represent community health nurses on the national level, have carried on the tradition of the NOPHN. Both have published documents that delineate the essence of community–public health nursing practice and that clarify the role of specialty prepared community health nurses in the delivery of health care (ANA, 1986; APHA, 1996).

The ANA's and APHA's definition of community–public health nursing practice can be found in the boxes on the following page. The ANA's definition of community health nursing is currently under revision. It is anticipated

The American Nurses Association's Definition of Community Health Nursing

Community health nursing practice promotes and preserves the health of populations by integrating the skills and knowledge relevant to both nursing and public health. The practice is comprehensive and general, and is not limited to a particular age or diagnostic group; it is continual, and is not limited to episodic care. . . .

Community health nursing practice promotes the public's health. The programs, services, and institutions involved in public health emphasize promotion and maintenance of the population's health, and the prevention and limitation of disease . . . While community health nursing practice includes nursing directed to individuals, families, and groups, the dominant responsibility is to the population as a whole.

From American Nurses Association, Council of Community Health Nurses: *Standards of community health nursing practice*, Pub No. CH-10 Kansas City, Mo., 1986, ANA, pp. 1-2.

The Canadian Public Health Association's Definition of Community Health/Public Health Nursing

Community health/public health nursing is an art and a science that synthesizes knowledge from the public health sciences and professional nursing theories. Its goal is to promote and preserve the health of populations and is directed to communities, groups, families and individuals across their life span, in a continuous rather than episodic process.

Community health/public health nurses play a pivotal role in identifying, assessing and responding to the health needs of given populations. They work in collaboration with, among others, communities, families, individuals, other professionals, voluntary organizations, self-help groups, informal health care providers, governments and the private sector.

From Canadian Public Health Association (CPHA): *Community health/public health nursing in Canada: preparation and practice*, Ottawa, Ontario, 1990, CPHA, p. 3.

The American Public Health Association's Definition of Public Health Nursing

Public health nursing is the practice of promoting and protecting the health of populations using knowledge from nursing, social, and public health sciences.

Public health nursing practice is a systematic process by which:

- The health and health care needs of a population are assessed in order to identify sub-populations, families, and individuals who would benefit from health promotion or who are at risk of illness, injury, disability, or premature death;
- A plan for intervention is developed with the community to meet identified needs that takes into account available resources, the range of activities that contribute to health and the prevention of illness, injury, disability, and premature death;
- The plan is implemented effectively, efficiently, and equitably;
- Evaluations are conducted to determine the extent to which the interventions have an impact on the health status of individuals and the population;
- The results of the process are used to influence and direct the current delivery of care, deployment of health resources, and the development of local, regional, state, and national health policy and research to promote health and prevent disease.

From APHA, Public Health Nursing Section: *The definition and role of public health nursing, a statement of APHA public health nursing section*, Washington, D.C., 1996, APHA, pp. 1-2.

that this revised definition will be published during the second half of 1997 and that the population-focused nature of community health nursing practice will be strengthened in this updated statement. Standards for practice are presented in selected chapters throughout the text to illustrate the scope of services community health nurses provide when they work with a variety of at-risk populations (e.g., school-age children, the elderly, home health care clients, and clients needing rehabilitation services).

The emphasis in community health nursing, promoting the health of the community, has not changed over time. In 1912 the NOPHN stated in its constitution that "the object of this organization shall be to stimulate responsibility for the health of the community" (NOPHN, 1975, p. 27). This goal is reaffirmed by both the ANA and the APHA. The importance of this goal is recognized worldwide. For example, the Canadian Public Health Association's definition for community–public health nursing (see the box above) articulates this responsibility for nurses in Canada. The World Health Organization also highlights this responsibility in documents describing community health nursing practice (WHO, 1974, 1978, 1985).

UNIQUENESS OF COMMUNITY HEALTH NURSING PRACTICE

Community health nursing's philosophy and scope of practice distinguish this practice field from other specialty areas in nursing. Community health nurses focus on providing *preventive* health services, as opposed to curative care, to enhance the health of individuals, families, and groups within the community. Nursing service to individuals is viewed within the context of the family. It is recognized that the health of individuals can affect the health of all family members and that the family provides an environment that influences the health of its members. The family is seen as a natural unit of service (Figure 2-1). It is also seen as a significant entry point from which to identify community

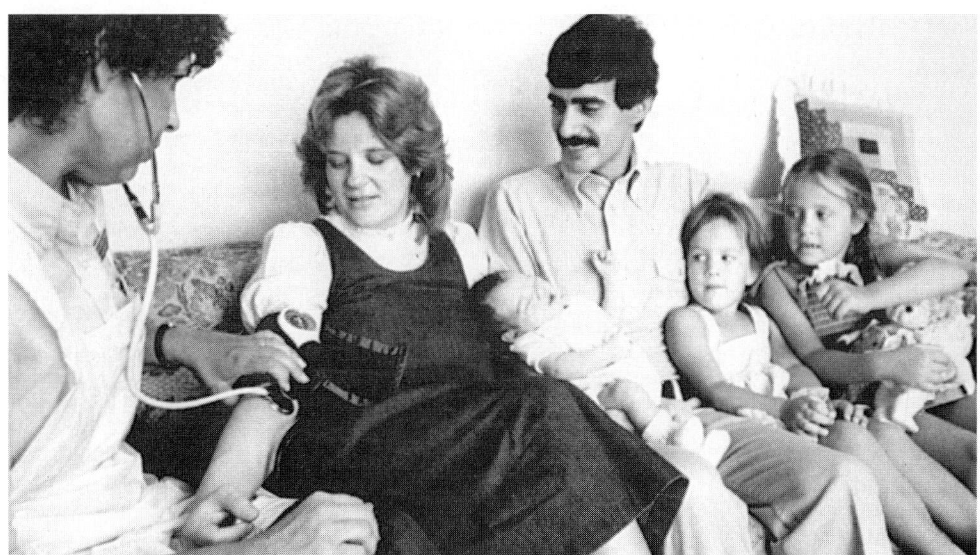

Figure 2-1 The family is seen as the natural unit of service in community health nursing practice. During a home visit, the community health nurse determines the health status of all family members and assesses family dynamics as well. *(Courtesy Genesee Region Home Care Association, Rochester, New York.)*

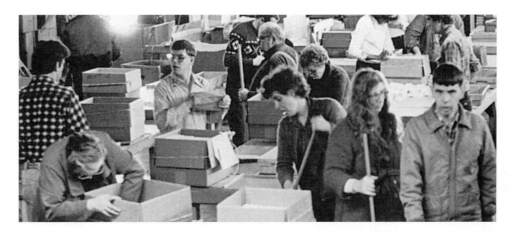

Figure 2-2 Aggregates as well as individuals and families are *clients* in community health nursing practice. An aggregate is a group of individuals who have in common one or more personal or environmental characteristics (Williams, 1977). Community health nurses focus on identifying at-risk aggregates in the community to target resources more effectively. Individuals who are retarded, for example, make up a high-risk aggregate. Persons in this population group often need an array of community services to strengthen their self-care capabilities. *(Courtesy Sunshine Workshop, a nonprofit voluntary agency sponsored by the Association of Retarded Citizens in Knox County, Tennessee. Photographer, Mary Louise Peacock.)*

strengths, needs, and resources related to the delivery of health care services.

Community health nursing practice is comprehensive and general, not limited to a particular age group or diagnostic group (ANA, 1986, p. 2). Community health nurses work with clients across the life span. They are committed to improving *the health of the community* by identifying subpopulations (Figure 2-2), families, and individuals who would benefit from health promotion or who are at risk of illness, injury, disability, and premature death (APHA, 1996, p. 1). Determining specific populations at risk facilitates the identification of individuals and families at risk.

The World Health Organization defined three necessary components of community health nursing that continue to delineate the uniqueness of this nursing specialty (WHO, 1974):

- Accepting responsibility for ensuring that needed health services are provided in the community. This

Essential Features of Contemporary Nursing Practice

Definitions of nursing frequently acknowledge four essential features of contemporary nursing practice:

- Attention to the full range of human experiences and responses to health and illness without restriction to a problem-focused orientation;
- Integration of objective data with knowledge gained from an understanding of the patient or group's subjective experience;
- Application of scientific knowledge to the processes of diagnosis and treatment; and,
- Provision of a caring relationship that facilitates health and healing.

American Nurses Association (ANA): *Nursing's social policy statement*, Washington, D.C., 1995, American Nurses Publishing, p. 6.

Classic Definition of Public Health

Public health is the science and art of preventing disease, prolonging life, and promoting physical and mental health and efficiency through organized community efforts focused toward

- Maintaining a sanitary environment;
- Controlling communicable diseases;
- Providing education regarding principles of personal hygiene;
- Organizing medical and nursing services for early diagnosis and treatment of disease; and
- Developing social machinery to ensure everyone a standard of living adequate for health maintenance, so organizing these benefits as to enable every citizen to realize his birthright of health and longevity.

From Winslow C-EA: *Man and epidemics*, Princeton, N.J., 1952, Princeton University Press, p. 60.

does not imply that community health nurses provide these services. Rather, it focuses attention on the need for nurses to participate in community assessment efforts that identify community health concerns and health planning activities that develop intervention strategies for addressing these concerns.

- The care of vulnerable groups in a community is a priority. A major reason for involvement in the health care of populations at risk is their vulnerability. The long involvement of community health nursing in the care of mothers, children, and disadvantaged groups is based on this belief.
- The client (individual, family, group, or community) must be a partner in planning and evaluating health care.

Community health nursing is a *synthesis of nursing and public health* practice. Community health nurses use the knowledge and skills of professional nursing and the philosophy, content, and methods of public health when delivering services in the community. Essential features of contemporary nursing practice are identified in the box above. "The nursing profession remains committed to the care and nurturing of both healthy and ill people individually or in groups and communities" (ANA, 1995, p. 6). However, "the extent to which individual nurses engage in the total scope of nursing practice is dependent on their educational preparation, experience, roles, and the nature of the patient populations they serve" (ANA, p. 12). Public health preparation helps community health nurses to extend their scope of practice to populations and communities. This includes the philosophy, content, and methods of epidemiology, biostatistics, social policy, health planning, public health organization and administration, and public health law.

The classic definition of public health is presented in the box, above right. The values reflected in this definition have guided public health and community health nursing practice over time and are reflected in the United States' current vision for public health (see the box on the following page). Community health nursing and public health professionals "generate organized community efforts for the purpose of promoting health and preventing disease" (IOM, 1988).

A MODEL FOR COMMUNITY HEALTH NURSING PRACTICE

White's (1982) conceptual model for public health nursing practice graphically depicts the essential elements of this specialty area (Figure 2-3). This model visualizes the interrelationships between the determinants of health and public health nursing practice priorities, dynamics, and interventions. The scope of practice is very broad, extending from "one-to-one nursing intervention to a global perspective of world health" (White, p. 528). As indicated previously, extending practice to address the needs of populations is a distinguishing feature of community health nursing.

Determinants of Health

White's model illustrates that health or illness results from the interplay of multiple factors. She identifies four categories of determinants—human/biological, social, environmental, and health care system—that influence the level of wellness among individuals, families, populations, and communities. Implicit in this model is the belief that having an understanding of the multidimensional nature of health assists the community health nurse in planning health promoting interventions (White, 1982). Chapters 6 and 11 examine the determinants of health in greater detail.

Practice Priorities

"The overall focus of public health nursing is achieving and maintaining the public's health—at all times" (White, 1982, p. 528). To accomplish this goal, commu-

Public Health in America

Vision
Healthy People in Healthy Communities
Mission
Promote Physical and Mental Health and Prevent Disease, Injury, and Disability

PUBLIC HEALTH
- Prevents epidemics and the spread of disease
- Protects against environmental hazards
- Prevents injuries
- Promotes and encourages healthy behaviors
- Responds to disasters and assists communities in recovery
- Assures the quality and accessibility of health services

ESSENTIAL PUBLIC HEALTH SERVICES
- Monitor health status to identify community health problems
- Diagnose and investigate health problems and health hazards in the community
- Enforce laws and regulations that protect health and ensure safety
- Inform, educate, and empower people about health issues
- Mobilize community partnerships to identify and solve health problems
- Link people to needed personal health services and assure the provision of health care when otherwise unavailable
- Evaluate effectiveness, accessibility, and quality of personal and population-based health services
- Assure a competent public health and personal health care workforce
- Develop policies and plans that support individual and community health efforts
- Research for new insights and innovative solutions to health problems

From Eilbert KW, Barry M, Bialek R, Garuf M: Measuring expenditures for essential public health services, Washington, D.C., 1996, Public Health Foundation, p. 4.
Source: Essential Public Health Services Work Group of the Public Health Functions Steering Committee.
Membership:
American Public Health Association
Association of State and Territorial Health Officials
National Association of County and City Health Officials
Institute of Medicine, National Academy of Sciences
Association of Schools of Public Health
Public Health Foundation
National Association of State Alcohol and Drug Abuse Directors
National Association of State Mental Health Program Directors
U.S. Public Health Service
Centers for Disease Control and Prevention
Health Resources and Services Administration
Office of the Assistant Secretary for Health
Substance Abuse and Mental Health Services Administration
Agency for Health Care Policy and Research
Indian Health Service
Food and Drug Administration
National Institutes of Health

nity health nurses assist clients in keeping well. They also help them to prevent disease occurrence and to minimize the consequences of disease and poor health (White). In community health nursing, the emphasis is on three practice priorities—preventing, promoting, and protecting. Preventive strategies ranging from health promotion to rehabilitation are used by the nurse in the community.

Prevention is the primary focus of community health nursing intervention. This focus entails a continuum of activities essential for preventing disease, prolonging life, and promoting health. These activities have traditionally been grouped under three levels of prevention: primary, secondary, and tertiary (Leavell, Clark, 1965, p. 21). *Primary prevention* deals with health-promoting activities and specific protection from health problems. "Disease prevention or specific protection begins with a threat to health—a disease or environmental hazard—and seeks to protect as many people as possible from harmful consequences of that threat" (USDHEW, 1979, p. 119). Providing immunizations for populations across the life span is an example of a disease preventing nursing intervention.

"Health promotion begins with people who are basically healthy and seeks the development of community and individual measures which can help them to develop lifestyles that can maintain and enhance the state of well-being" (USDHEW, 1979, p. 119). Health-promoting strategies work well in situations where one wants to decrease risks for disease by changing lifestyle patterns. Teaching caregivers of ill clients stress management techniques, or providing "Healthy Heart" meals in employee cafeterias, are examples of health promotion strategies. The World Health Organization (WHO) institutionalized the concept of health promotion through the development of the *Charter for Health Promotion*. The WHO views health promotion as "a process of advocacy for health, encouraging a healthy lifestyle and mediating be-

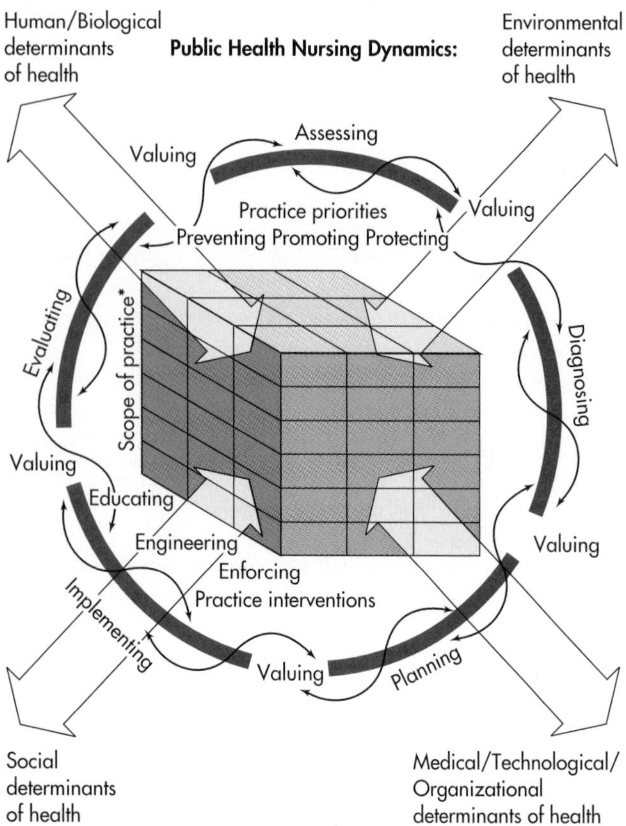

Figure 2-3 A public health nursing conceptual model. The determinants of the health framework presented are modified from those in *Healthy people: the Surgeon General's report on health promotion and disease prevention,* 1979. (From White MS: *Construct for public health nursing,* Nurs Outlook 30:529, 1982.)

tween different interests in society in the pursuit of health. Health promotion means building healthy public policy, creating supportive personal skills, and orienting health services" (Turner, 1986).

Secondary prevention, or health maintenance, involves activities aimed at early diagnosis, prompt treatment, and disability limitation. Identification of health needs, health problems, and clients at risk is inherent in secondary prevention. Conducting a health risk appraisal, observing for poor maternal-infant bonding, and reinforcing the need to carry out regular breast self-examination are examples of secondary prevention activities.

Tertiary prevention has rehabilitation as its major focus. Rehabilitation activities assist clients in reaching their maximum potential. The nurse who teaches a client with arthritis how to rest at intervals throughout the day is implementing a tertiary prevention activity. Assisting a client who has had a cerebrovascular accident to continue with a physical and speech therapy regimen is also carrying out aspects of tertiary prevention.

Practice Dynamics

White's (1982) model reflects that the community health nurse uses two key processes to identify health promoting and disease prevention needs among client populations and to establish priorities for community health nursing intervention. These are the *nursing process* and the *valuing process*. The nursing process is used to assess and diagnose client needs and to plan, implement, and evaluate effective nursing interventions. This process is used in community health nursing to build healthy communities (see Chapter 13) as well as to deliver nursing services to individuals and families (see Chapter 9).

Valuing, the second dynamic process in White's model, guides nursing interventions and decision making and influences the development of goals and priorities for care. Valuing is "the process of assigning or determining the worth or merit of something" (White, 1982, p. 529). The influence that valuing has on decision making becomes particularly evident during times of scarce resources. When resources are limited, professionals must critically examine their beliefs about practice and target resources so that they are used effectively and efficiently. Community health professionals place a high priority on targeting resources for at-risk aggregates in the community (APHA, 1996). Their overall focus is "nursing for the health of the community." Identifying aggregates at risk and planning services to meet their needs benefits the community as a whole. *Aggregates at risk are those who engage in certain activities or who have certain characteristics that increase their potential for contracting an illness, injury, or health problem.* Individuals who smoke, for example, constitute an aggregate at high risk for developing cancer. The at-risk concept is basic to public health practice. It guides epidemiological study of health and disease occurrence. It also provides a framework for assessing the health status of clients across the continuum of practice and for developing health promoting intervention. This concept is discussed further in Chapter 11.

Nursing Interventions

According to White (1982), community health nursing interventions fall into three major categories: education, engineering, and enforcement. *Educative* nursing actions help clients to voluntarily acquire knowledge essential for understanding healthy functioning, to develop attitudes that foster preventive health behaviors, and to establish practices conducive to effective living. Educative strategies are commonly used in community health nursing practice. For example, community health nurses help families learn about normal growth and development and child care, conduct discussions related to sexuality issues in the school setting, and distribute health education materials in clinics, industrial plants, and other community health settings. Nurses visiting clients whose care is being reimbursed by Medicare also help clients to learn about their health concerns. They may, for example, teach clients about their many medications, including why, when, and how to take them. They may also teach accurate wound care to clients and their families.

Because the community health nurse believes that clients and families are in charge of their own lives and will ultimately make the decisions that influence their own health, education is considered the most strategic intervention. Community health nurses work on the principle that when people are given a fish, their hunger is cured for several days. When people are taught how to fish their hunger is cured for many days. This concept is emphasized throughout the text, as are strategies to assist nurses in incorporating it into their practice.

Engineering strategies focus on environmental modification for the purpose of eliminating or managing environmental risk factors that affect healthy living. Campaigning against television advertisements that promote alcohol and cigarette use, conducting clinics for the treatment of sexually transmitted diseases, promoting actions to eliminate safety hazards in a schoolyard, and creating a system to help elderly clients safely take their many medications, are examples of engineering nursing interventions.

Enforcement interventions are actions that impose regulatory controls and are designed to prevent disease, promote health, and protect society from harmful substances and conditions. Enforcement actions encourage the passage of regulations and legislation, such as seat belt, helmet, and drug abuse laws, that mandate health-promoting behaviors. Laws may also mandate that high-risk clients with tuberculosis (the drug-addicted, those with failed TB treatment, the homeless, and those who have problems understanding the disease) take their pills under direct observation.

To intervene effectively in the community health setting, the nurse must engage in political activity. The political arena is where health care decisions are made for the public as a whole. Sound public policy is needed to eliminate or manage environmental risk factors, prevent disease, and promote public health. Political activism is emphasized in Chapters 14 and 25.

The dynamics and dimensions in White's model (Figure 2-3) stress the value of preventive activities. Preventing, promoting, and protecting are practice priorities. This model illustrates the community health nurse's use of the nursing process on the individual and aggregate level to provide preventive health services, and the multiple dimensions or determinants of health that must be addressed to successfully enhance individual and group health. It also illustrates the use of a range of intervention strategies, including political activism, to dilute or eliminate negative health determinants in the environment.

HEALTHY PEOPLE 2000 MANDATE GUIDES PRACTICE

The *Healthy People 2000* mandate, the nation's vision for improving the health of the nation, provides a framework for identifying populations at risk and for developing prevention strategies that address population-focused needs. This mandate identifies a national strategy for increasing the span of *healthy* life among Americans, reducing health disparities, and achieving universal access to preventive health care services. It establishes directives for addressing the prevention of major chronic illnesses, injuries, and infectious disease. These directives target population groups that are at highest risk of premature death, disease, and disability and promote a comprehensive strategy for achieving improvements in health that are possible through prevention (USDHHS, 1991).

The *Healthy People 2000* mandate challenges professionals and the American public to establish specific goals and objectives for improving health in local communities. This mandate emphasizes building healthy communities that provide a nurturing environment for individuals, families, and populations. It articulates the importance of developing preventive interventions that address the needs of at-risk populations across the life span. It provides a framework for helping communities to target scarce resources and to develop public policies that promote health and prevent disease.

Healthy People 2000 objectives will be used throughout this text to assist the reader in identifying major health needs among population groups across the life span and in formulating strategies for addressing these needs. Community health nurses nationwide are using the *Healthy People 2000* document (USDHHS, 1991) to identify community needs and to develop health programs that effectively and efficiently reach populations at risk. Innovative initiatives are being developed at the local level to address health concerns identified by community residents. These initiatives provide exciting opportunities for an interdisciplinary cadre of health care professionals.

HEALTH FOR ALL MANDATE

"What unites people around public (community) health is the focus on society as a whole, the community, and the aim of optimal health status" (IOM, 1988, p. 39). This is the theme that guides community health action at all levels of national and international government. In 1978 158 countries attending the International Conference on Primary Health Care, held in Alma-Ata, USSR, set for themselves a common goal, "Health for All by the Year 2000" (WHO, 1978). In committing themselves to this goal, countries did not mean that by the year 2000 disease and disability would no longer exist. The focus was placed on all people having *access to health services* that would assist them in leading socially and economically productive lives (Mahler, 1979). "The goal of Health for All by the Year 2000 is a vision founded on social equity; on the urgent need to reduce the gross inequality in the health status of people in the world, in developed and developing countries, and within countries" (Maglacas, 1988).

The Declaration of Alma-Ata specifies that primary health care is the key vehicle for attaining the "health for all" goal. Primary health care is a blend of essential health services, personal responsibility for one's own health, and health-promoting action taken by the community. It must include at least the following eight components (WHO, 1988, p. 23):

- Education concerning prevailing health problems and the methods of preventing and controlling them
- Promotion of food supply and proper nutrition
- An adequate supply of safe water and basic sanitation
- Maternal and child health care, including family planning
- Immunization against the major infectious diseases
- Prevention and control of locally endemic diseases
- Appropriate treatment of common diseases and injuries
- Provision of essential drugs

Primary health care facilitates client entry into the health care system, promotes integrated and coordinated services, requires client participation in the program planning and evaluation process and in policy making, and promotes self-reliance and self-determination (WHO, 1978). Community health nurses promote these types of services, activities, and values.

What is the status of "Health for All By the Year 2000"? "What is generally very clear is that every country, every member state of WHO has done something toward the attainment of 'health for all'. But unfortunately the level of achievement tends to be very unbalanced" (Little, 1992). Developing countries have basic concerns, such as food and water, and thus there has been a limited expansion of health budgets in many countries. Health care for all is a target. Nurses as primary health care providers continue to play an instrumental role in making this happen.

No one discipline can address all of the health needs in the community. That is why community health nurses stress the importance of multidisciplinary planning. Multidisciplinary planning and cooperation can facilitate community diagnosis (Chapter 13) and health planning (Chapter 14). It also promotes effective and efficient use of resources.

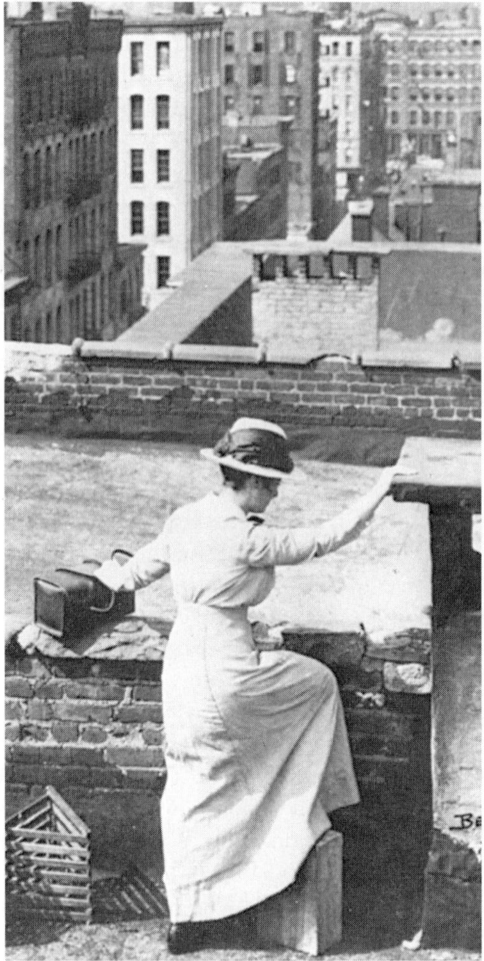

Figure 2-4 Community health nurses traditionally have gone into a variety of community settings to serve individuals, families, and groups. In this picture, a Henry Street nurse is climbing over a tenement roof on New York's Lower East Side to visit her clients in the home. Today, community health nurses usually do not climb over rooftops. They do, however, reach out to clients in all types of settings (e.g., homes, schools, rural clinics, neighborhood health centers, and sheltered workshops). *(Courtesy Visiting Nurse Service of New York City.)*

SETTINGS, WORK FORCE, AND ROLES

Community health nurses implement a variety of roles in the practice setting and provide a broad range of services aimed at promoting individual and aggregate health. They work in diverse health and health-related organizations. Changing health care delivery trends have resulted in a need for increased numbers of nurses who can function in the community setting. It is anticipated that there will be a massive expansion of primary care in ambulatory and community settings by the end of the century (Pew Health Professions Commission, 1995).

Settings in which Community Health Nurses Function

An exciting aspect of community health nursing is the existence of varied settings and modalities for practice. Community health nurses were first employed by visiting nurse associations, where they responded to the needs of people at greatest risk by nursing the sick in their homes and by providing instruction to both manage illness and remain well (Figure 2-4). With the increase of home care this remains an important avenue. They have also been employed by health departments or other tax-supported agencies, visiting nurse associations or other non–tax-supported agencies, schools, and occupational health programs.

State and local health departments are mandated to protect the health of the community and, therefore, to provide a broad range of services that address the needs of groups across the life span. Visiting nurse associations primarily emphasize the delivery of home health care or bedside nursing services. Health programs in schools and occupational settings mainly serve a specific segment of the community. School-age children are the focus in school health programs, whereas the well adult is the target of service in the occupational health setting. Migrant health clinics, prisons, rural and urban nursing centers, homeless shelters, senior citizen centers, neighborhood health centers, and churches are other settings in which the community health nurse works and where services are targeted for specific aggregates. In the evolving health care system, community health nurses are also working in managed care organizations and care management agencies established to assist clients in accessing needed health care services.

All of these settings have the following elements in common: an emphasis on independent practice by the practitioner; an understanding that the physical and social environment is critical to the state of health; and a focus on the concept that clients need to be taught how to fish rather than simply being given a fish to cure their hunger. Although the concepts of community assessment and intervention are less common in home health practice, where currently only illness care is reimbursed, there are encouraging signs that home health agencies are also realizing that it is at the community level that problems are both caused and solved (Green, Driggers, 1989; Walcott-McQuigg, Ervin, 1992; Zerwekh, 1992).

The Public Health Nursing Section of the American Public Health Association (1996) has provided guidelines to assist nurses in expanding their community-focused efforts when they are working in private, voluntary, or nonofficial agencies. Often these types of agencies only serve a specific segment of the community, such as clients who need home health care services or individuals and families in a specific church or school district. In these settings the APHA recommends that nurses first analyze the needs of clients served by the organization and then extend their scope of service to individuals/families within the community who are eligible for service but have not availed themselves of the care offered (APHA, p. 9). This "targeted outreach" helps "the nurse to move away from solely meeting the needs of consumers as individually presented and toward practicing public (community) health nursing for all individuals or families within the population group or program focus" (APHA, p. 9).

Size of the Work Force in Community Health Nursing

The earliest known count of public health nurses in the United States was reported in 1901 by Harriett Fulmer at the International Congress of Nurses in Buffalo, N.Y. At that time there were 58 public health nursing organizations employing about 130 nurses. By 1912 Mary Gardner found that approximately 3000 nurses were engaged in delivering community health nursing services. In 1992 there were approximately 250,000 registered nurses working in public/community health settings, representing almost 14% of the registered nurse work force in the United States. Of these nurses, about 37% worked in home health care settings, 27% worked in official health departments and community centers, 20% worked in schools, and 17% worked in other settings such as occupational health (almost 8%) (USDHHS, 1993). Between 1988 and 1992 the number of registered nurses employed by home health care agencies almost doubled (USDHHS). It is forecasted that one out of every 10 nurses will be employed in home care by 2005 (Shindul-Rothschild, Berry, Long-Middleton, 1996).

Roles and Functions of Community Health Nurses in a Managed Care Environment

"The overarching goal of health care reform, whether led by the private sector or by state or federal government, should be to improve the health and quality of life of the American people, while constraining costs" (Gordon, Baker, Roper, Omenn, 1996). A recent Institute of Medicine (1988) report on *The Future of Public Health* identified three core public health functions that need to be implemented to achieve this goal. These are *assessment, policy development,* and *assurance*. Briefly summarized, these functions involve assessing the health status of the community, promoting the development of comprehensive health policies, and assuring constituents that services necessary to achieve agreed-upon goals are provided, by encouraging actions by other entities, by requiring such action through regulation, or by providing services directly (IOM). Assurance also involves determining "a set of high-priority personnel and communitywide health services that governments will guarantee to every member of the community" (IOM, p. 8).

Community health nurses are implementing the core public health functions to address the needs of clients across the continuum of practice. They are assessing the health status of individuals, families, populations, and communities. They are also participating in the development of health policies (e.g., standards of care, health regulations, and public policy) that promote health and prevent disease. Additionally, they are providing services to clients across the age continuum and are working in partnership with communities to ensure that every member of the community has access to essential health services (Conley, 1995). It is anticipated that in the evolving managed health care environment, community health nurses will be less involved in providing personal health services on the individual and family levels of practice and more involved in population-focused care. This will

Selected Roles Assumed by Community Health Nurses

ADVOCATE

Community health nurses facilitate clients' efforts in obtaining needed health services and in negotiating an appropriate care management plan. They also promote community awareness of significant health problems, lobby for beneficial public policy, and stimulate supportive community action for health.

CAREGIVER

Community health nurses provide care to individuals, families, and vulnerable populations in a variety of settings (e.g., churches, safe houses for domestic violence victims, homes, homeless shelters, migrant health camps, and worksites). This care includes a range of activities such as hands-on physical care, educating a client about his or her health problems, and screening for undiagnosed health conditions.

CARE MANAGER

Community health nurses help clients to make decisions about appropriate health care services and to achieve service delivery integration and coordination. They advocate for services when needed and make referrals as necessary.

CASEFINDER

Community health nurses conduct targeted outreach to identify clients in need of service and to assist clients in accessing appropriate care. They also observe for clients who may have potential or actual service needs during their daily course of activities.

COUNSELOR

Community health nurses are often in a unique position to help clients cope with normative and nonnormative stressors that could lead to crises and to adapt to changes in the environment. When assuming this role, they help clients to express emotions and feelings, to clarify facts in the situation, to confront the stress in manageable doses, and to accept assistance if needed.

EDUCATOR

Community health nurses apply the principles of teaching and learning to promote positive health action and to facilitate behavioral change. They use these principles to help clients across the age continuum to learn about new events and healthy functioning and to apply acquired knowledge.

EPIDEMIOLOGIST

Community health nurses use the epidemiological method to analyze health problems among population groups and to develop population-focused interventions.

GROUP LEADER

Community health nurses use the group process to provide targeted preventive services and to manage caseload responsibilities. Through group process, community health nurses are able to assist small client or community groups to learn new knowledge and skills, to support group members during stressful times, or to problem-solve around issues important to the community.

HEALTH PLANNER

Community health nurses use the health planning process to develop, implement, and evaluate health services for populations at risk. This process is used to provide community-wide or population-specific health services.

MANAGER

Community health nurses are responsible for managing caseload demands in an effective and efficient manner. They are also often responsible for managing problems and activities of other members of the health care team.

vary in local communities across the country based on community need and the availability of health care resources. This will also vary based on the mission and goals of specific community health nursing agencies. For example, the mission and goals of official public health agencies focus on population-focused care, whereas home health agencies are oriented towards the provision of personal health services.

A variety of roles are assumed by nurses in providing community health nursing services (Green, Driggers, 1989; Gulino, La Monica, 1986; Riportella-Muller, Selby, Salmon et al, 1991). A partial listing of the types of roles community health nurses commonly implement across settings is displayed in the box above. In the rapidly changing health care environment some of these roles may undergo significant transformation. For example, in a managed care system community health nurses are expected to identify client need and to justify appropriate service requirements. This implies that the care manager must increasingly become a business negotiator. Although role responsibilities may change rapidly, this change may bring new opportunities for improving and expanding service delivery. Community health nurses have the knowledge and skills to assume expanded role responsibilities in integrated health care systems.

SERVICES PROVIDED BY COMMUNITY HEALTH NURSES

To achieve their goals, community health nurses provide multiple and diverse direct and indirect client services. Direct client services usually involve a personal relationship between the nurse and client (who can be a person, a family, an aggregate, or the community). Teaching, hands-on bedside care, health risk appraisal, counseling, health planning with consumers, and the delivery of clinic services are examples of direct client services. Indirect client services

A View *from the* Field: A Day in the Life of a Community Health Nurse

Her first stop by 8 AM each day is at her desk in the health department to pick up messages from the day before, make phone calls, and plan her day's schedule.

After morning coffee with the other nurses, which offers time for comparisons, she starts her calls.

"Sometimes you've had a dark day and you need input, you need to talk to someone," she explains. "I could get depressed if I allowed myself, but I realize whose problem it is. It's not my problem. It's only my place to help when I'm accepted."

Many calls start with a request from a school or another public health nurse, or Charlene's own case finding.

Her first stop on a gray, cheerless day recently was a happy one, to visit a new baby. Paul Daniel Conner had spent 2 months in a hospital nursery after being born prematurely, weighing only 3 pounds, 7 ounces. Now 2½ months old, he had adjusted easily to his mother's style in the 2 weeks he has been home.

"He's a perfect baby," says his mother, Julie. "He doesn't ever cry." But she does have a few questions, written on a scrap of paper.

"I was surprised how easy it has been. I've been just really relaxed with him," she tells Charlene.

The routine on a visit to a new baby includes leaving a sheaf of pamphlets for the mother's spare-time reading. Topics include first aid, exercises for the mother, feeding, birth control, and descriptions of the free services offered by the health department.

Charlene advises Mrs. Conner not to put Paul Daniel to bed with a bottle.

"A baby will get a pool of milk, juice or Kool-Aid in its mouth that causes tooth decay. I see children with nothing but little brown stubs left of their teeth," she explains.

"You can use your blender to make baby food from table food, then freeze it in an ice cube tray and put it in a bag. But be sure to freeze it."

The telephone number for the Western Michigan Poison Center and instructions on taking a baby's temperature are all part of the routine which ends with a full examination of the baby and measuring its height and weight.

Charlene tells Mrs. Conner she can take her baby to the health department's well-baby clinic, in the Belmont area, for children from birth to school age.

"It's one of your benefits as a taxpayer. You can take the baby in for his shots, but continue to see the doctor."

The idea appeals to Mrs. Conner. She takes the information, the telephone number she would use for an appointment.

"You can call me anytime," Charlene says as she leaves. "I'm usually in early in the morning."

Few newborns in Kent County are seen by a public health nurse. Many don't need it; more probably do. All it would take is a call—from the hospital, from the mother, or even from a relative.

"There are many out there I'm not getting, mothers who are having problems adjusting to a new baby, who didn't like children or babies before and now overcompensate," Charlene explains.

A stop at West Oakview School is squeezed in before the students' lunch break to check a girl with bites on her arms and legs (probably flea bites from a cat, Charlene thinks) and a progress report from a class for emotionally impaired youngsters.

At North Oakview School, after lunch, Charlene calls in to her office for messages. Then she visits a "readiness room" for 5- to 7-year-olds taught by Ann Westerhof.

"If Charlene didn't come in once a week, I don't know what I'd do," Mrs. Westerhof exclaims. "She's the go-between for me and the families. She helps me know what I can and can't do."

The "star" of this visit is Jim Fragale, 6, who is sporting a new brace, an unusual contraption with a tripod base and straps that keep his legs bent to aid healing of the hip joints.

The cause of Jim's hip problem is unknown, Charlene explains. "The ball joint of the hip softens, then starts coming back. But the regeneration is dependent on rest and nutrition."

Jim had a little trouble balancing when he was first fitted with the brace, and even fell backwards, Mrs. Westerhof explains. "And he was a little embarrassed by it at first. But now he can show the other students tricks they can't do."

Charlene's link was knowing what agency to contact to make the brace a reality. "So many times, parents can't afford the treatment needed, and Char knows how to get it," Mrs. Westerhof adds.

From the young to the old—that switch in thinking is typical for public health nurses.

Twice a month, Charlene is in charge of the well-baby clinic in Belmont. She sees humanity at its beginnings there, in the tots brought in for free care—routine physical examinations by a doctor, immunizations, and advice for parents.

Although the wait can be long, the time can be used to ask a public health nurse about the little doubts, those questions that seem too insignificant for the doctor.

From Haradine J: Public health nurse makes a difference, *Grand Rapids Press*, December 3, 1978, pp. 29-33.

Continued

A View from the Field A DAY IN THE LIFE OF A COMMUNITY HEALTH NURSE—cont'd

"I thought he'd outgrow it by this time. I guess he won't," one mother was overheard commenting to one of the three nurses staffing the clinic.

These chats, informal and friendly, offer help on parenting to start the young out right.

When the young, at 14 or 15, stumble along the way, Charlene and the other public health nurses are there, just a telephone call away.

Sometimes it's the child's problem, and sometimes it's the parent's, spreading over to the child. "Rare is the teenager who will say, 'Hey, I've got a problem,'" Charlene notes. "Some social workers do refer kids to me.

"We see some child abuse cases and we see neglect, which is so hard to prove. It's insidious and camouflaged. Sometimes the parents are too wrapped up in themselves, or it might be a lack of resources, of money.

"We have to know what help is available from the different agencies."

The old pose a different problem, when loneliness and loss have taken their toll. Charlene pulls into a driveway along the Grand River, next to a small house with a tidy yard at 4566 Abrigador Trail NE. It's a call to the other end of life.

"They say I'll live to be 90, but I don't care to," says Josephine Robbins as Charlene takes her blood pressure.

"I know that," Charlene replies, acceptingly, as she removes the blood pressure cuff from the arm of the woman, who is 80.

The youngest of seven, Josephine says, "The others, they're all gone. My sister was 92."

Her husband, Lloyd, died in March. "What do I have to live for?" she asks.

In answer to Charlene's questions on her health, she reports only "a catch in my side" now and then. But she takes "just a little Lydia Pinkham's and it goes away."

An active woman now very lonely and anxious, Josephine looks forward to the weekly nurse visit. "You're not taking any of those pills, are you?" Charlene asks in a warning tone.

"No, I threw them out." A neighbor had given Josephine two drugs, Librium (a tranquilizer) and nitroglycerine (a heart drug), saying, "They always helped me. Maybe they'll help you."

Charlene had become aware of them on her last visit when she had asked what medications Josephine was taking.

Josephine worries about getting her things in order, her will, her records and being able to pledge her eyes and kidneys before she dies. "They said I had to come down and sign in front of two witnesses, but I can't get down there," she tells the nurse. Charlene explains, "Not necessary; just witnesses, here in your home."

Besides the decisions for her will, on the who and what of all she owns, Josephine must finish the mural she is painting on one wall, then paint a scene in a window and refinish some furniture. And then. . . .

"There's just an awful lot of red tape," the gray-haired woman comments sadly. "I'm never going to be through."

The public health nurse visits often when the need is great, then as the crisis eases, the visits taper off, to make time and room for someone else with other pressing needs.

Days are filled with joy and sadness. Charlene believes she gets as much as she gives in her 8-5 job. "I need people. I see myself as a helping person and they are fulfilling to me."

But in public health the rewards are seldom quick in coming. "You see something grow. You see a person who has never had any self-confidence make strides.

"I'm really in preventive medicine," Charlene says. "By educating others and by my intervention, I believe I'll make a difference."

include such things as record keeping, talking to a community agency about available resources to meet client needs, and supervising the care provided by a home health aide.

Provided are two Views from the Field that chronicle a day in the life of two community health nurses: Charlene is employed by a county health department, and John is employed by a large voluntary visiting nurses' association. The stories illustrate the range of services provided by nurses in various community settings.

The community health nurses in these two stories illustrate several important concepts in community health nursing. The community health nurse is a generalist and serves all population groups. She or he works in the client's setting, using principles of primary, secondary, and tertiary prevention. The community health nurse also serves population groups in clinics and schools; concepts from the public health sciences of biostatistics, epidemiology, and administration help the nurse to identify needs of these aggregates.

The range of services provided by community health nurses is extensive. Although some community health nurses focus on addressing the needs of a specific segment of the population, such as John Roethke, who is working with clients who need home health care services, all community health nurses extend themselves to promote the development of a

A View *from the* Field — A Day in the Life of a Visiting Nurse

Shortly before noon on yet another 90-plus-degree September day, John Roethke is praising automobile air-conditioning as he navigates the streets of West Philadelphia in search of a particular shopping center.

A few minutes later he finds it and, more importantly, the pay phone he uses to inform his next patient that he's just around the corner.

When Roethke pulls up to Derrick Smith's building at the Court Apartments in Yeadon, a family member already has a third-floor window open. Smith and his aunt have trouble climbing the three flights of stairs, so they have devised a ritual: Roethke calls when he gets close, honks his horn when he arrives, and they toss him the front-door key from the third floor.

Just another day for a home health care nurse.

Before joining the Visiting Nurse Association of Greater Philadelphia, Roethke worked in the trauma center at Albert Einstein Medical Center and as an emergency room nurse manager at Parkview Hospital.

"I thought I'd be bored silly working in home care after being in emergency rooms for so long." the 34-year-old Bethlehem native says. "But that hasn't happened. I'm working with a lot of high-tech equipment and teaching patients how to use it. It really astounds me that I'm teaching a 78-year-old woman how to work a CADD pump."

The computer-assisted delivery device, the size of a transistor radio, pumps medication into a patient's veins at a preset rate.

"It sounds kind of corny, but patients really do better at home where they are in familiar surroundings," Roethke says. "Hospitals in the 21st century won't be anything like they are today. They'll have an emergency room, a huge outpatient department and intensive-care units for surgery and that's it. Everything else will be home care."

Roethke's work day begins around 8 AM, when he contacts patients to let them know when he will be coming by.

His first stop on this oppressively hot day is in South Philadelphia, a few blocks from where Connie Mack Stadium once stood. The patient, 72-year-old Early Yearwood, suffers from cardiomyopathy—his heart is having a difficult time pumping fluid to his kidneys.

Roethke, who at 6-foot-6 is not the prototype nurse, attracts a few curious stares as he lifts his bag from the car's trunk.

Inside, Early and his wife, Mary, are watching a television game show. The lights are off and two fans are oscillating in the heat.

"How do you feel today, Earl?" Roethke asks, as he checks Yearwood's blood pressure.

"Bad," he responds.

For a half-hour Roethke examines Yearwood and administers 50 milligrams of Lasix, a treatment for cardiomyopathy. At the same time he quizzes Yearwood's wife on how and when she should change Yearwood's bandages. Home health aides are available to help patients get out of bed and dressed, but the idea, Roethke explains, is to have the family do as much as it can. If a nurse thinks the family can't handle the responsibility, a recommendation will be made to return the patient to the hospital.

Though Yearwood is stoic for most of the visit, Roethke gets him to smile occasionally.

"Now, no jogging around the block," Roethke says, as he packs up his equipment.

"I don't think I could do that," Yearwood answers with a grin.

On the way to his next patient, Derrick Smith, Roethke tells of two events that lead him to home health care.

He is going through a divorce and has joint custody of his children. Working as a home health care nurse allows him to set his own schedule so he can spend more time with his three daughters.

He also had the experience of becoming a patient after getting stuck with a needle and contracting hepatitis B.

"When you become a patient they just don't strip away your clothes, they strip away your dignity," Roethke says. "I'm not trying to come down hard on the hospitals because they have a tremendous job to do."

But it made him an advocate for home care.

Roethke says he is unconcerned about visiting patients in high-crime areas, but he agrees maybe he should be.

"Some of the other nurses told me, in the drug-infested areas the drug dealers know you're there to care for the elderly in the neighborhood and they leave you alone," he says. "I don't bank on that, but I never had any problems."

Smith, the 44-year-old Yeadon patient, also suffers from cardiomyopathy.

"This is great," Smith says of being treated at home. "I've been in the hospital so much for so long. I don't want to go back."

"I've seen so much improvement." Roethke spent 40 minutes with Smith, checking his vital signs and administering about 200 milligrams of Lasix, seemingly oblivious to Smith's niece and nephew playing and yelling just a few feet away.

From George J: For John Roethke, the job of visiting nurse is anything but dull, *Philadelphia Business Journal*, October 7, 1991, pp. 1, 3-4.

Continued

A View from the Field: A Day in the Life of a Visiting Nurse—cont'd

Before he leaves, the children hug Roethke, wrapping their arms around his knees.

"People are always giving you food or little gifts. It's amazing," Roethke says. "They're welcoming you into their home. When I worked in the emergency room it was often on patients who didn't want to be there. They'd fight you. If I didn't get called a MF at least once a shift I didn't feel loved."

Roethke's third visit on this day is a marked departure from the first two. His patient, Shirley Channick, lives in the Valley Forge Towers in King of Prussia.

The key isn't tossed out the window. The maid lets him in after a security guard buzzes him through the lobby.

Channick has rheumatoid arthritis and an infection stemming from a hip replacement. Her arthritis keeps Channick from administering medication to herself, so she is being treated with antibiotics delivered by a CADD pump.

Roethke's next stop is the office, where he will spend hours tackling the Medicare and Medicaid forms the job generates.

"I thought I'd find it difficult to work in long-term care where you don't always see improvement," he says. "I haven't found that to be the case. Maybe I should stop looking."

system of care that addresses population-focused needs. Additionally, community health nurses in all settings collaborate with other community agencies to ensure that needs of clients across the age continuum are addressed. Community health nursing is "nursing for the community's health."

Summary

Community health nursing is a synthesis of nursing and public health practice applied to promoting and preserving the health of populations (ANA, 1986). The community health nurse's philosophy and scope of practice distinguishes her or him from other nurses in the practice setting. Community health nurses serve individuals and aggregates (groups of people) across the life span on a continuing basis. Their major goal is to protect and promote the health of the community. Prevention is their primary focus in nursing practice. Identifying at-risk populations within the community assists community health nurses to effectively and efficiently provide preventive health care services.

Community health nurses work in a variety of settings and implement multiple roles such as casefinder, educator, group worker, and health planner. Changing health care delivery trends have increased the demand for community-based services and, in turn, the number of qualified community health nurses. The excitement of this specialty area lies in its diversity.

Critical Thinking Exercise

The definition of community health nursing states that it is a synthesis of nursing and public health practice. Discuss examples from the stories about a day in the life of a community health nurse and a day in the life of a visiting nurse (pp. 39-42) where elements of public health/community health nursing are practiced.

REFERENCES

American Nurses Association (ANA): Council of Community Health Nurses: *Standards of community health nursing practice*, Pub No. CH-10, Kansas City, Mo., 1986, ANA.

American Nurses Association (ANA): *Nursing's social policy statement*, Washington, D.C., 1995, American Nurses Publishing.

American Public Health Association (APHA), Public Health Nursing Section: *The definition and role of public health nursing in the delivery of health care*, Washington, D.C., 1981, The Association.

American Public Health Association (APHA), Public Health Nursing Section: *The definition and role of public health nursing, a statement of APHA public health nursing section*, Washington, D.C., 1996, APHA.

Association of Community Health Nursing Educators (ACHNE): *Essentials of baccalaureate nursing education for entry level community health nursing practice*, Louisville, Ky., 1990, ACHNE.

Beery WL, Greenwald HP, Nudelman PM: Managed care and public health: building a partnership, *Public Health Nurs* 13:305-310, 1996.

Brainard A: *Organization of public health nursing*, New York, 1921, Macmillan.

Canadian Public Health Association (CPHA): *Community health/public health nursing in Canada: preparation and practice*, Ottawa, Ontario, 1990, CPHA.

Conley E: Public health nursing within core public health functions: "back to the future," *J Public Health Management Practice* 1(3):1-8, 1995.

Courtney R, Ballard E, Fauver S et al: The partnership model: working with individuals, families, and communities toward a new vision of health, *Public Health Nurs* 13:177-186, 1996.

Eilbert KW, Barry M, Bialek R et al: Measuring expenditures for essential public health services, Washington, D.C., 1996, Public Health Foundation, p. 4.

Essential Public Health Services Work Group: Public health in America, *The Nation's Health* pp. 1, 3, Dec. 1994.

Fitzpatrick ML: *The National Organization for Public Health Nursing, 1912-1952: development of a practice field*, New York, 1975, National League for Nursing.

Gardner MS: Typewritten Reminiscences, Feb. 5, 1948, NOPHN Archive Microfilm H25. In Fitzpatrick ML, ed: *The National Organization for Public Health Nursing, 1912-1952: development of a practice field*, New York, 1975, National League for Nursing, p. 17.

George J: For John Roethke, the job of visiting nurse is anything but dull, *Philadelphia Business Journal*, October 7, 1991, pp. 1, 3-4.

Goeppinger J: Primary health care: an answer to the dilemmas of community nursing, *Public Health Nurs* 1:129-140, 1984.

Gold M, Sparer M, Chu K: Medicaid managed care: lessons from five states, *Health Affairs* 15:153-166, 1996.

Gordon RL, Baker EL, Roper WL, Omenn GS: Prevention and the reforming U.S. health care system: changing roles and responsibilities for public health, *Annu Rev Public Health* 17:489-509, 1996.

Green JL, Driggers B: All visiting nurses are not alike: home health and community health nursing, *J Community Health Nurs* 6:83-93, 1989.

Gulino C, La Monica G: Public health nursing: a study of role implementation, *Public Health Nurs* 3:80-91, 1986.

Haradine J: Public health nurse makes a difference, *Grand Rapids Press*, December 3, 1978, pp. 29-33.

Institute of Medicine (IOM), Committee for the Study of the Future of Public Health: *The future of public health*, Washington, D.C., 1988, National Academy Press.

Koopman JS: Comment: emerging objectives and methods in epidemiology, *AJPH* 86:630-632, 1996.

Leavell HR, Clark EG: *Preventive medicine for the doctor in his community: an epidemiological approach*, ed 3, New York, 1965, McGraw-Hill.

Little C: Health for all by the year 2000: where is it now? *Nurs Health Care* 13(4):198-204, 1992.

Maglacas AM: *Health for all*, Paper presented at a conference on international health, Ann Arbor, Mi., September 1988, University of Michigan.

Mahler H: What is health for all? *World Health*, November 1979, p. 3-5.

McNeil E: Transition in public health nursing, *U Michigan Medical Center J* 33:286-291, 1967.

National Organization for Public Health Nursing (NOPHN): Constitution of the National Organization for Public Health Nursing, Article 2, 1912, Wald: New York Public Library folder: NOPHN No. 1. In Fitzpatrick ML, ed: *The National Organization for Public Health Nursing, 1912-1952: development of a practice field*, New York, 1975, National League for Nursing, p. 27.

Pew Health Professions Commission: *Critical challenges: revitalizing the health professional for the twenty-first century*, San Francisco, 1995, UCSF Center for the Health Professions.

Riportella-Muller R, Selby ML, Salmon ME et al: Specialty roles in community health nursing: a national survey of educational needs, *Public Health Nurs* 8:81-89, 1991.

Salmon ME: Public health policy: creating a healthy future for the American public, *Fam Community Health* 18:1-11, 1995.

Shea S: Community health, community risks, community action, *Am J Public Health* 82(6):785-787, 1992.

Shindul-Rothschild J, Berry D, Long-Middleton E: Where have all the nurses gone? Final results of AJN's patient care survey, *Am J Nurs* 96:25-37, 1996.

Turner J: Charter for health promotion, *Lancet* 2:1407, 1986.

U.S. Department of Health, Education and Welfare (USDHEW): *Healthy people: the Surgeon General's report on health promotion and disease prevention*, Washington, D.C., 1979, Public Health Service.

U.S. Department of Health and Human Services (USDHHS): *Healthy People 2000: national health promotion and disease prevention objectives, full report, with commentary*, Washington, D.C., 1991, Public Health Service.

U.S. Department of Health and Human Services (USDHHS): *Registered nurse population 1992: findings from the National Sample Survey of Registered Nurses*, Washington, D.C., 1993, Division of Nursing, Health Resources and Services Administration.

Walcott-McQuigg J, Ervin NE: Stressors in the workplace: community health nurses, *Public Health Nurs* 9(1):65-71, 1992.

White MS: Construct for public health nursing, *Nurs Outlook* 30:527-530, 1982.

Williams CA: Community health nursing: what is it? *Nurs Outlook* 24:250-254, 1977.

Winslow C-EA: *Man and epidemics*, Princeton, N.J., 1952, Princeton University Press.

World Health Organization (WHO): *Community health nursing*, 1974 WHO Expert Committee Report 558, Geneva, 1974, WHO.

World Health Organization (WHO): *Alma-Ata 1978: primary health care: report of the International Conference on Primary Health Care*, Alma-Ata, USSR, Geneva, 1978, WHO.

World Health Organization (WHO): *A guide to curriculum review for basic nursing education: orientation to primary health care and community health*, Geneva, 1985, WHO.

World Health Organization (WHO): *Four decades of achievement: highlights of the work of WHO*, Geneva, 1988, WHO.

Zerwekh JV: Community health nurses: a population at risk, *Public Health Nurs* 9:1, 1992.

Zotti ME, Brown P, Stotts RC: Community-based nursing versus community health nursing: what does it all mean? *Nurs Outlook* 44:211-217, 1996.

SELECTED BIBLIOGRAPHY

Archer SE: Synthesis of public health science and nursing science, *Nurs Outlook* 30:442-446, 1982.

Barnes D, Eribes C, Juarbe T et al: Primary health care: a confusion of philosophies, *Nurs Outlook* 43:7-16, 1995.

Bracht N, ed: *Health promotion at the community level*, Newbury Park, Ca., 1990, Sage.

Capuzzi C: Families and community health nursing. In Hanson SMH, Boyd ST, eds: *Family health care nursing: theory, practice, and research*, Philadelphia, 1996, F.A. Davis.

Consensus conference on the essentials of public health nursing practice and education, HRSA 84-564 (POLP), Rockville, Md., 1985, Health Resources and Services Administration.

Duffy M, Pender N, eds: *Conceptual issues in health promotion: report of proceedings of a Wingspread Conference*, Racine, Wi., 1987, Sigma Theta Tau.

Hanchett E: *Nursing frameworks and community as client: bridging the gap*, Norwalk, Ct., 1988, Appleton & Lange.

Kenyon V, Smith E, Hefty LV et al: Clinical competencies for community health nursing, *Public Health Nurs* 7:33-39, 1990.

Maglacas AM: Health for all: nursing's role, *Nurs Outlook* 36:66-71, 1988.

Misener TR, Alexander JW, Blaha AJ et al: National delphi study to determine competencies for nursing leadership in public health, *Image J Nurs Sch* 29:47-51, 1997.

Shamansky SL, Clausen CL: Levels of prevention: examination of the concept, *Nurs Outlook* 28:104-108, 1980.

Stevens PE, Hall JM: Applying critical theories to nursing in communities, *Public Health Nurs* 9(1):2-6, 1992.

Whall AL: The family as the unit of care in nursing: a historical review, *Public Health Nurs* 3:240-249, 1986.

Williams A, Wold JL: Healthcare for the future: caring for populations in alternative settings, *Nurs Educ* 21:23-26, 1996.

Williams CA: Beyond the Institute of Medicine report: a critical analysis and public health forecast, *Fam Community Health* 18:12-23, 1995.

Zerwekh J: A family caregiving model for public health nursing, *Nurs Outlook* 39:213-217, 1991.

Zerwekh J: Going to the people—public health nursing today and tomorrow, *AJPH* 83:1676-1678, 1993.

Zerwekh J, Primomo J, Deal L, eds: *Opening doors: stories of public health nursing*, Olympia, Wa., 1992, Washington State Department of Health.

3

Community as Partner

Objectives

Upon completion of this chapter, the reader should be able to:

1. Define the term *community.*
2. Discuss the concept of community as partner.
3. Discuss the meaning of community as client.
4. Describe the service areas of a community.
5. Discuss the functions of a community.
6. Discuss community dynamics.
7. Define the term *aggregate.*
8. Discuss the healthy communities initiative.
9. Discuss some health problems of rural communities.
10. Differentiate between a community's normal line of defense and its flexible line of defense.
11. Discuss the relevance of community assessment to community health nursing practice.

> There can be no health without community: that sense of mutual values and goals held by people regardless of geographic boundaries and their collective responsibility for nurturing their biophysical environment.
>
> DR. NANCY MILIO (1990)

As discussed in Chapter 2, the uniqueness of community health nursing lies in the fact that nurses in this specialty area care for the "community" and their practice is community oriented. Community health nurses work in partnership with communities to promote health. They view the community as client and work toward ensuring equal access to health services for everyone, "health for all."

In its definition of community health nursing, the American Nurses Association has said that nursing efforts to promote and maintain health in the community entail the understanding and application of (1) concepts of public health and community; (2) skills of community organization and development; and (3) nursing care of selected individuals, families, and groups for health promotion, health maintenance, health education, and coordination of care (ANA, 1986, p. 1). This chapter presents the concepts of community-as-partner and community-as-client, defines the term *community*, and discusses community dynamics and nursing care of aggregates in the community. Chapters 13 and 14 build on this material and discuss how community assessment, diagnosis, and health planning processes assist public health professionals in working with communities.

COMMUNITY AS PARTNER

Today more than ever before nurses are working in partnership with communities to promote health. This partnership means that the nurse does not decide what community health priorities and actions should be, but works collaboratively with communities to build on their strengths and to facilitate community empowerment. "To be empowered means that one (community, family, individual) has the knowledge, skills and capacity for effective and self-determined action" (Courtney, 1995, p. 370; Courtney, Ballard, Fauver et al, 1996, p. 180).

Empowerment is a proactive, participatory change process that encourages people and organizations in communities to use their skills and resources in collective action to improve the quality of life within the community (Israel, Checkoway, Schulz, Zimmerman, 1994). A partnership is a union of people focused on collective action for a common endeavor or goal. Increasingly, the importance of developing partnerships to promote collective action for enhancing quality of life is recognized. From a community health perspective a partnership would focus on improving the health of the community.

Building on the work of Goeppinger and Shuster (1988) and experience from their community Partnership Primary Care Project, Courtney, Ballard, Fauver, Gariota, and Holland (1996) have expanded the concept of partnership. They see a partnership as "the negotiated sharing of power between health professionals and individual, family, and/or community partners. These partners agree to be involved as active participants in the process of mutually determining goals and actions that promote health and well-being. The ultimate goal of the partnership process is to enhance the capacity of individual, family and community partners to act more effectively on their own behalf" (p. 180). This definition reflects several key characteristics of a client/professional partnership: negotiated power, mutual goal setting, active versus passive client participation, and mobilization of a client's capacity for effective, self-determined action. Courtney, Bullard, Fauver, et al, have found in their experience that, although partnerships are valuable, some clients may not want to engage in a partnership relationship, and this decision must be respected.

Community action partnerships recognize the value of community representatives and health care providers working together to create health care systems that are user-friendly, accessible, culture-sensitive, and responsive to community needs (Pender, 1996, p. 296). They involve developing networks of people to take action for health, promote broad-based community participation, promote equity in health, and focus on what is best for the total community (Flynn, 1994, p. 55). The community's right to identify health problems and their solutions is recognized, and provider-community alliances are developed (Milio, 1992, p. 24). Viewing the community as partner has the nurse and the community working collaboratively to promote health. The "Healthy Communities" initiatives discussed later in this chapter involve nurses working in partnership with communities to promote health and improve the quality of life within the community.

COMMUNITY AS CLIENT

Conceptualizing community as client can be difficult for the nurse. In the acute care setting nursing care is often provided to individuals and families, but not as often to aggregates or communities. Moving to a community focus requires understanding the value of aggregate- and community-oriented practice. As our health care system becomes more integrated across the continuum of care, the need for such an understanding becomes essential. The majority of health care will be community based by the turn of the century. Health care professionals in all settings will need an understanding of community dynamics to succeed in the evolving health care environment.

The importance of the community-as-client concept has long been recognized in community health nursing practice. Lillian Wald, Mary Breckenridge, and other early community health nursing leaders realized that health problems, and their solutions, were deeply embedded in the structure of the community. These leaders promoted the idea that the dominant responsibility of the community health nurse was to the population as a whole, the community (ANA, 1980; National Organization for Public Health Nursing, 1975).

Today this responsibility has been integrated into the American Nurses Association's definition of community health nursing practice and the American Public Health Association's definition for this specialty area (see Chapter 2). Nursing interventions in the community historically have focused on health promotion and disease prevention. Many of these interventions are directed toward aggregates at risk for health problems. The nurse works in partnership with the community to promote health.

DEFINING COMMUNITY

The concept of community is basic to public health practice and is a distinguishing feature of community health nursing (Turner, Chavigny, 1988, p. 118). The word *community* has been in common use since its Latin origin as *communitas*, and there are no less than 100 definitions for the word *communis*, from which *community* was derived (Shamansky, Pesznecker, 1981, p. 182). Communities are frequently defined within one of two frameworks: (1) geographical area or (2) relational (McMillan, Chavis, 1986, p. 6).

Geographical definitions look at communities in terms of legal or geopolitical jurisdictions such as cities, towns, municipalities, or census tracts. In the United States, official public health services are offered through the geopolitical units of state and local governments.

Relational definitions are more abstract and examine how a group of people interacts to achieve common goals. Relational definitions are often more real for the populace, who frequently do not limit their personal definition of community to geographical boundaries. With relational definitions the boundaries of communities overlap, and people often have membership in more than one community. An example of such overlapping boundaries is a person who lives in one community and works or receives health care in another.

Health, social, urban, and political scientists have defined community from several different perspectives, and nursing literature reveals diverse usages and definitions of the term *community*. Characteristics that have emerged as being essential to a definition of community are (1) people, (2) social interaction, (3) area, and (4) common ties (Hillery, 1955, pp. 118-119; Wellman, Leighton, 1988, p. 58). Although communities have many similarities, each community is uniquely different.

People in a community share things in common such as land, history, culture, heritage, and even destiny (MacIver, Page, 1949, pp. 8-10; Moore, 1996). A community is where people live, maintain their homes, earn their living, become educated, rear their children, and carry on day-to-day activities (Poplin, 1979, p. 8). A community can be defined in a very broad sense as a group of people living in an environment that has the ability to meet their major life goals and needs such as food, shelter, and socialization.

The American Public Health Association (1991, p. 444) has said that the term *community* implies an entity from which the nature and scope of a public health problem, as well as the capacity to respond to that problem, can be defined; and that, depending on the problem area and response capacity, the definition of community may vary. According to the Association, for most instances of public health the community is defined as a geopolitical unit such as a town, city, or county.

The definition of community used in this text is the World Health Organization (WHO) definition that is incorporated into the American Nurses Association's (1986) Standards of Community Health Nursing Practice. This definition states that a "community is a social group determined by geographical boundaries and/or common values and interests; community members know and interact with one another; the community functions within a particular social structure; and the community creates norms, values, and social institutions" (WHO, 1974).

The American Community

The American community has been studied since the early 1900s. Early researchers on the American community were usually social scientists and included MacIver (1917), Hillery (1955), Sanders (1958), and Warren (1955, 1966). Many of these early studies have become classics in the field and are still cited in today's social science and nursing literature. These early researchers recognized that there was a relationship between the community and the health of its members. One of them, Irwin T. Sanders, published in the community health nursing literature. His article "The Community: Structure and Function" appeared in *Nursing Outlook* (Sanders, 1963). For interested readers, *The Community: An Introduction to a Social System* (Sanders, 1958, 1966, 1975), *The Community in America* (Warren, 1963, 1972, 1978, 1987), and *Studying Your Community* (Warren 1955, 1965) are considered classic works on the American community.

Early research on the American community focused on the community as a natural area. This natural area is similar to the geographical definition of community mentioned earlier in this chapter. Contemporary research on community has been broadened to a natural network approach. The natural network approach is more relational in nature and takes into account the widening scope of resources and services necessary to maintain the health and social well-being of a community in today's technological, complex, and diverse society. It creates an awareness of contemporary community health concerns such as health disparities, access to resources, and resource distribution.

Communities as Social Units

Communities are social units and settings for social action. A community is the basic unit of social organization that transmits values, attitudes, and beliefs to its members (Arensburg, Kimball, 1972, p. 15). Community health nurses need to be aware of, and respect, the values, attitudes, and culture of the communities in which they work.

As a social unit, the community has a life within which individuals define their own lives (Moore, 1996). The community helps to provide its members a sense of who they are and where they are going and perpetuates the culture and heritage of the community. A community can be differentiated from other social units, such as groups, in that one's life can basically be lived within its bounds (Arensburg, Kimball, 1972, p. 17; MacIver, Page, 1949, pp. 8-10; Warren, 1978, p. 6). This is possible because of the various services and functions that the community provides and offers for its residents.

Communities as Part of a Larger Society

A community is part of, and has ties to, larger societies. These ties to the larger society are frequently on a county, state, regional, or national level. A community has patterns of communication and leadership that link it to the larger society and its resources. Patterns of communication and leadership are discussed later in this chapter.

In many communities health care resources are inadequate to meet the community's increasingly diverse health care needs, and people must go outside the community to the larger society to obtain the necessary health care. This is becoming increasingly evident in rural communities where health care resources are shrinking.

Community Autonomy

Some communities will have a greater sense of autonomy than others, and people will have varying degrees of loyalty to their communities. In some places a sense of community will exist, and in others it will not. Research has shown that a population base of 10,000 to 20,000 is preferred for maintaining a sense of community, that larger cities of up to 100,000 can still maintain this sense, and that cities or geographical areas larger than 100,000 often need to be broken down into target areas such as neighborhoods or districts to maintain a sense of community and provide effective health care delivery (Chamberlain, 1988, p. 302). Also, if a community has a relatively "mobile" or transient populace it may be difficult for a sense of community to exist because people do not stay in the community long enough to develop ties to it.

COMMUNITY DYNAMICS

Community dynamics occur as a result of interactions within the community and between the community and the larger society. These interactions are instrumental in determining what public health services are offered in the community and the level of community health, and for achieving healthy communities. Community dynamics involve interactions between the community's people, goals and needs, environment, service systems, patterns of communication, leadership, and community functions. Figure 3-1 is a flow chart that summarizes the information on community dynamics presented in this chapter and assists the reader in visualizing and conceptualizing the discussion that follows.

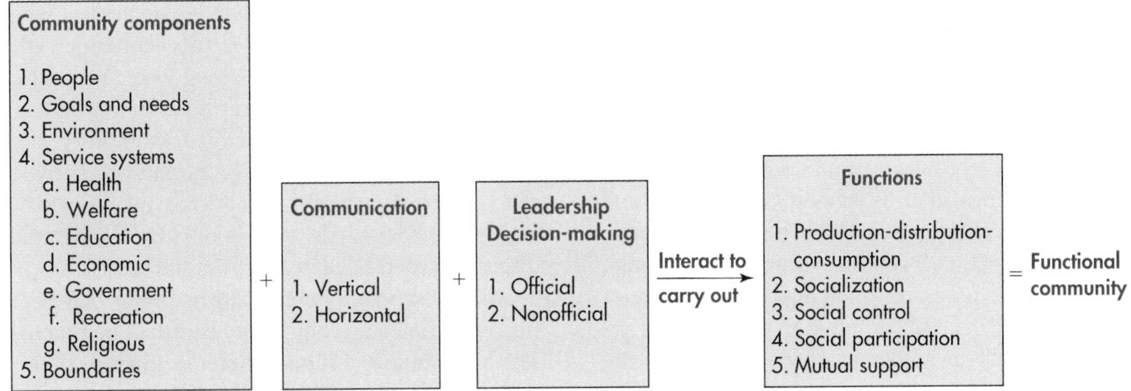

Figure 3-1 Community dynamics. *(Service systems data from Sanders IT:* The community: an introduction to a social system, *ed 2, New York, 1966, Ronald Press; communication and function data from Warren RL:* The community in America, *ed 2, Chicago, 1972, Rand-McNally.)*

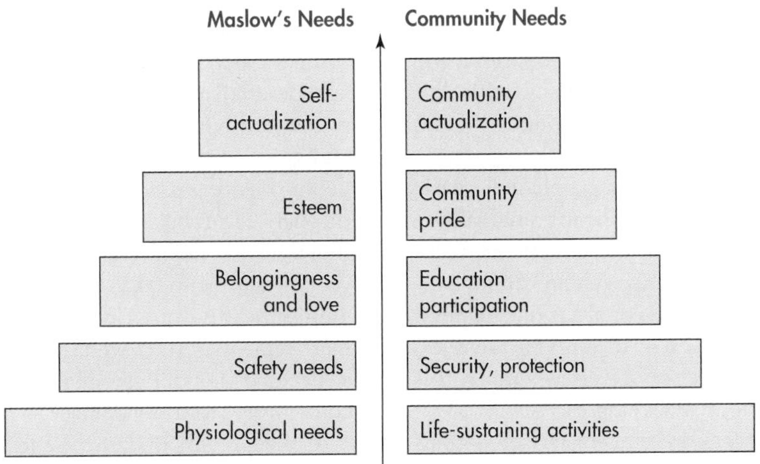

Figure 3-2 A comparison of Maslow's identification of basic needs of the individual with those of the community as a client. *(From Higgs ZR, Gustafson DD:* Community as client: assessment and diagnosis, *Philadelphia, 1985, F.A. Davis.)*

Components of a Community

Communities have the components of people, shared goals and needs, environment, service systems, and boundaries. Communities also have patterns of communication and leadership and carry out a variety of functions.

People are a community's most important resource: they are its essence and give the community its identity. They have responsibilities to the community, and the community has responsibilities to them.

Knowledge of the values, attitudes, and beliefs of the people in the community, and knowledge of basic community population characteristics such as cultural and ethnic backgrounds, age, sex, income level, and educational level, are essential for effective community health planning and action. For example, when analyzing a community in relation to age distribution, a nurse became aware that the community in which she worked was made up of young families and school-age children. This community would have different health care needs than a community of predominantly senior citizens. The Community Assessment in Chapter 13 gives parameters to use in gathering data on the people of a community.

Goals and needs of a community should be determined by its people. Each community has health goals and needs. Nurses are working with communities to help them determine their community health needs, establish health goals and action plans, and become healthier communities. Community health nurses' skills and competence make them a valuable resource in assisting the community to assess, set, and achieve its health goals. The nurse can also serve as an advocate for the community in obtaining the health care resources and services necessary to achieve these goals.

Community health goals and needs have been compared to Maslow's hierarchical order of basic needs (Higgs, Gustafson, 1985, p. 12; Meneshian, 1988, p. 116). Figure 3-2 shows a comparison of these needs.

Community environment has physical, biological, and sociocultural components. These components combine to make each community unique and have a major impact on the overall health of the community.

The physical environment of the community includes the geography, climate, terrain, natural resources, and structural entities (buildings such as schools, workplaces, and homes). The biological environment of the community includes various flora, fauna, bacteria, viruses, molds, fungi, toxic substances, and food and water supplies. The sociocultural environment of the community reflects culture, values, attitudes, and demographic characteristics of the people of the community.

These environments play a significant role in community health. For example, in many rural communities well water is the only source of fresh water. If this well water is contaminated or if children in these communities do not have regular fluoride treatments, community health problems can develop. Environmental health concerns such as contaminated food and water supplies, air pollution, and toxic chemicals pose serious problems to public health. Environmental health concerns for the community health nurse are discussed in Chapter 6.

Service systems of a community help people meet basic needs of daily living as well as specific health and welfare needs. These service systems are made up of numerous agencies and organizations. When a service system cannot provide all the services needed by the populace (e.g., a rural hospital that does not provide open heart surgery), members of the community must find the service elsewhere. In this way a "community of solution" is developed.

Sanders (1966, p. 170) viewed the major service systems of the community as (1) health, (2) social welfare, (3) educational, (4) economic, (5) governmental, (6) recreational, and (7) religious. These community service systems form a network of resources that deliver services to community members. Each system is crucial and in some way affects health.

Not all service systems have equal importance within the community, and sometimes they become out of balance with one another. An example of an imbalance in service systems is when the welfare system receives a disproportionate amount of the tax dollars, thus reducing the tax dollars available to other community systems such as education or health. Once this system equilibrium has been disturbed, it may never be restored, or it may take years to recover.

Also, service systems may have some form of authority over one another. For example, the religious system may influence the health practices of its members. The religious practices of fasting, eating or not eating certain foods, and prohibiting the use of certain health care services, such as general medical care, blood transfusions, and family planning methods, are examples of how religious beliefs make an impact on the health care delivery system.

Although the health system is the central focus for the community health nurse it is the economic system (economic sufficiency) that has long been recognized as the usual focus for the citizenry and leadership of the community (National Commission on Community Health Services, 1966, p. 7). Until a community's basic economic needs are met, it is not likely that people will work diligently on other needs, such as health. The health system is discussed separately later in this chapter.

All the service systems have a role to play in maintaining and promoting community health. The nurse should assess a community's service systems, identify their resources and services, discover how each fits into the overall structure of the community, and use them to promote health.

Boundaries of a community serve to regulate the exchange of energies between the community and its external environment. In general, boundaries may be concrete (definite, spatial) or conceptual (elusive, nonspatial). Concrete boundaries are more absolute and easier to see and to define. They include geographical boundaries (mountains, valleys, and deserts), political boundaries (cities, towns, counties, states, and nations), situational boundaries (home, school, and work), and combinations of these. For example, many public health services in the United States are provided through local health departments. The service areas of these health departments are usually determined by the geopolitical boundaries of cities, towns, or counties. Community health nurses working in these health departments must remember that even though their service area may be a specified geopolitical area, that area may not reflect "the community" for the populace.

Conceptual boundaries are less definite, more relational, and more flexible in nature. They often do not fit into a neatly defined space. They include boundaries such as interest area, problem solving, socially defined, or service area. Service-area boundaries are of special interest to the community health nurse. The health service area for a community is the area within which a health problem can be defined and solved. If the necessary health care resources do not exist within the community, a "community of solution" develops, and the health service area for the community expands outside its bounds. For example, many rural communities have serious gaps in the health care services available, and their service area boundary for health care may be enlarged to include other localities.

Community Communication Patterns

Communities have both horizontal and vertical patterns of communication (Warren, 1978, pp. 163-164). Vertical patterns of communication link the community to the larger society (state, national, and international); horizontal patterns of communication link the community to its people, environment, and systems. The strength and ease with which these patterns operate will largely determine the extent to which the community is able to be self-sufficient and provide for the needs of its membership. Horizontal patterns of communication greatly influence the internal dynamics of the community. This communication within the community transmits community culture, tradition, values, and attitudes from generation to generation and helps to preserve the community.

Community Leadership

The leadership and decision-making processes within a community critically influence how well that community will function. A community usually has official (elected and appointed) leadership such as a mayor or city council, school board, and school principals. This leadership is obvious to community members and other communities. However, much of a community's leadership is nonofficial (not elected or appointed).

Nonofficial community leadership is less obvious and may be more difficult to detect. However, this leadership often has more influence, power, and control over community action and decision making than the official leadership.

The local community religious leader to whom people may go for advice and guidance, and the wealthy philanthropist who heavily subsidizes community health activities, are examples of nonofficial leaders. Nonofficial leaders are often the "heroes" of the community, those whom people in the community revere and respect. It is frequently such people in the community to whom others turn for advice, emotional support, and assistance. The use of these nonofficial leaders in health education activities can aid in the adoption of health promotion behaviors (Wiist, Flack, 1990, p. 381).

The community health nurse will find it useful to identify community leaders and their health and welfare responsibilities. These leaders greatly influence what type of services will be available for the community. They can assist in making health a community priority and facilitate the implementation of health care services in the community. An example of such facilitation is a research study by Wiist and Flack (1990) that showed how the support of religious leaders in a community made a large-scale cholesterol education program possible and successful.

Some aspects of community life are controlled by leadership decisions made outside the community. These decisions are frequently in the form of state, federal, and international laws and regulations. The community must adhere to such legal decisions even though they may be in conflict with its values, attitudes, and ideology. Such health and welfare legislation is discussed throughout this text.

Community Functions

To provide for the life goals and needs of its population, the community carries out a number of functions. Warren (1978, pp. 171-212) gives the following functions of a community:

PRODUCTION-DISTRIBUTION-CONSUMPTION The community produces, distributes, and uses goods and services that are essential for meeting the health and welfare needs of its residents. This triad of activities involves extensive resource and service coordination.

SOCIALIZATION Socialization is the process by which prevailing knowledge, values, beliefs, customs, and behavior are transmitted to a community's members. It is a lifelong process that helps persons learn how to effectively relate in a social environment and to develop a philosophy of life.

SOCIAL CONTROL The community influences the behavior of its members through norms, regulations, and rules of social control. Social control has a legal component that is often enforced through law agencies, courts, and the government. It also has a social sanction component. Social control helps to safeguard and protect the community by providing mechanisms for safety and order.

SOCIAL PARTICIPATION People have basic needs for self-expression and self-fulfillment. These needs are largely met through interaction with others. This function provides opportunity for members of the community to communicate, socially interact, and obtain support. It helps community members to achieve psychosocial wellness. Social networks evolve through social participation.

MUTUAL SUPPORT Mutual support involves people lending assistance to one another. It is frequently offered through family, friends, neighbors, and religious groups, as well as official and private health and social service organizations within the community.

These functions provide for the services and activities necessary for everyday community life. The way in which a community carries out these functions affects how well the community health nurse will be able to meet the needs of the population. For example, if there is a gap in production-distribution-consumption, the community may not have the health resources to meet the health needs of its population. If people have not been socialized to value preventive health care, or if they have customs (such as religious fasting) that affect the delivery of health care services, the nurse's ability to implement preventive health care services can be hindered. If community health policy is inadequate, or if the health policy is not enforced, the health of the community may be in jeopardy. If the members of the community do not value social interaction and participation, the community's response to clinics, classes, and group activities may not be maximized. If a community does not offer sufficient mutual support, there may be few health and welfare assistance programs for community members in need of them, and it may be difficult to engage the community in partnership activities.

The Functional Community

The figure on community dynamics (Figure 3-1) illustrated how components of the community interact to create a functional, healthy community. Functional communities can identify, prioritize, and address community strengths and needs and are capable of problem solving and crisis resolution. Functional communities collaboratively work with health care professionals to increase and maintain community competence.

According to Warren (1988 pp. 413-418) a functional community has the following characteristics: people interact, participate, and have a degree of commitment to the community; the community has some autonomy from the larger society; people can confront their problems through concerted action (viability); decision making is relatively equally distributed throughout the population and not concentrated (power distribution); there is a balance of differences (degree of heterogeneity); and the degree of conflict is manageable.

Functional communities can become dysfunctional as a result of the impact of community stressors. Community stressors are tension-producing stimuli that have the potential to cause disequilibrium and can result in disruption in the community (Anderson, McFarlane, 1996, p. 172). They can arise from inside or outside the community and include natural disasters and economic crises. Stressors occur when service systems are unable to provide the necessary services for effective community functioning (e.g., the inability of a community to maintain a tax base sufficient to adequately operate the local health department). The reaction to these stressors may be reflected in community health statistics such as morbidity and mortality rates, crime statistics, and unemployment (Anderson, McFarlane, p. 172). When community stressors arise, the community needs to problem solve and work toward crisis resolution.

THE HEALTH SYSTEM AND THE COMMUNITY

As mentioned previously in this chapter, community service systems help a community to achieve its basic needs. The community service system of health is of major importance to the community health nurse. Health system resources include individuals and groups, private health practitioners, community health volunteers, hospitals, clinics, pharmacies, nursing homes, health departments, and departments of social services. The priority that the community places on health, and the resources it funds and allocates, will play a major role in the overall health of the community.

Health resources in the community are both governmental and private (see Chapter 4). The government (official) sector provides traditional public health services, such as communicable disease control, and preventive health services through official health departments. Private-sector provision of health care services often includes resources such as hospitals, outpatient clinics, private practitioner's offices, and service agencies such as the American Red Cross. In both the government and private sectors there are a variety of health care practitioners, including nurses, nurse practitioners, physicians, dentists, psychiatrists, psychologists, social workers, environmental health workers, ancillary health care personnel, and volunteers. Local health departments are an excellent source of information on community health resources and services.

A community has a level of health reached over time that is called its *normal line of defense* (Anderson, McFarlane, 1996, p. 169). This line of defense can include characteristics such as high immunity levels and low infant mortality and is contrasted with the community's flexible line of defense, which represents a state of health that is more dynamic or in flux owing to temporary stressors such as environmental disasters and epidemics (Anderson, McFarlane, p. 169). These lines of defense are used in partnership with communities for health planning, implementation, and evaluation.

Difficulties in the Community Health System

When analyzing the community health system, several concerns may become apparent. A major concern stressed in *Healthy People 2000* is that of access (see Chapter 5). Many Americans do not have access to appropriate health care services for reasons such as cost, transportation, and lack of an appropriate resource. Some people simply "fall through the cracks" in our health care system and do not receive appropriate health care. The working poor in our communities often have problems of access to health care as a result of being uninsured or underinsured.

Communication between the health care system and the other community systems has historically been weak (see Chapter 5). In many communities official local health departments have little contact with private health care resources and other official health and welfare resources. The health system of the community may have little communication with the people of the community, and partnerships for community health may not exist. With the current trend emphasizing coalition building for community action, more effective partnerships are emerging in many communities.

No one agency has statutory (legal) responsibility for managing the health resources in the community, and responsibilities for who manages what resource are often vague and unclear. Not only is the overall management of the health system weak, but the management skills of individual health practitioners may also be weak. Health practitioners frequently have not had educational experiences that prepare them to manage health care resources. Health care professionals must understand the principles of management if the health care system is to carry out its functions effectively, work in partnership with communities, and promote community health.

American communities have historically reacted better to disaster and catastrophic health events than to providing ongoing, preventive community health services. There is often indifference to a health problem if no serious, long-term, or personal effects are apparent. Also, the feeling within many American communities that the primary responsibility for health resides with official health depart-

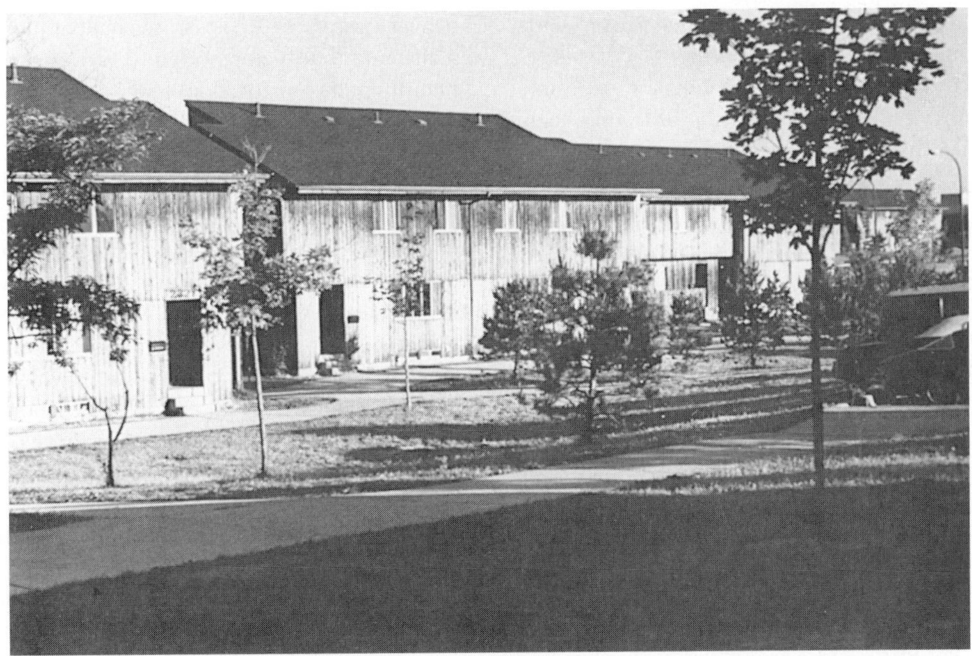

Figure 3-3 Residents of a university housing project for married students form an aggregate of persons who have shared personal and environmental characteristics. These families can be at risk because they can experience multiple stresses such as crowded living conditions, financial difficulties, and educational pressures.

ments and health care practitioners deters community involvement in health. Healthy community initiatives are necessary to assist communities to take responsibility for their own health.

AGGREGATES IN THE COMMUNITY

A community is made up of various aggregates. As discussed in Chapter 2, aggregates are groups of persons who have one or more shared personal or environmental characteristics (see Figure 3-3). Historically, community health nurses have provided services to aggregates based on age-related developmental tasks and at-risk characteristics. In these times of cost containment this historical approach has assumed new relevance. It can be much more cost-effective to serve a group of people than to work with people on an individual basis. Increasingly, community health activities are being provided to aggregates.

The developmental approach is based on the theory that individuals develop in their own way, yet conform to a common developmental pattern. It postulates that failure to accomplish developmental tasks at the appropriate time makes subsequent development more difficult. Erikson's (1978) eight stages of the life cycle (infancy, early childhood, play age, school age, adolescence, young adulthood, adulthood, and senescence) have been used widely in nursing. Using this approach, this text assists the reader in looking at services to aggregates such as preschool children, school-age children, adults, and the elderly, based on the developmental needs of each age group.

Aggregates can also be looked at from a risk perspective. Examples of aggregates at risk addressed in this text are adults who are disabled, persons with long-term care needs, persons with AIDS, teenage parents, homeless individuals and families, victims of domestic violence, individuals and families living in poverty, disadvantaged groups, and ethnic and racial minority groups. An at-risk perspective helps health care professionals to identify groups who have a high potential for mortality and morbidity.

Community health nurses use both the developmental and at-risk approaches as a foundation for assessing health strengths and needs, identifying health promotion activities for aggregates across the life span, and working in partnership with communities to develop health promotion strategies. The community health nurse's role in providing services to aggregates is discussed throughout this text. Assessing and planning services for aggregates in the community are discussed in Chapters 13 and 14. Working with groups in the community is discussed in Chapter 23.

HEALTHY COMMUNITIES

Public health has long recognized the importance of working with communities to resolve their problems (Hancock, 1987, p. 4). In the nineteenth century major public health achievements occurred in response to the appalling health conditions in communities, and contemporary public health initiatives are again focusing on improving the health of communities. Since the days of Lillian Wald community health nurses have worked in partnership with communities to make communities healthier places to live.

A classic report by the National Commission on Community Health Services (1966) issued the following goals for achieving healthy communities that are still to be fulfilled:

All communities of this nation must take the action necessary to provide comprehensive personal health services of high quality to all people in the community. These services should embrace those directed toward promotion of positive good health, application of established preventive measures, early detection of disease, prompt and effective treatment, and physical, social, and vocational rehabilitation of those with residual disabilities. This broad range of personal health services must be patterned so as to assure full and intelligent use by all groups in the community.

Healthy People 2000 envisioned establishing healthy communities through the commitment of individuals, agencies, and organizations at the community level (USDHHS, 1995, p. 143). It established an objective for communities to take part in community health promotion programs and developed a set of public health indicators to assist communities in assessing their general health status and progress in achieving community health (see Chapter 13). The document supported states in formulating and promoting statewide disease prevention and health promotion objectives that could be the blueprint for local initiatives and encouraged involvement from both the public and private sectors in healthy communities programs (USDHHS, pp. 143-145).

Having healthy communities has become a national and international goal, and healthy community initiatives are gaining impetus worldwide. Such initiatives use the previously discussed concept of "community-as-partner" to build on community strengths and facilitate community empowerment for health action. They make health a community priority, encourage shared responsibility for health community wide, involve local people, focus on hard-to-reach populations, and promote healthy public policies (Flynn, Rains, 1993, p. 24; Flynn, 1995, p. 6). The process for doing so is discussed in Chapters 13 and 14.

Dr. Beverly Flynn (1995) has noted, "Over the past few years, public health problems have pushed their way to the forefront of America's domestic agenda. From the halls of Congress to our living rooms, the media has focused attention on the debilitating effects of poverty, violence, and inadequate access to health care. In the face of these growing problems, many communities have pledged to enhance their quality of life by participating in Healthy Cities, an innovative, grassroots approach to health promotion and disease prevention" (p. 6). Such initiatives are taking place in more than 200 American communities.

Success in establishing healthy communities will mean change. It will require removal of racial, economic, organizational, and geographical barriers to the use of health services. It will require universal health coverage through health insurance and other prepayment plans. It will require a citizenry that is empowered to participate in all aspects of planning, implementation, and evaluation of healthy community initiatives.

Healthy Community Initiatives Worldwide

The idea for the contemporary healthy communities movement had its origins in Canada in 1984 and was endorsed by the Canadian Public Health Association. In 1986 the World Health Organization (WHO) actively endorsed such initiatives as part of its overall move toward "Health Care for All." Today WHO offers the "Healthy Communities Program." This program uses diverse community coalitions to assess their own health priorities, develop effective community health promotion actions, and promote community health (Sasenick, 1994, p. 56).

Healthy community initiatives put health on the agenda of local governments and create new structures and processes for achieving health (International Council of Nurses, 1991, p. 109). They challenge local communities to engage in collaborative problem solving to improve the quality of life, reduce disparities in health access and status, rethink approaches to health care delivery, and address factors that contribute to good health (Norris, 1993, p. 6; National Civic League, 1995, p. 1).

Such initiatives facilitate community empowerment processes for health action, focus on the community, involve citizen participation and problem solving, and strive to improve the quality of life (Flynn, Ray, Rider, 1994, p. 395). They respond to the unique health needs of each community and focus on primary prevention. Chapter 14 discusses such initiatives in relation to health planning.

Helping communities to develop strategies that address social and health problems and to consider the complex factors that contribute to wellness is an essential part of building healthy communities (Norris, Lampe, 1994, p. 2). Organized community effort to promote health and prevent disease is both valuable and effective (Institute of Medicine, 1988, p. 17). Communities are becoming increasingly sophisticated in their efforts to address preventive health needs (Eisen, 1994, p. 236).

Worldwide there are more than 1000 healthy communities initiatives (Nakajima, 1996). There may even be such an initiative in your own home town. Colorado, California, and Indiana have numerous initiatives, and more states are becoming actively involved. We can be proud that in the United States community health nurses have played an important role in the development of healthy communities. Some U.S. initiatives that facilitate healthy communities are presented.

PLANNED APPROACH TO COMMUNITY HEALTH (PATCH) The Centers for Disease Control and Prevention (CDC) sponsors PATCH. PATCH has been operating since 1986 and uses broad-based community advisory groups to promote community health (Flynn, 1994, p. 56). Essential elements of PATCH are local ownership and decision making; community partnerships; community members recommending goals using local health data; ranking health problems and setting objectives; carrying out interventions; and evaluating the program and interventions (Speers, 1992, p. 132). It was initially designed to strengthen state and local health departments' capacities to plan, implement, and evaluate community-based health promotion activities (Kreuter, 1992, p. 135). PATCH programs have often targeted rural and underserved communities (Green, Kreuter, 1992, p. 140). These programs have been implemented in 17 states and 50 communities (Speers, 1992, p. 132). For more information contact the Centers for Disease Control and Prevention, 1600 Clifton Rd NE, Atlanta, Georgia, 30333.

NATIONAL HEALTHY COMMUNITIES INITIATIVE This initiative was developed in 1989 by the National Civic League in cooperation with the U.S. Public Health Service. It promotes a collaborative community-based approach to health promotion (National Civic League, 1995). The National Civic League administers the Colorado Healthy Communities Initiative (HCI), the largest statewide initiative in the United States, and publishes the Healthy Communities Directory, Healthy Communities Resource Guide, and The Healthy Communities Handbook. The League also sponsors the "Healthy Communities Action Project," a training program to help community leaders develop innovative approaches to improving community health. For information on HCI and the Healthy Communities Action Project contact National Civic League, 1445 Market, Suite 300, Denver, Colorado, 80202-1728.

BUILDING HEALTHIER COMMUNITIES: THE UNITED WAY The United Way has played a significant role in helping America become a healthier nation and is committed to improving the health of the nation's citizens (Norris, 1993, pp. 17-18). The United Way is working to incorporate healthy community concepts through collaborative community problem solving, fundraising, allocations of funds, and provision of services (Norris, p. 18). For information on United Way healthy community initiatives contact United Way of America, 701 North Fairfax Street, Arlington, Virginia, 22314.

CITYNET HEALTHY CITIES This initiative was developed at the Institute of Action Research for Community Health of the Indiana University School of Nursing. A nurse, Dr. Beverly C. Flynn, is director of the institute and heads the WHO Collaborating Center in Healthy Cities. CITYNET fosters collaborative working relationships with universities, local health departments, hospitals, local government, arts and culture, business and industry, education, environment, media, religion, and other sectors of community life to promote health (Flynn, 1994, p. 55). This approach energizes individuals to enact positive change and develop healthier communities through analysis, consensus, social action, and health policies (Flynn, 1993, p. 15). "Healthy Cities Indiana" was the first "healthy cities" project in the United States. For information and materials on CITYNET and Healthy Cities Indiana contact CITYNET Healthy Cities, Institute of Action Research for Community Health, Indiana University School of Nursing, 1111 Middle Drive, NU 236, Indianapolis, Indiana, 46202.

COMMUNITY & INSTITUTIONAL ASSESSMENT PROCESS (CIAP) The Public Health Resource Group developed CIAP. CIAP uses epidemiological models and clinical indicators to estimate the health status factors that affect the utilization of inpatient and outpatient services in a community (Flynn, 1994, p. 56). It focuses on facilitating service development based on the needs of individual communities. For information contact Public Health Resource Group, 120 Exchange Street, Portland, Maine, 04101.

HEALTHY COMMUNITIES 2000: MODEL STANDARDS This is published by the American Public Health Association (APHA, 1991) and was developed in conjunction with the Centers for Disease Control, the Association of State and Territorial Health Officials, the National Association of County and City Health Officials, and the Association of Schools of Public Health. These standards are discussed in Chapter 5. The guidelines presented in the document assist U.S. communities in establishing achievable community health objectives in conjunction with the national health objectives in *Healthy People 2000*. The Association has also published *The Guide to Implementing Model Standards: Eleven Steps Toward a Healthy Community*.

Healthy community initiatives demonstrate that health is not just the responsibility of individuals or health professionals, but also is a mandate of the community as a whole (Flynn, 1993, p. 80). These initiatives are expanding rapidly and are making an impact on public health across the United States and throughout the world.

One important component of a community is neighborhoods. Many healthy community initiatives are using neighborhoods to promote health. To illustrate the significant influence of neighborhoods on the health of the community, a discussion of neighborhoods and health follows.

Neighborhoods and Health

Nurses have long recognized the importance of neighborhoods and health. Lillian Wald and the nurses of the Henry Street Settlement worked in neighborhoods in New York City. Mary Breckinridge and the nurses of the Frontier Nursing Service served many rural "neighborhoods." Mrs. Breckinridge's autobiography, *Wide Neighborhoods*, addressed the work of the service in helping to improve the health of these rural neighborhoods.

People may identify more closely with their neighborhood than with the community as a whole. Neighborhoods represent people with common values, attitudes, needs, concerns, and even history. They are playing an increasingly important role in health service provision and have many strengths that are conducive to promoting health. Neighborhood-based health initiatives provide health care

Classifications of Neighborhoods

INTEGRAL

The individuals in this setting have frequent face-to-face contacts. The norms, values, and attitudes of the neighborhood support those of the larger community. People are cohesive within the neighborhood but belong to other groups outside their area of residence. There is a form of power, authority, and leadership within this type of neighborhood which aids its members to reach out to the larger society for assistance when a problem arises that cannot be handled internally.

PAROCHIAL

People in this setting also have face-to-face contacts, but there is an absence of ties to the larger community. These neighborhoods tend to be protective of their status, to screen out values that do not conform to their own, and to enforce their own beliefs within the neighborhood. The power, authority, and leadership structure within this type of neighborhood encourages isolation from the larger community.

DIFFUSE

Neighbors within this type of environment interact infrequently with each other and have few ties with the larger community. There is often a lack of shared norms, values, and attitudes. A primary tie between these neighbors is geographic proximity to one another. There may be little or no leadership in these areas. When leadership exists, it is often not representative of the entire neighborhood, but is composed of an "elitist" leadership that ignores or subverts the values of most residents. Groups of residents, such as those living in a public housing unit, may be categorized and separated from the mainstream of the neighborhood.

STEPPING-STONE

This type of neighborhood is characterized by a rapid membership turnover and families who have a weak sense of identity with the neighborhood. Members are willing to give up the ties established in the neighborhood if other commitments arise; they strive to attain a higher social status. Residents of these areas do, however, have close ties to the larger community and do interact regularly with neighbors. Leadership is usually not effective because of the high rate of mobility; conflicts arise between the needs of the local neighborhood and the values of social mobility.

TRANSITORY

Members of this kind of neighborhood fail to participate in or identify with the local community. There is an emphasis on people keeping to themselves, because links with others may interfere with the goals of the individual and the family. There may be a widespread feeling of mistrust in this type of neighborhood.

ANOMIC

Such a neighborhood is completely disorganized; its residents lack participation in and a common identification with the neighborhood or the larger community. This neighborhood reflects mass apathy and is not likely to influence or alter the values of its residents through any form of socialization. There is little interaction between people within the neighborhood or between the neighborhood and the larger community, and leadership activity is largely lacking.

Warren DI: Neighborhoods in urban areas. In Warren RL, ed: *New perspectives on the American community*, ed. 3, Chicago, 1977, Rand McNally, pp. 224-237.

workers and citizens with small community units to work with, empower participants with a sense of ownership and involvement, and offer a mechanism for targeting resources to low-income and at-risk populations.

Having neighborhood health initiatives can ease barriers to utilization of services such as transportation, and coordination among agencies may be easier to negotiate in a neighborhood than in an entire community. Many neighborhood health initiatives offer services such as child care, interpreters, and use of neighborhood "community health volunteers." These volunteers are recruited from the community where the program is located, are trained to promote health, and are usually well received by the community (Sherer, 1994, p. 52). Overall, neighborhood health initiatives provide a level of social comfort that is conducive to health action (Eisen, 1994, p. 238).

Warren (1977, pp. 224-229) has classified neighborhoods to identify the differences between them. Descriptions of these classifications are given in the box above. Neighborhoods vary greatly in leadership, cohesiveness, and self-sufficiency; these variances have an impact on the health resources and services available.

Identifying the type of neighborhood in which nurses work can assist them to function in partnership with the community to meet health needs. For example, if a community health nurse is working in a parochial neighborhood, it would be important to work closely with neighborhood leaders in the delivery of health care services. The nurse may find that the parochial neighborhood readily becomes involved in providing services for its residents. However, there also may be more resistance in this neighborhood to health services proposed by the larger community, especially if they do not coincide with neighborhood values and beliefs. On the other hand, in an anomic neighborhood the community health nurse may find little neighborhood leadership and may need to assist in developing this leadership to facilitate health action. In addition, the nurse may find that the anomic neighborhood offers few services to its residents and that services need to be sought from outside the neighborhood. Whatever the type of neighborhood, its structure has implications for the activities of the community health nurse.

An enlightening example of a neighborhood health initiative is the community-based nursing model that addresses the specific health needs of the Mantua neighborhood in West Philadelphia.

> Mantua . . . is a neighborhood in West Philadelphia with a population of approximately 10,000; the majority of Mantua residents (94 percent) are African Americans, 65 percent live in single-parent households, and more than 50 percent are in families at or below the poverty level. The infant mortality rate is among the highest in Philadelphia—28 per 1000 live births. Only 38 percent of Mantua residents have finished high school, and only 5 percent have completed college. Despite the presence of a renowned medical facility only blocks away and several other fine hospitals nearby, significant numbers of residents do not obtain health care. (Whelan, 1995)

Whelan (1995) noted that 60% of the children screened in West Philadelphia had elevated lead levels (it was estimated that only 10% had been screened); only 30% of 2-year-olds in Mantua were fully immunized; almost 25% of Mantua births were to adolescents; 32.7% of the women in Mantua delayed prenatal care or had none at all; 21% of the women had low birth weight infants; and rates of gonorrhea and syphilis were many times the national average. Based on these maternal-child health indicators it was decided to develop a community-based health initiative in the Mantua neighborhood. The project's overall mission was to create a health care site that would minimize barriers to access, increase utilization of health services, and improve the health status of the community (Whelan, p. 186). Evaluation methods were used to measure whether Health Corner objectives had been met.

In the Mantua project, members of the community were the driving force in determining the appropriateness of services, and a "Neighborhood Advisory Council" was established. Services at the site included well-child care focusing on immunizations and lead screenings; services for adolescents focusing on sexually transmitted diseases screening and treatment; family planning; and walk-in pregnancy testing for women of all ages, with referrals to early prenatal care. Referral mechanisms and linkages between community agencies were developed and community health improved.

The project is a success story for community health partnerships. It received a U.S. Department of Health and Human Services "Secretary's Award for Innovations in Health Promotion and Disease Prevention." It is a model for others who are considering implementing neighborhood health initiatives.

Although neighborhoods in urban communities are frequently written about in the health literature, it is increasingly recognized that rural communities have significant health issues. Rural health initiatives are being developed across the nation to address these issues and improve rural health.

RURAL COMMUNITIES

Rural communities have unique health care needs. Access to health care in rural communities is impeded by poverty, inadequate transportation, large geographical distances, an aging population base, and rural economic decline (Orloff, Tymann, 1995, p. vii). Community health nurses have historically provided services to rural communities.

table 3-1 States with More Than 50% of Their Population Residing in Rural Areas*

State	Percentage of Population Residing in Rural Areas
Alaska	57.6%
Arkansas	60.5%
Idaho	80.4%
Iowa	54.2%
Kentucky	54.2%
Maine	63.9%
Mississippi	69.7%
Montana	75.8%
Nebraska	52.8%
New Mexico	51.6%
North Dakota	62.0%
South Dakota	71.3%
Vermont	76.9%
West Virginia	63.7%
Wyoming	71.0%

From Office of Technology Assessment (Congress of the United States): *Health care in rural America*, Washington, D.C., 1990, The Office, p. 39.
*Note: Kansas, New Hampshire, North Carolina, and Oklahoma have 40% or more of their population residing in rural areas.

What Is a Rural Community?

There is lack of consensus on how to define a rural community. Most frequently, communities are defined as rural based on population. A rural community is frequently defined as a community of less than 2500 residents. Recently the term "frontier" has been used to describe select rural communities with a population density of less than 6 people per square mile, as compared to between 6 to 100 per square mile for a rural community (Lee, 1991, pp. 10-11). Within rural communities, frontier communities have their own unique set of health needs and concerns.

Of the four major regions of the country, the South has the highest proportion of its population living in rural areas. Across the nation, 77% of counties are considered nonmetropolitan (Weinert, Burman, 1994, p. 66). States where 50% or more of the population is considered rural are listed in Table 3-1.

In the early 1800s approximately 90% of the U.S. population was rural; at the turn of the century that changed to about 60%, and today the rural population is about 27% (approximately 64 million) (Office of Technology Assessment, 1990, p. 38). Interestingly, nearly 15,000 towns have

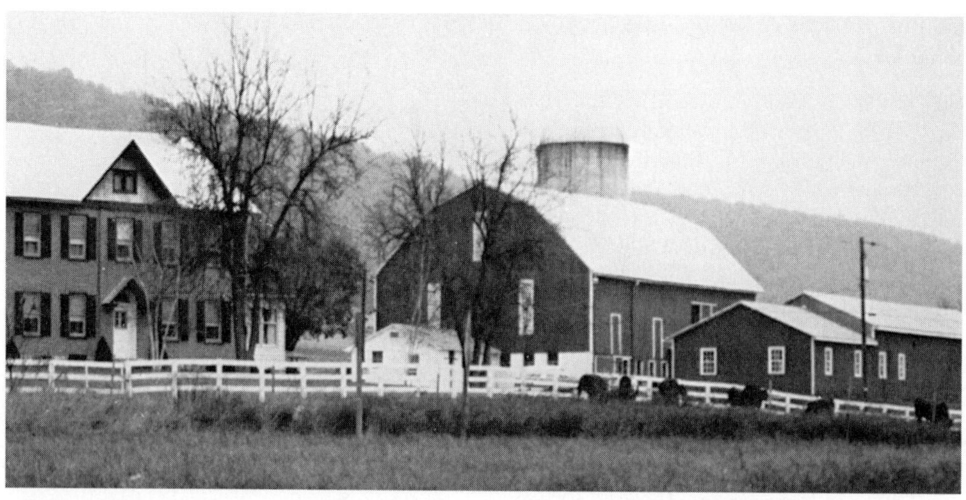

Figure 3-4 Some 64 million Americans live in rural communities. Residents in rural settings are regularly exposed to environmental hazards such as pesticides, water pollution, soil pollution, and toxic chemicals. Many rural Americans lack access to regular and emergency health care services. The shortage of health care in rural communities presents serious problems for many rural Americans, and public health efforts need to be strengthened in these communities. *(Courtesy Henry Parks.)*

a population of less than 2500 (Weinert, Burman, 1994, p. 66) (see Figure 3-4).

Rural communities are often described in terms of their major economic activity or focus, including farming, manufacturing, mining, government (e.g., military bases), federal lands, and retirement. The health status of a rural community is often directly related to the primary economic resource of the region (Bushy, 1991a, p. 133).

Health and the Rural Community

Nurses can be proud that they have played a major role in providing primary health care to rural families and communities (Bushy, 1990, p. 34). Mary Breckinridge, a nurse and midwife, founded the Frontier Nursing Service in rural Kentucky, and it is still operating today. Lillian Wald was one of the first to advocate for rural health services. In 1915 Wald wrote:

> In 1908 I began to urge that in a country dedicated to peace it would be fitting for the American Red Cross to consecrate its efforts to the upbuilding of life and the prevention of disaster . . . The concrete recommendation made was that the Red Cross should develop a system of visiting nursing in the vast, neglected country areas. This suggestion has been adopted and an excellent beginning made with a Department of Town and Country Nursing directed by a special Committee (p. 61).

The American Red Cross Rural Nursing Service was formally established in 1912, and the name was changed to Town and Country Nursing Service the following year (see Chapter 1). Wald's vision was that rural nursing services would become available across the nation. Although this vision was not actualized, the organized provision of rural nursing in the United States had been initiated. Today an awareness of populations at risk and the characteristics of rural communities assist the community health nurse in developing community partnerships for health and providing effective nursing services. The following discussion examines selected rural health statistics and needs.

SOCIOCULTURAL CHARACTERISTICS Rural communities differ from urban ones in a number of sociocultural characteristics, and researchers have consistently supported the existence of a unique rural culture (Bushy, 1991a, p. 134). A major characteristic of rural America is its social and economic diversity (Federal Office of Rural Health Policy [FORHP], 1993). In general, rural communities have fewer minority residents, lower incomes, poorer health, less education, and higher percentages of elderly people than their urban counterparts (Office of Technology Assessment [OTA], 1995, pp. 2, 40). Values prevalent in rural Americans are achievement, activity and work, traditional moral values and role orientation, group conformity, conservative political viewpoints, and a more religious nature (Lee, 1991, p. 15). Rural communities are generally slower than urban communities to change traditional values and attitudes (Bushy, 1991a, p. 134). Research has demonstrated that rural residents have greater resistance to outsiders and prefer to interact with people they know who are similar to themselves (Bushy, p. 136). Rural communities have higher rates of households of children living with both parents and have fewer households headed by women (OTA, 1990, p. 40).

Fewer minority Americans reside in rural areas than in urban areas, and 98% of rural residents are native born (OTA, 1990, p. 40). Exceptions to this minority status include communities with migrant farm workers and Native

Americans. In general, rural minorities are poorer than the rest of the rural population.

Rural communities are often more closely knit than urban communities and have stronger patterns of communication within the community. In contrast, urban communities are often known for the isolation that is evident when people living next to each other do not even know one another's names. Rural residents are more familiar with local government and leadership than their urban counterparts.

PERCEIVED HEALTH STATUS AND PRACTICES Research has shown that rural residents generally define health as the ability to work and to do what needs to be done (Long, 1993; Long, Weinert, 1989; Weinert, Burman, 1994; Weinert, Long, 1987). Such health beliefs are a determinant of health perception and health-seeking behaviors (Bushy, 1991a, p. 135).

Rural dwellers are more independent and self-reliant and resist accepting help or services, especially from those seen as "outsiders" or from agencies seen as national or regional "welfare" programs (Long, Weinert, 1989, p. 121). This self-reliance may delay them from seeking care until they are gravely ill (Weinert, Burman, 1994). The nurse "can anticipate greater acceptance and use by rural residents of an updated but old and trusted health care resource, rather than a new, professional, but 'outsider' service" (Long, Weinert, 1989, p. 124).

Health status indicators are often not favorable. Rural residents are less likely to use seatbelts regularly (resulting in higher motor vehicle fatality rates), less likely to exercise regularly, more likely to be obese, and less likely to use preventive screening services (OTA, 1990, p. 43). Public health problems such as AIDS, homelessness, mental illness, and family violence are evident in rural communities. However, rural communities often have fewer resources available to work with such conditions, and the more traditional value systems of the rural community can affect service provision to these aggregates at risk.

Little research has been done on the health of rural children and adolescents. Research has shown that children in rural areas have a higher rate of immunization than urban children (OTA, 1990, p. 43). Infant mortality rates are higher in rural areas than in urban. Each year almost 300 children die and another 23,500 are injured in farm-related accidents (FORHP, 1993).

Research on the prevalence of mental disorder in rural areas has largely been limited to looking at depression (Weinert, Burman, 1994, p. 74). This research has been inclusive and further research is needed. Rural Americans are more likely than their urban counterparts to use their primary health care provider for mental health as well as physical health care (Weinert, Long, 1990, p. 70). When they seek mental health therapy they are frequently only available for short-term therapy because of limited finances and work and distance constraints (Weinert, Long, p. 70).

Some Facts and Figures on Rural Communities

64 million Americans are living in rural areas—approximately one fourth of the U.S. population.

One in five rural Americans lives in poverty (of these, nearly 5 million are children).

The South has the highest proportion of its population living in rural areas, and in 15 states 50% or more of the population live in rural areas.

Fewer minority Americans reside in rural areas, and 98% of rural residents are native born.

Rural America is aging faster than America in general. Although the elderly account for 12% of the U.S. population as a whole, they account for 25.4% of the rural population.

More than 22 million rural Americans live in federally designated "Health Professions Shortage Areas."

Almost 8 million rural Americans have no health insurance, and another 4.5 million are underinsured.

Alcohol is by far the most widely abused drug in rural areas. Alcohol usage by rural children is increasing, and one third of rural children have had their first drink by the age of 10.

Alcohol treatment and arrest rates are higher in rural areas than in nonrural areas.

Data from USDHHS: *Prevention resource guide: rural communities*, Rockville, Md., 1991, USDHHS; Office of Technology Assessment, Congress of the United States: *Health care in rural America*, Washington, D.C., 1990, The Office; Federal Office of Rural Health Policy: *On creating a composite statistical picture of rural America*, Washington, D.C., 1993, U.S. Government Printing Office.

SUPPORT SYSTEMS Findings from several studies have indicated that rural persons prefer to use informal sources (e.g., family, neighbors, friends) for help and support in dealing with health problems rather than formal sources (e.g., hospitals or clinics) (Long, Weinert, 1989, p. 121). Even when they live at a great distance, family, neighbors, and friends are frequently relied on to assist with both diagnosing and treating health problems (Weinert, Long, 1993, p. 53; Weinert, Burman, 1994, p. 76). Formal health care providers are not trusted and are viewed as outsiders. Rural residents will often prefer the "old doc" whom they know over the new specialist who is unfamiliar (Long, Weinert, 1989, p. 121).

HEALTH DISPARITIES Rural residents have higher rates of long-term illness, disability, injury-related mortality, and fetal, infant, and maternal mortality than their urban counterparts (Goeppinger, 1993, p. 1; OTA, 1990, pp. 5-6; Weinert, Burman, 1994, p. 72; Weinert, Long, 1993, p. 47). The accompanying boxes give some interesting facts and figures on health in rural communities and resources for information on rural health.

The incidence of back problems is significantly higher in rural populations than in others (Weinert, Burman,

Rural Health Information Resources

National Rural Health Association
One West Armour Boulevard, Suite 301
Kansas City, MO 64111

Rural Information Center
U.S. Department of Agriculture
National Agricultural Library, Room 304
10301 Baltimore Boulevard
Beltsville, MD 20705-2351
1-800-633-7701

Office of Rural Health Policy
U.S. Department of Health and Human Services
5600 Fishers Lane, Room 14-22
Rockville, MD 20857

National Association for Rural Mental Health
P.O. Box 570
Wood River, IL 62095

National Rural Institute on Alcohol and Drug Abuse
University of Wisconsin, Eau Claire
Eau Claire, WI 54702-4004

Federal Programs to Enhance Rural Health Resources

National Health Service Corps provides placement services, scholarships, and educational loan repayment for physicians and other health professionals willing to serve in designated rural areas. It also provides grants to schools educating and training primary health care providers such as family practitioners and nurse practitioners.

Federal Area Health Education Centers Program links medical centers with rural practice sites to provide educational services and rural clinical experiences to students, faculty, and practitioners in a variety of health professions.

Community and Migrant Health Centers Grant Program promotes primary health care facilities in rural areas.

Rural Health Care Transition Grant Program provides grants to small rural hospitals for strategic planning and service enhancement.

From Office of Technology Assessment, Congress of the United States: *Health care in rural America*, Washington, D.C., 1990, The Office, p. 9.

1994, p. 72). Agricultural workers have some of the highest rates of occupational illness, injury, disability, and death in the nation. Rural communities have a higher rate of many communicable diseases than the general population (e.g., intestinal parasite diseases, tuberculosis, influenza, and pneumonia) but a lower rate of AIDS (Weinert, Burman, p. 72).

Rural residents consistently rate their physical health to be poorer than their urban counterparts (OTA, 1990). However, they rate their social health as stronger (Weinert, Burman, 1994, p. 68).

Alcohol and drug use in rural communities is on the rise. A study showed that almost 60% of a sample of rural sixth and seventh graders reported using alcohol (Long, Boik, 1993), and alcohol use in rural adolescents was significantly correlated with cigarette smoking (Sarvela, McClendon, 1987; Weinert, Burman, 1994, p. 73).

Fetal, infant, and maternal mortality rates are all higher in rural than urban areas (OTA, 1990, pp. 25-26). Contributing to these rates is the limited availability of obstetrical services and primary care providers in rural areas and the lower socioeconomic status and lack of medical insurance among rural residents.

ACCESS TO HEALTH CARE Access to services is a major problem for rural Americans. Distance from health care resources, lack of transportation, lack of health insurance, lack of primary care resources, and work schedules all contribute to this situation (Strategies, 1996, p. 101; Weinert, Long, 1993, p. 47). Also, an attitude of self-reliance, the rural work ethic, and lower literacy levels contribute to lower utilization of available health care resources (Bushy, 1991a, p. 137).

Interestingly, access barriers are generally not identified by rural families as a major deterrent to seeking primary health care (Bushy, 1991a, p. 136). Instead, rural families cite the fear of receiving insensitive treatment and fear that others may find out about the family's use of services as deterrents to using health services (Bushy, pp. 136-137).

Access to emergency medical services (EMS) for rural areas is becoming an increasing problem. It is difficult to deliver EMS to widely dispersed populations quickly, efficiently, and cost effectively. There are often shortages of EMS personnel in rural areas. Rural ambulance services find they cannot support themselves financially.

HEALTH CARE RESOURCES States rely heavily on the federal government for assistance in maintaining and expanding rural health resources (OTA, 1990, p. 9). Medicare and Medicaid dollars fund many rural health services. Selected federal programs to enhance rural health resources are noted in the box above. Some states are creating Offices of Rural Health to better provide for the health of their rural residents.

The number of rural hospitals declined 12% between 1980 and 1990 and this number is still declining (AHA study, 1990, p. 3). Many rural hospitals closed due to a shortage of registered nurses (Wakefield, 1990, p. 86). Rural areas rely heavily on satellite clinics, often offered through hospitals or health departments, to provide primary health care to residents. With scarce resources, some rural communities are networking with each other to provide health care services and health education programs (Hemman, McClendon, Lightfoot, 1995, p. 170).

Rural residents often have great distances to travel to access health care. Almost half of all rural counties in the United States do not have a public transportation system (FORHP, 1993). Also, poor roads in rural areas can increase the time it takes to travel to health care facilities.

HEALTH CARE PROVIDERS Getting health care providers to practice in rural settings has been difficult. More than 22 million rural Americans live in federally designated "Health Professions Shortage Areas," or areas that have a primary care provider-to-patient ratio of 1 to 3500 or worse—this involves more than 1800 underserved rural communities (FORHP, 1993). Rural areas have approximately one half the physicians that urban areas do, and many rural doctors are expected to retire or leave their practices in the near future (Wakefield, 1990, p. 87).

Additionally, shortages in public health professionals, psychologists, physical therapists, speech therapists, rehabilitation specialists, social workers, and other health care providers are drastically affecting the quality of health care available to rural communities. There are estimated shortages of at least 45,000 registered nurses, 1200 psychiatrists, and nearly 1000 dentists in rural areas (FORHP, 1993). Also, health care providers often do not receive much formal education on rural health.

AGING OF RURAL AMERICA Rural America is "aging" faster than America in general. Although the elderly account for 12% of the U.S. population as a whole, they account for 25.4% of the rural population (Wakefield, 1990, p. 85). Rural elderly have higher rates of poverty and report significantly poorer health than do their urban counterparts (Eggebeen, Lichter, 1993, p. 94).

ECONOMICS AND HEALTH The last two decades have witnessed rural economic decline and resulting concerns in the viability of the rural health care system. There is a higher incidence of poverty in rural populations, and one in five rural Americans lives in poverty (Wakefield, 1990, p. 85). Nearly 5 million rural children live in poverty (Vulnerable populations, 1991, p. 128). The rate of poverty in rural America is the highest it has been in nearly 20 years (Vulnerable populations, p. 128). The average rural family has a median income close to $10,000 less a year than an urban family (OTA, 1990, p. 40).

Economic barriers prevent many rural residents from receiving adequate health care. Almost 8 million rural Americans have no health insurance, and another 4.5 million are underinsured (FORHP, 1993). There are few large businesses and more small family businesses in rural areas. Urban communities tend to have more diverse economic activity than rural areas.

Nursing and the Rural Community

Nurses are frequently the sole health care provider for people living in rural areas, yet little has been written to guide their practice, and there is a lack of rural nursing research and theory (Long, Weinert, 1989, p. 113; Weinert, Long, 1991, p. 24). The health care needs of rural populations cannot be adequately met through the use of existing nursing models (Long, Weinert, 1989, p. 113). Research and literature on rural nursing is beginning to emerge. Bushy (1991) has edited a two-volume book, *Rural Nursing*, and Weinert and Long (1987, 1990, 1991) are developing a theoretical framework for rural nursing (see the box above).

As with other health care providers in rural areas, nurses must deal with a lack of anonymity and much greater role diffusion (needing to be a "jack of all trades") than providers in urban settings (Long, Weinert, 1989, p. 123). Rural nurses often see themselves as isolated from the professional mainstream and distanced from collegial support (Davis, Droes, 1993, p. 160; Long, Weinert, 1989, p. 124).

To develop nursing interventions for rural families there needs to be a better understanding of the support network (Weinert, Long, 1993, p. 47). Rural families can participate in and benefit from thoughtful assessment and collaboratively planned strategies to address their needs. According to Weinert and Long, "The establishment of trust, based on consistency, longevity of relationship, and sincere effort to

Rural Health Nursing Theory: Weinert and Long

KEY RURAL CONCEPTS IDENTIFIED

Work and health beliefs
Isolation and distance
Independence and self-reliance
Lack of anonymity
Outsider/insider
Oldtimer/newcomers

INITIAL RELATIONAL STATEMENTS

Rural dwellers define health primarily as the ability to work, to be productive, and to do usual tasks.

Rural dwellers are self-reliant and resist accepting help from those viewed as outsiders. Help, including health care, is usually sought through an informal rather than a formal system.

Health care providers in rural areas must deal with a lack of anonymity and much greater role diffusion than providers in urban or suburban settings.

From Long K, Weinert C: Rural nursing: developing the theory base, *Schol Inq Nurs Prac* 3(2):113-127, 1989; Weinert C, Long K: Understanding the health care needs of rural families, *Family Relations* 36:450-455, 1987; Weinert C, Long K: Rural families and health care: refining the knowledge base, *J Marriage Fam Rev* 15 (1):57-75, 1990; and Weinert C, Long K: The theory and research base for rural nursing practice. In Bushy A, ed: *Rural nursing*, vol 1), Newbury Park, Ca., 1991, Sage; as cited in Weinert C, Burman ME: Rural health and health-seeking behaviors. In Fitzpatrick JJ, Stevenson JS, eds: *Annual Review of Nursing Research*, vol 12, New York, 1994, Springer, p. 82.

understand and appreciate the specific rural culture is an essential first step in implementing interventions with rural families" (p. 53).

Long and Weinert (1989) have also noted that "nurses who enter rural communities must allow for extended periods prior to being accepted. Involvement in diverse community activities such as civic organizations and recreational clubs may assist the nurse in being known and accepted as a person. In rural communities acceptance as a health care professional is often tied to personal acceptance. Rural communities are not appropriate practice settings for nurses who prefer to maintain entirely separate professional and personal lives" (p. 124).

Nurses must rise to the challenge of adapting community-based health care to rural areas. This involves a blending of the formal network with the existing informal system, since rural residents are unlikely to use a new, more formal health care service in place of an established informal resource (Weinert, Long, 1990, p. 65). Nurses in rural areas should focus on establishing collaborative relationships with community leaders and work in partnership with these leaders. Mutual respect between local leaders and health care professionals is necessary (Weinert, Long, p. 65).

Nurses can help to provide rural populations with the information necessary to make appropriate decisions about self-care and health care. Nurses can provide instruction, support, and relief to family members and neighbors, who are often the primary care providers for the sick.

To function in rural settings the nurse needs to be a generalist but understand change theory and leadership techniques. The rural nurse must also understand techniques for accessing diverse information and networks (Long, Weinert, 1989, p. 125).

Future Directions for Rural Health

New and innovative ways need to be developed to bring health care to rural Americans and improve their access to health care. Nurse practitioners have played a unique role in provision of rural health services through independent practice and working with rural health centers. However, more health care professionals are needed to practice in rural communities.

An expanded knowledge and theory base for rural nursing practice needs to be developed (Bushy, 1991b, p. 304). A priority for nurse researchers is the development of rural nursing theory and a knowledge base relevant to the health care needs of rural populations (Weinert, Burman, 1994, p. 84). Recent federal initiatives have facilitated rural health and rural nursing research. The Agency for Health Care Policy and Research (AHCPR) has initiated a rural health research agenda that encourages research in areas such as access to services, supply of health professionals, health care delivery, primary health care, health promotion and disease prevention, technology, and services to special rural populations (e.g., minorities, the elderly, persons living in poverty, persons with HIV/AIDS, the homeless, children, and pregnant women) (AHCPR). AHCPR and the National Institute for Nursing Research jointly invite applications for research grants to study ways of improving the health and well-being of vulnerable populations living in rural areas.

It has been proposed by some that rural nursing become a specialty area within community health nursing, and this may happen in the future. Currently, challenging opportunities exist in the rural practice setting. Community and migrant health centers (see Chapter 22) are bringing primary care services to numerous underserved populations. Mobile clinics are delivering care to remote areas with significant success. Innovation in service delivery is being encouraged through federal grants to rural communities and has resulted in highly successful outreach programs. Nurses are bringing services to the home, schools, worksites, and other community-based settings in rural communities around the world (Randall, 1995).

INTERNATIONAL COMMUNITIES

International health is everyone's concern, and nurses are involved in numerous international health activities. As an outcome, international health can be viewed in terms of worldwide morbidity and mortality. As a process, people, organizations, technology, and resources work together to promote international health. Morbidity and mortality are important indicators of world health and differ greatly among nations. Some diseases are endemic in one country and epidemic in another (see definitions in Chapter 11). Worldwide the incidence of tuberculosis, AIDS, malaria, and waterborne diseases is increasing, and developing nations have much different health problems than developed nations. Examining international health statistics provides information about health status and trends in the world and the United States and assists in developing strategies to promote world health (see information on international health in Chapters 11 and 15).

It is a small world after all, and we must preserve the environment and protect the world from threats to health. In terms of impact, diseases and conditions such as pollution and water shortages in one country can readily affect other countries. For example, ozone depletion and the polluting of the air and seas contribute to the destruction of the global environment (see Chapter 6). The impact of disease transmission, as exemplified with the worldwide AIDS epidemic, has helped people to understand that one nation cannot afford to look at health conditions as other people's problems—they are our problems too.

Numerous agencies discussed in this text have an international health role. The Centers for Disease Control and Prevention (CDC), the World Health Organization, the United Nations Children's Fund (UNICEF), and the American Public Health Association (APHA) are discussed in Chapter 5, and the American Red Cross is discussed

A View *from the* Field — A TOWN IN BRAZIL

by Barbara Young

With less than two years' experience of field public health nursing in the inner cities of Columbus and Dayton, Ohio, I was assigned the position of head nurse for a federal health post in the southern part of the state of Bahia in Brazil. The town where I would spend over two years, Ibicarai, had a population of 20,000 inhabitants, mostly poor. There was also a small upper class comprised of professionals and merchants. The middle class was almost nonexistent. The lower class were those who worked on the cacao plantations or did menial and domestic work. The major ethnic makeup of Ibicarai was a blend of the descendants of the original Tupi-Guandani Indian, Portuguese, and African. Lebanese and Syrians made up a small minority.

My home was of white stucco-type construction. Mud was packed between a lattice of upright sticks. White coating was painted over the dried mud. The floors were packed clay. My water source was a well in the back yard. The wood shack outhouse was "out Back" and consisted of a raised platform with a hole in it. Time magazine was my favorite toilet paper because it was softer than the local variety. Cooking was done on my built-in charcoal stove. Refrigerators only existed at the local "vendas" where you could buy cold beer. Refrigerators were the status symbol. I had no such status. I learned that fresh meats should be purchased early in the morning and added to the daily black bean pot if you had fresh meat at all.

The federal public health post to which I was assigned stood in the center of town. Each weekday, the people would walk into town from the five surrounding barros (neighborhoods), and I would assist with triage at the front door of the clinic. Those most in need were seen first. These were usually sick babies. Some less acute patients were told to return the next day. It was always difficult for me to see those patients who were turned away because I knew they had to walk miles to get to the clinic. My assignment included the supervision of four visitadoras (visiting nurses) and three attendants (aides to the clinic). I communicated in Portuguese, assisted with the triage, supervised the intravenous medications, supervised the local midwives and, generally, made this a healthier community!

The public health issues of this community were enormous. There were shoeless children with bloated abdomens. Although women enjoyed their social time together as they washed clothes against rocks in the river that ran through town, the river played a role in the life cycle of the schistosome, the parasite causing schistosomiasis.

Family planning existed only for the rich who could afford to purchase "the pill" at the local pharmacy. The local bishop, the fifteenth child in a large family, prohibited me from responding to requests for family planning. A woman in a distant barro died of tetanus poisoning after childbirth. In another barro, a woman died of placenta previa, partially because the nearest hospital was an hour away. My neighbor across the street swallowed her wedding band in a misguided attempt to abort an unwanted pregnancy. The local daily diet consisted mainly of black beans, rice, and farina, a grainy substance of little nutritive value. Tropical fruits were abundant. Only wealthier families could add meat and vegetables to the bean pot.

How could one American public health nurse make a difference? It seemed overwhelming. Clearly, any change in this scene would take a great deal of time. It would take the commitment of many people. It would involve the education of the population. It would include the political leaders. Where would I begin?

The midwives came to the health post to receive free supplies. We scheduled their visit for supplies to coincide with a "refresher" class. I went with the visitadoras to walk to distant barros to visit new mothers. We talked of nutrition. We encouraged the consumption of tropical fruits and vegetables rich in vitamins. Although I felt these visits were useful, I was obsessed with a concern about the contaminated river. The river, which ran behind the poorest homes, was used for washing family clothes and dishes. Women needed the social interaction with friends, but they did not need schistosomiasis and the resultant liver disease.

Luiz, a young man with a fifth-grade school education, came to our home one evening. He was an organizer. If we could help him and teach him what to do, he would help set up a literacy program. His participation provided the opportunity to use the rather radical teaching method of the exiled Brazilian Secretary of Education, Paulo Friere: "Train the Trainer." We began by teaching Luiz. He then taught ten young women who had graduated from high school. With the mayor's backing, we set up classes all over the city. The plantation workers came to class in their cleanly pressed clothes after a day in cacao groves. I remember one class including the following: "panela (pan). A utensil used to boil water to prevent disease." In this way, the teachers introduced health principles along with the literacy.

Two days after Christmas, hard rains began. The river rose and topped the bridge from the camp. Water cov-

From Zerwekh J, Young B, Primono J, Deal L, eds: *Opening doors: stories of public health nursing*, Olympia, Wa., 1992, Washington State Department of Health, pp. 131-135. Used with permission.

Continued

A View from the Field: A TOWN IN BRAZIL—cont'd

ered the roads and isolated the town. I was told that this was the "20-year flood waters." Twenty percent of the town's houses, particularly those belonging to the poor who lived along the river, were washed away or severely damaged. Families took refuge in church and school buildings. The three Italian Sisters of Charity and I collaborated to make visits to the homeless families. We obtained medical help when needed. We worked with city officials to avoid the possibility of a typhoid outbreak. Immunizations were given. Then we began to plan for the rebuilding.

Two and one-half years after I arrived in the town, it was time to prepare to leave. Peace Corp volunteers met in Rio de Janerio for a debriefing from the state department and we wanted to know, before we returned to the United States, how we would know if our presence had made a difference? The reply from the state department official was this: "You may never know, but twenty years from now, someone may cast an important vote due to your work here. You must believe that your work here has made a difference."

It was almost twenty years later that I decided to return to Ibicarai. When I drove into town with Luiz as my guide, we first went to the barro where Luiz had lived. The streets were paved. Street lighting was provided by a rural electrification project. His mother's home had running water from a city water system. A Coca-Cola bottling plant on the outskirts of the barro provided jobs. Close to the town there was a beautiful new bus station with bright yellow Mercedes buses proudly moving in and out of stalls. An attractive woman in an orange attendant's dress saw me from across the lobby.

"Are you Dona Barbara?"

"Yes," I said, feeling a lump in my throat.

Tearfully hugging me, she said, "I prayed that you would return some day."

in Chapter 6. The APHA publication *Control of Communicable Diseases Manual*, now in its 16th edition, is the classic text on the world's communicable diseases and should be part of every community health nurse's library.

Nursing and International Health

Lillian Wald and the Henry Street Settlement Nurses worked with U.S. immigrants in New York City to promote health. They realized the importance of looking at culture in relation to health practices and beliefs and strove to provide culturally sensitive care. Today nursing organizations such as the International Council of Nurses (ICN), the Transcultural Nursing Society, Sigma Theta Tau, the American Nurses Association (ANA), and the National League for Nursing (NLN) all recognize the importance of international health and offer a variety of publications and services in the area. In its position statement on cultural diversity in nursing practice the ANA (1996) states, "Ethnocentric approaches to nursing practice are ineffective in meeting health and nursing needs of diverse cultural groups of clients. Knowledge about cultures and their impact on interactions with health care is essential for nurses in a clinical setting, education, research or administration" (p. 89).

Nurses need to be concerned about world health and involved in international health activities. The experience of one international nurse is given in the View from the Field. This nurse's story illustrates the contributions nurses can make worldwide. Nurses must understand and value diversity and promote world health. In today's world people are all inextricably linked.

COMMUNITY ASSESSMENT

The community health nurse is in the unique position of working with the community on a day-to-day basis. The nurse provides services in homes, schools, clinics, industry, and other settings and has multiple opportunities to collect community health data and to comprehensively assess the community. Chapter 13 addresses the community assessment process, and community assessment is briefly addressed here in relation to assisting the nurse in conceptualizing both the community as client and as partner.

The Committee for the Study of the Future of Public Health (Institute of Medicine, 1988, p. 7) recommended that every public health agency regularly and systematically collect, assemble, analyze, and make available information on the health of the community. In community health partnerships assessment data is gathered as a collaborative effort. A community assessment provides a "window" through which to view the community. It provides the means for looking at community strengths, problems, and potential problems. It can identify aggregates at risk and gaps in community resources. It is the basis for community health planning and service provision.

It can be difficult for both neophytes and experienced professionals to collect all of the data that must be obtained when doing a community assessment. Community assessment tools can help professionals to collect and organize community data. Stein and Eigsti (1982) have developed a tool to assist the practitioner in doing an initial, brief community assessment. This tool is based on a set of master categories that characterize community data. It provides observational information about a community's environment, mode of functioning, and social and health resources. Because community health nurses collect these data while driving through or walking around in a community, this form of community assessment has been termed a "windshield" survey of the community. A windshield assessment provides a beginning database about a community.

Community assessment tools will vary in their comprehensiveness. An in-depth comprehensive assessment tool that assists health agencies to obtain a comprehensive profile of a community is presented in Appendix 13-1. Other community assessment tools and frameworks from which nurses can assess the community are found in Allor (1983), Anderson and McFarlane (1996), Caretto and McCormick (1991), Clark (1986), Edelman and Mandle (1990), Hanchett (1988), Martin (1988), Meneshian (1988), Rauckhorst, Stokes, and Mezey (1980), Rodgers (1984), and Ruffing-Rahal (1987). White and Valentine (1993) developed an innovative computer-assisted video instructional program for community assessment. Through knowledge gained from a community assessment, the community health nurse has a database for community diagnosis and health planning (see Chapters 13 and 14).

Illustrative of how community assessment can assist in health planning was a project conducted by a local health department in a rural community. A group of community health nurses carried out a community assessment of their rural county. The nurses found that a major health problem was traffic deaths among males 16 to 24 years of age; the death rates for this age group were significantly higher than the expected death rates for the age group. After careful data analysis, factors contributing to this were determined to be narrow, winding, two-lane roads with no shoulders; an image among the young rural males that fast cars were "macho"; no recreational facilities except bars; unlighted roads; and the necessity of driving very long distances to employment sites. These data pointed out the urgent need for a traffic safety program, which was initiated in the local high school.

Community assessments can help communities determine community strengths and resources, and provide direction for the community in relation to health (Sasenick, 1994, p. 56). Community assessment assists in seeing the links among primary health care, health and social service programs, and the health and welfare needs of the community (White, Valentine, 1993, p. 349). Community assessment processes can help communities across our nation to identify and address disparities in service delivery.

Summary

The community is the client for the community health nurse. Each community is unique and has its own health care needs. Developing a conceptual understanding of the word *community*, community dynamics, and how health problems are assessed and solved within the community are crucial in caring for the community. Nurses work in partnership with diverse communities to promote health. Today communities across the country are putting health on their agendas and working to build healthier communities. Nurses gather information about the communities in which they work, they "assess" the community to identify health problems and needed resources, and they build on community strengths to promote health action.

Working with individuals, families, and aggregates at risk becomes far more exciting when the community health nurse understands community concepts. This knowledge, coupled with flexibility in meeting the changing and diverse health needs of the community, facilitates the achievement of healthy communities.

CRITICAL *Thinking Exercise*

Look at the beginning of the chapter where the term *community* was defined and discussed. Conceptualize in your mind the community you lived in during high school or the community you live in now. Look at this community in terms of some of the major components of community dynamics, such as service systems, communication patterns, leadership, and community functions. What were some of the major values held by this community? What were/are some of the major strengths of this community? What were some of the health needs of this community? How could a nurse work collaboratively with a community to build on these strengths and facilitate community empowerment?

REFERENCES

Agency for Health Care Policy and Research (AHCPR): *Health services research on rural health: grant announcement*, Rockville, Md., 1994, AHCPR.

AHA study reports changes, trends in 1980s, *Reflections* 16(2):3, 1990.

Allor MT: The "community profile," *J Nurs Educ* 22:12-17, 1983.

American Nurses Association (ANA), Community Health Nursing Division: *Conceptual model of community health nursing*, Pub No CH-10, Kansas City, Mo., 1980, The Association.

American Nurses Association (ANA): *Standards of community health nursing practice*, St. Louis, 1986, ANA.

American Nurses Association (ANA): *American Nurses Association position statement on cultural diversity in nursing practice*, Washington, D.C., 1996, ANA.

American Public Health Association (APHA): *Healthy communities 2000: model standards. Guidelines for implementing the year 2000 national health objectives*, Washington, D.C., 1991, The Association.

Anderson ET, McFarlane JM: *Community-as-partner: theory and practice in nursing*, Philadelphia, 1996, Lippincott.

Arensburg CM, Kimball ST: *Culture and community*, Gloucester, Ma., 1972, Peter Smith.

Bushy A: Rural determinants in family health: considerations for community nurses, *Fam Comm Health* 12(4):29-38, 1990.

Bushy A, ed: *Rural nursing*, vols 1 & 2, Newbury Park, Ca., 1991, Sage.

Bushy A: Rural determinants in family health: considerations for community nurses. In Bushy A, ed: *Rural nursing*, vol 1, Newbury Park, Ca., 1991a, Sage, pp. 133-145.

Bushy A: Meeting the challenges of rural nursing research. In Bushy A, ed: *Rural nursing*, vol 2, Newbury Park, Ca., 1991b, Sage, pp. 304-318.

Caretto VA, McCormick CS: Community as client: a "hands-on" experience for baccalaureate nursing students, *J Comm Health Nurs* 8(3):179-189, 1991.

Chamberlain RW: *Beyond individual risk assessment: community-wide approaches to promoting the health and development of families and children—conference proceedings*, Washington, D.C., 1988, National Center for Education in Maternal and Child Health

Christianson JZ: *A community data base record,* unpublished Master of Public Health thesis, Houston, Tx., 1977, University of Texas Health Science Center.

Clark CC: *Wellness nursing: concepts, theory, research and practice*, New York, 1986, Springer, pp. 287-290.

Courtney R: Community partnership primary care: a new paradigm for primary care, *Public Health Nurs* 12:366-373, 1995.

Courtney R, Ballard F, Fauver S et al: The partnership model: working with individuals, families, and communities toward a new vision of health, *Public Health Nurs* 13:177-186, 1996.

Davis DJ, Droes NS: Community health nursing in rural and frontier counties, *Nurs Clin North Am* 28(1):159-169, 1993.

Edelman CL, Mandle CL: *Health promotion throughout the lifespan*, ed 2, St. Louis, 1990, Mosby, pp. 139-143.

Eggebeen DJ, Lichter DT: Health and well-being among rural Americans: variations across the lifecourse, *J Rural Health* 9(2):86-98, 1993.

Eisen A: A survey of neighborhood-based, comprehensive community empowerment initiatives, *Health Educ Q* 21(2):235-252, 1994.

Erikson EH: *Childhood and society*, ed 2, New York, 1978, Norton.

Federal Office of Rural Health Policy (FORHP): *On creating a composite statistical picture of rural America*. Washington, D.C., 1993, U.S. Government Printing Office.

Fitzpatrick JJ, Stevenson JS, eds: *Annual review of nursing research*, vol 12, New York, 1994, Springer.

Flynn BC: Healthy cities: the future of public health. Restructuring how we live, *Health Care Trends Transit* 4(3):12-18, 80, 1993.

Flynn BC: Partnerships for health, *Health Care Forum J* 37(3):55-56, 73, 1994.

Flynn BC: Healthy Cities: building partnerships for healthy public policy, *Nurs Policy Forum* 1(6):6-9, 20-25, 1995.

Flynn BC, Rains JW: Establishing community coalitions for prevention: health cities Indiana. In Knollmueller RN, ed: *Prevention across the lifespan: healthy people for the 21st century*. Washington, D.C., 1993, American Nurses Association, pp. 21-30.

Flynn BC, Ray DW, Rider MS: Empowering communities: action research through healthy cities, *Health Educ Q* 21(3):395-405, 1994.

Goeppinger J: Health promotion for rural populations: partnership interventions, *Comm Health* 16(1):1-10, 1993.

Goeppinger J, Shuster G: Community as client: using the nursing process to promote health. In Stanhope M, Lancester J, eds: *Community health nursing*, ed 2, St Louis, 1988, Mosby.

Green LW, Kreuter MW: CDC's planned approach to community health as an application of PRECEED and an inspiration for PROCEED, *J Health Educ* 23(3):140-147, 1992.

Hanchett ES: *Nursing frameworks and community as client*, Norwalk, Ct., 1988, Appleton & Lange.

Hancock T: Healthy Cities: the Canadian project, *Health Promotion* 26(2):2-4, 27, 1987.

Hemman EA, McClendon BJ, Lightfoot SF: Networking for educational resources in a rural community, *J Contin Educ Nurs* 26(4):170-173, 1995.

Higgs ZR, Gustafson DD: *Community as client: assessment and diagnosis*, Philadelphia, 1985, FA Davis.

Hillery GA Jr: Definitions of community: areas of agreement, *Rural Sociol* 20(2):118-120, 1955.

Institute of Medicine: *The future of public health,* Washington, D.C., 1988, National Academy Press.

International Council of Nurses: Cities in distress: a rescue strategy, *Int Nurs Rev* 38(4):105-117, 1991.

Israel BA, Checkoway B, Schulz A, Zimmerman M: Health education and community empowerment: conceptualizing and measuring perceptions of individual, organizational and community control, *Health Educ Q* 21(2):149-170, 1994.

Kreuter MW: PATCH: its origin, basic concepts, and links to contemporary health policy, *J Health Educ* 23(3):135-139, 1992.

Lee HJ: Definitions of rural: a review of the literature. In Bushy A, ed: *Rural nursing,* vol 1, Newbury Park, Ca., 1991, Sage, pp. 7-20.

Long KA: The concept of health: rural perspectives, *Nurs Clin North Am* 28:123-130, 1993.

Long KA, Boik R: Predicting alcohol use in rural children: a longitudinal study, *Nurs Res* 42:79-86, 1993.

Long KA, Weinert C: Rural nursing: developing the theory base, *Scholar Inq Nurs Pract* 3(2):113-127, 1989.

MacIver RM: *Community*, London, 1917, MacMillan.

MacIver RM, Page CH: *Society: an introductory analysis*, New York, 1949, Rinehart.

Martin A: Community assessment: the cornerstone of effective marketing, *Pediatr Nurs* 14:50-53, 1988.

McMillan DW, Chavis DM: Sense of community: a definition and theory, *J Comm Psychol* 14:6-23, 1986.

Meneshian S: Nursing assessment of a community. In Caliandro G, Judkins B, eds: *Primary nursing practice*, Glenview, Ill., 1988, Scott, Foresman, pp. 111-118.

Milio N: Healthy cities: the new public health and supportive research, *Health Prom Int* 5(4):291-297, 1990.

Milio N: Stirring the social pot: community effects of program and policy research, *J Nurs Adm* 22(2):24-29, 1992.

Moore T: *Conversation on the philosophy of community*, Knoxville, Tn., April 26, 1996, University of Tennessee, College of Nursing.

Nakajima H: World Health Day 1996: Healthy Cities for better life, *World Health* 49:3, 1996.

National Civic League: *National Civic League: a century of community building*, Denver, 1995, The League.

National Commission on Community Health Services: *Health is a community affair*, Cambridge, Ma., 1966, Harvard University Press.

National Organization for Public Health Nursing (NOPHN): Constitution of the National Organization for Public Health Nursing, Article 2, 1912, Wald: New York Public Library folder: NOPHN No. 1. In Fitzpatrick ML, ed: *The National Organization for Public Health Nursing, 1912-1952: development of a practice field*, New York, 1975, National League for Nursing.

Norris T: *The healthy communities handbook*, Denver, 1993, National Civic League.

Norris T, Lampe D: Healthy communities, healthy people, *Natl Civ Rev* 83(3):2-11, 1994.

Office of Technology Assessment (OTA), Congress of the United States: *Health care in rural America*, Washington, D.C., 1990, The Office.

Office of Technology Assessment (OTA), Congress of the United States: *Impact of health reform on rural areas: lessons from the states*, Washington, D.C., 1995, The Office.

Orloff TM, Tymann B: *Rural health: an evolving system of accessible services*, Washington, D.C., 1995, National Governor's Association.

Pender N: *Health promotion in nursing practice*, Stanford, Ct., 1996, Appleton & Lange.

Poplin DC: *Communities: a survey of theories and methods of research*, ed 2, New York, 1979, Macmillan.

Randall T: *The outreach sourcebook: rural health demonstration projects 1991 to 1994*, Rockville, Md., 1995, Federal Office of Rural Health Policy.

Rauckhorst LM, Stokes SA, Mezey MD: Community and home assessment, *J Gerontol Nurs* 6:319-327, 1980.

Rodgers SS: Community as client—a multivariate model for analysis of community and aggregate health risk, *Public Health Nurs* 1:210-222, 1984.

Ruffing-Rahal MA: Resident/provider contrasts in community health priorities, *Public Health Nurs* 4:242-246, 1987.

Sanders IT: *The community: an introduction to a social system*, New York, 1958, Ronald Press.

Sanders IT: *The community: an introduction to a social system*, ed 2, New York, 1966, Ronald Press.

Sanders IT: *The community: an introduction to a social system*, ed 3, New York, 1975, Ronald Press.

Sanders IT: The community: structure and function, *Nurs Outlook* 11:642-645, 1963.

Sasenick, SM: How healthy is your community? *Health Care Forum J* 37(3):56, 1994.

Sarvela P, McClendon E: Correlates of early adolescent peer and personal substance use in rural northern Michigan, *J Rural Health* 9:57-62, 1987.

Shamansky SL, Pesznecker B: A community is . . . , *Nurs Outlook* 29:182-185, 1981.

Sherer JL: Neighbor to neighbor, *Hosp Health Netw* 68(20):52-56, 1994.

Speers M: PATCH: preface, *J Health Educ* 23(3):132-133, 1992.

Stein KZ, Eigsti DG: Utilizing a community data base system with community health nursing students, *J Nurs Educ* 21:26-32, 1982.

Strategies to improve rural health, *Public Health Rep* 111(2):101, 1996.

Turner JG, Chavigny KH: *Community health nursing: an epidemiologic perspective throughout the nursing process*, Philadelphia, 1988, Lippincott.

United States Department of Health and Human Services (USDHHS): *Prevention resource guide: rural communities*, Rockville, Md., 1991, USDHHS.

United States Department of Health and Human Services (USDHHS): *Healthy People 2000 midcourse review and 1995 revisions*, Rockville, Md., 1995, USDHHS.

Vulnerable populations. In Bushy A, ed: *Rural nursing*, vol 1, Newbury Park, Ca., 1991, Sage, pp. 127-132.

Wakefield MK: Health care in rural America: a view from the nation's capital, *Nurs Econ* 8(2):83-89, 1990.

Wald L: *The house on Henry Street*, New York, 1915, Henry Holt.

Warren DI: Neighborhoods in urban areas. In Warren RL, ed: *New perspectives on the American community*, ed 3, Chicago, 1977, Rand McNally, pp. 224-237.

Warren RL: *Studying your community*, Chicago, 1955, Rand McNally.

Warren RL: *The community in America*, Chicago, 1963, Rand McNally.

Warren RL: *Studying your community*, Chicago, 1965, Rand McNally.

Warren RL: *Perspectives on the American community*, Chicago, 1966, Rand McNally.

Warren RL: *The community in America*, ed 2, Chicago, 1972, Rand McNally.

Warren RL: *The community in America*, ed 3, Chicago, 1978, Rand McNally.

Warren RL: *The community in America*, ed 4, Chicago, 1987, Rand McNally.

Warren RL: The good community—what would it be? In Warren RL, Lyon L, eds: *New perspectives on the American community*, ed 5, Chicago, 1988, Rand McNally, pp. 412-419.

Weinert C, Burman ME: Rural health and health-seeking behaviors. In Fitzpatrick JJ, Stevenson JS, eds: *Annual review of nursing research*, vol 12, New York, 1994, Springer, pp. 65-92.

Weinert C, Long KA: Understanding the health care needs of rural families, *Family Relations* 36:450-455, 1987.

Weinert C, Long KA: Rural families and health care: refining the knowledge base, *J Marr Fam Rev* 15(1):57-96, 1990.

Weinert C, Long KA: The theory and research base for rural nursing practice. In Bushy A, ed: *Rural nursing*, vol 1, Newbury Park, Ca., 1991, Sage, pp. 21-38.

Weinert C, Long KA: Support systems for the spouses of chronically ill persons in rural areas, *Fam Community Health* 16(1):46-54, 1993.

Wellman B, Leighton B: Networks, neighborhoods, and communities: approaches to the study of the community question. In Warren RL, Lyon L, eds: *New perspectives on the American community*, Chicago, 1988, Dorsey, pp. 57-72.

Whelan E-M: The Health Corner: a community-based nursing model to maximize access to primary care, *Public Health Rep* 110(2):184-188, 1995.

White JE, Valentine VL: Computer assisted video instruction and community assessment, *Nurs Health Care* 14(7):349-353, 1993.

Wiist WH, Flack JM: A church-based cholesterol education program, *Public Health Rep* 105(4):381-388, 1990.

World Health Organization (WHO): *Community health nursing: report of a WHO expert committee*, Technical Report Series No. 558, Geneva, 1974, The Organization.

Zerwekh J, Young B, Primono J, Deal L, eds: *Opening doors: stories of public health nursing*, Olympia, Wa., 1992, Washington State Department of Health.

SELECTED BIBLIOGRAPHY

Agency for Health Care Policy and Research (AHCPR): *Rural health care research: impacting vulnerable populations: Grant announcement*, Rockville, Md., 1991, AHCPR.

American Nurses Association (ANA): *A guide for community-based nursing services*, Kansas City, Mo., 1985, ANA.

Anderson ET, McFarlane JM: *Community as client: application of the nursing process*, Philadelphia, 1988, Lippincott.

Anderson ET, McFarlane JM, Helton A: Community-as-client: a model for practice, *Nurs Outlook* 34:220-224, 1986.

Bracht N: *Health promotion at the community level*, Newbury Park, Ca., 1990, Sage.

Breckinridge M: *Wide neighborhoods: a story of the Frontier Nursing Service*, New York, 1952, Harper and Row.

Chalmers K, Kristajanson L: The theoretical basis for nursing at the community level: a comparison of three models, *J Adv Nurs* 14:569-574, 1989.

Dunn AM, Decker SD: Community as client: appropriate baccalaureate- and graduate-level preparation, *J Comm Health Nurs* 7:131-139, 1990.

Eigsti DG, Stein KZ, Fortune M: The community as client for continuity of care, *Nurs Health Care* 3:251, 1982.

Farley S: The community as partner in primary health care, *Nurs Health Care* 14(5):224-249, 1993.

Goldstein G, Kickbusch I: A healthy city is a better city, *World Health* 49:4-6, 1996.

Hanchett ES: *Nursing frameworks and community as client*, Norwalk, Ct., 1988, Appleton & Lange.

Neufeld A, Harrison MJ: The development of nursing diagnoses for aggregates and groups, *Public Health Nurs* 7(4):251-255, 1990.

Pender NJ, Barkauskas VH, Hayman L, et al: Health promotion and disease prevention: toward excellence in nursing practice and education, *Nurs Outlook* 40(3):106-112, 1992.

Ruybal SE, Bauwens E, Fasla MJ: Community assessment: an epidemiological approach, *Nurs Outlook* 23:365-368, 1975.

Sanders IT: Health in the community. In Freeman HE, Levine S, Reeder LG, eds: *Handbook of medical sociology*, ed 3, Englewood Cliffs, N.J., 1979, Prentice Hall, pp. 412-433.

Selvy ML, Tuttle DM: Community health assessment and program planning in the nurse practitioner curriculum: evaluation of a guided design learning module, *Public Health Nurs* 4:160-165, 1987.

Sills GM, Goeppinger J: The community as a field of inquiry in nursing. In Werly HH, Fitzpatrick JJ, eds: *Annual review of nursing research,* vol 3, New York, 1985, Springer, pp. 4-23.

Stoner MH, Magilvy JK, Schultz PR: Community analysis in community health nursing practice: the GENESIS model, *Public Health Nurs* 9(4):223-227, 1992.

Wallerstein N, Bernstein E: Introduction to community empowerment, participatory education, and health, *Health Educ Q* 21 (2):141-148, 1994.

Warren RL: Observations on the state of community theory. In Warren RL, Lyon L, eds: *New perspectives on the American community,* ed 5, Chicago, 1988, Rand McNally, pp. 84-86.

Warren RL: The community in America. In Warren RL, Lyon L, eds: *New perspectives on the American community,* ed 5, Chicago, 1988, Rand McNally, pp. 152-157.

4

U.S. Health and Welfare Legislation and Services

OBJECTIVES

Upon completion of this chapter, the reader should be able to:

1. Summarize the development of health and welfare practices in the United States.
2. Discuss the purpose and mandates of significant health and welfare legislation in the United States.
3. Explain how the Social Security Act and the Public Health Service Act have influenced health and welfare practices in the United States.
4. Discuss how health and welfare legislation affects community health nursing practice.
5. Discuss U.S. health care spending.
6. Explain methods of health care financing in the United States.
7. Differentiate between private and government health and welfare services.
8. Give an overview of the health and welfare systems in the United States.
9. Discuss current issues in health and welfare reform in the United States.
10. Discuss the concept of managed care.

> We have left undone those things which we ought to have done and we have done those things which we ought not to have done, and there is no health in us.
>
> BOOK OF COMMON PRAYER

Chapter 1 discussed the evolution of community health nursing in the United States. The legislation and services discussed in this chapter help to ensure for many Americans access to health care and an adequate standard of living. This chapter presents the historical evolution of U.S. health and welfare practices and discusses health and welfare legislation, services, and programs. Chapter 5 explores the organization of health and welfare services on the federal, state, and local levels.

Clients with whom the community health nurse works use programs presented in this chapter, such as Old Age, Survivors, and Disability Insurance; Temporary Assistance to Needy Families; Supplemental Food Program for Women, Infants, and Children; Food Stamps; Unemployment Insurance; and Supplemental Security Income. They also use different payment and organizational systems presented, such as Medicaid, Medicare, private insurance, HMOs, PPOs, POSs, and IPAs. Nurses need to educate clients about services and programs, assist clients in using them, and understand how legislation enables their provision.

THE EVOLUTION OF HEALTH AND WELFARE PRACTICES

Health and welfare practices have evolved over time. Across civilizations, early public health practices focused on controlling communicable disease. Early societies used communicable disease control measures such as isolation (often in the form of quarantine or banishment), burial of the dead, and protection and conservation of food and water supplies to promote health.

Egyptians of 1000 BC were possibly the healthiest of all ancient civilized people (Pickett, Hanlon, 1990, p. 21). They practiced rigorous personal hygiene measures; isolated lepers; had elaborate sewage, drainage, and water-supply systems; and used pharmaceutical preparations and surgical treatments. The Romans practiced public health measures that included provision of public sanitation services, including the removal of garbage and rubbish; protection of the public water supply; and supervision of public food and housing (Pickett, Hanlon, p. 22). As early as 1500 BC the Hebrews had a written hygienic code in Leviticus that dealt with personal and community hygiene (Pickett, Hanlon, p. 21).

Public health has a proud history. Public health measures have prevented countless deaths, helped to control communicable disease, and improved the quality of life. Throughout the history of public health, two major factors have determined how problems were solved: the level of scientific and technical knowledge, and the content of public values and popular opinions (Institute of Medicine, 1988, p. 1).

An examination of the historical evolution of health and welfare legislation and services in the United States demonstrates that their development was reactionary rather than preventive in nature. Historically, health and welfare programs have been decentralized and operate at all levels of government, as well as in the private sector. It was not until 1980 that U.S. national health objectives were developed. Unfortunately, public health in the United States is often taken for granted, and areas in which there were great strides, such as provision of safe drinking water, communicable disease control, smoking cessation, and teen pregnancy prevention, are beginning to slip backward.

EUROPEAN INFLUENCE ON U.S. HEALTH AND WELFARE POLICY

European influence has been singled out because of the significant impact it had on the development of U.S. health and welfare policy. Health and welfare policies in the United States reflect a background that is European, primarily English, in origin.

Europe was not always a pacesetter in public health practices. Europeans of the Middle Ages (500-1500 AD) did not follow many of the health practices of previous times and cultures. They allowed refuse to accumulate in streets and dwellings, dumped human waste into public water supplies, improperly stored and prepared foods, often ignored personal hygiene, and allowed child labor. These practices did little to promote health.

During this time epidemics of cholera, smallpox, typhoid, plague, and diphtheria raged. In the 1300s bubonic plague nearly exterminated the human race, reportedly killing up to half of the world's population (Pickett, Hanlon, 1990, p. 24). Epidemics of such magnitude have never been seen since, and public health practices evolved to control communicable diseases.

During the Middle Ages a number of beliefs prevailed that affected health and welfare practices. *Divine causation*, the belief that conditions reflect the will and judgment of God, flourished and greatly influenced provision of health and welfare services. Conditions such as poverty, illness, and disability were often viewed as having divine causation rather than societal causation; and the sick, disabled, and poor were largely ignored as a public responsibility. *Self-help*, the belief that it was the responsibility of individuals or their responsible relatives to assume provision for care, was the prevailing policy. During this period poverty was often equated with crime, and beggars, vagrants, and the disabled could be physically punished, imprisoned, or sent to poorhouses. When assistance was given, it was usually church sponsored and took the form of food and shelter. There was little governmental involvement in issues of public health and welfare. When governmental involvement occurred it was often in response to economic depressions, wars, natural disasters, epidemics, and mass public indignation. It was an economic depression that brought about the Elizabethan Poor Law of 1601.

The Elizabethan Poor Law of 1601

A severe economic depression in England spurred the enactment of the Elizabethan Poor Law of 1601. Large-scale involuntary unemployment and the fear of insurrection stimulated the government to provide welfare aid (Coll, 1969, p. 5). This law granted the right to assistance through taxation and established three major categories of dependent people: the vagrant, the involuntarily unemployed, and the helpless (Coll, p. 5). The last two categories were deemed the "worthy" poor. The helpless included widows, the disabled, and dependent children. Poor law concepts included the following:

1. *Local administration*. It was the responsibility of local government to aid those in need. The locality decided who would receive aid and the amount and type of aid. Aid was frequently administered through the church.
2. *General aid*. General aid, usually in the form of food and shelter, was available to the worthy poor.
3. *Responsible relatives*. Relatives could be held responsible for the financial support of other family members.
4. *Restrictive residence*. The locality of the individual's origin was responsible for the financial support of the individual. An indigent who migrated from his or her locality of origin could be returned to it.
5. *Individual means test*. Aid was administered on an individual basis through determination of means and needs. Local jurisdictions exercised the right to use moral qualifications to determine who was worthy of assistance.
6. *Minimal subsistence*. A recipient was to receive no more assistance than necessary to exist.
7. *Compulsory work or service*. Work or service by the recipient was often compulsory to obtain assistance, and refusal to work could be a punishable crime. Workhouses for the indigent were commonplace.
8. *Funding through taxation*. Funds to administer the poor law were raised through local taxes.

The Elizabethan Poor Law was a forerunner of U.S. welfare policy, and *all* of the original 13 colonies adopted it in some form. Following poor law tradition, the United States left administration of assistance programs largely under local control, implemented responsible relative clauses, administered means tests, provided minimal subsistence, generally mandated work or service, imposed restrictive residency, and derived welfare revenues through taxation. Restrictive residency laws are now unconstitutional in the United States. However, many original poor law concepts are part of contemporary health and welfare policy. A report written in England more than 200 years ago has provided the impetus for U.S. public health policy.

The Chadwick Report

In 1832 the British Parliament appointed a royal commission to revise the poor law, and in 1834 the revisions were implemented. Edwin Chadwick was a member of this commission and later, in 1842, published the *Report of the Labouring Population and on the Means of Its Improvement*, often referred to as the Chadwick Report. The report detailed the unsanitary conditions in which the laborers lived and the lack of proper refuse disposal, contaminated water supplies, high rates of morbidity and mortality, and generally poor living conditions of the laboring population.

At the time of Chadwick's report, one half of the children of working-class parents died before their fifth birthday, and in large English cities the average age of death for laborers was 16, compared to 22 for tradesmen and 36 for the gentry (Richardson, 1887, cited in Pickett, Hanlon, 1990, p. 26). Chadwick's report helped to bring about the passage of the English Public Health Act of 1848, the establishment of a General Board of Health, and the writing of the Shattuck Report in the United States in 1850.

THE DEVELOPMENT OF U.S. HEALTH AND WELFARE POLICY

The word *health* was left out of the U.S. constitution, and each state was made responsible for legislating its own health laws and providing for the health of its citizens. Recognition of the need for control of communicable disease and the beliefs of divine causation, self-help, and minimal government intervention prevailed in the United States. Federal intervention in public health and welfare assistance programs was almost nonexistent in early America. A major impetus to developing U.S. public health policy was the Shattuck Report.

The Shattuck Report

This report was the forerunner of contemporary U.S. public health policy. The Shattuck Report was written in 1850 by Lemuel Shattuck, a teacher, statistician, and legislator. The report recommended measures such as the creation of state and local boards of health; collection of vital statistics; supervision of housing, factories, sanitation, and foods; procurement of immunizations; community health control measures; and school health and health education. The majority of Shattuck's recommendations are still accepted today as sound public health practice.

Before the report, local boards of health had begun to emerge in the United States. Some of the earliest were in Baltimore, Maryland (1798); Charleston, South Carolina (1815); Philadelphia, Pennsylvania (1818); and Providence, Rhode Island (1832). Following the Shattuck Report, the number of boards of health expanded. In 1869 Massachusetts established the first state board of health in line with Shattuck's recommendations (Pickett, Hanlon, 1990, p. 32). These state and local boards of health were the forerunners of today's state health authorities (SHAs) and local health departments (LHDs).

Development of Voluntary Agencies

When the term *voluntary* is used in relation to health and welfare services, it can be somewhat confusing. *Voluntary* refers to private, nonprofit resources that are not under the auspices of federal, state, or local government; are not tax supported; have no legal powers; and rely heavily on donations, endowments, grants, and fees-for-service as funding mechanisms. Voluntary resources traditionally represent people doing for people and a willingness to help others. These resources usually have a large volunteer staff.

Voluntary agencies have a long and distinguished history. By the 1870s voluntary organizations were emerging to work with health and welfare issues in the United States. In 1872 the American Public Health Association (APHA) was founded; its first president was Dr. Stephen Smith. Today it remains one of our foremost public health organizations, helping to protect and promote the nation's health.

In 1882 one of our country's best-known voluntary organizations, the American Red Cross, was founded by Clara Barton. In 1892 the Anti-Tuberculosis Society of Philadelphia, a forerunner of today's American Lung Association, was established. Other voluntary organizations continued to develop. Concurrently, private profit-making health organizations were emerging, some of which have made significant contributions to public health practice (Figure 4-1). Today there are thousands of voluntary health and welfare organizations in the United States.

At the same time, institutions and almshouses (poorhouses) were the major form of welfare assistance in this country. Such residential facilities often separated the poor, disabled, frail elderly, mentally ill, and mentally retarded from the rest of the population. Concurrently, voluntary organizations such as associations for retarded citizens and mental health organizations arose to help meet the needs of these aggregates in a more effective way.

Today nurses work extensively with voluntary agencies in the community. Voluntary organizations remain an important part of U.S. health and welfare service provision. This voluntary tradition is to be applauded. Voluntary resources are discussed further in Chapter 5.

The Volunteer Tradition

The United States has the strongest volunteer tradition of any country in the world. One state, Tennessee,

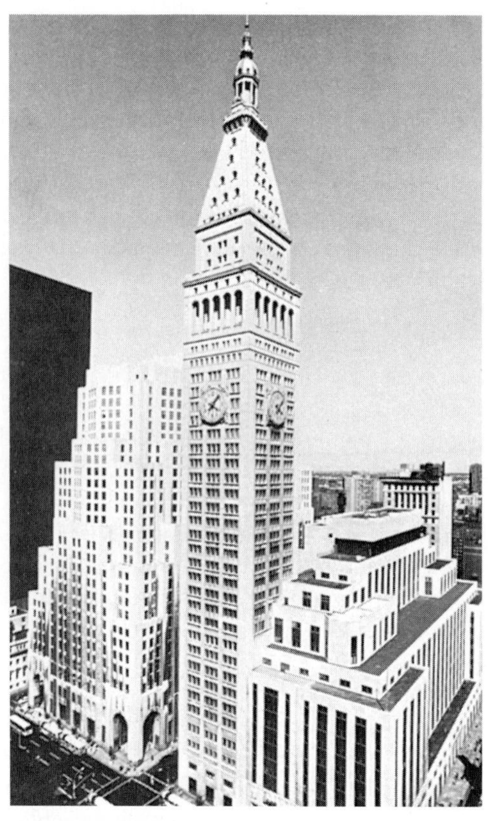

Figure 4-1 Lillian Wald contracted with the Metropolitan Life Insurance company for the provision of public health nursing services to its subscribers. The company is still providing public health services today. *(Photo courtesy Metropolitan Life Insurance.)*

is nicknamed the "Volunteer State." The American volunteer tradition has early roots. Early American settlers were often trying to break from the traditional and sometimes oppressive influences of church and state from which they came. In general, they were mistrustful of governmental intervention into matters of personal and public health and welfare. People helped each other, charities developed, and voluntary organizations emerged.

The United States went through what has been termed by some social and health researchers as the *voluntaristic period.* This was the time between the Civil War and 1935, and it was during this period that many voluntary agencies were founded. The passage of the Social Security Act of 1935 signaled governmental involvement in the provision of health and welfare services and eliminated some of the need for voluntary organizations.

Volunteers are often the backbone of a voluntary agency. They work throughout the community in settings such as shelters for the homeless, safe houses for battered women and children, schools, and local health department clinics. They provide direct services, raise funds, act as advocates, serve on boards of directors, and assist administration. Volunteers provide many important services. It is commendable that millions of Americans are involved in volunteer work each year.

Volunteers bring a human, caring element to service provision. They should be treated with respect and given appropriate, meaningful roles. In working with volunteers, the nurse works to promote an environment that fosters positive working relationships.

Establishing Government Involvement in the Delivery of Health and Welfare Services

As noted previously, the word *health* was left out of the U.S. Constitution, and issues of health and welfare were left primarily to the states. Federal involvement in these issues emerged slowly and cautiously.

The federal Marine Hospital Service was established in 1798. In 1879 a National Board of Health was established; this Board was short-lived and disbanded in 1883. Today there is no National Board of Health in the United States. In 1912 the Marine Hospital Service became the United States Public Health Service (USPHS). The system of federal grants-in-aid to states originated in 1919 and supplied revenue to states for health and welfare programs. At that time federal government involvement in matters of public health and welfare was minimal.

By 1919 all states had a government branch dealing with health, often known as the state department of public health, and many states had a government branch dealing with welfare, often a state department of social services. State public health programs focused on the control of communicable disease and maternal-child health, since these were the primary public health problems of the era. State welfare assistance programs focused on providing services to widows, dependent children, and the indigent elderly. State welfare insurance programs, in the form of workers' compensation, began to evolve in 1911.

THE GREAT DEPRESSION The Great Depression started with the stock market crash of 1929 and peaked in 1933 when 13 million persons, 25% of the work force, were unemployed, and 19 million persons were on state relief rolls. Neither private nor government-funded health and welfare programs could handle the demands created by this event. Possibly no other single event has had such an impact on U.S. health and welfare policy.

The Great Depression showed the general public that anyone could become poor. It dealt a mortal blow to the belief of divine causation, because many people whom the general public believed were not deserving of poverty became impoverished. States and the general public put considerable pressure on the federal government to assist those in need. Economic times were desperate for millions of Americans.

A major concern that emerged out of the Depression was a large, young, and restless unemployed workforce. New jobs were hard to generate, and many jobs were held by older workers with seniority. Across the country demonstra-

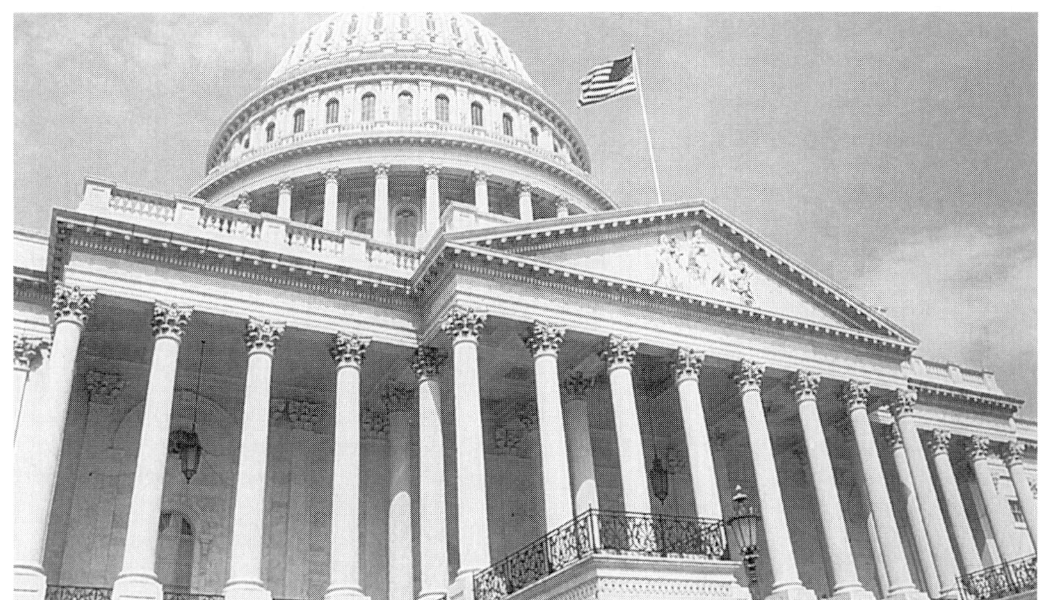

Figure 4-2 The Capitol Building, Washington, D.C. Public health professionals need to monitor proposed laws to ensure that the health care needs of clients are met.

tions and protests took place to bring about government intervention to help ease the economic distress.

At this time there was no mandatory retirement age and few retirement pension plans. The idea of mandatory retirement of workers, with the retiree being eligible for a government pension, emerged. Such retirement benefits became part of the Social Security Act of 1935 and helped quiet the general unrest of the American people.

THE SOCIAL SECURITY ACT OF 1935 Out of the Depression, under the presidency of Franklin D. Roosevelt, came the federal Social Security Act of 1935. The passage of the Social Security Act gave the United States the dubious distinction of being the last major industrial nation to develop a federal welfare program.

The Social Security Act established insurance programs (contributory) and assistance programs (noncontributory). Contributory programs are financed through both taxation and individual contributions, whereas assistance programs are financed only through taxation. It consolidated federal welfare programs under one law and is a landmark piece of legislation, possibly the most important one of our time. Since 1935 the Social Security Act has been amended numerous times to incorporate other health and welfare programs. It is one of many legislative acts that is important for the community health nurse to understand and is discussed in depth later in this chapter.

U.S. HEALTH AND WELFARE LEGISLATION

Each year numerous laws with health and welfare implications are enacted, and many existing laws are amended (Figure 4-2). Health and welfare legislation should be examined in terms of its administration, funding, services offered, clients served, service delivery, and quality control.

The responsibility to implement this legislation is often dispersed over several agencies at the federal, state, and local levels, with a resulting diffusion of responsibility and accountability (Institute of Medicine, 1988, p. 115).

An in-depth perspective on laws can be obtained by reading materials specific to each piece of legislation in the *United States Code—Congressional and Administrative News* and the *United States Statutes at Large*. An understanding of this legislation is needed for the community health nurse to assist clients in obtaining services, identify gaps in the delivery of health and welfare services, and work in partnership with communities to promote health.

Major Health and Welfare Legislation

Several acts of legislation had a major impact on the development of health and welfare policy and practices in the United States. The nurse needs to be aware of this legislation because it has significant impact on the availability of health and welfare services. When nurses examine new legislation, they will often find that it is an amendment to an existing law rather than an entirely new law, and that amendments to a law can significantly alter it. Federal laws are designated *public law* and are followed by the number of the congressional session and the sequential number of the law.

The Social Security Act of 1935 and the Public Health Service Act of 1944 are two of the most significant pieces of U.S. legislation ever enacted (Gerber, McGuire, 1995, p. 266). Many new laws are amendments to these two acts, and they provide numerous health and welfare services for clients.

1965: The Turning Point in Health Law in the United States

1. Drug Abuse Control Amendments of 1965 (PL 89-74).
2. Federal Cigarette Labeling and Advertising Act (PL 89-92).
3. Mental Retardation Facilities and Community Mental Health Centers Construction Act Amendments of 1965 (PL 89-105).
4. Community Health Services Extension Amendments of 1965 (PL 89-109).
5. Health Research Facilities Amendments of 1965 (PL 89-115).
6. Water Quality Act of 1965 (PL 89-234).
7. Heart Disease, Cancer and Stroke Amendments of 1965 (PL 89-239).
8. The Clean Air Act Amendments and Solid Waste Disposal Act of 1965 (PL 89-272).
9. Health Professions Educational Assistance Amendments of 1965 (PL 89-290).
10. Medical Library Assistance Act of 1965 (PL 89-291).
11. The Appalachian Regional Development Act of 1965 (PL 89-4).
12. The Older Americans Act (PL 89-73).
13. The Social Security Amendments of 1965 (PL 89-97).
14. The Vocational Rehabilitation Act Amendments of 1965 (PL 89-333).
15. The Housing and Urban Development Act of 1965 (PL 89-117).

From Forgotson EH: 1965: the turning point in health law—1966 reflections, *Am J Public Health* 57(6):934-935, 1967.

Major Social Security Act Programs

ORIGINAL PROGRAMS

Aid to the Blind (AB)
Old Age Assistance (OAA)
Aid to Dependent Children (ADC)
Old Age Insurance (OAI)
Unemployment Insurance

SUBSEQUENT PROGRAMS

1939: Old Age and Survivors Insurance (OASI)—*replaces* OAI
1950: Aid to the Permanently and Totally Disabled (APTD)
Aid to Families of Dependent Children (AFDC)—*replaces* ADC
1956: Old Age, Survivors, and Disability Insurance (OASDI)—*replaces* OASI
1965: Medicaid and Medicare
1972: Supplemental Security Income (SSI)—*replaces* three programs: AB, OAA, APTD
1996: Temporary Assistance to Needy Families (TANF)*—replaces AFDC

*The name of this temporary assistance program will vary from state to state (e.g., Family Independence Program in Michigan). It is anticipated that further state welfare reform legislation will be passed throughout the rest of the century. However, emphasis in future state legislation will continue to remain on providing assistance on a temporary basis and on assisting families to achieve independence.

The year 1965 has been called the turning point in U.S. public health law and federal involvement in matters of public health (Forgotson, 1967, p. 934). During 1965 at least 15 important laws relating to health were passed. The box above lists those laws. Discussion of some major U.S. health and welfare legislation follows.

SOCIAL SECURITY ACT OF 1935 (PUBLIC LAW 74-721) AS AMENDED The Social Security Act of 1935 provided for the general welfare by establishing a system of federal old-age benefits and by enabling the states to make adequate provision for aged persons, blind persons, dependent and crippled children, maternal and child welfare, and the administration of state unemployment compensation laws. This act established a Social Security Board and mechanisms for raising revenue for retirement income and welfare purposes. The Social Security Act was a giant step toward safeguarding the health and welfare of Americans. When the act was passed in 1935 it included both welfare insurance and welfare assistance programs. Original and subsequent programs under the act are listed in the box above right. Table 4-1 lists the major programs of the Social Security Act and their source of administration. Table 4-2 lists some major amendments to this act.

Determination of eligibility for social security *assistance* programs is handled through a number of federal, state, and local agencies. Temporary Assistance to Needy Families (TANF) and Medicaid are often applied for at state departments of human services.

Determination of eligibility for social security *insurance* programs is handled through local branches of the federal Social Security Administration. Social Security Administration offices are located throughout the country, and representatives are sent to communities in which there are no offices. Applications for the insurance programs of Old Age, Survivors, and Disability Insurance (OASDI) and Medicare, as well as the assistance program of Supplemental Security Income (SSI), can be made at these federal offices.

Today nearly every American family is involved with the Social Security Act in some form. Employers, employees, and the self-employed pay into the insurance programs of the act. Almost 95% of all U.S. workers contribute to these programs. The social security insurance protection, OASDI, earned by workers stays with them even in a new job or residence. The contributions made by a worker determine the amount and type of benefits.

table 4-1 Some Major Social Security Act Programs and Their Source of Administration

Type of Benefits	Type of Programs: Federal Programs*	State-Federal Programs†	Federal-State Programs‡
Welfare insurance (cash benefit)	Old Age, Survivors, and Disability Insurance (OASDI)	Unemployment Insurance [Department of Labor, Department of the Treasury]	None
Welfare assistance (cash benefit)	None	Temporary Assistance to Needy Families (TANF) [Social Security Administration]	Supplemental Security Income (SSI)
Health insurance	1. Medicare A—hospital insurance, prepaid through social security contributions 2. Medicare B—medical insurance, individual premium required	None	None
Health assistance	None	1. Medicaid [Health Care Financing Administration] 2. Miscellaneous maternal and child health programs (i.e., services to crippled children, PRESCAD)	None

*Administered federally through the Social Security Administration and/or the Health Care Financing Administration.
†Administered through the state government. Federal sharing agency may be indicated in brackets by program.
‡Administered federally through the Social Security Administration. State sharing agency or agencies will vary in each state.
Note: Programs such as workers' compensation, general assistance, and food stamps are not provided for under the Social Security Act of 1935 and are discussed later in this chapter.

PUBLIC HEALTH SERVICE ACT OF 1944 (PUBLIC LAW 78-410) AS AMENDED The Public Health Service Act of 1944 consolidated and revised the laws relating to the Public Health Service and has since served to consolidate national public health legislation. It is the major piece of public health legislation in the country but inexplicably does not have administration over the Medicaid and Medicare programs of the Social Security Act.

This act incorporates legislation about health care personnel, health facility construction and modernization, and services to specific population groups. Over the years this law has been frequently amended to provide financing for traineeships for health care professionals (e.g., nurse training acts); grants-in-aid to schools of public health; construction of community mental health centers and facilities; national comprehensive health planning and resource development; the development of health maintenance organizations; health services for migratory workers; family planning services and communicable disease control; emergency medical services; and research and facilities for the prevention and control of conditions such as heart disease, cancer, stroke, kidney disease, sudden infant death syndrome, arthritis, Cooley's anemia, sickle cell anemia, AIDS, and diabetes mellitus. Amendments such as the Heart Disease, Cancer, and Stroke Amendments gave research and service priority to some of the leading causes of death in this country. Table 4-3 lists some major amendments under this act.

CIVIL RIGHTS ACT OF 1964 (PUBLIC LAW 88-352) Most states and many municipalities have enacted civil rights laws that forbid discrimination and ensure constitutional rights. Federal civil rights legislation was enacted in the United States in 1866, 1870, and 1871. Contemporary civil rights acts were enacted in 1957, 1960, 1964, and 1968. In 1980 the Civil Rights of Institutionalized Persons Act (Public Law 96-247) was enacted.

Of all the civil rights legislation, the Civil Rights Act of 1964 is often considered to be the most significant; it was designed to ensure fair and equal treatment for all. The act forbade discrimination on the basis of race or sex in public accommodations, public facilities, and public education. It also enforced the constitutional right to vote. It established the Commission on Equal Employment Opportunity and attempted to ensure fair employment practices. If a state or local government is found to be practicing discrimination, the federal Attorney General can sue to have that state's revenue-sharing funds cut off. The Civil Rights Restoration Act of 1987 (Public Law 100-259) clarified and enlarged the scope of the coverage of this act.

ECONOMIC OPPORTUNITY ACT OF 1964 (PUBLIC LAW 88-452) The Economic Opportunity Act of 1964 was designed

table 4-2 Selected Amendments: Social Security Act of 1935

Year	Amendment
1939	*Social Security Amendments* provided for the payment of insurance benefits to qualifying survivors of workers. The insurance program under the act now was Old Age and Survivors Insurance (OASI).
1950	*Social Security Amendments of 1950* provided for federal aid to states for financial assistance to people who were disabled under Aid to the Permanently and Totally Disabled. Under a new title, Title XIV, Aid to Dependent Children was broadened to include the relative with whom the child was living and became known as Aid to Families with Dependent Children.
1956	*Social Security Amendments of 1956* provided disability insurance benefits for qualifying disabled individuals and reduced to 62 the age at which benefits could be paid to women (The Social Security Amendments of 1961, Public Law 87-64, would make this the age for men also). The insurance portion of the act now was Old Age, Survivors, and Disability Insurance (OASDI).
1963	*Maternal and Child Health and Mental Retardation Planning Amendments* assisted states and communities in preventing mental retardation through expansion and improvement of maternal child health and crippled children's programs.
1965	*Social Security Amendments of 1965* established Medicare (Title XVII) and Medicaid (Title XIX). These were landmark pieces of legislation and marked the advent of major federal government involvement in health care delivery. Medicare greatly influenced the expansion of home health care services.
1967	*Social Security Amendments of 1967* consolidated maternal and child health and crippled children programs under one authorization and provided for funding of family planning services. Established the Early, Periodic, Screening, and Development Testing (EPSDT) under Medicaid and allowed Medicaid recipients free choice in the selection of qualified medical facilities and practitioners.
1972	*Social Security Amendments of 1972* mandated the establishment of Professional Standard Review Organizations (PSROs) in health care. Established the assistance program of Supplemental Security Income (SSI) to replace the categorical assistance programs of Old Age Assistance, Aid to the Blind, and Aid to the Permanently and Totally Disabled. This change provided for more nationally uniform payment levels to qualifying individuals and set a minimum level of payment. Health insurance coverage for the disabled was made available under Medicare.
1977	*Social Security Act—Rural Health Clinic Amendments* provided payment for rural health clinic services and allowed for direct reimbursement for nursing services in these settings.
1982	*Tax Equity and Fiscal Responsibility Act of 1982* set forth a system of prospective payment for Medicare services called Diagnostic-Related Groups (DRGs).
1984	*Child Support Enforcement Amendments of 1984* amended the act to allow *mandatory* income withholding and other improvements in the child support enforcement program so that children in the United States who are in need of assistance in securing financial support from their parents will receive such assistance. Included provisions for increasing the availability of federal parent locator services to state agencies, collection of past-due support from federal tax refund, and the inclusion of medical support in child support orders.
1985	*Consolidated Omnibus Budget Reconciliation Act of 1985 (COBRA)* amended the act to extend Medicaid coverage for prenatal and postnatal care to low-income women in two-parent families where the primary breadwinner is unemployed, expanded Medicaid services available under home- and community-based services waivers, and permitted states to offer hospice services to the terminally ill as a Medicaid benefit.
1986	*Omnibus Budget Reconciliation Act of 1986 (OBRA)* amended the Social Security Act under Medicaid to allow states to have the option of expanding coverage for pregnant women, infants up to age 1, and children up to age 5 who had incomes below the federal poverty level; required states to continue Medicaid coverage to disabled individuals who lost their eligibility for SSI assistance as a result of work earnings; clarified Medicaid coverage policies with regard to aliens and homeless individuals; and gave states the option of expanding Medicaid coverage for respiratory care services in the home.
1988	*Family Support Act of 1988* reformed the federal welfare system and revised the AFDC program to emphasize work and child support. Established child support programs, job opportunities, and basic skills and training programs. Established a federal requirement that welfare recipients seek employment, and required that each state establish an education, training, and work (NETWork) program. Established rules regarding recipient rights.
1996	*Personal Responsibility and Work Opportunity Reconciliation Act of 1996* (commonly known as the "Welfare Reform Bill") amended the Social Security Act to reform the federal welfare system. It imposes a 5-year lifetime limit on welfare benefits and changes AFDC to temporary assistance to needy families (TANF). It also restricts benefits for legal immigrants.

table 4-3 Selected Amendments: Public Health Service Act of 1944

Year	Amendment
1946	*Hospital Survey and Construction Act,* often called the Hill-Burton Act. Authorized grants to states for construction of health care facilities.
1962	*Migrant Health Act* authorized grants to family clinics for migratory workers.
1964	*Nurse Training Act* provided funding for nursing education and construction of nursing schools.
1968	*Health Manpower Act* extended and improved programs relating to the training of nursing, health professions, and allied health professions.
1970	*Communicable Disease Control Amendments* authorized grants for communicable disease control, vaccination assistance, and studies to determine community-based communicable disease programs designed to contribute to national protection against tuberculosis, venereal disease, rubella, measles, poliomyelitis, diphtheria, tetanus, pertussis, and other selected communicable diseases. *Family Planning Services and Population Research Act* established population research and voluntary family planning programs that would promote public health and welfare by expanding, improving, and better coordinating the family planning services and populations research activities of the federal government.
1971	*Nurse Training Act* provided for training increased numbers of nurses through construction grants to schools of nursing and student loan guarantees, advanced training traineeships, scholarships, loan repayment and forgiveness, and capitation grants. Prohibited sex discrimination in student selection for awards. *Health Maintenance Organization Act* provided assistance for the establishment and expansion of HMOs.
1974	*National Health Planning and Resource Development Act* authorized the development of national health policy and effective state and area health planning resources development programs. Established health service areas and health systems agencies and required state health planning and development agencies.
1977	*Rural Health Clinics Act* established rural health clinics in underserved sections of the country.
1981	*Omnibus Budget Reconciliation Act* enacted many budget and program cuts under the Public Health Service Act. It revised health planning policy, eliminated Public Health Service Hospitals at the end of fiscal year 1981, consolidated many of the categorical programs of the act into block grants to states, but left in place categorical funding for immunizations, tuberculosis, venereal disease, family planning, and migrant health.
1988	*Health Omnibus Programs Extension Act* created a new title to the act, Title XIV: Health services with respect to acquired immune deficiency syndrome (AIDS). This new title provided comprehensive AIDS services. Extended nurse traineeships and health professions education.
1990	*Home Health Care and Alzheimer's Disease Amendments* authorized demonstration projects for home health care services on Alzheimer's disease, established the Task Force on Aging Research to implement research on the aging process and on diagnosis and treatment of disease, disorders, and disability related to aging to assist the aged individual in retaining independence. *Year 2000 Health Objectives Planning Act* established a program of grants to states for the development of state plans for meeting the objectives established by Healthy People 2000.
1992	*Preventive Health Amendments* placed major emphasis by the federal government on preventive health and primary prevention activities. Changed the name of the Centers for Disease Control to Centers for Disease Control and Prevention. Provided for more comprehensive services to Migrant Health Centers in the areas of maternal and child health and community education. Provided for international exchange programs for public health officials from the United States and abroad who are interested in working in another country.

to mobilize the human and financial resources of the nation to combat poverty. It included work training and study programs, established the Office of Economic Opportunity, authorized Volunteers in Service to America (VISTA), the Job Corps, Upward Bound, Neighborhood Youth Corps, Head Start, neighborhood health centers, and community action programs. An impetus to antipoverty programs, it also incorporated urban and rural community action programs and assistance to small businesses and work experience programs.

OLDER AMERICANS ACT OF 1965 (PUBLIC LAW 89-73) This act was passed to provide assistance in the development of programs to help older Americans. It provided grants to states for community planning and services and for training and research in the field of gerontology and aging. It established the Administration on Aging, which is now part of the Department of Health and Human Services. This act gave national attention to the needs of the elderly, established state and local agencies on aging, and facilitated services to older Americans. It is discussed extensively in Chapter 20.

NATIONAL ENVIRONMENTAL POLICY ACT (PUBLIC LAW 91-190) This is one of the best known and most significant pieces of U.S. environmental health legislation. It established national environmental policy and authorized formation of the Environmental Protection Agency (EPA). Environmental health legislation is discussed in depth in Chapter 6.

OCCUPATIONAL SAFETY AND HEALTH ACT OF 1970 (PUBLIC LAW 91-956) The Occupational Safety and Health Act is the most comprehensive piece of legislation on occupational health and safety in the United States. Championed by organized labor, its intent is to protect the health of the worker, and it made worker health a public concern. The United States was the last major industrial nation to enact such a law. This act is discussed in depth in Chapter 18.

REHABILITATION ACT OF 1973 (PUBLIC LAW 93-112) The Vocational Rehabilitation Act of 1920 (Public Law 66-236) was an outgrowth of the health care needs evidenced by veterans after World War I and was a forerunner of the 1973 act. The Rehabilitation Act of 1973 replaced the 1920 act but retained its major components. This act extended and revised the authorization of grants to states for vocational rehabilitation services; emphasized services to persons with severe disabilities; expanded federal responsibilities and training programs; defined services necessary for rehabilitation programs; established the National Architectural and Transportation Barriers Board to enforce legislation designed to remove architectural barriers for persons who are severely disabled; and began affirmative action programs to facilitate employment for them. This act is discussed further in Chapter 19.

EDUCATION FOR ALL HANDICAPPED CHILDREN ACT OF 1975 (PUBLIC LAW 94-142) This act amended the Education of the Handicapped Act (Public Law 90-247). Through it the federal government took an active role in ensuring the educational rights of people who are handicapped. The law helps to provide free, public education for children who are handicapped (see Chapters 15 and 16). Before its passage, many American children had been denied access to the public educational system because they were handicapped. Periodically the government has tried to deregulate the act and to become less involved in protecting these educational rights, but active lobbying by parent groups and professionals has prevented this.

STEWART B. MCKINNEY HOMELESS ASSISTANCE ACT (PUBLIC LAW 100-77) This act dealt with the increasing problem of homelessness in America and provided urgently needed assistance to improve the lives of the homeless, with special emphasis on elderly persons, the disabled, and families with children. It established the Interagency Council on the Homeless, Emergency Food and Shelter Program National Board, Emergency Food and Shelter Grants, Supportive Housing Demonstration Program, Primary Health Services and Substance Abuse Services Grant Program, and Food Assistance for the Homeless Food Stamp Program. It authorized emergency food supplies for the homeless, HUD programs for emergency shelter, supportive housing, programs for primary health care, substance abuse services, community mental health care, adult education for the homeless, education for homeless children and youth, job training for the homeless, and studies of homelessness among youth and Native Americans.

INDIVIDUALS WITH DISABILITIES EDUCATION ACT OF 1990 (PUBLIC LAW 101-476) This act was formerly known as the Education for All Handicapped Children Act (just discussed). It mandates a free and appropriate public education for all children and youth with disabilities. Supreme Court decisions relating to this act have mandated that for certain services and benefits a noncategorical rather than a disease-specific approach be applied, which means that children with serious disabilities will not be denied services even when their specific disease or condition is not specified on an eligibility list.

AMERICANS WITH DISABILITIES ACT (PUBLIC LAW 101-336) The Americans with Disabilities Act was signed into law on July 26, 1990. The act is one of the most significant pieces of legislation in this country to help guarantee the rights of the nation's 43 million disabled citizens. It includes a new definition of disability and helped to ensure equal access and opportunity in employment, transportation, education, public accommodations, and telecommunications. This landmark act increased the opportunity for people who are disabled to be integrated into the mainstream of society. It is further discussed in Chapter 19.

YEAR 2000 HEALTH OBJECTIVES PLANNING ACT (PUBLIC LAW 101-582) This act amended the Public Health Service Act of 1944. It established a program of grants to states for the development of state plans for meeting the objectives established by *Healthy People 2000*.

PREVENTIVE HEALTH AMENDMENTS OF 1992 (PUBLIC LAW 102-531) This act amended the Public Health Service Act of 1944. It emphasized and mandated major federal involvement in preventive health and primary prevention activities. It changed the name of the Centers for Disease Control to Centers for Disease Control and Prevention (CDC). The act authorized prevention programs, including injury control; lead poisoning; preventable infertility from sexually transmitted diseases; vaccination services; screening and detection programs for breast, cervical, and prostate cancer; and international cooperation in preventive health measures. Further, the act provided for more comprehensive maternal and child health services and community education programs in Migrant Health Centers, and established the National Foundation for the Centers for Disease Control and Prevention. The purpose of the foundation is to promote the public's health and support and implement activities for the prevention and control of diseases, disorders, injuries, and disabilities. Foundation activities include (1) programs of fellowships for state and local public health officials to work and study in association with the CDC, (2) international exchange programs for public health officials who are interested in working in a foreign country, (3) studies, projects, and research on prevention, (4) forums for government officials and private entities to exchange information, (5) meetings, conferences, courses, and training workshops, (6) programs to improve the collection and analysis of data on the health status of various populations, and (7) programs for writing, editing, printing, and publishing books and materials.

FAMILY AND MEDICAL LEAVE ACT (PUBLIC LAW 103-5) This law requires covered employers to provide up to 12 weeks (during a 1-year period) of unpaid, job-protected leave to "eligible" employees for family and medical reasons including the birth or adoption of a child; care of an ill child, spouse, or parent; or the employee's own illness. The employer must provide adequate protection of the employee's employment and health benefits during the leave. Upon return from FMLA leave, most employees must be restored to their original or equivalent positions with equivalent pay and benefits; and the use of such leave cannot result in the loss of any employment benefit that accrued before the leave. The U.S. Department of Labor investigates FMLA violations, and employees may bring civil action against employers for violations of the law.

STATE WORKERS' COMPENSATION ACTS The state workers' compensation acts are the oldest form of government health and welfare insurance in this country. The first state act was legislated in 1911, and by 1948 all states had such acts. The federal government provides workers' compensation benefits for federal employees. Workers' compensation programs vary greatly from state to state in the amount of cash and health care benefits provided. State workers' compensation laws are usually administered by the state labor department or an independent workers' compensation agency. Workers' compensation is discussed further under insurance programs in this chapter.

THE U.S. HEALTH CARE SYSTEM

Comprehensive health services exist in the United States, but they are unequally distributed, fragmented, and expensive. Almost any health care service is available in the United States, but these services may be neither accessible nor affordable. Amazingly, the average life expectancy of Americans continues to increase, the death rate is historically low, and the infant mortality rate continues to decline. Sometimes we make advances in spite of ourselves. However, compared to other developed nations, the United States lags behind on many indicators of health.

There is great complexity and diversity in the U.S. health care delivery system. This presents major problems for nurses when they attempt to educate clients about health care resources and coordinate services (the organization of health and welfare services is discussed in Chapter 5).

Millions of Americans are uninsured or underinsured. It is estimated that 40 million Americans do not have health insurance. The accompanying box gives information on the uninsured and underinsured in the United States. Figure 4-3 shows the percent of people in the United States who are uninsured by age.

A Look at the Uninsured and Underinsured in the United States—Who Are They?

- Almost 15% of the U.S. population, or 40 million people, are uninsured; more people than at any time since the passage of Medicare and Medicaid in 1965.
- About 86% of the uninsured are employed workers and their families.
- Men are more frequently uninsured than women.
- Young adults are the age group most likely to be uninsured.
- 5 million young women have insurance policies that exclude maternity care.
- Many senior citizens are underinsured since Medicare only pays for about 50% of their medical expenses.
- The poor are more likely than other socioeconomic groups to be uninsured: 22% of families with incomes of less than $25,000 are uninsured, while only 8% of families with incomes of greater than $50,000 are uninsured.
- 33% of Hispanic Americans and 20% of African-Americans are uninsured as compared to 10.7% of the white population.
- Today there are 50 to 70 million Americans who, due to inadequate health insurance coverage, could likely become bankrupt or suffer severe financial distress in the event of a major illness.
- Professionals are not exempt from being uninsured: there are almost 30,000 uninsured physicians, more than 300,000 uninsured teachers/professors, and almost 53,000 uninsured clergy. However, no legislators are uninsured.

Data from Himmelstein DU, Woolhandler S: *The national health program chartbook*, Cambridge, Mass., 1992, The Center for National Health Program Studies, Harvard Medical School/Cambridge Hospital, pp. 3-7, 13; White House Domestic Policy Council: *Health Security: The President's Report to the American People*, Washington, D.C., 1993, U.S. Government Printing Office; National Center for Health Statistics: *Health, United States, 1994*, Hyattsville, Md., 1995, U.S. Public Health Service.

Ensuring accessibility to preventive health care services has become a national health goal. Even when preventive services are available, many people do not use them (barriers to use of services are discussed in Chapter 10). Preventive services such as free or low-cost immunization clinics are available throughout the country, yet many children and adults are not adequately immunized. Many preventable conditions such as heart disease, cancer, stroke, injuries, HIV infection, alcoholism, drug abuse, low birth weight infants, and communicable diseases continue to occur in the United States at great personal and economic expense (National Center for Health Statistics, 1995). Of the approximately half-million Americans who die of cancer each year, it is estimated that more than 115,000 could have been saved if they had utilized early diagnosis and treatment services (American Cancer Society, 1996, p. 1).

Preventive services are too important to be ignored! Yet health care is still sought and offered in this country

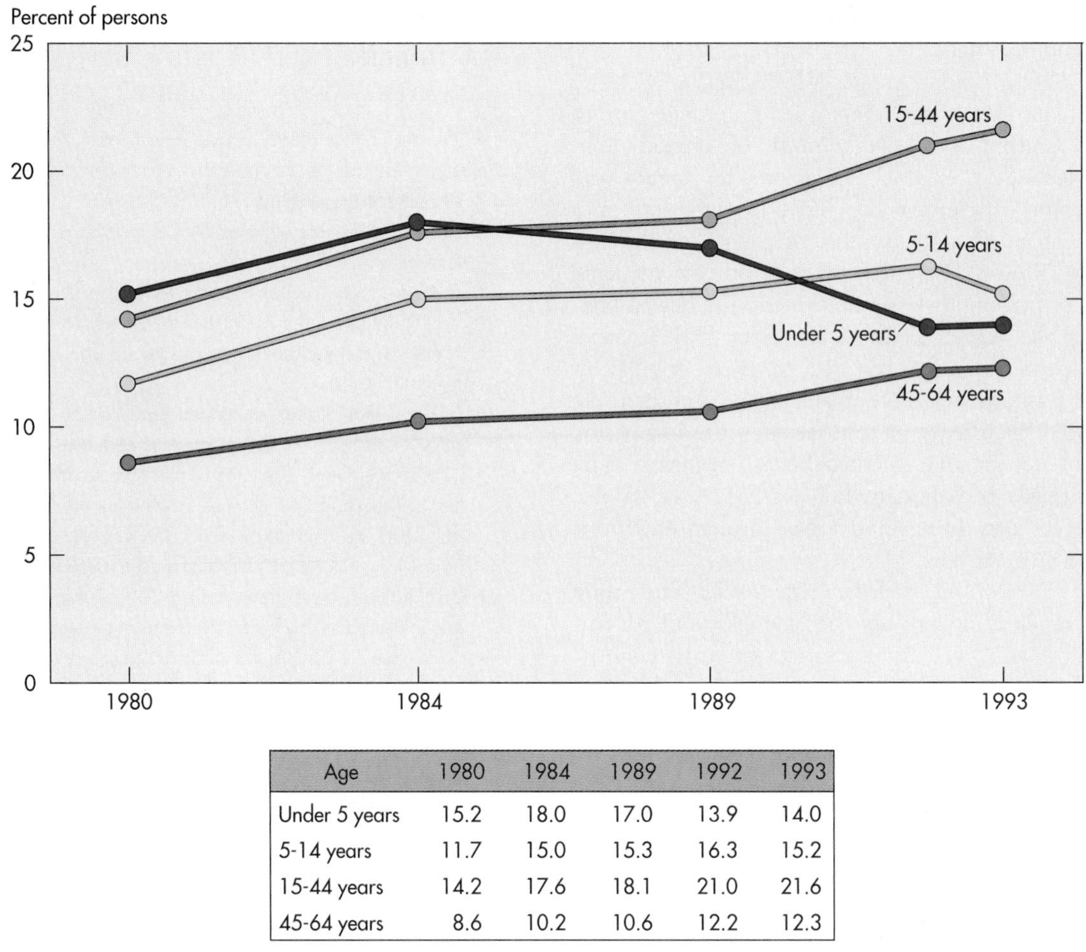

Age	1980	1984	1989	1992	1993
Under 5 years	15.2	18.0	17.0	13.9	14.0
5-14 years	11.7	15.0	15.3	16.3	15.2
15-44 years	14.2	17.6	18.1	21.0	21.6
45-64 years	8.6	10.2	10.6	12.2	12.3

Figure 4-3 Percentage of persons under 65 years of age who are uninsured, by age. *(From National Center for Health Statistics:* Health, United States, 1994, *Hyattsville, Md., 1995, U.S. Public Health Service, p. 35.)*

primarily on a "treatment" rather than a preventive basis. The CDC estimates that nearly half the premature deaths among Americans could have been avoided by changes in individual behaviors and another 17% by reducing environmental risks—almost 1 million American deaths each year are preventable (USDHHS, 1995, pp. 3-4). Americans are taking a serious look at our present health care system. Some interesting facts on this system are in the following box.

Health Care Facilities and the Health Care Work Force

Health care resources in the United States are fragmented, unequally distributed, and increasingly expensive. Presently there is little coordination between health care resources, and not all Americans have equal access to health care.

The United States has an abundance of health care facilities. There are thousands of state and local health departments and countless private agencies who provide health care services. There are 5619 acute-care hospitals, 547 long-term hospitals, and 17,685 nursing homes in the United States (NCHS, 1995, pp. 211-212, 265). Of these acute-care and long-term hospitals, 334 are federally owned, 3260 are nonprofit, 790 are for-profit, and 1682 are run by state and local governments (NCHS). The trend is toward for-profit ownership of these facilities.

The number of acute-care hospitals has been steadily declining over the last 20 years, especially in rural areas. It is predicted that by the end of this century as many as half of the nation's hospitals will close and there will be a massive expansion into primary care in ambulatory and community settings (Pew Health Professions Commission, 1995, p. i). This has great implications for community health nursing practice because the site of care is increasingly the community.

Government ownership of hospitals includes armed forces hospitals, prison hospitals, state long-term psychiatric care facilities and facilities for the mentally retarded, state university medical school hospitals, and city and county hospitals for the indigent. The U.S. government closed its Public Health Service hospitals at the end of fiscal year 1981.

Some Interesting Facts About the U.S. Health Care System*

- The United States spends approximately $1 trillion a year on health care.
- The United States spends more on health care than the education and defense budgets put together.
- Every year the United States spends more money on health care. In 1965 the federal government spent 4% of its budget on health care—today it spends almost 20%.
- Without health care reform, spending on health care will jump from 14% of the Gross Domestic Product (GDP) to 19% by the year 2000.
- Health care fraud accounts for approximately 10% of national health expenditures (almost $100 billion a year).
- Only 1% of the U.S. health care budget is spent on public health. Approximately 94% is spent on secondary and tertiary care—a treatment rather than a prevention model.
- The United States spends more than any other industrialized nation on health care.
- The United States and South Africa are the only industrialized countries without a form of national health insurance guaranteeing "health for all."
- The United States ranks 22nd worldwide in infant mortality. This is almost twice as high as Japan and almost 40% higher than Canada.
- Forty million Americans do not have health insurance. The working poor make up the majority (86%) of uninsured and underinsured Americans.
- Health care costs add about $1100 to the cost of every car made in America.
- Without health care reform, workers will lose almost $600 a year in wages by the year 2000. If health care reform had occurred 20 years ago, today's workers would be earning over $1000 a year more in wages.
- Health expenditures are one of the leading causes of bankruptcy in the United States.
- Failure to control overall health care spending will make it difficult, if not impossible, to bring the federal budget into balance. Americans can no longer afford their present health care system!

Modified from Maternal and Child Health Bureau: *Child Health USA '95*, Washington, D.C., 1996, U.S. Government Printing Office; National Center for Health Statistics: *Health, United States, 1994*, Hyattsville, Md., 1995, U.S. Public Health Service; White House Domestic Policy Council: *Health Security: The President's Report to the American People*, Washington, D.C., 1993, U.S. Government Printing Office; General Accounting Office: *Health care reform*, Washington, D.C., 1993, GAO; Zarate AO: *International mortality chartbook: levels and trends, 1955-91*, Hyattsville, Md., 1994, Public Health Service.

*Actual numbers change yearly but are used here to illustrate concerns about the nation's current health care system. These concerns are providing an impetus for health care reform.

Research studies have consistently shown that rural and inner-city areas have a significantly smaller health work force than suburban areas and that affluent areas have more health care resources than areas where there are high levels of poverty. The government offers financial incentives to universities that make a commitment to increase their output of health practitioners who will serve in areas with shortages of health care personnel and students who will practice in such areas.

Presently more than 10 million people are employed in health care occupations in the United States (NCHS, 1995, p. 192). Health care is one of the nation's biggest businesses, and employment in the health care industry is growing more rapidly than civilian employment in general. For every 10,000 Americans there are approximately 24 physicians, 74 registered nurses, 6 dentists, 6 pharmacists, and 10 optometrists in practice today (NCHS). There are almost 2 million registered nurses in the United States. Almost two thirds of physicians practicing in the United States today are specialists.

It is predicted that by the end of this century there will be a surplus of 100,000 to 150,000 physicians as the demand for specialty care shrinks, a surplus of 200,000 to 300,000 registered nurses as hospitals close, and a surplus of 40,000 pharmacists as drug dispensing becomes more automated (Pew Health Professions Commission, 1995, p. i). At the same time the need for public health professionals will increase and primary care providers and nurses can help to fill this need. The competencies needed for health professionals in the future are discussed in Chapter 25.

Health Care Cost

In general, health care in the United States is disproportionately inflationary and expensive. Rising health expenditures have placed an increased burden on federal, state, and local government budgets. In 1965 expenditures for health care amounted to 4% of federal government expenditures, and today that number has skyrocketed to almost 20% (NCHS, 1995, p. 31).

Despite decades of policy aimed at reducing health care costs, U.S. health care spending increases every year. Health care spending has reached almost $1 trillion each year in the United States (14% of the gross domestic product [GDP], or $3299 per person per year (NCHS, 1995, p. 6). Most developed nations have been able to stabilize their health spending at less than 10% of their GDP.

The United States spends more on health care than any other country in the world and often has less to show for it. The United States ranks 22nd in infant mortality, 16th in mortality for males and 14th in mortality for females

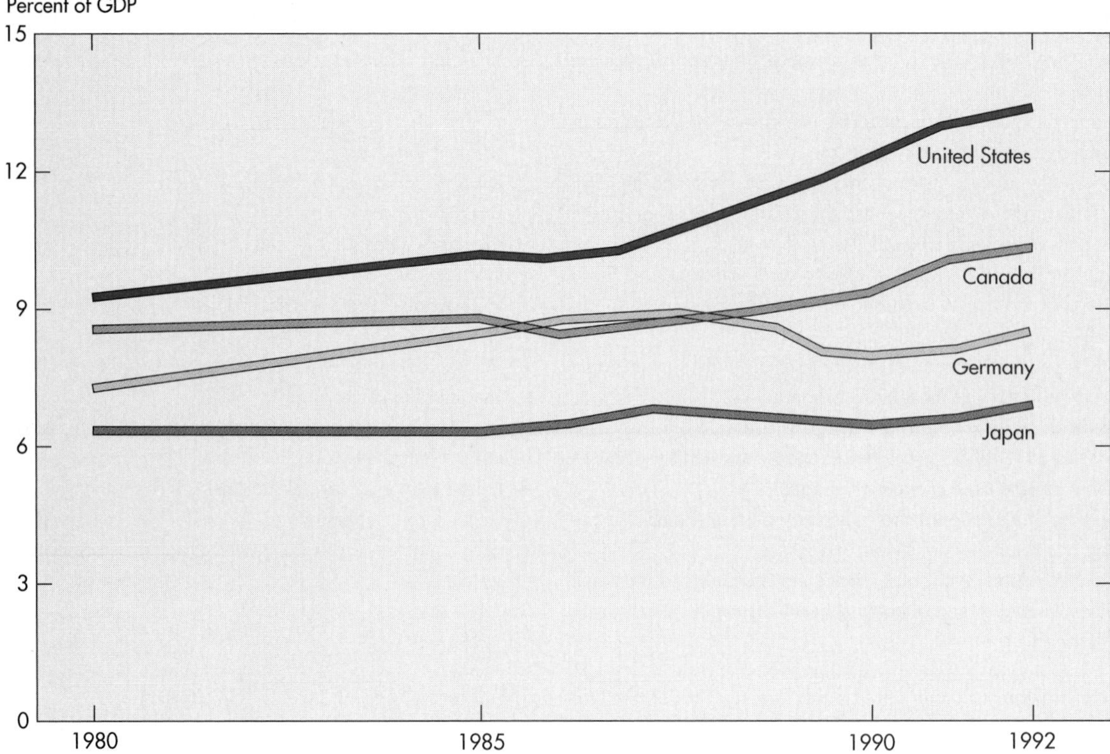

Figure 4-4 Health expenditures as a percentage of gross domestic product: selected countries. *(From National Center for Health Statistics:* Health, United States, 1994, *Hyattsville, Md., 1995, U.S. Public Health Service, p. 30.)*

(Maternal and Child Health Bureau, 1996; Zarate, 1994). Figure 4-4 compares health expenditures of the United States and selected countries related to GDP.

The rise in national health expenditures from 1940 to 2000 are shown in Table 4-4. The figures are astounding; measures need to be enacted to contain costs! Failure to control overall health care costs will make if difficult, if not impossible, to bring the federal budget into balance (GAO, 1993, p. 4).

Many people do not use health care services because they are unable to afford them. The nation is presently looking at ways to reform the health care system to decrease costs, enhance access to services, improve service coordination, make services more equitable, and focus more on preventive services.

Health Care Reform

After looking at the facts in the box on the previous page, it is easy to see that the U.S. health care system needs reform. In 1993 President Clinton's *Health Security Act* proposed a national health program. That legislation did not pass. Single-payer national health programs such as Canada's have been proposed but have not been legislated (Clancy, Himmelstein, Woolhandler, 1993, p. 30). Health care professionals must monitor carefully all proposed national health programs to ensure that they actually provide the services needed by the population as a whole.

table 4-4 National Health Expenditures—United States: Selected Years

Year	Cost (Rounded to Nearest Billion)	Per Capita Cost	Percent of GNP
1940	$ 4	$ 29	4
1950	$ 13	$ 80	4.5
1960	$ 27	$ 143	5.3
1970	$ 74	$ 346	7.4
1980	$ 251	$1068	9.3
1990	$ 697	$2680	12.6
2000	$1616	$5712	16.4

From National Center for Health Statistics: *Health, United States, 1994,* Hyattsville, Md., 1995, U.S. Public Health Service, pp. 219, 223.

Among present proposals for achieving cost containment two strategies are prominent: managed competition and direct controls (GAO, 1993, p. 13). Direct controls involve governmental regulation; managed competition may or may not use governmental regulation. The use of managed competition in both private and governmental programs has increased dramatically. Government regulations are increasingly controlling the costs in government-funded programs. Government-funded health care programs such as Medicare use direct controls to dictate the size of payments under the program and the types of services allowed.

The American Public Health Association (APHA) has championed the platform of "Health Care for All" in the United States by the year 2000. The American Nurses Association has developed a national health care agenda, *Nursing's Agenda for Health Care Reform*, that advocates access, quality, and services at affordable costs. The agenda has been endorsed by more than 40 nursing organizations and calls for (1) a basic core of essential health care services available to everyone (universal coverage); (2) a restructured health care system focusing on consumers and their health, with services to be delivered in convenient sites by the most appropriate provider; (3) use of primary care providers, including nurse practitioners, clinical nurse specialists, and certified nurse midwives; and (4) a shift from the predominant focus on illness and cure to an orientation toward wellness and care (ANA, 1991). In addition, the ANA agenda proposes stringent cost-containment mechanisms, a federally defined standard package of essential health care services, insurance reform, case management for clients with continuing care needs, and provisions for long-term care. Nursing is promoting new models of health care delivery that emphasize wellness and care versus illness and cure.

State governments feel the need to establish reforms because they have a major stake in financing and providing health care; an average 20% of a state's budget goes to fund health care programs (GAO, 1992, p. 15). Many states are developing plans that will reduce health care costs and at the same time provide all state residents with access to health care coverage by blending public and private funding to provide this access (GAO, p. 24).

The Pew Health Professions Commission (1995, p. i; O'Neil, 1993) predicts that by the year 2000 there will be a new American health care system. Characteristics of this emerging health care system are given in the accompanying box. The Commission further predicts that this evolving system will be as follows:

- More managed with better integration of services and financing;
- More accountable to those who purchase and use health services;
- More aware of and responsive to the needs of enrolled populations;
- More innovative and diverse in how it provides for health;
- More inclusive in how it defines health;
- Less focused on treatment and more concerned with education, prevention, and care management;
- More oriented to improving the health of the entire population; and
- More reliant on outcomes data and evidence.

Characteristics of the Emerging Health Care System

Orientation toward health
Population perspective
Intensive use of information
Focus on the consumer
Knowledge of treatment outcomes
Constrained resources
Coordination of services
Reconsideration of human values
Expectations of accountability
Growing interdependence

From Pew Health Professions Commission: *Critical challenges: revitalizing the health professions for the twenty-first century*, San Francisco, Ca., 1995, UCSF Center for the Health Professions, p. 2.

Managed competition, or "managed care," is a key feature of health care reform. Managed care is both a structure and a process. From a structural perspective managed care establishes organizational and financing mechanisms for delivery of services. From a process perspective a care management process is emphasized. Managed care as a process is discussed in Chapter 10 and managed care as a structure is discussed here.

Managed Care

Managed care has rapidly gained national acceptance as a strategy for ensuring accessible, effective care at affordable cost (Masso, 1995, p. 46; Richards, 1996, p. 13). An important purpose of managed care is to keep people healthy (Shamansky, 1996, p. 161).

There is no universally accepted definition of managed care, and the term is used to refer to a wide variety of prepayment "capitation" plans (Hicks, Stallmeyer, Coleman, 1993, p. 1). Traditionally, health care reimbursement has focused on a fee-for-service system in which health care services are paid for as billed. *Capitation* is the acceptance of a prepaid, per-person payment for specified health services. The provider manages the clients' care, referring them to additional covered services as necessary, and agrees to provide services for a fixed prepayment regardless how many services are used and how many referrals are made (Gillis, Thomas, 1996). Capitation can reduce the use of unnecessary tests, services, and procedures and is part of many managed care plans.

Managed care began in the 1930s when prepaid group plans were established. Managed care organizations pay for and provide services. These plans provide comprehensive health care services and focus on prevention. Managed care is characterized by the following:

- Direct service provision to enrollees on a prepayment basis, with each enrollee paying a fixed amount regardless of the volume or expense of the services used.

- A defined package of benefits.
- Service provision through physicians, nurses, and other health care providers who are under contractual agreement with the managed care organization. Subscribers are limited to usage of the health workers employed by the plan, unless they choose a point-of-service plan (discussed later in this chapter) in which they have a different level of benefits based on their choice of a participating or nonparticipating provider.
- Comprehensive general practitioner services that include both inpatient and outpatient care and have an emphasis on preventive health practices.
- Internal, self-regulatory mechanisms to ensure quality of care and cost control.

The accompanying box provides some additional information on managed care. States are looking to managed care to control rising health care costs. Almost all states are operating or developing Medicaid managed care programs. About 25% of the nation's Medicaid recipients are enrolled in managed care plans, and this percentage increases daily (Children's Defense Fund, 1996, p. 21; Hsu, 1995). For example, Tennessee obtained a Medicaid waiver to offer TennCare, a managed care program. Under TennCare recipients select a health care provider from a number of health maintenance organizations (HMOs). Managed care is cost effective, provides for care management and continuity, and emphasizes preventive care. One familiar form of managed care is the HMO. HMOs and other methods of health care financing will be discussed later in this chapter.

Today more than 100 million Americans are enrolled in managed care organizations (HIAA, 1995, p. 7). Managed care is the trend of the future. It will continue to grow because of its popularity with insurance carriers, employers, and the government as an effective way to control health care costs, eliminate unnecessary care, keep people well, and provide health care more efficiently (Commonwealth Fund, 1995; Johnson, 1995, p. 45). However, managed care is not a quick fix to the nation's health care problems.

Recently concerns have emerged with the managed care delivery system (Bowman, 1996). Research has shown that managed care organization enrollees had concerns about their plan's access to services and quality of care (Commonwealth Fund, 1995; Davis, Collins, Schoen, Morris, 1995), and fears have been expressed that people's health will be given less importance than costs and profits (Hsu, 1995). Questions such as, "Do the managed care organizations consistently act in the best interests of the client? Will health care providers be restricted in telling patients about treatment options? Will health care providers be criticized for acting as client advocates?" and "Will certain expensive procedures be 'rationed'?" are left to be answered. Also, because it is designed primarily to cut costs and serve those already insured, the managed care structure does not always translate well when applied to the populations traditionally served by public health (Managed care, 1996).

A Look at Managed Care

THEORY

Patients receive care through a single "seamless" system as they move from wellness to sickness back to wellness again. Continuity of care, prevention, and early diagnosis are stressed.

WHAT IS MANAGED?

Who: Provider network
What: Services covered
Where: Site of service
When: Duration of treatment

HOW IS CARE MANAGED?

Provider selection
Quality assurance
Care management/utilization management
Patient and staff education and feedback
Financial arrangements

Modified from Gillis L, Thomas D: *Developing clinical systems for working in a managed care environment,* Washington, D.C., June 7-9, 1996, Conference on Health Care for the Homeless.

METHODS OF HEALTH CARE FINANCING IN THE UNITED STATES

The methods of health care financing in the United States are diverse, complicated, and confusing. Both government and private sector resources provide methods of health care financing.

To help make this diverse system of financing clearer, a discussion of financing methods follows: the box on the following page summarizes methods of health care financing. Keep in mind that future methods of financing health care in the United States may be significantly different, and it is anticipated that an increasing number of Americans will be enrolled in managed care plans.

Individual Payment (Direct, Out of Pocket)

Individual payment for health care services is exactly what it says—the individual pays for the health care directly. For the millions of Americans who are uninsured and underinsured, individual payment is a hard reality, and they often seek only treatment and crisis health care. Such health behaviors present serious consequences for both personal and community health.

Direct payment accounts for more than $20 billion each year, or $2920 per person (NCHS, 1995, p. 229). It is interesting to note that payment for hospital expenses amounts to 2.8% of out-of-pocket expenses, and 33% of out-of-pocket

Methods of Health Care Financing in the United States

INDIVIDUAL PAYMENT (direct, out-of-pocket)

HEALTH INSURANCE

1. Government: Medicare, Workers' Compensation
2. Private: Blue Cross–Blue Shield, commercial insurance, self-insurance, health maintenance organizations (HMOs), preferred provider organizations (PPOs), and point-of-service organizations (POSs)

HEALTH ASSISTANCE

1. Government: Medicaid, Maternal-Child Health (MCH) Programs
2. Private: Numerous services offered by voluntary, community, agencies, and individuals, such as the American Heart Association, the American Lung Association, local churches, and individual donations

HEALTH SERVICE PROGRAMS

1. Government: Programs for veterans, military personnel, merchant marines, Native Americans on reservations, native Hawaiians, and federal employees
2. Private: On-site employee health services and group health maintenance centers

Forms of Health Insurance Coverage in the United States

HOSPITAL

Insurance that covers the cost of inpatient hospital services

SURGICAL

Insurance that covers physicians' fees for surgical care

REGULAR MEDICAL

Insurance that pays for physicians' fees for nonsurgical care; there are usually maximum benefit amounts for specified services

MAJOR MEDICAL

Insurance that provides benefits for most types of medical expenses and usually supplements an existing insurance program, frequently has maximum benefit limits, and is subject to deductibles and coinsurance

SPECIALTY

Insurance that provides payment for the cost of specified services such as dental care and mental health

DISABILITY

Insurance that protects against wages lost from disability; may provide long-term or short-term benefits

CATASTROPHIC

Insurance that protects against the high cost of acute or long-term illness that would otherwise not be covered by insurance

expenses go for nursing home care (NCHS, p. 230). When out-of-pocket expenses become excessive it can place the individual and family at great financial risk, and many Americans file for bankruptcy each year as a result of health care costs. A form of health care financing that helps to protect the individual and family from the financial risk of health care is health insurance.

Health Insurance

Health insurance is a contractual agreement between an insurer and an insuree for the payment of specified health care costs. Health insurance is administered by both government and private agencies. Private health insurance programs serve the majority of the American people, whereas government programs are limited largely to serving the aged and disabled.

Most health insurance programs cover hospital and surgical costs. Many insurance plans do not include regular medical, major medical, disability, or dental insurance. Some insurance plans do not cover the cost of prescription medications or health care equipment. The box, above right, illustrates some general forms of health insurance coverage. Most people are vulnerable to the cost of long-term health care and catastrophic illness. Chapter 21 examines this problem and the actions needed to correct it.

The rising costs of health insurance are prompting employees to limit the services covered. Even with health insurance, many people are involved in some form of individual payment because of insurance deductibles, premiums, fixed payments, and uncovered expenses. A *deductible* is a set expense that must be paid by the insuree before the insurer will reimburse for services (e.g., $500 deductible). A *premium* is the monthly amount that an insuree pays for an insurance plan. *Fixed payments* are arrangements whereby only a specified amount for a health service is paid by the insurer, regardless of the cost to the client (e.g., $600 for antepartal care). *Uncovered services* are services that the insurer does not pay for, leaving payment to the insuree (e.g., prescription drugs under Medicare).

GOVERNMENT HEALTH INSURANCE Government health insurance did not exist in any significant form until 1965, with the passage of Medicare under the Social Security Act. There are two major forms of government health insurance: (1) Medicare and (2) workers' compensation programs. Medicare is a federal program, and workers' compensation is a state program.

MEDICARE. Medicare is a federal health insurance program for aged and disabled persons created by the 1965 amendments to the Social Security Act. It is the largest health insurance program in the United States today. People apply for Medicare at local branches of the federal Social Security Administration.

An excellent publication describing the Medicare program, *The Medicare Handbook*, is updated yearly by the Health Care Financing Administration. The Social Security Administration publishes *Guide to Health Insurance for People with Medicare*, which can be obtained free of charge by calling the administration's toll-free number, 1-800-638-6833. Medicare has two parts: Medicare A and Medicare B.

Medicare A insures almost 37 million aged and disabled Americans at a cost to the federal government of almost $104 billion a year (Social Security Administration [SSA], 1995, p. 320). It is a hospital insurance program, financed through individual Social Security contributions. In addition to inpatient hospital care, Medicare A covers selected posthospitalization home health care services such as skilled nursing care, physical or speech therapy, and hospice care. It sets limits on the number of hospital and extended care facility days that will be covered and is subject to yearly changes in services and deductibles.

Medicare B is a voluntary supplemental medical insurance program. In 1995 the monthly premium was $46.10, and some health care reform proposals are advocating significantly increasing this premium. Examples of services covered are physicians' services and selected services by clinical psychologists, certified nurse anesthetists, nurse practitioners, clinical social workers, dentists, podiatrists, optometrists, and chiropractors; emergency treatment; outpatient physical therapy and speech therapy; specified equipment; radiation therapy; and other services on a qualifying basis. It excludes coverage for prescription drugs, glasses, dentures, hearing aids, yearly physical examinations, dental care, and routine foot care. Because of these exclusions, many persons 65 and older have obtained supplemental private health insurance "Medigap" policies (these policies are discussed in this chapter under private health insurance).

WORKERS' COMPENSATION. Workers' compensation was the first form of social and health insurance to develop widely in the United States. It is established by state law and is state administered. It provides both cash benefits and medical care to workers who have an occupational illness or injury and survivor benefits to the dependents of workers whose deaths resulted from job-related accidents or occupational diseases (SSA, 1995, p. 113).

Almost 90% of the U.S. work force is covered by workers' compensation (SSA, 1995, p. 346). Benefits paid under workers' compensation programs amount to almost $43 billion dollars a year (approximately $18 billion is for medical expenses) (SSA, p. 346). Programs are almost exclusively financed by employers, but some new state laws require nominal contributions by the employee for hospital and medical benefits.

The amount of the cash benefit awarded is related to the degree and permanence of the injury, the worker's earnings, and the number of the worker's dependents. Each state sets a minimum and maximum payment range for workers' compensation benefits. Workers' maximum wage replacement averages about 67% of their take-home earnings before taxes. This reduction in pay causes financial hardship for families, in addition to the other adjustments the family is making in relation to the disability.

Benefits are awarded regardless of who is at fault for the occurrence. Loss of ability to work is generally a criterion for awarding benefits. If the worker is injured on the job but suffers no loss of ability to work, such as with certain types of hearing loss, the injury may not be compensable. In some states workers may receive benefits only for a specified period of time, and there may be waiting periods before the compensation can begin. However, if the condition appears to be permanent, most states provide for the payment of weekly benefits for life or the entire period of disability (SSA, 1995, p. 114).

PRIVATE HEALTH INSURANCE The ancient Chinese may have had the first form of health insurance based on the custom of paying the doctor when in good health and discontinuing payment during periods of illness, and the Greeks and Romans offered some early forms of health insurance (HIAA, 1995, p. 1). Some consider the program started by Montgomery Ward and Company in 1911, which provided weekly benefits for the company's sick or injured employees, the first group health insurance plan in the United States (HIAA, p. 1).

In 1929 a group of teachers contracted with Baylor Hospital in Dallas, Texas to provide specific health services at a predetermined cost (HIAA, 1995, p. 2). The monthly premium was 50 cents, and the Baylor Plan offered 21 days of semiprivate care at Baylor Hospital in Dallas, Texas (Wilner, Walkley, O'Neill, 1978, pp. 138-139). Out of this plan emerged the Blue Cross–Blue Shield concept of 1939. In 1940 less than 10% of the civilian population was covered by private health insurance (HIAA, 1983, p. 13). Today almost 70% of the population (more than 180 million Americans) are covered by private health insurance, and this insurance pays more than $253 billion a year in claims (HIAA, 1995, p. 41).

Health insurance plans are often provided as part of employee work benefits. The most common forms of health insurance in this country are the traditional (fee-for-service) plans of Blue Cross–Blue Shield, commercial insurance, and self-insurance, and the managed care insurance plans of HMOs, PPOs, independent practice associations (IPAs), and POS plans. In traditional plans people can usually see any doctor and use any hospital; in managed care plans these options are limited. Forms of health insurance are discussed below.

MEDIGAP. Medigap is private insurance that helps pay for health care services not covered under Medicare A and B. It is voluntary insurance that many older Americans purchase. The Omnibus Budget Reconciliation Act of 1990 (PL 101-508) required that standards for Medigap policies include an open enrollment period for new Medicare bene-

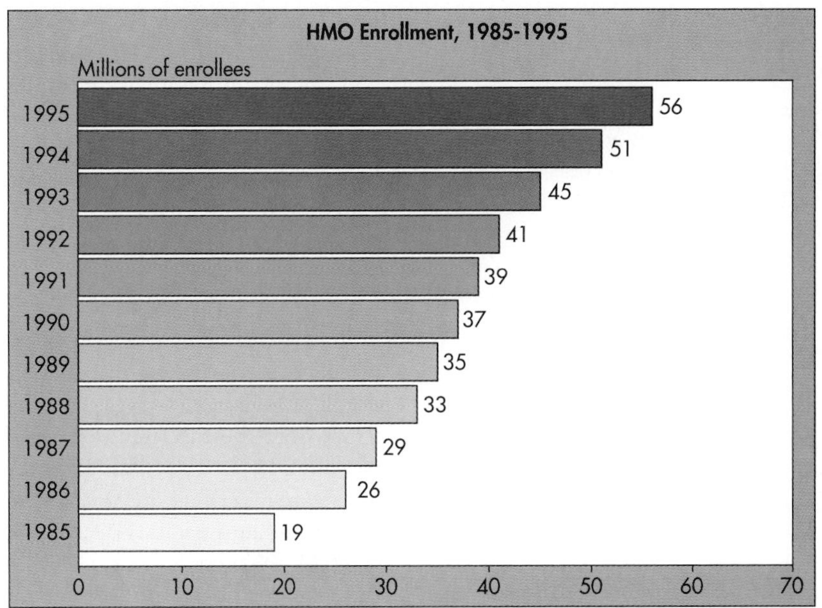

Figure 4-5 HMO enrollment, 1985-1995. *(From Health Insurance Association of America:* Source book of health insurance data, 1995, *Washington, D.C., 1995, The Association, p. 34.)*

ficiaries aged 65 or older, forbade insurers to deny coverage or discriminate in the price of the policy, required that the policy could not be canceled or a renewal refused solely on the basis of the health of the policyholder, and mandated usage of the same format, language, and definitions in all Medigap policies (SSA, 1993, p. 47).

BLUE CROSS–BLUE SHIELD ORGANIZATIONS. Blue Cross–Blue Shield organizations are nonprofit (voluntary) health insuranceorganizations serving both individuals and groups. Blue Cross is the hospital component, and Blue Shield is the major medical component. These organizations pay almost $62 billion in insurance benefits and insure almost 66 million Americans annually (HIAA, 1995, pp. 40-41). The organizations are tax-exempt and exist through specific state legislation. The state insurance commissioner usually has powers of regulation over these programs, with rate increases being subject to public hearings and approval by the commissioner. They are allowed to contract with providers of service for agreed-upon fees, and payment is made directly to the service provider.

COMMERCIAL INSURANCE. Commercial insurance is provided by private profitmaking organizations. These organizations provide health insurance for almost 83 million Americans and cover services similar to those offered under Blue Cross–Blue Shield plans. Commercial insurers compete with Blue Cross–Blue Shield and have pioneered several types of health insurance coverage now common to other carriers, including major medical care, prescription drugs, and posthospitalization home care services. Commercial insurers contract with clients for prepaid premiums and benefits. Clients are expected to pay the service provider and are reimbursed by the insurer for the agreed-upon cost.

SELF-INSURANCE. Self-insurance was stimulated by the passage of the Employee Retirement Income Security Act of 1974 (HIAA, 1978, p. 20). Under this act, corporations and organizations can establish self-funded, nonprofit health plans and escape the taxes and regulations of state insurance laws. This is the method of insurance for more than 60 million Americans (HIAA, 1995, p. 41).

HMOS. HMOs are a form of managed care and are the most rapidly growing method of health insurance in the United States today. The term *health maintenance organization* was coined to emphasize the positive health promotion and primary prevention focus (Hicks, Stallmeyer, Coleman, 1993, p. 2). The Health Maintenance Organization Act of 1973 (Public Law 93-222), an amendment to the Public Health Service Act of 1944, aided in HMO development and authorized the Department of Health and Human Services to set minimal standards for them to be federally certified (Randal, 1995, p. 11). Historically, HMOs have operated as a prepayment (capitation) and managed care system that focused on prevention, cost-containment, and comprehensive service provision. HMOs can be nonprofit or for-profit, with the nonprofit organizations being in the minority (Randal, p. 11).

Today there are almost 600 HMOs in the United States insuring more than 51 million Americans (20% of the insured population) (HIAA, 1995, p. 33). Figure 4-5 shows the steady increase in HMO enrollment since 1985. States with the most residents insured by HMOs are California (38.3%), Oregon (37.5%), Maryland (36.2%), and Arizona

Types of HMOs

STAFF MODEL

The traditional HMO model, with salaried physicians who serve HMO insurees at HMO facilities. Insurees are covered only when they use HMO doctors and hospitals. This plan offers the greatest potential for controlling usage and costs.

GROUP MODEL

Similar to the staff model, but the HMO pays a physician group a negotiated, capitation rate. If they occur, referrals to nonparticipating physicians are usually paid out of this capitation.

NETWORK MODEL

The HMO contracts with two or more independent group practices to provide services and pays a fixed monthly fee per enrollee (capitation). The group decides how fees will be distributed to individual physicians.

INDEPENDENT PRACTICE ASSOCIATIONS (IPA)

Care providers have contracts with the PPO to provide health care services to insurees for a set fee schedule. Members are covered only when using IPA doctors and designated hospitals. Physicians usually maintain their own offices and may contract with more than one plan.

MIXED

A mixed model combines two or more of these models into one HMO.

Data from Health Insurance Association of America: *Source book of health insurance data, 1995*, Washington, D.C., 1995, The Association, p. 31; Randal J: Managed care reshapes health care delivery, *SAMHSA News* III(3): 10-11, 14, Summer 1995; Hicks LL, Stallmeyer JM, Coleman JR: *Role of the nurse in managed care*, Washington, D.C., 1993, American Nurses Publishing, pp. 13-20.

(35.8%) (HIAA, p. 29). Medicaid and Medicare enrollees participating in HMOs are increasing.

HMOs provide a wide range of health care services for a specified group (enrolled, defined population) at a fixed, prepaid cost (capitation rate). They are distinguished from the traditional fee-for-service system by combining the delivery and financing of health care services into one health care delivery system (Hicks, Stallmeyer, Coleman, 1993, p. 2). In general, an HMO member is financially covered for health services only if the member receives them from providers participating in the plan (site-of-service restrictions) or if they are preauthorized to receive services from a provider outside the plan (Hicks, Stallmeyer, Coleman, p. 2). It is these site-of-service restrictions that are least attractive to HMO subscribers and have spurred the development of other prepaid services such as PPOs. The various types of HMOs are presented in the accompanying box.

PPOs. Preferred provider organizations are another form of managed care. They began to develop in the 1980s and offer the subscriber more flexibility in choosing service providers than do HMOs. These rapidly growing plans lack universal definition, falling somewhere between an HMO and traditional health insurance. In these plans a limited number of physicians (often hospitals and other health care providers may be included) become "preferred providers" by contracting with an insurer who agrees to pay them to care for its subscribers on a fee-for-service basis, but at prenegotiated discount rates (Randal, 1995, p. 11). Providers accept the negotiated PPO fee payment in full and do not bill patients for additional amounts (Hicks, Stallmeyer, Coleman, 1993, p. 3). Listings of approved providers are given to subscribers, who are expected to use the PPO-approved service providers. When the insuree strays from the PPO network of providers, he or she will pay more in out-of-pocket expenses (Randal, 1995, p. 11). There are more than 1100 PPOs in the United States serving 45 million people (HIAA, 1995, p. 22).

Point-of-Service (POS) plans. POS plans are sometimes referred to as HMO-PPO hybrids. They use a network of selected contracted, participating providers. Under this plan subscribers usually select a primary care physician who controls referrals for medical specialists (HIAA, 1995, pp. 32-33). These plans are not as well established or used as the HMO and PPO options. For higher premiums and copayments members can use nonHMO health services.

National Health Insurance

The United States is the only major industrial nation in the world not to have national health insurance. Theodore Roosevelt proposed national health insurance as early as 1912, but his efforts were unsuccessful (Harrington, 1989, p. 214). Possibly the closest that early attempts came to enacting a national health program was in 1938. In that year President Franklin D. Roosevelt called a *National Health Conference* in Washington, D.C. At the conference a national health program was discussed and Annie Goodrich, a nurse and former Dean of the School of Nursing at Yale University, spoke in favor of a national program and stated that the strongest agent in such a program was the nurse (Kalisch, Kalisch, 1982, pp. 137-138). Following the conference public interest in a national health program rose, but World War II entered the picture and priorities shifted to the war effort (Kalisch, Kalisch, pp. 139-140). Following World War II, President Harry Truman attempted to legislate a nationwide system of health insurance stating that "the real cost of medical services and the need for them cannot be measured merely by doctors' bills and medical bills. The real cost to society is in unnecessary human suffering and the yearly loss of hundreds of millions of working days" (Kalisch, Kalisch, p. 142). Once again legislation failed to be passed. Numerous presidents since have unsuccessfully attempted to have national health insurance enacted.

As recently as 1993 President Clinton proposed the *Health Security Act*, but the act did not pass. Health care reform legislation, including proposals for national health insurance, continue to be introduced in Congress. Proposed

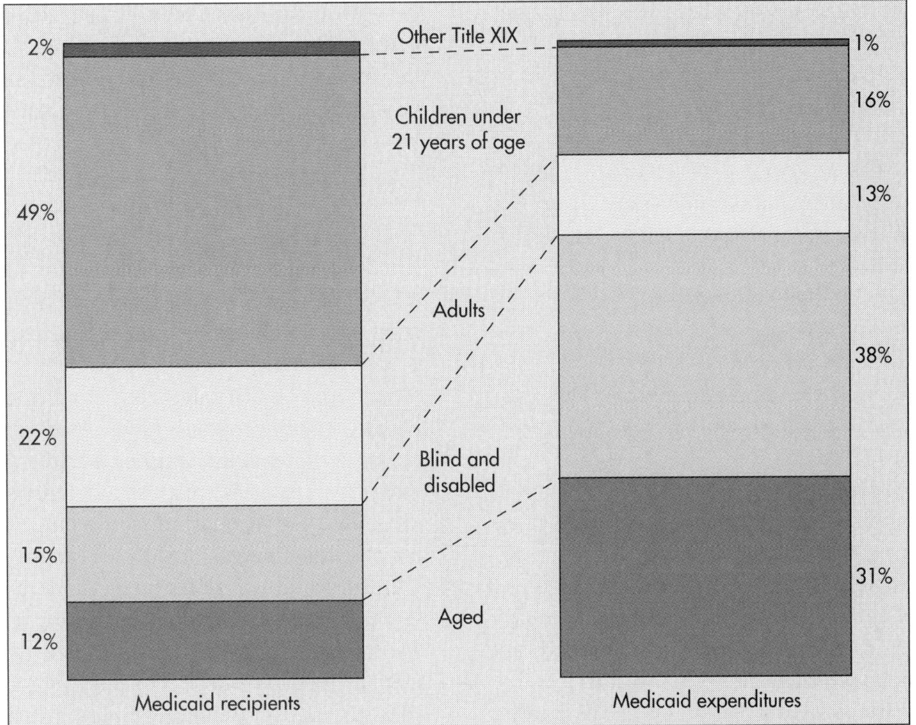

Notes: Other Title XIX includes some participants in the Supplemental Security Income program and other people deemed medically needy in participating states. Children under the age of 21 years includes children in the Aid to Families with Dependent Children (AFDC) program. Adults are those in families with dependent children and include those in the AFDC (now TANF) program. Percentages do not add to 100 because of rounding.

Figure 4-6 Medicaid recipients and expenditures by basis of eligibility. *(From National Center for Health Statistics:* Health United States, 1994, *Hyattsville, Md., 1995, U.S. Public Health Service, p. 42.)*

programs have varied as to whether they would be federally or privately administered, who would be covered, what would be covered, how they would be funded, and what quality control measures would be taken. As discussed previously in this chapter, the United States is in desperate need of health care reform.

Health Assistance

Health assistance programs provide health services to qualifying individuals without contributions or premium payments. Generally the individual does not participate in cost-sharing for the services (e.g., government programs such as Medicaid).

GOVERNMENT HEALTH ASSISTANCE The major government health assistance programs are the Medicaid and a number of maternal-child health programs. These programs are noncontributory in nature (the recipient does not pay premiums or make contributions).

MEDICAID. Medicaid was created by the same 1965 Social Security Act amendments that created Medicare. It is a federal-state entitlement program that provides health services for the medically indigent (people who are unable to meet their health care expenses and who fall within specified economic guidelines). People who are on Temporary Assistance to Needy Families (TANF) and Supplemental Security Income (SSI) are automatically eligible for Medicaid but must apply for it. Medicaid is the largest program providing health care services to America's poor. However, only about half of those with income below the poverty level receive Medicaid (Landers, 1995, p. 7).

Approximately 40 million people are enrolled in the program at a cost of more than $135 billion (SSA, 1995, p. 338). Medicaid payments for institutional and community-based long-term care are more than $46 billion each year (SSA, p. 338). Federal cost-sharing for the program varies from 50% to 83%, depending on the state's economic status (SSA, p. 105). Figure 4-6 shows Medicaid recipients and expenditures based on age.

States are looking to managed care to lower their Medicaid costs, and about one third of the Medicaid population is now enrolled in managed care plans, most of them in traditional HMOs (Managed care, 1996, p. 1). States are presently in the process of evaluating these plans in terms of access and quality of care (Managed care, p. 6).

Within broad federal guidelines each state (1) establishes its own eligibility standards, (2) determines the type, amount, duration, and scope of services, (3) sets the rate of payment for services, and (4) administers its own Medicaid program (SSA, 1995, p. 103). Programs vary greatly from state to state in relation to covered services. The 1996 "Welfare Reform Law" places restrictions on public services for legal immigrants.

To receive federal funds the state Medicaid program must offer certain basic services, which are as follows:

- Inpatient hospital services
- Outpatient hospital services
- Prenatal care
- Physician services
- Nursing facility services for individuals age 21 or older
- Home health care for persons eligible for skilled-nursing services
- Family planning services and supplies
- Rural health clinic services
- Laboratory and x-ray services
- Pediatric and family nurse-practitioner services
- Certain federally qualified ambulatory and health center services
- Nurse-midwife services
- Early and periodic screening, diagnosis, and treatment (EPSDT) for children under the age of 21

Some people are eligible for both Medicaid and Medicare and are called "dual eligibles." The state's Medicaid program can pay the Medicare premiums for such individuals, and Medicaid supplements the Medicare coverage with services not available under Medicare, such as prescriptions, hearing aids, eyeglasses, and long-term care. Unfortunately, many people eligible for this dual status are not participating because they are not aware that they are eligible. For the medically indigent, Medicaid helps pay for nursing home care.

MATERNAL-CHILD HEALTH (MCH) PROGRAMS. These programs traditionally have been a major source of funding for activities that are carried out by local health departments to meet the needs of high-risk mothers and children. These activities include the nutrition and health programs for women, infants, and children (WIC), medical or dental care, and comprehensive preventive medical care services through centers such as PRESCAD (Preschool, School-Age, and Adolescent). These services are discussed more extensively in Chapter 15. The monies appropriated for these programs now are largely available through federal block grants.

PRIVATE HEALTH ASSISTANCE Health assistance in the private sector is primarily of a voluntary, nonprofit nature. This volunteerism is prevalent, with many people donating time, money, and effort to help procure health services for others. Candy stripers in the local hospital, volunteer respite workers, and readers for the blind are examples of volunteers who are helping clients to obtain health care services. The dedicated leadership, financial support, and personal service of volunteers and voluntary agencies (non–tax-supported) have greatly aided the health care delivery system in this country.

Service groups such as the American Cancer Society, American Diabetes Association, American Heart Association, Associations for Retarded Citizens, Lions' Clubs, Rotarians, Goodfellows, Knights of Columbus, church groups, and Visiting Nurse Associations provide cash and service benefits in the health field. A majority of U.S. hospitals operate on a voluntary, nonprofit basis. When the best hospitals in the United States are selected every year, it is these voluntary, nonprofit hospitals that make it to the top of the list (The Honor Roll, 1995, p. 52).

Health Service Programs

Some government and private health service programs are administered through an organization for the benefit of specific employees or service groups. These programs often encompass a combination of insurance and assistance benefits.

Government programs have been generally established to meet the health care needs of specific population groups. Health service programs have existed for veterans, military personnel, merchant marines, Native Americans on reservations, native Hawaiians, and federal employees. These programs vary in relation to the type of services and benefits offered. Changes in these programs may occur with the Clinton administration's health care reform.

Private service programs are often part of a benefit package for employees in the work setting. In addition to payment of employee health insurance premiums, many industries provide on-grounds employee health services. These services are usually preventive and treatment-oriented for work-related disease and disability.

THE U.S. WELFARE SYSTEM

The primary task of the welfare system is to alleviate the economic hardships of the most disadvantaged. Welfare programs reflect an effort to ensure a basic standard of living and to promote social well-being. Like the health care financing system, the welfare system is complex. In this text programs are arbitrarily divided into welfare insurance and assistance programs. The benefits provided under insurance (contributory) programs have historically been better than those provided under assistance (noncontributory) programs. The box on the next page outlines welfare insurance and assistance programs. Many people who use welfare assistance programs live in poverty.

Poverty

Poor health status is strongly associated with low family income. Unfortunately, the percentage of Americans living in poverty is on the rise. In 1980 13% of Americans lived in poverty; today that percentage has risen to over 15% (SSA, 1995, p. 163). Today more than 39 million Americans live in poverty, including 15 million children. There is a great discrepancy in poverty among ethnic groups in the United States. For example, 54% of American children of Puerto Rican descent, 46% of black children, 40% of Hispanic children, and 17% of white children live in poverty (poverty is further discussed in Chapter 12) (SSA, p. 164).

In all states except Alaska and Hawaii, a family of one is considered to be living in poverty if family income is $7470 or less. This amount is added to in increments of $2560 for

U.S. Welfare Insurance and Assistance Programs

WELFARE INSURANCE

Government

1. Old Age, Survivors, and Disability Insurance (OASDI)
2. Unemployment insurance
3. Worker's compensation

Private

WELFARE ASSISTANCE

Government

1. Temporary Assistance to Needy Families (TANF)
2. Supplemental Security Income (SSI)
3. Food Stamps
4. Supplemental Food Program for Women, Infants, and Children (WIC)
5. General assistance

Private

each additional household member. So, for a family of four, a yearly income of $15,150 or less would be considered to be living in poverty (Alaska: 1 person family = $9340/increment of $3200; Hawaii: 1 person family = $8610/increment of $2940) (SSA, 1995, p. 167).

Welfare Reform

"The welfare reform bill of 1996 (Personal Responsibility and Work Opportunity Reconciliation Act of 1996, PL 104-193), signed into law by President Clinton, makes the most dramatic changes in federal anti-poverty programs in six decades" (Hasson, 1996, p. 6A). This bill reflects a significant philosophical shift in thinking about welfare assistance in the United States. It ends a 61-year guarantee of federal aid and imposes a 5-year lifetime limit on welfare benefits. It also reduces spending on food stamps, bars most federal aid to future legal immigrants for 5 years, and makes it more difficult for select children to receive federal disability payments. It is anticipated that full implementation of the provisions of the "Welfare Reform Bill of 1996" in every state could take years (Hasson, p. 6A).

States lead the way in welfare reform. Unable to wait for the federal government to establish welfare reform guidelines, many states had enacted their own welfare reform legislation before the passage of the 1996 national welfare reform bill. In an attempt to cut welfare costs and balance budgets, states continue to look at ways to reform their welfare systems. In 1995-1996, Indiana, Massachusetts, North Dakota, Wyoming, and Oklahoma lead the ranks in states that have reduced the number of families on TANF—each of these states had at least a 25% drop in their welfare population (Welch, 1996, A1).

Most states are participating in federally granted welfare waivers to initiate "experimental" welfare programs. States are setting age limits on when someone could start receiving TANF benefits, limiting the amount of time that a family could be on the welfare program, excluding from coverage children who are born after the family goes on assistance, tightening up work requirements, encouraging teenage mothers to stay in school by offering bonuses or reducing benefits if they drop out, and working to move families to self-sufficiency.

Wisconsin's revolutionary welfare-to-work law is designed to do away with welfare in the state by requiring able-bodied parents to work or begin job training. Wisconsin's governor, Tommy Thompson, calls the state plan the "blueprint for ending welfare in America" (Thompson, 1996, p. 15A). The program will replace TANF with "Wisconsin Works," offering job placement and training for almost 80% of the states' welfare families by fall 1997 (Eggleston, 1996, p. A-5). Assistance will no longer be an entitlement but will be offered in return for work. Participants would be limited to 2 consecutive years with a 5-year maximum and will pay part of child and health care on a sliding scale. The program hopes to end traditional welfare in Wisconsin and make families self-sufficient.

In Michigan, recent welfare reform provisions included that a teen parent had to live with adult supervision in order to receive cash assistance; within a week after eligibility is determined a recipient would have to attend a job finding session; recipients would have to spend 20 hours a week in job training, at work, or performing community service (this increases to 35 hours a week by the year 2002); and mothers with newborns would have to begin looking for a job or take classes in parenting or child development once the infant is 13 weeks old (Pyen, 1995, p. A-1). At the same time Michigan's Department of Social Service is being renamed the Family Independence Agency.

More and more states are expected to implement such initiatives. Welfare in the United States is expected to change drastically in the next decade. Public health and special population group advocates, such as the Children's Defense Fund and the Black Crusade for Children, are concerned that this trend could increase the health disparities among Americans and restrict resources to children (BCCC, 1996; Children's Defense Fund, 1996).

Welfare Insurance

Welfare insurance programs are contributory. The individual or someone on behalf of the individual, such as the employer or the government, pays a premium, and benefits are awarded by virtue of these past premium contributions. Welfare insurance programs are found in both the government and private sectors.

GOVERNMENT WELFARE INSURANCE The federal government became extensively involved in welfare insurance programs with the passage of the Social Security Act in 1935. Discussed earlier in this chapter, this act and its amendments are the basis for many federal government

Origin of the Term "Social Security"

Abraham Epstein is the person generally recognized as introducing the term "Social Security." He was a national leader in the social welfare movement in the first half of this century. Epstein authored three books. The most well known is *Insecurity, a Challenge to America* (1933).

From 1918 to 1927 Epstein served as the research director of the Pennsylvania Commission on Old Age Pensions and was instrumental in having the state adopt an old-age assistance law in 1923. When Epstein realized that the Pennsylvania Commission would not be continued, he decided to establish a national organization to boost public support for social legislation such as state old-age assistance and pension programs. In 1927 he founded the American Association for Old Age Security. In 1933 he changed the name of his organization to the American Association for Social Security.

When Epstein was asked by Wilbur Cohen, later Secretary of the Department of Health, Education, and Welfare, why he chose the term "Social Security," he explained that at the time Germany was using the term "Social Insurance" and England was using the term "Economic Security," and he did not want to use either of these. Epstein responded that he wanted a term to convey a program that not only provided economic security for workers, but the type of security that would promote the welfare of society as a whole. In a letter to Cohen, Epstein stated, "I was convinced that no improvement in the conditions of labor can come except as the security of the people as a whole is advanced."

It was Epstein's term "Social Security" that became the title of one of our country's landmark pieces of legislation, the Social Security Act of 1935. It is a term that has become a household word and denotes economic security to millions of Americans.

From Origin of the term "Social Security," *Social Security Bulletin* 55(1):63-64, 1992.
Original article based on letters:
1. Cohen to Abraham Epstein, March 3, 1941, Abraham Epstein Papers, Columbia University Library, New York.
2. Epstein to Wilbur J. Cohen, March 4, 1941, Abraham Epstein Papers, Columbia University Library, New York.
3. Frankel to Wilbur J. Cohen, October 1949, Abraham Epstein Papers, Columbia University Library, New York.

welfare insurance programs today. State governments also provide welfare insurance. A discussion of the major government welfare insurance programs follows.

Old Age, Survivors, and Disability Insurance (OASDI). OASDI is commonly called "Social Security." A history of the term Social Security is given in the above box.

OASDI is a Social Security Act program that provides cash benefits to a qualified worker and his or her family when the worker retires in old age, becomes severely disabled, or dies. Eligibility is based on the amount of time worked and the amount of contributions made to the program. The principles that have historically guided benefit provision with the program are given in the box at right. Social Security benefits are applied for at local offices of the federal Social Security Administration. In 1995 the SSA became an independent agency and is no longer part of the Department of Health and Human Services.

OASDI is the largest income maintenance program in the country and is administered by the Social Security Administration (SSA). Presently almost 43 million Americans receive OASDI benefits, totaling more than $316 billion in benefits each year (SSA, 1995, p. 169-170).

Employers, employees, and the self-employed pay mandatory contributions into OASDI. The maximum amount of taxable earnings and worker contribution is updated each year. Employer and worker contributions to OASDI have steadily increased over the years. Table 4-5 illustrates the maximum annual worker taxable earnings and contributions to OASDI for selected years from 1937 to 1995.

Old Age, Survivors, and Disability Insurance (OASDI): Program Principles

WORK RELATED

Benefits grow out of the individual's own work history. The amount of cash benefits the worker and his/her family receive is related to work earnings and contributions and the amount of time worked.

NO MEANS TEST

Benefits are a qualifying insured worker's right and are paid regardless of other income.

CONTRIBUTORY

During work years, workers pay Social Security taxes (FICA) to finance benefits. These taxes are routinely deducted from employee earnings. In this way workers "contribute" to the program.

UNIVERSAL COMPULSORY COVERAGE

95% of the U.S. workforce is covered under OASDI. Coverage is universal and compulsory.

RIGHTS DEFINED BY LAW

A person's rights to OASDI benefits are clearly defined in federal law.

From Schwartz D, Grundmann H: Social Security programs in the United States—old age, survivors and disability insurance, *Social Security Bulletin* 54(9):6, 9-10, 1991.

table 4-5 Maximum Annual Worker Taxable OASDI Earnings and Annual Contributions

Year	Maximum Annual Worker Taxable Earnings	Maximum Worker Annual Contributions
1937	$ 3,000	$ 30.00
1953	$ 3,600	$ 54.00
1963	$ 4,800	$ 162.00
1973	$10,800	$ 464.40
1983	$35,700	$1,704.68
1993	$57,600	$3,225.60
1994	$60,060	$3,723.72
1995	$61,200	$3,894.40

From Social Security Administration: *Annual statistical supplement to the Social Security Bulletin, 1995*, Washington, D.C., 1995, The Administration, p. 51.

table 4-6 Projected Year of Retirement with Full OASDI Benefits: Based on Year Person Becomes 62

If you are an OASDI eligible worker who becomes 62 in:		
2000	you can retire with full benefits at	65 and 2 months
2001		65 and 4 months
2002		65 and 6 months
2003		65 and 8 months
2004		65 and 10 months
2005-2016		66
2017		66 and 2 months
2018		66 and 4 months
2019		66 and 6 months
2020		66 and 8 months
2021		66 and 10 months
2022 and over		67

From Social Security Administration: *Annual Statistical Supplement to the Social Security Bulletin, 1995*, Washington, D.C., 1995, The Administration, p. 53.

The *old age insurance* part of the program provides the worker with retirement income. More than 31 million people receive OASDI retirement insurance benefits, and the average monthly benefit for a retired worker is $697 (SSA, 1995, p. 170). Presently more than 36,000 centenarians receive Social Security (SSA, p. 169).

Full Social Security retirement benefits have historically begun at age 65. However, the retirement age under the program is gradually being raised to 67, and people can start to receive benefits as early as age 62. Starting to receive benefits earlier than age 65 means that the amount of cash benefits is permanently reduced. If a worker delays retirement past age 65, certain financial rewards and incentives accrue through age 70. If a worker returns to work after beginning retirement benefits, there is a limit on the amount that the worker can earn if he or she still wants to collect Social Security retirement benefits. The Social Security Administration publishes a free booklet, A *Guide to Social Security Retirement Benefits*, which can be obtained by calling 1-800-772-1213. For the age at which persons can retire and receive full OASDI benefits, see Table 4-6.

The *survivors' insurance* component of the act provides benefits to the family of a deceased or disabled qualifying worker. Ninety-five percent of American children and their surviving parent are eligible for benefits should the family breadwinner die. The Social Security Administration publishes a booklet, A *Guide to Social Security Survivors Benefits*, which can be obtained free of charge by calling the administration.

The *disability insurance* component of the act provides benefits to qualifying persons under 65 years of age on the basis of medical evaluations and the person's continued inability to work. After age 65 the disabled worker can apply for the old-age component of the insurance program. More than 3 million disabled workers receive benefits under OASDI, with average monthly benefits of $661.70 (SSA, 1995, p. 173). The Social Security Administration publishes a free booklet, A *Guide to Social Security Disability Benefits*.

Figure 4-7 gives the average monthly benefits for all OASDI programs. Figure 4-8 illustrates OASDI beneficiaries by type of benefit. The U.S. Social Security system is coordinated with the social security systems of various countries to help ensure benefits to people who have lived and worked in other nations. The United States presently has Social Security agreements with 17 nations: Austria, Belgium, Canada, Finland, France, Germany, Greece, Ireland, Italy, Luxembourg, the Netherlands, Norway, Portugal, Spain, Sweden, Switzerland, and the United Kingdom.

Unemployment Insurance. This insurance was one of the original components of the act. It is a state-federal program that provides benefits to regularly employed members of the labor force who are involuntarily unemployed and who are able and willing to seek employment. States decide who administers the program, the amount and duration of the benefits, eligibility requirements, and disqualification criteria.

All contributions collected for this program must be deposited in the unemployment trust fund of the U.S. Treasury Department. To be eligible for benefits the worker must remain registered to work and must actively seek employment while collecting benefits. Most states provide a maximum of 26 weeks of benefits each year. For workers who have exhausted state benefits, a federal program of 13 weeks of extended benefits is available during times of high unemployment, for a total of 39 weeks (SSA, 1995,

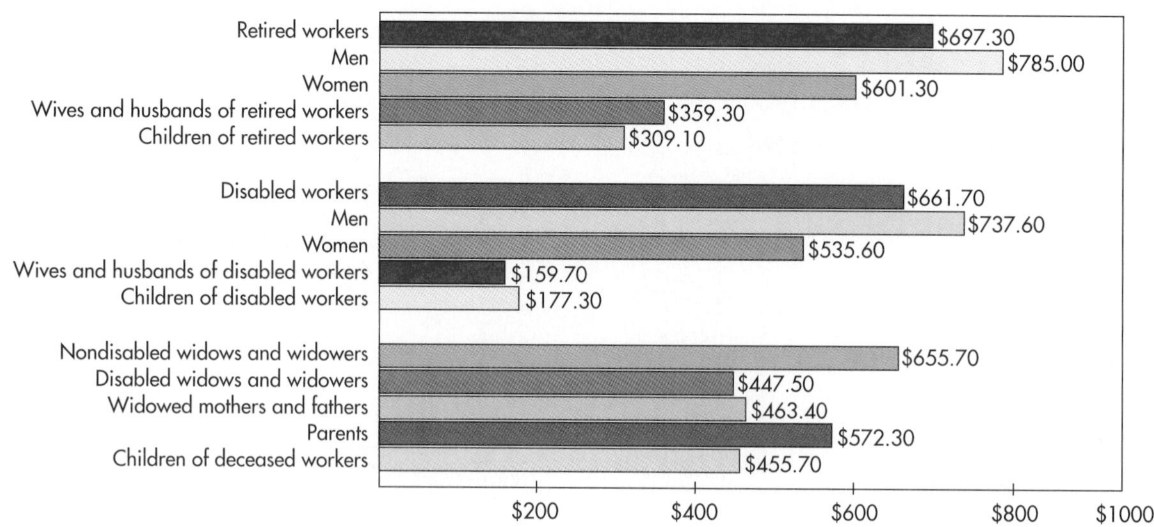

Figure 4-7 Average OASDI benefit amounts, by type. (*From Social Security Administration:* Annual Statistical Supplements to the Social Security Bulletin, 1995, *Washington, D.C., 1995, The Administration, p. 173.*)

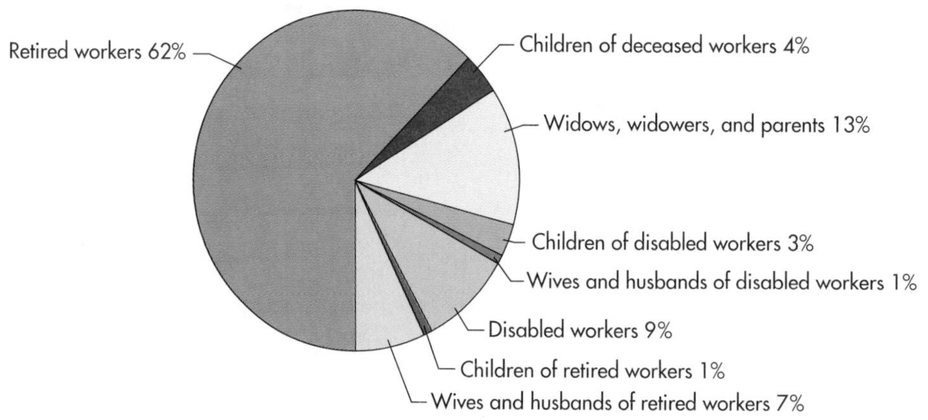

Figure 4-8 OASDI beneficiaries by type of benefit. (*From Social Security Administration:* Annual Statistical Supplements to the Social Security Bulletin, 1995, *Washington, D.C., 1995, The Administration, p. 171.*)

p. 111). If employment has not been found when unemployment benefits are exhausted, the family is often left without means of financial support and will begin to look at available state or local assistance programs or job training programs.

Program benefits vary greatly from state to state. Almost 110 million workers are insured under state unemployment insurance programs; more than 3 million workers collect unemployment benefits each year, with an average weekly benefit amount of $182 (SSA, 1995, p. 343).

WORKERS' COMPENSATION. This insurance has already been discussed under the legislative section on state workers' compensation and the health insurance section in this chapter. Refer to those sections for information on this program. Workers' compensation provides cash benefits and health care benefits for insured workers.

PRIVATE WELFARE INSURANCE Private welfare insurance, often in the form of income replacement insurance, is available through a number of agencies. Major forms of private welfare insurance include retirement and disability insurance. Many of these programs are obtained through the workplace, whereas others are purchased individually by the consumer. Millions of American workers are covered by private retirement insurance through their place of employment. The Retirement Income Security Act of 1974 helped to safeguard the financial integrity of these private retirement programs.

Welfare Assistance Programs

Welfare assistance programs are noncontributory or minimally contributory programs for qualifying indigent individuals, and they provide cash and service benefits (e.g., food,

Applying for Government Welfare Assistance

When applying for government welfare assistance an applicant is generally asked to provide some or all of the following information:

- Proof of residence
- Proof of gross income from all sources for all household members
- Record of all property, including savings accounts, checking accounts, bonds, and land owned
- Record of house payments or rent and also insurance and taxes
- Record of utility bills
- Record of current medical and dental expenses
- Birth dates and social security numbers of household members
- Records of child support and alimony
- Proof of tuition and other required educational expenses
- Records of child care payment for employment or training purposes

shelter, and clothing). They exist largely as a result of state and federal legislation and are locally administered. Once a person's eligibility for a categorical government welfare assistance program has been determined, he or she usually receives cash benefits, social service benefits, and medical benefits through Medicare or Medicaid. Welfare assistance programs include both government and private programs.

GOVERNMENT WELFARE ASSISTANCE Government welfare assistance programs provide subsistence benefits for those without other resources. Applicants often apply for these programs through local departments of social service or through the Social Security Office, depending on the program. Information that is often requested of applicants is given in the accompanying box. Some major categorical government welfare assistance programs include TANF and SSI. Other government assistance programs include general assistance, food stamps, and WIC. These programs are discussed below.

TEMPORARY ASSISTANCE TO NEEDY FAMILIES (TANF). TANF, formerly known as Aid to Families with Dependent Children (AFDC), is a state-federal program established by the Personal Responsibility and Work Opportunity Act of 1996 (PL 104-193), commonly known as the welfare reform bill. This program provides financial aid on a *temporary* basis (a 5-year lifetime limit was imposed by PL 104-193) and helps parents to become self-sufficient through welfare-to-work programs.

Families usually apply for TANF at local branches of the state department of human or social services. Recently some states have changed the name of their official department of human or social services (e.g., Family Independence Agency) and the name of the TANF program (e.g., Family Independence Program) to reflect the changing philosophical focus in the U.S. welfare system, which is to provide the type of assistance needed for families to become independent in fulfilling family functions.

Any U.S. citizen can apply for TANF. Starting in August of 1996, legal immigrants were barred from receiving TANF and some other types of welfare assistance (e.g., Medicaid) for the first 5 years after entering the United States. Some categories of immigrants (e.g., Cuban-Haitian entrants) and some welfare assistance programs (e.g., emergency Medicaid and child nutrition programs) are exempt from this bar (National Immigration Law Center, 1996).

TANF families are eligible for food stamps and Medicaid, but they must apply for them. Even when food stamp monies are taken into account, TANF families are below the poverty level of income. These families frequently need other types of community assistance such as referrals for clothing, housing, and furniture.

An "employability" plan is developed for TANF families. Provisions of PL 104-193 will cut off aid to the states unless half of their welfare recipients move into jobs. It is anticipated that "many states will not be able to find enough jobs and will need time to set up job training and public sector jobs" (Hasson, 1996, p. 6A). The impact of the sweeping welfare reform changes is unknown. Activists for poor children and needy families are concerned about the future of needy people in the United States.

SUPPLEMENTAL SECURITY INCOME (SSI). SSI is federal-state assistance provided for under the Social Security Act, federally administered through the Social Security Administration. The objective for establishing this program was to develop a uniform national minimum cash income program to provide aid to the indigent aged, blind, and disabled. The federal SSI payment standard is $458 per month for an individual and $687 per month for a couple (SSA, 1995, p. 295). More than 6.2 million people receive SSI each year (SSA, p. 295). The 1996 welfare reform bill makes it more difficult for children who have mental problems to receive federal disability payments.

Federal monetary benefits under the program remain constant throughout the nation and are adjusted to reflect Social Security cost-of-living increases. Forty-eight states supplement the program with additional cash benefits. State supplementary benefits vary and may be made directly to the beneficiary or paid through the federal Social Security Administration. Adults are usually the beneficiaries of SSI, but a child may be eligible if he or she suffers from an impairment that is expected to last a year or longer, such as mental retardation, terminal illness, or blindness. Applications for SSI are made at local branches of the federal Social Security Administration offices. Qualifying United States citizens and legally admitted aliens are eligible. The Social Security Administration publishes a free booklet, *A Guide to the Supplemental Security Income Program*.

FOOD STAMPS. Food stamps were begun on a pilot basis in 1961 to improve the nutritional adequacy of low-income individuals and families. It was formally established by the Food Stamp Act of 1964. It is a federal-state program under state administration; the federal sharing agency is the Department of Agriculture. Application is made at the local office of the state department of human or social services. Persons qualify on the basis of financial need, and people on TANF and SSI are automatically eligible. The 1996 welfare reform bill has provisions that will reduce spending on food stamps by $28 billion over 6 years (1996-2002) and that limit benefits to able-bodied individuals without children (Hasson, 1996, p. 6A).

An eligible family of four persons receives approximately $386 per month in food stamps (SSA, 1995, p. 359). The average food stamp recipient has approximately $1 worth of food stamps to use for each meal ($97 per person per month). Each year more than 27 million Americans take part in this program at an annual cost to the government of almost $24 billion (SSA, p. 359).

Food stamps are available across the nation. Coupons are given and are used like money at participating stores. Food stamps can be used only to purchase edible items; no imported foodstuffs, alcoholic beverages, or tobacco products can be bought with them. They must be used by the person to whom they were issued (not transferrable). Most grocery stores accept food stamps.

SUPPLEMENTAL FOOD PROGRAM FOR WOMEN, INFANTS, AND CHILDREN (WIC). WIC is a federal nutrition and health assistance program authorized under the Child Nutrition Act of 1966 and administered at the federal level by the Food and Nutrition Service of the U.S. Department of Agriculture. Local nonprofit health and welfare agencies apply to their respective states to qualify for funds from this program, and presently there are almost 9000 approved local WIC sites in the United States. Most local health departments are WIC sites.

WIC is designed to help pregnant and postpartum women, infants, and children up to 5 years of age who have been identified by health professionals as being at nutritional risk and who meet certain age and income requirements. The program includes food distribution, health assessment, and *mandatory* nutrition education. Participants receive vouchers that are redeemable at participating grocery stores for items such as infant formula, cereal, and juices; milk; cereals; and cheese. The WIC program has been very successful in promoting adequate nutrition and nutrition education. Many of the families on the community health nurse's caseload receive WIC.

Families apply for WIC at any designated WIC site. If a family is receiving food stamps, participation in WIC does not affect their food stamp eligibility. WIC serves 5.4 million people each year at a cost of $2.6 billion (approximately $30.17 per person each month) (SSA, 1993, p. 73). More than 40% of infants born in the United States participate (SSA, p. 73).

OTHER NUTRITION PROGRAMS. Other nutrition programs in which the federal government is involved are school lunch programs, school breakfast programs, school milk programs, needy family commodity foods, and food programs for the elderly. The school breakfast and lunch programs have done a lot to improve the nutritional status of America's children and provide millions of meals each year.

GENERAL ASSISTANCE. General assistance, or "direct assistance," is a state and locally funded and administered program offered in 36 states. No federal monies are involved. The program is often administered through the state Department of Human or Social Services. General assistance is usually in the form of cash assistance, vouchers, or payments to vendors. This is often the only form of government assistance available for individuals who are poor but who do not qualify for TANF, unemployment insurance, OASDI, or SSI. In many states general assistance is limited to emergency relief (e.g., a catastrophic event such as a flood), short-term relief, and burial benefits. Any citizen can apply. Approximately one million people receive general assistance in the United States each year (SSA, 1993, p. 75).

LOW-INCOME HOME ENERGY ASSISTANCE PROGRAM. This program provides eligible households with funds for heating and cooling costs and for weather-related and supply shortage emergencies. On the federal level the program is administered by the Department of Health and Human Services. States make payments directly to eligible households or to home energy suppliers on behalf of eligible households. Payments may be provided in vouchers, cash, fuel, or prepaid utility bills. Almost $1.5 billion is appropriated by Congress for the program each year (SSA, 1993, p. 74). This program has provided valuable assistance to many older and disabled Americans.

PUBLIC HOUSING AND OTHER ASSISTED HOUSING. Starting in the late 1930s the federal government has provided leadership and a commitment to providing decent, safe, sanitary, and affordable housing for all Americans (SSA, 1993, p. 75). The Department of Housing and Urban Development (HUD) is the federal agency responsible for federally administering public housing programs for low-income families. Today many public housing units are in poor repair, in unsafe neighborhoods, and tend to segregate low-income families. However, public housing reform is being considered, and the old high-rise tenements for the poor may soon be replaced with a system that promotes modern homes in mixed-income neighborhoods and a universal voucher system that families can use toward rent for any qualifying housing. A number of housing programs presently exist.

Public, low-rent housing units (more than 1.4 million units) are available to low-income families with children and people who are elderly or disabled. The units are owned, managed, and administered by a local Public Housing Agency. Rental charges are set by federal statute, usually

State Departments of Human Service: Selected Services

- *Health and welfare assistance programs* (e.g., TANF, Food Stamps, Medicaid): Helping families to meet basic needs
- *Adoption services:* Accepting and placing children for adoption, recruiting adoptive families, and supporting and evaluating the adoption placement
- *Foster care:* Funding, licensing, and monitoring
- *Day care:* Licensing, monitoring, and maintaining a listing of such placements
- *Counseling:* Counseling individuals and families with problems to strengthen family functioning and to help prevent family breakdown
- *Chore services:* Paying part or all of the cost for unskilled help with household tasks, personal care, home maintenance, or other activities for qualifying aged and disabled
- *Education or training:* Providing funds and counseling services so that persons can improve their job skills through education and training programs
- *Employment:* Helping people find jobs
- *Family planning:* Providing information and referral to appropriate agencies
- *Homemaking:* Teaching people about home management
- *Housing:* Subsidizing low-income housing and keeping lists of appropriate low-income housing
- *Information and referral:* Helping people learn about community services
- *Mental health treatment and rehabilitation:* Providing services to persons with mental health problems through community mental health agencies
- *Money management:* Helping people learn to budget
- *Placement:* Helping place youth and adults in appropriate living facilities with follow-up (often in the form of foster care)
- *Problem services:* Investigating reports of abuse and neglect and providing counseling services to prevent recurrence of such problems, counseling services for runaway youth, housing in emergency situations, and protection of aging clients and children from abuse and neglect (protective services)

at 30% of the monthly adjusted income of the recipient's household. The federal government spends almost $3 billion each year to subsidize these units and another $1.4 billion to maintain them (SSA, 1993, p. 75).

Rental assistance programs are limited to very low-income families. Such programs account for federal outlays of $12.3 billion and cover 2.8 million housing units (SSA, 1993, p. 76). These programs are designed to give families the opportunity to lease rental housing that is suitable to the family's needs. In the Rental Assistance Program the family is free to locate a suitable dwelling unit that meets program housing quality standards. The family usually pays 30% of their income toward the rent (maximum amounts are set on the price of the rental unit). In the Rental Voucher Program the monthly assistance payments are based on the difference between a standard for the area (not the actual rent) and 30% of the family's monthly adjusted income. In the voucher program families pay more than 30% of their income towards the rent if they select a unit that rents above the payment standard, or less than 30% if the unit rents below the payment standard. There is no maximum rent to the owner as in the rental certificate program. In the Moderate Rehabilitation Program eligibility and tenant requirements are the same as in the Rental Certificate Program. However, assistance under the program is limited to buildings that have been made accessible for people who are disabled.

Housing programs for the homeless are administered by the Department of Housing and Urban Development. Housing for the Homeless programs cover emergency, transitional, and permanent housing and cost the federal government $450 million each year (SSA, 1993, p. 76). Safe Havens (for battered women) and rural Housing Homeless Assistance were authorized by the federal government, but no monies were appropriated for them.

Supportive housing programs include Supportive Housing for the Elderly and Supportive Housing for Persons with Disabilities. These programs pay for the building of special housing units to be made available to low-income elderly and disabled persons. The federal government pays out over $500 million for such programs each year (SSA, 1993, p. 77).

OTHER STATE AND LOCAL GOVERNMENT SERVICES. In addition to the programs discussed, many state and local governments offer a number of other welfare services. These services are listed in the above box.

PRIVATE WELFARE ASSISTANCE Following its volunteer tradition, the United States is one of the few countries in the world to offer such a magnitude of private welfare assistance programs. Historically the provision of social services and educational programs has been an important aspect of the private sector (Kerns, Glanz, 1991, p. 4). The private sector has played a significant and valuable role in the provision of social welfare programs to local communities in the United States. Provision of such services costs private social welfare agencies more than $730 billion a year and represents about 40% of the nation's social welfare expenditures (Kerns, 1992, p. 61).

A census survey involving a sample representing 106,000 social service agencies and establishments found numerous services are frequently provided by private welfare agencies in the areas of individual and family services, residential care, recreation and group work, civic and social activities, and job training and rehabilitation. Examples of these services are given in the box on the following page. Most of these services involve short-term

Services Frequently Provided by Private Welfare Agencies

INDIVIDUAL AND FAMILY SERVICES
Counseling and referral services to families and children, family service agencies, adoption services, advocacy, emergency and disaster services, child day care services, and senior citizens services

RESIDENTIAL CARE
Group foster homes, halfway homes, and shelters for the homeless

RECREATION AND GROUP WORK
Such as YMCA, YWCA, Boy Scouts, and Girl Scouts

CIVIC AND SOCIAL ACTIVITIES
Provided by organizations such as Rotarians, Goodwill Industries, Lions Clubs, Jaycees, and churches

JOB TRAINING AND VOCATION REHABILITATION
Sheltered workshops, vocational rehabilitation agencies, and skill training centers

From Kerns WL, Glanz MP: Private social welfare expenditures, 1972-88, *Social Security Bulletin* 54(2):2-11, 1991, p. 6.

(acute) relief but do not provide long-term assistance for chronic problems.

Summary

Over the ages health and welfare practices and services have evolved. We have come a long way in developing public health knowledge and technology. However, good public health practices are not always followed, and public health is often taken for granted.

Early public health and welfare services were usually voluntary and were sponsored by churches and local organizations. In this country the Shattuck Report was the impetus behind the development of public health practice and the forerunner of contemporary public health policy and practice.

In the United States the federal government was slow to get involved in health and welfare service provision. Two pieces of legislation that set the stage for government involvement were the Social Security Act of 1935 and the Public Health Service Act of 1944. The health and welfare programs of the Social Security Act have been enlarged over the years and provide many of the services that are used by the clients of community health nurses today. Legislation in the 1980s and 1990s has significantly affected the provisions of these acts and the availability of funding for health and welfare services. Today legislation is being proposed to reform the health care system and control health care costs.

Health and welfare services are found at all three levels of government—federal, state, and local—and in the private sector. These services are complicated, diverse, and often poorly coordinated. Keeping up with government services is facilitated by knowledge of legislation and ordinances. Keeping up with private-sector health and welfare services requires diligent effort on the part of the nurse because these services vary greatly from locality to locality.

Forty million Americans do not have health insurance, and even more are underinsured. Many Americans do not have access to necessary health services. For many community health nursing clients, basic welfare needs such as food and shelter are a higher priority than health needs; health needs may not be viewed as a priority until the nurse can assist the client in meeting existing welfare needs.

Knowledge of health and welfare legislation and services is essential when nursing a community. Such knowledge will equip the community health nurse to more effectively deal with client situations encountered daily in the practice setting. Through this knowledge nurses can help clients become aware of the services available and use these services to enhance the clients' quality of life. The nurse needs to work in partnership with other health care professionals, local leadership, service groups, and organizations to promote health.

CRITICAL *Thinking Exercise*

This chapter gives community health nurses an overview of the depth and scope of health and welfare services available to people in the United States. What were your thoughts as you read the chapter? Were you overwhelmed? Interested in what will occur with health and welfare reform? Disenchanted with delivery? All of these? Many services were presented in this chapter. Think about a client you have served and the practical use of the service information presented. What services could the client be eligible for? How might health and welfare reform help or hinder this client?

We are indebted to Professor Dorothy Donabedian, colleague and friend, whose efforts have stimulated both student and faculty awareness of the health and welfare systems as they apply to community health nursing practice. Her enthusiasm, encouragement, and suggestions in this work have been greatly appreciated.

REFERENCES

American Cancer Society: *Cancer facts and figures—1996*, New York, 1996, The Society.

American Nurses Association (ANA): *Nursing's agenda for health care reform*, Kansas City, Mo., 1991, The Association.

Black Community Crusade for Children (BCCC): *Leave no child behind*, Washington, D.C., 1996, BCCC.

Bowman L: House panel told about woes of managed care, *The Knoxville News-Sentinel*, May 31, 1996, p. A12.

Children's Defense Fund: *The state of America's child yearbook, 1996*, Washington, D.C., 1996, The Fund.

Clancy CM, Himmelstein DU, Woolhandler S: Questions and answers about managed competition, *Health/PAC Bulletin* 23:30-32, 1993.

Coll BD: *Perspectives in public welfare: a history*, Washington, D.C., 1969, U.S. Government Printing Office.

Commonwealth Fund: *Managed care: the patient's perspective*, New York, 1995, The Fund.

Davis K, Collins KS, Schoen C, Morris C: Choice matters: enrollees' views of their health plans, *Health Affairs* Summer:100-112, 1995.

Eggleston R: Wisconsin riding wave of welfare reform, *USA Today*, May 20, 1996, p. A-5.

Forgotson EH: 1965: the turning point in health law—1966 reflections, *Am J Public Health* 57(6):934-946, 1967.

General Accounting Office (GAO): *Health care reform*, Washington, D.C., 1993, GAO.

General Accounting Office (GAO): *Access to health care: states respond to growing crisis*, Washington, D.C., 1992, GAO.

Gerber DE, McGuire SL: Understanding contemporary health and welfare services: the Social Security Act of 1935 and the Public Health Service Act of 1944, *Nurs Outlook* 43:266-272, 1995.

Gillis L, Thomas D: *Developing clinical systems for working in a managed care environment*, Washington, D.C., June 7-9, 1996, Conference on Health Care for the Homeless.

Harrington C: A national health care program: has its time come? *Nurs Outlook* 36:214-216, 225, 1989.

Hasson J: Welfare enters new world, *USA Today* August 23, 1996, p. 6A.

Health Insurance Association of America (HIAA): *Source book of health insurance data 1977-78*, Washington, D.C., 1978, The Association.

Health Insurance Association of America (HIAA): *Source book of health insurance data 1983-84*, Washington, D.C., 1983, The Association.

Health Insurance Association of America (HIAA): *Source book of health insurance data 1995*, Washington, D.C., 1995, The Association.

Hicks LL, Stallmeyer JM, Coleman JR: *Role of the nurse in managed care*, Washington, D.C., 1993, American Nurses Publishing.

Himmelstein DU, Woolhandler S: *The national health program chartbook*, Cambridge, Ma., 1992, The Center for National Health Program Studies, Harvard Medical School/Cambridge Hospital.

Hsu I: Health care evolution at the state level: the growth of Medicaid managed care, *HPDP Communicator*, Winter:5, 1995.

Institute of Medicine—Committee for the Study of the Future of Public Health: *The future of public health*, Washington, D.C., 1988, National Academy Press.

Johnson EA: The public's future perspective on managed care, *Health Care Manage Rev* 20(2):45-47, 1995.

Kalisch BJ, Kalisch PA: *Politics of nursing*, Philadelphia, 1982, Lippincott.

Kerns WL: Private social welfare expenditures, 1972-90, *Social Sec Bull* 55(3):59-66, 1992.

Kerns WL, Glanz MP: Private social welfare expenditures, 1972-88, *Social Sec Bull* 54(2):2-11, 1991.

Landers T: Medicaid managed care: a brief analysis, *J NY State Nurses Assoc* 26(3):7-11, 1995.

Managed care and public health struggling to coexist, *The Nation's Health* May/June:1,6,7, 1996.

Masso AR: Managed care and alternative-site health care delivery, *J Health Care Management* 1:45-51, 1995.

Maternal and Child Health Bureau: *Child health USA '95*, Washington, D.C., 1996, U.S. Government Printing Office.

National Center for Health Statistics (NCHS): *Health, United States, 1994*, Hyattsville, Md., 1995, United States Public Health Service.

National Immigration Law Center: *Overview of benefit restrictions to immigrants in 1996 welfare and immigration laws*, Washington, D.C., 1996, The Center.

O'Neil EH: *Health professions education for the future: schools in service to the nation*, San Francisco, 1993, Pew Health Professions Commission.

Origin of the term "Social Security," *Social Sec Bull* 55(1):63-64, 1992.

Pew Health Professions Commission: *Critical challenges: revitalizing the health professions for the twenty-first century*, San Francisco, 1995, UCSF Center for the Health Professions.

Pickett G, Hanlon JJ: *Public health administration and practice*, ed 9, St. Louis, 1990, Mosby.

Pyen CW: Will new welfare work? *Ann Arbor News*, December 7, 1995, A-1.

Randal J: Managed care reshapes health care delivery, *SAMSHA News* III(3):10-11, 14, Summer 1995.

Richards SD: Managed care 101, *Nurs Policy Forum* 2(3):13, 1996.

Richardson BW: *The health of nations, a review of the works of Edwin Chadwick*, vol 2, London, 1887, Longmans, Green & Co.

Schwartz D, Grundmann H: Social Security programs in the United States—old age, survivors, and disability insurance, *Social Sec Bull* 54(9):6-19, 1991.

Shamansky S: Yet another treatise on managed care, *Public Health Nurs* 13(3):161-162, 1996.

Shattuck L: *Report of the Sanitary Commission of Massachusetts*, Cambridge, Ma., 1948, Harvard University Press (originally published by Dutton & Wentworth in 1850).

Social Security Administration (SSA): *Annual statistical supplement to the Social Security Bulletin, 1995*, Washington, D.C., 1995, The Administration.

Social Security Administration (SSA): *Understanding Social Security*, Washington, D.C., 1993, The Administration (SSA Publication No. 05-10024).

The Honor Roll, *U.S. News* 119(4):52, July 24, 1995.

Thompson T: If you don't work, you don't get paid in Wisconsin, *USA Today*, May 28, 1996, p. 15A.

U.S. Department of Health and Human Services (USDHHS): *Healthy people 2000: national health promotion and disease prevention objectives, full report, with commentary*, Washington, D.C., 1991, U.S. Government Printing Office.

U.S. Department of Health and Human Services (USDHHS): *Healthy People 2000: midcourse review and 1995 revisions*, Washington, D.C., 1995, U.S. Government Printing Office.

Welch WM: Is innovation or economic boom behind change? *USA Today*, May 29, 1996, A1-2.

White House Domestic Policy Council: *Health security: the President's report to the American people*, Washington, D.C., 1993, U.S. Government Printing Office.

Wilner DM, Walkley RP, O'Neill EJ: *Introduction to public health*, ed 7, New York, 1978, Macmillan.

Zarate AO: *International mortality chartbook: level and trends, 1955-91*, Hyattsville, Md., 1994, Public Health Service.

SELECTED BIBLIOGRAPHY

American Association for Retired Persons (AARP): *Health care America: meeting America's health care needs*, Washington, D.C., 1992, The Association.

American Public Health Association: *A national health program for all of us: the American Public Health Association's Guide to the Health Care Reform Debate*, Washington, D.C., undated, The Association.

Bernstein NR: *APHA, the first one hundred years*, Washington, D.C., 1972, American Public Health Association.

Corning PA: *The evolution of Medicare . . . from idea to law*, Research Report No. 29, Washington, D.C., 1969, U.S. Department of Health, Education, and Welfare, Social Security Administration, Office of Research and Statistics.

Eliot MM: The Children's Bureau, fifty years of public responsibility for action in behalf of children, *Am J Public Health* 52(4):576-591, 1962.

Furman B: *A profile of the United States Public Health Service, 1798-1948*, Washington, D.C., 1973, National Library of Medicine.

Hanlon JJ, Rogers F, Rosen G: A bookshelf on the history and philosophy of public health, *Am J Public Health* 50(4):445-458, 1960.

Health Resources Administration: *Health in America: 1776-1976*, Washington, D.C., 1976, United States Public Health Service.

Ravenel MP: *A half century of public health: jubilee historical volume of the American Public Health Association*, New York, 1921, American Public Health Association.

Rosenberg CE: *Origins of public health in America: selected essays 1820-1855*, New York, 1972, Arno Press.

Smillie WG: The national board of health, 1879-1883, *Am J Public Health* 33(8):925-930, 1943.

Social Security Administration: *The social security handbook*, Washington, D.C., 1995, U.S. Government Printing Office.

Trattner W: *From poor law to welfare state*, ed 3, New York, 1984, Free Press.

U.S. General Accounting Office (GAO): *Medicaid: states' turn to managed care to improve access and control costs*, March 1993, GAO.

Winslow C-EA: *The evolution and significance of the modern public health campaign*, New Haven, 1984, Yale University Press (originally published in 1923).

5

Healthy People 2000: Organization of U.S. Health and Welfare Resources

Objectives

Upon completion of this chapter, the reader should be able to:

1. State the "levels" and "sectors" into which health care is organized and delivered in the United States.
2. Discuss the *Healthy People* initiative.
3. List the three major national goals of *Healthy People 2000.*
4. Explain the core public health functions of local, state, and federal government.
5. Discuss the major agencies of the U.S. Department of Health and Human Services (USDHHS).
6. Describe patterns of organizational structure between state health authorities (SHAs) and local health departments (LHDs).
7. Discuss service functions of SHAs and LHDs.
8. Discuss federal, state, and local government welfare organization.
9. Identify private health and welfare resources on the federal, state, and local level.

The intent of this chapter is to assist the nurse in becoming familiar with the Healthy People initiative; year 2000 national health objectives; federal, state, and local health and welfare agencies; public health in the United States; and core public health functions. The organization of health and welfare resources is discussed, and key agencies on the federal, state, and local levels are presented.

HEALTHY PEOPLE 2000: PROVIDING FOR THE PUBLIC'S HEALTH

The word *health* was left out of the U.S. Constitution. The federal government bases its involvement in matters of health and welfare on the Preamble to the Constitution, which charges it with providing for the general welfare of the people. Public health has historically been the responsibility of the individual states and is provided for through state constitutions, legislation, and public health codes. Since 1980 the United States has had national health objectives, and across the nation individuals, health and welfare agencies, and all levels of government are working to achieve them.

The *Healthy People* Initiative

In 1979, under the presidency of Jimmy Carter, the Surgeon General of the United States issued a landmark report that started the Healthy People Initiative. It is called *Healthy People: The Surgeon General's Report on Health Promotion and Disease Prevention*, often referred to as *Healthy People*. This report analyzed the leading causes of death in the United States and suggested that many of these deaths are preventable. It is estimated that approximately half of all U.S. mortality was due to unhealthful behavior, one fifth to environmental hazards, one fifth to human biological factors, and one tenth to inadequacies in the health care system. *Healthy People* shaped national health policy for the oncoming decade (1980-1990) and was the first in a series of documents that would outline national health priority areas, goals, and objectives. Major documents in this initiative are discussed in this chapter, and are listed in the box on the next page.

Healthy People established broad national health goals targeted for achievement in 1990 and issued a challenge to the nation to accomplish them. It launched an unprecedented initiative to promote healthful lifestyles and improve the health of Americans, and called on all levels of government, professionals, and lay people to undertake a venture that promised to reduce preventable death and disability across the life span (USDHHS, 1986, p. v). This preventive, life span approach to health established goals

HEALTHY PEOPLE 2000 Major Documents

USDHEW: *Healthy people: the Surgeon General's report on health promotion and disease prevention,* Washington, D.C., 1979, U.S. Government Printing Office. (Commonly called *Healthy People*)

USDHHS: *Promoting health/preventing disease: objectives for the nation,* Washington, D.C., 1980, U.S. Government Printing Office.

USDHHS: *The 1990 health objectives for the nation: a midcourse review,* Washington, D.C., 1986, U.S. Government Printing Office.

USDHHS: *Healthy people 2000: national health promotion and disease prevention objectives, full report, with commentary,* Washington, D.C., 1991, U.S. Government Printing Office. (Commonly called *Healthy People 2000*)

From USDHHS: *Healthy People 2000: midcourse review and 1995 revisions*, Washington, D.C., 1995, U.S. Government Printing Office.

under the areas of healthy infants, healthy children, healthy adolescents and young adults, healthy adults, and healthy older adults, as well as special at-risk aggregates across the life span.

Healthy People established three target areas: preventive health services (priority areas: family planning, pregnancy and infant care, immunizations, sexually transmissible diseases, and blood pressure control); health protection (priority areas: toxic agent control, occupational safety and health, accidental injury control, fluoridation of community water supplies, and infectious agents control); and health promotion (priority areas: smoking cessation, reduction of the misuse of alcohol and drugs, stress control, and improvement of nutrition, exercise, and fitness).

Promoting Health/Preventing Disease: Objectives for the Nation was published in 1980. It set forth 226 specific objectives necessary for attaining the broad national health goals established in *Healthy People*. Objectives were established in each of the 15 priority areas and were to be attained by the year 1990.

The *1990 Health Objectives for the Nation: A Midcourse Review* was published in 1986. This review provided Americans with an assessment of how the nation was doing in its decade-long quest to improve the nation's health status.

The midcourse review showed that the nation was on its way to achieving nearly half of the 226 objectives, that about one fourth were unlikely to be achieved, and that in some cases the trend was away from reaching the 1990 targets (USDHHS, 1986, p. iii). The review found reductions in both smoking and per-capita alcohol consumption, increased use of automobile seat belts, and reduced death rates from strokes, cirrhosis, and traffic accidents. However, it showed that Americans had regressed in the areas of weight control, illicit drug use, control of violent behavior, teenage pregnancy, infant health, family planning, physical fitness and exercise, provision of safe water, and control of sexually transmitted diseases.

Because of the different data gathering and reporting mechanisms in individual states, it was often difficult to obtain information on how well each state was doing in meeting *Healthy People* objectives. A report 2 years later by the Public Health Foundation (PHF) (PHF, 1988) found that states did not always have the information necessary to evaluate their progress toward the 1990 objectives and that state public health surveillance and information systems were insufficient. Having adequate surveillance systems would become a priority area in *Healthy People 2000*.

Healthy People 2000: The Initiative Continues

Healthy People 2000: National Health Promotion and Disease Prevention Objectives, often referred to as *Healthy People 2000*, "provides a vision for achieving improved health for all Americans" (USDHHS, 1995, p. 2). Published in 1991, it became the flagship of the initiative, building on the efforts of *Healthy People*, and shaping U.S. health policy for the next decade (1990-2000). It is the product of a national effort involving almost 300 national organizations, state health authorities, the Institute of Medicine, the National Academy of Sciences, and the U.S. Public Health Service.

Healthy People 2000 outlines broad national health goals and almost 300 national health objectives under 22 priority areas (including 7 new ones). It focuses on prevention and working in partnership with communities to promote health. National health objectives are organized under three categories that identify the type of preventive intervention involved: health promotion, risk reduction, and services and protection (USDHHS, 1995, p. 273). Objectives were included that address aggregates at highest risk of illness and premature death, including low-income families, minority groups, and persons with disabilities. They emphasize prevention of disability and morbidity; improving general health status; and inclusion of more screening interventions for early detection of asymptomatic disease and conditions (USDHHS, p. 272). The following boxes give an overview of the national goals, age-related objectives, and priority areas of *Healthy People 2000*.

Full achievement of these goals and objectives is dependent on a health system reaching all Americans and integrating personal health care and population-based public health (USDHHS, 1995, p. 2). The Year 2000 Health Objectives Planning Act (Public Law 101-582) established a program of grants to states for the development of state plans for assisting communities in meeting national health objectives. It is important for nurses to be aware of the priority areas in *Healthy People 2000* and implement nursing interventions that can help achieve national health objectives. Many of the local health agencies that the nurse works with will be involved in activities to meet these objectives and facilitate healthy communities.

HEALTHY COMMUNITIES 2000: MODEL STANDARDS *Healthy Communities 2000: Model Standards* (1991) was developed by the American Public Health Association, National Association of County Health Officials, Centers for Disease Control and Prevention, and the Association for State and Territorial Health Officials. The Health Services Extension Act of 1977 (Public Law 95-83) mandated the development of model standards for community preventive health services in American communities. These model standards encompass all of the priority areas and national objectives in *Healthy People 2000* and assist communities in establishing community health objectives (APHA, 1991, p. ix). The federal government encourages state health authorities (SHAs) and local health departments (LHDs) to use these standards.

YEARLY UPDATES Each year the federal government publishes updates that outline the progress being made toward achieving the year 2000 health objectives. The most comprehensive of these updates has been the midcourse review and revisions done in 1995.

HEALTHY PEOPLE 2000: MIDCOURSE REVIEW AND 1995 REVISIONS This document outlined the progress that the country had made toward the year 2000 objectives and revised some objectives. In developing the midcourse review, lead agencies were guided by the criteria given in the box on the following page (USDHHS, 1995, pp. 272-273). The review stated that families, schools, worksites, and community programs all provide important preventive health opportunities and called for renewed commitment to improving the nation's health, stating:

> *Healthy People 2000* cannot be accomplished by the Federal Government alone. Leadership must come from institutions and individuals throughout the Nation. Each person makes decisions about how fast to drive, whether to wear a safety belt, what to eat, and how much alcohol to drink. In families, parents have the opportunity to promote health and encourage healthy habits for their children. Community organizations—schools, religious institutions, and voluntary organizations—can become more actively engaged in promoting health. Employers can make worksites healthy. This midcourse review offers not only a report to the Nation on progress to date, or a blueprint for what is possible by the year 2000, but it outlines opportunities to renew the Nation's commitment to making a difference in the health of its citizens as the 21st century approaches. (USDHHS, p. 5)

The midcourse review found that progress had been made toward 50% of the objectives, 18% were moving away from the target, 3% showed no change, and tracking data were not available for 29% (USDHHS, 1995, p. 12). Some areas that were moving away from target and had a higher incidence than expected included number of overweight Americans, teen pregnancies, violent and abusive behavior, occupational work-related injuries, low birth weight infants, disability related to chronic conditions, pneumonia and

HEALTHY PEOPLE 2000 National Health Goals

- Increase the span of healthy life for Americans
- Reduce health disparities among Americans
- Achieve access to preventive services for all Americans

From USDHHS: *Healthy people 2000: national health promotion and disease prevention objectives, full report, with commentary*, Washington, D.C., 1991, U.S. Government Printing Office, p. 6.

HEALTHY PEOPLE 2000 Age-Related Objectives

HEALTHY INFANTS AND CHILDREN

Reduce the death rate for children by 15 percent to no more than 28 per 100,000 children aged 1 through 14, and for infants by approximately 30 percent to no more than 7 per 1,000 live births. (Baseline: 33 per 100,000 for children in 1987 and 10.1 per 1,000 live births for infants in 1987)

HEALTHY ADOLESCENTS AND YOUNG ADULTS

Reduce the death rate for adolescents and young adults by 15 percent to no more than 85 per 100,000 people aged 15 through 24. (Baseline: 99.4 per 100,000 in 1987)

HEALTHY ADULTS

Reduce the death rate for adults by 20 percent to no more than 340 per 100,000 people aged 25 through 64. (Baseline: 423 per 100,000 in 1987)

HEALTHY OLDER ADULTS

Reduce to no more than 90 per 1,000 people the proportion of all people aged 65 and older who have difficulty in performing two or more personal care activities (a reduction of about 19 percent), thereby preserving independence. (Baseline: 111 per 1,000 in 1984-85)

From USDHHS: *Healthy people 2000: national health promotion and disease prevention objectives, full report, with commentary*, Washington, D.C., 1991, U.S. Government Printing Office, pp. 562, 571, 579, 587.

HEALTHY PEOPLE 2000 Priority Areas with Responsible Agencies

HEALTH PROMOTION

1. Physical activity and fitness
   - President's Council on Physical Fitness and Sports
2. Nutrition
   - National Institutes of Health
   - Food and Drug Administration
3. Tobacco
   - Centers for Disease Control and Prevention
4. Alcohol and other drugs
   - Alcohol, Drug Abuse, and Mental Health Administration
5. Family planning
   - Office of Population Affairs
6. Mental health and mental disorders
   - Alcohol, Drug Abuse, and Mental Health Administration
7. Violent and abusive behavior
   - Centers for Disease Control and Prevention
8. Educational and community-based programs
   - Centers for Disease Control and Prevention
   - Health Resources Services Administration

HEALTH PROTECTION

9. Unintentional injuries
   - Centers for Disease Control and Prevention
10. Occupational safety and health
    - Centers for Disease Control and Prevention
11. Environmental health
    - National Institutes of Health
    - Centers for Disease Control and Prevention
12. Food and drug safety
    - Food and Drug Administration
13. Oral health
    - National Institutes of Health
    - Centers for Disease Control and Prevention

PREVENTIVE SERVICES

14. Maternal and infant health
    - Health Resources and Services Administration
15. Heart disease and stroke
    - National Institutes of Health
16. Cancer
    - National Institutes of Health
17. Diabetes and chronic disabling conditions
    - National Institutes of Health
    - Centers for Disease Control and Prevention
18. HIV infection
    - National AIDS Program Office
19. Sexually transmitted diseases
    - Centers for Disease Control and Prevention
20. Immunization and infectious diseases
    - Centers for Disease Control and Prevention
21. Clinical preventive services
    - Health Resources and Services Administration
    - Centers for Disease Control and Prevention

SURVEILLANCE AND DATA SYSTEMS

22. Surveillance and data systems
    - Centers for Disease Control and Prevention

From USDHHS: *Healthy people 2000: national health promotion and disease prevention objectives, full report, with commentary*, Washington, D.C., 1991, U.S. Government Printing Office, p. 659.

HEALTHY PEOPLE 2000 Criteria Guiding Midcourse Review

Credibility—Objectives should be realistic and should address the issues of greatest priority.

Public comprehension—Objectives should be understandable and relevant to a broad audience, including those who plan, manage, deliver, use and pay for health services.

Balance—Objectives should be a mixture of outcome and process measures, recommending methods for achieving changes and setting standards for evaluating progress.

Measurability—Objectives should be quantified.

Continuity—Year 2000 objectives should be linked to the 1990 objectives where possible but reflect the lessons learned in implementing them.

Compatibility—Objectives should be compatible where possible with goals already adopted by Federal agencies and health organizations.

Freedom from data constraints—The availability or form of data should not be the principal determinant of the nature of the objectives. Alternate and proxy data should be used when necessary.

Responsibility—The objectives should reflect the concerns and engage the participation of professionals, advocates, and consumers as well as State and local health departments.

From USDHHS: *Healthy people 2000: midcourse review and 1995 revisions*, Washington, D.C., 1995, U.S. Government Printing Office, pp. 272-273.

Public Health: What It Does

Focuses on primary prevention
Leads the development of sound health policy and planning
Educates people about health risks and health promotion
Prevents epidemics
Protects the environment, workplaces, housing, food, and water
Enforces laws and regulations that protect health and ensure safety
Promotes healthy behaviors
Links people to needed personal health services
Monitors the health status of the population
Mobilizes community action for health
Responds to disasters
Assures the quality, accessibility, and accountability of medical care
Targets high-risk and hard-to-reach populations with clinical services
Maintains diagnostic laboratory services
Collects health statistics
Researches to develop new insights and innovative solutions

Modified from U.S. Public Health Service: *For a healthy nation: returns on investment in public health*, Washington, D.C., 1994, USDHHS.

The Public Health Approach

Defines the health problem
Identifies the risk factors associated with the problem
Develops community-level interventions to control or prevent the causes of the problem
Implements interventions to improve the health of the population
Monitors interventions to assess their effectiveness

From U.S. Public Health Service: *For a healthy nation: returns on investment in public health*, Washington, D.C., 1994, USDHHS, p. 5.

influenza deaths, and financial barriers to preventive health services (USDHHS, pp. 15-17).

PUBLIC HEALTH IN THE UNITED STATES

The evolution of public health in the United States was discussed in Chapter 4. Public health practices have provided the foundation for significant improvements in both health and life expectancy. The accompanying boxes outline what public health does and the public health approach. The health care system and the public health system have taken separate paths toward the goal of limiting disease, disability, and premature death (Pearson, Spencer, Jenkins, 1995, p. 24). Historically, public health has been a stronghold for primary prevention while the health care system in general has focused on a "treatment" model (USPHS, 1994, p. 3).

The diversity of health and welfare resources in the United States makes it notable among countries of the world for its complicated policy relationships between levels of governments and its interweaving of private and public sector activity to maintain the public's health (Institute of Medicine, 1988, p. 37). In the government sector public health functions are carried out by the federal Department of Health and Human Services, state health authorities (SHAs), and local health departments (LHDs). Under the Constitution individual states have primary responsibility for ensuring the public health. In this present era of health care reform it will be interesting to see what the future holds for public health.

The Future of Public Health

The Future of Public Health is a landmark report on public health in the United States. Published in 1988 by the Institute of Medicine's (IOM) Committee for the Study of the Future of Public Health, this report examined the status of public health in the United States and provided a futuristic view for the public health system. The Committee broadly defined the mission of public health to be "the measures that we as a society take collectively to provide the conditions that ensure the people's health" (IOM, 1988, p. 17).

After careful study of the public health system the Committee concluded that the nation had lost sight of its public health goals and that the public health system was in disarray and a threat to the health of the nation (IOM, 1988, p. 191). This Committee found that decision making in public health is frequently driven by crises and the concerns of organized interest groups rather than by comprehensive analysis or the objective of enhancing the quality of life (IOM, p. 5). Some barriers cited to promoting public health included the lack of consensus on the mission of public health, inequities in public health services, problems in relationships among the several levels of government, the poor public image of public health, and fragmented decision making (IOM, p. 108). The Committee stated that public health resources have become so fragmented and diverse that deliberate action is often difficult if not impossible (IOM, p. 1).

The Committee stated that an impossible responsibility has been placed on America's public health resources "to serve the basic health needs of entire populations, while at the same time averting impending disasters, providing personal health care to those rejected by the rest of the health system, and to take on the new public health problems while confronting the old" (IOM, 1988, pp. 2, 138). According to the committee, public health in the United States requires that threats to the public health be successfully countered, including immediate crises such as the AIDS epidemic and access to health and welfare services for the indigent; enduring problems such as injuries, chronic illness, teen pregnancy, control of high blood pressure, smoking, and substance abuse;

and growing challenges such as the aging of the population, homelessness, and environmental health (IOM, pp. 19-30).

The Committee concluded that the American public has slackened its public health vigilance and come to take for granted the successes of public health, such as control of communicable disease and provision of safe food and water. The Committee stated that it is no wonder the American public health system is in trouble—*the wonder is that the system has done so much, for so long, with so little* (IOM, 1988, p. 2). The committee developed a list of core public health functions.

Core Public Health Functions

In *The Future of Public Health* core functions in ensuring public health were determined to be assessment, policy development, and assurance (IOM, 1988, pp. 7-8, 41-42, 141-142). These functions exist at all levels of government, and the government's role in ensuring these core functions includes:

Assessment. Regularly and systematically collect, assemble, analyze, and make available information on the health of the community, including statistics on health status, community health needs, and epidemiological and other studies of health problems. This is a governmental function that cannot be delegated.

Policy development. Exercise responsibility to serve the public interest in the development of comprehensive public health policies by promoting use of the scientific knowledge base in decision-making about public health and by leading in the development of public health policy. Agencies must take a strategic approach, developed on the basis of a positive appreciation for the democratic political process.

Assurance. Ensure constituents that services necessary to achieve agreed-upon goals are provided, either by encouraging actions by other entities (private or public sector), by requiring such action through regulation, or by providing services directly. Involve the general public and key policymakers in determining a set of high-priority personal and community-wide health services that governments will guarantee to every member of the community. This guarantee should include subsidization or direct provision of high-priority personal health services for those unable to afford them.

Public Health and Health Care Reform

Health care reform was discussed in Chapter 4. When reviewing proposals for health care reform it is important to look at the role of public health. Proposals need to incorporate public health provisions as part of a national health plan. Despite its centrality to the well-being of Americans, public health funding is jeopardized (USPHS, 1994, p. ii). Health care reform needs to ensure adequate funding for public health activities.

Historically, insufficient funds have been devoted to public health. In 1932 the United States spent $1 per person, 3.4% of the national health care expenditures, on public health (Committee on the Costs of Medical Care, 1932, p. 118; Koplin, 1990, p. 420). Today those numbers have changed to $34 per person but amount to only 1% of national health care expenditures (USPHS, 1994, p. 42). Over the past two decades public health funding has declined approximately 25% (USPHS, p. 3); during this same period many public health problems have emerged or increased. Public health is grossly underfunded in the United States!

A strengthened public health system is vital as our nation confronts challenges to the health of the public (USPHS, 1994, p. ii). Public health must retain its leadership role in primary prevention, and health care reform needs to provide sufficient resources to support and strengthen the public health system (USPHS, p. 43).

FEDERAL GOVERNMENT: HEALTH AND WELFARE FUNCTIONS AND ORGANIZATION

The United States has a wealth of health and welfare resources, the scope of which is not seen elsewhere in the world. The organization of these resources is diverse and complicated (see the box below for the organization of these resources). In addition to the core functions of public health previously discussed, each level of government has unique public health responsibilities. The federal government's public health responsibilities include the following (Institute of Medicine, 1988, p. 9):

- Support knowledge development and dissemination through data gathering, research, and information exchange
- Establish nationwide health objectives and priorities, and stimulate debate on interstate and national public health issues
- Provide technical assistance to help states and localities determine their own objectives and to carry out action on national and regional objectives

Organization of Health and Welfare Services: United States

THREE LEVELS

Federal
State
Local

TWO SECTORS

Public (governmental)
Private*

*Private-sector resources can be nonprofit or for-profit (proprietary) agencies.

- Provide funds to states to strengthen state capacity for services, especially to achieve an adequate minimum capacity, and to achieve national objectives
- Ensure actions and services that are in the public interest of the entire nation, such as control of AIDS and similar communicable diseases, interstate environmental actions, and food and drug inspection

Table 5-1 gives examples of some functions and activities of the federal government in relation to public health and welfare. Today almost all federal level agencies are involved in matters of health and welfare in some way. However, the single most important agency in matters of health and welfare is the U.S. Department of Health and Human Services (USDHHS). Most of the health and welfare functions of the federal government are coordinated and administered through this department.

U.S. DEPARTMENT OF HEALTH AND HUMAN SERVICES

This department assumed a cabinet-level position on April 11, 1953, as the Department of Health, Education, and Welfare (DHEW). In 1980 the DHEW split into the U.S. Department of Health and Human Services (USDHHS) and the Department of Education. The USDHHS is the department most involved with the nation's human resources and concerns, and it touches the lives of more Americans than any other federal agency. It is charged with safeguarding the health and welfare of the nation.

The secretary of the department advises the President on health, welfare, and income security issues. In 1995 the Department went through a major reorganization (Figure 5-1 depicts the organization of the USDHHS). Major components of the USDHHS are discussed here, using information from the U.S. Government Manual.

U.S. Public Health Service

The U.S. Public Health Service (USPHS) is the oldest, and possibly the best known, of the department's agencies. It was established in 1798 as the Marine Hospital Service and became the PHS in 1912. Under the direction of the Surgeon General it carries out the mandates of the Public Health Act of 1944 and is charged with protecting and advancing the nation's physical and mental health.

Under the reorganization that occurred, PHS agencies became USDHHS operating divisions that report directly to the Secretary. These operating divisions, along with the Office of Public Health and Science (OPHS), constitute the "reorganized" PHS. On the USDHHS organizational chart the OPHS is under the Assistant Secretary for Health. Through PHS initiatives activities such as broad-based public health assessments will be conducted and population-based, clinical, preventive health services will be encour-

table 5-1 FEDERAL GOVERNMENT HEALTH AND WELFARE FUNCTIONS

FUNCTIONS	SELECTED ACTIVITIES
Assessment and planning	Includes a number of ongoing national assessments and collection planning of health and welfare statistics. Health planning activities include setting national health objectives and assisting states in their implementation. Stimulates debate on national health and welfare issues.
Assurance	Involves periodic evaluation of progress toward national health objectives and monitoring of the quality and effectiveness of national public health programs. Provides technical assistance and funds to states and localities to promote health and welfare.
Policy development	Includes enacting the necessary health and welfare legislation and making adequate appropriations for implementing legislative mandates.
Personal and community health	Carries out extensive personal and community health services, including services in the *Healthy People 2000* priority areas, providing direct services to special population groups (e.g., Native Americans, Native Hawaiians, military personnel, rural Americans, and migrant workers). Supports programs such as VISTA, community mental health centers, rural health centers, and senior citizen centers.
International health and welfare	Is a member of and supports international health and welfare organizations including the United Nations, WHO, and the Peace Corps. Participates in foreign aid, international disaster relief, environmental health, and world peace and human rights activities.
Education and training	Supports knowledge development and dissemination. Subsidizes grants and loans for education and training of health and welfare professionals. Provides grants-in-aid to schools of public health and is involved in health education and public health programs. Offers numerous health and welfare publications at low or no cost to the general public. Maintains numerous national clearinghouses, which distribute educational materials, and the U.S. Government Printing Office.
Research	Subsidizes research for the advancement of health and welfare. The National Institutes of Health conduct rigorous research programs and collaborate on international research. The National Institute of Nursing Research is one of these national institutes.

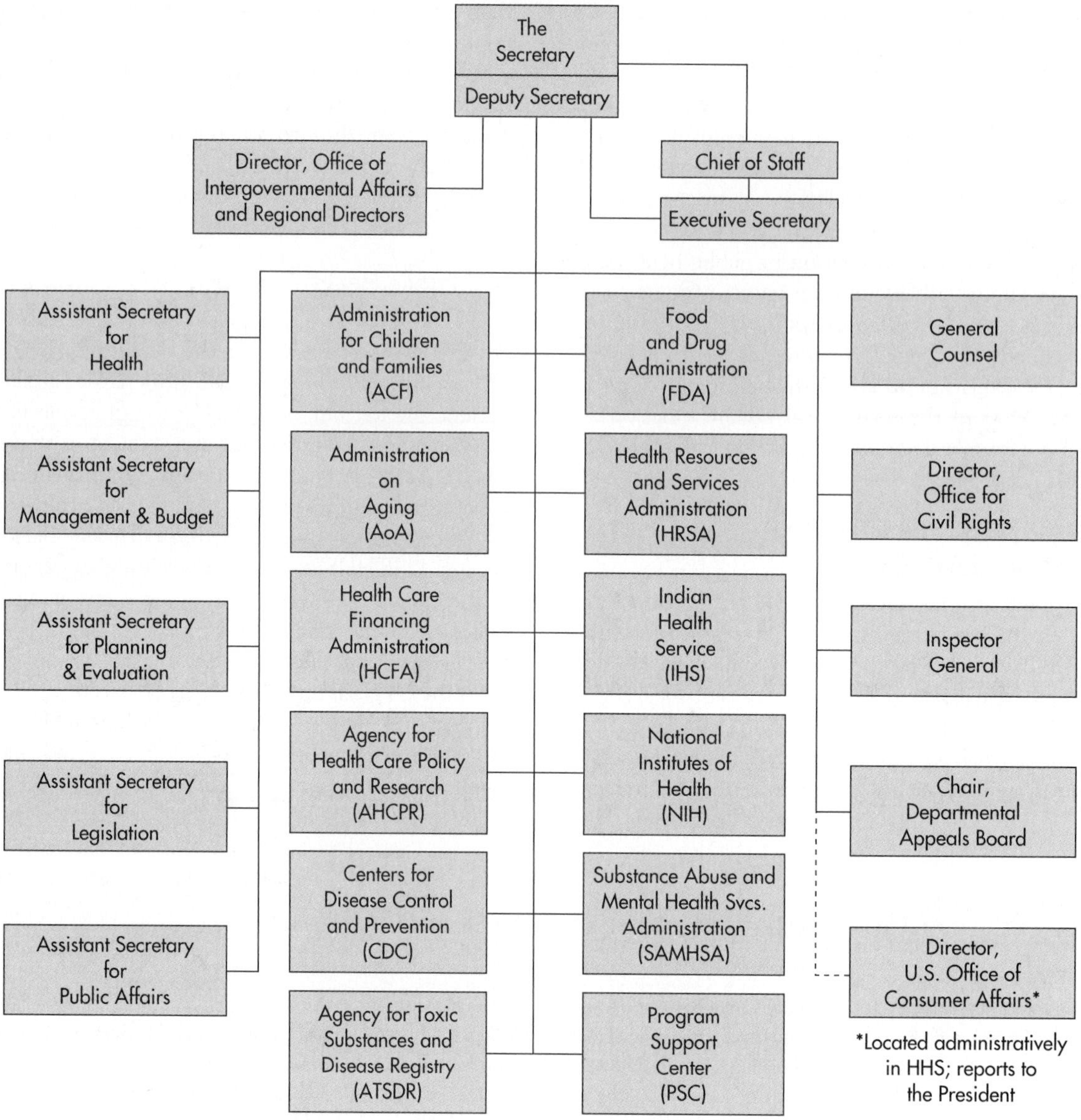

Figure 5-1 Organization of the U.S. Department of Health and Human Services. *(From U.S. Department of Health and Human Service:* Organizational chart, *Washington, D.C., 1996, The Department.)*

aged and coordinated (Shalala, 1995, p. 2). The PHS provides leadership in areas of women's health, minority health, emergency preparedness, population affairs, international and refugee health, disease prevention and health promotion, physical fitness, HIV/AIDS policy, and public health research.

Administration for Children and Families

The Administration for Children and Families (ACF) was created April 15, 1991. It provides numerous services to children, families, persons who are developmentally disabled, and Native Americans. It administers state grant programs, community service programs, Head Start, services for wayward youth, Child Abuse Prevention and Treatment Act provisions, Child Support Enforcement Act provisions, and refugee resettlement programs.

Administration on Aging

The Administration on Aging (AoA) was created by the Older Americans Act of 1965 and is the principal agency designated to implement programs of this act. It develops policies, plans programs to promote the health and welfare of older Americans, and administers grants to states to establish state and community programs for older persons.

Health Care Financing Administration

The Health Care Financing Administration (HCFA) was created by the Department of Health, Education, and Welfare reorganization of March 8, 1977, and oversees the administration of Medicare, Medicaid, and federal quality control measures designed to improve the delivery of health care services. Chapters 4, 14, and 21 address issues handled by this agency.

Agency for Health Care Policy and Research

The Agency for Health Care Policy and Research (AHCPR) was established in 1989. It is the lead agency for health services and health care delivery research. It is the only federal agency charged with producing and disseminating information about the quality, medical effectiveness, and cost of health care. Some priorities include reducing health care costs, improving access to and quality of health care, and developing models for health care reform.

Centers for Disease Control and Prevention

The Centers for Disease Control was established in 1973. In 1992 its name was changed to Centers for Disease Control and Prevention, but the acronym (CDC) remained the same. It is the federal agency charged with protecting the public's health. It includes 11 operating components: (1) Epidemiology Program Office, (2) International Health Program Office, (3) National Immunization Program Office, (4) Public Health Practice Program Office, (5) National Center for Prevention Services, (6) National Center for Environmental Health, (7) National Center for Injury Prevention and Control, (8) National Institute for Occupational Safety and Health (NIOSH), (9) National Center for Chronic Disease Prevention and Health Promotion, (10) National Center for Infectious Diseases, and (11) National Center for Health Statistics. Some major program components focus on communicable disease prevention and control, health promotion, chronic disease prevention, occupational safety and health, public health emergencies, and international health. The Centers also coordinate the use of rare therapeutic and immunoprophylactic agents and direct and enforce national quarantine measures.

Food and Drug Administration

The Food and Drug Administration (FDA) was formally established in 1931. Its activities are directed toward protecting the health of the nation against impure and unsafe food, drugs, and cosmetics. Major divisions include (1) Office of Operations, (2) Center for Drug Evaluation and Research, (3) Center for Biologic Evaluation and Research, (4) Center for Food Safety and Applied Nutrition, (5) Center for Veterinary Medicine, (6) National Center for Devices and Radiological Health, (7) National Center for Toxicological Research, (8) Regional Operations, (9) Office of Policy, (10) Office of External Affairs, and (11) Office of Management Systems.

Agency for Toxic Substances and Disease Registry

The Agency for Toxic Substances and Disease Registry (ATSDR) was established on April 19, 1983. Its Disease Registry provides leadership and direction to activities designed to protect the public and workers from the adverse effects of exposure to hazardous substances in storage sites that are released in fires, explosions, or transportation accidents. It assists the Environmental Protection Agency (EPA) in identifying hazardous wastes that need to be regulated. It carries out the health-related responsibilities of the Comprehensive Environmental Response, Compensation and Liability Act of 1980, the Resource Conservation and Recovery Act, and provisions of the Solid Waste Disposal Act.

Health Resources and Services Administration

The Health Resources and Services Administration (HRSA) was established in 1982. It has leadership responsibility for issues relating to access, equity, quality, and cost of health care. The administration supports states and communities in their efforts to plan and deliver health care, especially to underserved populations. It strengthens the public health system by working with state and local public health agencies and oversees management of the federal initiative to combat infant mortality. It provides leadership in improving the education, distribution, quality, and utilization of the nation's health professionals. HRSA funds AIDS demonstration and training projects, administers the National Organ Transplant Act, processes claims submitted under the National Vaccine Injury Compensation Program, monitors rural health issues, provides care for Hansen's disease patients, and works to address the special health needs of populations in U.S. border regions and immigrant populations.

Indian Health Service

The Indian Health Service (IHS) provides a comprehensive system of health care to Native Americans and Alaskan Natives in cooperation with the Native American tribes. Its goal is to raise the health status of Native Americans and Alaskan natives to the highest level possible. The IHS assists Native American tribes in developing health programs by providing consultation, training, and health planning activities.

National Institutes of Health

The National Institutes of Health (NIH) is the principal biomedical research agency of the federal government. The goal of NIH is to improve the health of the nation through increasing the understanding of processes affecting human health, disability, and disease; advancing knowledge concerning the health effects of interactions between humans and the environment; developing methods of preventing, diagnosing, and treating disease; and disseminating research findings. Institutes in the NIH include: (1) National Cancer Institute, (2) National Heart, Lung, and Blood Institute, (3) National Institute of Diabetes and Digestive and Kidney Disease, (4) National Institute of Allergy and Infectious Diseases, (5) National

Institute of Child Health and Human Development, (6) National Institute on Deafness and Other Communicative Disorders, (7) National Institute of Dental Research, (8) National Institute of Environmental Health Science, (9) National Institute of Neurological Disorders and Stroke, (10) National Eye Institute, (11) National Institute on Aging, (12) National Institute of Arthritis and Musculoskeletal and Skin Diseases, (13) National Institute of General Medical Sciences, (14) National Institute of Alcohol Abuse and Alcoholism, (15) National Institute on Drug Abuse, (16) National Institute of Nursing Research, and (17) National Institute of Mental Health. The NIH also includes the National Library of Medicine, National Center for Research Resources, National Center for Human Genome Research, Clinical Center, Division of Computer Research and Technology, Fogarty International Center, and the Division of Grants.

Substance Abuse and Mental Health Services Administration

The Substance Abuse and Mental Health Services Administration (SAMHSA) provides national leadership for the prevention and treatment of addictive and mental disorders. SAMHSA strives to improve access and reduce barriers to high-quality, effective treatment and prevention programs for individuals, families, and communities. It supports strategies to prevent the abuse of alcohol and other drugs.

SOCIAL SECURITY ADMINISTRATION

The Social Security Administration (SSA) was originally established on July 16, 1946 when its predecessor, the Social Security Board, was abolished. The Social Security Independence and Program Improvement Act of 1994 made the administration an independent agency of the federal government as of March 31, 1995. Before becoming an independent agency it had been part of the USDHHS.

The administration oversees the OASDI and SSI programs of the Social Security Act of 1935. It is responsible for studying health care needs and poverty in the United States, assigns social security numbers, and maintains individual records of social security earnings.

The SSA includes 10 regional offices (Boston, New York, Philadelphia, Atlanta, Chicago, Dallas, Kansas City, Denver, San Francisco, and Seattle), over 1300 local offices across the country, and is the major federal agency dealing with social welfare programs. Local offices have responsibility for informing people about SSA programs, assisting in filing and processing claims, and helping claimants file appeals. Requests can be made to local offices for information on social security. The administration can be contacted at 1-800-772-1213 for information and programs and publications.

OTHER FEDERAL INVOLVEMENT IN HEALTH AND WELFARE

On the federal level numerous agencies have health and welfare functions. The Veterans' Administration provides hospital, nursing home, and outpatient medical and dental care to eligible veterans of military service; coordinates veteran compensation, pension, and assistance programs; and provides rehabilitation training for disabled veterans. Other federal health and welfare involvement includes the Endangered Species Committee, United States Information Agency, Architectural and Transportation Barriers Compliance Board, Commission on Civil Rights, the Tennessee Valley Authority, Disability Rights Council, President's Committee on Physical Fitness, and President's Committee on Employment of People with Disabilities. All U.S. cabinet-level departments provide services that relate to the improvement of national and international health and welfare conditions.

Cabinet-Level Involvement

Cabinet-level departments are extensively involved in provision of health and welfare services to the American public. One cabinet-level department, the Department of Health and Human Services, has already been discussed. All cabinet-level departments sponsor research, education, and training opportunities. The following box looks at cabinet-level involvement in health and welfare activities.

Two important government agencies that do not have cabinet status are the Corporation for National and Community Service and the Environmental Protection Agency (the EPA is discussed in Chapter 6). The federal government is also involved in numerous international health activities.

Corporation for National and Community Service

The corporation was established by the National and Community Service Act of 1993. It fosters civic responsibility and strengthens the ties that bind us together as a people. The corporation's mission is to develop and support an ethic of service in America and mobilize Americans of all backgrounds in volunteer, community-based service. In exchange for 1 or 2 years of service, volunteers receive service education awards of up to $4,725 per year to repay college loans or help finance their their college education. The corporation is divided into three major divisions: AmeriCorps (programs: AmeriCorps*USA, AmeriCorps* National Civilian Community Corps, AmeriCorps* VISTA), Learn and Serve America (programs: School-Based and Community-Based Programs, Higher Education Programs), and National Senior Service Corps (programs: Retired and Senior Volunteer Program [RSVP], Foster Grandparent Program, Senior Companion Program). It is headquartered in Washington, D.C., and can be reached at 1-800-942-2677.

Cabinet-Level Involvement: United States

Department of Agriculture. Sets and enforces food and drug standards. Offers nutrition education and training and works to minimize hunger and malnutrition in the United States. Its national food programs include food stamps, National School Lunch Program, School Breakfast Program, Special School Milk Program, senior citizen nutrition programs, Commodity Supplemental Food Program, and Supplemental Food for Women, Infants, and Children program (WIC). Maintains the National Agricultural Library, conducts agricultural research, operates cooperative extension services, and offers international food assistance programs. Its Forest Service oversees the national forest system (more than 191 million acres).

Department of Commerce. Promotes national economic development and encourages technological advancements. Its Bureau of the Census collects and disseminates data about the economy of the country and the characteristics of population groups; census information is discussed more thoroughly in Chapter 13. It maintains a national measurement system.

Department of Defense. Provides the military forces necessary to deter war and to protect the national security. Administers the health and medical care services for military forces as well as civilian dependents of service personnel. Operates the National Civil Defense Program.

Department of Education. Safeguards the nation's educational system. Oversees bilingual education, educational civil rights, education of people who are disabled, and vocational and adult education. Offers services to the nation's schools.

Department of Energy. Provides the framework for a comprehensive national energy plan. Is responsible for energy conservation and regulations, radioactive waste management, environmental restoration, cleanup of inactive waste sites, and nuclear energy and weapons. Ensures that departmental programs are in compliance with environmental safety and health regulations.

Department of Health and Human Services. This department has been discussed separately in this chapter. It is the lead federal agency in matters of health and welfare.

Department of Housing and Urban Development. Is the principal agency concerned with national housing needs and fair housing opportunities. Provides public low-income housing and oversees the development and modernization of impoverished communities, the establishment of new communities, and emergency shelter grants. (Some of the housing programs under the department were discussed in Chapter 4.)

Department of the Interior. Is the nation's major environmental conservation agency, responsible for protecting our natural resources. Implements policies for the protection of the environment pursuant to the National Environmental Protection Act of 1969, and enforces laws concerning flood plains, wetlands, and endangered species. Assists communities in environmentally sound land use. Is responsible for preserving historic places and national parks (has jurisdiction over 270 million acres of public land). Its Bureau of Indian Affairs promotes improvement of health and welfare conditions for Native Americans.

Department of Justice. Protects the health and welfare of the American public by enforcing federal laws. Is instrumental in protecting civil rights, prosecutes high-level narcotic and drug offenders, and is involved in programs to help reduce homicide, violence, and drug addiction in the United States. Represents the United States in litigation involving environmental health and public lands and natural resources. Its Bureau of Prisons is responsible for all health, food, and sanitation services in federal prisons.

Department of Labor. Promotes the health and welfare of workers and strives to improve working conditions of Americans. Helps to protect the economic future and retirement security of working Americans and is the national guardian of a vast private retirement and welfare benefit system. Administers provisions of a variety of federal labor laws, including the Occupational Safety and Health Act of 1970, the Job Training and Partnership Act of 1982, and the Employment Retirement Income Security Act of 1974. Coordinates federal compensation and unemployment programs and enforces safety standards and fair employment practices. Activities of the department's Occupational Safety and Health Administration and the Mine Safety and Health Administration focus on promoting worker health and safety. Oversees workers' compensation legislation and black lung benefits. Compiles statistics about the American work force.

Department of State. Assists the President in formulating foreign policy, carries out foreign aid and trade agreements, assists in improving the quality of life in underdeveloped countries, is an advocate of international human rights, and is involved in international law enforcement. Is responsible for refugee programs, international travel, passports, and representing our country abroad. Develops, administers, and staffs a worldwide primary health care system for department employees and their eligible dependents residing abroad.

Department of Transportation. Enforces certain air, land, and water standards in relation to interstate transport. Its U.S. Coast Guard is responsible for guarding the American coastline, promoting boating safety, and enforcing the federal Water Pollution Control Act and other laws relating to protection of the marine environment. Its National Highway Traffic Safety Administration is charged with reducing morbidity and mortality on U.S. highways, conducts programs aimed at reducing traffic accidents, and compiles transportation statistics. Its Federal Aviation Administration develops and implements programs and regulations to control aircraft noise, sonic booms, and other environmental effects of civil aviation. Sets and enforces regulations for the safe interstate transportation of hazardous materials. Oversees transportation related to civil emergencies.

Department of the Treasury. Assists other government agencies in preventing illegal drug traffic and illegal possession of firearms, alcoholic beverages, and tobacco products through the U.S. Customs Service and the Bureau of Alcohol, Tobacco, and Firearms.

Modified from Office of the Federal Register: *U.S. government manual 1995-96*, Washington, D.C., 1995, U.S. Government Printing Office.

International Involvement

The United States is involved with a number of agencies, groups, and governments on an international level to maintain and improve health, welfare, and environmental conditions throughout the world. Several intergovernmental agreements, especially in relation to disease control, trade, immigration, world peace, and respect for basic human rights, have been developed to enhance the well-being of all people.

UNITED NATIONS The United States is extensively involved in international health and welfare issues through the United Nations (UN). This international assembly is dedicated to promoting welfare, peace, and health. Two major UN-sponsored groups with which the United States works are the World Health Organization and the United Nations' Children's Fund.

WORLD HEALTH ORGANIZATION Efforts to organize international health activities took place between 1851 and 1909, when a series of meetings known as the International Sanitary Conferences occurred. These meetings were the precursor to the International Office of Public Health in 1909 (Pickett, Hanlon, 1990, p. 74). In 1948 the World Health Organization (WHO) was created as part of the United Nations. However, any nation can belong to WHO without being a member of the United Nations. A major goal of WHO is to achieve international cooperation for health throughout the world.

WHO focuses much of its international health activity on the control of communicable disease and maternal and child health. It sets international quarantine measures, collects epidemiological data, is actively involved in coordinating international AIDS research and information, and is a clearinghouse for international health information. WHO is also concerned with worldwide health standards and practices, standardizing international health regulations, providing statistical and health education services, promoting research, and training health workers. WHO publishes international health statistics and documents worldwide outbreaks of disease. The headquarters of WHO is located in Geneva, Switzerland.

UNITED NATIONS' CHILDREN'S FUND The United Nations' Children's Fund (UNICEF) attempts to meet the emergency and ongoing needs of children, particularly children in developing countries. It has improved maternal and child health by combating malnutrition (through food programs), preventing and controlling communicable diseases (through immunization and treatment programs), and providing food, shelter, and other basic welfare needs. UNICEF works closely with WHO to promote health and welfare services for at-risk mothers and children throughout the world.

PEACE CORPS The Peace Corps was established in 1961 and was made an independent agency by the International Security and Development Act of 1981. Americans of all ages and from all walks of life serve as volunteers in the Peace Corps. The Corps is charged with promoting a better understanding of the American people and promoting world peace and friendship by helping to meet the needs of other countries.

Thousands of Peace Corps volunteers serve in Central and South America, the Caribbean, Africa, Asia, the Pacific, Europe, Russia, the Ukraine, and the Baltics. Volunteers work in areas of education, agriculture, health, environment, and small business and urban development. Community projects incorporate the skills of volunteers with the resources of the host country and international assistance programs. To increase international understanding, Corps volunteers make presentations in U.S. elementary, junior high, and senior high schools. Main headquarters are in Washington, D.C., and can be reached at 1-800-424-8580.

STATE AND LOCAL GOVERNMENT: PUBLIC HEALTH SERVICES RELATIONSHIP

Each state is responsible for providing for the health of its residents, has a public health code that authorizes public health activities, and has a state health authority (SHA) that deals with health. Most SHAs have local affiliates. The SHA and local health department (LHD) are official government agencies that are supported by taxes and provide health services to the general public. State public health codes establish what type of administrative relationship exists between SHAs and LHDs.

Administrative Relationships Between SHAs and LHDs

Historically three organizational patterns have characterized the administrative relationships between SHAs and LHDs: (1) the SHA has direct administrative authority over the LHD; (2) the local government operates the LHD and has direct administrative authority over it; the SHA provides consultation; or (3) shared control, where the state has some authority, such as appointing local health officers or budget approval, and the LHD is autonomous in other areas. SHAs usually share in the cost of LHD services, but the cost-sharing ratio varies greatly. LHDs provide many direct services to clients, whereas SHAs are more involved in indirect service provision. Services provided by SHAs and LHDs vary; some common service areas are discussed here.

Service Functions of SHAs and LHDs

An overall goal of state health authorities and local health departments is to enhance personal and community health. This is done through provision of public health services in the categories found in the following box. These service functions are discussed for both SHAs and LHDs in this chapter.

STATE HEALTH AUTHORITY (SHA)

The U.S. Constitution empowers state governments to protect the health and welfare of their citizens. States are the central authorities in the nation's public health system and have the primary responsibility for public health (Institute of Medicine, 1988, p. 8). The state health authority (SHA) is the agency or department dealing with health on the state level. The structure of SHAs differs from state to state. Figure 5-2 is an organizational chart depicting how a SHA might be organized.

The Institute of Medicine's Committee for the Study of the Future of Public Health recommended that, in addition to the core functions of assessment, policy development, and assurance previously discussed, the public health duties of states should include the following (Institute of Medicine, 1988, p. 12):

- Assessment of health needs in the state based on statewide data collection
- Assurance of an adequate statutory base for health activities in the state
- Establishment of statewide health objectives, delegating power to local health departments (LHDs) as necessary and holding them accountable
- Assurance of statewide efforts to develop and maintain essential personal, educational, and environmental health services, provision of access to necessary services, and problem solving for public health
- Guarantee of a minimum set of essential health services
- Support of local service capacity, especially when disparities exist in local ability to raise revenue and/or administer programs

There are 55 state and territorial health agencies. Thirty-three states have an independent SHA, and the remainder have a "superagency" where health, welfare, environmental health, and/or mental health are combined into one agency—similar to the USDHHS (PHF, 1995a, p. 1) (Figure 5-3). A major drawback to superagencies is the blending of services in one agency with the possibility of one detracting from another and having little emphasis placed on issues of health. The Institute of Medicine's Committee for the Study of the Future of Public Health (1988, p. 152) recommended that public health be organizationally separate from welfare, but that the agencies maintain close and cooperative ties.

Approximately nine SHAs combine public health with mental health, and six combine public health with environmental health (PHF, 1995a, p. 1). Forty-four SHAs are designated as the state crippled children's agency, and eight are the state Medicaid agency (PHF, 1995a, p. 1).

Service Functions of SHAs and LHDs

1. Administrative
2. Communicable disease control
3. Personal health (maternal-child health and adult health)
4. Environmental health and safety
5. Occupational health
6. Vital statistics
7. Laboratory
8. Health education and training
9. Research
10. Emergency and special medical

State Public Health Code

Each state authorizes specific public health services through its legislated public health code. All of these codes include policies on communicable disease control and the

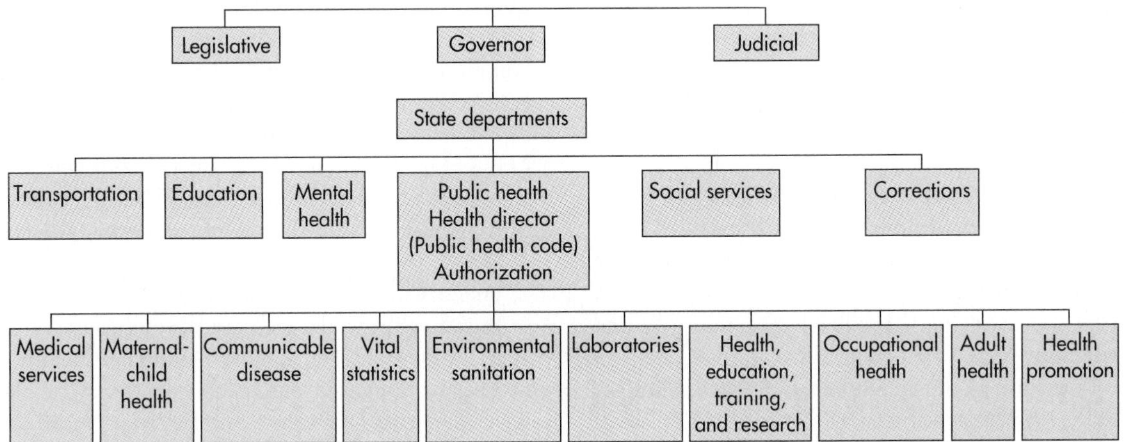

Figure 5-2 Organizational chart of a state health authority (SHA).

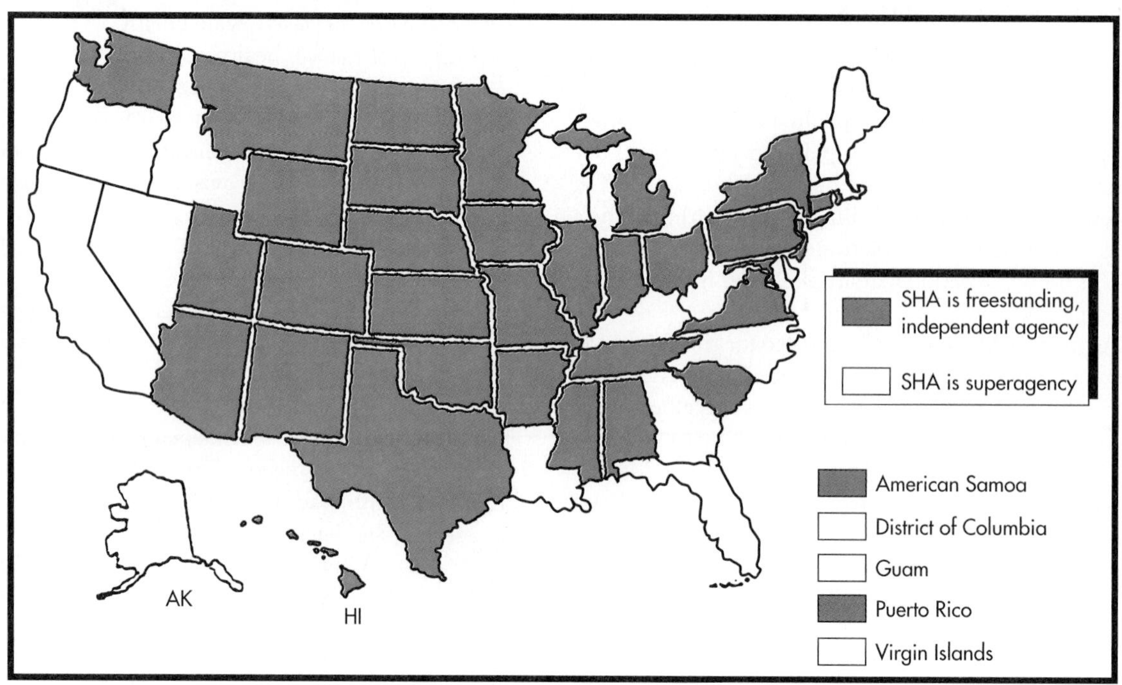

Figure 5-3 State health authorities (SHAs) that are organized as freestanding independent agencies. *(From Public Health Foundation: SHAs—freestanding agencies v. superagencies,* Public Health Macroview *7(1):1, 1995, p. 1.)*

collection of vital statistics. These codes designate what administrative relationship exists between SHAs and LHDs. The SHA can delegate responsibility for certain health activities mandated in the code to LHDs, but ultimate responsibility for the activity rests with the state.

Chief Executive

The chief executive of a SHA is often called the health officer or director. State health officers are frequently physicians who are political appointees. The average term of service is 2 years; greater continuity of leadership in such positions is needed (Institute of Medicine, 1988, p. 148). Less than half of SHA health officers have public health training or experience. Some states are now requiring graduate education in public health (Institute of Medicine, p. 174).

Spending

SHAs spend \$11.3 billion each year (PHF, 1995b, p. 2). SHA spending is financed primarily from state (41%) and federal funds (32%) (PHF, 1995b, p. 2). A comparison of SHA and LHD expenditures is shown in Figure 5-4, SHA spending by source of funds is shown in Figure 5-5, and SHA spending by type of program is shown in Figure 5-6. Recently states have not been a stable source of funding for SHAs (PHF, 1992, p. 2). Faced with deteriorating fiscal conditions and decreases in state funding, many SHAs are trimming their budgets and cutting back on services offered (PHF, p. 2).

Service Functions

The state health authority is charged with furnishing the leadership and funding to meet state public health needs. It carries out this charge through the service functions described in the following sections.

ADMINISTRATIVE Assessment, policy development, and assurance are core functions of SHAs. In the area of policy development, states provide the legal, statutory basis for public health practice in their public health codes. SHAs are often involved in setting and enforcing state environmental health standards and legislation (see Chapter 6). Representatives of the SHA meet regularly with state legislators, congressmen, politicians, health professionals, and community action groups to develop public health legislation responsive to the needs of the people in the state. States may delegate enforcement of public health law to LHDs, but this function is overwhelmingly assigned to states in the public health codes. The SHA may take action against a LHD that is not adhering to state health policies.

Assessment and assurance activities include assessment of state health needs, program development, ongoing program evaluation, and quality assurance. Health planning activities are carried out in conjunction with the federal government and local communities to promote community health and meet *Healthy People 2000* objectives.

Consultation services are provided to LHDs and other health agencies. The state health department advises local

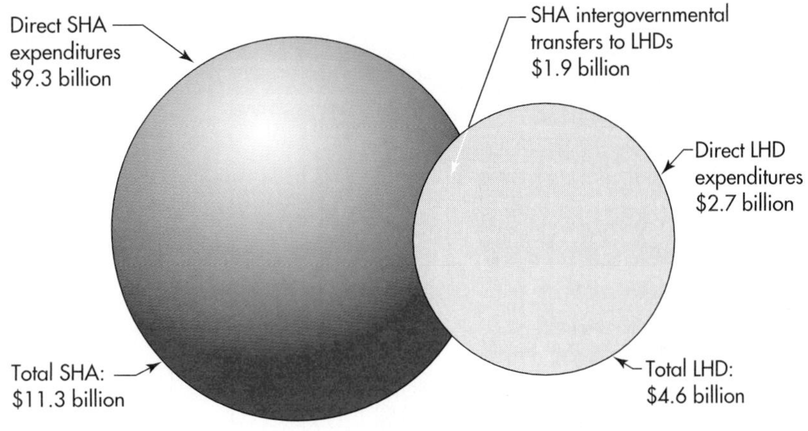

Figure 5-4 State health authority and local health department spending. *(From Public Health Foundation: State health agency and local health department spending in 1991 by source of funds,* Public Health Macroview *7(1):2, 1995, p. 2.)*

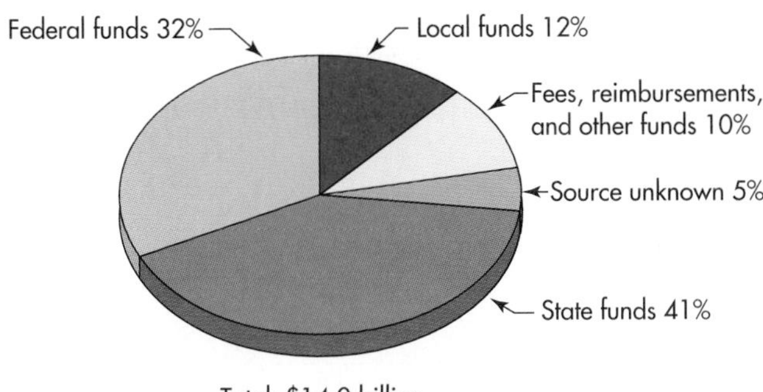

Figure 5-5 State health authority (SHA) spending by source of funds. *(From Public Health Foundation: State health agency and local health department spending in 1991 by source of funds,* Public Health Macroview *7(1):2, 1995, p. 2.)*

health departments on health planning and programs, budget, and personnel policies. Consultants are available in such fields as maternal-child health, nutrition, epidemiology, community health nursing, mental health, occupational health, and environmental health. These consultant activities are usually well utilized and are a major state health department service.

Administration of federally aided programs is an important function of state health authorities. The federal government provides funding for health programs, many through block grants. Federal monies often provide programs and services in areas such as health education/risk reduction, communicable disease, cardiovascular disease, emergency medical services, sex offenses, rodent control, epidemiology, environmental health, and immunizations. Prevention Block Grant monies fund many health programs. Figure 5-7 shows how these grant monies are spent by states.

Coordination of federal, state, and local health programs and services is another function assumed by the SHA. Data are compiled on available health resources and services offered throughout the state and nation.

Personnel policies, including hiring and promotional guides, job descriptions, grievance procedures, and personnel manuals, are developed by the SHA. SHAs may assist LHDs in obtaining staff members. In some states the state health department establishes the qualifications for local health officers.

CONTROL OF COMMUNICABLE DISEASE Communicable disease control is a major service function of SHAs. The state establishes immunization policies, quarantine measures, and communicable disease guidelines. States often provide laboratory diagnostic services and supply LHDs with biologics such as vaccines. Recent outbreaks of immunizable childhood communicable diseases such as measles and rubella, a rise in cases of tuberculosis, and the AIDS epidemic dramatically illustrate the importance of communicable disease control as a function of SHAs. Communicable disease control is often taken for granted by the general public, but continuous, comprehensive efforts are needed to control communicable disease in our nation's communities!

PERSONAL HEALTH SERVICES Personal health services are considered direct services delivered to individuals, except those related to environmental health. States are usually not heavily involved in direct provision of personal health services. LHDs are generally the service providers in this area. Generally the state's role in personal health involves the administration of federal block grant monies, consultation, and evaluation services. In some states SHAs provide services to special populations such as people who are mentally ill or mentally retarded, migrants, workers (occupational health services), and children with disabilities.

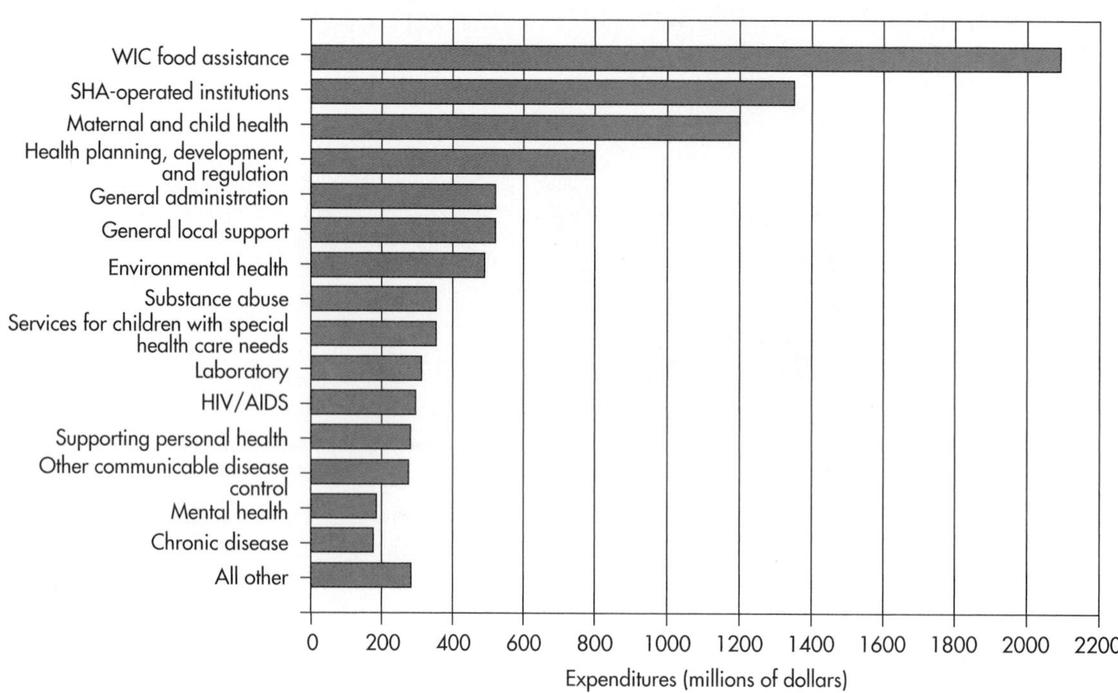

Figure **5-6** State health authority (SHA) spending by type of program. *(From Public Health Foundation:* 1991 public health chartbook, *Washington, D.C., 1991, The Foundation.)*

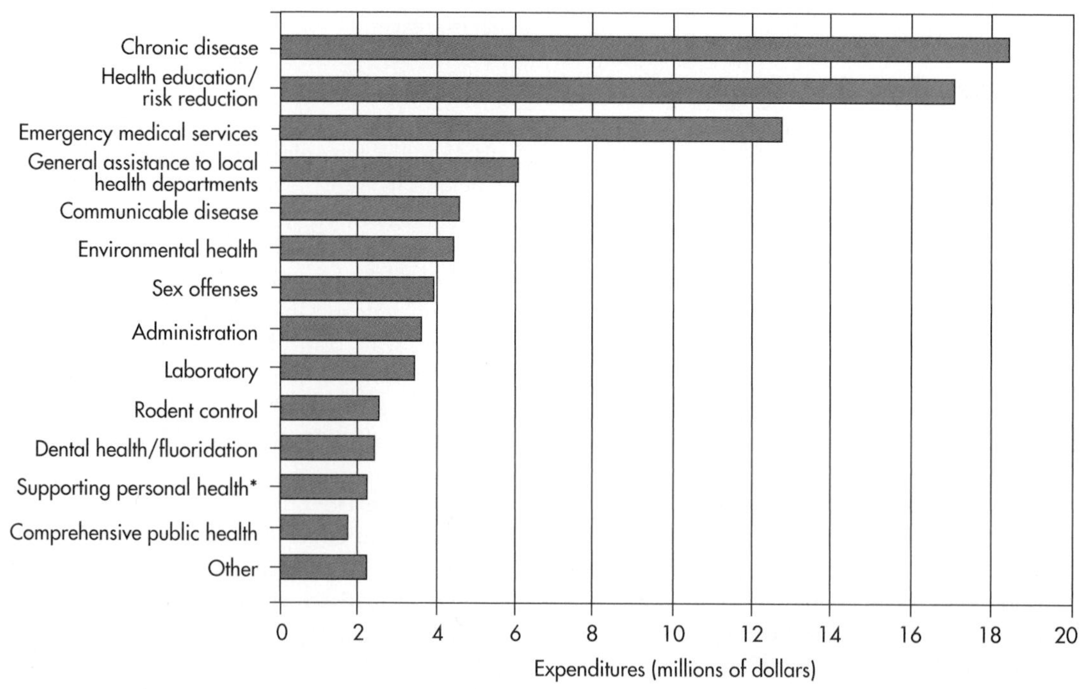

*Includes epidemiology, home health services, and field service nursing.

Figure **5-7** Prevention block grant spending by type of service. *(From Public Health Foundation:* 1991 public health chartbook, *Washington, D.C., 1991, The Foundation).*

OCCUPATIONAL HEALTH State health officials are assuming a more prominent role in occupational health and safety. However, SHAs are the lead agency for occupational health in only five states: New Jersey, New Mexico, North Dakota, Rhode Island, and Texas (PHF, 1991a). State occupational safety and health standards must be equal to or exceed federal standards. A number of states code occupational information on death certificates; some states collect data about parental occupation on birth certificates to help pinpoint causes of congenital malformations and disorders; and a few states have registries for occupational diseases. Chapter 18 provides information on occupational health in the United States.

VITAL STATISTICS Vital statistics are collected by the SHA, and many states have centers for health statistics. States develop standardized forms, including certificates of birth, death, fetal death, marriage, and epidemiological reporting forms. The state disseminates statistical information to individuals and agencies, including the National Center for Health Statistics. The SHA has an abundance of information about the health status of its population and the health resources within the state (see Chapter 13).

LABORATORY SERVICES Laboratory services are operated by most SHAs. LHDs and private physicians often use these services in providing care to clients. There is usually no fee, or a minimal fee, to the public for laboratory analysis of reportable communicable diseases. The laboratory also certifies vaccines and other biologics. The diagnostic services rendered are primarily in relation to communicable disease control and environmental sanitation.

HEALTH EDUCATION AND TRAINING Education, training, and research are carried out by the SHA. The state promotes the development of new health knowledge through the support of state colleges, universities, and research agencies; the development of training and inservice programs for SHA and LHD personnel; and involvement in research activities. SHAs are valuable resources when health information is needed.

SHAs promote community health education activities and provide health information to the general public, often in the form of printed materials, classes, videos, and public service announcements. Recently some states have expanded their health education activities to include paid advertising. When using radio and television SHAs have tried to have ads air when target groups were watching or listening. The ad campaigns have been effective and have primarily addressed tobacco and drug use and AIDS. In an ad campaign in Minnesota, 55% of the target group members recalled at least one billboard, 70% recalled at least one radio ad, and more than 95% recalled at least one TV ad; in a California campaign the recall rate was approximately 70% to 75% (PHF, 1991b, p. 3). The U.S. Public Health Service has recommended that more SHAs investigate the use of paid advertising to address public health issues (PHF, 1991b, p. 3).

RESEARCH State health departments promote the development of new health care research. They carry out research studies and subsidize research activities. Research funds need to be increased; however, these funds are often the first monies included in budget cuts.

EMERGENCY AND SPECIAL MEDICAL SERVICES Special medical services include the provision of hospital and institutional services for chronic or long-term conditions such as mental retardation, mental illness, and tuberculosis. In the event of emergencies such as epidemics and natural disasters, emergency services ensure that the necessary public health care is made available to the community in need.

Staff

The SHA is headed by a chief executive (health officer or other title) who is usually appointed by the governor; this person is traditionally a physician. Other staff members include administrators, clerical workers, and consultants in fields such as community health nursing, occupational health, mental health, epidemiology, statistics, maternal-child health, health education, and nutrition. SHAs have legal counsel available to them, often through the state attorney general's office. States may have regional directors who serve as intermediaries between their regions and the state department. Most SHA personnel, except for the chief executive, are civil service employees.

Community health nurses are a valuable part of SHA staffs. They are hired to provide consultant services and help to establish state health policies, particularly in relation to maternal-child health and adult health services. They work closely with LHDs to improve the quality of care delivered to individuals, families, and aggregates at risk. Generally, community health nurses who work for state health departments are prepared at the master's or doctoral level and have community health nursing experience.

LOCAL HEALTH DEPARTMENT (LHD)

The Public Health Foundation's definition of a local health department (LHD) is displayed in the box on the next page. There are nearly 3000 local health departments in the United States (PHF, 1991c, p. 1). According to this definition, no local health departments exist in five states: Arkansas, Delaware, Rhode Island, Vermont, and Virginia (PHF, 1991c, p. 142). When LHDs do not exist, public health services are offered through the state or territorial health authority.

The Institute of Medicine's Committee for the Study of the Future of Public Health recommends that, in addition to the core public health functions (see the section on federal government functions in this chapter), LHDs also be responsible for the following activities (Institute of Medicine, 1988, pp. 9-10):

- Assessment, monitoring, and surveillance of local health problems and needs and resources for dealing with them.

Definition of a Local Health Department

Local health department (LHD): an official (governmental) public health agency which is, in whole or in part, responsible to a substate governmental entity or entities. An entity may be a city, county, city-county, federation of counties, borough, township, or any other type of substate governmental entity. A local health department must:

- Have a staff of one or more full-time professional public health employees (e.g., public health nurse, sanitarian);
- Deliver public health services;
- Serve a definable geographic area; and
- Have identifiable expenditures and/or budget in the political subdivision(s) it serves.

From Public Health Foundation: *Public health agencies 1991: an inventory of programs and block grant expenditures*, Washington, D.C., 1991c, The Foundation, p. 148.

- Policy development and leadership fostering local involvement and a sense of ownership, emphasizing local needs, and advocating equitable distribution of public resources; and complementary private activities commensurate with community needs.
- Assurance that high-quality services, including personal health services, needed for the protection of public health in the community are available and accessible to all persons; that the community receives proper consideration in the allocation of federal, state, and local resources for public health; and that the community is informed about how to obtain public health, including personal health, services, or how to comply with public health regulations.

The LHD is the basic unit for the delivery of public health services, and most Americans benefit directly or indirectly from LHD services. It has responsibility for a specific jurisdiction, often a geopolitical jurisdiction such as a city, town, or county. In the United States many LHDs are organized on either a county or city level.

Administration

LHDs usually have a board of health and a health officer. Each LHD will establish its own organizational pattern. An example of an organizational structure for a local health department is given in Figure 5-8.

Funding

Local health departments receive their funding from a number of sources, with the largest percentage coming from local tax dollars. The Public Health Foundation (PHF) has for many years had the responsibility of compiling national statistics on the funding of state and local health departments. Recently PHF funding has been cut, and national statistics on LHD funding are becoming difficult to obtain. The most recent statistics show that, nationally, LHDs spend over $4.1 billion (PHF, 1991c, p. 3). See Figure 5-9 for local health department spending by source of funds.

Service Functions

Just as each LHD establishes its own organization, each determines its own services and methods of service provision. Traditionally LHDs have offered personal and environmental health services. Personal health services offered by LHDs have focused on maternal-child health and control of communicable disease, including immunization services, tuberculosis and sexually transmitted disease clinics, well-baby clinics, school health services, chronic disease programs, family planning, and home care.

Traditionally most LHDs have not actively engaged in the provision of ongoing primary care services. LHD provision of primary care services to disadvantaged populations has been more popular in the southeastern part of the country (PHF, 1989). The Institute of Medicine Committee has cautioned that provision of such service may drain vital resources away from population-wide services, that the U.S. public health system is inadequately equipped to address these needs, and that this provision of primary care may pose a threat to the maintenance of important disease prevention and health promotion efforts (Institute of Medicine, 1988, pp. 13, 152-153). The committee endorsed the idea that the ultimate responsibility for ensuring equitable access to health care for all rests with the federal government. However, many people in this country remain medically underserved, and primary care services being provided at reasonable cost through local health departments may be part of the health care reform of the future.

Many people in the community are not aware of the services available at their LHD. A major role of the community health nurse is to familiarize the public about LHD programs and services. The people of the community support the LHD with their tax dollars and, in return, it has many services available to them.

Local health departments have functions similar to those carried out by the state health department, but the services they provide are more direct. Direct services offered by local health departments are extensive.

ADMINISTRATIVE The administrative functions of the local health department are identical in coverage to those implemented by the state health department, but the specific services vary.

Assessment, policy development, and assurance are core functions of LHDs. These functions involve ongoing community assessment and the promulgation and enforcement of local health standards, regulations, and policies. The standards established by a LHD usually relate to public food handling, storage, preparation, and disposal and to public water supplies, including wells, septic systems, and pools or lakes at recreational facilities. LHDs also supervise and license local health facilities such as

- People of the County
  - Board of Commissioners
    - Board of Health
      - Health Officer
        - Medical Director
          - Epidemiologist
        - Medical Advisory Committee
        - Director of Environmental Health
          - Sanitarians
        - Health Planner and Evaluator
        - Director of Health Education
          - Health Educators
        - Director of Public Health Nursing
          - Clinic Supervisors
            - Family Planning / Well Baby Clinic Staff
              - Adult Health
          - Field PHN Supervisors
            - Field Public Health Nurses
          - Special Services Coordinator
            - W.I.C. and Crippled Children Staff
        - Business Manager
          - Personnel Staff / Bookkeeper / Secretaries / Maintenance
        - Chief of Statistical Services
          - Statisticians

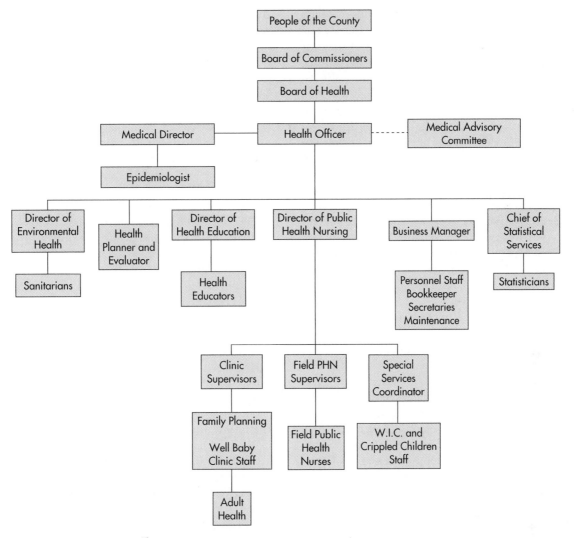

Figure 5-8 Organizational chart of a local health department.

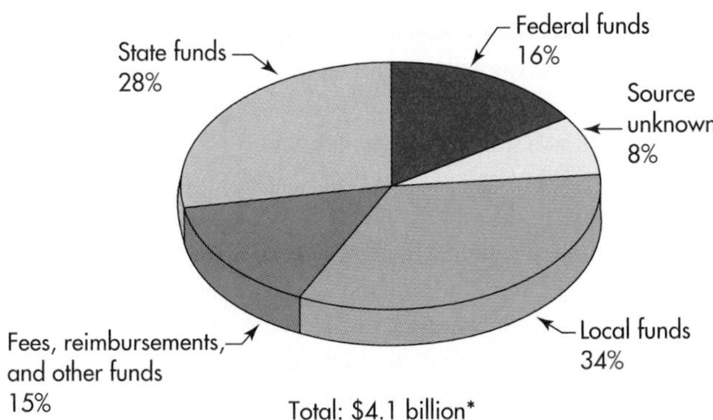

*Includes $1.8 billion in intergovernmental transfers from state health agencies.

Figure 5-9 Local health department spending by source of funds. *(From Public Health Foundation:* 1991 public health chartbook, *Washington, D.C., 1991, The Foundation.)*

hospitals, nursing homes, and restaurants, and carry out ongoing programs.

Legislation is guided and influenced by the LHD, often in the form of local ordinances and codes. LHDs make their communities' public health needs known to the state legislature and influence state public health legislation. It is imperative that local health departments assume leadership in the formulation of public health policy, because they are the direct service providers and have first-hand knowledge of client needs. If local health departments do not become involved in policy making, important preventive health care services may be lacking in a community.

Consultation services are offered by the LHD to groups, organizations, and individuals. These activities usually involve consulting services from community health nurses, environmental engineers, nutritionists, and epidemiologists.

Consultation in relation to state and local health policy, environmental safety, communicable disease control, and personal health services is offered in a variety of community settings, including schools, industry, hospitals, nursing homes, and community service groups within the health department's jurisdiction.

Coordination is an important function of the LHD. It involves working cooperatively with local health agencies and helps to minimize duplication of services, eliminate unnecessary services, facilitate case management, and aid in the provision of the greatest number of services at the least amount of cost and community effort. Interagency planning is essential in providing coordinated, comprehensive community health programs and services. The LHD often provides leadership for resource coordination and development with the local community. Community involvement is encouraged, and consumers are involved in looking at the provision of health services. Consumer participation is discussed in Chapters 13 and 14.

Health planning activities include working in partnership with communities to determine public health needs and plan appropriate health intervention strategies (see Chapter 14). The LHD also participates in statewide health planning activities.

Personnel policies, promotion guides, position descriptions, grievance policies, and manuals are developed by local health departments to facilitate effective personnel management. Staff turnover and job satisfaction are often related to how well an organization is managed (see Chapter 23). Some position descriptions and qualifications, such as health officer, may be determined by the SHA, and some health departments use state services to recruit qualified personnel. Many local health department employees are civil service employees, and personnel policies will reflect civil service guidelines.

CONTROL OF COMMUNICABLE DISEASE Communicable disease control is a major emphasis of the LHD. Each local health authority, in conformity with regulations of higher authority (state, national, and international), will determine what diseases are to be routinely and regularly reported, who is responsible for reporting, the nature of the reports, and the manner in which the reports are to be forwarded (Benenson, 1995, p. xxiii). Reportable communicable diseases that are required by international health regulations are cholera, plague, smallpox, yellow fever, and those diseases under surveillance by WHO: louseborne typhus fever and relapsing fever, paralytic poliomyelitis, viral influenza, and malaria (Benenson, p. xxiv).

Communicable diseases reportable to the LHD will vary, and their selection is often dependent on the severity and frequency of the disease. Some communicable diseases will be reported on the basis of individual cases, and some only if epidemics occur. Some commonly reportable individual cases of communicable diseases are viral hepatitis, infectious hepatitis, rubella, salmonellosis, venereal syphilis, diphtheria, gonorrhea, leprosy, rubeola, meningococcal meningitis, Q fever, rabies, shigellosis, tetanus, tuberculosis, typhoid, and whooping cough.

The communicable disease services of LHDs include prevention, case finding, early diagnosis, and treatment. Many LHDs operate sexually transmitted disease, tuberculosis, and immunization clinics at little or no cost to the general public. The department makes epidemiological studies of suspected or reported cases of communicable disease, and the community health nurse is actively involved in this follow-up (see Chapter 11).

The health department provides other communicable disease measures, such as enforcing quarantines; conducting public food, water, and refuse disposal inspections; and maintaining communicable disease statistics. The environmental health division is extensively involved in these measures. Continuing surveillance and prevention of communicable diseases is an important LHD activity. It is too easy to become lax about this surveillance when there has been no recent outbreak of disease.

PERSONAL HEALTH SERVICES Personal health services are a major component of LHD services. They include both maternal-child and adult health activities. Programs in dental health, substance abuse, accident prevention, and nutrition are essential to an effective program of personal health services (Pickett, Hanlon, 1990). To carry out these services the health department offers an extensive array of clinics, classes, and home visit services.

School health is a major component of personal health services. Community health nurses implement nursing interventions in schools, including health education, counseling, screening programs, and direct nursing care. Nurses are frequently involved in hearing, vision, and scoliosis screening programs to identify children who have health needs and facilitate early diagnosis and treatment. School health services and the role of the school nurse are discussed in Chapter 16.

Many other maternal-child health services are provided by the LHD. Clinic services include family planning, immunization, sexually transmitted disease control, and well-child check-ups. A variety of other services are offered, including classes for expectant and new parents and home visits to follow up on antepartal and postpartum clients, children with disabilities, and high-risk mothers and infants. Counseling and health teaching in relation to immunizations, growth and development, and community resources are a few examples of the types of services provided by community health nurses when they make home visits. In addition, programs such as the Supplemental Food Program for Women, Infants, and Children (WIC), dental health, and hearing-vision programs are often provided by the LHD.

Nursing interventions in relation to adult health involve clinics, classes, and home visit services. The nurse provides direct care to clients in immunization, family planning, primary care, and sexually transmitted disease clinics. Nursing interventions include health education activities about chronic conditions such as heart disease, diabetes, cancer, epilepsy, arthritis, stroke, alcoholism, and drug abuse; and teaching about primary prevention, early diagnosis and treatment, and community resources. Community health nurses teach classes and conduct screening activities (e.g., blood pressure, breast cancer, and geriatric multiphasic screening) at the health department and in community settings such as schools, churches, and industry. The community health nurse works closely with community resources to assist the adult in meeting health care needs. Major goals of the community health nurse when working with adult clients are to enhance their self-care capabilities and promote health.

ENVIRONMENTAL HEALTH Many of the public health successes we have had in the past in controlling communicable disease have come about as a result of effective environmental health practices (e.g., safe water management, safe sewage disposal). Traditionally health departments have been involved in environmental health as it relates to air and water quality, land use, environmental safety, building codes and safety, noise pollution, waste management, sanitation, food quality and protection, and vector and animal control. Environmental concerns dealing with radiation control and toxic and hazardous substances have recently emerged. Environmental health is discussed in Chapter 6.

OCCUPATIONAL HEALTH The Occupational Safety and Health Act of 1970 allows states to establish their own occupational safety and health administrations. Occupational health activities are largely conducted on the state level and are not routinely carried out by LHDs. However, some industries are contracting with local health departments to provide diagnostic and screening programs and assist with recordkeeping. Some occupational health nurses, especially those in small industries, are seeking consultation from the nursing staff in the local health department for the development of health policies and procedures and the management of clinic facilities. Although this would seem to be a natural area for LHDs, there has been little involvement by them in the past.

VITAL STATISTICS Vital statistics are collected by LHDs and used for health planning purposes. The LHD keeps statistics on births, deaths, and reportable communicable diseases, maintains registers of individuals known to have specific communicable diseases where carrier states exist (typhoid), conducts morbidity and mortality surveys as necessary, and maintains records on jurisdictional health facilities. The LHD may even issue birth and death certificates to people within its jurisdiction.

LABORATORY SERVICES Laboratory services are provided by the LHD. However, many do not have their own laboratories and use state facilities. Laboratory services may be extended to hospitals, clinics, and private practitioners on a contractual, fee-for-service basis. Laboratory services include water analysis, serology, urology, parasitology, identification of microorganisms, x-ray services for tuberculosis control, sanitation laboratory services, and metabolic and genetic screening for conditions such as phenylketonuria (PKU) and sickle cell anemia. These services are essential for communicable disease control and environmental sanitation and safety, as well as for the treatment of genetic and metabolic disorders and genetic counseling related to these conditions.

HEALTH EDUCATION AND TRAINING Education and training are a part of LHD services. Health educators are often hired by LHDs to coordinate health education activities. The LHD provides health education services directly to individual clients, develops and carries out community health education programs, distributes health education materials, provides classes, and serves as a health information center.

Training activities largely involve staff inservice and continuing education programs. Some health departments offer tuition reimbursement for employees who take university course work in public health or related fields as a staff benefit.

RESEARCH LHDs engage in research to promote the health of aggregates at risk and the community and to strengthen the health care delivery system. Research is carried out by a variety of staff members and can be done in conjunction with program evaluation studies.

Research activities often include morbidity, mortality, and program evaluation studies. State health departments are usually more actively involved in research, but increasingly LHDs are recognizing the need for such activity. Research studies related to service effectiveness and cost containment are especially emphasized at the local level. Staff should be encouraged to engage in research, and research activities should be an ongoing function of the agency.

EMERGENCY AND SPECIAL MEDICAL SERVICES Special and emergency medical services offered by the LHD usually involve catastrophic medical care during a natural disaster or an epidemic, compulsory hospitalization through judicial admissions for acute communicable diseases such as tuberculosis, and care for those involved in serious environmental accidents (e.g., hazardous chemical spills or contamination). Health department personnel are also involved in health planning activities designed to meet the emergency needs of community citizens. In order to carry out these diverse functions and meet emergency and special needs, LHDs employ staff members from a variety of disciplines.

Staff

Staff will vary from one LHD to another. The minimum staff includes (1) a health officer, (2) a community health nurse, (3) an environmental engineer (sanitarian), and (4) a clerk. Additional personnel include statistician, epidemiologist, health educator, physical therapist, occupational

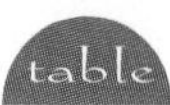

5-2 Historically Recommended Staff-to-Community Ratio

Staff	Population
Health officer/medical personnel	1:50,000
Sanitarians (environmental engineers)	1:15,000
Community health nurses	1:5,000
Office personnel (clerk)	1:15,000

Data from Hanlon JJ, McHose F: *Design for health*, ed 2, Philadelphia, 1971, Lea & Febiger, p. 56.

health specialist, nutritionist, dentist, dental hygienist, veterinarian, and social worker. To provide comprehensive community health services, a basic multidisciplinary staff is necessary. Table 5-2 shows the historically recommended staff-to-community population ratio.

These ratios often are not achieved in many local communities. However, estimating the number of community health personnel needed in a local area is not as simple as previously thought. Multiple factors, such as current health problems in the community and the type and supply of health professionals in an area, influence workforce planning. LHDs must establish staffing priorities based on available resources and needs.

HEALTH OFFICER Traditionally a health officer was a physician with public health training who was licensed to practice in the state. Today many health officers are still physicians, but the field is opening up to other health professionals such as nurses and public health administrators. If the health officer is not a physician, a medical director is hired to provide medical direction and consultation for LHD programs. The health officer administers the agency; prepares and submits budgets; appoints and hires personnel; takes part in program planning, implementation, and evaluation; and serves as a consultant to health department staff and community agencies. The health officer is responsible for seeing that all divisions in the local health department are run efficiently and in a cost-effective manner.

COMMUNITY HEALTH NURSE Community health nurses carry out a variety of health activities, which are discussed throughout this text. Community health nurses use a synthesis of nursing and public health theory to promote community health. They are the backbone of the personal health services of the health department and are extensively involved in most health department programs. The types of services offered by the nursing division in a LHD vary, depending on the work force available and other community resources that have been developed to meet the health care needs of community citizens.

Many LHDs use nurse practitioners to run clinics such as antepartal, sexually transmitted diseases, family planning, and WIC. If the LHD has a home care program the community health nurses will be used to provide skilled nursing care in the home. Community health nurses are extensively involved in health education activities and conduct a variety of classes (e.g., expectant parent classes, diabetic classes, and family planning information sessions).

Baccalaureate preparation is recommended for entry-level positions in community health (ANA, 1986; Anderson, Meyer, 1985; Jones, Davis, Davis, 1987). Baccalaureate-prepared nurses are required to have community health nursing content during their educational preparation and have a strong background in the human and social sciences.

ENVIRONMENTAL ENGINEER The environmental engineer (sanitarian) is responsible for the elimination or reduction of hazards in the environment. Environmental engineers apply principles of public health, toxicology, health, education, law enforcement, and industrial health and use practical and technical measures to eliminate or control environmental health problems. They have historically been members of LHD staffs; their efforts have facilitated communicable disease control and promoted a safe and healthy environment.

SUPPORT STAFF Many other people may be employed by LHDs, including social workers, lab technicians, practical nurses, home health aides, and clerical staff. A clerk/secretary is usually responsible for maintaining the records and schedules of the health department. Clerical and support staff are very important; without them it is difficult to effectively and efficiently manage health department services.

STATE AND LOCAL GOVERNMENT WELFARE ORGANIZATION

The provision of welfare assistance and insurance programs in every state and locality is legally mandated as a result of the Social Security Act of 1935. The primary purpose of official governmental welfare agencies is to assist indigent individuals in meeting their basic needs of food, shelter, and clothing. Benefits provided by these agencies are usually in the form of cash, food, or shelter.

Official welfare services are organized in much the same manner as official health services. There is a state-level department, usually a state department of social or human services, that establishes rules and regulations, sets guidelines for service provision, and administers services. Local branches of this state department provide direct services to clients.

Local departments of social services administer state-subsidized programs such as Temporary Assistance to Needy Families, food stamps, General Assistance, and Medicaid. Protective services for children and adults are often administered through departments of social service. Old Age, Survivors & Disability Insurance (OASDI) and Supplemental Security Income (SSI) are administered by the federal government through local Social Security Administration offices. For further discussion of state and local governmental welfare services and programs see Chapter 4.

PRIVATE HEALTH AND WELFARE ORGANIZATION

The United States abounds in private health and welfare resources. Historically there has been limited coordination between private and government resources, and there is no central coordination of private health and welfare resources. As we move toward a partnership model in service delivery, an increasing number of cooperative ventures are being established between all types of agencies in the community. Private resources can be classified as either for-profit or nonprofit.

Private for-profit health and welfare services include an increasing number of hospitals, a large percentage of nursing homes, health and welfare professionals in private practice, pharmacies, health business companies (medical equipment companies, hospital supplies), and proprietary social service agencies. These services are available on a fee-for-service basis and are organized primarily as companies and independent businesses.

Private nonprofit resources are often voluntary resources. They are not mandated by any law and provide services on a nonprofit basis. They are represented by individuals, professional societies, service organizations, agencies, and facilities. Their services augment official (government) services. Voluntary resources are uniquely American. Individual voluntary efforts (volunteerism) have likely been with us since this country was founded.

Voluntary efforts have provided services that otherwise would not have been possible. The accompanying box briefly summarizes the characteristics of voluntary resources in the United States. Figure 5-10 depicts one voluntary agency, the American Red Cross. See Chapters 1 and 4 for additional discussion of voluntary agencies.

The functions of voluntary, nonprofit health agencies were studied in the classic Gunn-Platt Report. The functions of these agencies were described as pioneering and include exploration of and surveying for unmet needs, demonstration, education, supplementation of official activities, guarding of citizens' interest in health, promotion of health legislation, planning and coordination, and development of well-balanced community health programs (Gunn, Platt, 1945). These functions have not altered over time and are becoming increasingly more significant in this era of federal cost containment.

Millions of Americans volunteer their services to assist health and welfare programs each year. Operating funds for voluntary resources come largely from individual contributions, fees for service, membership dues, investment earnings, sales of goods and publications, bequests, grants, and contracts for service. Fund-raising is of vital importance to these organizations, and monies are often raised through donations. One voluntary service agency, the United Way, represents a large number of local voluntary resources with one central fund-raising campaign. Giving to the United Way campaign means giving to many voluntary resources with one donation. The federal government has encouraged private philanthropic giving to voluntary organizations by permitting contributions to be deducted from personal and corporate income tax.

Voluntary Resources: Characteristics, Classifications, and Examples

CHARACTERISTICS

Voluntarily organized

Governed by a board of directors that includes lay and/or professional members

Have no legal powers

Receive support primarily from voluntary contributions, fees for service, third party payers, and grants

Usually provide services to a defined geographical location

CLASSIFICATIONS

Professional societies

American Nurses Association (ANA), American Public Health Association (APHA)

Service agencies

Visiting Nurse Association (VNA), American Cancer Society, American Red Cross, Alcoholics Anonymous, Rockefeller Foundation, United Community Services

Facilities

Universities, public museums, and libraries

Individuals

Local communities have many private health and welfare resources. The Visiting Nurse Association and home health care programs are discussed in the next section, because home health care is becoming one of the major responsibilities of nurses in the community setting (see Chapter 21). Limiting discussion to these types of private health and welfare organizations is not meant to imply that other private agencies do not provide a valuable service to the community.

Home health care agencies are often administered by an executive director or chief executive officer (CEO) who operates under a board of directors if it is a nonprofit, voluntary agency (e.g., VNA), or owners of the company if it is a proprietary agency. Both VNAs and home health care agencies are primarily staffed and administered by nurses. An organizational chart of a VNA is given in Figure 5-11. Chapter 21 discusses the organization of all types of home health care agencies.

Visiting Nurse Associations (VNAs)

Visiting Nurse Associations are especially significant voluntary organizations in community health. VNAs began with the Women's Branch of the New York City Mission, organized in 1877 to teach hygiene in the homes of the

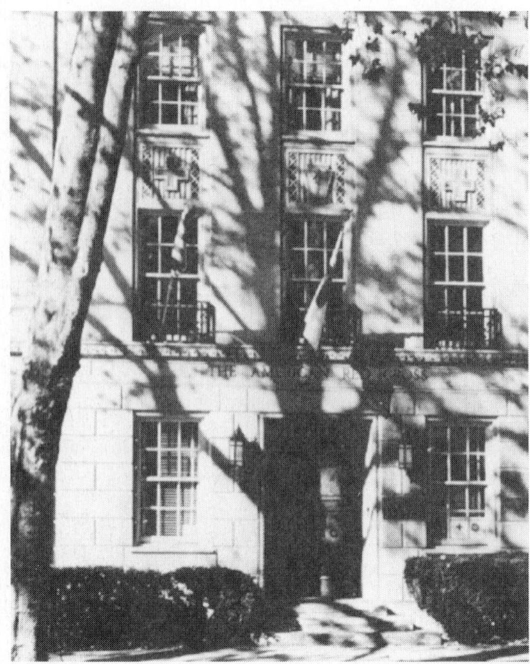

Figure 5-10 For over 100 years the American Red Cross, a voluntary, nonprofit organization, has initiated the development and provision of health and welfare services. Established originally to assist and support military men and their families during times of war and to aid victims of disasters, this agency continues to make significant public health contributions. Some of its current efforts include the provision of selected health and welfare services based on community need. The American Red Cross continues to provide relief for disaster victims and to serve military families. Local chapters of this organization can be found in most major cities across the United States. *(Courtesy Henry Parks, photographer.)*

disadvantaged. VNAs have been discussed in Chapter 1. Historically they have been organized as private, nonprofit, voluntary agencies. VNAs primarily make home visits to people who are in need of skilled nursing and augment the health education and clinic services of the LHD. Over the years there has been coordination and cooperation between VNAs and LHDs, and in some instances combined agencies were formed. Combination agencies consolidate a LHD and a VNA under one administrative structure.

In contrast to the health department, the program emphasis of the VNA is usually on secondary and tertiary preventive activities rather than on primary prevention. However, staff nurses do engage in primary prevention counseling as they provide skilled nursing care. For example, they discuss accident prevention when they assist clients with mobility.

Home Health Care Agencies

Home health care agencies are organized in both the private for-profit and nonprofit sectors. The organization of home health agencies differs from that of local health departments. As with VNAs, they deliver skilled nursing services to individuals in their homes. Shortened hospital stays have rapidly increased the need for such agencies, with people being discharged into the community still in need of nursing care. Clients who use the services of home health care agencies are often elderly, disabled, or recently discharged from a hospital setting. These programs are rapidly growing in numbers, largely in the private, for-profit sector. An emerging trend is for local hospitals to start their own home health care agency. Home health care is discussed in depth in Chapter 21.

COORDINATION OF HEALTH AND WELFARE RESOURCES

The United States has great diversity in health and welfare resources. Lack of coordination among these resources presents a multitude of problems for both providers and recipients of service. Providers of service may become frustrated because they find it difficult to learn about the resources available and effect change in the system. Recipients of service are frustrated because they are not aware of resources, do not understand how to use them, and often receive fragmented care. A major role of the community health nurse is to explain and coordinate community services. Lack of resource coordination can adversely affect the quality of care delivered to clients, as demonstrated in the following case scenario.

CASE *Scenario*

John Falta, age 19, was in a motorcycle accident that necessitated an amputation below the right knee. He was hospitalized for 6 weeks and upon discharge was referred to a local VNA for skilled nursing services, the Office of Vocational Rehabilitation for rehabilitation training, and the Department of Social Services for assistance with his medical expenses. In addition, a physical therapist from the hospital saw John on a weekly basis at home, and a volunteer from a local amputee self-help group visited him regularly to help him adapt to the changes that had occurred in his life. Each of these health and welfare resources provided a valuable service, but because they were not initially coordinated John found it difficult to understand why so many people were involved in his care. He told the visiting nurse that he was confused and depressed about the onslaught of so many "helping agencies" and the different goals that had been set for him. The nurse suggested that a conference be arranged between John, his family, and the involved resources; John agreed that this was necessary. The conference helped to coordinate John's care and stimulated John's involvement in the rehabilitation process. Because he had a clearer picture of what was happening, his depression decreased

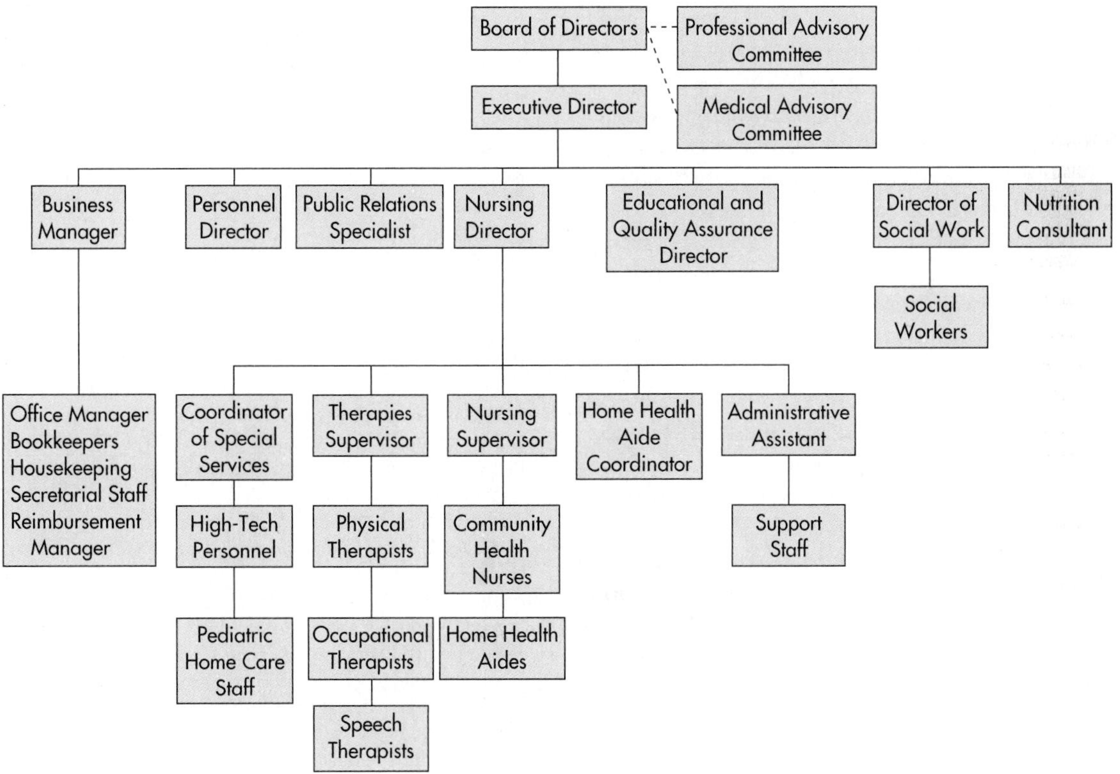

Figure 5-11 Organizational chart of a visiting nurse association.

and he actively participated in establishing goals for his future.

It is not uncommon to encounter clients like John Falta in community health nursing practice. Health and welfare personnel meet too infrequently to plan for coordinated service delivery. When such meetings do occur, they are often arranged to deal with individual client problems rather than to plan for coordinated preventive health and welfare resources and services.

A classic example of lack of coordination between health and welfare systems in this country is the administration of the government health insurance program of Medicare and the health assistance program of Medicaid. These programs are locally administered by agencies that traditionally are not considered to be health agencies: the Social Security Administration and state departments of social service. Official and private health agencies have little input into, control over, or administration of these two major governmental health programs. The case study of John Falta also evidenced such lack of coordination; health care and welfare professionals were not communicating with one another or with professionals from other systems.

Lack of coordination of services has been evident in all sectors of our health and welfare systems for decades. The National Commission on Community Health Services (1966, p. 132) identified minimal coordination between official (government) and private health care agencies. The National Health Planning and Resource Development Act of 1974 (Public Law 93-641) was passed to improve the delivery and coordination of government health care services to all segments of the population. However, in 1981 the Omnibus Budget Reconciliation Act was passed, which ended the federal mandate for Public Law 93-641 planning. It is now hoped that federal block grant program funding will improve the coordination of services (see Chapter 14).

Community health nurses are in a unique position to influence coordination of care on both an individual level with clients and a community level with health planners. On an individual level community health nurses are frequently the primary providers in the home setting. At this level one of their major functions is coordination of community resources for the families they visit. The John Falta case illustrates this. On a community level, community health nurses are currently writing grants to obtain block grant funding for community health services. The holistic philosophy of community health nurses provides them with the skills needed to integrate service delivery issues.

Summary

The Institute of Medicine's Committee for the Study of the Future of Public Health found that public health is a vital function that is in trouble in the United States. Public health agencies have many challenges to face, including AIDS, chronic disease, an aging population, leadership, financing, policy development, funding, and access to service.

The nation as a whole needs to make a concerted effort to ensure the stability of the public health system. The federal government has taken a leadership role in establishing national health objectives and supporting model public health standards. Americans must not be lax in their public health practices or attempt to divest themselves of public health issues. Public health cannot be taken for granted!

The community health nurse needs to be aware of national health objectives and model standards and be at the forefront of health care reform. The nurse must understand how health and welfare resources are organized to enhance service delivery, familiarize clients with the service delivery system, link clients to services, and facilitate client care. Nurses must be able to work in partnership with communities to promote public health and to facilitate community empowerment for health. They must instill in people the belief that public health is too important to be neglected or taken for granted.

CRITICAL *Thinking Exercise*

Local health departments (LHDs) all over the United States have historically provided public health services to local communities, and as national health care reform emerges these agencies could play a major role in service provision. Envision new and innovative ways for these LHDs to provide services to the community. How could existing LHD services be expanded? What new services could LHDs provide? What services do they need to provide to facilitate meeting the *Healthy People 2000* goals and objectives, and how could these services be funded? How do you see the nursing role(s) in community health service delivery?

REFERENCES

American Nurses Association (ANA): *Standards of community health nursing practice,* Washington, D.C., 1986, American Nurses Publishing.

American Public Health Association (APHA): *Healthy communities 2000: model standards. Guidelines for community attainment of the year 2000 national health objectives,* ed 3, Washington, D.C., 1991, The Association.

Anderson E, Meyer AT: *Consensus conference on the essentials of public health nursing practice and education,* Rockville, Md., 1985, USDHHS, Public Health Service.

Benenson AS, ed: *Control of communicable diseases manual,* ed 16, Washington, D.C., 1995, American Public Health Association.

Committee on the Costs of Medical Care: *Medical care for the American people,* Chicago, 1932, University of Chicago Press.

Gunn SM, Platt PS: *Voluntary health agencies: an interpretative study,* New York, 1945, Ronald Press.

Hanlon JJ, McHose F: *Design for health,* ed 2, Philadelphia, 1971, Lea & Febiger.

Institute of Medicine (IOM), Committee for the Study of the Future of Public Health: *The future of public health,* Washington, D.C., 1988, National Academy Press.

Jones DC, Davis JA, Davis MC: *Public health nursing education and practice* (Accession number HRP-0909092), Springfield, Va., 1987, National Technical Information.

Koplin AN: The future of public health: a local health department view, *J Public Health Policy* 11:420-437, 1990.

National Commission on Community Health Services: *Health is a community affair,* Cambridge, Ma., 1966, Harvard University Press.

Office of the Federal Register: *United States government manual, 1995/96,* Washington, D.C., 1995, U.S. Government Printing Office.

Pearson TA, Spencer M, Jenkins P: Who will provide preventive services? The changing relationships between medical care systems and public health agencies in health care reform, *J Public Health Manage Prac* 1(1):16-27, 1995.

Pickett G, Hanlon JJ: *Public health administration and practice,* ed 9, St. Louis, 1990, Mosby.

Public Health Foundation (PHF): *Status report: state progress on 1990 health objectives for the nation,* Washington, D.C., 1988, The Foundation.

Public Health Foundation (PHF): Survey shows wide variation in LHD reporting, *Public Health Macroview* 2(3):2, 1989.

Public Health Foundation (PHF): *1991 public health chartbook,* Washington, D.C., 1991a, The Foundation.

Public Health Foundation (PHF): Paid advertising—a powerful tool for SHAs, *Public Health Macroview* 4(2):3, 1991b.

Public Health Foundation (PHF): *Public health agencies 1991: an inventory of programs and block grant expenditures,* Washington, D.C., 1991c, The Foundation.

Public Health Foundation (PHF): Budget woes force SHAs to make cuts, *Public Health Macroview* 5(1):2, 1992.

Public Health Foundation (PHF): SHAs—freestanding agencies v. superagencies, *Public Health Macroview* 7(1):1, 1995a.

Public Health Foundation (PHF): State health agency and local health department spending in 1991 by source of funds, *Public Health Macroview* 7(1):2, 1995b.

Shalala D: *New role for the assistant secretary of health,* Washington, D.C., 1995, USDHHS (memo to staff).

U.S. Department of Health, Education, and Welfare (USDHEW): *Healthy people: the Surgeon General's report on health promotion and disease prevention,* Washington, D.C., 1979, U.S. Government Printing Office.

U.S. Department of Health and Human Services (USDHHS): *Promoting health/preventing disease: objectives for the nation,* Washington, D.C., 1980, U.S. Government Printing Office.

U.S. Department of Health and Human Services (USDHHS): *The 1990 health objectives for the nation: a midcourse review,* Washington, D.C., 1986, U.S. Government Printing Office.

U.S. Department of Health and Human Services (USDHHS): *Healthy people 2000: national health promotion and disease prevention objectives, full report, with commentary,* Washington, D.C., 1991, U.S. Government Printing Office.

U.S. Department of Health and Human Services (USDHHS): *Organizational chart,* Washington, D.C., 1996, USDHHS.

U.S. Department of Health and Human Services (USDHHS): *Healthy people 2000: midcourse review and 1995 revisions,* Washington, D.C., 1995, U.S. Government Printing Office.

U.S. Public Health Service (USPHS): *For a healthy nation: returns on investment in public health,* Washington, D.C., 1994, USDHHS.

SELECTED BIBLIOGRAPHY

Cohen WJ: Current problems in health care, *N Engl J Med* 281:193-197, 1969.

DeLaw N, Greenberg G, Kinchen K: A layman's guide to the U.S. health care system, *Health Care Financing Rev* 14:151-169, 1992.

Elders MJ: Macroviewpoint: prescription for America's youth, *Public Health Macroview* 5(1):6, 1992.

Harmon RG: Macroviewpoint: partners for the 1990s public health and primary care, *Public Health Macroview* 4(1):6, 1991.

Kennedy EM: *In critical condition: the crisis in American health care*, New York, 1973, Pocket Books.

Larsen BL: Macroviewpoint: chronic disease control in the '90s—making prevention count, *Public Health Macroview* 4(2):6, 1991.

Lorsch RL: *State and local politics: the entanglement*, Englewood Cliffs, N.J., 1983, Prentice-Hall.

Miller CA, Gilbert B, Warren DG, et al: A survey of local public health departments and their directors, *Am J Public Health* 67:931-939, 1977.

Oberle MW, Magenheim MS: Healthy People 2000 and community health planning, *Annu Rev Public Health* 15:259-275, 1994.

Public Health Foundation: SHA staffing declines 8% from 1979-1985, *Public Health Macroview* 1(4):5, 1988.

Public Health Foundation: Progress on the Healthy People 2000 objectives: healthy children, *Public Health Macroview* 4(1):4-5, 1991.

Public Health Foundation: Progress on the Healthy People 2000 objectives: nutrition, *Public Health Macroview* 4(2):4-5, 1991.

Public Health Foundation: Progress on the Healthy People 2000 objectives: HIV/AIDS, *Public Health Macroview* 5(1):4-5, 1992.

Remington RD: The future of public health—two years of progress, *Public Health Macroview* 3(5):6, 1990.

Stevens RH: A case study of public health nursing directors in state health departments, *Public Health Nurs* 12:432-435, 1995.

Stoto MA: Public health assessment in the 1990s, *Annu Rev Public Health* 13:59-78, 1994.

6

Environmental Health and Disaster Nursing

Objectives

Upon completion of this chapter, the reader should be able to:

1. Discuss environmental health as a public health concern.
2. Discuss the origins of environmental health in the United States.
3. Be aware of the *Healthy People 2000* national health objectives that relate to environmental health.
4. Describe the nurse's role in environmental health.
5. Name three major pieces of environmental health legislation in the United States.
6. Discuss the role of federal, state, and local governments in environmental health.
7. Discuss selected environmental diseases.
8. Discuss areas of environmental concern.
9. Discuss the phases of disaster management.
10. Describe the nurse's role in disasters.

We did not inherit the earth from our ancestors.
We borrow it from our children.

OLD PENNSYLVANIA DUTCH SAYING

Environmental health was one of the earliest public health concerns. Maintenance of safe food and water, proper sewage disposal, and interment of the dead became matters of law and custom. Archaeologists and historians have indicated that the Minoans (3000-1430 BC) and the Myceneans (1430-1150 BC) built drainage systems, toilets, and water-flushing systems (Pickett, Hanlon, 1990, p. 21). About 1500 BC the Hebrews had a written hygienic code with environmental practices, Athenians of 1000-400 BC had elaborate environmental sanitation measures, and early Egyptians constructed drainage systems and earth privies for sewage (Pickett, Hanlon, p. 21).

During the Middle Ages, 500 to 1500 AD, many of these earlier environmental health practices were ignored, and epidemics of leprosy, typhus, and bubonic plague ravaged the civilized world (Kalisch, Kalisch, 1995, p. 11). In the mid-1300s bubonic plague, known as the Black Death, killed as many as 60 million people (Kalisch, Kalisch, p. 12). Bubonic plague is spread by rodents and their fleas, and when left untreated has a case fatality rate of 50% to 60% (Benenson, 1995, p. 353). Diseases and conditions related to environmental factors are not a thing of the past; they are with us today and will continue to emerge.

In fact, the link between the environment and health is becoming increasingly evident, and environmental health continues to be a primary public health concern. In *Healthy People* the Surgeon General stated that "there is virtually no major chronic disease to which environmental factors do not contribute, either directly or indirectly" (USDHEW, 1979, p. 105) and noted that 20% of the deaths in the United States can be attributed to such environmental factors as pollution and toxic chemicals. The PEW Health Professions Commission (Shugars, O'Neil, Bader, 1991, p. 44) noted that the twentieth century has created countless environmental health problems that contribute to illness and chronic disease.

ENVIRONMENTAL HEALTH IN THE UNITED STATES

Environmental health has biological, chemical, physical, and sociological components and includes the immediate and future conditions in which people live. Definitions of environmental health are identified in the box on the next page.

In the colonial United States (1607-1797) little attention was paid to community hygiene and sanitation, and there was almost a complete lack of community organization for health services (Smillie, 1955, pp. 15, 72). During

Environmental Health Defined

ENVIRONMENTAL HEALTH: THE SCIENCE

The systematic development, promotion and conduct of measures that modify or otherwise control those external factors in the indoor and outdoor environment which might cause illness, disability or discomfort through interaction with the human system.

ENVIRONMENTAL HEALTH FROM A PERSONAL HEALTH PERSPECTIVE

Freedom from illness or injury related to exposure to toxic agents and other environmental conditions that are potentially detrimental to human health.

From USDHHS: *Evaluating the environmental health workforce* [HRP #0907160], Rockville, Md., 1988, USDHHS, p. 11.
From Institute of Medicine (Committee on Enhancing Environmental Health Content in Nursing Practice, Pope AM, Snyder MA, Mood LH, eds): *Nursing, health and the environment: strengthening the relationship to improve the public's health*, Washington, D.C., 1995, National Academy Press, p. 15.

this time epidemics of cholera, smallpox, yellow fever, measles, dysentery, influenza, pneumonia, scarlet fever, diphtheria, malaria, and syphilis continually recurred (Smillie, pp. 21-60). Although such epidemics were attributed to environmental health hazards such as inadequate ventilation, overcrowding, impure water, and inadequate housing, little was done to improve these conditions (Clark, 1972, pp. 30-36).

Early regulations that had an impact on environmental health included a 1610 Virginia law that stated no man or woman dare throw out water or suds from foul clothes into the open street, clean pots or kettles within twenty feet of a well or pump, or do the necessities of nature within a quarter mile of the town (Smillie, 1955, p. 61). Those who violated the law could be whipped and punished (Smillie, p. 61). Early environmental measures were often more concerned with the aesthetics of the environment than with related health consequences, and environmental practices frequently were directed at keeping the environment "sightly" and controlling "ill airs."

Early measures to control contagious disease in the United States often involved the use of isolation and quarantine (Smillie, 1955, p. 62); quarantine was accepted by the general public as a legitimate governmental function (Hill, 1976, p. 9). Sanitary police enforced quarantine measures and special "quarantine" physicians were employed to make home visits (Clark, 1972, pp. 8-10). As early as 1796 the federal government passed a quarantine act to enforce health and quarantine regulations at U.S. ports of entry.

The beginnings of organized environmental health activities in the United States started with the Shattuck Report in 1850 (see Chapter 4). This report made numerous recommendations regarding environmental sanitation and emphasized the need for controlling overcrowded housing, providing safe factories and buildings, ensuring food and water sanitation, and vaccinating against disease (Smillie, 1955, p. 252). Some early environmental sanitation activities in the United States included safeguarding community water supplies; proper sewage, refuse, and waste disposal; food and milk sanitation; disinfection and fumigation during epidemics; pest and vector control; and building safety. These activities produced great strides in environmental health and would become functions of state and local boards of health (Smillie, pp. 340-375).

When the American Public Health Association (APHA) was founded in 1872, only three states (California, Massachusetts, and Virginia) and the District of Columbia had established boards of health. Dr. Stephen Smith, APHA's first president and one of its founders, wrote *The City That Was*, a shocking description of the unsanitary conditions prevailing in New York City. He was a staunch supporter of environmental health activities (Ravenel, 1921, p. 32), and APHA had a strong focus on environmental health issues. The National Board of Health (1879-1883) instituted many environmental health activities in an effort to control epidemics and communicable disease.

In this century environmental health activities have expanded from a focus on sanitation and controlling communicable disease to include protecting and preserving the environment in which we live. Efforts by the American people have helped to preserve the environment, including establishment of state and national park systems, and to protect endangered wildlife. State health authorities and local health departments have consistently been involved in environmental health activities (see Chapter 5). The role of the federal government in environmental health is discussed later in this chapter. Some U.S. environmental health activities are listed in the following box.

ENVIRONMENTAL HEALTH AND THE *HEALTHY PEOPLE 2000* NATIONAL HEALTH OBJECTIVES

National objectives for environmental health were established in 1980. These objectives were based on data presented in *Healthy People* (USDHEW, 1979), and were projected to be achieved by 1990. Progress toward almost 75% of the 1990 environmental health objectives could not be measured because states did not have adequate environmental surveillance and monitoring systems (USDHHS, 1992, pp. 68, 103).

Healthy People 2000 listed environmental health as one of 22 priority areas and reestablished national environmental health objectives (see the box on p. 129). These objectives challenged the nation to promote environmental health and preserve the global environment. They focused on improving state-based environmental surveillance and monitoring systems, providing safe drinking water, reducing human exposure to toxic agents, improving the environment by effective solid waste disposal, eliminating immediate risks from

Selected U.S. Environmental Health Activities

The Shattuck Report was published in 1850 and outlined numerous environmental health activities necessary to ensure community health.

In 1872 the American Public Health Association was founded and became an advocate for environmental health activities.

On September 10, 1875, the first U.S. conservation organization, the American Forestry Association, was established. This organization remains active today.

On September 25, 1890, Yosemite Park was established by the U.S. Congress in an effort to preserve our natural lands and forests.

The Wilderness Society was founded on January 21, 1935. It remains an important conservation policy group that works primarily on issues involving federal public lands (national forests, national parks, national wildlife refuges). The group was instrumental in persuading Congress to create a national wilderness system.

The National Wildlife Federation was founded on February 5, 1936, and has the largest membership of any U.S. conservation organization. Its publications include *National Wildlife, International Wildlife,* and the children's magazines *Your Big Backyard* and *Ranger Rick.*

Rachel Carson published the environmental classic *Silent Spring* in 1962. This book about the effects of pesticide use is considered by many to have provided the impetus for the modern environmental movement in the United States.

In 1964 America's first permanent national wilderness system was established.

In 1970 the first annual Earth Day was held. On Earth Day professionals and the lay public focus on activities to promote an awareness of the environment, address environmental health issues, and develop strategies to preserve the environment.

On December 2, 1970, the Environmental Protection Agency (EPA) was established.

In 1979 *Healthy People* assessed environmental health in the United States, and national health objectives relating to environmental health were written in 1980.

In 1989 *50 Simple Things You Can Do to Save the Earth* was published. It sold more than 1.5 million copies. A sequel has now been published.

In 1990 more than 200 million people around the world celebrated the 20th anniversary of Earth Day.

In 1991 *Healthy People 2000* established environmental health as a national health priority area and set national environmental health objectives.

In 1995 *Healthy People 2000: Midcourse Review and 1995 Revisions* gave the nation an update on progress toward environmental health objectives.

hazardous waste sites, and improving household management of recyclable materials and toxic waste.

Progress toward achieving these objectives was mixed. Surveillance data show that the nation has actually regressed in the percentage of Americans who have safe drinking water—90% of the population in 1980, approximately 80% in 1990 (USDHHS, 1992, p. 66), and only 68% in 1995 (USDHHS, 1995, p. 82). An increasing number of U.S. lakes and rivers are becoming polluted, and the number of waterborne disease outbreaks from infectious agents and chemical poisoning has increased (USDHHS, p. 82).

Data and revisions on other objectives show that substantial progress has been made in reducing blood lead levels, decreasing the amount of toxic agents released into the environment, increasing the percentage of Americans that live in counties that meet EPA standards for air pollution (rising from 50% to almost 77%), and increased use of recycling (USDHHS, 1995, pp. 82-83). Slight progress has been made toward Americans testing their homes for radon, states adopting construction standards to minimize radon levels, and states requiring disclosure of radon concentrations in the sale of property (USDHHS, p. 82). In 1995 an objective was added to reduce the proportion of children aged 6 and younger who are regularly exposed to tobacco smoke at home (USDHHS, p. 217).

THE NURSE AND ENVIRONMENTAL HEALTH

The environment has been a central concept in the domain of nursing since the days of Florence Nightingale. Environment is a core concept in Nightingale's model of nursing, and it was her contention that the environment could be altered in such a way as to improve conditions and assist in curing the patient (Selanders, 1993). Nightingale's regard for the patient's environment is traced to her work with soldiers in the Crimea where she partially attributed their sickness and death to unsanitary environmental conditions. She stressed the importance of developing sanitary codes for hospitals and identified five factors for nurses to consider in optimizing the physical environment of the ill person: (1) pure air, (2) pure water, (3) efficient drainage, (4) cleanliness, and (5) light (Nightingale, 1869). As the *Healthy People 2000* objectives show, these factors are considered important today.

Lillian Wald, the founder of public health nursing and the Henry Street Nursing Settlement in 1893, was well aware of environmental health issues and the effect they had on community health. She regularly admonished anyone who did not observe city sewage and sanitation laws, and established milk stations to provide safe milk for infants and children (Coss, 1993, pp. 134, 137; Wald, 1915). To help children get away from the environmental pollutants and hazards of the city she built playgrounds and started "fresh air" camps in the country.

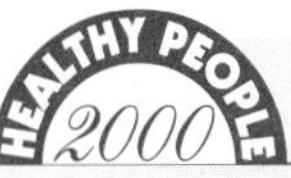

Objectives for Environmental Health

1. Reduce asthma morbidity, as measured by a reduction in asthma hospitalizations to no more than 160 per 100,000 people.
2. Reduce the prevalence of serious mental retardation among school-aged children to no more than 2 per 1,000 children.
3. Reduce outbreaks of waterborne disease from infectious agents and chemical poisoning to no more than 11 per year.
4. Reduce the prevalence of blood lead levels exceeding 15 μg/dL and 25 μg/dL among children aged 6 months through 5 years to no more than 300,000 and zero respectively.
5. Reduce human exposure to criteria air pollutants, as measured by an increase to at least 85 percent in the proportion of people who live in counties that have not exceeded any Environmental Protection Agency standard for air quality in the previous 12 months.
6. Increase to at least 40 percent the proportion of homes in which homeowners/occupants have tested for radon concentrations and that have either been found to pose minimal risk or have been modified to reduce risk to health.
7. Reduce human exposure to toxic agents by decreasing the release of hazardous substances from industrial facilities: 65 percent decrease of substances on the Department of Health and Human Services list of carcinogens, and a 50 percent reduction in the substances on the Agency for Toxic Substances and Disease Registry (ATSDR) priority list of the most toxic chemicals.
8. Reduce human exposure to solid waste–related water, air, and soil contamination, as measured by a reduction in average pounds of municipal solid waste produced per person each day to no more 4.3 pounds before recovery and 3.2 pounds after recovery.
9. Increase to at least 85 percent the proportion of people who receive a supply of drinking water that meets the safe drinking water standards established by the Environmental Protection Agency.
10. Reduce potential risks to human health from surface water, as measured by an increase in the proportion of assessed rivers, lakes, and estuaries that support beneficial uses, such as consumable fish and recreational activities.
11. Perform testing for lead-based paint in at least 50 percent of homes built before 1950.
12. Expand to at least 35 the number of states in which at least 75 percent of local jurisdictions have adopted construction standards and techniques that minimize elevated indoor radon levels in those new building areas locally determined to have elevated radon levels.
13. Increase to at least 30 the number of states requiring that prospective buyers be informed of the presence of lead-based paint and radon concentrations in all buildings offered for sale.
14. Eliminate significant health risks from National Priority List hazardous waste sites, as measured by performance of clean-up at these sites sufficient to eliminate immediate and significant health threats as specified in health assessments completed at all sites.
15. Establish curbside recycling programs that serve at least 50 percent of the U.S. population and continue to increase household hazardous waste collection programs.
16. Establish and monitor in at least 35 states' plans to define and track sentinel environmental diseases *(sentinel environmental diseases include lead poisoning, other heavy metal poisoning, pesticide poisoning, carbon monoxide poisoning, heatstroke, hypothermia, acute chemical poisoning, methemoglobinemia, and respiratory diseases triggered by environmental factors).*
17. Reduce to no more than 20 percent the proportion of children aged 6 and younger who are regularly exposed to tobacco smoke at home.

RELATED NATIONAL HEALTH OBJECTIVES: FOOD SAFETY

1. Reduce infections caused by key foodborne pathogens to incidences of no more than:

Salmonella species	16/100,000
Campylobacter jejuni	25/100,000
Escherichia coli 0157:H7	4/100,000
Listeria monocytogenes	0.5/100,000

2. Reduce outbreaks of infections due to *Salmonella enteritidis* to fewer than 25 outbreaks yearly.
3. Increase to at least 75 percent the proportion of households in which principal food preparers routinely refrain from leaving perishable food out of the refrigerator for over 2 hours and wash cutting boards and utensils with soap after contact with raw meat and poultry.
4. Extend to at least 70 percent the proportion of states and territories that have implemented model *Food Code 1993* for institutional food operations and to at least 70 percent the proportion that have adopted the new uniform food protection code that sets recommended standards for regulation of all food operations.

From USDHHS: *Healthy People 2000: midcourse review and 1995 revisions*, Washington, D.C., 1995, U.S. Government Printing Office, pp. 213-218.

Mary Breckinridge, the founder of the Frontier Nursing Service in 1925, used environmental health principles in her work (Breckinridge, 1952; Salazar, Primomo, 1994; Wilkie, Moseley, 1969, p. 131). In planning to build a rural hospital she took into consideration that the building site have a source of clean water, be at a safe distance from outdoor privies that could contaminate wells, be away from noise, and have adequate light (Wilkie, Moseley, p. 131).

Modern nursing scholars still consider the concept of environment to be central to the development of nursing knowledge and maintenance of health. Nurses are well positioned to help ameliorate the adverse impact of environmental hazards on the health of individuals and communities (Bellack, Musham, Hainer et al, 1996, p. 74; Institute of Medicine, 1995, p. 15). Today a major focus in community health nursing is examining the interrelationship of environment, health, and disease.

The Role of the Nurse in Environmental Health

Historically, nursing environmental health activities were limited to the immediate environment (e.g., hospital) or the family home (Neufer, 1994, p. 156). Community health nurses care for clients with conditions that originate in the environment, including injuries and illnesses resulting from disasters and exposure to toxic wastes, chemicals, and water and air pollution; malnutrition; and overcrowding. They apply their skills in nursing process by identifying and analyzing possible environmental health hazards and developing appropriate nursing interventions (Neufer, Narkunas, 1994, p. 329).

Although nurses are involved in environmental health activities there is a lack of literature and research on the subject. A review of the nursing research literature from 1961 to 1990 showed only 53 articles that addressed the environment (Kleffel, 1991, p. 43). A review of the literature from 1990-1994 showed 14 nursing research reports directly related to environmental health (Institute of Medicine, 1995, p. 110). More research needs to be done in relation to nursing interventions and environmental health, and environmental health content should be routinely integrated into nursing curriculum (American Association of Colleges of Nursing, 1993; Institute of Medicine, 1995, p. 6; Snyder, Ruth, Sattler, Strasser, 1994, p. 326). Recently the National Institutes of Health has offered fellowships for nurses to gain additional training in environmental health sciences.

Nursing actions are directed toward promoting health by reducing environmental risks and preserving the earth's environment. Nurses need to acquire the knowledge and skills to recognize and treat environmentally induced disease, become advocates for environmental issues, conduct environmental assessments and research, and work in partnership with communities to prevent and minimize environmental hazards and disasters (Bellack, Musham, Hainer et al, 1996, p. 75; Worthington, Cary, 1993). Nurses are involved in environmental health activities as professionals and as concerned citizens. They work collaboratively with environmental health specialists to reduce the incidence of environmental diseases and conditions.

NURSING ORGANIZATIONS A specialty organization, Nurses for Environmental and Social Responsibility, is dedicated to educating nurses and the public about actual and potential threats to human and environmental health. An environmental health nursing philosophy from this organization is in the accompanying box.

The *American Holistic Nurses Association* has developed a position statement in support of a healthful environment (Schuster, 1990, p. 27), and the *International Council of Nurses* (ICN) has developed a position statement that delineates the nurse's role in safeguarding the environment. The ICN position statement is given in the box on the next page. The ICN has addressed the need for nurses to assist in environmental health education activities, environmental surveillance, multidisciplinary environmental health activities, and formulating environmental health policy and legislation. ICN also proposes that nurses form collaborate community relationships for environmental health, and be actively involved in environmental health research.

Environmental Health Nursing Philosophy

Believing that human beings and the physical environment, both as open systems, are continuously exchanging matter and energy with one another, Environmental Health Nursing (EHN) is concerned with the effects of environmental degradation on human health. EHN's goal is to decrease, avoid, or eliminate environmental exposures which are determined by research and consensus in the scientific community to constitute an unacceptable risk to human health.

EHN maintains the basic tenants of the nursing profession—promotion and restoration of health and the prevention of illness using the nursing process—assessment, planning, implementation, and evaluation—in this expanded arena.

In assessing the environmental conditions to identify existing or potential exposures associated with the health of the community, EHN integrates knowledge from the natural and behavioral sciences. EHN collaborates with industry, government agencies, and other scientific disciplines, and the public.

EHN believes that individuals and communities have a right to know the environmental risks to which they are exposed, as well as a right to participate in decisions of risk acceptance. To assist the community in logical decision making, EHN interprets research and communicates risks of exposures to the community.

EHN assesses communities' perception of risk and helps them cope with disturbances in their environment which they perceive have diminished their health. EHN teaches changes in life style that can decrease, avoid, or eliminate exposures. EHN assists communities in interfacing with agencies and industry in planning and implementing efforts to reduce exposures.

When involved in planning and implementation efforts to remove or prevent exposures, EHN considers: research findings, perception of risk, susceptible populations, law, and the cost-benefit ratio in decision making.

From Portman C: Environmental health nursing philosophy, *Nurses for Environmental and Social Responsibility Newsletter* 1(3):3, 1995.

The Nurse's Role in Safeguarding the Human Environment

The preservation and improvement of the human environment has become increasingly important for humankind's survival and well-being. The vastness and urgency of the task places on every individual and every professional group the responsibility to participate in the efforts to safeguard humankind's environment, and to conserve the world's resources, to study how their use affects humankind and how adverse effects can be avoided.

THE NURSE'S ROLE IS TO:

Help detect ill effects of the environment on the health of man, and vice-versa.

The nurse should:

- apply observational skills for the detection of ill effects of environment on the individual;
- observe individuals in all settings for effects of pollutants in order to advise on protective and/or curative measures;
- record and analyze observations made of ill effects of environment and/or pollutants on individuals;
- be informed and report observations of the ecological consequences of pollutants and their adverse effects on the human being.

Be informed and apply knowledge in daily work with individuals, families and/or community groups as to the data available on potential health hazards and ways to prevent and/or reduce them.

The nurse should be informed about:

- the studies and identification of the environmental problems at local, national, and international levels;
- their effects on man;
- the standards for the protection of the human organism, especially from pollutants;
- ways to prevent and/or reduce health hazards.

Be informed and teach preventive measures about health hazards due to environmental factors as well as about conservation of environmental resources to the individual, families and/or community groups.

The nurse can:

- request and attend continuing education programs about the study of the environment and the application of this knowledge in daily life and work;
- provide health education for both the general public and health personnel in order to create awareness of environmental issues and to involve the public with environmental management and control;
- apply knowledge in areas where nursing intervention may prevent or reduce health hazards;
- report on steps taken to control the significant environmental problems of the area.

Work with health authorities in pointing out health care aspects and health hazards in existing human settlements and in the planning of new settlements.

Nurses can:

- participate in exchange of information and experience about similar environmental problems with authorities in other areas;
- cooperate with health authorities in the preparation of programs to enable national and local authorities to influence their own environments;
- participate in the promotion of legislation to improve health care and reduce/prevent health hazards, and encourage the enforcement of such legislation where/when appropriate;
- participate in national/local pre-disaster planning; and cooperate in international programs in case of disasters in other countries.

Assist communities in their action on environmental health problems.

The nurse can assist communities in programs to:

- reduce harmful pollutants (chemical, biological or physical, e.g. noise) in air, soil, water and food by industries or other human efforts;
- improve nutrition;
- encourage family planning;
- assess environmental factors in work situations and pursue activities for the elimination or reduction of hazards;
- educate the general public and all levels of nursing personnel in environmental and other health hazards, especially those related to unacceptable levels of contamination.

Participate in research providing data for early warning and prevention of deleterious effects of the various environmental agents to which man is increasingly exposed; and research conducive to discovering ways and means of improving living and working conditions.

The nurse, as principal investigator or in collaboration with other nurses or related professions, can carry out epidemiological and experimental research designed to provide data for:

- early warning for prevention of health hazards;
- improving living and working conditions;
- monitoring the environmental levels of pollutants;
- measuring the impact of nursing intervention on environmental hazards.

From International Council of Nurses: *The nurse's role in safeguarding the human environment: position statement,* Geneva, Switzerland, 1986, The Council.

STANDARDS OF PRACTICE No specific standards of practice for environmental health nursing exist. The box on the next page lists the general environmental health competencies for nurses recommended by the Institute of Medicine's Committee on Enhancing Environmental Health Content in Nursing Practice. Committee recommendations for nursing practice, education, and research in relation to environmental health are given in the box on page 133.

ENVIRONMENTAL HEALTH LEGISLATION

The Social Security Act of 1935 serves as umbrella legislation, consolidating U.S. social welfare legislation under one

General Environmental Health Competencies for Nurses

I. BASIC KNOWLEDGE AND CONCEPTS

All nurses should understand the scientific principles and underpinnings of the relationship between individuals or populations, and the environment (including the work environment). This understanding includes the basic mechanisms and pathways of exposure to environmental health hazards, basic prevention and control strategies, the interdisciplinary nature of effective interventions, and the role of research.

II. ASSESSMENT AND REFERRAL

All nurses should be able to successfully complete an environmental health history, recognize potential environmental hazards and sentinel illnesses, and make appropriate referrals for conditions with probable environmental etiologies. An essential component of this is the ability to access and provide information to patients and communities, and to locate referral sources.

III. ADVOCACY, ETHICS, AND RISK COMMUNICATION

All nurses should be able to demonstrate knowledge of the role of advocacy (case and class), ethics, and risk communication in patient care and community intervention with respect to the potential adverse effects of the environment on health.

IV. LEGISLATION AND REGULATION

All nurses should understand the policy framework and major pieces of legislation and regulations related to environmental health.

From Institute of Medicine (Committee on Enhancing Environmental Health Content in Nursing Practice, Pope AM, Snyder MA, Mood LH, eds): *Nursing, health, and the environment: strengthening the relationship to improve the public's health*, Washington, D.C., 1995, National Academy Press, p. 5.

law; the Public Health Service Act of 1944 does the same for public health legislation. However, there is no umbrella legislation for environmental health, and numerous environmental health laws exist. The scope of this legislation, and its lack of consolidation, makes it difficult and time consuming to locate and become knowledgeable about environmental health.

Environmental legislation has tended to be reactive and responsive to the demands and crises of the moment rather than preventive (Rabe, 1990, p. 320). The environmental awareness that evolved in the United States in the 1960s marked the advent of numerous pieces of legislation. An overview of selected environmental health legislation in the United States is given in the box on page 134. As a result of this legislation American industry and government are spending more than $100 billion each year to protect the environment (General Accounting Office [GAO], 1993, p. 4).

Environmental legislation is diverse and encompasses areas such as the Superfund (the environmental fund created to finance the cleanup of hazardous substances), water and air quality, toxic substances in the environment, pesticides, soil conservation, solid waste disposal, radiation, ocean dumping, environmental research, noise pollution, endangered species, and nuclear waste. The *National Environmental Policy Act* (Public Law 91-190) of 1969 is one of the most significant, and best-known, pieces of U.S. environmental health legislation. This act established the Environmental Protection Agency (EPA).

THE ROLE OF FEDERAL, STATE, AND LOCAL AGENCIES IN ENVIRONMENTAL HEALTH

Many of the public health successes that have occurred in relation to communicable disease control, improving the quality of life, and reducing mortality across the life span (especially infant mortality) have come about as a result of environmental health practices. The private sector has been involved in environmental health activities, often from the standpoint of serving as an advocate for safeguarding and preserving the nation's lands and wildlife. Traditionally the federal government has enacted national environmental health legislation, while state health authorities (SHAs) and local health departments (LHDs) have been involved in direct provision of environmental health services, policies, and regulations.

Federal Government and Environmental Health

The federal government is involved in promoting environmental health, and some major agencies of the federal government are discussed here (executive branch and other federal agency involvement in environmental health activities is described in Appendix 6-1). The federal government assists in protecting the public from the adverse consequences of exposure to harmful environmental agents and protecting and preserving the nation's natural resources. The federal government is involved in direct provision of emergency and disaster services, but direct provision of day-to-day environmental health services is usually carried out through state health authorities (SHAs) and local health departments (LHDs).

ENVIRONMENTAL PROTECTION AGENCY The EPA, a freestanding agency of the federal government, was created on December 2, 1970 and has regional offices across the nation. It is the federal government's foremost environmental agency and is the single largest employer of environmental health professionals in the world. The agency's mission is to control and abate environmental pollution.

The EPA is well-known for its efforts to protect and enhance the American environment and enforce national environmental health legislation. It works to control and abate pollution in the areas of air, water, solid waste, noise, radiation, and toxic substances, and manages the Superfund toxic waste cleanup program. It is mandated to mount an integrated, coordinated attack on environmental pollution in cooperation with state and local governments. The EPA

Recommendations on Environmental Health and Nursing Practice, Education, and Research

NURSING PRACTICE

Environmental health should be reemphasized in the scope of responsibilities for nursing practice.

Resources to support environmental health content in nursing practice should be identified and made available.

Nurses should participate as members and leaders in interdisciplinary teams that address environmental health problems.

Communication should extend beyond counseling individual patients and families to facilitating the exchange of information on environmental hazards and community responses.

Nurses should conduct research regarding the ethical implications of occupational and environmental health hazards and incorporate findings into curricula and practice.

Although the environment as a domain in nursing has not been well developed it is an important aspect of nursing practice and research.

NURSING EDUCATION

Environmental health concepts should be incorporated into all levels of nursing education.

Environmental health content should be included in nursing licensure and certification examinations.

Expertise in various environmental health disciplines should be included in the education of nurses.

Environmental health content should be an integral part of lifelong learning and continuing education for nurses.

Professional associations, public agencies, and private organizations should provide more resources and educational opportunities to enhance environmental health in nursing practice.

NURSING RESEARCH

Multidisciplinary and interdisciplinary research endeavors should be developed and implemented to build the knowledge base for nursing practice in environmental health as it relates to the practice of nursing.

The number of nurse researchers should be increased to prepare to build the knowledge base in environmental health as it relates to the practice of nursing.

Research priorities for nursing in environmental health should be established and used by funding agencies for resource allocation decisions and to give direction to nurse researchers.

Current efforts to disseminate research findings to nurses, other health care providers, and the public should be strengthened and expanded.

From Institute of Medicine (Committee on Enhancing Environmental Health Content in Nursing Practice, Pope AM, Snyder MA, Mood LH, eds): *Nursing, health, and the environment: strengthening the relationship to improve the public's health*, Washington, D.C., 1995, National Academy Press, pp. 10-11.

coordinates and supports research and antipollution activities and disseminates information on safeguarding the environment.

FEDERAL EMERGENCY MANAGEMENT AGENCY The Federal Emergency Management Agency (FEMA) was established in 1979 and reports directly to the White House. It is the central federal agency for emergency planning, preparedness, and response, working closely with state and local governments and the American Red Cross to prepare for disasters and minimize the loss of life and property when disasters strike.

FEMA's numerous activities include producing training programs, publications, and technical guidance; managing the President's Disaster Relief Fund (which is the source of most federal funding assistance after major disasters); sponsoring the U.S. Fire Administration; carrying out national emergency management and multihazard response planning; doing flood-plain management and dam safety; planning for emergencies at commercial nuclear power plants and military chemical stockpile sites; providing emergency food and shelter; ensuring federal government continuity during national security emergencies; and coordinating federal response to the consequences of major terrorist incidents.

NATIONAL CENTER FOR ENVIRONMENTAL HEALTH The National Center for Environmental Health (NCEH) is part of the U.S. Department of Health and Human Services. The mission of the NCEH is to promote health and quality of life by preventing and controlling disease, injury, and disability related to interactions between people and their environment outside the workplace (NCEH, 1995, p. 1). It carries out activities related to the health effects of environmental hazards (including birth defects and developmental disabilities) and works extensively with childhood lead poisoning prevention, improving air pollution and respiratory health, improving environmental health surveillance programs, and providing technical assistance to the National Park System in matters of environmental health. The center collaborates with state and local health departments, federal and state regulatory agencies, research institutions, private groups, and international organizations to promote environmental health.

AGENCY FOR TOXIC SUBSTANCES AND DISEASE REGISTRY The Agency for Toxic Substances and Disease Registry (ATSDR) is part of the U.S. Department of Health and Human Services. It assists the federal government in registering toxic substances and providing information about community health risks. The ATSDR has been discussed in Chapter 5.

State Government and Environmental Health

State health authorities (SHAs) historically have been involved in environmental health activities and provide

Selected Environmental Health Legislation: United States*

1948 *Water Pollution Control Act (Public Law 80-845)*—Authorized the Public Health Service to help states develop water pollution control programs and to aid in the planning of sewage treatment plants.

1963 *Clean Air Act (Public Law 88-206)*—Authorized direct grants to states and localities for air pollution control; provided for federal enforcement of interstate air pollution; directed major research efforts for control of motor vehicle exhaust, removal of sulfur from fuel, and the development of air quality criteria.

1965 *Solid Waste Disposal Act (Public Law 89-272)*—Established a program of grants to states to develop solid waste disposal programs.

1966 *Disaster Relief Act of 1966 (Public Law 89-769)*—Authorized assistance to U.S. communities suffering a major natural disaster. Significant amendments in 1970.

1969 *National Environmental Policy Act (Public Law 91-190)*—One of the best-known and most significant pieces of U.S. environmental health legislation. Established national environmental policy and authorized formation of the Environmental Protection Agency (EPA).

1970 *Environmental Education Act (Public Law 91-516)*—Authorized the establishment of education programs to encourage public understanding of policies and environmental activities designed to enhance environmental quality. Established the Office of Environmental Education.

Lead-Based Paint Poisoning Prevention Act (Public Law 91-695)—Provided federal assistance to help cities and communities combat lead-based paint poisoning. Established demonstration and research projects.

1973 *Endangered Species Act (Public Law 93-205)*—The first federal law to protect endangered and threatened species of U.S. fish, wildlife, and plants.

1974 *Safe Drinking Water Act (Public Law 93-523)*—Amended the Public Health Service Act to require the Environmental Protection Agency to set national drinking water standards and to aid states and localities in enforcement.

1976 *Toxic Substances Control Act (Public Law 94-469)*—Regulated toxic chemicals already in existence and tried to prevent new hazardous chemicals from entering the market. Required EPA to test existing hazardous chemicals, gather and disseminate information about these chemicals, and prevent future chemical risks by premarket screening and tracking. An overall goal of the act was to prevent unreasonable injury to individual health or harm to the environment associated with the manufacture, processing, distribution, use, or disposal of hazardous chemical substances.

1980 *Asbestos School Hazard Detection and Control Act (Public Law 96-270)*—Established a program for the inspection of schools to detect the presence of hazardous asbestos materials; provided for loans to states or local educational agencies to contain or remove hazardous asbestos materials from schools and replace such materials with suitable building materials.

Comprehensive Environmental Response, Compensation and Liability Act of 1980 (Public Law 96-510)—Known as the "Superfund," this act provided for liability, compensation, cleanup, and emergency response for hazardous substances released into the environment and cleanup of inactive hazardous waste disposal sites. The EPA was to oversee the programs of the act. It established the Agency for Toxic Substances and Disease Registry and the Hazardous Substance Response Trust Fund.

1990 *Global Change Research Act of 1990 (Public Law 101-606)*—Required the establishment of a United States Global Change Research program aimed at understanding and responding to global change. Encouraged international discussion toward protocols in global change research.

Environmental Research Geographic Local Information Act (Public Law 101-617)—Provided a method of locating private and governmental research on environmental issues by specific geographic locations. The EPA will identify major environmental research relating to a specific geographical area, compile and maintain the research, and make it available to the public. The EPA is authorized to enter into contractual agreements to obtain the data.

America the Beautiful Act of 1990 (Public Law 101-624)—This act was Title XII, Subtitle C of the Food, Agriculture, Conservation and Trade Act of 1990. Authorized the President to designate a private nonprofit foundation to be eligible for a grant to be used to create public awareness and a spirit of volunteerism in relation to tree-planting projects in U.S. communities and urban areas.

Global Climate Change Prevention Act of 1990 (Public Law 101-624)—This act was Title XIV of the Food, Agriculture, Conservation and Trade Act of 1990. Established, within the Department of Agriculture, a global climate change program to coordinate all issues and activities relating to climate change including policy analysis and research.

*Note: Many of these acts are frequently amended.

many environmental health services (see Chapter 5). Some SHAs administer federal environmental health legislation. The Clean Air Act is administered by 10 SHAs, the Clean Water Act by 9, the Safe Drinking Water Act by 27, the Resource Conservation and Recovery Act by 11, and the Superfund by 11 (Public Health Foundation [PHF], 1991).

The SHA is the lead environmental agency in 10 states (PHF, 1991). In the other 40 states a separate state level agency, such as the *Department of Environment*, is the lead environmental agency. This trend toward removing environmental health authority from SHAs has led to diffuse patterns of responsibility, lack of coordination, and inadequate handling of environmental problems (Institute of Medicine, 1988, p. 150). The state agency in charge of environmental health activities will collect information on environmental pollution in local communities, maintain an environmental disease registry, take part in environmental monitoring activities, and provide consultation to LHDs.

Local Government and Environmental Health

Local health departments (LHDs) have traditionally offered numerous environmental health services to the local communities that they serve (see Chapter 5). Such services are often provided through the department's environmental engineers or sanitarians. Community health nurses work cooperatively with them to implement nursing interventions.

Environmental health personnel work to prevent, eliminate, and control environmental hazards through various environmental health programs (USDHHS, 1988, p. 3). LHDs are often responsible for testing community water and air, overseeing solid and hazardous waste disposal, performing food and restaurant inspections, monitoring noise pollution, ensuring sanitation of public swimming and recreational facilities, implementing vector (e.g. skunk, rat, and mosquito) control measures, and ensuring safe housing (Table 6-1).

Private Sector Environmental Health Activities

Shortly after the establishment in 1872 of Yellowstone, our first national park, the first private U.S. conservation organization, the American Forestry Association, was established. Other organizations such as the National Wildlife Federation, Sierra Club, Wilderness Society, World Wildlife Federation, Environmental Action, Greenpeace, Worldwatch Institute, and Nature Conservancy are actively involved in promoting international environmental health. These groups have many interesting magazines and publications (e.g., National Wildlife Federation publishes the magazines *National Wildlife*, *International Wildlife*, and for children *Your Big Backyard* and *Ranger Rick*). The efforts of the American Red Cross, an international voluntary agency, are discussed later in this chapter under disaster nursing.

Millions of Americans each year participate in activities to support the environment. In local communities people are taking part in environmentally safe activities and donating time to plant trees and clean up parks, lakes and rivers. Every year in the United States, on the third Saturday in September, people of all ages spend the day cleaning up trash from beaches and waterways—in one day removing more than 4 million pounds of garbage (No matter, 1996). Each year more than 200 million people around the world celebrate Earth Day on April 22. We can be proud of such efforts to support our environment—after all, there is only one earth!

Private corporations are helping too. Each year corporations across the nation make financial donations and sponsor environmental projects. One such project, *EarthQuest*, a traveling exhibit sponsored by the Ford Motor Company, the Hertz Corporation, and IBM, is a giant video game where children try to avoid Toxicus, the monster of waste, and learn about making choices that environmentally help the planet (Watch for, 1996). In another initiative, Target stores work cooperatively with the National Wildlife Federation to publish *EarthSavers*, a free newspaper available to children at their stores nationwide.

THE ENVIRONMENTAL HEALTH WORK FORCE

Almost 80% of all environmental health practitioners are employed by government agencies at the federal, state, and local levels (USDHHS, 1988, p. 3). The federal government is the largest employer of environmental health professionals in the United States (Sexton, Perlin, 1990, p. 913). For half a century the title *sanitarian* has been used to describe the environmental health practitioner who applies technical knowledge obtained from the biological and chemical sciences to promote and protect environmental health (USDHHS, 1988, p. 3). Nationwide, local health departments employ sanitarians to design and implement environmental health programs. Today more contemporary titles include *environmental engineer, environmental health specialist*, and *environmentalist*. Historically, the environmental health work force has focused on reducing the incidence of communicable diseases spread by vectors and contaminated food and water. It is estimated that more than 120,000 additional environmental health specialists are needed to meet the nation's demands (Gordon, 1990, p. 904).

Environmental Health Teamwork

Community health nurses work collaboratively with other health professionals on environmental health concerns. For example, interdisciplinary teams of personnel including nurses, sanitarians, and health educators work together to combat lead poisoning in children. On such a team the nurse might teach about lead poisoning prevention, complete risk assessments on targeted aggregates, do lead screenings in well-baby and WIC clinics, and participate in community education activities at a local health fair. The environmental health sanitarian may make joint home visits with the community health nurse to conduct an environmental assessment, complete mapping programs to identify clusters of cases within a local community, enforce housing codes to eliminate lead in the home environment, and participate in community education activities. The health educator may develop and organize community education activities. Together they might write grants to obtain funds for program development.

Another example of a cooperative interaction between nurses and environmental health personnel is their col-

table 6-1 Environmental Health Programs within Local Health Departments (LHDs)

Categories of Environmental Concern	Programs	Program Purpose
Air	Air quality management	To ensure a community air resource conducive to good health that will not injure plant or animal life or property and will be esthetically desirable
Water	Water supply sanitation	To ensure the provision of safe public and private water supplies, adequate in quantity and quality for every person
	Water pollution control	To ensure the cooperation with state water pollution control agencies and that surface and subsurface water supplies meet all state and local standards and regulations for water quality
Waste	Solid waste management	To ensure that all solid wastes are stored, collected, transported, and disposed of in a manner that does not create health, safety, or esthetic problems
	Liquid waste management	To ensure the treatment of liquid wastes in such a manner as to prevent problems of sanitation, public health nuisances, or pollution
	Toxic and hazardous waste management	To ensure that toxic and hazardous wastes are stored, collected, transported, and disposed of in a manner that does not create health or safety problems
Food	Food protection	To ensure that all people are adequately protected from unhealthful or unsafe food or food products. This necessitates a comprehensive food protection program covering every facility where food or food products are stored, transported, processed, packaged, served, or vended, and regulating sanitation, wholesomeness, adulteration, advertising, labeling weights and measures, and fill of containers
Recreational areas	Swimming pool sanitation and safety	To ensure the safety and sanitation of public, semipublic, and private swimming pools
	Recreational sanitation	To ensure that all public recreational areas are operated so as to prevent health and safety problems
Product safey	Consumer product safety	To ensure that all people are adequately protected from unhealthful or unsafe substances or products in the home, business, and industry
Radiation	Radiation control	To prevent unnecessary or hazardous radiation exposure from the transportation, use, or disposal of all types of radiation-producing devices and products
Occupational	Occupational health and safety	To ensure, in cooperation with state officials, the health and safety of workers in places of employment through controlling relevant environmental factors
Vectors	Vector control	To control all insects, rodents, and other animals that adversely affect health, safety, or comfort
Noise	Noise pollution control	To prevent hazardous or annoying noise levels in residential, business, industrial, and recreational structures and areas
Accidents	Environmental injury prevention	To influence or regulate planning, design, and construction in such a manner as to reduce the possibility of accidents through proper management of the environment
Buildings	Housing sanitation, safety, and rehabilitation	To ensure programs that will provide decent, safe, and healthful housing for all people
	Institutional sanitation, safety, and rehabilitation	To ensure that institutions such as hospitals, schools, nurseries, jails, and prisons are operated so as to prevent sanitation and safety problems

Modified from American Public Health Association: Position paper on the role of official local health agencies, *Am J Public Health* 65:189-193, 1975; and USDHHS: *Evaluating the environmental health workforce* (HRP#0907160), Rockville, Md., 1988, USDHHS, p. 3.

laboration in conducting epidemiological investigations of serious outbreaks of foodborne diseases such as botulism and salmonella. During these investigations both disciplines interview affected persons, investigate sources of contamination, and may conduct house-to-house surveys to identify ill people (see Chapter 11). Nurses are becoming increasingly involved in aggregate and community-based environmental health activities and aware of the importance of environmental health. Individually and as part of a team, community health nurses must have an active role in environmental health issues (Neufer, 1994, p. 156).

SELECTED ENVIRONMENTAL DISEASES

Most environmental illnesses and injuries are caused by physical, chemical, biological, or sociological hazards. Many of these environmental diseases are highly preventable (Landrigan, 1992, p. 941). Physical hazards include radiation, dust, vibration, noise, heat, and cold. Chemical hazards include toxicants, irritants, asphyxiants, poisons, carcinogens, mutagens, and teratogens. Biological hazards include infectious agents such as bacteria, viruses and protozoa, plants, insects, fungi, and molds. Sociological hazards include stress, violence, and inadequate housing. Many of these hazards enter the environment through direct discharge into air or water, inadequate landfills, and dumping sites.

Environmental etiology is evident in numerous diseases and conditions including cancer, genetic damage, birth defects, neurological effects, psychological disorders, liver disease, infectious diseases, injuries, and lung disease (Rabe, 1990, p. 318). In this century significant strides have been made in controlling environmentally linked diseases such as malaria, yellow fever, typhoid fever, cholera, dysenteries, and milkborne and foodborne diseases. However, lead poisoning, environmental cancers and lung diseases, and waterborne, foodborne, soilborne, and vectorborne diseases are still very prevalent.

For today's nurse addressing environmental health requires a systematic assessment of air, soil, surface water, and groundwater quality, and the related public health implications of toxic chemicals in the environment (Neufer, 1994, p. 156). To aid in determining environmental etiology an environmental health history should be routinely taken by the nurse as part of a client's health history. This environmental history includes the information in the accompanying box.

SELECTED ENVIRONMENTAL HISTORY INFORMATION

- Occupation of family members and potential hazards in the work setting
- Building materials used and stored in the home (e.g., asbestos)
- Source of water
- Source of fresh fruits and vegetables
- Home heating system
- Home pesticide use
- Contact with pets
- Hobbies (especially hobbies that might increase exposure to chemicals, sunlight, or waste products)
- Types of industry in the neighborhood
- Known exposures to lead or other chemicals
- Vector exposure
- Exposure to known or suspected sources of contaminated air, soil, or water

Waterborne Diseases

The provision of safe water is a major environmental health challenge. Unless water quality is substantially upgraded, it will continue to be a threat to national and international public health. Some scientists believe that perhaps 80% of all the illnesses in the world could be prevented if people had access to safe water supplies (Nadakavukaren, 1995, p. 611). Waterborne diseases are a result of water that is biologically and/or chemically polluted (water pollution is discussed later in this chapter). The CDC and the EPA have a collaborative surveillance system for collecting and reporting data on U.S. waterborne disease outbreaks.

Worldwide, access to safe drinking water is an increasing problem (1.2 billion people do not have safe drinking water). Accessibility to safe drinking water has decreased in the United States; it is estimated that more than 30% of the population does not have safe drinking water (USDHHS, 1995, p. 82). Improving the integrity of the water supply and control of waterborne disease is addressed in *Healthy People 2000* objectives. As the safety of their drinking water becomes less sure, Americans are spending more than $3 billion each year on bottled water (Nadakavukaren, 1995, p. 629). Interestingly, a recent congressional committee investigation found that 31% of bottled waters marketed in the United States exceeded the maximum allowable levels for microbial contamination (Nadakavukaren, p. 629).

Agents responsible for waterborne diseases include parasites such as protozoa, bacteria such as *Salmonella* and *Shigella*, viruses, and chemicals (e.g. lead, nitrates, copper). Waterborne diseases include typhoid, cholera, polio, hepatitis, and bacterial dysentery. The most frequent conditions caused by waterborne pathogens are gastroenteritis, giardiasis, and chemical poisoning (USDHHS, 1995, p. 318).

People living in rural areas, or areas where untreated well water is used, are at greater risk for contracting waterborne diseases than people using city water. Thousands of individual cases of waterborne diseases are reported each year, and the number of waterborne epidemics has recently increased in the United States. In 1993 in Milwaukee a waterborne epidemic caused by a protozoan parasite, *Cryptosporidium*, sickened more than 400,000 people and resulted in an estimated 104 deaths and 4000 hospitalizations (Morris, Naumova, Levin, Munasinghe, 1996, p. 237). Deaths often occur among immunosuppressed persons.

Many waterborne disease go undiagnosed and untreated. Waterborne pathogens are suspected to be responsible for as many as 30 million cases of waterborne disease each year in the United States (Morris, Naumova, Levin, Munasinghe, 1996, p. 237). Worldwide more than 250 million cases of waterborne diseases are reported annually, and each year 3 million young children die from waterborne diarrheal diseases (Nadakavukaren, 1995, p. 611). As water quality decreases the incidence of waterborne diseases can be expected to increase.

In many countries a heavy financial burden is placed on families because they must buy drinking water. In Port-au-Prince, Haiti, 20% of a typical slum-dweller's household budget is spent on purchasing drinking water. Egypt is a classic example of a country that is almost entirely dependent on water resources beyond its own borders, and the potential for "water wars" looms in the Middle East (Nadakavukaren, 1995, pp. 544, 549-550).

Foodborne Diseases

Estimates on the frequency of foodborne illness in the United States range from 12 to 81 million cases each year and cost the country billions of dollars (Nadakavukaren, 1995, p. 346). Worldwide, foodborne diseases are very prevalent, especially in developing countries—but they can happen anywhere. In Japan, food poisoning caused by *Escherichia coli* sickened more than 6000 children after they ate school-prepared lunches—the same strain of bacteria that just a few years before affected 500 people who ate undercooked hamburgers in the state of Washington (Wasson, 1996, 9A).

Healthy People 2000 has objectives to reduce infections caused by foodborne pathogens, reduce the incidence of outbreaks of foodborne diseases, and increase the percentage of American households where safe food handling occurs. Factors that may be implicated in outbreaks of foodborne illness include improper holding temperatures for food, inadequate cooking, contaminated equipment, contaminated food, and infected food handlers. There are hundreds of known causes of foodborne illness. However, the etiology of many foodborne outbreaks is unknown. For those of known etiology the greatest number (approximately two thirds) are bacterial in origin, about one fifth are chemical, and the remainder are viral or parasitic (Blumenthal, 1985, pp. 32-33). Causative agents include *Staphylococcus aureus, Bacillus cereus, Clostridium perfringens, Escherichia coli, Helicobacter pylori, Salmonella,* and *Shigella* (Benenson, 1995). Consumer tips for safe foodhandling are given in the accompanying box.

Contributors to foodborne disease are *food contaminants*. These contaminants include dirt, hairs, animal feces, fungi, insect fragments, pesticide residues, and traces of chemical substances (Nadakavukaren, 1995, p. 330). Growth hormones in meat and poultry and pesticide residues on fruits and vegetables are well-known food contaminants. The Food and Drug Administration (FDA) has established "Defect Action Levels" that specify the maximum limit of contamination the agency permits before legal action is taken to remove the product from the market (Nadakavukaren, p. 330).

Consumer Tips for Safe Food Handling

When You Shop. Buy cold food last, get it home fast.

When You Store Food. Keep it safe; refrigerate and freeze fresh meat, poultry, or fish immediately if you can't use it within a few days.

When You Prepare Food. Keep everything clean; wash hands in hot soapy water before preparing food and after using the bathroom, changing diapers, and handling pets; avoid contact between raw and cooked food; protect food from insects, rodents, and other animals.

When You're Cooking. Cook thoroughly. Generally cook red meat to 160° F and poultry to 180° F.

When You Serve Food. Never leave it out over 2 hours; use clean dishes and utensils; pack lunches and picnics in insulated carriers with a cold pack.

When You Handle Leftovers. Use small containers for quick cooling of the leftover food and remove stuffing from meats and poultry.

When You Reheat. Bring sauces, soups, and gravy to a boil, and heat other leftovers to 165° F.

Kept It Too Long? When in doubt, throw it out!

Modified from U.S. Department of Agriculture: *A quick consumer guide to safe food handling* (Home and Garden Bulletin No. 248), Washington, D.C., 1995, The Department.

Soilborne Diseases

Soilborne parasitic diseases are the most common infectious diseases in the world and are primarily transmitted by the fecal-oral route (Blumenthal, 1985, p. 41). In tropical climates half of the population may actually be infected with *Ascaris lumbricoides* (Benenson, 1995, p. 55). Prevalence of this large roundworm infection is greatest in children 3 to 8 years old (Benenson, p. 55). A single female *Ascaris* can produce 200,000 eggs per day (Benenson, p. 56)!

Hookworm is widely endemic in tropical and subtropical countries (Benenson, 1995, p. 241), and millions of persons are infected with hookworm worldwide. Pinworm is the most common worm infection in the United States, with prevalence highest in school-age children and infection often occurring in more than one family member (Benenson, p. 170). Climate helps to make these infections more prevalent in the southeastern United States. Community health nurses regularly assess for exposure to soilborne diseases when working with children.

Vectorborne Diseases

A *vector* is a nonhuman carrier of disease organisms that can transmit these organisms directly to humans. Vector transmission is an indirect form of biological or mechanical disease transmission. *Mechanical transmission* includes the disease spread by a crawling or flying insect (e.g., mosquitoes, ticks, and houseflies) that does not require multiplication or development of the transmitted organism (Benenson, 1995, p. 544). *Biological transmission* involves multiplication (propagation) or development of the organism before the vector transmits the infective agent (Benenson, p. 544).

table 6-2 SOME INSECT VECTORS AND DISEASES TRANSMITTED BY THEM

VECTOR	DISEASE	PATHOGEN
MOSQUITOES		
Anopheles sp.	Malaria	*Plasmodium* sp. (protozoa)
Culex sp.	Filariasis	*Wuchereria bancrofti* and *Brugia malayi* (nematodes)
Culex sp.	Encephalitis	Arbovirus
Aedes aegypti	Yellow fever	Arbovirus
Aedes aegypti	Dengue	Arbovirus
BITING FLIES		
Deer fly	Filariasis	*Loa loa* (nematode)
Black fly	River blindness	*Onchocerca volvulus* (nematode)
Tsetse fly	Sleeping sickness	*Trypanosoma gambiense* and *T. rhodesiense* (protozoa)
Sandfly	Kala-azar	*Leishmania donovani*
	Tropical ulcer	*Leishmania tropica*
	Cutaneous leishmaniasis	*Leishmania mexicana*
	Espundia	*Leishmania braziliensis* (protozoa)
	Phlebotomus fever	Arbovirus
OTHER INSECTS		
Gnats	Filariasis	*Mansonella ozzardi* (nematode)
Rat flea	Plague	*Yersinia pestis* (bacteria)
	Murine typhus	*Rickettsia mooseri*
Body louse	Epidemic typhus	*Rickettsia prowazekii*
	Trench fever	*Rickettsia quintana*
Tick	Rocky Mountain spotted fever	*Rickettsia rickettsii*
Tick	Colorado tick fever	Arbovirus
Tick	Lyme disease	*Borrelia burgdorferi*
Mite	Rickettsialpox	*Rickettsia akari*

Modified from Blumenthal DS, ed: *An introduction to environmental health*, New York, 1985, Springer, p. 35.

As with waterborne and foodborne disease, vectorborne illness has a higher prevalence in developing nations. Health professionals' lack of training in the etiology, diagnosis, and treatment of such diseases has hampered international diseases control efforts (Kurz, 1990, p. 51). The use of protective clothing and insect and tick repellants can help prevent these diseases. The use of insecticides and mosquito control measures has decreased the occurrence of vectorborne diseases worldwide. Some insect vectors and the diseases transmitted by them are given in Table 6-2. The vectorborne diseases of malaria, yellow fever, Lyme disease, and Rocky Mountain spotted fever are briefly discussed.

Malaria and *yellow fever* are two well-known vectorborne diseases transmitted by mosquitoes. Malaria is still a major illness in many tropical and subtropical areas. Yellow fever was prevalent in the United States until the early 1900s. It was an epidemic of this disease originating in the port of New Orleans that precipitated the formation of a National Board of Health in 1879. Yellow fever occurs primarily in tropical regions and remains an important health problem in West Africa (Kurz, 1990, p. 46). It occurs most frequently among young adult males who are occupationally exposed in forests (Benenson, 1995, p. 520).

Lyme disease is a vectorborne disease transmitted by ticks. It was diagnosed in 1975 in Lyme, Connecticut after the Connecticut State Health Department was notified of an abnormally high incidence of juvenile arthritis, a relatively rare condition. Epidemiologists investigated and found that the causative agent was a spirochete bacterium, *Borrelia burgdorferi*, and was transmitted to humans, dogs, and horses by the bite of an infected deer tick. There are three stages of Lyme disease. The first is a spreading red rash that begins as a red bump at the site of the tick attachment and expands outward in a circular fashion. It is often accompanied by headache, fever, chills, backache, and fatigue. If the disease is not treated it can progress to the second stage, where there may be evidence of central nervous system dysfunction, muscle pain, and cardiac abnormalities. The third stage can begin months or years after the initial lesion and usually involves recurrent bouts of arthritis, often in the knees. Vaccines for the disease are in advanced stages of development (CDC, 1996, p. 49). Almost 12,000 cases of this disease occur each year in the United States (CDC, p. 46).

Rocky Mountain spotted fever is a vectorborne disease transmitted by ticks. It seldom occurs in the Rocky Mountains but is common in the Southeast. Its causative agent is *Rickettsia rickettsii*. Symptoms include fever, severe headache, chills, deep muscle pain, malaise, and frequently a rash that starts on the extremities and spreads to the rest of the body. No vaccine is available for the disease, but it is believed that one attack may result in lifelong immunity.

Zoonoses

Zoonoses are infections transmitted under natural conditions from vertebrate animals to humans (Benenson, 1995). Methods of transmission include inhalation, ingestion, and animal bites. Some of the better known zoonoses are *rabies*, *toxoplasmosis*, and *cat scratch fever*.

Rabies is probably the best known of the zoonoses. The causative agent is a virus. No treatment is successful for rabies once symptoms occur, and it is almost always fatal. It is estimated that 40,000 rabies deaths occur worldwide each year (Benenson, 1995, p. 383). Animals can be vaccinated for rabies; however, many wild and domestic animals are infected with the rabies virus. The most effective rabies prevention is the immediate and thorough cleansing with soap or detergent and flushing with water of all wounds caused by an animal bite or scratch (Benenson, p. 383). Rabies immune globulin and/or vaccine is used as indicated.

The infectious agent for toxoplasmosis is *toxoplasma gondii*, a protozoa, and the definitive host is cats. Primary infection during pregnancy can result in fetal brain damage, hydrocephaly, microcephaly, or death. The infectious agent for cat scratch fever is *Bartonella benselae*, a bacteria, and domestic cats are the reservoir.

Lead Poisoning

Lead poisoning is a major environmental health disease and one of this country's important environmental health problems. A strong national effort is in place to reduce lead in American homes and eradicate childhood lead poisoning (USDHHS, 1991, p. 66; USDHHS, 1995, p. 81). An estimated 3 million children younger than 6 years of age (15% of all U.S. children in this age group) have elevated blood lead levels (Maternal and Child Health Bureau, 1995, p. 29), and the potential for lead poisoning in this age group is even greater since more than 13 million American preschoolers live in homes contaminated with lead-based paint (Snyder, Ruth, Sattler, Strasser, 1994). The Agency for Toxic Substances and Disease Registry estimates that 400,000 children are at risk of being born with lead poisoning each year because their mothers have elevated blood lead levels (Nadakavukaren, 1990, p. 28). More than 1 million American workers may be exposed to lead in the workplace (ATSDR, 1994, p. 428).

Lead poisoning has been documented throughout history, and some historians theorize that it was one of the conditions leading to the fall of the Roman Empire. Many wealthy and influential Romans could afford to have water piped to their homes and to eat from expensive glazed dishes. These water pipes often contained lead, as did the finishes and glazes used on dishes and tableware. The effects of this exposure could have resulted in children of the ruling class being unable to meet their full mental potential and in adults evidencing neurotoxicity, bizarre behavior, stillbirth, and sterility.

Lead poisoning was a serious problem in the early days of the American auto industry because many auto workers placed lead in the doors and frames of automobiles. They inhaled lead throughout the day and ingested lead when they sat around the assembly line to eat their meals. Research studies on lead poisoning in the auto industry, done by Dr. Carey P. McCord of the University of Michigan, resulted in regulations to protect workers from lead inhalation, protective measures for workers, and the first lunchrooms and cafeterias in industry—places for workers to eat that were away from lead particles (McCord, 1976).

Lead can be inhaled, ingested, or transmitted in utero. It is an extremely toxic substance to the cardiovascular, renal, reproductive, and neurological systems (Preventing lead poisoning, 1992, p. 1). Exposure to high levels of lead is potentially fatal. Symptoms of lead poisoning include listlessness, pallor, loss of appetite, irritability, behavioral changes, and growth and developmental delays (see Chapter 15). Even low levels of exposure can cause central nervous system damage, hearing impairments, and growth deficits (USDHHS, 1991, p. 14).

Children absorb more than 50% of the lead they ingest, and young children are especially vulnerable to the effects of lead (Preventing lead poisoning, 1992, p. 1). If a calcium or iron deficiency exists, even more lead will be absorbed from the gastrointestinal tract (Preventing lead poisoning, p. 1). Lead poisoning in children is often contracted from lead in paint, ducts, water, gas fumes, and soil. It is especially prevalent in inner-city areas where high concentrations of lead exist in soil and air near heavily traveled roadways and in old buildings that may have been painted with lead paint before 1950. Recently the U.S. Consumer Product Safety Division has cited dangerous levels of lead in imported vinyl miniblinds and banned further imports of them (Cohen, 1996, D1). Upon exposure to light and heat the blinds deteriorate and lead dust accumulates. Washing will not prevent the deterioration and people are being urged to dispose of them. Unfortunately, millions of American homes may have these blinds and not even be aware of the danger.

In 1971 Congress passed the Lead-Based Paint Poisoning Prevention Act, which banned the usage of lead-based paint in interior paints and on furniture and toys. Major gains have been made in understanding and treating lead poisoning, and the average amount of lead ingested daily by U.S. children has dramatically decreased (Bourgoin, Evans, Cornett et al, 1993, p. 1155). However, lead poisoning is still a problem for children and adults.

The American Nurses Association has stated that "childhood lead poisoning is the most common preventable pediatric health problem in the United States" but it is epidemic among American children (ANA, 1996, p. 193). ANA's position statement supports lead poisoning prevention activities to reduce children's blood lead levels.

Healthy People 2000 has an objective to reduce the prevalence of blood lead levels exceeding 15 μg/dl and 25 μg/dl among American children 6 months through 5 years of age. The National Center for Environment Health conducts studies on lead poisoning and works to eradicate childhood lead poisoning in the United States. The federal government has published *The Nature and Extent of Lead Poisoning in Children in the United States: A Report to Congress* (ATSDR, 1988) and the *Strategic Plan for the Elimination of Childhood Lead Poisoning* (CDC, 1991). Casefinding and eliminating sources of lead poisoning in the home and community is a major challenge for community health nurses.

Environmental Lung Diseases

Environmental pollutants in the air contribute to numerous lung diseases, including bronchial asthma, acute respiratory conditions and irritations, pneumoconiosis, allergic alveolitis, and lung cancer. Reducing human exposure to air pollutants such as ozone, carbon monoxide, nitrogen dioxide, sulfur dioxide, environmental tobacco smoke, and particulates is important in reducing the incidence of environmentally linked lung diseases included lung cancer, mesothelioma, emphysema, and asthma. (Environmental tobacco smoke is discussed more in this chapter under indoor air pollution and in Chapter 17, and occupational lung diseases are discussed in Chapter 18.) The EPA estimates that at least 150,000 serious respiratory ailments among young children are caused each year by exposure to environmental tobacco smoke (Nadakavukaren, 1995, p. 229).

Asthma has been linked to passive inhalation of smoke and other environmental pollutants and affects approximately 10 million Americans (USDHHS, 1991, p. 317). Childhood asthma is a major health problem that has recently had increasing rates of morbidity and mortality, and children with asthma have shown marked improvements when their parents quit smoking. Asthma incidence rises in the summertime, with peak levels of atmospheric ozone, and with year-round increase in nitrogen oxides in the air (Landrigan, 1992, p. 942). In inner cities asthma is the leading cause of hospital admissions for children 5 to 15 years old, with asthma rates highest among black and Hispanic children (Landrigan, p. 942).

Although air quality has improved significantly in recent years, fewer than 50% of Americans live in counties that meet all the EPA air quality standards (EPA, 1990). Significant gains have been made in reducing air pollution from motor vehicles and other sources; additional gains are needed to promote the public's health.

Environmental Cancers

In 1775 Sir Percival Pott, an English physician, made an association between cancer of the scrotum in chimney sweeps and exposure to soot, an early determination of an environmental carcinogen. Cancer is the second leading cause of death in the United States and, although the etiology of many cancers is unknown, some cancers are linked to environmental carcinogens. Today the relationships between smoking and lung cancer, radon and lung cancer, exposure to the sun and skin cancer, asbestos and malignant mesothelioma, and occupational cancers (see Chapter 18) are well known. Other environmental carcinogens include x-rays, pesticides, coal tars, and some air pollutants (including a number of chemicals found in tobacco smoke).

Environmental tobacco smoke has been estimated to account for 30% of all cancers in the United States (USDHHS, 1991, p. 72). By the year 2000 an estimated 300,000 American workers will have died of diseases caused by asbestos-related lung cancer and malignant mesothelioma (Landrigan, 1992, p. 941). An increasing risk with asbestos is the number of school children exposed to it as a result of insulation in older school buildings. The EPA estimates that approximately 20,000 cases of lung cancer each year occur as a result of radon exposure (USDHHS, 1991, p. 322). Environmental exposures to carcinogens are generally preventable.

Birth Defects

Birth defects are technically not an environmental disease, but they are conditions that are being increasingly linked to environmental factors. Birth defects are the leading cause of death in infants. Approximately 150,000 infants are born each year in the United States with birth defects (Nadakavukaren, 1995, p. 204). Embryos that are genetically normal may be seriously damaged by environmental hazards—teratogens that cause birth defects. Fetal vulnerability is most acute from the 18th day after conception to the 60th day, with a peak around the 30th day (Nadakavukaren, pp. 205, 212). Spina bifida, blindness, deafness, mental retardation, and phocomelia are some examples of birth defects known to have linkages to environmental teratogens. When infants survive birth defects they are usually left with chronic, lifelong, debilitating problems that often prevent them from living independent lives. Some known human teratogens are given in Table 6-3.

PRESERVING THE ENVIRONMENT

People have added to the destruction of the global environment. However, increasing concern about global environmental conditions and the ability of the planet to maintain future generations has resulted in many initiatives to preserve and protect Earth's environment. Polls have put environmental issues at the top of Americans' concerns, along with AIDS, crime, and drugs (Schuster, 1990, p. 26). Environmental issues are a part of every major political campaign, and Americans are demanding ecologically sound products, legislation, and activities. People are working together to protect the environment and make the

table 6-3 SOME KNOWN HUMAN TERATOGENS

TERATOGEN	EFFECT
IONIZING RADIATION	
X-rays	Central nervous system disorders, microcephaly, eye problems, mental retardation
Nuclear fall-out	
PATHOGENIC INFECTIONS	
German measles	Congenital heart defect, deafness, cataracts
Syphilis and herpes simplex type 2	Mental retardation, microcephaly
Cytomegalovirus	Kidney and liver disorders, pneumonia, brain damage
Toxoplasmosis	Fatal lesions in the central nervous system
DRUGS AND CHEMICALS	
Thalidomide	Phocomelia
Methyl mercury	Mental retardation, sensory and motor problems
DES	Vaginal cancer in girls, genital abnormalities in boys
Dioxin	Structural deformities, miscarriages
Anesthesia	Miscarriages, structural deformities
Alcohol	Mental retardation, growth deficiencies, microcephaly, facial irregularities
Cigarette smoke	Low birth weight, miscarriage, stillbirth
Dilantin	Heart malformations, cleft palate, harelip, mental retardation, microcephaly
Valproic acid	Spina bifida
Accutane	Cardiovascular abnormalities, deformation of the ear, hydrocephaly, microcephaly
Tegison	Same effects as Accutane

From Nadakavukaren A: *Our global environment: a health perspective*, ed 4, Prospect Heights, Il., 1995, Waveland Press, p. 205.

world a healthier place to live. Some contemporary environmental health concerns are discussed here.

Greenhouse Effect

We are in the process of changing the earth's atmosphere. Natural greenhouse gases in the atmosphere form a blanket around the earth that keeps the planet warm. These natural gases are predominantly carbon dioxide, methane, and nitrous oxide. When technological gases (especially carbon dioxide) thicken this blanket, they trap heat around the earth and result in global warming. Carbon emissions from burning fossil fuel have more than tripled throughout the world over the past half-century (Flavin, Tunali, 1995, p. 10). Eventually the temperature of the earth's surface will warm enough to cause climatic and environmental changes that can be detrimental to health.

Scientists estimate that by 2050 the earth's temperature could increase by as much as four degrees centigrade (Wittkopf, Kegley, 1990, p. 33). This would be as great a change as the drop of four degrees centigrade that caused the last Ice Age (Doll, 1992, p. 939). Many scientists fear that rising temperatures will melt polar ice caps, raise ocean levels, flood and destroy coastal areas and wetlands, alter weather patterns and change rain distribution, increase the frequency of droughts, cause massive wildfires, and create deserts. Climate changes resulting from global warming can result in "habitats on the move" for humans, plants, and animals and the creation of conditions more conducive to the spread of many communicable diseases.

Climate changes as a result of global warming can result in dramatic changes in food production and create "environmental refugees" when food becomes scarce. In addition to food shortages, such warming can result in the extension of areas favorable to vectorborne and parasitic diseases; an increase in communicable diseases; increased incidence of fungal skin diseases, skin cancer, skin rashes, heat stroke, and exhaustion; and patterns of human migration that can result in overcrowding and other unfavorable social conditions. The enlargement of tropical climates would bring malaria, encephalitis, yellow fever, and other insectborne disease to formerly temperate climates.

Air Pollution

Air pollution results when one or more chemicals exist in the air in concentrations high enough to harm plants, animals, or humans. Particulate matter and excess heat and noise are considered to be air pollutants also.

Air pollution has always occurred through natural occurrences in the environment, including volcanoes, forest fires, pollination, dust storms, and swamp gas. Historically, concern for the effects of air pollution on public health dates back to at least the thirteenth century, when government commissions were established in England to investigate sources of air pollution and "the fouling of air" (Blumenthal, Greene, 1985, p. 117). The Industrial Revolution greatly added to the problem of air pollution, and gas-powered vehicles, power plants, and industry continue to contribute to this problem today. Early community efforts to minimize air pollution in the United States included local regulations to control unpleasant "airs," limiting outdoor burning, and controlling smoke.

The Clean Air Acts of 1970, 1977, 1990, and 1994 have worked to reduce air pollution in the United States and mandated establishment of national ambient air quality standards for suspended particulates, sulfur oxides, carbon monoxide, nitrogen oxide, artificial ozone, hydrocarbons, and lead. An example of how this legislation assists communities in cleaning up their air is seen in Rothschild, Wisconsin. When students in Rothschild began suffering from asthma attacks brought on by sulfur dioxide emissions from a local paper mill, parents protested, the EPA used the Clean Air Act to enforce mill emission standards, and the number of school children experiencing medical emergencies from asthma declined (Monks, 1996, p. 27).

The American Lung Association sponsors Clean Air Week each year in May and tries to educate the American public about the importance of clean air and respiratory health. However, according to the Environmental Protection Agency 164 million Americans (66% of the U.S. population) live in areas where the Clean Air Standard is exceeded (CDC, 1993, p. 302). An air pollution success story is that of Chattanooga, Tennessee. The city's air was so polluted in the 1950s that when women wearing nylon stockings walked outside their legwear would sometimes disintegrate (Glick, 1996, p. 44). The citizens of Chattanooga engaged in a successful environmental clean-up, and today the city is a model for others trying to recover from air pollution.

Healthy People 2000 addresses the need for more American cities to comply with these standards. The Centers for Disease Control and Prevention (CDC) recognize that, in order for this to occur, additional educational methods focused on air pollution control and improved coordination between health and environmental agencies is needed (CDC, 1993, p. 303). Air pollution is often classified as indoor or outdoor.

Indoor Air Pollution

Indoor air pollution is a significant concern and may pose a greater risk to human health than outdoor air pollution. Levels of 11 common pollutants can be found in the average American home at concentrations up to 5 to 70 times greater than they are found outdoors (Miller, 1996, p. 438). Indoor air pollution is often caused by radon, tobacco smoke, infectious agents, allergens, combustion smoke (e.g., furnaces, fireplaces, and woodstoves), household chemicals, pesticides, and building materials (e.g., asbestos and formaldehyde-treated products). It causes symptoms such as dizziness, headaches, coughing, sneezing, nausea and vomiting, burning eyes, and chronic fatigue. Indoor air pollutants frequently cause acute and chronic respiratory infections and conditions, allergic reactions, headaches, and cancer.

Some buildings are considered "sick" because of indoor air pollution and can result in people suffering from "sick building syndrome." According to the World Health Organization this syndrome is characterized by eye, nose, and throat irritation; a sensation of dry mucous membranes and skin; erythema; mental fatigue; headache; a high frequency of airway infections and cough; hoarseness; wheezing, itching, and nonspecific hypersensitivity; and nausea and dizziness (Jaakkola, Tuomaala, Seppanen, 1994, p. 422). A sick building is suffering from indoor air pollution severe enough to cause symptoms, illness, and even death of its occupants. Newer buildings are more likely to be sick because of reduced air exchange to save energy and emission of chemicals from new carpeting and furniture (Miller, 1996, p. 439). The EPA estimates that at least 17% of the 4 million commercial buildings in the U.S. are "sick"—including the EPA's Washington, D.C. headquarters (Miller, p. 439)!

Research conducted by the National Aeronautics and Space Administration (NASA) has indicated that the use of houseplants can actually help to absorb contaminants in the air; they use plants as part of the biological life support system aboard orbiting space stations (Why clean, 1990, p. 1F). NASA found that plants help to remove benzene, formaldehyde, and carbon monoxide and put oxygen back into the environment.

RADON Radon is a colorless, odorless, cancer-producing gas formed by radioactive decay of the radium and uranium found in natural soil. Since the 1980s radon has been recognized as a serious form of indoor air pollution and a national health problem. The EPA has ranked radon as one of the most dangerous cancer risks in the environment. It is the second leading cause of lung cancer in the United States, responsible for up to 30,000 deaths each year (EPA, 1993, p. 2). Radon can be found all over the United States, but some areas are "hot spots" for radon.

Radon particles are carried deep into the lung where they release small bursts of energy and damage lung tissue, resulting in possible lung damage, lung disease, and lung cancer. Lung damage from radon has no early warning symptoms. Smokers are much more vulnerable to the effects of radon and have higher death rates from it than nonsmokers (EPA, 1992, p. 12).

The EPA estimates that 4 to 5 million American homes and up to 20% of American schools (11 million students) have elevated radon levels (Miller, 1996, p. 442). Radon silently seeps into American homes, schools, and businesses through cracks in basement walls, floors, and foundations; joint spaces between walls and floors; well water; and openings around pipes and sump pumps. The box on the following page shows how radon can hide undetected in the American home. Elevated radon levels in buildings pose health threats, but there are simple, inexpensive ways to fix a radon problem. EPA recommends that homeowners across the nation test their homes for radon. If a home has a radon problem and the home has well water, the well should be tested for radon too. Has your home been tested?

Is Radon Gas Hiding in Your Home?

When Stanley Watras walked into the Limerick nuclear power plant near Philadelphia on a December morning in 1984 he started radiation-detection alarms ringing. It was determined that the radioactive contamination on Watras had come from outside the nuclear facility, and Watras' home was checked for possible sources of radiation contamination.

To everyone's amazement, tests revealed that the Watras home had levels of radon gas approximately 1000 times higher than normal. Investigators estimated that the Watras family was receiving radiation exposure equivalent to 455,000 chest x-rays a year just by living in their house. The Watras family had been unaware of the radon in their home.

Further investigation showed that radon was "hiding" in thousands of American homes. It was determined that large sections of eastern Pennsylvania, New Jersey, and New York, which are underlain by a uranium geological formation, had thousands of homes where elevated levels of radon existed. Is radon gas hiding in your home?

Modified from Nadakavukaren A: *Our global environment: a health perspective*, ed 4, Prospect Heights, Il., 1995, Waveland Press, p. 503.

The federal government is trying to educate the American public to the dangers of radon, and every state has a state radon office. The Environmental Protection Agency has numerous publications on radon, including *A Citizen's Guide to Radon*, and children's publications on radon, such as *Learning About RADON: a Part of Nature*. To get more information on radon and to find out about state radon offices phone 1-800-SOS-RADON.

ENVIRONMENTAL TOBACCO SMOKE (ETS) ETS is a major indoor air pollutant and health risk. ETS is a complex mixture of more than 4000 chemicals, many of which are toxic or carcinogenic (EPA, 1993, p. 13). The EPA estimates that approximately 3000 lung cancer deaths occur each year in the United States as a result of ETS (EPA, p. 13). Children's lungs are especially susceptible to the harmful effects of ETS. Conditions such as bronchitis, pneumonia, asthma, and acute respiratory infections occur up to twice as often during the first 2 years of life in children who are exposed to ETS, and there is strong evidence of increased middle ear infections, reduced growth, and reduced lung function (EPA, p. 13). The more smoking in the home, the higher the prevalence of respiratory symptoms (Murdock, 1991, p. 12). The Occupational Safety and Health Administration is considering a ban on workplace smoking (Kerbel, 1995, p. 49).

OTHER INDOOR AIR POLLUTANTS These pollutants include biological air pollutants, volatile organic compounds (VOCs), and combustion products. According to the EPA (1993), examples of biological air pollutants are dust, mites, molds, and animal dander; VOCs include benzene, carbon tetrachloride, and formaldehyde; and combustion products include carbon monoxide, nitrogen dioxide, and sulfur dioxide. Biological agents are known to cause infections, hypersensitivity, and toxicoses (EPA, p. 14). VOCs can be found in paint, upholstery, spray cans, copy machine toners, and clothing, and their health effects include irritation of the eyes and respiratory system, liver and kidney damage, cancer, and birth defects (EPA, p. 14). Combustion products are derived primarily from malfunctioning heating devices and motor vehicle emissions from garages or loading docks; they produce symptoms similar to influenza and include fatigue, nausea, dizziness, headaches, tachycardia, and cognitive impairment (EPA, p. 14). For more information on indoor air pollutants call the EPA's Indoor Air Quality Information Clearinghouse at 1-800-438-4318.

Outdoor Air Pollution

Outdoor, or "ambient," air pollution is prevalent in the United States. Major ambient air pollutants are carbon oxides, sulfur oxides, nitrogen oxides, volatile organic compounds (e.g., methane, benzene, and formaldehyde), suspended particles, photochemical oxidants (e.g., ozone and hydrogen peroxide), radioactive substances, heat, and, noise.

Smog is a combination of the words *smoke* and *fog* and is a major form of outdoor air pollution. All major American cities suffer from some level of smog. It is more prevalent in industrial areas with dense population, large numbers of motor vehicles, and a sunny, dry climate. The Los Angeles metropolitan area suffers the worst levels of smog in the nation (The 27th environmental, 1995, p. 36). Smog harms plants, animals, and people. It has been blamed for numerous outbreaks of respiratory illness and distress in addition to crop losses and deforestation (pine trees are very susceptible).

Outdoor air pollution can result in such health conditions as lung cancer, bronchial asthma, acute respiratory illnesses/conditions, and skin and eye conditions. Lung damage from polluted air is a risk for millions of Americans. Air pollution also damages agriculture, vegetation, and property, creates aesthetic problems, and affects the economy in terms of property damage and loss, morbidity, mortality, and absenteeism from work.

Ozone Depletion

An invisible layer of natural ozone shields and protects the earth's surface against ultraviolet radiation. People are destroying this natural ozone shield by use of chlorofluorocarbons (CFCs) and other man-made chemicals. CFCs are compounds made up of carbon, chlorine, and fluorine. They are routinely used in refrigeration and air conditioning (e.g., freon), aerosol sprays, and cleaning agents; 750,000 metric tons of CFCs are used annually worldwide (Elmer-Dewitt, 1992, p. 64). CFCs deplete the ozone layer when they rise into the stratosphere and their chlorine atoms react with ozone. International agreements have been put in place to phase out CFC use by the year 2000 (Lemonick, 1992, p. 60).

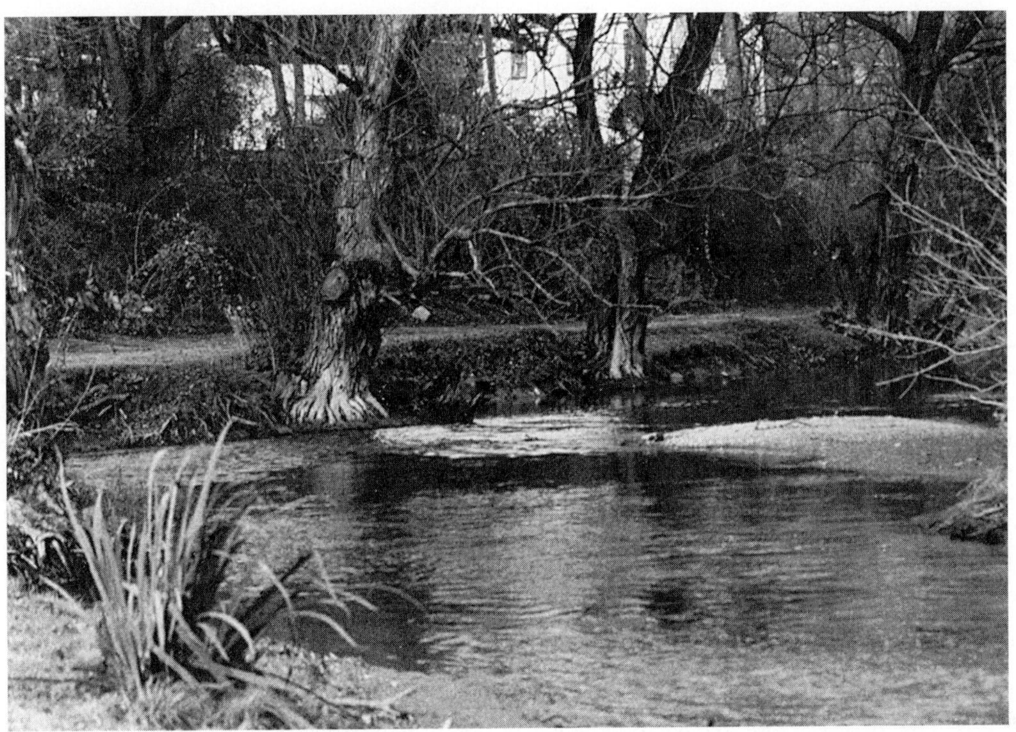

Figure 6-1 Safeguarding our natural resources is a major public health need. Despite our modern technology, our nation has not been able to control disease outbreaks related to environmental pollutants. In recent years there has been a dramatic rise in the number of disease outbreaks from contaminated water. *(Courtesy Henry Parks, photographer.)*

Sherwood Rowland, at the University of California at Irvine, issued the first ozone depletion alert in 1974 (Lemonick, 1992, p. 62). A hole in the ozone layer over Antarctica was confirmed in 1985, and another over the North Pole in 1988 (Miller, 1996, p. 318). Now researchers have found signs of ozone depletion in North America (Snider, 1993, A1). Worldwide, ozone levels continue to decline. Fifty-four million Americans live in areas that do not meet the federal ozone standard (The 27th environmental, 1995, p. 36).

Holes in the ozone layer deplete our natural protection from the sun, making it increasingly important to wear sunglasses, protective clothing, and sunscreen when exposed to the sun for prolonged periods. It is crucial to minimize the time spent in the sun during the peak period of 10 AM to 3 PM, minimize sunbathing, and avoid being in the sun for long periods of time. Ozone depletion is a health hazard. It is expected to result in increased incidence of skin cancer and accelerated skin aging, eye cataracts, mutations in DNA, immune system weakening, depletion of food crops by interference with the process of photosynthesis, and phytoplankton depletion (phytoplankton is important in the ocean food chain). Scientists are also concerned about the possible effects of ozone depletion on climate.

Water Pollution

The human body's dependence on a regular intake of water is second only to its need for oxygen (Nadakavukaren, 1995, p. 544). As amazing as it may seem, less than 3% of the Earth's water is fresh, and only 1% is suitable for drinking. Americans use almost 100 billion gallons of fresh water every day, much more than other countries (Loehr, 1989, p. 26).

Water is a renewable resource, but in the near future water supply could become a serious crisis in many areas of the United States. Water resources in the United States are not evenly distributed; areas in the Pacific Northwest can receive 80 inches of rainfall annually, whereas the driest state, Nevada, may receive less than 10 inches annually. Even where there are abundant sources of water, serious problems result if that water is unfit for human consumption. We need to conserve and protect our nation's water supplies (Figure 6-1).

Existing U.S. water supplies are rapidly being polluted and depleted. According to the EPA, 30% of the nation's rivers and 42% of its lakes are polluted, 40% of the nation's fresh water is unusable, and toxic chemicals are still being discharged into the nation's waters (The 27th environmental, 1995, p. 38).

Sources of potential water pollution are construction activities, industrial wastes, human and animal wastes, landfill waste, accidental spills, mining operations, leaking underground storage tanks, agricultural waste and runoff, fallout of airborne pollutants, urban street runoff, fertilizers, and pesticides. Homeowners add to groundwater contamination through the use of septic tanks and by dumping household chemicals down the drain or on the ground. Household septic tanks are used by almost 30% of the U.S. population, account for 3.5 billion gallons of waste being introduced into the soil each day, and have the potential to add to water pollution (Loehr, 1989, p. 26).

In less-developed countries millions of people do not have access to safe drinking water. Each year millions of people worldwide become ill and die from preventable waterborne diseases such as polio, typhoid, cholera, hepatitis, and bacterial dysentery. The United States has set a goal that 85% of the population will have safe drinking water by the year 2000 (USDHHS, 1995, p. 215). Nurses should encourage families using well water to have their water checked on a regular basis.

Hazardous Waste

Hazardous wastes pose serious health problems. The *Resource Conservation and Recovery Act* defined hazardous waste as any discarded material that may pose a substantial threat or potential danger to human health or the environment. Such wastes have properties that make them hazardous to human health such as toxicity, flammability, explosiveness, radioactivity, reactivity, corrosiveness, and communicability (the presence of pathogens). The EPA estimates that each year one metric ton of hazardous waste is produced for every U.S. citizen.

An increasing number of hazardous waste sites in the U.S. are prompting communities to become more concerned about environmental health issues (Neufer, Narkunas, 1994, p. 329). Improper disposal of hazardous industrial waste has lead to Superfund legislation, numerous health problems, communities being evacuated and relocated, and community coalitions for environmental health. Recently an environmentally sound process called *bioremediation* has been used to devour waste products and unwanted hazardous waste materials. In bioremediation special bacteria are used to break down hazardous waste into nonhazardous compounds. Such safe, innovative methods to deal with hazardous waste materials need to be developed and encouraged.

Nurses need to be aware of hazardous wastes in the community, consider whether community members have been exposed, and determine the effect on public health (Neufer, Narkunas, 1994, p. 334). Hazardous and toxic wastes have been linked to deaths, poisoning, acute and chronic illness, cancer, birth defects, blindness, and sterility. In 1992 two 9-year-old Tampa boys were killed while playing inside a municipal waste bin located behind an industrial firm (Nadakavukaren, 1995, p. 668). The bin contained toxic chemical wastes, and officials concluded that the boys had died as a result of inhalation of toxic fumes. Love Canal in New York and countless other incidents have been examples of the effects of hazardous wastes on human life and health.

Acid Rain

Acid rain is the falling of acids and acid-forming compounds from the atmosphere to earth. Sulfur dioxide is the primary component of acid rain. It mixes with nitrogen oxides in the atmosphere to chemically form sulfuric acid and nitric acid. These acids fall back to earth in the form of acid rain or snow. Rain that had a pH value almost equivalent to that of battery acid once fell on Wheeling, West Virginia (Miller, 1996, p. 436)! Areas along the Appalachian Mountains can have rain that has the acidic content of lemon juice! Acidic lakes, rivers, and streams can upset the ecological balance needed to sustain fish, plant, and animal life.

Electric utilities are responsible for the majority of sulfur dioxide emissions in the United States. You can help prevent acid rain by conserving energy. It is estimated that the effects of acid rain in the United States cost up to $10 billion a year (Miller, 1996, p. 437). Acid causes dermatological conditions, kills aquatic life, can result in crop depletion, results in the loss of plant and animal diversity, and harms the health of humans.

Loss of Biological Diversity

Extinction is forever! Once a plant, animal, or insect species is gone we can never get it back. It is estimated that animal and plant species will become extinct at a rate of 50,000 species a year during the next few decades—the greatest mass extinction since the die-off of the dinosaurs (Raven, 1995, p. 38). Unfortunately, we are living through the greatest extinction event of the last 65 million years. For the first time in millions of years species are vanishing more rapidly than new ones are evolving (Nadakavukaren, 1995, p. 179).

To protect endangered species, the Endangered Species Act of 1973 was passed. It gave the United States one of the most far-reaching laws ever enacted by any country to prevent the extinction of imperiled animals and plants. More than 760 native mammals, birds, reptiles, crustaceans, plants, and other life forms were officially protected. In addition, more than 500 foreign species are now protected under the act. The U.S. Fish and Wildlife Service of the Department of Interior is charged with protecting American wildlife and endangered species.

Conservation biologists estimate that each day 50 to 200 species of plants and animals become extinct worldwide (Miller, 1996, p. 639)! If poaching, animal exploitation, environmental pollution, and destruction of critical habitats continue at the present rate, within the next few decades up to two million of the world's plant, animal, and insect species could be lost forever (Nadakavukaren, 1995,

p. 179). The World Wildlife Foundation has launched a global endangered seas campaign to rebuild depleted fish supplies and implement solutions to destruction of the sea environment (WWF, 1996b). Government and private efforts to save endangered species are to be applauded.

Plants are especially important to health—more than 60% of the world's people depend directly on plants for their medicines, and plants play a role in the derivation of the top 20 pharmaceutical products sold in the United States (Raven, 1995, p. 40). Preserving critical habitats and land is crucial to preserving plant and animal species.

We need to remember that everything in nature is interlinked. Species diversity is a major determinant of ecological stability and human survival. As we lose plant and animal species we increase the risk of our own extinction. With the loss of each plant species we could possibly be losing a cure for AIDS, cancer, or numerous other diseases or conditions.

Garbage and Solid Waste

The United States has the dubious distinction of being the world's biggest solid waste producer. With only 4.5% of the world's population, Americans produce 33% of the world's solid wastes—11 billion tons each year (Miller, 1992, p. 519). Trash and solid waste have become major national problems. American households and businesses throw away 200 million tons of garbage a year, more than 4 pounds per person each day.

Where to put garbage and solid waste is becoming a big problem. More than two thirds of the nation's landfills have closed since the late 1970s, and many of those remaining will be full in the near future (Beck, Hager, King et al, 1989, p. 67). Trash, landfills, piles of refuse, and unsightly, unsanitary conditions are becoming a regular part of the American landscape; "America the beautiful" may soon be a phrase from the past.

Today the three Rs of waste control are *Reuse*, *Recycle*, and *Reduce*. Americans need to practice the three Rs more. Recycling is becoming more popular in the United States, but still less than 20% of U.S. solid waste is recycled. Recycling has gone from a necessary burden of government to revenue-producing "big business" (Young, 1996, p. 246). For example, New York City expects to earn almost $25 million from selling its newsprint in 1996; and Madison, Wisconsin is receiving $23 per ton for its recyclables—close to $1 million a year (Young, p. 246).

Using "reusables" and reducing the amount of garbage and solid waste has been slow to gain momentum in the United States; just look at how disposable items are used in everyday life—including health care settings. The best way to manage garbage and waste is to not produce it in the first place. Garbage and solid waste produce health risks such as the possibility of soil and water pollution, spread of communicable disease, and accidental illness and injury.

Desertification

According to the United Nations Environment Programme (UNEP), desertification is one of the most serious global environmental problems (Stopping, 1996, p. 194). Most desertification occurs naturally at the edges of existing desert as a result of dehydration of the top layers of soil, but desertification can also result from overgrazing, improper soil management and use of water resources, and deforestation. Worldwide, three million square miles (an area the size of Brazil, or 12 times the size of Texas) have become desert during the past 50 years. Each year 23,000 square miles become desert (an area the size of West Virginia), and an estimated 63% of rangelands and 60% of rainfed cropland are threatened by desertification (Miller, 1996, p. 518). In the American Southwest overgrazing is largely responsible for the formation of Arizona's Sonoran Desert (Nadakavukaren, 1990, p. 138).

Once land has become desert it is difficult to reclaim. Restoration efforts often involve reforestation. Loss of land previously used for food production has a direct impact on nutrition and quality of human life. Also, migration of people and animals resulting from "habitats on the move" can result in overcrowding and other undesirable social conditions.

Wetlands Destruction

U.S. wetlands are rapidly being depleted and destroyed. These wetlands include swamps, marshes, ponds, river bottoms, flood plains, and ponds. Until recently many wetland areas were seen as nuisances because of water accumulation and insects, and many wetlands were drained for agricultural, industrial, and residential purposes. However, environmentalists and the general public are now recognizing their value, and legislation has been passed to preserve and protect remaining wetlands.

Over half of America's wetlands are gone. We have built on wetland flood plains and have made many cities vulnerable to flooding. Recent flooding along the Mississippi River has shown this to be true and demonstrated the serious loss of life and property destruction that can occur in floods. In relation to health, wetlands serve as "living filters" for purifying contaminated surface waters (Nadakavukaren, 1995, pp. 174-175) and, when left intact, serve as natural floodplains.

Deforestation

Ralph Waldo Emerson (1836) said, "In the woods, is perpetual youth . . . In the woods, we return to reason and faith." Emerson believed that the outdoors offered a cleansing of both mind and spirit and that through nature people can find knowledge and self-discovery (Seeing beauty, 1996, p. 50). Unfortunately our woods are being rapidly depleted, and the beauty of many forests is lost forever. Protected state and national forests are helping to save trees. However, even protected forests are threatened by pollution (Davis, 1996, A1).

The World Wildlife Fund has launched a global campaign to protect the world's forests. It is encouraging nations to set aside as protected areas at least 10% of their representative original forests and work to slow forest loss and degradation (WWF, 1996c). Such activities are essential considering that an area the size of Austria is deforested each year (Wittkopf, Kegley, 1990, p. 32). In many underdeveloped countries forests are being cleared and burned to make way for farms and industry. In the United States it takes over 500,000 trees to supply Americans with their Sunday papers each week (The Earthworks Group, 1990). Although trees are a renewable resource, like water, they are renewable at a slow rate.

Carbon dioxide is removed from the atmosphere by green plants during photosynthesis. Cutting down forests destroys the natural process of removing carbon dioxide from the atmosphere. Deforestation accelerates global warming and results in "habitats on the move" and loss of plant and animal life (Wittkopf, Kegley, 1990, p. 32).

Rainforests are forests that receive at least 100 inches of rain each year (Rainforests, 1990, p. 3). Tropical rainforests are located in a narrow region near the equator in Africa, South and Central America, and Asia. Haiti has lost all of its original primary forest, and Bangladesh has lost 95% of its original tropical rainforest (Hinrichsen, 1994, p. 38). Once there were more than 5 billion acres of rainforest; today there is less than half that amount (Rainforests, 1990, p. 3).

Although rainforests make up only 6% to 7% of the Earth's surface, over half of the world's plant, animal, and insect species live in them (Myers, 1992, p. 282). If the current rate of rainforest destruction continues, up to two million species of plants, animals, and insects will become prematurely extinct in the next 30 years—presently we are losing 74 species per day, and the rate is accelerating (Nadakavukaren, 1995, p. 179).

One in four pharmaceuticals has components from a rainforest plant, and 70% of the plants identified by the National Cancer Institute as being helpful in the treatment of cancer are found only in the rainforests. Rainforests include plants from which analgesics, antibiotics, heart drugs, cancer drugs, hormones, diuretics, tranquilizers, laxatives, dysentery treatments, and anticoagulants are made (Carr, Pederson, Ramaswamy, 1996, p. 135). Examples of plants that are pharmaceuticals are the serpentine root (reserpine) used in tranquilizers, Mexican yam (diosgenin) for infertility drugs, cinchona tree (quinine) for malaria, and rosy periwinkle (vincristine and vinblastine) to fight cancer (Carr, Pederson, Ramaswamy, p. 135).

Energy Depletion

The United States has the distinction of being the world's largest energy user and waster. At least 43% of all energy used in the United States is unnecessarily wasted, and this waste equals all the energy consumed by two thirds of the world's population (Miller, 1996, pp. 333-334).

Major sources of U.S. energy are the nonrenewable resources of petroleum, coal, and natural gas. Renewal sources of energy include thermal, electric, hydroelectric, wind, solar (photovoltaic cells), geothermal, and biomass power—they account for only about 10% of U.S. energy use each year (Kozloff, 1994).

The largest users and wasters of energy in the United States are energy-inefficient buildings, factories, and vehicles. Every winter the energy equivalent of all the oil that flows through the Alaskan pipeline in a year leaks through American windows (The Earthworks Group, 1990). Such unnecessarily wasted energy has been estimated to cost about twice as much as the annual U.S. federal budget deficit, or more than the entire military budget.

Overpopulation

The human species has had a population explosion in the last 50 years. Overpopulation contributes to depletion of natural resources and increased sewage and solid wastes. The world population is more than 5.6 billion, and it is expected to reach 11 billion by the year 2050 (Miller, 1996, p. 4). Millions of people in the world are hungry or malnourished and lack safe drinking water.

Overpopulation places a strain on world food supplies and causes overcrowding and unsafe health conditions. Population growth is already outstripping food production and water supply. Already more than 900 million people in developing countries do not get enough calories to maintain normal levels of physical development, and 36% of preschool children in developing countries are below expected weight for their age (Brown, 1995). Poverty, malnutrition, overcrowding, increased susceptibility to disease, and shortened life span are all health-related conditions that are affected by overpopulation.

DISASTER NURSING

Throughout history natural and manmade disasters have disrupted food and water supplies and sanitation, causing communicable disease, injury, illness, and death. Media coverage of disaster events such as 1992's Hurricane Andrew, the 1995 Oklahoma City bombing, and recent droughts and floods has shown the public the devastating effects that disasters impose on human life, property, and the environment. A common denominator in these disaster and emergency situations is nursing's immediate response (Mikulencak, 1993).

Legislation has been enacted to provide federal assistance to individuals and communities to aid recovery from devastation caused by disasters to human life and property. The Disaster Relief Act of 1966 (Public Law 89-769) was a landmark piece of legislation that affected disaster relief efforts. In addition to providing disaster funds this law mandated a Disaster Assistance Study. In response to this study the Disaster Relief Act of 1970 (Public Law 91-606) was passed. This act repealed previous disaster relief legislation, with the exception of Section 302 of the 1966 Act,

Defining Emergency and Major Disaster

EMERGENCY

Any hurricane, tornado, storm, flood, high water, wind-driven water, tidal wave, tsunami, earthquake, volcanic eruption, landslide, mudslide, snowstorm, drought, fire, explosion, or other catastrophe in any part of the United States which requires Federal emergency assistance to supplement State and local efforts to save lives and protect property, public health and safety or to avert or lessen the threat of a disaster.

MAJOR DISASTER

Any hurricane, tornado, storm, flood, high water, wind-driven water, tidal wave, tsunami, earthquake, volcanic eruption, landslide, mudslide, snowstorm, drought, fire, explosion, or other catastrophe in any part of the United States which in the determination of the President, causes damage of sufficient severity above and beyond emergency services by the Federal Government, to supplement the efforts and available resources of States, local governments, and disaster relief organizations in alleviating the damage, loss, hardship, or suffering caused thereby.

From U.S. Congress: *Disaster Relief Act Amendments of 1974* (Public Law 93-288), Section 102.

that pertained to providing disaster assistance to public educational facilities.

The Disaster Relief Act of 1970 defined *disaster* and provided direction for coordinating disaster assistance, ranging from early disaster warnings to relocation. The Disaster Relief Act Amendments of 1974 (Public Law 93-288) distinguished between the terms *disaster* and *emergency*. These definitions still provide the basis on which a catastrophic environmental event is declared a disaster. The definition that Congress uses to identify a major disaster is given in the above box. The Amendments of 1974 expanded coverage under the act, clarified the administration of disaster relief efforts, mandated immediate federal disaster relief, and provided for long-term economic assistance for disaster areas.

FEMA (1986) describes two types of disasters: natural and technological (manmade). According to FEMA *natural disasters* include droughts, earthquakes, tsunamis, forest fires, landslide and mudslides, blizzards, hurricanes, tornadoes, floods, and volcanic disruptions; and *technological disasters* include hazardous substance accidents (e.g., chemicals, toxic gases), radiological accidents, dam failures, resource shortages (e.g., food, electricity, and water), structural fire and explosions, and domestic disturbances (e.g., terrorism, bombing, and riots). FEMA provides general guidelines in four disaster management phases for each natural or technological disaster.

Although little can be done to prevent natural disasters, much can be done to prevent technological disasters. The United Nations (UN) declared the 1990s as the "International Decade for Natural Disaster Reduction," with emphasis on disaster prevention and preparedness (Bates, Dynes, Quarantelli, 1991; Pickens, 1992). Consistent with the UN declaration, The World Health Organization (WHO) developed a checklist to aid disaster preparedness efforts (Pickens). It is important to remember that "the most important community resource in a disaster is individual preparedness" (Garcia, 1985, p. 229).

The American Red Cross

Since 1881, when Clara Barton founded the American Red Cross (ARC), the organization has provided emergency services for casualties from natural and manmade disasters such as wars, famines, earthquakes, epidemics, floods, and organized blood drives (Oates, 1996). Today there are more than 1 million trained American Red Cross volunteers across the country (ARC, 1990). The ARC is known all over the world for its disaster relief efforts. All ARC disaster relief assistance is free (ARC, 1993).

The Red Cross is not a government agency, but it is chartered by Congress to provide special services to members of the U.S. Armed Forces and disaster victims. It provides disaster assistance, publications and training, and works with FEMA to develop guidelines for community disaster preparation (ARC, 1990; FEMA, 1993). There are local offices of the ARC across the country. These offices have numerous publications for families to use to prepare for disasters, as well as publications, videos, and services of interest to the nurse. The box on the next page lists some publications available from the Red Cross. An especially helpful publication for individuals and families is the Emergency Preparedness Checklist, which is a joint FEMA and ARC (1993) publication. Nurses work with the Red Cross and other agencies in all phases of disaster management.

Phases of Disaster Management

FEMA (1986) describes four disaster management phases: mitigation, preparedness, response, and recovery, which serve as a model for community disaster preparations and nursing interventions (see Figure 6-2). Some preparedness, response, and recovery activities by local communities and the American Red Cross are given in Table 16-4.

MITIGATION Disaster mitigation "includes any activities that prevent a disaster, reduce the chance of a disaster happening, or reduce the damaging effects of unavoidable disasters" (FEMA, 1986, p. 1.6). Nurses have a key role in disaster mitigation by working with local, state, and federal agencies in identifying disaster risks and developing disaster prevention strategies through extensive public education in disaster prevention and readiness. Effective mitigation includes recognizing and preventing potential technological disasters and being adequately prepared should such events occur.

To plan effectively for disaster prevention the nurse needs to have community assessment information (see Chapter 13), including knowledge of community resources (e.g., emergency services, hospitals, and clinics), community health personnel (e.g., nurses, doctors, pharmacists, emergency medical teams, dentists, and volunteers), community government officials, and local industry. In disaster mitigation the nurse also needs to consider community climate and terrain conducive to disasters such as floods, tornadoes, hurricanes, and earthquakes. Planning for disasters requires leaders be aware of resources, prepared to mobilize resources, and able to prevent chaos and confusion (Dinerman, 1990).

Selected Publications Available from the American Red Cross

Are You Ready? Your Guide to Disaster Preparedness, FEMA H-34, 1993.
Emergency Preparedness Checklist, ARC #4471, 1993.
Emergency Food and Water Supplies: A Family Protection Brochure, FEMA-215, 1992.
Helping Children Cope With Disaster, ARC #4499, 1993.
Your Family Disaster Supplies Kit, ARC #4463, 1992
Are Your Ready for an Earthquake? ARC #4455, 1990.
Are You Ready For a Winter Storm? ARC #4464, 1991.
After a Flood: The First Steps, ARC #4476, 1992.
Fire, ARC #4456, 1993.
Flood, ARC #4458, 1992.
Hurricane, ARC #4454, 1994.
Safe Living in Your Manufactured Home, ARC #4465, 1991.
Tornadoes: A Preparedness Guide, ARC #5002, 1993.
Thanks to the Disaster Leave Law: This Could Be You, ARC #5047, 1994.
The Disaster Services Human Resources System, ARC #4420, 1986.
Thunderstorms and Lightening: A Preparedness Guide, ARC #5001, 1994.
Winter Storms: A Guide to Survival, ARC #4467, 1991.

PREPAREDNESS Preparedness "includes plans or preparations made to save lives and to help response-and-rescue operations" (FEMA, 1986, p. 1.6) in the event of a natural or technological disaster. Nurses have a key role in maximizing the health and safety of all individuals affected by a disaster. Community health nurses have skills in triage and crisis intervention and are involved in acute care, triage, first aid, rescue and evacuation procedures, managing life-threatening events, recognizing and preventing communicable illnesses, assessment, and provision of immediate health care needs during disaster impact.

Disaster preparedness involves developing plans for rescue, evacuation, caring for disaster victims, training disaster response personnel, and gathering resources, equipment, and materials necessary for coping with disaster (ARC, 1993; Martin, 1994). Community-focused planning skills are discussed in Chapter 14. Establishing an effective public communication system is essential for successful disaster emergency communication and community safety (Rattien, 1990; Sikich, 1996). Making anticipatory provisions for food, water, clothing, shelter, and medicine is also an important preparedness activity. It is crucial for the nurse to understand effective disaster preparedness. Through community assessment nurses can identify disaster risks and collaborate in developing disaster plans for the particular disaster risks (e.g., tornado, chemical spills, floods, earthquakes, and explosions).

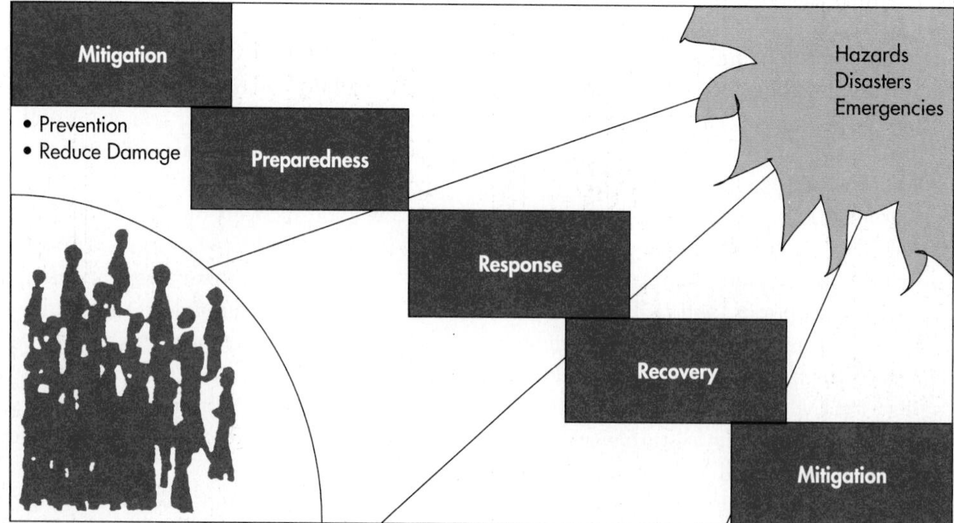

Figure 6-2 **Phases of disaster management.** *(From Federal* Emergency Management Agency *[FEMA]: Emergency management U.S.A., Washington, D.C., 1986, FEMA, p. 1.5.)*

RESPONSE Response "includes actions taken to save lives and prevent further damage in a disaster or emergency situation" (FEMA, 1986, p. 1.6) and puts predisaster planning services into action (ARC, 1993; FEMA, 1986). Nurses work with community disaster teams in emergency rescue and care operations with a focus on lessening the effect on victims. This includes triage of disaster victims, providing immediate health care (e.g., first aid), providing food and shelter, maintaining effective channels of communication, and minimizing chaos and panic.

In disaster response a primary concern for nurses is safety; safety for themselves, the rescue team, and victims. Nurses are involved in promoting not only safety and physical health, but also the mental health of all involved in the disaster. The nurse works to reduce fear, panic, and hysteria by encouraging victims to express their fears and concerns. Helping people to cope with the disaster situation involves

table 6-4 Disaster Management Responsibilities: Preparedness, Response, and Recovery

Red Cross	Other Voluntary Organizations	Business and Labor Organizations	Local Government
PREPAREDNESS			
• Participates with government in developing and testing community disaster plan. Designates persons to serve as representatives at government emergency operations centers and command posts. • Develops and tests local Red Cross disaster plans. • Identifies and trains personnel for disaster response. • Collaborates with other voluntary agencies in developing and maintaining a local Voluntary Organizations Active in Disaster group to promote cooperation and coordinate resources for disasters. • Works with business and labor organizations to identify resources and people for disaster work. • Educates the public about hazards and ways to avoid, prepare for, and cope with their effects. • Acquires material resources needed to ensure effective response.	• Collaborate in developing and maintaining a local Voluntary Organizations Active in Disaster group to identify roles, resources, and plans for disasters. • Identify and train personnel for disaster response. • Identify community issues and special populations for consideration in disaster preparedness. • Make plans to continue to serve regular clients following a disaster. • Identify facilities, resources, and people to serve in time of disaster. • Educate specific client groups on disaster preparedness.	• Develop disaster plans for business locations and integrate their plans with the community disaster plan. • Develop procedures to facilitate continuity of operations in time of disaster. • Develop plans for assisting business employees following a disaster. • Identify union and business facilities, resources, and people that may be able to support community disaster plans. • Provide volunteers, financial contributions, and in-kind gifts to the Red Cross and other voluntary organizations to support disaster preparedness. • Educate employees and union members about disaster preparedness.	• Coordinates the development of the community plan and conducts evaluation exercises. • Trains staff to carry out the plan. • Passes legislation to mitigate the effects of potential disasters. • Designs measures to warn the population of disaster threats. • Conducts building safety inspections. • Develops procedures to facilitate continuity of public safety operations in time of disaster. • Identifies public facilities, resources, and public employees for disaster work. • Educates the public about disaster threats in the community and safety procedures.
RESPONSE			
• Operates shelters. • Provides feeding services. • Provides individual and family assistance to meet immediate emergency needs. Services include providing the means to purchase groceries, clothing, and household items.	• Provide services that are identified in predisaster planning. • Provide regular services to ongoing client groups.	• Take action to protect employees and ensure the safety of the facility. • Advise public safety forces of hazardous conditions.	• Provides for coordination of the overall relief effort. • Advises the public on safety measures such as evacuation. • Provides public health services.

From American Red Cross: *Disasters happen*, Washington, D.C., 1993, American Red Cross.

Continued

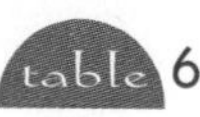 6-4 Disaster Management Responsibilities: Preparedness, Response, and Recovery—cont'd

Red Cross	Other Voluntary Organizations	Business and Labor Organizations	Local Government
• Provides Disaster Health Services, including mental health support. • Handles inquiries from concerned family members outside the area. • Coordinates relief activities with other agencies, business, labor, and government. • Informs the public of services available. • Seeks and accepts contributions from those wishing to help.	• Identify unanticipated needs and provide resources to meet those needs. • Act as advocates for their client groups. • Coordinate services with all other groups involved with the disaster response. • Seek and accept donations from those wishing to help.	• Identify resources like union halls, generators, and heavy equipment that are available to support the disaster response. • Provide volunteers, financial contributions, and gifts of goods and services to the relief effort.	• Provides fire and police protection to the disaster-affected area. • Inspects facilities for safety and health codes. • Provides ongoing social services for the community. • Repairs public buildings, sewage and water systems, streets, and highways.

RECOVERY

- During recovery, all of the segments represented here pull together with one goal—the restoration of the economic and civic life of the community.
- Government takes the lead in rebuilding roads, bridges public works, and buildings, and providing services to citizens.
- Business returns to operation to provide economic support to the community.
- Voluntary agencies, including the Red Cross, work together to identify and meet the remaining needs of individuals and families.
- The Red Cross remains available to support those with long-term needs by helping people access vital services and apply for assistance from local, state, and federal disaster programs. However, if such relief assistance is not available, the Red Cross can also provide assistance to promote the recovery of individuals.
- All of the groups involved work in partnership with the people affected by disasters, who are ultimately responsible for their own recovery.

caring, listening, encouraging people to express their feelings, and providing emotional support to the victims and their families.

RECOVERY Recovery "includes actions taken to return to a normal, or even safer, situation following a disaster" (FEMA, 1986, p. 1.6). The recovery period may last for an extended period of time. The goal of recovery is to prevent debilitating effects and restore personal, economic, and environmental health and stability to the community (ARC, 1993). Disaster relief activities can range from local, state, regional, national, and international efforts.

Shock, depression, and grief are common occurrences in a disaster. During the recovery phase the mental health services have a key role. From a mental health viewpoint, a number of emotional reactions occur in phases in relation to a disaster (see the following box).

Rescue personnel should be included in the mental health efforts of the recovery process. Prevention and control of stress among emergency workers is important. Rescuers are vulnerable to emotional crises in relation to disaster events (Craft, 1996) and as a result debriefings are important interventions for rescue personnel (Stuhlmiller, 1996).

Community health nurses have unique skills for assisting communities in planning for disaster relief efforts and addressing problems that occur during a disaster. Community health nurses' knowledge of community resources, community assessment and organization, epidemiology, health planning, and family health promotion provides a background for organizing and participating in community relief efforts. This knowledge is discussed in Chapters 8, 13, and 14.

Nursing Role in Disasters

Although all health care workers are essential in disaster preparedness (Pickens, 1992), nurses play important roles in planning and implementing disaster relief efforts, preventing technological disasters, and addressing problems that occur during a disaster, such as the physical and emotional stress of disaster victims (see Figure 6-3). Nurses have key leadership roles in disaster preparation and response (Komnenich, Feller, 1991). The American Nurses Association and the American Red Cross have cited the need for more RNs to be trained for disaster relief (Turner, 1993, p. 3). During a disaster many environmental health problems emerge (see Figure 6-4).

Phases of Emotional Reaction During a Disaster

From a mental health viewpoint, work with victims of disasters has suggested a classification related to emotional reactions:

- *Heroic phase*
  This phase appears at the time of the disaster and is characterized by people working together to save each other and their property. Excitement is intense, and people are concerned with survival.
- *Honeymoon phase*
  This is a relatively short (2 weeks to 2 months) postdisaster period in which the victims feel buoyed and supported by the promises of governmental and communal help and see an opportunity to reconstitute quickly. Optimism continues high, losses are counted, and plans to reestablish are made.
- *Disillusionment phase*
  Lasting anywhere from several months to a year or more, this phase contains unexpected delays and failures which emphasize the frustration from bureaucratic confusion. Victims turn to rebuilding their own lives and solving their own individual problems.
- *Reconstruction phase*
  This phase may last for several years. It is characterized by a coordinated individual and community effort to rebuild and reestablish normal functioning.

From Farberow NL, Gordon NS: *Manual for child health workers in major disasters*, Washington, D.C., 1986, USDHHS (Substance Abuse and Mental Health Services Administration), p. 3.

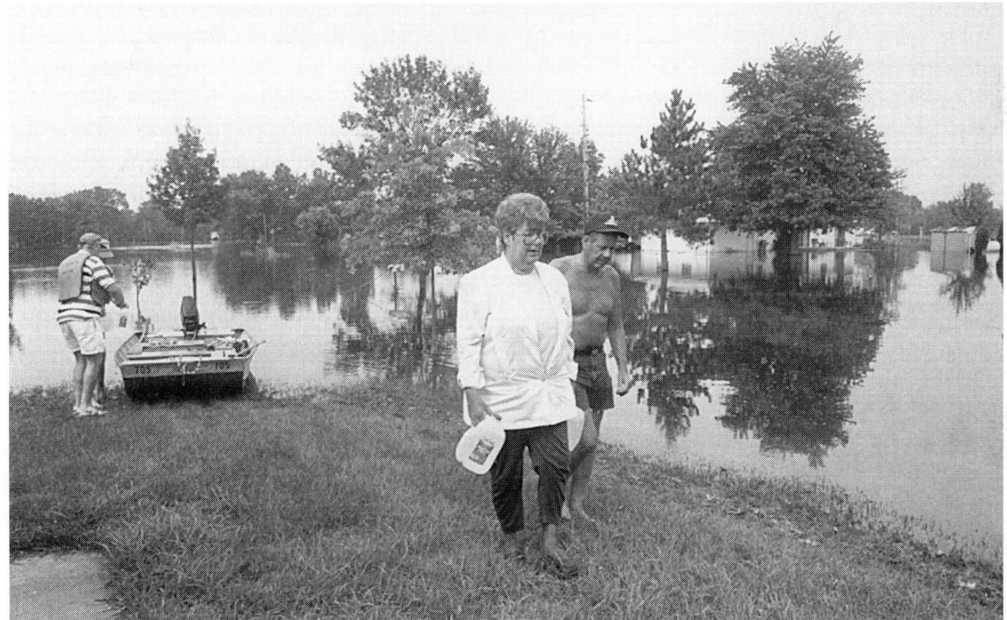

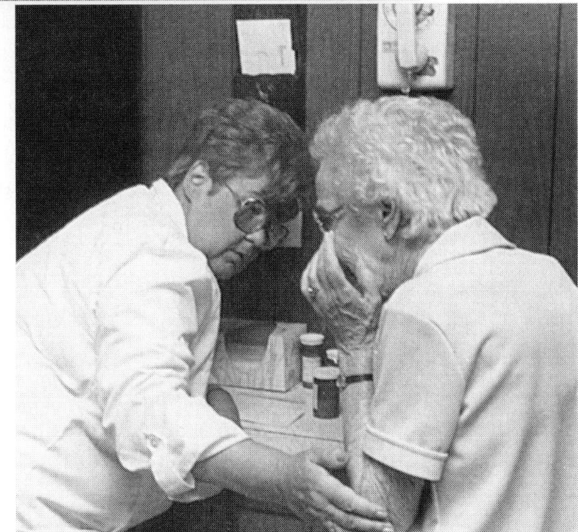

Figure 6-3 A nurse/disaster planner boats out to flooded areas and assists an 86-year-old widow who refused to leave her home until conditions became extremely severe. Nurses functioning in situations such as these need to use crisis intervention skills to help these individuals and families cope with the stresses they are experiencing. *(Courtesy Kathy Kuper.)*

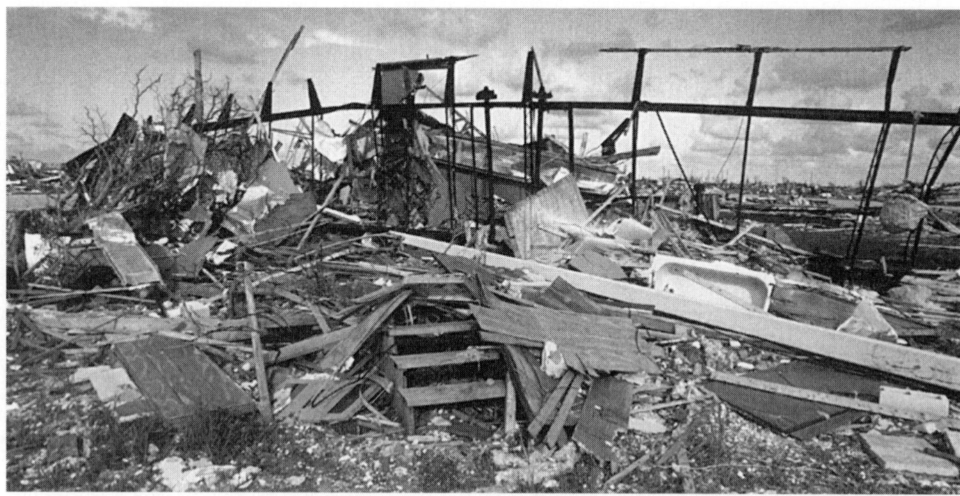

Figure 6-4 Hurricanes and other environmental disasters cause many community-wide health problems. *(Courtesy U.S. Department of Agriculture.)*

Nurses have the responsibility to collaborate with community agencies and officials to recognize and reduce disaster risks and maximize the health and safety of individuals involved in disaster crises. Community disaster strategies for nurses are given in the box on the next page. Nursing's role in a disaster varies according to the type and magnitude of the disaster.

In this decade of disaster reduction, the American Nurses Association has made concerted efforts to collaborate with the American Red Cross, federal and civilian agencies, and nursing specialty organizations to enhance nurses' contributions in disaster management (Turner, 1993). These collaborative efforts proved timely for nurses' responses during the 1995 Oklahoma bombing disaster (Canavan, 1996; Craft, 1996). An agency that nurses often work closely with in providing disaster relief is the American Red Cross.

During recovery efforts nurses may make numerous referrals for physical and emotional support services and treatment for victims and their families (Clunn, 1996). Recovery encompasses dealing with many disaster effects such as loss of life, income, and home. As a result of a disaster food and water supplies can become contaminated, and communicable disease and other conditions, such as domestic violence and depression, can become rampant.

Summary

Environmental health is a primary public health concern. Environmental health problems exist worldwide and cause problems such as communicable disease, respiratory conditions, cancer, poverty, and ecological disturbances in the environment. Manmade and natural disasters in recent years have caused tremendous economic instability and extensive personal suffering in communities across the United States and the world.

Healthy People 2000 has directed attention toward dealing with environmental concerns in the United States by establishing specific environmental health objectives. Worldwide, nurses are being encouraged to safeguard the human environment. Specific environmental health roles for nurses have been identified, and community health nurses have unique skills to deal with environmental health issues. Environmental health legislation supports public health professionals in their efforts to resolve environmental health problems.

Florence Nightingale was aware of the importance of the environment in nursing, and nurse scholars today reinforce this importance. The environment cannot be overlooked in the provision of nursing care. Nurses need to embrace the historical role of environmental health activities in preventing communicable disease, as well as take an advocacy role in relation to preserving the global environment. We all need to focus on preserving and protecting that which we cannot create. Remember that pollution is not only unhealthy, it is difficult to eradicate, and extinction is forever!

CRITICAL *Thinking Exercise*

Examine the local community in which you live. What types of environmental hazards exist? What types of environmental disasters have occurred or have the potential to occur in this community? What are some of the agencies that have responded or would respond to a disaster? What disaster provisions has the community made? Describe some of the activities you see nurses being responsible for in a disaster. What actions could the nurse take to promote environmental health?

Community Disaster Strategies for Nurses*

ASSESS THE COMMUNITY

Is there a current community disaster plan in place?
What previous disaster experiences has the community been involved with locally, statewide, nationally?
How is the local climate conducive to disaster formation (e.g., hurricanes, tornadoes, blizzards)?
How is the local terrain conducive to disaster formation (e.g., earthquakes, flood, forest fires, avalanches, mudslides)?
What are the local industries?
Are there any community hazards (e.g., toxic waste and chemical spills, industrial or agricultural pollutants, mass transportation problems)?
What personnel are available for disaster interventions (e.g., nurses, doctors, dentists, pharmacist, clergy, volunteers, emergency medical teams)?
What are the locally available disaster resources (e.g., food, clothing, shelter, pharmaceutical)?
What are the local agencies and organizations (e.g., hospitals, schools, churches, emergency medical, Red Cross, etc.)?
What is immediately available for infant care (e.g., formula, diapers), care of the elderly and disabled?
What are the most salient chronic illnesses in the community that will need immediate attention (e.g., diabetes, arthritis, cardiovascular)?

DIAGNOSE COMMUNITY DISASTER THREATS

Determine actual and potential disaster threats (e.g., toxic waste spills, explosions, mass transit accidents, hurricanes, tornadoes, blizzards, floods, earthquakes, etc.).

COMMUNITY DISASTER PLANNING

Develop a disaster plan to prevent or deal with identified disaster threats.
Identify local community communication system.
Identify disaster personnel, including private and professional volunteers, local emergency personnel, agencies, and resources.
Identify regional backup agencies, personnel, etc.
Identify specific responsibilities for various personnel involved in disaster coping and establish a disaster chain of command.
Set up an emergency medical system and chain for activation.
Identify location and accessibility of equipment and supplies.
Check proper functioning of emergency equipment.
Identify outdated supplies and replenish for appropriate readiness.

IMPLEMENT DISASTER PLAN

Focus on primary prevention activities to prevent occurrence of man-made disasters.
Practice community disaster plans with all personnel carrying out their previously identified responsibilities (such as emergency triage, providing supplies such as food, water, medicine, crises and grief counseling, etc.).
Practice using equipment, obtaining and distributing supplies.

EVALUATE EFFECTIVENESS OF DISASTER PLAN

Critically evaluate all aspects of disaster plans and practice drills for speed, effectiveness, gaps, and revisions.
Evaluate the disaster impact on community and surrounding regions.
Evaluate response of personnel involved in disaster relief efforts.

*See Chapters 3 and 13 for specific guidelines for community assessment.

The authors would like to acknowledge the efforts of Ella M. Brooks in the writing of this chapter.

REFERENCES

Agency for Toxic Substances and Disease Registry (ATSDR): *The nature and extent of lead poisoning in children in the United States: a report to Congress*, Washington, D.C., 1988, USDHHS.

Agency for Toxic Substances and Disease Registry (ATSDR): Lead toxicity, *AAOHN J* 43(8):428-440, 1994.

American Association of Colleges of Nursing: *Addressing nursing's agenda for health care reform*, Washington, D.C., 1993, The Association.

American Nurses Association (ANA): *American Nurses Association position statement on lead poisoning and screening: compendium of American Nurses Association position statements*, Washington, D.C., 1996, The Association.

American Public Health Association (APHA): Position paper on the role of official local health agencies, *Am J Public Health* 65:189-193, 1975.

American Red Cross (ARC): *A history of helping others*, Washington, D.C., 1990, ARC.

American Red Cross (ARC): *Disaster happens*, Washington, D.C., 1993, ARC.

American Red Cross (ARC) and Federal Emergency Management Agency (FEMA): *Emergency preparedness checklist*, Pub. #4471, Washington, D.C., 1993, ARC.

Bates F, Dynes R, Quarantelli EL: The importance of the social sciences to the international decade for natural disaster reduction, *Disasters* 15(3):288-289, 1991.

Beck M, Hager M, King P et al: Buried alive, *Newsweek* November 27, 1989, pp. 66-76.

Bellack JP, Musham C, Hainer A et al: Environmental health competencies: a survey of U.S. nurse practitioner programs, *J Nurs Educ* 35(2):74-81, 1996.

Benenson AS, ed: *Control of communicable diseases manual*, ed 16, Washington, D.C., 1995, American Public Health Association.

Blumenthal DS, ed: *An introduction to environmental health*, New York, 1985, Springer.

Blumenthal DS, Greene M: Air pollution. In Blumenthal DS, ed: *An introduction to environmental health*, New York, 1985, Springer.

Bourgoin BP, Evans DR, Cornett JR et al: Lead content in 70 brands of dietary calcium supplements, *Am J Public Health* 83(8):1155-1160, 1993.

Breckinridge M: *Wide neighborhoods: a story of the Frontier Nursing Service*, New York, 1952, Harper and Brothers.

Brown LR: Reassessing the earth's population, *Society* May/June:7-10, 1995.

Canavan K: Nurses' heroism reflects essence of profession: ANA, Red Cross recognize 10 nurses for selfless deeds, *Am Nurse* 28(4):1, 18-19, 1996.

Carr TA, Pederson HL, Ramaswamy S: Rain forest entrepreneurs. In Allen JL, ed: *Environment: annual edition 96/97*, Guilford, Ct., 1996, Dushkin.

Centers for Disease Control and Prevention (CDC): Populations at risk from air pollution—United States, 1991, *Morb Mortal Wkly Rep* 42(16):301-304, 1993.

Centers for Disease Control and Prevention (CDC): *A strategic plan for the elimination of childhood lead poisoning*, Atlanta, Ga., 1991, USDHHS.

Centers for Disease Control and Prevention (CDC): Lyme disease—United States, 1995, *Morb Mortal Wkly Rep* 45(23):46-49, 1996.

Clark HG: Origins of public health in America: superiority of sanitary measures over quarantines. An address delivered before the Suffolk District Medical Society at its third Anniversary meeting, Boston, April 24, 1852. In Rosenberg CE, ed: *Medicine and society in America*, New York, 1972, Arno Press.

Clunn P: The nurse's kit for survivors, *Reflections* 22(1):8-9, 1996.

Cohen JS: Lead danger prompts vinyl miniblind alert, *USA Today*, June 25, 1996, D1.

Coss C: Lillian D. Wald: progressive activist, *Public Health Nurs* 10(3):134-138, 1993.

Craft M: The many graces of Oklahoma nurses, *Reflections* 22(1):10-13, 1996.

Davis M: Pollution, funds are top concerns about Smokies, *The Knoxville News-Sentinel*, June 25, 1996, A1, A3.

Dinerman N: Disaster preparedness: observations and perspectives, *J Emerg Nurs* 16(4):252-254, 1990.

Doll R: Health and the environment in the 1990s, *Am J Public Health* 82(7):923-941, 1992.

Elmer-Dewitt P: How do you patch a hole in the sky that could be as big as Alaska? *Time* 139(7):64-65, February 17, 1992.

Environmental Protection Agency (EPA): *Characterization of municipal solid wastes in the United States: 1990 update*, Washington, D.C., 1990, EPA.

Environmental Protection Agency (EPA): *A citizen's guide to radon: the guide to protecting yourself and your family from radon*, ed 2, Washington, D.C., 1992, U.S. Government Printing Office.

Environmental Protection Agency (EPA): *Radon: the health threat with a simple solution. A physician's guide*, Washington, D.C., 1993, EPA.

Farberow NL, Gordon NS: *Manual for child health workers in major disasters*, Washington, D.C., 1986, USDHHS (Substance Abuse and Mental Health Services Administration).

Federal Emergency Management Agency (FEMA): *Emergency management U.S.A.*, Document No. HS-2, Washington, D.C., 1986, FEMA.

Federal Emergency Management Agency (FEMA): *Are you ready? Your guide to disaster preparedness*, Document H-34 #8-0908, Washington, D.C., 1993, FEMA.

Flavin C, Tunali O: Getting warmer: looking for a way out of the climate impasse, *World Watch* March/April:10-19, 1995.

Garcia LM: *Disaster nursing: planning, assessment and intervention*, Rockville, Md., 1985, Aspen.

General Accounting Office (GAO): *Environmental protection issues*, Washington, D.C., 1993, GAO.

Glick D: Cinderella story, *Natl Wildlife* 34(2):42-46, 1996.

Gordon LJ: Who will manage the environment? *Am J Public Health* 80(8):904-905, 1990.

Hill L: Health in America: a personal perspective. In U.S. Department of Health, Education, and Welfare: *Health in America 1776-1976*, DHEW Pub. No (HRA) 76-616, Washington, D.C., 1976, U.S. Government Printing Office, pp. 3-15.

Hinrichsen D: Putting the bite on planet earth, *International Wildlife* September/October:36-45, 1994.

Institute of Medicine (Committee for the Study of the Future of Public Health): *The future of public health*, Washington, D.C., 1988, National Academy Press.

Institute of Medicine (Committee on Enhancing Environmental Health Content in Nursing Practice, Pope AM, Snyder MA, Mood LH, eds): *Nursing, health, and the environment: strengthening the relationship to improve the public's health*, Washington, D.C., 1995, National Academy Press.

International Council of Nurses: *The nurse's role in safeguarding the human environment: position statement*, Geneva, Switzerland, 1986, The Council.

Jaakkola JJK, Tuomaala P, Seppanen OL: Air recirculation and sick building syndrome: a blinded crossover, *Am J Public Health* 84(3):422-428, 1994.

Kalisch PA, Kalisch BJ: *The advance of American nursing*, Boston, 1995, Little, Brown.

Kerbel WS: Indoor air quality: taking a second look at blueprints, *Occup Health Saf* 64(1):47-49, 72, 1995.

Kleffel D: Rethinking the environment as a domain of nursing knowledge, *Adv Nurs Sci* 14(1):40-51, 1991.

Komnenich P, Feller C: Disaster nursing. In Fitzpatrick JJ, Taunton RL, Jacox AK: *Annual review of nursing research*, volume 9, New York, 1991, Springer, pp. 123-134.

Kozloff KL: Renewable energy technology: an urgent need, a hard sell, *Environment* November:4-9, 25-31, 1994.

Kurz X: The yellow fever epidemic in Western Mali, September-November 1987: why did epidemiological surveillance fail? *Disasters* 14(1):46-54, 1990.

Landrigan R: Commentary: environmental diseases—a preventable epidemic, *Am J Public Health* 82(7):941-943, 1992.

Lemonick MD: The ozone vanishes, *Time* 139(7):60-63, February 17, 1992.

Loehr RC: Groundwater contamination—the problem and potential solutions, *National Forum* 69(1):26-28, 1989.

Martin F: Volunteering for disaster nursing, *Imprint* 41(2):45-46, 1994.

Maternal and Child Health Bureau: *Child health USA '94*, Washington, D.C., 1995, USDHHS.

McCord CP: Conversation with author regarding industrial lead poisoning, Ann Arbor, Mi., 1976, University of Michigan.

Mikulencak M: RNs begin relief efforts in flood-devastated Midwest, *Amer Nurse* September 1993, p. 3.

Miller GT: *Living in the environment*, ed 8, Belmont, Ca., 1992, Wadsworth.

Miller GT: *Living in the environment: principles, connections and solutions*, ed 9, Belmont, Ca., 1996, Wadsworth.

Monks V: Environmental regulations: who needs them? *Natl Wildlife* 34(2):24-31, 1996.

Morris RD, Naumova EN, Levin R, Munasinghe RL: Temporal variation in drinking water turbidity and diagnosed gastroenteritis in Milwaukee, *Am J Public Health* 86(2):237-242, 1996.

Murdock BS, ed: *Environmental issues in primary care*, Minneapolis, Mn., 1991, Minneapolis Department of Health.

Myers N: Guest essay: tropical forests and their species, going, going . . . ? In Miller GT: *An introduction to environmental science: living in the environment*, ed 7, Belmont, Ca., 1992, Wadsworth.

Nadakavukaren A: *Man in the environment: a health perspective*, ed 3, Prospect Heights, Ill., 1990, Waveland Press.

Nadakavukaren A: *Our global environment: a health perspective*, ed 4, Prospect Heights, Ill., 1995, Waveland Press.

National Center for Environmental Health (NCEH): *National Center for Environmental Health information book*, Washington, D.C., 1995, USDHHS.

Neufer L: The role of the community health nurse in environmental health, *Public Health Nurs* 11(3):155-162, 1994.

Neufer L, Narkunas D: Hazardous substance releases at the community level, *AAOHN J* 42(7):329-335, 1994.

Nightingale F: *Notes on nursing: what it is and what it is not*, New York, 1869, Dover.

No matter where you live, you can help clean up our coasts, *Earth-Savers* Summer:2-3, 1996.

Oates S: A woman of valor: Clara Barton and the Civil War, *Reflections* 22(1):16-17, 1996.

Office of the Federal Register: U.S. government manual 1995-96, Washington, D.C., 1995, U.S. Government Printing Office.

Pickens S: The decade for natural disaster reduction: the role of health care workers, *Nurs Health Care* 13(4):192-195, 1992.

Pickett G, Hanlon JJ: *Public health administration and practice*, ed 9, St. Louis, 1990, Mosby.

Portman C: Environmental health nursing philosophy, *Nurses for Environmental and Social Responsibility Newsletter* 1(3):3, 1995.

Preventing lead poisoning, *Health Watch* 12(1):1-3, 1992.

Public Health Foundation (PHF): *1991 Public health chartbook*, Washington, D.C., 1991, The Foundation.

Rabe B: Environmental health policy. In Pickett G, Hanlon JJ: *Public health administration and practice*, ed 9, St. Louis, 1990, Mosby, pp. 317-330.

Rainforests, *Kids for Saving Earth News* Fall 1990, p. 3.

Rattien S: The role of the media in hazard mitigation and disaster management, *Disasters* 14:36-45, 1990.

Raven P: A time of catastrophic extinction: what we must do, *The Futurist* September/October:38-41, 1995.

Ravenel MP: *A half century of public health: jubilee historical volume of the American Public Health Association*, New York, 1921, American Public Health Association.

Salazar MK, Primomo J: Taking the lead in environmental health: defining a model for practice, *AAOHN J* 42(7):317-324, 1994.

Schuster EA: Earth caring, *Adv Nurs Sci* 13(1):25-30, 1990.

Seeing beauty: thoughts from Emerson, *Int Wildlife* 26(4):50, 1996.

Selanders LC: *Florence Nightingale: an environmental adaptation theory*, Newbury Park, 1993, Sage.

Sexton K, Perlin SA: The federal environmental health workforce in the United States, *Am J Public Health* 80(8):913-920, 1990.

Shugars DA, O'Neil EH, Bader JD: *Healthy America: practitioners for 2005*, Durham, NC, 1991, The Pew Health Professions Commission.

Sikich G: *Emergency management planning handbook*, New York, 1996, McGraw-Hill.

Smillie WG: *Public health: its promise for the future*, New York, 1955, Macmillan.

Snider M: Ozone loss measured over North America, *USA Today* April 22, 1993, A1.

Snyder M, Ruth V, Sattler B, Strasser J: Environmental and occupational health education, *AAOHN J* 42(7):325-328, 1994.

Stopping the dry destruction. In Allen JL, ed: *Environment: annual edition 96/97*, Guilford, Ct., 1996, Dushkin.

Stuhlmiller C: Studying the rescuers, *Reflections* 22(1):18-19, 1996.

The Earthworks Group: *Simple things you can do to save the earth: 1991 tip a day calendar*, New York, 1990, Andrews and McNeel.

The 27th environmental quality review, *Natl Wildlife* 33(2):34-41, 1995.

Turner EA: ANA, Red Cross cite need for more RNs to be trained for disaster relief, *Amer Nurse*, September 1993, p. 3.

United States Department of Agriculture: *A quick consumer guide to safe food handling* (Home and Garden Bulletin No. 248), Washington, D.C., 1995, The Department.

United States Department of Health, Education and Welfare (USDHEW): *Healthy people*, Washington, D.C., 1979, U.S. Government Printing Office.

United States Department of Health and Human Services (USDHHS): *Evaluating the environmental health workforce* (HRP #0907160), Rockville, Md., 1988, USDHHS.

United States Department of Health and Human Services (USDHHS): *Healthy people 2000: national health promotion and disease prevention objectives for the nation, full report, with commentary*, Washington, D.C., 1991, U.S. Government Printing Office.

United States Department of Health and Human Services (USDHHS): *Health United States 1991 and prevention profile*, Washington, D.C., 1992, U.S. Government Printing Office.

United States Department of Health and Human Services (USDHHS): *Healthy people 2000: midcourse review and 1995 revisions*, Washington, D.C., 1995, U.S. Government Printing Office.

Wald L: *The house on Henry Street*, New York, 1915, Henry Holt and Company.

Wasson N: *E. coli* illness fells 6,000 children, *USA Today*, July 18, 1996, 9A.

Watch for EarthQuest at a museum near you! *EarthSavers*, Summer: 1, 1996.

Why clean air lovers are becoming indoor-houseplant lovers, *USA Today*, January 26, 1990, 1F.

Wilkie KE, Moseley ER: *Frontier nurse Mary Breckinridge*, New York, 1969, Julian Messner.

Wittkopf ER, Kegley CW: Our imperiled environment: impediments to a global response, *Natl Forum* 70(1):32-35, 1990.

World Wildlife Fund (WWF): WWF launches global endangered seas campaign, *Focus* 18(3):1, 1996b.

World Wildlife Fund (WWF): WWF launches global campaign to protect world's forests, *Focus* 18(4):1, 1996c.

Worthington K, Cary A: Primary health care: environmental challenges, *Am Nurse* 25(10):10-11, 1993.

Young JE: The sudden new strength of recycling. In Allen JL, ed: *Environment: annual review 96/97*, Guilford, Ct., 1996, Dushkin.

SELECTED BIBLIOGRAPHY

Brown L: Six pressing environmental concerns, *Natl Forum* 70(1): 8-11, 1990.

Cleveland H: Introducing the global commons, *Natl Forum* 70(1):4-7, 1990.

Durkin MS, Khan N, Davidson LL et al: The effects of a natural disaster on child behavior: evidence for posttraumatic stress, *Am J Public Health* 83(11):1549-1553, 1993.

Graves JS: Emotional aftermath of a major earthquake, *AAOHN J* 43(2):95-100, 1995.

Public health and the global environment (Editorial), *Can J Public Health* 81(1):3-4, 1990.

Reed PG, Zurakowski TL: Nightingale revisited: a visionary model for nursing. In Fitzpatrick JJ, Whall AL: *Conceptual models of nursing*, ed 2, Norwalk, Ct., 1989, Appleton and Lange, pp. 33-47.

Rycroft RW: Acid rain: air quality, global change, or what? *Natl Forum* 70(1):40-42, 1990.

Schuster EA, Brown CL: *Exploring our environmental connections*, New York, 1995, National League for Nursing.

The marine mammal exemption program: what it does, what it does not, *Marine Conservation News* 5(3):12, Autumn 1993.

Udall JR: Global warming, *Natl Forum* 70(1):36-39, 1990.

United States Department of Health and Human Services (USDHHS): *Human problems in major disasters: a training curriculum for emergency medical personnel* (DHHS Pub. # ADM 90-1505), Washington, D.C., 1990, USDHHS.

United States Department of Health and Human Services (USDHHS): *Prevention and control of stress among emergency workers* (DHHS Pub. # ADM 90-1497), Washington, D.C., 1990, USDHHS.

United States Department of Health and Human Services (USDHHS): *Disaster response and recovery: a handbook for mental health professionals* (DHHS #SMA 94-3010), Washington, D.C., 1994, USDHHS.

United States Department of Health and Human Services (USDHHS): *Psychosocial issues for children and families in disasters* (DHHS Pub. # SMA 95-3022), Washington, D.C., 1995, USDHHS.

7

Family Assessment and Cultural Diversity: Concepts and Tools

Objectives

Upon completion of this chapter, the reader should be able to:

1. Construct a personal definition for the term *family.*
2. Identify variations in family structure in the United States.
3. Describe the cultural diversity among American families.
4. Discuss the meaning of the phrase *the family is the unit of service.*
5. Explain how the use of a theoretical framework for family study promotes family-focused nursing practice.
6. Discuss the structural and process parameters for family assessment and their relevance to community health nursing practice.
7. Discuss how cultural factors influence health and health behaviors.
8. Formulate guidelines for completing a cultural assessment.
9. Describe tools used to facilitate the family assessment process.

The ancient trinity of father, mother, and child has survived more vicissitudes than any other relationship. It is the bedrock underlying all other family structures. Although more elaborate family patterns can be broken from without or may even collapse of their own weight, the rock remains. In the Götterdammerung which otherwise science and overfoolish statesmanship are preparing for us, the last man will spend his last hours searching for his wife and child.

LINTON *(1959, P. 52)*

Despite the fact that major social, demographic, and economic changes have altered traditional family structures and lifestyles in the past three decades, families remain one of the central institutions in the United States (Fine, 1992). Even though traditional family forms have changed as a result of such events as divorce, single parenthood, and a growing number of mothers in the work force, the family is still the basic social unit in society. "Families are America's most precious resource and most important institution. The strength of our families is the key determinate of the health and well-being of our nation, of our communities, and of our lives as individuals" (White House Conference on Families, 1978, p. 286).

As we approach the twenty-first century, child advocates are reconfirming the importance of the family in providing a healthy start for children. However, they are recognizing that rapid societal changes are making it more difficult for many families to provide a nurturing environment. All Americans are being urged to help eliminate societal conditions that increase a family's vulnerability to stress and crises.

"On June 1, 1996, over 250,000 people of every race, faith, age, and state gathered at the Lincoln Memorial to Stand For Children in the largest and most uplifting demonstration of commitment to children in American history" (Children's Defense Fund, 1997, p. xvii). This national mobilization effort was a day for spiritual, family, and community renewal. It was a call for action to help children by strengthening families and communities. Nurses play a vital role in promoting family and community wellness.

THE AMERICAN FAMILY: CULTURALLY AND STRUCTURALLY DIVERSE

Diversity and *change* are the terms that best describe today's American family. Cultural backgrounds, socioeconomic levels, and family structures differ nationwide. The two-parent nuclear family unit—mother, father, and child(ren)—established through the legal sanction of marriage is less

Select Family Lifestyles in the United States

TRADITIONAL FAMILY STRUCTURES

- *Nuclear family*—legally married couple with children in a common household with one or both partners gainfully employed.
- *Reconstituted nuclear family*—blended or stepfamily household with children with one or both partners gainfully employed.
- *Dyadic nuclear family*—childless, legally married couple with one or both partners gainfully employed. Family may never have had children or children may be "launched."
- *Single-parent family*—one-parent family as a consequence of divorce, abandonment, or separation. Parent may or may not be working.
- *Single adult*—living alone, usually with a career, who may or may not desire to marry.
- *Three-generation family*—extended family with three or more generations living in a common household.
- *Kin network*—nuclear households or unmarried members living in close geographical proximity and operating within a reciprocal system of exchange of goods and services.

NONTRADITIONAL FAMILY STRUCTURES

- *Binuclear family*—coparenting and joint custody family system where the child is part of two nuclear households.
- *Unmarried single family*—one-parent family where marriage is not desired or possible.
- *Unmarried couple family with children*—usually a commonlaw marriage.
- *Voluntary childless nuclear family*—a legally married couple who have chosen not to have children.
- *Heterosexual cohabiting family*—unmarried couple living together.
- *Commune family*—household of more than one monogamous couple with children, sharing common facilities and resources; socialization of children is a group activity.
- *Lesbian/gay family*—a male or female couple living together with or without children.

Modified from Sussman MB, chairperson: *Changing families in a changing society: 1970 White House Conference on Children*, Forum 14 report, Washington, D.C., 1971, U.S. Government Printing Office, pp. 228-229; Macklin ED: Nontraditional family forms. In Sussman MB, Steinmetz SK, ed: *Handbook of marriage and the family*, New York, 1987, Plenum Press, pp. 317-353.

prevalent, and alternative family forms are more common and more accepted, as shown in the above box. The box on the next page presents select trends that have altered traditional family patterns.

Household composition has changed significantly in the past several decades (Figure 7-1). Although the number of U.S. households has almost doubled in less than 40 years, the share of households headed by married couples has fallen from 74% to 55%. During this same period the proportion of children living with one parent more than doubled and household size has shrunk from an average of 3.3 persons to 2.6 persons (see the box on p. 161) (Francese, 1996).

In 1995 there were almost 99 million households in the United States. Of these, 70% were family households, which was a 10% drop from 1980. It is projected that by the year 2010 there will be 115 million households. It is also anticipated that the overall composition of households will shift (Figure 7-2, p. 162), reflecting a decreasing proportion of family households with children and increasing proportions of family households having no children and people living alone. Aging cohorts of empty-nest, post–World War II baby boomers will influence this shift (Day, 1996).

The wide variety of ethnic and racial groups in the United States enriches the diversity of family life (Figure 7-3, p. 163). It is projected that the U.S. population will become more diverse by race and Hispanic origin. By the middle of the twenty-first century it is anticipated that the black population will almost double, the Asian and Pacific Islander population will increase to more than five times its current size, and the Hispanic-origin population will triple its current size. After 1995 it is predicted that the Hispanic-origin population will add more people to the nation than any other cultural group (U.S. Bureau of the Census, 1993, p. 5).

Future fertility and immigration will significantly influence the country's population characteristics in the next 60 years. It is projected that births will slowly decline until the year 2000, but after the year 2015 there will be more births every year than ever before in American history (Day, 1993). Since 1980 approximately 27% to 29% of the nation's population growth has been the result of net international migration, and it is anticipated that immigration will be higher in the future (U.S. Bureau of the Census, 1993, pp. 3, 5). Between 1980 and 1990 the foreign-born in the United States increased by 40.4%, from 14.1 million to 19.8 million persons. The number of foreign-born persons in the United States in 1990 was the largest number of foreign-born individuals in the history of the United States. Between 1980 and 1990 European immigration decreased and Latin American and Asian immigration increased significantly (Table 7-1, p. 163).

With increasing diversity and change, new opportunities and challenges have emerged for families and society. For example, men are increasingly enjoying the opportunities associated with parenthood (Figure 7-4, p. 164) and women are valuing the career options available to them in the job market. However, the institutions that make up American society have been slow to adapt to these changes (Levitan, Conway, 1990; Tiedje, Darling-Fisher, 1996). As women

Selected Trends That Have Altered Traditional Family Patterns in the United States

INCREASE IN DIVORCE*

- Number of currently divorced persons more than quadrupled between 1970 and 1995.
- Almost 9% of all adults ages 18 and over were divorced in 1995.
- Although the rate of divorce is beginning to stabilize, there were over 17 million divorced persons in the United States in 1995.
- Rise in percentage divorced differed by race between 1970 and 1995: the proportion of white adults divorced rose from approximately 3% to 8%; black adults divorced rose from about 4% to 11%; Hispanic adults divorced rose from about 4% to 8%.

LATER MARRIAGES AND INCREASE IN NEVER-MARRIED

- The median age at first marriage has risen more than 3 years for men and women between 1975 and 1994.
- Married-couple households dropped from 75% of all households in 1960 to 54% in 1995.
- Number of never-married persons more than doubled between 1970 and 1994, from 21 to 44 million.

RISE IN MOTHER-CHILD FAMILIES

- The proportion of children living with one parent more than doubled between 1970 and 1994.
- Almost 90% of children in a one-parent home live with the mother.
- Demographers estimate that half of all children will live in mother-child families at some time in their lives.
- Black children (57%) are more likely to be living with one parent than white children (21%) and children of Hispanic origin (32%).

GROWING NUMBER OF MOTHERS IN THE LABOR FORCE

- Today, both parents are working in one out of two married-couple families, which is significantly different from 1940, when only one out of seven married women worked out of the home.
- Sixty-two percent of women with preschool-age children were in the labor force in 1995.
- The percentage of mothers with children aged 6 to 17 working in the civilian labor force rose from 52% in 1975 to 76% in 1995.

LONGER LIFE EXPECTANCY AND INCREASE IN NUMBER OF ELDERLY

- An American child born in 1994 can be expected to live, on the average, over 75 years, which is a significant improvement over the 47-year life expectancy of persons born in 1900.
- The elderly population increased 11-fold from 1990 to 1994, compared with only a 3-fold increase for those under age 65.
- Racial and ethnic diversity within the elderly population will continue to increase in the twenty-first century.

Data from Cherlin A, Furstenberg F: The American family in the year 2000. In Cornish E, ed: *The 1990s and beyond*, Bethesda, Md., 1990, World Future Society; Maternal and Child Health Bureau: *Child health USA '95*, Washington, D.C., 1996, U.S. Government Printing Office; U.S. Bureau of the Census: *How we're changing: demographic state of the nation: 1996*, Washington, D.C., 1996, U.S. Government Printing Office; U.S. Bureau of the Census: *65+ in the United States*, Washington, D.C., 1996, U.S. Government Printing Office; U.S. Bureau of the Census: *Statistical abstract of the United States: 1996*, ed 116, Washington, D.C., 1996, U.S. Government Printing Office.
*The number divorced is a count of currently divorced and not yet married.

move into the workforce, families often need to deal with complicated child care and elder care arrangements and have to coordinate family and work roles and intergenerational relationships.

In the coming years, society must address child care and elder care concerns as well as issues such as increasing poverty, the dramatic rise in premarital childbearing, out-of-control health care costs, and maintaining the viability of social support organizations as volunteer workers become less available (Hooyman, 1992; Levitan, Conway, 1990; Spanier, 1989). Social policy must take into consideration the needs of varying family forms and lifestyles, because the American family is changing.

DEFINING THE FAMILY

What actually constitutes a family is no longer easy to define. Various family organizational structures have made the concept of the family an elusive one, open to numerous definitions depending on one's value system. The traditional definition of this term—a group of two or more persons related by blood, marriage, or adoption who reside together—is no longer adequate for understanding and studying the needs of the American family. A much broader definition is needed to portray the significant commitments individuals can make to each other, even though they choose an alternative family form (e.g., a cohabiting or gay/lesbian relationship) outside of the bonds of marriage. A family in its broadest sense is *a group of two or more persons related by blood, marriage, adoption, or emotional commitment who have a permanent relationship and who work together to meet life goals and needs*.

Practitioners in the helping professions must remain flexible in their interpretation of the word *family* so that social policies that enhance the growth of all types of families are developed. Families who are not legally bound together by marriage have the same needs as families who are.

Number of Households and Size of Households in the United States: 1960 to 2010

Households In—		Persons per Household In—	
1960	53 million	1960	3.30
1970	63 million	1970	3.14
1980	81 million	1980	2.76
1990	93 million	1990	2.63
1995	99 million	1995	2.62
2010	115 million (projected)	2010	2.53 (projected)

From Day JC: *Projections of the number of households and families in the United States: 1995 to 2010*, U.S. Bureau of the Census, current population reports, series P 25-1129, Washington, D.C., 1996, U.S. Government Printing Office, p. 8; U.S. Bureau of the Census: *Statistical abstract of the United States: 1996*, ed 116, Washington, D.C., 1996, U.S. Government Printing Office, p. 59.

They need financial resources, social and educational opportunities, and health services to meet their basic needs. Denying them options to strengthen their family life does not strengthen our nation and is not sensitive to their needs.

Practitioners in the helping professions must also carefully identify their attitudes and values about family life. Although community health nurses may not choose a particular mode of living for themselves, their personal preferences should not influence their clinical judgments about the adequacy of family functioning. Data collected from the family should be the key factor the community health nurse uses to determine family strengths and needs. A single-parent mother, for instance, may be meeting the needs of her child much more appropriately than a married couple who are having endless conflicts in their marriage. Assumptions about how well a family is providing for its members should not be made solely on the basis of the family's organizational structure.

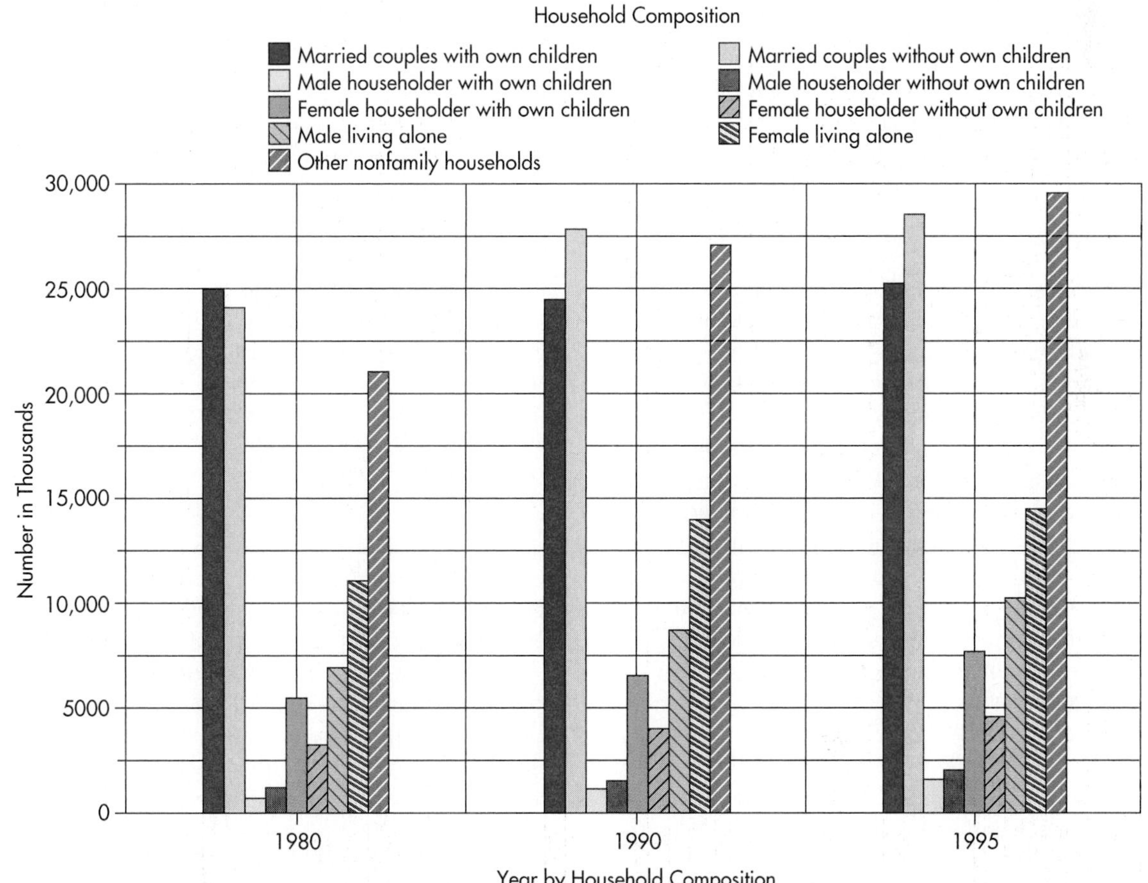

Figure 7-1 Household composition in the United States: 1980-1995. *(Modified from U.S. Bureau of the Census:* Statistical abstract of the United States: 1996, *ed 116, Washington, D.C., 1996, U.S. Government Printing Office, p. 59.)*

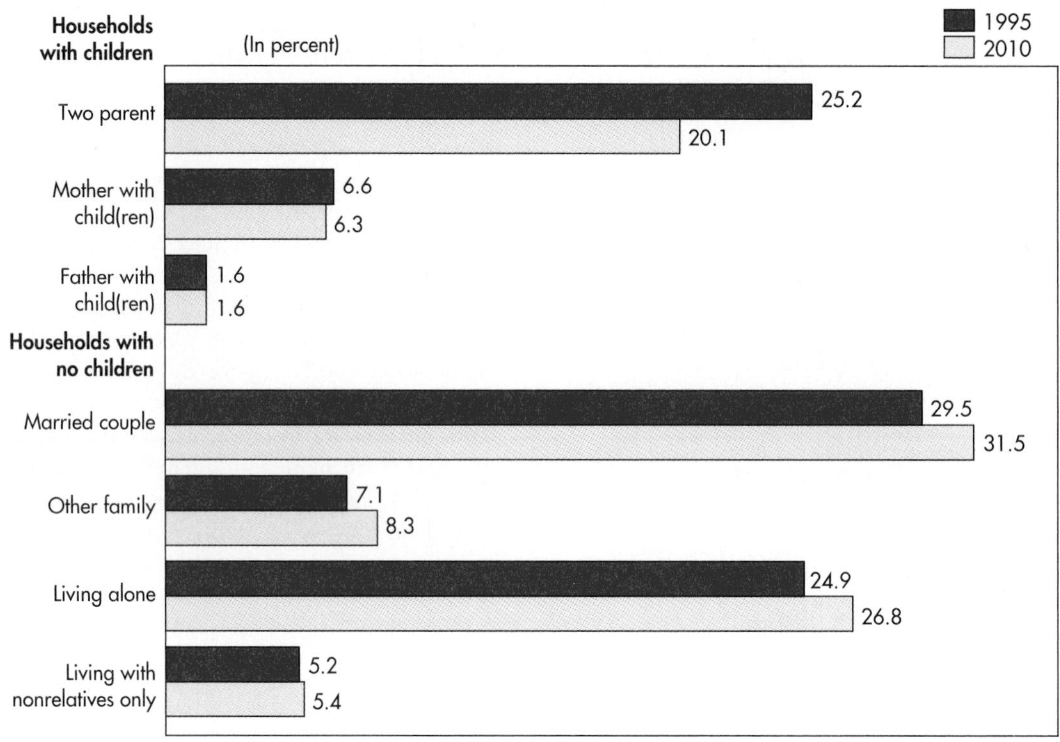

Figure 7-2 Projections of changing household composition: 1995 and 2010. *(From Day JC:* Projections of the number of households and families in the United States: 1995 to 2010, *U.S. Bureau of the Census, current populations reports, series P 25-1129, Washington, D.C., 1996, U.S. Government Printing Office, p. 11.)*

THE FAMILY AS A UNIT OF SERVICE

Despite the changing nature of the American family, community health nurses still subscribe to the philosophy that the family is the basic unit of service in community health nursing practice. They believe that the family, as the major socializing unit of society, determines how its individual members relate and act in our culture. They recognize that the family greatly influences the beliefs, values, attitudes, and health behaviors of its members and realize that the health of individual family members affects the health of the entire family unit. They see that the family provides support and encouragement at times of stress and joy. They value the role the family has in facilitating the physical and psychosocial growth of its members.

Ronald Peterson (1978) put into very simple but impressive terms the significance of the family in promoting the growth of its individual members. He presented the following concept of the family at a national conference on the chronic mentally ill client:

> A family is a place where I think a lot of things go on. You really don't feel you're being "raised," that people are doing things to you, to raise you. Your life seems "real" and most of the time, almost everything that happens to you, you talk about it. Sometimes you have good news, sometimes you have bad news. But most of the time, it's just talking about what is going on.
>
> It's a place you go from, to the doctor or to the hospital or the dentist, or school, or to the movies or to a job. But it's a place where you belong, where you somehow learn a lot. You change I'm sure, but usually without knowing it. And you certainly are not looked at as a patient or one who is being rehabilitated. You don't get discharged or terminated, and even when you grow up and get a job of your own and move away, it's a place you keep in touch with and visit. There's always an interest, and that's what makes the difference.

Families do make a difference. They provide supportive and nurturing services in a way no other social institution does. Families influence health beliefs and attitudes even when they are not physically present. They often extend themselves much further in providing assistance than would friends or health care professionals. It is for these reasons that community health nurses believe in the family-centered approach to nursing care.

Historical Perspectives

Historically the family-centered approach to community health nursing practice grew out of the recognition that the physical care of an individual client could not be divorced from all other aspects of a client's functioning. Innovative community health nursing leaders of the early 1900s recognized that a preventive, holistic approach to the delivery of

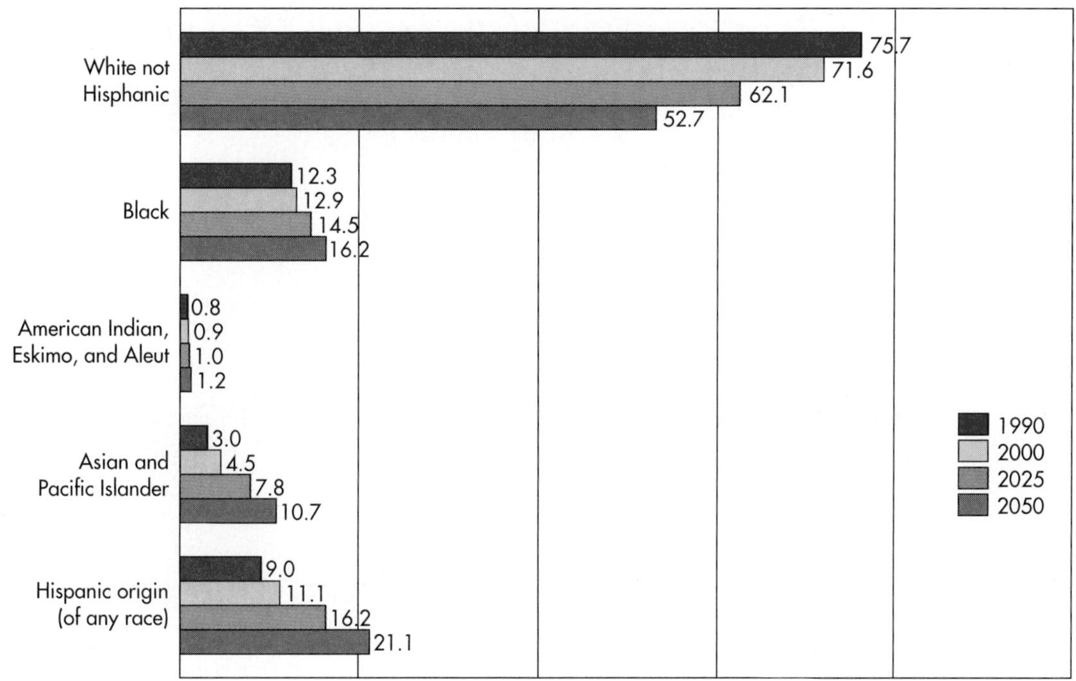

Figure 7-3 Race and Hispanic origin populations in the United States, percent of the total population: 1990, 2000, 2025, 2050. *(From U.S. Bureau of the Census:* Population profile of the United States: 1993, *current population reports, series P23-185, Washington, D.C., 1993, U.S. Government Printing Office, p. 5.)*

table 7-1 National Origins of the Foreign-Born Population in the United States: 1980 and 1990

Of the 14.1 million foreign-born in the United States in 1980 and the 19.8 million foreign-born in 1990—

Foreign-Born	1980	1990
European	36.6%	22.0%
Asian	18.0%	25.2%
Mexican	15.6%	21.7%
Caribbean	8.9%	9.8%
Central American	2.5%	5.7%
South American	4.0%	5.2%
African	1.4%	1.8%
Other countries	13.0%	8.6%

From U.S. Bureau of the Census: *Population profile of the United States: 1993*, current population reports, series P23-185, Washington, D.C., 1993, U.S. Government Printing Office, p. 40.

nursing services was essential if the health of an individual, the family, and the community was to be maintained and enhanced. They saw the need to work with the family and the community in order to achieve their goals with individual clients.

The concept of family-centered care has evolved over time. Initially emphasis was on analyzing how the family could assist its members to achieve health and well-being. Gradually the enhancement of the health and well-being of the entire *family unit* became the primary objective for community health nursing visits, with a focus on examining family dynamics and identifying the health status of all family members.

Clinical practice and research has sufficiently demonstrated over time the value of the family-centered approach to community health nursing practice. "The family constitutes perhaps the most important social context within which illness occurs and is resolved. It consequently serves as a primary unit in health and medical care" (Litman, 1974, p. 495). The family influences the development of health behavior, the use of health services, and health outcomes for individuals (Danielson, Hamel-Bissell, Winstead-Fry, 1993; Friedman, 1992; Loveland-Cherry, 1996).

Although the family-centered approach to nursing care is valued, it is not fully realized in the clinical setting. Lack of knowledge regarding family processes, federal legislation that financially supports individual services, insufficient criteria for judging family health, and heavy caseload demands impede nurses' efforts to implement family care. However, a renewed focus on the family is emerging as institutional health care is significantly decreasing and home care is rapidly growing.

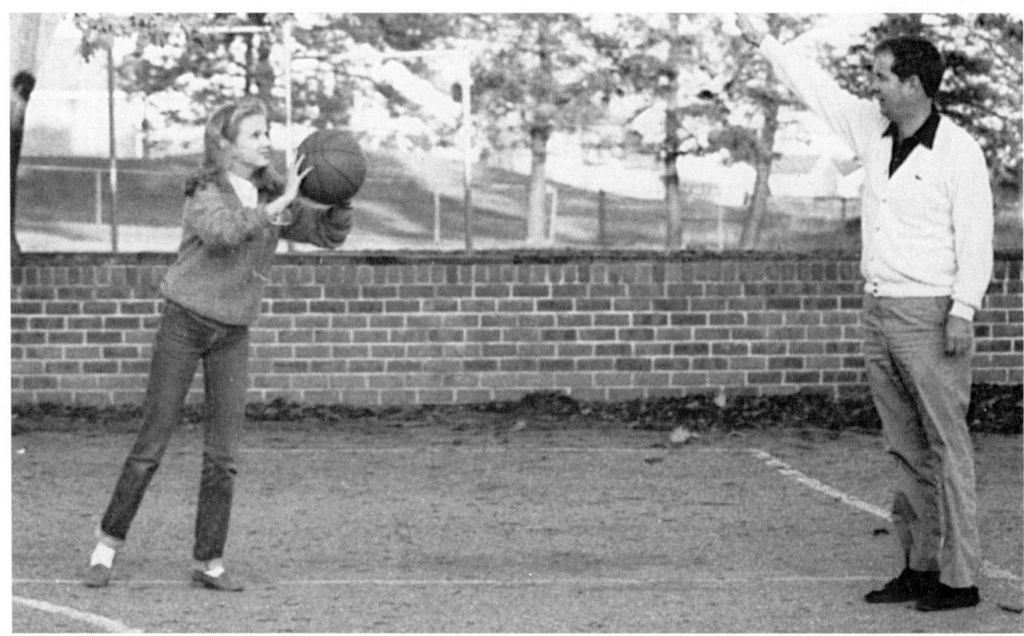

Figure 7-4 Increasingly, fathers are becoming more involved in parenting and are significantly influencing a child's socialization. *(Courtesy Henry Parks, photographer)*

Community health nursing leaders of the past were truly creative and innovative. They were far ahead of their time when they subscribed to the belief that family care was a key principle in community health nursing practice. It was not until the 1950s that most professional disciplines actually began to focus attention on working with families rather than with individual clients. It was only at this time that social scientists initiated systematic theory building in relation to family processes.

Knowledge gained about family functioning since the 1950s has made it easier for nurses to analyze family strengths and needs and to intervene appropriately with families. Theoretical frameworks that have emerged from the study of the family assist nurses in organizing the family assessment process and in identifying the range of variables essential for understanding family relationships. To successfully implement family-centered care, the community health nurse must internalize the belief that working with the family as a unit is important.

THEORETICAL FRAMEWORKS FOR FAMILY NURSING

Use of a theoretical framework for guiding the family assessment process is essential in the clinical setting. A theory—"a set of relatively specific and concrete concepts and propositions that describe, explain, or predict something of interest" (Whall, Fawcett, 1991, p. 4)—helps the practitioner to assess family structure and process in an organized and logical fashion. Theories provide boundaries to consider when collecting data about client situations and facilitate the synthesis of data so family strengths, needs, and interventions can be identified. When a theoretical framework is lacking, it is difficult to group data and to identify relationships between all of the variables that influence family health.

The family can be analyzed from multiple perspectives. Duvall and Miller (1985), who partially listed the kinds of family studies currently being conducted, identified 16 disciplines (e.g., anthropology, demography, history, law, and public health) involved in family study. Burr and Leigh (1983) found at least 19 disciplines, including nursing, that shared an interest in developing a knowledge base related to the family. The field of family study has had an interdisciplinary focus since its origin. An interdisciplinary focus adds depth to family analysis because concepts about several facets of family life are synthesized.

"The development of *explicit* family nursing theory is just beginning" (Artinian, 1991, p. 53). The original thrust of the major nursing theorists was centered on the individual. Recent expansion of some of the major conceptual models of nursing (e.g., King, Neuman, Rogers, and Roy) to include a focus on the family is evident and is providing an explicit impetus for formal family nursing theory development (Loveland-Cherry, 1996; Whall, Fawcett, 1991). The Family Nursing Continuing Education Project, a 3-year project begun in 1987, was designed to foster a nationwide network of family nurses who hoped to achieve a common knowledge and research base for their practice (Krentz, 1989).

"Theoretical frameworks from other disciplines have guided the evolution of family nursing science" (Hanson, Boyd, 1996, p. 43). "Family theories developed in disciplines other than nursing provide direction for identifying characteristics of optimal families" (Loveland-Cherry, 1996, p. 24). Illustrative of this is the developmental framework that emerged from theorists in the social sciences. The developmental framework delineates life-cycle stages and specific family tasks that need to be accomplished during each stage. Families that are able to achieve their stage-specific developmental tasks while maintaining the integrity of the family unit and promoting the growth of individual family members have been defined as healthy, or optimal, families (Loveland-Cherry).

Select theoretical frameworks from the social sciences that are particularly relevant to family nursing are briefly summarized below. These frameworks were first outlined by Hill and Hansen (1960) in their classic writing during the 1960s. Practitioners generally find that an eclectic approach, or one that integrates concepts from several frameworks, best meets their needs when completing a family assessment. When nurses conduct a family assessment, emphasis is on identifying the health promotion needs of the family.

Structural-Functional Approach

The structural-functional framework was developed by social scientists from sociology and social anthropology. It views the family as a social system that interacts with other social systems within society. It focuses on the analysis of family interplay between collateral systems such as school, work, or health care worlds and the transactions between the family and its subsystems (husband-wife dyad, sibling cliques, and personality systems of individual family members). With this approach emphasis is on examining the functions society performs for the family, as well as the functions the family performs for society and its individual family members. In addition, this framework looks at how the structure (organizational parameters) of systems affects family functioning (Hill, Hansen, 1960). The family in the structural-functional approach is seen as open to outside influences and transactions.

The structural-functional approach to family study helps the practitioner to systematically assess family structure and function. A family's structure (organization) influences what is viewed as important to the family and facilitates or inhibits the family's ability to carry out its functions. The family carries out several functions to promote family growth, to provide a nurturing environment for individual family members, and to meet the needs of society.

Friedman (1992) has identified five family functions that are especially important for nurses to consider when assessing and intervening with families. These are (1) the *affective* function, which addresses the psychological needs of family members, including the need for companionship and love; (2) the *socialization and social placement* function, which helps children to prepare for and assume adult social roles; (3) the *reproductive* function, which ensures the continuity of the family across generations and society survival; (4) the *economic* function, which involves securing adequate resources for survival and decision-making processes focused on the appropriate allocation of these resources; and (5) the *health care* function, which entails obtaining physical necessities such as food, shelter, and clothing and health care for all family members (Friedman, pp. 75-77).

The structural-functional approach provides a meaningful framework for guiding family assessment in the clinical setting. The broad scope of this framework allows for the analysis of the multiple environmental forces that influence family functioning in addition to family interactions and transactions (Aldous, 1978, p. 14). The changing nature of the American family makes it increasingly critical for the practitioner to examine the interplay between the family and its external environment. Many functions once assumed primarily by the family system, such as child-rearing responsibilities, are now being shared by collateral systems in the community.

Interactional Approach

Frequently labeled as the *symbolic* interactional frame of reference, this approach comes from sociology and social psychology. The interactionalist views the family as a unity of interacting personalities within which individual family members occupy a position or positions, such as husband-father, wife-mother, and daughter-sister. A cluster of roles—such as provider, homemaker, companion, and sex partner—are assigned to each of these positions, and a set of social norms or behavioral role expectations is perceived for each of these roles by the individual fulfilling them. Perceptions about role expectations emerge from an individual's self-concept and from an individual's reference group. As each individual carries out the various roles, role expectations are retained, modified, or discarded based upon the reactions of others within the family environment (Aldous, 1978, pp. 10, 14).

Interactionalists view the family as being relatively closed to outside systems. Family members are seen as actors and reactors who interact with their environment through symbolic communication. As a reactor, an individual does not simply respond to stimuli from the external environment. Symbolic communication evolving from the self and the environment helps individuals interpret and select the environment to which they respond. Based on this assumption, interactionalists stress that investigators or clinicians must see the world from the point of view of the individual (Stryker, 1964, pp. 134-135).

The interactional framework emphasizes analysis of the internal aspects of family functioning but neglects the family's relationships with other social systems. This framework identifies how relationships with others affect an individual's functioning. In addition to role analysis, interactionalists examine communication, decision-making and problem-solving processes, conflict, reactions to stress, and other family situations such as divorce and domestic violence that are influenced by family interactions and interactive processes (Aldous, 1978; Hill, Hansen, 1960). This approach helps the practitioner to identify if family interactions promote or inhibit effective family functioning.

Developmental Approach

Concepts from various disciplines and approaches (rural sociology, child psychology, human development, sociology, and structural-functional and interactional approaches) were synthesized to create the developmental approach to family study. This approach looks at family development throughout its generational life cycle. It examines developmental tasks and role expectations for children, parents, and the family as a unit and traces these change during a series of specific stages in the family life cycle (Hill, Hansen, 1960).

Duvall has focused her scholarly efforts on defining normal family development. She identified eight stages in the two-parent, nuclear family life cycle that highlight critical periods of family growth, development, and change (Duvall, Miller, 1985). These stages address family events related to the comings and goings of family members: marriage, birth and rearing of children, launching children from the household, and retirement and death (Carter, McGoldrick, 1988). The developmental framework helps practitioners to assess what a given family is going through at any particular time and provides a basis for forecasting role transition issues throughout a family's life span (Duvall, Miller, 1985). This, in turn, aids the professional in predicting potential educational and resource needs of families. For example, new childbearing families often desire information about child care and growth and development patterns of children and may need help in obtaining adequate supplies for infant care. Additionally, they frequently need assistance in achieving a balance between family and personal needs. Reconciling conflicting developmental tasks and needs of various family members is a major task for childbearing families (Carter, McGoldrick, 1988; Duvall, Miller, 1985).

In recent years family theorists have focused attention on examining how variables such as changing family structures, social and economic factors, and cultural and ethnic differences influence the family life cycle. Family life-cycle patterns have changed dramatically as a result of the lower birth rates, longer life expectancy, the changing role of women, postponment of marriage, and the increasing divorce and remarriage rate (Carter, McGoldrick, 1988). To address these changes, Carter and McGoldrick have added an additional stage to the family life cycle. They begin the new family life cycle at the stage of young adulthood (Table 7-2). This is in contrast to the traditional sociological depiction of the family life cycle, which commences at courtship or marriage. During the young adulthood, or "between families," stage young men and women formulate personal life goals and differentiate themselves from their family of origin. In the past this phase was never considered necessary for women, because "their identities were determined primarily by their family functions as mother and wife" (Carter, McGoldrick, p. 11).

When using the developmental framework for guiding family assessment, practitioners should realize that there are major variations in the family life cycle. Socioeconomic and cultural factors influence the timing (Table 7-3) of the life cycle phases and the importance given to different life cycle transitions (Fulmer, 1988; McGoldrick, 1988). For example, funerals are a significant occurrence for African-American and Irish families, who go to considerable expense to bury their loved ones. In contrast, Italian and Polish families place the greatest emphasis on weddings and often celebrate this occurrence over a considerable period of time (McGoldrick). The professional who understands that there are significant variations in the family life-cycle can more effectively evaluate family functioning during critical transition periods.

Systems Approach

First introduced by biologist Ludwig von Bertalanffy (1968), systems theory is currently used by many disciplines. General systems theory is a science of wholeness; an underlying assumption of system theory is the belief that the whole is greater than the sum of its parts. From a family perspective, this implies that the family unit has a unique character that is different from that of its individual parts (family members) (Boss, 1988). However, change in one part of the family system affects the system as a whole, as well as all individual family members. For example, when a family member becomes ill and is unable to carry out his or her role responsibilities, the whole family unit needs to change to successfully cope with the demands of the stress encountered.

A system consists of two or more connected components or subsystems that form an organized whole and that interact with each other to achieve desired goals. A family is a social system of interdependent members (components) possessing two fundamental system features: *structure*, or organization, and *function*, or interaction. Family members engage in continual interaction according to roles and norms that evolve over time and make it possible for the family to survive and achieve desired goals (Janosik, Green, 1992).

An input-process-output feedback model (Figure 7-5) is frequently used to depict the structural relationships of a system. In simplistic terms, this model illustrates that all systems have *inputs*, or resources that, when *processed*, help the system to achieve its goals, or *outputs*. The processing of inputs (resources) received from the environment requires a series of dynamic, interrelated transactions. These transactions link together the environment, the system inputs, and the system outputs. Transactions or processes used by

table 7-2 The Stages of the Family Life Cycle

Family Life Cycle Stage	Emotional Process of Transition: Key Principles	Second-Order Changes in Family Status Required to Proceed Developmentally
1. Leaving home: single young adults	Accepting emotional and financial responsibility for self	Differentiation of self in relation to family of origin Development of intimate peer relationships Establishment of self re work and financial independence
2. The joining of families through marriage: the new couple	Commitment to new system	Formation of marital system Realignment of relationships with extended families and friends to include spouse
3. Families with young children	Accepting new members into the system	Adjusting marital system to make space for child(ren) Joining in childrearing, financial, and household tasks Realignment of relationships with extended family to include parenting and grandparenting roles
4. Families with adolescents	Increasing flexibility of family boundaries to include children's independence and grandparents' frailties	Shifting of parent-child relationships to permit adolescent to move in and out of system Refocus on midlife marital and career issues Beginning shift toward joint caring for older generation
5. Launching children and moving on	Accepting a multitude of exits from and entries into the family system	Renegotiation of marital system as a dyad Development of adult-to-adult relationships between grown children and their parents Realignment of relationships to include in-laws and grandchildren Dealing with disabilities and death of parents (grandparents)
6. Families in later life	Accepting the shifting of generational roles	Maintaining own and/or couple functioning and interests in face of physiological decline; exploration of new familial and social role options Support for a more central role of middle generation Making room in the system for the wisdom and experience of the elderly, supporting the older generation without overfunctioning for them Dealing with loss of spouse, siblings, and other peers and preparation for own death. Life review and integration

Modified from Carter B, McGoldrick M, eds: *The changing family life cycle: a framework for family therapy*, ed 2, New York, 1988, Gardner Press, p. 15.

families to maintain healthy family functioning are discussed in a later section of this chapter.

The feedback mechanism is a major attribute of a system. This mechanism assists the family system in identifying its strengths and needs and in evaluating how well it is accomplishing its goals. Feedback provides data essential for effective adaptation to internal and external system changes. It provides information that helps the system to select corrective actions when problems exist. A system needs a mechanism that facilitates the sharing of both positive and negative feedback. A family system that discourages negative input often remains static or develops ineffective family patterns.

No system can function in a vacuum. The environment in which a system exists greatly influences how the system is able to function. The environment imposes constraints (e.g., rules that require school attendance or prohibit drinking and driving) on the family system and provides resources for effective family functioning. However, every system has filtering mechanisms, or *boundaries*, that regulate the flow of energy to and from the environment and be-

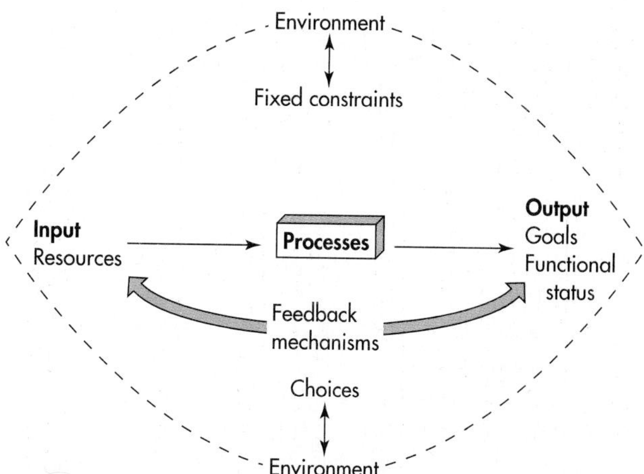

Figure 7-5 Structural arrangements of a system. *(Modified from Clemen [Parks] SJ: Introduction to health care facility: food services administration, University Park, Pa., 1974, Pennsylvania State University Press, p. 24.)*

table 7-3 Comparison of Family Life Cycle Stages

Age	Professional Families	Low-Income Families
12-17	Prevent pregnancy Graduate from high school Parents continue support while permitting child to achieve greater independence	First pregnancy Attempt to graduate from high school Parent attempts strict control before pregnancy. After pregnancy, relaxation of controls and continued support of new mother and infant
18-21	Prevent pregnancy Leave parental household for college Adapt to parent-child separation	Second pregnancy No further education Young mother acquires adult status in parental household
22-25	Prevent pregnancy Develop professional identity in graduate school Maintain separation from parental household. Begin living in serious relationship	Third pregnancy Marriage—leave parental household to establish stepfamily Maintain connection with kinship network
26-30	Prevent pregnancy Marriage—develop nuclear couple as separate from parents Intense work involvement as career begins	Separate from husband Mother becomes head of own household within kinship network
31-35	First pregnancy Renew contact with parents as grandparents Differentiate career and child-rearing roles between husband and wife	First grandchild Mother becomes grandmother and cares for daughter and infant

Modified from Fulmer R: Lower-income and professional families: a comparison of structure and life cycle process. In Carter B, McGoldrick M, eds: *The changing family life cycle: a framework for family therapy*, ed 2, New York, 1988, Gardner Press, p. 551.

tween family subsystems. Boundaries in a system are not physical barriers. Rather, they are abstract entities such as norms, values, attitudes, and rules that inhibit or facilitate human transactional processes between systems.

Energy transport is crucial to the survival of any system. An effectively functioning family system uses energy to obtain resources from the outside, to process resources to achieve its goals, and to release outputs into the environment. "The most important factor governing the amount of energy needed is the rate of utilization of energy within the system itself. Systems with high levels of activity utilize large quantities of energy, and therefore must receive greater amounts of input from the environment in order to meet their energy demands" (Friedman, 1992, p. 118). Family systems that are ineffectively dealing with stress and crisis frequently lack the energy to obtain input from the environment.

A system that exchanges energy and resources with other systems is an open system. "Depending on the nature of family boundaries, a family system may be fully open, entirely closed, or somewhere in between" (Janosik, Green, 1992, p. 13). Families generally interact with the environment to obtain resources (e.g., information, financial, and health care) necessary for family growth and survival and to reduce stress within the family system. "The key to successful family adaptation is selective permeability of family boundaries" (Friedman, 1992, p. 119). This implies that a family can be too open or too closed. Boundary maintenance issues are addressed further in a later section of this chapter.

Systems theory provides a framework for family assessment that is consistent with the holistic nature of humankind and professional practice. It offers a logical way to integrate all of the factors that influence family functioning and link the family together into a meaningful whole. It provides a humanistic philosophy of professional care that negates individual blame and addresses family strengths as well as needs. "Approaching the family as a system in which parents, children, extended family members, and the community influence each other in reciprocal ways means that whatever occurs is a shared responsibility" (Janosik, Green, 1992, p. 15).

USE OF THEORETICAL FRAMEWORKS

Table 7-4 summarizes select characteristics of the four family theories just discussed. Since only an introductory description was presented, the reader will find it useful to explore the literature in depth when selecting a conceptual framework for guiding practice. Of particular interests is literature that helps readers to examine the application of concepts in nursing practice (Bomar, 1996; Friedman, 1992; Hanson, Boyd, 1996; Whall, 1991; Wright, Leahey, 1994).

It is important to remember that no one theoretical framework focuses attention on all aspects of family functioning. An example is a situation in which a nurse visits a young married couple in their twenties who have just had their first child. Using a developmental framework, the nurse would direct his or her evaluation of family health on

table 7-4 SELECT CHARACTERISTICS OF FOUR FAMILY THEORIES

THEORY	FOCUS OF ANALYSIS	ADVANTAGES	DISADVANTAGES
Structural-functional	Family interplay between collateral systems Transactions between the family and its subsystems	Allows for analysis of the multiple forces that influence family functioning. Handles well family interactions and transactions	Family and its individual family members are considered to be reactive, passive elements of systems. Deals poorly with social change processes and dynamics
Interactional	Internal aspects of family functioning, including role analysis, communication, decision-making, problem-solving and conflict resolution processes, reactions to stress, and other family dynamics (e.g., divorce and domestic violence) influenced by family interactions	Views family members as having control over their environment (e.g., family members interpret and select the environment to which they respond). Focuses on seeing the world from the client's perspective	Neglects family relationships with other systems
Developmental	Accomplishment of individual and family developmental tasks throughout the generational life cycle. Change in the family system over time	Highlights critical periods of family growth and development. Keeps the traditionally defined family in focus throughout its life span. Recognizes and helps to predict what a given family is experiencing at any particular time	Data that examine socioeconomic, cultural, and ethnic variations in the family life cycle are limited
Systems	Analysis of the family as a whole. Interdependence of the various parts of the family system and change. Interactions of the family system and its external environment	Unites scientific thinking across disciplines. Provides a holistic perspective for analyzing family functioning that negates blame. Allows for analysis of family relationships with other systems and environmental influences on health. Examines family change and adaptation processes	Complex theory can make it difficult for an inexperienced practitioner to fit all family dynamics into the specific categories defined within the system

how well the family and individual members were accomplishing stage-specific development tasks. On the other hand, systems-oriented nurses would focus their analysis on how the change in the family system (the addition of a new family member) has affected system functioning as a whole (e.g., its resources and goals, family processes, subsystems—especially the spouse relationships—and the family's interactions with its external environment).

Community health nurses generally use a combination of several theoretical frameworks to guide the family assessment process. This is appropriate because client situations vary and because no one framework explains all family phenomena. In the clinical setting it is essential for the nurse to examine the multiple aspects of family functioning, including the family's relationships with other social systems and its interactions with the environment; an effective management plan can be developed only after all of these areas have been assessed.

PARAMETERS TO CONSIDER DURING THE FAMILY ASSESSMENT PROCESS

During the family assessment process, parameters related to both family structure and process should be considered regardless of the theoretical framework used to guide family assessment. These parameters assist the nurse in obtaining a holistic view of the family, helping the nurse to identify how the family is organized and how it interacts to carry out family functions.

Structural Parameters for Family Assessment

Structural components of a family are those variables that provide organization for the family system. They assist the family in coordinating their activities so that family and individual needs are met. Briar (1964), in his classic article on family organization, identified eight major structural characteristics of families: (1) division of labor, (2) distribution of power and authority, (3) communication, (4) boundaries of the family's world, (5) relations with other groups and systems, (6) ways of obtaining and giving emotional support, (7) rituals and symbols, and (8) a set of personal roles. These, as well as cultural values and attitudes and religious beliefs, are described below. Briar's delineation of the structural components of a family continues to be consistent with recent notions about the structural parameters of family life.

Division of Labor

Families allocate leadership responsibilities for maintaining their household in a variety of ways. Some follow traditional norms, with the man assuming major responsibility for the provider role and the woman the homemaker role, regardless of the other role responsibilities each person has in the partnership. Some divide tasks according to their likes and dislikes or the level of competence each person has in relation to a particular task. Others share responsibilities equally, based on the demands each person has from other role positions.

Cultural background is an important variable to consider when the nurse examines family role performance. Ethnicity significantly influences the development of attitudes about the division of labor within the family unit. For example, within the traditional nuclear family, it is common for Navajo Indian (Hanley, 1991) and Italian (Bowen, 1991) women to be responsible for the domestic duties associated within the home and for the men from these ethnic groups to be responsible for any outside work needed to maintain the family and its home. However, *intracultural diversity* also exists, and individuals may not practice or possess all the characteristics of the ethnic group with which they identify (Fong, 1985).

Families who rigidly define either the provider or homemaker role tend to experience more stress when family members are unable to perform their expected tasks than do families who have a flexible division of labor (Beavers, 1977; Lewis, Beavers, Gossett, Phillips, 1976; Otto, 1963; Pratt, 1976). It is also extremely difficult for families with rigid patterns of functioning to mobilize new coping mechanisms when experiencing a crisis. Health care professionals, for instance, often observe confusion and disorganization when a spouse dies. This confusion is heightened if the man or woman has not been prepared to deal with the demands of daily living. Assuming responsibilities for tasks one is not accustomed to performing is difficult at any time, but especially when one is experiencing a crisis.

Identifying how the division of labor is handled by a family helps the community health nurse to understand the stresses family members are experiencing when changes have occurred. Role strain results when families do not take into consideration that role responsibilities change over time. Mothers, for example, are often confronted with excessive role demands after the birth of a child. This is especially true if husbands do not share the responsibility for housekeeping and child care tasks. Role strain also occurs when family members are unable to perform the activities related to a given role. This is particularly noticeable when role modifications are needed because of the prolonged absence of one family member. Absences that are a result of illness, divorce, separation, or vocational responsibilities frequently require drastic modifications in a family's division of labor and result in role strain.

All family members can experience role strain when the division of labor is inappropriately balanced. Children may be required to assume adult responsibilities excessive for their age and level of growth and development. This most often occurs during times of crisis or when parents have not assumed adult leadership responsibilities required to maintain their household. It is important for community health nurses to recognize that children experience role strain when they assume parental functions, and to avoid reinforcing role-reversal patterns. It is easy to praise a child who is functioning beyond his or her chronological age. This praise, however, may support the continuance of family patterns that are unhealthy and that adversely affect a child's emotional growth and development.

Distribution of Power and Authority

Power was conceptualized by Bredemeir and Stephenson (1965) as "the capacity to carry out, by whatever means, a desired course of action despite the resistance of others and without having to take into consideration their needs. When power is institutionalized through respect, fear, esteem, or position, it is referred to as authority" (p. 50).

Several variables affect who will have power in the family system. The position of power can be *culturally* prescribed, usually with the father being in a position of authority by virtue of his role as a male. This is frequently seen in Spanish-American and Asian cultures, where male dominance is the norm. Power can also be *situationally* prescribed when family members do not necessarily follow cultural norms but develop a power structure based on their circumstances and personal interactions. The continuum of family power based on cultural and situational variables ranges from complete dominance to complete absence of power, both of which can produce ineffective family patterns. Complete dominance by one family member poses a threat to the self-esteem of other family members and makes it difficult for individuals to resolve the independence-dependence conflicts that arise during adolescence and young adulthood. Complete absence of power in a family system tends to produce confusion, disorganization, and chaos. Vulnerable families frequently exhibit power structures on either end of the continuum. In healthy families power is frequently shared by adult members and children are involved in the decision-making process.

Understanding the relationship between issues of power and decision making is essential to effect permanent changes within a family system. If the power and authority structure of a family is ignored, nursing interventions are often inappropriate and place additional stress on family members who lack the power to make decisions about needed health actions. Family members who have power must be consulted if changes in health behavior are to occur. One community health nurse, for instance, realized after several home visits to a Spanish-American family that the only way she would influence the family to obtain needed surgery for their 4-year-old preschooler was to talk with the child's father. Although the mother stated frequently that she felt it was important for her son to have surgery, no action was taken. When the mother was questioned regarding her husband's perceptions of this matter, the nurse discovered that he felt surgery was unnecessary and that he was the one who made the final decision about needed health care.

In situations where the dominant family member is temporarily immobilized, it is extremely important for the community health nurse to recognize that the family may reassign the dominant position to the nurse. Because of the nurse's professional status, families under stress may initially allow a nurse to assume a position of authority within the family structure. They may follow the nurse's suggestions without questioning the pros and cons to reduce their level of stress. These suggestions may not necessarily be appropriate for the family. Taking over decision making for a family is not therapeutic.

Communication Patterns

Verbal and nonverbal interactions within a family usually display significant regularities or patterns. Norms involving what is shared and not shared with whom are implicitly, if not explicitly, known by all family members. Messages are provided in a variety of ways to let family members know how to communicate within and outside the family system.

The ability to communicate accurately and effectively is essential to all aspects of family functioning because communication is an integral part of daily living. It helps the family to carry out its functions, to meet the needs of individual family members, and to move toward achieving its goals.

Communication is an extremely complex process, involving not only what is said but also how it is said and the *behavioral interactions* that occur during the course of a conversation. An individual can communicate even when verbal information is not shared. Watzlawick, Beavin, and Jackson (1967) noted that because all behavior in an interactional situation has message value, it is impossible for a person not to communicate. They believe that "activity or inactivity, words or silence, all have message value which influence others; others, in turn, cannot avoid responding to these communications and are thus, themselves communicating" (p. 49). Even silence conveys a message to an individual who is sharing thoughts, ideas, or feelings.

Communication-oriented theorists believe that family communication patterns need to be analyzed along several dimensions (Haley, 1971; Jackson, 1968; Satir, 1972; Watzlawick, Beavin, Jackson, 1967). Verbal, nonverbal, and behavioral processes should be observed to identify the content of communication, how the content is shared and received, and linguistic characteristics that influence interpretation of communication.

CONTENT OF COMMUNICATION What actually is conveyed is known as the *content* of communication. Observations should be made to determine what is being shared and what is not. It is not unusual for individuals to feel uncomfortable about sharing information concerning personal topics such as sexuality, finances, and troubled relationships with significant others. A health care professional needs to "listen between the lines" to help clients verbalize areas of concern beyond those that are explicitly expressed.

TRANSMISSION OF CONTENT How content is shared can significantly influence its meaning to the receiver. The sharing of content does not necessarily convey to the receiver accurate information or help the receiver to understand the message a person is attempting to send. Content becomes functional when there is clarity of thought, organization of ideas, and accuracy and completeness of facts. It is difficult for the receiver to understand what is being said when information is being withheld or unintentionally not shared, when too much information is shared in an unorganized manner, or when conflicting messages are being conveyed. These problems tend to distort reality and confuse the listener. They can lead to a lack of responsiveness or hostile interchange.

BEHAVIORAL INTERACTIONS How an individual responds, either verbally or nonverbally, during a conversation provides clues to others about how this individual views what is being said and how he or she regards the sender or receiver. Body mannerisms, eye contact, silence or responsiveness to content, vocal characteristics, and ways of eliciting information all provide behavioral messages that guide the course of a conversation. Behavioral messages are often far more meaningful from a positive or negative perspective than verbal content. They may provide *double-level messages* "with the voice saying one thing and the rest of the person saying something else" (Satir, 1972, p. 60). Healthy families tend to share fewer double-level messages than unhealthy families.

INTERPRETATION OF COMMUNICATION How content and behavioral interactions are interpreted varies from one individual to another. Perceptions about messages being conveyed are influenced by several factors, including things such as previous experiences between the sender and receiver, the motivations of the persons involved in the communication process, feelings about oneself, and current stresses being experienced. For example, families who have low self-esteem frequently find it difficult to interpret messages positively; praise is often not heard or negated.

The interpretation of messages is a key factor that determines the difference between effective and ineffective communication. When assessing family communication patterns, it is essential to notice if the content of communication, feelings, and behavioral transactions are accurately perceived. When healthy communication patterns exist, family members seek clarification if they do not understand the content, and they validate their interpretations of feelings and behavioral interactions.

MODES OF COMMUNICATION DURING STRESS Satir (1975) noted that individuals use five major transactional modes to communicate when they are under stress. These are placating, blaming, super-reasonable, irrelevant, and congruent (Table 7-5). Congruent transactions are the most functional. When the other transactional modes of communication become patterned, psychosomatic and other illnesses often result (Satir).

When nurses work with families under stress, they help these families to clarify the facts in the situation, to express feelings and emotions, and to avoid fault-finding or blame. The content of communication and behavioral interactions are frequently distorted during times of stress and crisis. Chapter 8 elaborates on family assessment and intervention when stress and crisis exists.

LINGUISTIC CHARACTERISTICS OF COMMUNICATION Families have varying dialects or language differences based on their cultural background, their socialization process, and their geographical location. It is essential for a community health nurse to note these differences because they may adversely influence the communication process. Generally, clients are more than willing to help a health care professional understand language differences if the professional shows genuine interest in learning about them.

Cultural differences among families are reflected in all aspects of verbal and nonverbal communications. Gestures, posture, facial expression, eye contact, touch, vocabulary, grammatical structure, voice qualities, and silence all send important messages to members of a specific ethnic group. For example, in some cultures (Mexican and some Native American) touch is considered magical and healing; in other cultures, such as the Vietnamese, touch produces anxiety because it is believed that the soul can leave the body on physical contact (Giger, Davidhizar, 1995; Roccereto, 1981). During the family assessment process it is important to determine whether there are cultural behaviors or styles of communication that the client practices. The bowing of the head to show respect in the traditional Japanese culture and speaking softly in the Southeast Asian culture are examples of these behaviors (Fong, 1985).

The primary goal of observing family communication patterns is to determine if the patterns established by a particular family are functional; that is, do they help the family to carry out its functions, to relate effectively to the environment, to meet the needs of individual family members, and to achieve its goals? It is important to remember that ways of achieving functional communication between family members can vary from one family to another.

Boundaries of the Family World

Boundary development and maintenance is essential for family survival and growth. Families must have effective filtering mechanisms so that the exchange of energies corresponds to the needs of the family. Energy exchanges that occur too rapidly or too slowly can be disruptive to the family system. Families need to bring inputs into their system and release outputs into the environment so that they can carry out their functions. However, they also need to limit the amount of input from the environment to prevent system overload and to limit the release of outputs to prevent energy depletion.

table 7-5 Modes of Communication during Stress

Communication Mode	Description
Placating	Family members outwardly agree with each other to avoid conflict in the family unit. There is an inconsistency between what a family member outwardly shares and what is inwardly felt.
Blaming	Family members fear assuming accountability for their feelings and actions and, thus, resort to fault-finding, blaming behaviors and other ineffective communication patterns to hide their insecurities.
Super-reasonable	Family members avoid the sharing of feelings and emotions by focusing on intellectual issues during the communication process. Avoidance of feelings and emotions makes it difficult to address ineffective family functioning and to reduce anxiety in the family system.
Irrelevant	Family member's mode of communication is illogical from the perspective of what is happening in the family environment. Irrelevant communication patterns affect the flow of a conversation, as well as problem-solving and decision-making processes.
Congruent	Family member's mode of communication is consistent between what the individual outwardly shares and what is inwardly felt and is logical in relation to what is happening in the environment.

Modified from Satir V: You as a change agent in helping families to change. In Satir V, Stachowiak J, Taskman H, eds: *Helping families to change*, New York, 1975, Jason Aronson, pp. 141-149.

The rate of energy flow between the family and the environment must vary in order for the family to maintain the integrity of its system. Families who do not adjust their energy flow to correspond to their current circumstances have difficulty handling stress and change. In times of family stress and change, limiting the exchange of inputs and outputs conserves energy needed to carry out activities of daily living. A new mother or father, for instance, may need to reduce working hours (output) to conserve energy for child care activities and to provide emotional support for others in the family system.

It is not uncommon for community health nurses to work with families who are having difficulty adjusting energy flow to and from their family system. When boundaries are too open or too closed, not agreed upon, or ambiguous, stress occurs in the family system. Families dealing with these types of boundary maintenance issues find it difficult to achieve family goals and to adapt during periods of stress and crisis.

BOUNDARIES TOO OPEN Disorganized, multiproblem, and crisis-prone families tend to take little control over what enters or exists their environment. They have numerous outsiders (inputs), such as health care professionals or legal authorities, working with them, and often they do not set rules about how and when family members should interact outside the family system. These families usually come to the attention of health care professionals because their outputs are not acceptable to the suprasystem (community). It is not unusual for such families to be referred to the community health nurse when their children enter school, since frequently they lack the energy to fulfill the health requirements (immunizations and physical examinations) mandated for school entry. In these situations, families' energies are often used to deal with outsiders or crises while the needs of individual family members are neglected.

BOUNDARIES TOO CLOSED Some families allow few inputs to cross their boundaries. They isolate themselves from the larger community, and as a consequence may not obtain the resources needed for family growth. Families from differing cultural backgrounds or families who have members with a mental or physical handicap, for example, may limit inputs from the environment because they fear that their differences will not be accepted. Conflicts between these families and their environment arise when they do not release outputs (e.g., do not send their children to school) or when their outputs are inadequate (e.g., children are not prepared to handle environmental demands and pressures).

BOUNDARIES NOT AGREED UPON At times community health nurses find a discrepancy between the views of one family member and another regarding boundary maintenance. Families may have some boundaries that are well defined and others that are unclearly defined. For example, they may use community resources appropriately but may not agree on how often and when they should interface with friends and the extended family. In these situations it is important for the community health nurse to help family members to address their differences and to work toward a mutually satisfying solution. Lack of agreement on boundary maintenance issues can lead to conflict, disequilibrium, and system disintegration.

BOUNDARY AMBIGUITY Boss (1988) believes that boundary ambiguity is a major barrier to stress management in families. In simple terms, she defines boundary ambiguity as "not knowing who is in and who is out of the family" (p. 73). Two types of boundary ambiguity exist. Boundary ambiguity occurs when a family member is *physically absent with psychological presence* or *physically present with psychological absence* (Boss). When a member of the family is physically absent as a consequence of kidnapping, a run-away incident, or other situations (e.g., divorce) that the family cannot control, the family becomes preoccupied with the absent member. This preoccupation prevents grieving and family restructuring (Boss).

Family members are frequently physically present but psychologically absent when they have an illness such as alcohol addiction or Alzheimer's disease, or when work and other demands consume a significant amount of time (Boss, 1988). In these situations, the family is intact but family members find it difficult to work together to achieve important family goals or to carry out family functions.

Relations with Other Groups and Systems

The development of relationships with other groups, such as extended kin or neighbors, and other systems, such as church, school, or health care agencies, is directly related to the way the family handles its boundary maintenance functions. Family boundaries can facilitate or inhibit the establishment and maintenance of interpersonal relationships with others outside the family system. Families with rigid boundaries have few contacts with persons outside their family system; families with flexible boundaries evaluate their needs for social support.

When assessing family relationships outside the family system, it is important to look at the *type* of relationships they have, as well as the contact allowed. Interaction with numerous people does not necessarily mean that the family is meeting their support, companionship, and growth needs. Some families develop relationships that involve more giving than receiving. In these situations, family energies are devoted to helping others but the family receives little support in return. In other families interactions with others in the environment are not evaluated and may result in negative outcomes. For example, children may encounter legal difficulties when no controls are placed on their relationships with people who engage in illegal activity such as drug selling.

Ways of Obtaining and Giving Emotional Support

Families need to achieve a balance between their relationship with others and their relationship with family members. If the family excludes itself from its external environment, they may lack support during times of stress and crisis. If, on the other hand, the family devotes all its energy to helping others, it is highly unlikely that the family will be able to meet the emotional needs of individual family members.

Families meet their emotional needs in a variety of ways. They develop norms that regulate sources of support, provide guidelines for giving support, and define when support will be given. When assessing the ways a family obtains and gives emotional support, it is important to examine who receives emotional support and when and how it is given.

DISTRIBUTION OF EMOTIONAL SUPPORT All family members need support, encouragement, and praise. If support is not evenly distributed, family members may seek support from their environment or isolate themselves from the family system. Or they may withdraw and limit contact with others outside the family, as well as within the family system.

How an individual member is viewed by other family members greatly affects the amount of emotional support this individual receives. Family norms and rules and the emotional maturity of the family influence how well individual members will be accepted by others in the family system. Individual members who do not conform to family norms usually receive less support than those who do. Illustrating this is the teenager from a family with high educational aspirations who does not share these same views and decides not to go to college. This teenager very quickly receives a message from the family that this is an inappropriate decision. If she or he does not alter these views, the family may withdraw its support.

WHEN AND HOW EMOTIONAL SUPPORT IS PROVIDED Some families provide emotional support only during times of stress and crisis. Other families provide this type of support on a regular basis or neglect the emotional needs of family members all together. All human beings need ongoing emotional care and nurturing. "Having at least one strong intimate relationship is an important predictor of good health" (Heaney, Israel, 1997, p. 186). Family members who lack consistent emotional support often experience physical or psychosocial difficulties. Frequently, individuals who do not receive effective support from the family system will seek this support from others in the external environment.

Families use both verbal and nonverbal communication to provide emotional support for their members. Some families share support spontaneously, whereas others are more reserved with their emotional interchanges. Neither pattern of functioning is right or wrong. The important thing to consider during the family assessment process is the perceptions of family members concerning the quality of emotional support they are receiving. Chapter 8 discusses how perceptions influence an individual's interpretation of what is occurring in their environment.

Set of Personal Roles

Every family has the task of organizing its roles in a way that helps the family to achieve its goals and to carry out its functions. No one role-allocation pattern works for all families. Families must allocate and differentiate roles in a manner that facilitates their functioning.

Personal roles as well as family roles evolve when families organize their role structure. Some common examples of personal roles are "the 'baby' in the family; the 'good' child; the 'bad' child; the scapegoat; the strict parent; and the 'sickest' member of the family. Such roles, even when they emerge fortuitously, can become patterned very quickly. As a result, the person may be 'locked' in the role, with important consequences for how others will treat him and what they will expect of him" (Briar, 1964, p. 254). When assessing family dynamics it is extremely important to identify how personal role allocation has influenced the behavior of all family members. The "sick" member of the family, for example, is often not allowed to do things that he or she is capable of doing. Frequently family members "take care" of this person so well that he or she never learns how to function independently.

Rituals and Symbols

Family rituals and symbols come from two major sources. Some are adopted from the culture as a whole or a subculture within the wider culture. Others develop from human transactional processes that have occurred within the family system (Briar, 1964).

Family rituals and symbols develop around multiple aspects of family life. They help family members and outsiders to identify what the family views as important. They provide structure for activities of daily living and for special occasions.

Examples of the types of rituals and symbols that develop in family systems are shared in Table 7-6. Although some of

table 7-6 EXAMPLES OF RITUALS AND SYMBOLS IN FAMILY SYSTEMS

RITUAL/SYMBOL	EXAMPLES
Mealtime activity	Designating times for meals, seating arrangements during meals, and conversation shared
Naming of family members	Giving nicknames to all family members or naming children after specific relatives
Holiday events	Serving specific types of food (Figure 7-6) or carrying out certain kinds of activities such as religious ceremonies (Figure 7-7)
Religious observances	Saying prayers at mealtime or bedtime or engaging in specific activities when a family member dies

the rituals within a family appear very similar to societal ones, family rituals usually have some very specific, unique characteristics.

Family rituals and symbols are extremely significant and are usually valued highly by families. They are often continued even when individual family members do not view them as important. Frequently pressure is placed on family members to conform to family rituals and symbols until the entire family unit alters its views about them.

Cultural Values and Attitudes

Numerous factors influence the biological, psychosocial, and spiritual development of all human beings. Human growth and development begins with genetic characteristics inherited from parents but then branches off in different directions as one interacts with one's environment. Within this environment, caring and nurturing by significant others greatly affects how growth progresses and what decisions are made about handling activities of daily living. Through environmental conditioning people learn patterns of behavior that influence how they relate to others, how they act in social situations, and how they make decisions about significant issues. Because these patterns of behavior provide stability and security, they are not easily altered; they continuously influence the direction of one's life. They shape beliefs and values that provide a foundation for future decision making.

Culture is the term used to describe the values, attitudes, and patterns of behavior that are transmitted to all individuals in a particular social environment. Social scientists have defined culture in many ways, but most of these definitions have three central themes: (1) beliefs, values, and patterns of behavior are learned and passed on from one generation to the next; (2) culture provides a prescription for daily living and decision making; and (3) the components of a culture are valued by members of the culture and are considered to be right and not open to questioning.

Every culture has a schema, composed of specific components, that shapes such things as family structure, dietary habits, religious practices, the development of art, music, and drama, ways of communicating, dress, and health behavior (Figures 7-6 and 7-7). A culture schema, for instance, affects how one perceives health and illness and when and from whom one seeks health care. For example, because the Jewish culture values the sacredness of human life and health, members of this particular cultural group have traditionally respected health care providers and have engaged in activities to restore health, regardless of the expense. The value the Jewish culture places on health is reflected in a favorite Yiddish parting phrase, *Sei gesund*, "be well" (Kensky, 1977). In contrast to the health values held by the Jewish culture are the beliefs and values transmitted

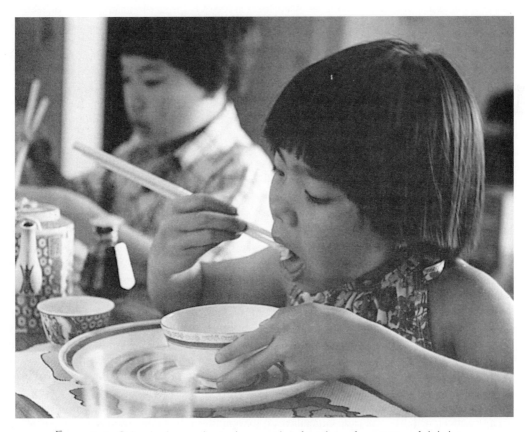

Figure 7-6 Cultural values and attitudes provide a foundation for activities of daily living.

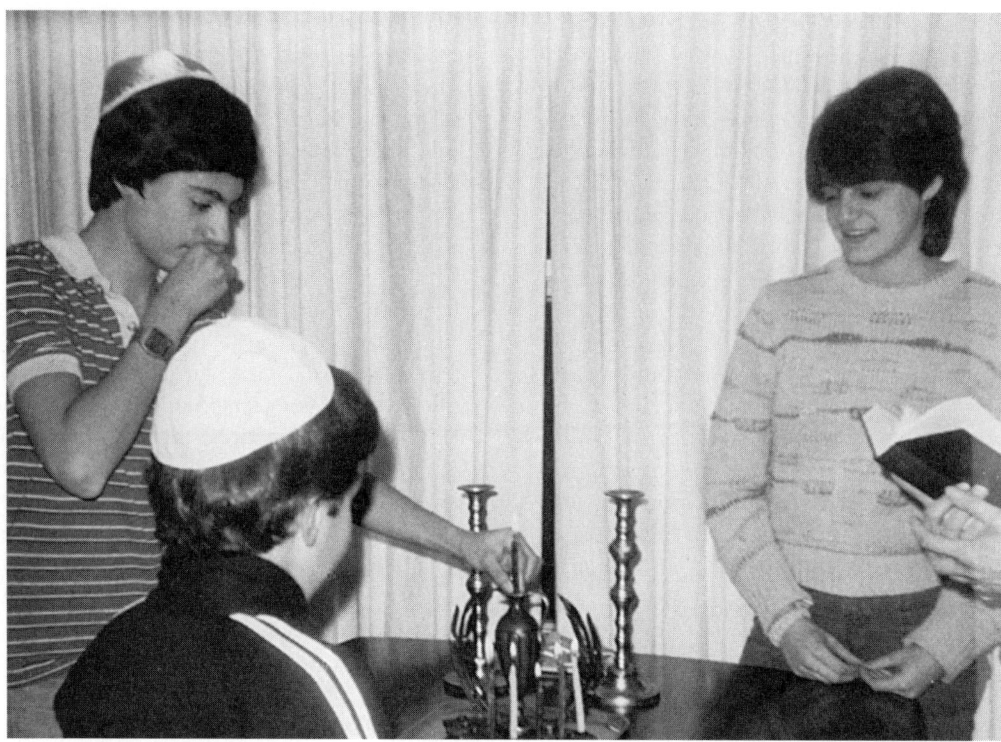

Figure 7-7 For centuries, religious systems have significantly influenced the development of customs and rituals within family systems and have preserved and transmitted these traditions from one generation to another. Hanukkah, a festive Jewish holiday lasting for 8 days in early December, has been celebrated for centuries in memory of the rededication of the temple of Jerusalem under the Maccabees in 164 BCE. Hanukkah is a celebration of freedom: freedom to practice one's own religion. It is a joyous time that includes a symbolic lighting of candles, the sharing of gifts, and the serving of special foods.

by the Mexican-American culture. Many individuals from this culture are influenced by a folk system that encourages the use of folk medicine and supports the belief that one has very little control over one's life; it is felt that supernatural forces cause disease and that one can do very little to prevent illness. Mexican healers, *curanderos(as)*, rather than health care professionals are used by some Mexican-American families when health care services are needed (Baca, 1973; Prattes, 1973; Samora, 1978).

A rich diversity of cultural values and attitudes exists in our nation. In community health nursing practice, encountering clients who have beliefs that differ from those of the health care professional is a common occurrence. For a community health nurse to work effectively with such clients, he or she must develop an appreciation for the inherent worth of different cultural patterns. This involves a process that not only increases knowledge about various cultural schemata but also increases acceptance of all human beings.

Developing cultural sensitivity in clinical practice enriches and broadens the nurse's approach to diverse families and can lead to a more effective delivery of care. Crucial to this process is being aware of one's own cultural background. Health care professionals are influenced by their own social conditioning, which has a long-lasting effect on everything they do. Social conditioning can positively or negatively influence the therapeutic relationship. Cultural patterns subtly influence the professional's perceptions about the appropriateness of a family's health beliefs, practices, and family relationships.

CULTURAL VARIATIONS. Select characteristics of some ethnic and racial groups are presented in Table 7-7. They illustrate cultural variations in relation to health beliefs and practices, family relationships, and communication processes. *However, nurses must understand that there are also intracultural variations based on socioeconomic factors and generational differences within groups* (Fong, 1985; Wong, 1995).

Cherry and Giger (1995) discuss intracultural variations in how African-Americans view descriptive terminology regarding their race. They have determined that some African-American individuals and groups encourage the use of the term *Black Americans*, whereas others prefer the term *African-Americans*. The latter term brings together the cultural heritage of Africa and America, whereas the emphasis in the former term is on biological and racial identity (Cherry, Giger, p. 165). In keeping with these findings and what is commonly used in the literature, the term *African-American* will be used throughout this text with the following exceptions: where necessary to preserve the integrity of another author's work, and where there is a specific intent to delineate between black and nonblack biological and racial variations.

When learning about specific cultural beliefs it is best to seek information from members of the particular culture being studied. Many cultural patterns are not written or recorded. Most, in fact, are transmitted from one generation to another through oral communication and behavioral transactions. Even when receiving input from individuals who represent a given cultural group, it is extremely important to remember that not all individuals within a cultural group have similar characteristics. Knowledge about cultural values and attitudes helps nurses to identify factors to consider when collecting data about family functioning. This knowledge, however, *never* replaces the need to obtain specific data from individual families during the assessment process. When working with families in the community setting, a cultural assessment should be done to determine their unique characteristics and needs.

Cultural assessments assist nurses in individualizing family care. When conducting a cultural assessment, community health nurses need to focus on collecting basic cultural data that identify major family values, beliefs, customs, and behaviors that influence and relate to health needs, health care practices, and family attitudes about health and illness, health care providers, and health care systems (Orque, Bloch, Monrroy, 1983; Tripp-Reimer, Brink, Saunders, 1984, p. 79). According to Tripp-Reimer, Brink, and Saunders, "basic cultural data include: ethnic affiliation, religious preference, family patterns, food patterns, and ethnic health care practices" (p. 79).

Appendix 7-1 displays a cultural assessment tool developed by Bloch (1983) to facilitate cultural assessments in the clinical setting. This tool identifies content areas such as race, language and communication processes, and nutritional variables to be considered when making a cultural assessment. Orque, Bloch, and Monrroy (1983) and Giger and Davidhizar (1995) examine factors to consider when providing nursing care for specific ethnic groups. Referring to these writings will help the reader to plan appropriate nursing interventions when working with families from different ethnic groups.

When using a cultural assessment guide, it is important to remember that a barrage of questions related to the cultural content areas on this tool is inappropriate. This type of interviewing inhibits communication and adversely affects the nurse-client relationship. When collecting data during the assessment phase of the nursing process, the community health nurse focuses on building a therapeutic relationship. The Giger and Davidhizar (1995) textbook provides some valuable guidelines to consider when collecting cultural data.

Religious Beliefs

Cultural values and attitudes are often shaped and maintained by religious systems. From earliest times religious systems have preserved and transmitted traditions from one generation to another, and have greatly influenced the development of norms for social behavior. Spiritual beliefs valued by these systems have provided a foundation for moral behavior in societies; they have also helped to maintain order and cohesiveness in social groups.

Despite major changes in religious systems in the past two decades, spiritual beliefs still affect the lives of most individuals. They influence such things as contraceptive practices, dietary habits, developmental transitions through rites of passage, selection of marriage partners, reactions to health and illness, and the development of customs and rituals (see Figure 7-7). Table 7-8 presents select religious beliefs that affect nursing care.

Spiritual beliefs of clients are often neglected in the clinical setting. Involving spiritual leaders in a client's care and allowing clients to verbalize their feelings about their religious values can strengthen the relationships between health care professionals and clients and can promote effective decision-making about needed health care services. Religious beliefs frequently comfort distressed individuals and help them cope with illness and crisis.

Process Parameters for Family Assessment

Basic to the understanding of family functioning is the analysis of family processes. Family processes are methods used by families to determine how their structure evolves, how decisions are made, and how the family carries out its functions to maintain stability and to promote growth within the family unit. Parameters to consider when assessing family processes can be found in the accompanying box.

Family health is a function of process rather than outcome. It is family process that helps the family manage stress, survive crises, deal with conflict, and organize itself so that it can achieve its goals. Usually, however, a family comes to the attention of the health care professional because its outputs are inadequate or because the family perceives difficulty in meeting its goals. When assessing family functioning it is extremely important to examine process

Text continues on p. 180.

Select Process Parameters to Consider during Family Assessment

- How the family integrates its role relationships
- How the family uses information from the environment
- How the family adapts to change within the family system and its environment
- How the family deals with conflict or disagreement
- How the family maintains the integrity of the family unit
- How the family promotes the personal autonomy of family members

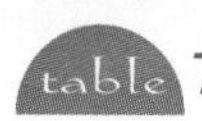

7-7 Selected Cultural Characteristics Related to Health Care of Children and Families

Cultural Group	Health Beliefs	Health Practices
ASIANS		
Chinese	A healthy body viewed as gift from parents and ancestors and must be cared for Health is one of the results of balance between the forces of *yin* (cold) and *yang* (hot)—energy forces that rule the world Illness caused by imbalance Believe blood is source of life and is not regenerated *Chi* is innate energy Lack of chi and blood results in deficiency that produces fatigue, poor constitution, and long illness	Goal of therapy is to restore balance of yin and yang Acupuncturist applies needles to appropriate meridians identified in terms of yin and yang Acupressure and *tai chi* replacing acupuncture in some areas *Moxibustion* is application of heat to skin over specific meridians Wide use of medicinal herbs procured and applied in prescribed ways Folk healers are herbalist, spiritual healer, temple healer, fortune healer Meals may or may not be planned to balance hot and cold Milk intolerance relatively common Use of condiments (e.g., monosodium glutamate and soy sauce) may create difficulty with some diet regimens (e.g., low-salt diets)
Japanese	Three major belief systems: *Shinto* religious influence Humans inherently good Evil caused by outside spirits Illness caused by contact with polluting agents (e.g., blood, corpses, skin diseases) Chinese and Korean influence Health achieved through harmony and balance between self and society Disease caused by disharmony with society and not caring for body Portuguese influence Upholds germ theory of disease	Believe evil removed by purification Energy restored by means of acupucture, acupressure, massage, and moxibustion along affected meridians *Kampō* medicine—use of natural herbs Believe in removal of diseased parts Trend is to use both Western and Oriental healing methods Care for disabled viewed as family's responsibility Take pride in child's good health Seek preventive care, medical care for illness May avoid some food combinations (e.g., milk and cherries, watermelon and crab) and believe pickled plums to have special properties Lactose intolerance relatively common
Vietnamese	Good health considered to be balance between yin and yang Believe person's life has been predisposed toward certain phenomena by cosmic forces Health believed to be result of harmony with existing universal order; harmony attained by pleasing good spirits and avoiding evil ones Belief in *am duc,* the amount of good deeds accumulated by ancestors Many use rituals to prevent illness Practice some restrictions to prevent incurring wrath of evil spirits	Family uses all means possible before using outside agencies for health care Fortune-tellers determine event that caused disturbance May visit temple to procure divine instruction Use astrologer to calculate cyclical changes and forces Regard health as family responsibility; outside aid sought when resources run out Certain illnesses considered only temporary (such as pustules, open wounds) and ignored Seek generalist health healers May use special diets to prevent illness and promote health Lactose intolerance prevalent
Filipinos	Believe God's will and supernatural forces govern universe Illness, accidents, and other misfortunes are God's punishment for violations of His will Widely accept "hot" and "cold" balance and imbalance as cause of health and illness	Some use amulets as a shield from witchcraft or as good luck pieces Catholics substitute religious medals and other items

Sources: Anderson, Fenichel, 1989; Clark, 1981; DeSantis, 1988; Geissler, 1994; Giger, Davidhizar, 1991; Holland, Sweeney, 1985; Hollingsworth, Brown, Brooten, 1980; Orgue, Bloch, Monrroy, 1983; Randall-David, 1989.
Modified from Wong DL: *Whaley and Wong's nursing care of infants and children*, ed 5, St. Louis, 1995, Mosby, pp. 56-61.

Family Relationships	Communication	Comments
Extended family pattern common Strong concept of loyalty of young to old Respect for elders taught at early age—acceptance without questioning or talking back Children's behavior a reflection on family Family and individual honor and "face" important Self-reliance and self-restraint highly valued; self-expression repressed Males valued more highly than females; women submissive to men in family	Open expression of emotions unacceptable Often smile when do not comprehend	Do not react well to painful diagnostic workup; are especially upset by drawing of blood Deep respect for their bodies and believe it best to die with bodies intact; therefore may refuse surgery Believe in reincarnation Older members fear hospitals; often believe hospital is a place to go to die Children sometimes breast-fed for up to 4 or 5 years*
Close intergenerational relationships Family provides anchor Family tends to keep problems to self Value self-control and self-sufficiency Concept of *haji* (shame) imposes strong control; unacceptable behavior of children reflects on family Many adopt practices of contemporary middle class Concern for child's missing school may result in sending to school before fully recovered from illness	Issei—born in Japan; usually speak Japanese only Nisei, Sansei, and Yonsei have few language difficulties New immigrants able to read and write English better than able to speak or understand it Make significant use of nonverbal communication with subtle gestures and facial expression Tend to suppress emotions Will often wait silently	Generational categories: Issei—1st generation to live in U.S. Nisei—2nd generation Sansei—3rd generation Yonsei—4th generation Issei and Nisei—tolerant and permissive childrearing until 5 or 6, then emphasis on emotional reserve and control Cleanliness highly valued Time considered valuable and used wisely Tendency to practice emotional control may make assessment of pain more difficult
Family is revered institution Multigenerational families Family is chief social network Children highly valued Individual needs and interests are subordinate to those of family group Father is main decision maker Women taught submission to men Parents expect respect and obedience from children	Many immigrants are not proficient in speaking and understanding English May hesitate to ask questions Questioning authority is sign of disrespect; asking questions considered impolite Use indirectness rather than forthrightness in expressing disagreement May avoid eye contact with health professionals as a sign of respect	Consider status more important than money Children taught emotional control Time concept more relaxed—consider punctuality less significant than other values (i.e., propriety) Place high value on social harmony
Family is highly valued, with strong family ties Multigenerational family structure common, often with collateral members as well Personal interests are subordinated to family interests and needs Members avoid any behavior that would bring shame on the family	Immigrants and older persons may not be able to speak or understand English	Tend to have a fatalistic outlook on life Believe time and providence will solve all

*Most Asian cultures consider the child 1 year old at the time of birth. Traditional Chinese custom adds 1 year on January 1 regardless of the birthday—a child born in December is 2 years old the next January.

Continued

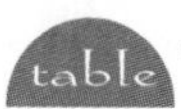

7-7 Selected Cultural Characteristics Related to Health Care of Children and Families—cont'd

Cultural Group	Health Beliefs	Health Practices
Blacks	Illness classified as: Natural—affected by forces of nature without adequate protection (e.g., cold air, pollution, food and water) Unnatural—evil influences (e.g., witchcraft, voodoo, hoodoo, hex, fix, rootwork); symptoms often associated with eating Believe serious illness sent by God as punishment (e.g., parents punished by illness or death of child) Believe serious illness can be avoided May resist health care because illness is "will of God"	Self-care and folk medicine very prevalent Folk therapies usually religious in origin Attempt home remedies first; poorer people do not seek help until illness serious Usually seek help from: "Old lady"—woman in community with a common knowledge of herbs; consulted regarding pediatric care Spiritualist—has received gift from God for healing incurable diseases or solving personal problems; strongly based in Christianity Priest (voodoo priest/priestess)—most powerful healer Root doctor—meets need for herbs, oils, candles, and ointments Prayer is common means for prevention and treatment Lactose intolerance relatively common
Haitians†	Illnesses have a supernatural or natural origin Supernatural illnesses are caused by angry voodoo spirits, enemies, or the dead, especially deceased ancestors Natural illnesses are based on conceptions of natural causation: Irregularities of blood volume, flow, purity, viscosity, color, and/or temperature (hot/cold) Gas (*gaz*) Movement and consistency of mother's milk Hot/cold imbalance in the body Bone displacement Movement of diseases Health is maintained by good dietary and hygienic habits	Health is a personal responsibility Foods have properties of "hot"/"cold" and "light"/"heavy" and must be in harmony with one's life cycle and bodily states Natural illnesses are treated by home remedies first Supernatural illness treated by healers: voodoo priest *(houngan)* or priestess *(mambo),* midwife *(fam saj),* and herbalist or leaf doctor *(dokte fey)* Amulets and prayer used to protect against illness due to curses or willed by evil people
HISPANICS		
Mexicans (Latinos, Chicanos, Raza-Latinos)	Health beliefs have strong religious association Believe in body imbalance as a cause of illness, especially imbalance between *caliente* (hot) and *frio* (cold) or "wet" and "dry" Some maintain good health is a result of "good luck"—a reward for good behavior Illness prevented by performing properly, eating proper foods, and working proper amount of time; accomplished through prayer, wearing religious medals or amulets, and sleeping with relics at home Illness is a punishment from God for wrongdoing, forces of nature, and the supernatural	Seek help from *curandero* or *curandera,* especially in rural areas Curandero(a) receives his/her position by birth, apprenticeship, or a "calling" via dream or vision Treatments involve use of herbs, rituals, and religious artifacts Practice for severe illness—make promises, visit shrines, offer medals and candles, offer prayers Adhere to "hot" and "cold" food prescriptions and prohibitions for prevention and treatment of illness

†This section was written by Lydia DeSantis, RN, PhD.

variables as well as outcomes desired by a family; family processes frequently need to be altered before desired outcomes can be reached.

Direct observation of the family system is the best way to gain an understanding of family processes. This is especially true during times of crisis, because it is during these periods that functional or dysfunctional behaviors become more evident. Decision-making and communication patterns should be analyzed carefully in an assessment of family processes. Chapter 8 presents the concepts

Family Relationships	Communication	Comments
Strong kinship bonds in extended family; members come to aid of others in crisis Less likely to view illness as a burden Augmented families common (unrelated persons living in same household) Place strong emphasis on work and ambition Sex-role sharing among parents Elderly members respected Maternal grandparent strong influence	Alert to any evidence of discrimination Place importance on nonverbal behavior May use nonstandard English or "black English" Use "testing" behaviors to assess personnel in health care situations before seeking active care Best to use simple, direct, but caring approach	High level of caution and distrust of majority group Social anxiety related to tradition of humiliation, oppression, and loss of dignity Will elect to retain dignity rather than seek care if values are compromised Strong sense of peoplehood High incidence of poverty Black minister a strong influence in black community Visits by family minister are sought, expected, and valued in helping to cope with illness and suffering
Maintenance of family reputation is paramount Lineal authority supreme; children in a subordinate position in family hierarchy Children valued for parental social security in old age and expected to contribute to family welfare at an early age Children viewed as "gifts from God" and treated with indulgence and affection	Recent immigrants and older persons may speak only Haitian creole May prefer family/friends to act as translators and confidants Often smile and nod in agreement when do not understand Quiet and gentle communication style and lack of assertiveness lead health care providers to falsely believe they comprehend health teaching and are compliant Will not ask questions if health care provider is busy or rushed	Will use biomedical and ethnomedical (folk) systems simultaneously Resistant to dietary and work restrictions Adherence to prescribed treatments directly related to perceived severity of illness
Traditionally men considered breadwinners and key decision makers in matters outside the home; women considered homemakers Males considered big and strong *(macho)* Strong kinship; extended families include *compadres* (godparents) established by ritual kinship Children valued highly and desired, taken everywhere with family Many homes contain shrines with statues and pictures of saints Elderly treated with respect	May use nonstandard English Some bilingual; many only speak Spanish May have a strong preference for native language and revert to it in times of stress May shake hands or engage in introductory embrace Interpret prolonged eye contact as disrespectful	High degree of modesty—often a deterrent to seeking medical care and open discussions of sex Youngsters often reluctant to share communal showers in schools Relaxed concept of time—may be late for appointments More concerned with present than with future and therefore may focus on immediate solutions rather than long-term goals Magicoreligious practices common May view hospital as place to go to die

Continued

of stress and crisis and examines some of the factors that affect decision making when people are distressed. Parameters to observe when looking at family communication patterns have been discussed previously in this chapter. Classic writings by Ackerman (1959, 1970), Bowen (1973), Haley (1971), Jackson (1968), Minuchin (1974), Satir (1972), and Watzlawick, Beavin, and Jackson (1967) provide an in-depth analysis of family processes and are very useful references for practitioners who view the family as their unit of service.

table 7-7 Selected Cultural Characteristics Related to Health Care of Children and Families—cont'd

Cultural Group	Health Beliefs	Health Practices
Puerto Ricans	Subscribe to the "hot-cold" theory of causation of illness Believe some illness caused by evil spirits and forces	Infrequent use of health care systems Seek folk healers—use of herbs, rituals Consult spiritualist medium for mental disorders *Santeria* is system, and practitioners are called *santeros* Treatments classified as "hot" or "cold"
Cubans[‡]	Prevention and good nutrition are related to good health	Diligent users of the medical model Eclectic health-seeking practices, including preventive measures, and, in some instances, folk medicine of both religious and nonreligious origins; home remedies; in many instances seek assistance of santeros and spiritualists to complement medical treatment Nutrition is important; parents show overconcern with eating habits of their children and spend a considerable part of the budget on food; traditional Cuban diet is rich in meat and starch; consumption of fresh vegetables added in U.S.
Native Americans (numerous tribes)	Believe health is state of harmony with nature and universe Respect of bodies through proper management All disorders believed to have aspects of supernatural Violation of a restriction or prohibition thought to cause illness Fear of witchcraft May carry objects believed to guard against witchcraft Theology and medicine strongly interwoven	Medicine persons: Altruistic persons who must use powers in purely positive ways Persons capable of both good and evil—perform negative acts against enemies Diviner-diagnosticians—diagnose but do not have powers or skill to implement medical treatment Specialists—use herbs and curative but nonsacred medical procedures Medicine persons—use herbs and ritual Singers—cure by the power of their song obtained from supernatural beings; effect cures by laying on of hands Lactose intolerance relatively common

[‡]This section was written by Mercedes Sandaval, PhD.

Characteristics that reflect dysfunctional processes in a family unit are presented in the box on page 190. These behaviors were identified by the North American Nursing Diagnosis Association (NANDA), a national organization established to develop standard nursing diagnoses for the profession. Having an understanding of these behaviors assists the community health nurse in identifying families who need nursing intervention.

TOOLS THAT FACILITATE THE FAMILY ASSESSMENT PROCESS

A community health nurse can use a variety of tools to facilitate family assessment. Some of these tools are discussed below. They are designed to help the practitioner elicit data about certain aspects of family structure, function, and process and to aid the health professional in determining major family concerns, needs, and strengths. Assessment tools, however, are only guides, and before using them one needs to have an understanding of family theory and of communication processes that enhance effective nurse-client relationships.

Family Assessment Guides

Many community health agencies have developed family assessment guides so that staff members can focus attention on family functioning in addition to the health status of

Family Relationships	Communication	Comments
Family usually large and home centered—the core of existence Father has complete authority in family—family provider and decision maker Wife and children subordinate to father Children valued—seen as a gift from God Children taught to obey and respect parents; corporal punishment to ensure obedience	May use nonstandard English Spanish speaking or bilingual Strong sense of family privacy—may view questions regarding family as impudent	Relaxed sense of time Pay little attention to *exact* time of day Suspicious and fearful of hospitals
Strong family ties with mother and father kinships Children supported and assisted by parents long after becoming adults Elderly cared for at home	Most are bilingual (English/Spanish) except for segments of the senior population	In less than 30 years Cubans have been able to obtain a higher standard of living than other Hispanic groups in U.S. Have been able to retain many of their former social institutions: bilingual and private schools, clinics, social clubs, the family as an extended network of support, etc. Many do not feel discriminated against nor harbor feelings of inferiority with respect to Anglo-Americans or "mainstream" population
Extended family structure—usually includes relatives from both sides of family Elder members assume leadership roles	Most continue to speak their Indian language, as well as English Nonverbal communication	Time orientation—present Respect for age Going to hospital associated with illness or disease; therefore may not seek prenatal care, since pregnancy viewed as natural process Tend to take time to form an opinion of professionals Sexual matters not openly discussed with members of opposite sex

individual family members. Appendix 7-2 is an example of such a tool. When completed it provides a quick visual summary of family strengths, family behaviors that need to be altered, and anticipated guidance needs.

Generally, family assessment guides examine both the family's relationships with its environment and its internal functioning. It is extremely important when designing guides to facilitate the data collection process to take into consideration the need to identify both effective and ineffective behaviors within a family system. It is easy to focus only on family problems. When this is done, ineffective family functioning may be overemphasized. This can lead to frustration, discouragement, and a feeling of hopelessness. Nurses who are unable to see family strengths "burn out" quickly; families who never receive positive feedback for what they are handling well question their ability to adequately maintain themselves and often become dependent on others for decision making.

A family assessment guide should be consistent with one's philosophy of practice. For example, in the community health setting, nurses firmly believe that a preventative health approach is important. This belief would be operationalized if staff members were encouraged to discern anticipatory guidance needs and then to plan nursing interventions that may prevent future health problems. An assessment guide that identifies the need to

Text continues on p. 189.

table 7-8 Selected Religious Beliefs That Affect Nursing Care

Beliefs about Birth and Death	Beliefs about Diet and Food Practices	Beliefs Regarding Medical Care	Comments
ADVENTIST (SEVENTH-DAY ADVENTIST; CHURCH OF GOD)			
Birth: Opposed to infant baptism Baptism in adulthood	Meat prohibited in some groups No alcohol, coffee, or tea	Some believe in divine healing and practice anointing with oil and use of prayer May desire communion or baptism when ill Believe in man's choice and God's sovereignty Some oppose hypnosis as therapy	Sabbath: Saturday for many Accept Bible literally
BAPTIST (27 GROUPS)			
Birth: Opposed to infant baptism Believers baptized by immersion as adults *Death:* Counsel and prayer with clergy, family, patient	Some groups discourage coffee, tea, and alcohol	"Laying on of hands" (some) May encounter some resistance to some therapies, such as abortion Believe God functions through physician Some believe in predestination; may respond passively to care	Fundamentalist and conservative groups accept Bible as inspired word of God
BLACK MUSLIM			
Birth: No baptism *Death:* Carefully prescribed procedure for washing and shrouding dead	Prohibit alcohol, pork, and foods traditional among American blacks (e.g., corn bread, collard greens)	Faith healing unacceptable Always maintain personal habits of cleanliness	General adherence to Moslem tenets overlaid, in many instances, by antagonism to whites, especially Christians and Jews Do not indulge in activities (such as sleeping) more than is necessary to health
BUDDHIST CHURCHES OF AMERICA			
Birth: No infant baptism Infant presentation *Death:* Last rite chanting often practiced at bedside soon after death Priest should be contacted	No requirements or restrictions Some sects are strictly vegetarian Discourage use of alcohol and drugs	Illness believed to be a trial to aid development of soul; illness due to Karmic causes May be reluctant to have surgery or certain treatments on holy days Cleanliness believed to be of great importance Family may request Buddhist priest for counseling	Optimistic outlook; teach ways to overcome fears, anxieties, apprehension
CHURCH OF CHRIST SCIENTIST (CHRISTIAN SCIENCE)			
Birth: No baptism *Death:* No last rites	No requirements or restrictions	Deny the existence of health crisis; see sickness and sin as errors of mind that can be altered by prayer Oppose human intervention with drugs or other therapies; however, accept legally required immunizations	Many desire services of practitioner or reader; will sometimes refuse even emergency treatment until they have consulted a reader Unlikely to donate organs for transplant

From Wong DL: *Whaley and Wong's nursing care of infants and children*, ed 5, St. Louis, 1995, Mosby, pp. 51-55.
Sources: Carpenito, 1992; Conley, 1990; personal communications.

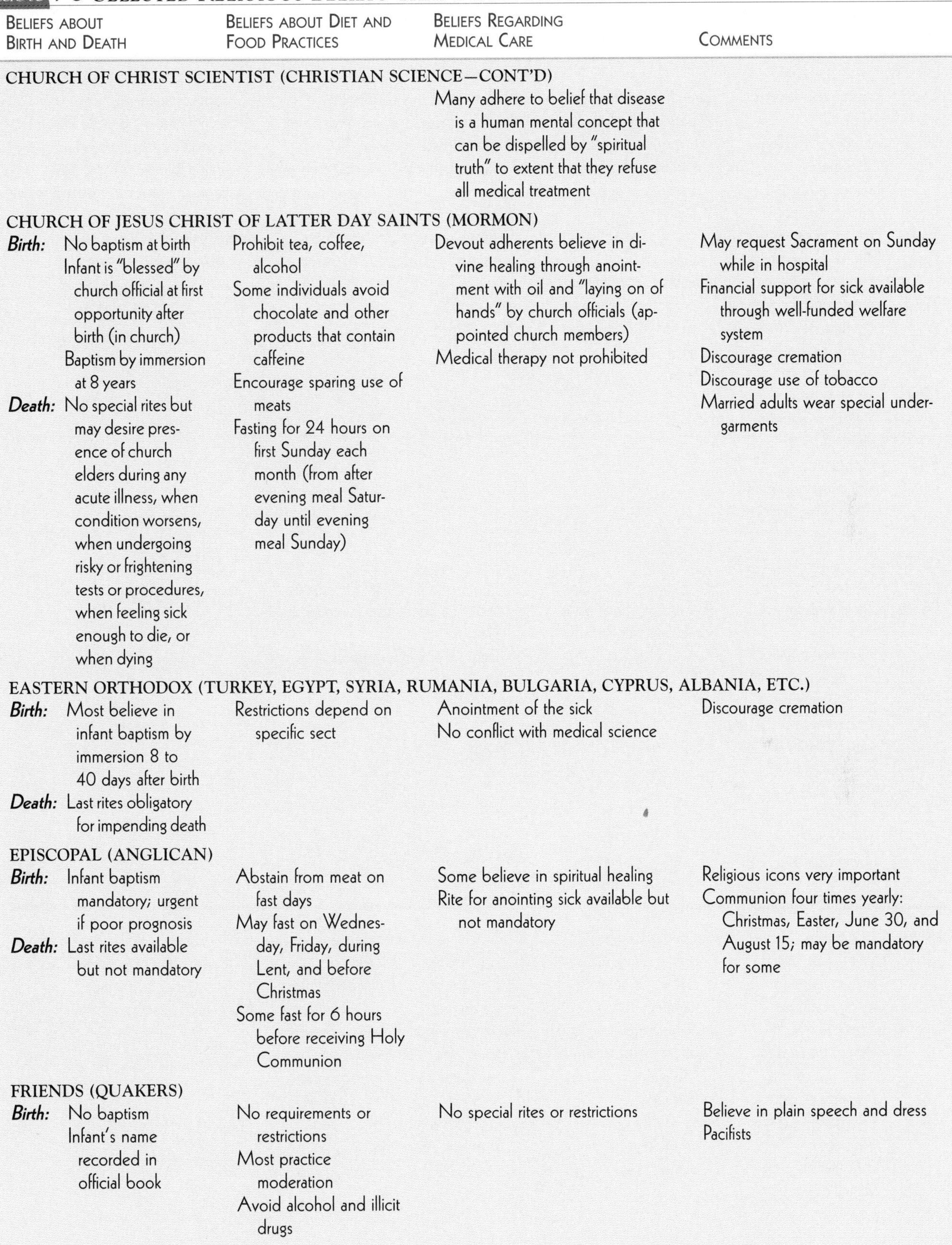

table 7-8 Selected Religious Beliefs That Affect Nursing Care—cont'd

Beliefs about Birth and Death	Beliefs about Diet and Food Practices	Beliefs Regarding Medical Care	Comments
CHURCH OF CHRIST SCIENTIST (CHRISTIAN SCIENCE—CONT'D)			
		Many adhere to belief that disease is a human mental concept that can be dispelled by "spiritual truth" to extent that they refuse all medical treatment	
CHURCH OF JESUS CHRIST OF LATTER DAY SAINTS (MORMON)			
Birth: No baptism at birth Infant is "blessed" by church official at first opportunity after birth (in church) Baptism by immersion at 8 years ***Death:*** No special rites but may desire presence of church elders during any acute illness, when condition worsens, when undergoing risky or frightening tests or procedures, when feeling sick enough to die, or when dying	Prohibit tea, coffee, alcohol Some individuals avoid chocolate and other products that contain caffeine Encourage sparing use of meats Fasting for 24 hours on first Sunday each month (from after evening meal Saturday until evening meal Sunday)	Devout adherents believe in divine healing through anointment with oil and "laying on of hands" by church officials (appointed church members) Medical therapy not prohibited	May request Sacrament on Sunday while in hospital Financial support for sick available through well-funded welfare system Discourage cremation Discourage use of tobacco Married adults wear special undergarments
EASTERN ORTHODOX (TURKEY, EGYPT, SYRIA, RUMANIA, BULGARIA, CYPRUS, ALBANIA, ETC.)			
Birth: Most believe in infant baptism by immersion 8 to 40 days after birth ***Death:*** Last rites obligatory for impending death	Restrictions depend on specific sect	Anointment of the sick No conflict with medical science	Discourage cremation
EPISCOPAL (ANGLICAN)			
Birth: Infant baptism mandatory; urgent if poor prognosis ***Death:*** Last rites available but not mandatory	Abstain from meat on fast days May fast on Wednesday, Friday, during Lent, and before Christmas Some fast for 6 hours before receiving Holy Communion	Some believe in spiritual healing Rite for anointing sick available but not mandatory	Religious icons very important Communion four times yearly: Christmas, Easter, June 30, and August 15; may be mandatory for some
FRIENDS (QUAKERS)			
Birth: No baptism Infant's name recorded in official book	No requirements or restrictions Most practice moderation Avoid alcohol and illicit drugs	No special rites or restrictions	Believe in plain speech and dress Pacifists

Continued

table 7-8 Selected Religious Beliefs That Affect Nursing Care—cont'd

Beliefs about Birth and Death	Beliefs about Diet and Food Practices	Beliefs Regarding Medical Care	Comments
GREEK ORTHODOX			
Birth: Baptism considered important Performed 40 days after birth If not possible to baptize by sprinkling or immersion, church allows child baptism "in the air" by moving child in the form of a cross as appropriate words are said ***Death:*** Last rites, administration of Sacrament of Holy Communion Should be performed while dying person is still conscious	Church-prescribed fast periods—usually occur on Wednesday, Friday, and during Lent; consist of avoiding meat and (in some cases) dairy products If health compromised, priest may be contacted to convince family to forego fasting	Each health crisis handled by ordained priest; deacon may also serve in some cases Holy Communion administered in hospital Some may desire Sacrament of the Holy Unction performed by priest	Oppose euthanasia Believe every reasonable effort should be made to preserve life until termination by God Discourage autopsies that may cause dismemberment Prefer burial to cremation
HINDU			
Birth: No ritual ***Death:*** Special prescribed rites Priest pours water into mouth of dead child, ties a thread around neck or wrist to signify blessing (should not be removed) Family washes body and is particular about who touches body	Many dietary restrictions Beef and veal not eaten Some strict vegetarians	Illness or injury believed to represent sins committed in previous life Accept most modern medical practices	Cremation preferred
ISLAM (MUSLIM/MOSLEM)			
Birth: No baptism ***Death:*** Patient must confess sins and beg forgiveness before death; family should be present Family washes and prepares body, then turns it to face Mecca Only relatives and friends may touch body	Prohibit all pork products and any meat that is not ritually slaughtered Daylight fasting practiced during ninth month of Muhammadan year (Ramadan) Strict Muslims do not use alcohol or mind-altering drugs	Faith healing not acceptable unless psychologic conditions of patient is deteriorating; performed for morale Ritual washing after prayer; prayer takes place five times daily (on rising, midday, afternoon, early evening, and before bed); during prayer, face Mecca and kneel on prayer rug	Older Muslims often have a fatalistic view that may interfere with compliance to therapy May oppose autopsy

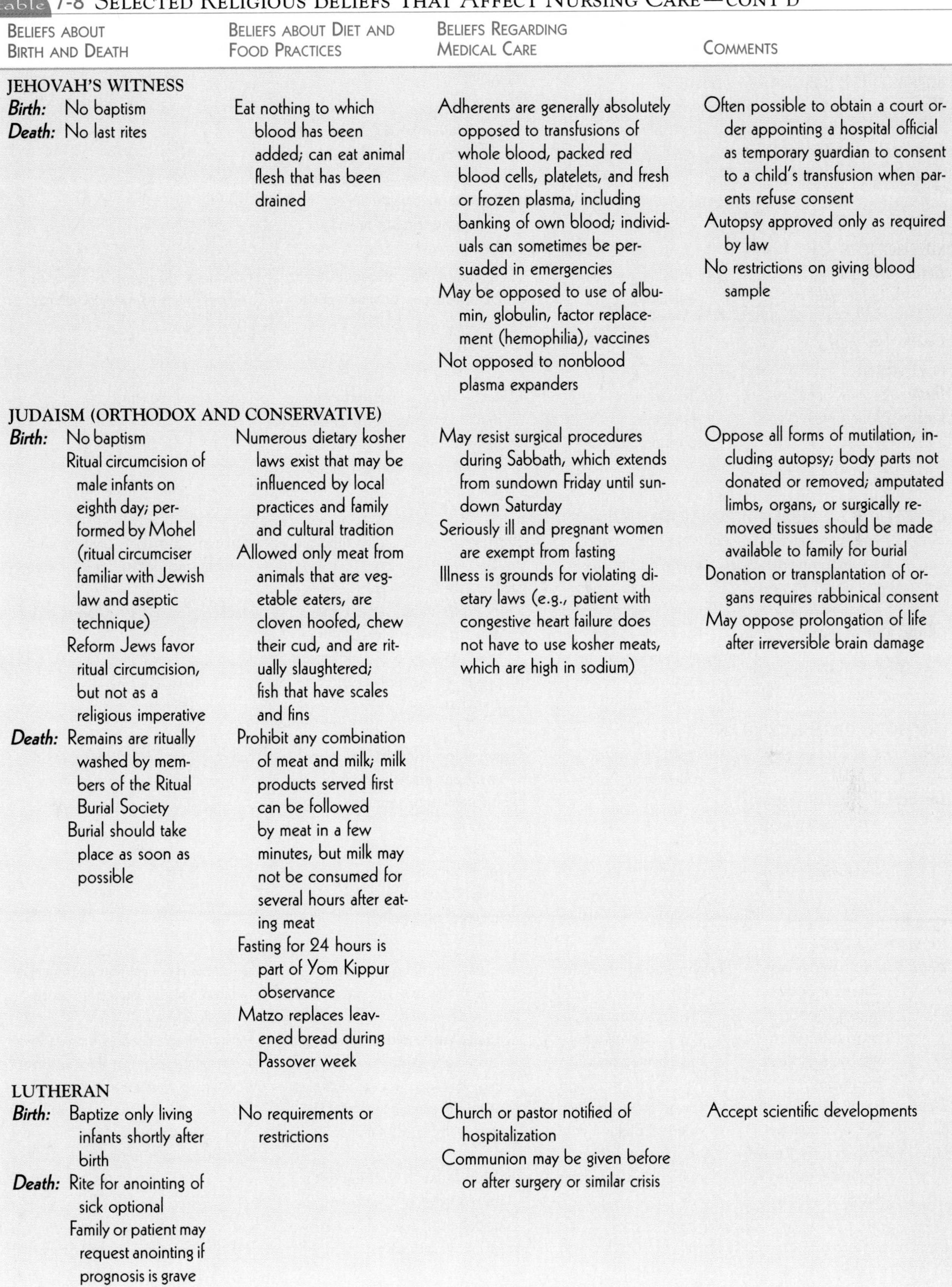

table 7-8 SELECTED RELIGIOUS BELIEFS THAT AFFECT NURSING CARE—CONT'D

Beliefs about Birth and Death	Beliefs about Diet and Food Practices	Beliefs Regarding Medical Care	Comments
JEHOVAH'S WITNESS			
Birth: No baptism ***Death:*** No last rites	Eat nothing to which blood has been added; can eat animal flesh that has been drained	Adherents are generally absolutely opposed to transfusions of whole blood, packed red blood cells, platelets, and fresh or frozen plasma, including banking of own blood; individuals can sometimes be persuaded in emergencies May be opposed to use of albumin, globulin, factor replacement (hemophilia), vaccines Not opposed to nonblood plasma expanders	Often possible to obtain a court order appointing a hospital official as temporary guardian to consent to a child's transfusion when parents refuse consent Autopsy approved only as required by law No restrictions on giving blood sample
JUDAISM (ORTHODOX AND CONSERVATIVE)			
Birth: No baptism Ritual circumcision of male infants on eighth day; performed by Mohel (ritual circumciser familiar with Jewish law and aseptic technique) Reform Jews favor ritual circumcision, but not as a religious imperative ***Death:*** Remains are ritually washed by members of the Ritual Burial Society Burial should take place as soon as possible	Numerous dietary kosher laws exist that may be influenced by local practices and family and cultural tradition Allowed only meat from animals that are vegetable eaters, are cloven hoofed, chew their cud, and are ritually slaughtered; fish that have scales and fins Prohibit any combination of meat and milk; milk products served first can be followed by meat in a few minutes, but milk may not be consumed for several hours after eating meat Fasting for 24 hours is part of Yom Kippur observance Matzo replaces leavened bread during Passover week	May resist surgical procedures during Sabbath, which extends from sundown Friday until sundown Saturday Seriously ill and pregnant women are exempt from fasting Illness is grounds for violating dietary laws (e.g., patient with congestive heart failure does not have to use kosher meats, which are high in sodium)	Oppose all forms of mutilation, including autopsy; body parts not donated or removed; amputated limbs, organs, or surgically removed tissues should be made available to family for burial Donation or transplantation of organs requires rabbinical consent May oppose prolongation of life after irreversible brain damage
LUTHERAN			
Birth: Baptize only living infants shortly after birth ***Death:*** Rite for anointing of sick optional Family or patient may request anointing if prognosis is grave	No requirements or restrictions	Church or pastor notified of hospitalization Communion may be given before or after surgery or similar crisis	Accept scientific developments

Continued

table 7-8 Selected Religious Beliefs That Affect Nursing Care—cont'd

Beliefs about Birth and Death	Beliefs about Diet and Food Practices	Beliefs Regarding Medical Care	Comments
MENNONITE (SIMILAR TO AMISH)			
Birth: No baptism in infancy Baptism during early or middle teens	No requirements or restrictions	No illness rituals Deep concern for dignity and self-determination of individual that would conflict with shock treatment or medical treatment affecting personality or will	
METHODIST			
Birth: No baptism at birth; performed on children or adults *Death:* No ritual	No requirements or restrictions	Communion may be requested before surgery or similar crisis	Encourage donations of body or body parts to medical science
NAZARENE			
Birth: Baptism optional *Death:* No last rites	No requirements or restrictions Alcohol prohibited	Church official administers communion and laying on of hands Adherents believe in divine healing but not exclusive of medical treatment	Cremation permitted
PENTECOSTAL (ASSEMBLY OF GOD, FOUR-SQUARE)			
Birth: No baptism at birth Baptism by complete immersion after age of accountability *Death:* No last rites	Abstain from alcohol, eating blood, strangled animals, or anything to which blood has been added Some individuals may resist pork	No restrictions regarding medical care Deliverance from sickness is provided for in atonement; may pray for divine intervention in health matters and seek God in prayer for themselves and others when ill	Some insist illness is divine punishment; most consider it an intrusion of Satan Practice glossolalia (speaking in tongues)
ORTHODOX PRESBYTERIAN			
Birth: Infant baptism by sprinkling *Death:* Last rites not a sacramental procedure; scripture reading and prayer	No requirements or restrictions	Communion administered when appropriate and convenient Blood transfusion accepted when advisable Pastor or elder should be called for ill person Believe science should be used for relief of suffering	Full forgiveness granted for any illness connected with a sin
ROMAN CATHOLIC			
Birth: Infant baptism mandatory; especially urgent in poor prognosis, when it may be performed by anyone *Death:* Rite for anointing of sick is mandatory Family or patient may request anointing if prognosis is grave	Fasting (eating only one full meal and no eating between meals) and abstaining from meat mandatory on Ash Wednesday and Good Friday; fasting optional during Lent; no meat on Fridays during Lent as general rule	Encourage anointing of sick, although this may be interpreted by older members of church as equivalent to old terminology "extreme unction" or "last rites"; they may require careful explanation if reluctance is associated with fear of imminent death Traditional church teaching does not approve of contraceptives or abortion	Family may request that major amputated limb be buried in consecrated ground Transplant accepted as long as loss of organ does not deprive donor of life or functional integrity of body Autopsy acceptable Religious articles important

table 7-8 SELECTED RELIGIOUS BELIEFS THAT AFFECT NURSING CARE—CONT'D

BELIEFS ABOUT BIRTH AND DEATH	BELIEFS ABOUT DIET AND FOOD PRACTICES	BELIEFS REGARDING MEDICAL CARE	COMMENTS
ROMAN CATHOLIC—CONT'D			
	Children and most hospital patients exempt from fasting Some older Catholics may adhere to older rule of no meat on Friday		
RUSSIAN ORTHODOX			
Birth: Baptism by priest only ***Death:*** Traditionally after death arms are crossed, fingers set in a cross	No meat or dairy products on Wednesday, Friday, and during Lent	Cross necklace is important and should be removed only when necessary and replaced as soon as possible Adherents believe in divine healing, but not exclusive of medical treatment	Opposed to autopsy, embalming, or cremation
UNITARIAN UNIVERSALIST			
Birth: Some practice infant baptism; most consider it unnecessary ***Death:*** No ritual	No requirements or restrictions	Most believe in general goodness of their fellow humans and appreciate expression of that goodness by visits from clergy and fellow parishioners during times of illness	Cremation preferred to burial Believe in fully living this life as they know and understand it

address anticipatory guidance issues supports staff in implementing a preventative approach to practice.

Family assessment tools are only helpful when the practitioner has the theoretical background to use them. Knowledge of role theory, cultural values and attitudes, family decision making, and concepts of stress and crisis is essential for effective use of an assessment guide. Assessment tools can never replace an understanding of theories that analyze family functioning or that describe how nurse-client interactions affect the therapeutic process.

Genograms

A genogram is a tool that aids the community health nurse in collecting generational information about family structure and processes. It visually portrays to the nurse and the family how the family has evolved. It very quickly helps the community health nurse to identify the relationships between family members, the health status of individual family members, and the family's reactions to sociocultural and spiritual variables that have affected their lives.

Figure 7-8 is a partial genogram constructed by a community health nurse during her sixth home visit to the Z. family. Before completing the genogram the nurse had been helping the family to deal with their feelings about the son's recent diagnosis of allergies and had identified a discrepancy in how each parent viewed the son's health status. Wondering whether this was related to previous life experiences, the nurse believed that a genogram could help her and the family to address how social conditioning can influence perceptions of health and illness. The nurse was able to trace each parent's attitudes about health and illness and discovered that all family members had unresolved feelings about the death of two children in the family. These feelings distorted the mother's perceptions about the seriousness of the son's health problems. Genograms can help family members to focus more clearly on current stressful events and gain an appreciation for how past events influence present health problems.

Genograms schematically depict a family tree. A family tree drawn by a professional differs from one drawn by a family in that the professional uses theory as a basis to elicit data about family structure, function, and process. The interview process is the most critical component to consider when completing a genogram. If information concerning child-rearing practices, health beliefs and attitudes, significant social data, and traditions passed on from one generation to another is not assessed, the genogram has little meaning. Completing the actual

NANDA Nursing Diagnosis: Altered Family Processes (Specify)*

DEFINITION

Inability of family system (household members) to meet needs of members, carry out family functions, or maintain communications for mutual growth and maturation.

DEFINING CHARACTERISTICS

- Inability of family members to relate to each other for mutual growth and maturation
- Failure to send and receive clear messages
- Poorly communicated family rules, rituals, symbols; unexamined myths
- Unhealthy family decision-making processes
- Inability of family members to express and accept wide range of feelings
- Inability to accept and receive help
- Does not demonstrate respect for individuality and autonomy of members
- Rigidity in functions and roles
- Fails to accomplish current (or past) family developmental tasks
- Inappropriate (nonproductive) boundary maintenance
- Inability to adapt to change
- Inability to deal with traumatic or crisis experience constructively
- Parents do not demonstrate respect for each other's views on child-rearing practices
- Inappropriate (nonproductive) level and direction of energy
- Inability to meet needs of members (physical, security, emotional, spiritual)
- Family uninvolved in community activities

ETIOLOGICAL OR RELATED FACTORS

- Situational crisis or transition (e.g., alcoholism of a member)
- Developmental crisis or transition

From Gordon M: *Manual of nursing diagnosis, 1997-1998*, St. Louis, 1997, Mosby, p. 377.

*This is a broad taxonomic category. Specify the processes that are altered.

drawing of a genogram takes minimal skill; focusing the conversation on relevant aspects of family functioning requires not only interviewing skill but also knowledge of family dynamics.

Eco-Map

An eco-map is another tool used by health care professionals that schematically portrays factual data about family relationships. It helps the family and the nurse to visually analyze a family's interactions with its external environment. Presented in Figure 7-9 is an eco-map developed by Dr. Ann Hartman for workers in a child welfare practice (Hartman, 1978). Based on a systems theoretical framework, Hartman's tool examines boundary-maintenance aspects of family functioning. It dramatically illustrates the amount of energy used by a family to maintain its system, as well as the presence or absence of situational supports and other family resources.

An eco-map helps families to identify how their energies are being used and when relationships with the external environment are positively or negatively influencing family functioning. For example, if a family's flow of energy as depicted on the eco-map reflects only an outward directional process (→→→), the family may have difficulty providing a nurturing environment for family members and in achieving its goals.

It is impossible to function effectively in the community health setting without looking at how the family interfaces with its external environment. The eco-map enhances the community health nurse's ability to gain this type of information. It is an especially useful tool because it summarizes on one page family strengths, conflicts, and stresses in relation to its interactions with individuals and agencies outside the family system. Community health nurses have found the use of the eco-map particularly beneficial when clients are involved with numerous community systems or when clients perceive a lack of support from significant others.

Family-Life Chronology

Community health nurses may encounter families who are experiencing relationship problems, a situation that makes it difficult for them to concentrate on health concerns or to take needed health actions. These families can find it hard to examine objectively what is happening in their relationships or to make a decision about seeking counseling. Satir's (1967) family-life chronology model (Figure 7-10) helps the community health nurse and the family to identify interactive processes that have evolved. Families that have had long-standing relationship difficulties should be referred for counseling. However, it is not unusual for significant family stress (e.g., illness or financial difficulties) to strain family relationships. The family-life chronology can help these families to identify the strengths in their relationships over time and the need to alter family functioning to reduce stress.

A community health nurse cannot ignore relationship problems when working with families in their homes. Such difficulties can disrupt all parameters of family functioning and are often the key factor in preventing a family from taking needed health action. If these difficulties are ignored, nursing intervention strategies can be ineffective. Dealing with the symptoms of distress such as physical health problems, complaints about lack of time for leisure activities, or feelings of depression, rather than with the relationship difficulties themselves will not alter a family's

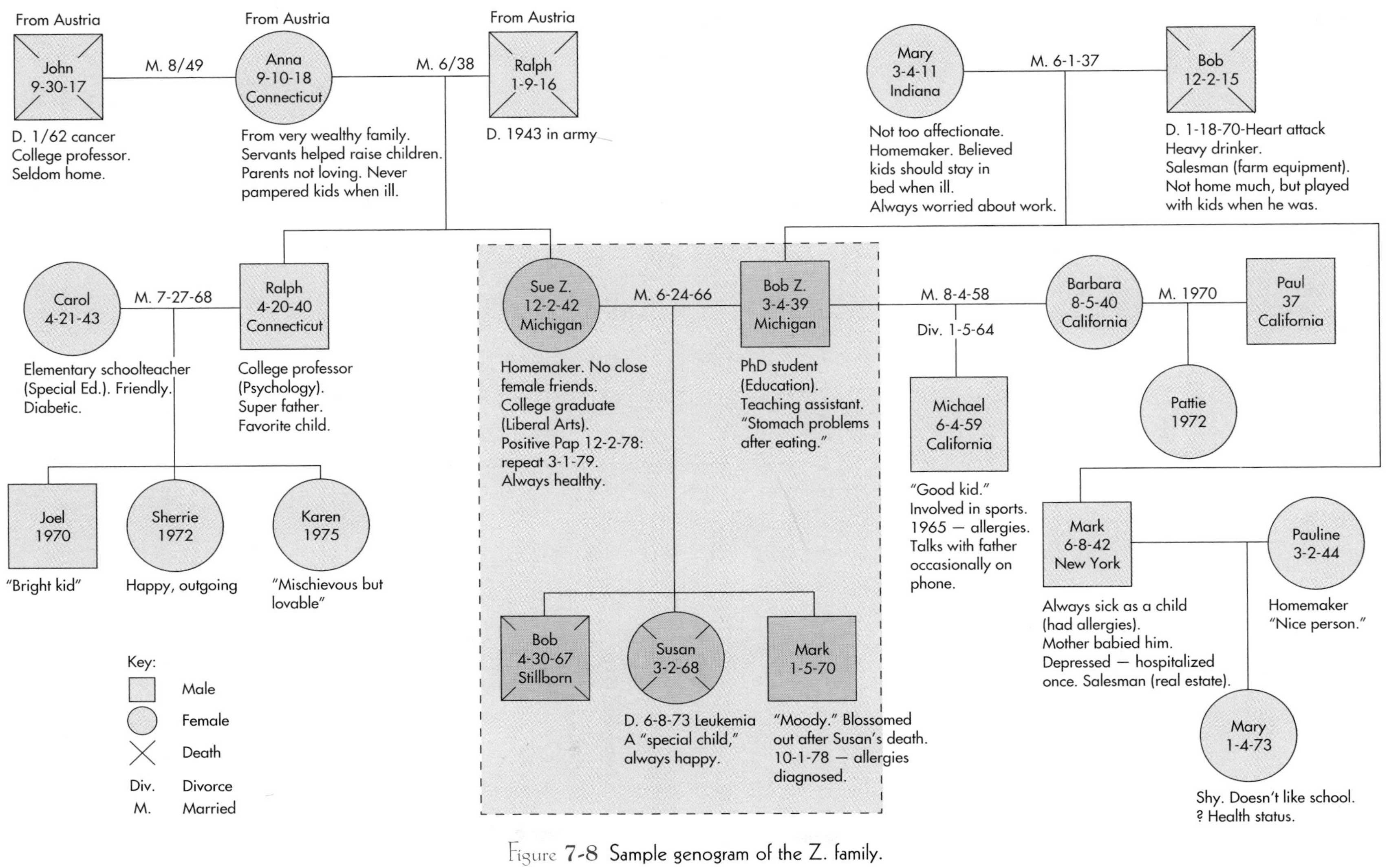

Figure 7-8 Sample genogram of the Z. family.

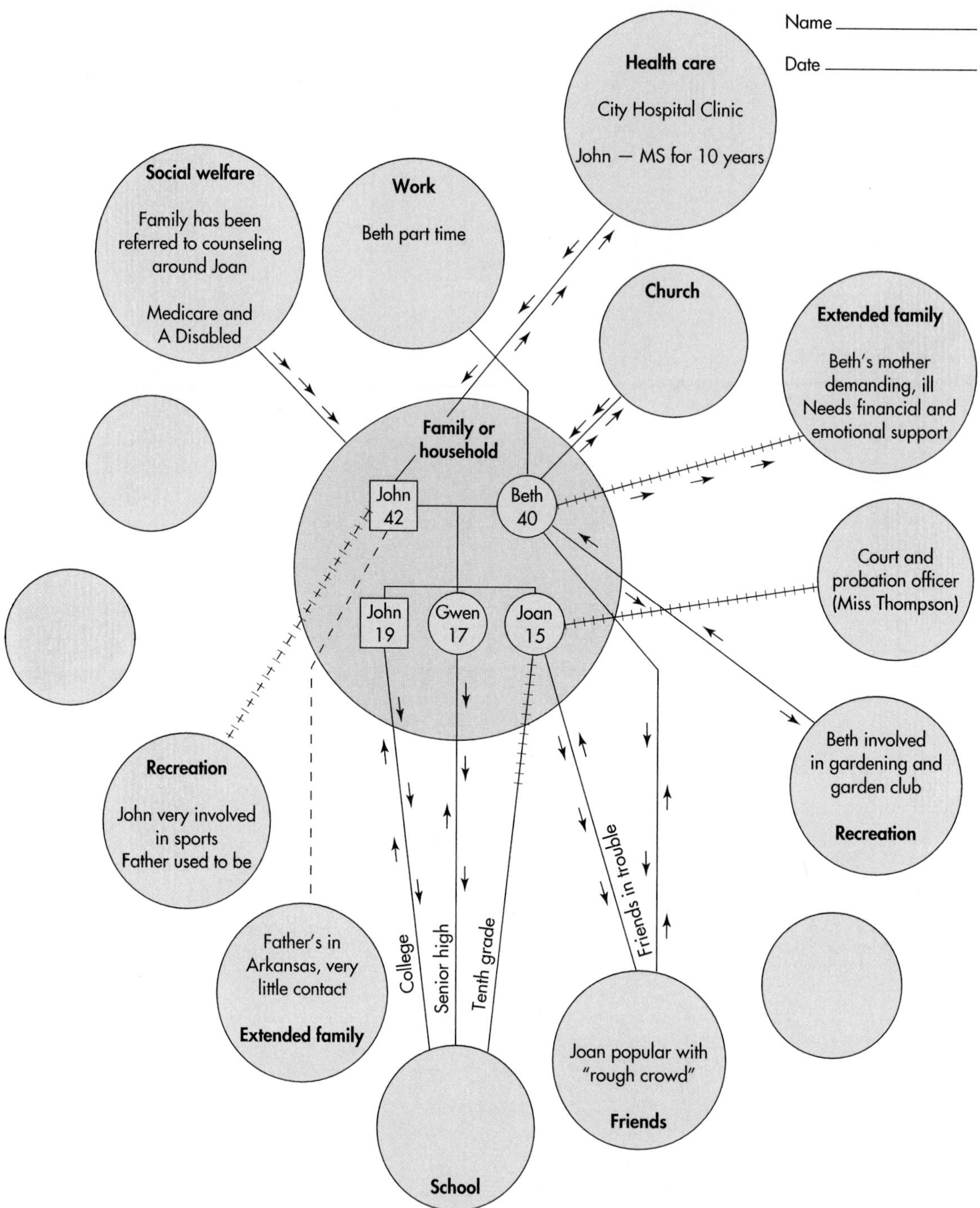

Figure 7-9 Eco-map. Fill in connections where they exist. Indicate nature of connections with a descriptive word or by drawing different kinds of lines: ——— for strong; --- for tenuous; ‡‡‡ for stressful. Draw arrows along lines to signify flow of energy, resources, etc. (→→→). Identify significant people and fill in empty circles as needed. *(From Hartman A: Diagrammatic assessment of family relationships,* Social Casework *59:470, 1978.)*

functioning in any lasting way. One mother, for example, complained to the community health nurse that she had no time for herself and that she found caring for three children, 4, 6, and 8 years old, very restrictive. Suggestions by the community health nurse on how she might care for her children and still have time for leisure activities were ignored. The mother finally shared with the nurse that her husband felt that "a woman's place was in the home. Even if I enrolled my 4-year-old son in a nursery school, I still could not get out of the house. My husband gets very

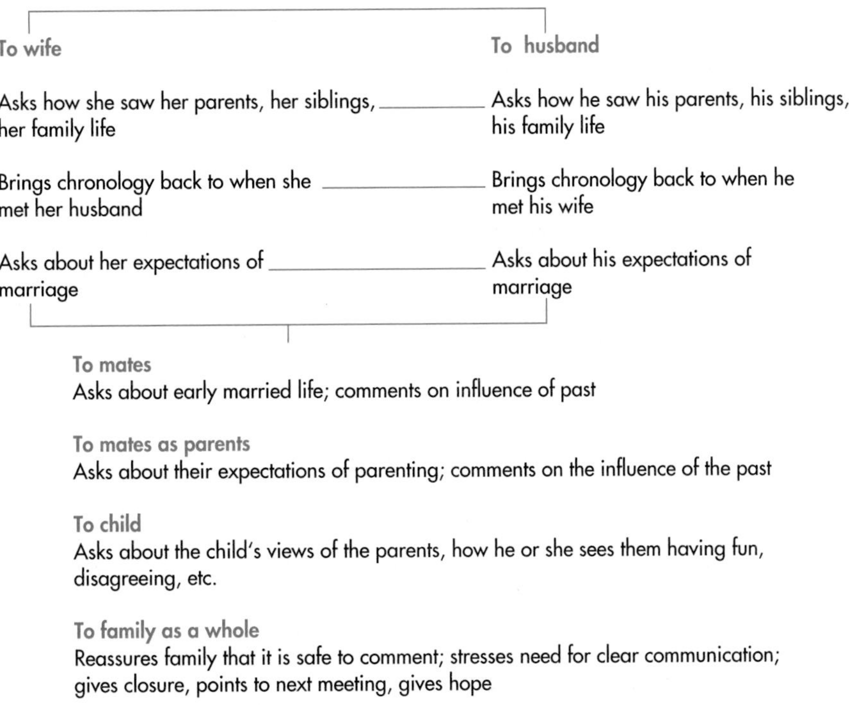

To mates
Asks about how they met, when they decided to marry, etc.
To wife
To husband
Asks how she saw her parents, her siblings, her family life
Asks how he saw his parents, his siblings, his family life
Brings chronology back to when she met her husband
Brings chronology back to when he met his wife
Asks about her expectations of marriage
Asks about his expectations of marriage

To mates
Asks about early married life; comments on influence of past

To mates as parents
Asks about their expectations of parenting; comments on the influence of the past

To child
Asks about the child's views of the parents, how he or she sees them having fun, disagreeing, etc.

To family as a whole
Reassures family that it is safe to comment; stresses need for clear communication; gives closure, points to next meeting, gives hope

Figure 7-10 Main flow of family-life chronology. *(From Satir V:* Conjoint family therapy: a guide to theory and technique, *Palo Alto, Ca., 1967, Science and Behavior Books, p. 135.)*

upset if I am gone from home without him." This woman was depressed and discouraged. Although she loved her children, she also wanted to explore adult interests. To fulfil this need she had to address relationship conflicts with her husband.

When addressing relationship difficulties with a family, it is important for the nurse to facilitate the development of effective family processes. This implies that the nurse avoids forming an alliance with an individual family member and encourages family members to find ways to discuss their differences. "Taking sides" in family conflicts is nontherapeutic and can adversely affect family functioning and the therapeutic relationship.

Videotaping

Videotaping is another tool which helps the community health nurse to assess individual and family functioning. Community health nurses find this tool especially useful when they want to assess family interactions and/or functional abilities of a family member. For example, videotaping can be used to examine how a disabled child is performing activities of daily living. Community health nurses use videotaping in this situation to observe simultaneously the actions of a child and family, as well as the functional capabilities of the client being assessed. It is important to observe both the client and significant others during a functional assessment, because behavior of significant others either inhibits or enhances functional development.

Videotaping provides specific data about family dynamics and a child's functional abilities that are often missed during a home visit. It is easy to overlook small accomplishments of a child when other activities are occurring in the environment. It is equally easy to miss nurse or family behaviors that adversely affect a child's performance. Families are usually receptive to videotaping, especially when the community health nurse explains that a more accurate evaluation of a child's abilities may be obtained through the use of this tool. Assuring them that confidentiality will be maintained also relieves their anxiety.

A videotaped child assessment can be very motivating to families because it dramatically illustrates a child's strengths and needs. Videotaping helps a family to identify positive and negative behaviors that are promoting or inhibiting a child's growth. The impact of seeing actual behaviors is not quickly forgotten.

A unique program, "A Star is Born," uses videotaping to help teenage parents to learn about child growth and development through the first year of life. This parent education program also helps mothers and fathers to identify how their interactions influence their child's emotional and physical development. The "A Star is Born" program is a creative way to help teenagers identify their strengths and needs in relation to parenting and to facilitate parent-infant bonding. It actively engages parents in the learning process and provides a way to role model effective parent-child interactions.

SUMMARY

Despite its changing nature, the family is still considered the basic unit of service in community health nursing settings. Historical evidence from clinical practice and research has sufficiently demonstrated that family-centered nursing services more effectively meet the needs of individuals, families, and communities than do services delivered only to individual clients. However, viewing the family from the traditional perspective is no longer appropriate because alternative family lifestyles and culturally diverse family forms are more prevalent in our society. The nuclear family unit is no longer the only acceptable form of family life.

It is essential for community health nurses to have an understanding of family theory in order to implement a family-centered preventive health approach to nursing care. Theory helps the practitioner to assess family structure, function, and process in an organized and logical fashion. It provides parameters to consider when collecting data about client situations. It assists in explaining the phenomena that are occurring within a family, which in turn helps one to plan effective intervention strategies.

Tools such as the genogram, the eco-map, and family assessment guides are available for facilitating the family assessment process. These tools do not, however, take the place of a genuine understanding of family dynamics. They only provide guidelines for the organization and collection of data.

CRITICAL *Thinking Exercise*

Given the following case situations, discuss how a nursing assessment from a holistic family perspective would differ from a nursing assessment directed toward the identified client (Sally Huling/Cissy Jones).

You are visiting Sally Huling, a 16-year-old teenager recently referred to the Visiting Nurse Association following her hospitalization for regulation of an unstable diabetic condition. Sally lives with her parents, a 10-year-old brother, and a 5-year-old sister in a four-bedroom, well-kept home in a middle-class neighborhood. While she was hospitalized both Sally and her family expressed anxiety about Sally's diabetic condition.

You are visiting Cissy Jones, age 2, who was referred for community health nurse follow-up by the nurse in the well-child clinic because of notable strabismus, and her family. The Jones family's income is minimal. They have inadequate furniture and clothing for their son, age 1 month. Although Mrs. Jones appears tired upon your first home visit, she is anxious to talk about resources for obtaining eye care for Cissy.

REFERENCES

Ackerman NW, ed: *The psychodynamics of family life: diagnosis and treatment of family relationships*, New York, 1959, Basic Books.

Ackerman NW, ed: *Family process*, New York, 1970, Basic Books.

Aldous J: *Family careers: developmental change in families*, New York, 1978, Wiley.

Anderson P, Fenichel D: *Serving culturally diverse families of infants and toddlers with disabilities*, Washington, D.C., 1989, National Center for Clinical Infant Programs.

Artinian NT: Philosophy of science and family nursing theory development. In Whall AL, Fawcett J: *Family theory development in nursing: state of the science and art*, Philadelphia, 1991, FA. Davis, pp. 43-54.

Baca JE: Some health beliefs of the Spanish speaking. In Reinhardt A, Quinn M, eds: *Family-centered community nursing: a sociocultural framework*, St. Louis, 1973, Mosby.

Beavers WR: *Psychotherapy and growth: a family systems perspective*, New York, 1977, Brunner/Mazel.

Bloch B: Bloch's assessment guide for ethnic/cultural variations. In Orque MS, Bloch B, Monrroy LSA, eds: *Ethnic nursing care: a multicultural approach*, St. Louis, 1983, Mosby, pp. 49-75.

Bomar PJ, ed: *Nurses and family health promotion: concepts, assessment, and interventions*, ed 2, Philadelphia, 1996, Saunders.

Boss P: *Family stress management*, Newbury Park, Ca., 1988, Sage.

Bowen M: Toward the differentiation of a self in one's own family. In Framo JL, ed: *Family interaction: a dialogue between family researchers and family therapists*, New York, 1973, Springer.

Bowen M: Italian Americans. In Giger JN, Davidhizar RE: *Transcultural nursing: assessment and intervention*, St. Louis, 1991, Mosby, pp. 293-314.

Bredemeir HC, Stephenson RN: *The analysis of social systems*, New York, 1965, Holt.

Briar S: The family as an organization: an approach to family diagnosis and treatment, *Soc Service Rev* 38:247-255, 1964.

Burr WR, Leigh GK: Famology: a new discipline, *J Marriage Family* 45:467-480, 1983.

Carpenito LJ: *Nursing diagnosis: application to clinical practice*, ed 4, Philadelphia, 1992, JB Lippincott.

Carter B, McGoldrick M, eds: *The changing family life cycle: a framework for family therapy*, ed 2, New York, 1988, Gardner Press.

Cherlin A, Furstenberg F: The American family in the year 2000. In Cornish E, ed: *The 1990s and beyond*, Bethesda, Md., 1990, World Future Society, pp. 23-30.

Cherry B, Giger JN: African-Americans. In Giger JN, Davidhizar RE: *Transcultural nursing: assessment and intervention*, ed 2, St. Louis, 1995, Mosby, pp. 165-203.

Children's Defense Fund: *The state of America's children, yearbook 1992*, Washington, D.C., 1997, The Fund.

Clark AL, ed: *Culture and child bearing*, Philadelphia, 1981, FA Davis.

Clemen (Parks) SJ: *Introduction to health care facility: food services administration*, University Park, Pa., 1974, Pennsylvania State University Press.

Conley L: Childbearing and childrearing practices in Mormonism, *Neonatal Network* 9(3):41-48, 1990.

Danielson C, Hamel-Bissell B, Winstead-Fry P: *Families, health and illness: perspectives on coping and intervention*, St. Louis, 1993, Mosby.

Day JC: *Population projections of the United States, by age, sex, race, and Hispanic origin: 1993 to 2050*, U.S. Bureau of the Census, current population reports, P 25-1104, Washington, D.C., 1993, U.S. Government Printing Office.

Day JC: *Projections of the number of households and families in the United States: 1995 to 2010*, U.S. Bureau of the Census, current population reports, series P 25-1129, Washington, D.C., 1996, U.S. Government Printing Office.

DeSantis L: Cultural factors affecting newborn and infant diarrhea, *J Pediatr Nurs* 3:391-398, 1988.

Duvall EM, Miller BC: *Marriage and family development*, ed 6, New York, 1985, Harper & Row.

Fine MA: Families in the United States: their current status and future prospects, *Family Relations* 41:430-434, 1992.

Fong CM: Ethnicity and nursing practice, *TCN* 7:1-10, 1985.

Francese P: The 100 millionth household, *American Demographics* 18:15-16, 1996.

Friedman MM: *Family nursing: theory and practice*, Norwalk, Ct., 1992, Appleton & Lange.

Fulmer R: Lower-income and professional families: a comparison of structure and life cycle process. In Carter B, McGoldrick M, eds: *The changing family life cycle: a framework for family therapy*, ed 2, New York, 1988, Gardner Press.

Geissler EM: *Pocket guide to cultural assessment*, St. Louis, 1994, Mosby.

Giger JN, Davidhizar RE: *Transcultural nursing: assessment and intervention*, St. Louis, 1991, Mosby.

Giger JN, Davidhizar RE: *Transcultural nursing: assessment and intervention*, ed 2, St. Louis, 1995, Mosby.

Gordon M: *Manual of nursing diagnosis 1997-1998*, St. Louis, 1997, Mosby.

Haley J, ed: *Changing families*, New York, 1971, Grune & Stratton.

Hanley CH: Navajo Indians. In Giger JN, Davidhizar RE: *Transcultural nursing assessment and intervention*, St. Louis, 1991, Mosby, pp. 215-240.

Hanson SM, Boyd ST: *Family health care nursing: theory, practice, and research*, Philadelphia, 1996, F.A. Davis.

Hartman A: Diagrammatic assessment of family relationships, *Social Casework* 59:465-476, 1978.

Heaney CA, Israel BA: Social networks and social support. In Glanz K, Lewis FM, Rimer BK, eds: *Health behavior and health education: theory, research and practice*, ed 2, San Francisco, 1997, Jossey-Bass.

Hill R, Hansen DA: The identification of conceptual frameworks utilized in family study, *Marriage Family Living* 22:299-311, 1960.

Holland S, Sweeney E: *Vietnamese children and families: the impact of culture*, Washington, D.C., 1985, Association for the Care of Children's Health.

Hollingsworth AO, Brown LP, Brooten DA: The refugees and childbearing: what to expect, *RN* 43:45-48, 1980.

Hooyman NR: Social policy and gender inequities in caregiving. In Dwyer J, Coward R, eds: *Gender, families, and elder care*, Newbury Park, Ca., 1992, Sage, pp. 181-201.

Jackson DD, ed: *Communication, family and marriage*, vol 1, Palo Alto, Ca., 1968, Science & Behavior Books.

Janosik E, Green E: *Family life; process and practice*, Boston, 1992, Jones & Bartlett.

Kensky AD: Cultural influences on the Jewish patient. In Clemen SA, Will M, eds: *Family and community health nursing: a workbook*, Ann Arbor, 1977, University of Michigan Press.

King IM: King's theory of nursing. In Clements IW, Roberts FB: *Family health: a theoretical approach in nursing care*, New York, 1983, Wiley, pp. 177-188.

Krentz LG: *Nursing of families and the health care delivery system: workshop proceedings*, Portland, Or., 1989, Oregon Health Sciences University.

Levitan SA, Conway EA: *Families in flux: new approaches to meeting workforce challenges for child, elder, and health care in the 1990s*, Washington, D.C., 1990, The Bureau of National Affairs.

Lewis J, Beavers R, Gossett JT, Phillips VA: *No single thread: psychological health in family systems*, New York, 1976, Brunner/Mazel.

Linton R: The natural history of the family. In Anshen RN, ed: *The family: its function and destiny*, revised ed, New York, 1959, Harper & Row.

Litman TJ: The family as a basic unit in health and medical care: a social-behavioral overview, *Soc Sci Med* 8:495-519, 1974.

Loveland-Cherry C: Family health promotion and health protection. In Bomar PJ, ed: *Nurses and family health promotion: concepts, assessments, and interventions*, ed 2, Philadelphia, 1996, Saunders, pp. 22-35.

Macklin ED: Nontraditional family forms. In Sussman MB, Steinmetz SK, ed: *Handbook of marriage and the family*, New York, 1987, Plenum Press, pp. 317-353.

Maternal and Child Health Bureau: *Child health USA '95*, Washington, D.C., 1996, U.S. Government Printing Office.

McGoldrick M: Ethnicity and the family life cycle. In Carter B, McGoldrick M: *The changing family life cycle: a framework for family therapy*, ed 2, New York, 1988, Gardner Press.

Minuchin S: *Families and family therapy*, Cambridge, Ma., 1974, Harvard University Press.

Neuman B: Family interventions using the Betty Neuman healthcare systems model. In Clements IW, Roberts FB: *Family health; a theoretical approach to nursing care*, New York, 1983, Wiley, pp. 177-188.

Orgue MS, Bloch B, Monrroy LSA: *Ethnic nursing care: a multicultural approach*, St. Louis, 1983, Mosby.

Otto H: Criteria for assessing family strengths, *Family Process* 2:329-338, 1963.

Peterson R: *What are the needs of the chronic mental patients?* Presented at the APA Conference on the Chronic Mental Patient, Washington, D.C., January 11-14, 1978.

Pratt L: *Family structure and effective health behavior: the energized family*, Boston, 1976, Houghton Mifflin.

Prattes O: Beliefs of the Mexican-American family. In Hymovich D, Barnard M, eds: *Family health care*, New York, 1973, McGraw-Hill.

Randall-David E: *Strategies for working with culturally diverse communities and clients*, Washington, D.C., 1989, Association for the Care of Children's Health.

Roccereto L: Selected health beliefs of Vietnamese refugees, *J Sch Health* 51:63-64, 1981.

Rogers ME: Science of unitary human beings: a paradigm for nursing. In Clements IW, Roberts FB: *Family health: a theoretical approach to nursing care*, New York, 1983, Wiley, pp. 255-278.

Roy C: Roy adaptation model. In Clements IW, Roberts FB: *Family health: a theoretical approach to nursing care*, New York, 1983, Wiley, pp. 255-278.

Samora J: Conceptions of health and disease among Spanish-Americans. In Martinez RH, ed: *Hispanic culture and health care; fact, fiction, folklore*, St. Louis, 1978, Mosby.

Satir V: *Conjoint family therapy: a guide to theory and technique*, Palo Alto, Ca., 1967, Science & Behavior Books.

Satir V: *Peoplemaking*, Palo Alto, Ca., 1972, Science & Behavior Books.

Satir V: You as a change agent in helping families to change. In Satir V, Stachowiak J, Taskman H, eds: *Helping families to change*, New York, 1975, Jason Aronson.

Spanier GB: Bequeathing family continuity, *J Marriage Family* 51(2): 3-13, 1989.

Stryker SL: The interactional and situational approaches. In Christensen HT, ed: *Handbook of marriage and the family*, Chicago, 1964, Rand McNally, pp. 125-170.

Sussman MB, chairperson: *Changing families in a changing society, 1970 White House Conference on Children*, Forum 14 report, Washington, D.C., 1971, U.S. Government Printing Office.

Tiedje LB, Darling-Fisher C: Fatherhood reconsidered; a critical review, *Res Nurs Health* 19:471-484, 1996.

Tripp-Reimer T, Brink PJ, Saunders JM: Cultural assessment: content and process, *Nurs Outlook* 32:78-82, 1984.

U.S. Bureau of the Census: *Population profile of the United States: 1993*, current population reports, series P23-185, Washington, D.C., 1993, U.S. Government Printing Office.

U.S. Bureau of the Census: *65+ in the United States*, Washington, D.C., 1996, U.S. Government Printing Office.

U.S. Bureau of the Census: *How we're changing: demographic state of the nation: 1996*, Washington, D.C., 1996, U.S. Government Printing Office.

U.S. Bureau of the Census: *Statistical abstract of the United States: 1996*, ed 116, Washington, D.C., 1996, U.S. Government Printing Office.

von Bertalanffy L: *General systems theory*, New York, 1968, George Braziller.

Watzlawick P, Beavin JH, Jackson DD: *Pragmatics of human communication: a study of interactional patterns, pathologies, and paradoxes*, New York, 1967, Norton.

Whall AL: Family system theory: relationship to nursing conceptual models. In Whall AL, Fawcett J: *Family theory development in nursing: state of the science and art*, Philadelphia, 1991, F.A. Davis, pp. 317-342.

Whall AL, Fawcett J: *Family theory development in nursing: state of the science and art*, Philadelphia, 1991, F.A. Davis.

White House Conference on Families, 1978, joint hearings before the subcommittee on Child and Human Development of the Committee on Human Resources, U.S. Senate and the Subcommittee on Select Education of the Committee on Education and Labor, House of Representatives, Ninety-fifth Congress, Washington, D.C., 1978, U.S. Government Printing Office.

Wong DL: *Whaley and Wong's nursing care of infants and children*, ed 5, St. Louis, 1995, Mosby.

Wright LM, Leahey M: *Nurses and families: a guide to family assessment and intervention*, ed 2, Philadelphia, 1994, F.A. Davis.

SELECTED BIBLIOGRAPHY

Allen ML, Brown P, Finlay B: *Helping children by strengthening families: a look at family*, Washington, D.C., 1992, Children's Defense Fund.

Bomar PJ: *Nurses and family health promotion: concepts, assessment, and interventions*, ed 2, Philadelphia, 1996, Saunders.

Friedman MM: *Family nursing: theory and practice*, Norwalk, Ct., 1997, Appleton-Century-Crofts.

Gilliss CL, Highley BL, Roberts BM, Martinson IM: *Toward a science of family nursing*, Menlo Park, Ca., 1989, Addison-Wesley.

Hanson SMH and Boyd ST: *Family health care nursing: theory, practice, and research*, Philadelphia, 1996, F.A. Davis.

Jung M: Family-centered practice with single-parent families, *Families in Society: J Contemporary Human Services* 77:583-591, 1996.

Kelly P: Family-centered practice with stepfamilies, *Families in Society: J Contemporary Human Services* 77:535-544, 1996.

Lapp CA, Diemert CA, Enestvedt R: Family-based practice discussion of a tool merging assessment with intervention, *Fam Community Health* 12:21-28, 1990.

Leininger M: Culture care theory, research, and practice, *Nurs Sci Q* 9:71-78, 1996.

Martin M, Henery M: Cultural relativity and poverty, *Public Health Nurs* 6:28-34, 1989.

McGoldrick M, Gerson R: *Genograms in family assessment*, New York, 1985, W.W. Norton.

Speer JJ, Sachs B: Selecting the appropriate family assessment tool, *Pediatr Nurs* 11:349-355, 1985.

Wagner GD, Alexander RJ: *Readings in family nursing*, Philadelphia, 1993, Lippincott.

Whall AL: The family as the unit of care in nursing: a historical review, *Public Health Nurs* 3:240-249, 1986.

Whall AL: *Family therapy theory for nursing: four approaches*, Norwalk, Ct., 1987, Appleton-Century-Crofts.

Wright LM, Leahey M: *Nurses and families: a guide to family assessment and intervention*, Philadelphia, 1994, F.A. Davis.

Zambrana RE: *Understanding Latino families: scholarship, policy, and practice*, Thousand Oaks, Ca., 1995, Sage.

8

Foundations for Family Intervention: Families Under Stress

OBJECTIVES

Upon completion of this chapter, the reader should be able to:

1. Discuss the concepts of stress and crisis as they relate to family functioning.
2. Describe factors that affect the outcome of a family crisis.
3. Identify characteristics that signal ineffective individual or family coping during periods of stress and crisis.
4. Differentiate between normative and nonnormative stressors and give examples of each type of stressor.
5. Describe general principles that the community health nurse should apply when giving constructive assistance to families during periods of stress and crisis.
6. Explain nursing intervention strategies used by community health nurses to promote effective family functioning during periods of stress and crisis.
7. Describe how culture influences perceptions of stress and crisis.

Accept me as I am so I may learn what I can become.

A major responsibility of the community health nurse is to help individuals and families handle stressful life events so that their energies can be used to achieve self-fulfillment and to develop a capacity to extend themselves to others. Some stress is normal and essential for life and growth. Stress provides the stimulus needed to adapt to the ever-changing conditions of life. Too much stress, however, prevents people from seeing what "they can become."

When he examined individual stress, Selye (1976, p. xv) found that any emotion or activity, whether it produces joy or sadness, causes stress. He noted that stressful life events often result in disease and unhappiness when individuals are not prepared to handle them. Persons frequently are not prepared to handle unexpected stressors, such as a new diagnosis of a chronic illness or the accidental death of a close family member. Individuals who encounter these types of stressors often do not recognize the signals of distress that reflect a need to mobilize different coping mechanisms.

From a family perspective, Boss (1988) defines stress "as pressure or tension in the family system. It is disturbance in the steady state of the family" (p. 12). This disturbance results from events or situations that have potential to cause change, and it is normal and even desirable at times (Boss). Stress is a dynamic state that can assist families in mobilizing stress management processes that promote growth for the family as a whole, as well as for individual family members. Boss contends that when addressing stress within a family system "the focus on the family system should not come at the expense of individuals within that system" (p. 19). However, she does believe that the stress level of the family unit, as well as individual family members, should be assessed when a change occurs in the family system. Both the family unit and individual family members may need assistance in coping with this change.

Community health nurses are in a key position to help individuals and families adapt to new or threatening life changes. In their work in the home and other settings they encounter clients who are experiencing various degrees of stress. Many times these clients have not had life experiences or exposure to knowledge that would assist them in altering patterns of functioning that intensify stress. Most parents, for instance, have not been prepared to handle children whose growth and development significantly deviate from the norm. Hence they experience heightened distress and are frequently open to professional intervention. Illustrative of this is the scenario encountered by a community health nurse when she visited the Slavovi family for the first time.

CASE *Scenario*

The Slavovi family was referred to the community health nurse for health supervision follow-up after the birth of their fourth child, Stephanie, who had multiple disabilities. Even though this was the family's first exposure to community health nursing service, Mr. and Mrs. Slavovi talked freely when the nurse visited. Both manifested high levels of anxiety and confusion about how to care for their newborn infant. Mr. and Mrs. Slavovi had always taken great pride in being good parents. Stephanie's physical and mental disabilities were particularly distressing to them: "We don't know how to help her. She continues to cry even when we hold her and seems to hurt all the time. Children need loving. Why doesn't Stephanie want us to hold her? We must be doing something wrong."

Having an understanding of the concept of stress helps the community health nurse to intervene more effectively with clients like the Slavovis. Stress theory provides the foundation for identifying signs and symptoms of distress and for recognizing potential stressors. It also provides clues about how to bring about change when a client's usual methods of coping are no longer effective.

THE STRESS PHENOMENON

Although the term *stress* dates back to the fourteenth century, Hans Selye's work on the physiological and psychological effects of stress on the human body (see the accompanying box) during the twentieth century played a major role in strengthening the scientific nature of this concept (Lazarus, Folkman, 1984). Selye (1976) defined stress as "the nonspecific response of the body to any demand" (p. 1). A demand that produces stress is known as a *stressor*. Selye noted that a stressor can produce unpleasant or disease-producing stress, known as *distress*, or good, pleasant, or curative stress, known as *eustress*.

A nonspecific set of responses in the nervous and endocrine systems alerts individuals to the occurrence of distress or eustress. According to Selye (1976), this set of responses evolves in three stages, which he labeled the general adaptation syndrome (GAS):

1. The *alarm reaction*, during which defense mechanisms are mobilized.
2. The *stage of resistance*, when adaptation is acquired because optimum channels of defense were developed.
3. The *stage of exhaustion*, which reflects a depletion of adaptation energy necessary to cope with prolonged and intensified stress. (p. 163)

Stress theory is based on the concepts of homeostasis (state of physiological balance) and adaptation. Because stress is an inherent and integral part of life, individuals must constantly readjust to maintain themselves. A state of balance is maintained when a person learns to recognize the signals of distress and then adapts or changes functioning to meet the demands of the stressor encountered. There are significant differences in how individuals respond to and cope with stress.

Lazarus's (1966) work on psychological stress highlighted the importance of examining individual responses to environmental demands and pressures. He believed that "although certain environmental demands and pressures produce stress in a substantial number of people, individual and group differences in the degree and kind of reaction are always evident" (Lazarus, Folkman, 1984, p. 22). For example, many people perceive job loss as a significant threat to their financial security, but some individuals view this event as a challenging opportunity for growth. This difference is influenced by a person's cognitive appraisal of a stressor event. "Psychological stress is a particular relationship between the person and the environment that is appraised by the person as taxing or exceeding his or her resources and endangering his or her well-being" (Lazarus, Folkman, p. 19). The factors that influence an individual's cognitive appraisal of a stressor event are discussed in a later section of this chapter.

Examples of Physiological and Psychological Signals of Stress

PHYSIOLOGICAL SIGNALS

Pounding of the heart
Dryness of the throat and mouth
Sweating
Frequent need to urinate
Diarrhea, indigestion, vomiting
Migraine headaches
Missed menstrual period
Loss of or excessive appetite
Increased smoking and alcohol and drug use
Increased use of legally prescribed drugs (e.g., tranquilizers or amphetamines)
Pain in neck or lower back

PSYCHOLOGICAL SIGNALS

General irritability, hyperexcitation or depression
Impulsive behavior, emotional instability
Overpowering urge to cry or run and hide
Inability to concentrate, flight of thoughts, and general disorientation
Floating anxiety
Trembling, nervous tics
Nightmares
Neurotic or psychotic behavior
Accident proneness

From Selye H: *The stress of life*, New York, 1976, McGraw-Hill, 174-177.

FAMILY STRESS

Boss (1988) believes that families "have a distinctive quality apart from the individuals making up the family" (p. 18). In keeping with this view, she assumes "that a family system has a character of its own and that this unity produces the variable, family perception" (p. 19). This perception influences the family's appraisal of stressful events or change in the family system and the coping processes mobilized by the family during periods of stress. Like individuals, there are significant differences in how families respond to and cope with stressor events in their environment.

In terms of the family, stress is manifested by ineffective family patterns, as well as by the occurrence of physiological and psychological signs and symptoms of stress in its individual family members. Strained communication patterns and difficulty carrying out activities of daily living are examples of ineffective family patterns that may result when a family is experiencing stress. Other examples are shared in Chapter 7.

All individuals and families have the capacity to deal with distress. However, in order to do so they need to learn the boundaries of stress that they can tolerate and the nurturing, coping, and adaptive resources that promote growth and homeostasis. Complex and dynamic interactions between multiple variables influence a family's abilities to effectively mobilize resources to prevent crisis. Hill (1949, p. 9; 1965), the father of family stress theory, illustrated this complexity in his classic ABCX model of family stress. He proposed that the interactions between the following factors influence whether a family under stress experiences a crisis:

A (the event and associated hardships) ⟶ interacting with **B** (the family's crisis-meeting resources, its role structure, flexibility, and previous history with crisis) ⟶ interacting with **C** (the definition the family makes of the event) ⟶ produces **X** (crisis).

Hill believed that a crisis-prone family was one who experienced stressor events with great frequency and severity (A), defined these events more frequently as crisis-provoking (C), had meager crisis-meeting resources (B), and had failed to learn from past experience with crises (Hill, 1965, p. 40).

Most family stress theorists have built on the work of Reuben Hill and confirm and expand his theories about the dynamic and complex nature of family stress and coping (Boss, 1987, 1988; McCubbin, McCubbin, 1987, 1991, 1993; McCubbin, Patterson, 1983, 1991). McCubbin and McCubbin (1993) have proposed that seldom is a single stressor at the root of family crisis; rather a "pile up of stressors" causes crisis situations in families. Family vulnerability to stress, "ranging from high to low, is determined by (1) the accumulation, or pile up, of demands on or within the family unit, such as financial debts, poor health status of relatives, and changes in a parent's work role or work environment, and (2) the trials and tribulations associated with the family's particular life-cycle stage with all of its demands and changes" (p. 28).

McCubbin, Thompson, and McCubbin (1996) focus on family change and adaptation over time and examine adaptation-oriented components during and beyond the initial crisis. They believe that a family's adjustment during periods of stress is influenced by several variables: (1) the severity of the stressor; (2) the pile up of stressors; (3) the family's perception of the stressors; (4) the family's established patterns of functioning; and (5) the family's abilities and capabilities to address and manage the stressor without introducing major changes in the family system (McCubbin, Thompson, McCubbin). Crisis usually results when new patterns of functioning or major changes in the family system are needed to deal with the demands of the stressor.

STRESSOR EVENTS

"A stressor event is an occurrence that is of significant magnitude to provoke change in the family system" (Boss, 1988, p. 36). Although stress and crisis are basically matters of individual perceptions, certain life events have frequently been found to increase a family's risk for stress and crisis. These events are viewed as normative or developmental, nonnormative or situational, or a combination of the two. Stressor events produce change in a family system that necessitates mobilizing the family's coping processes. *Stressor events lead to crisis only when the family is unable to adapt effectively to the changes brought about by the event* (Boss).

Normative stressors occur across the life spectrum. They relate to critical transition points in the course of normal human development that involve many physical, psychological, and social changes. These transition stages, such as entry into school, puberty, starting a career, moving from home (Figure 8-1), marriage, parenthood, middlescence, retirement, and facing one's own death from aging, promote change in a family system. Normative stressors were identified by the developmental family theorists (see Chapter 7). Although they are predictable, they often require significant role change and produce heightened stress. The role changes that occur during these *anticipated* events are discussed in Chapters 15 through 20.

Nonnormative stressors also occur across the life span, but they are usually *not anticipated* and frequently are highly stressful. Nonnormative stressors are events such as divorce, illness, accident, change in social status, cultural relocation, and premature death of a significant other. Since nonnormative stressor events often *occur suddenly* and *are unexpected*, individuals and families must deal with these events without benefit of anticipatory problem solving. This makes individuals and families more vulnerable to crisis or negative outcomes.

Sometimes normative and nonnormative stressor events occur simultaneously. When this happens, individual and family adjustment and adaptive energies become seriously overtaxed. Multiple stressors make it more difficult for persons to realistically appraise the changes that are occurring and to adjust their coping style to accommodate them. For example, a 5-year-old child who has recently changed cultural settings must deal with stresses related to school entry in addition to those related to living in a new environment. School entry in itself is often very traumatic. This, coupled with the pressures that result from relocation such as learning a different language, developing all new friendships, and adjusting to an unfamiliar lifestyle, can be overwhelming.

American families are experiencing a number of nonnormative stressors (see the box on the next page). Environmental conditions and lifestyle patterns are placing them at risk for situations such as domestic violence, criminal victimization, unexpected disasters, economic distress, and infectious diseases. Supportive family intervention can assist families in dealing with these stressors.

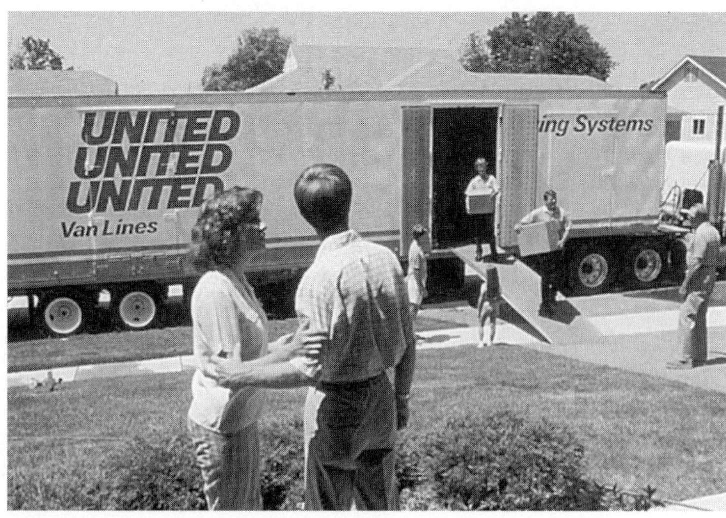

Figure 8-1 Moving is a normal transition event, but it can cause a great deal of stress. *(Courtesy United Van Lines.)*

Stress and Crisis Among America's Families

VICTIMS OF CRIME AND VIOLENCE[d]

- The United States ranks first among industrialized nations in violent death rates.
- Homicide and suicide claim more than 50,000 lives each year in the United States.
- Annually over 2 million people are injured by violent assaults.

WIDESPREAD UNINTENDED PREGNANCIES[a]

- Almost 60% of all pregnancies in the United States are unintended pregnancies.
- Annually, unintended pregnancy leads to approximately 1.5 million abortions in the United States.
- In 1990 about 44% of all births were the result of unintended pregnancy, with the proportion being significantly higher among women in poverty (60%), among black women (62%), among never-married women (73%), and among unmarried teenagers (86%).

POVERTY IS PREVALENT[b,e]

- In the United States a child is born into poverty every 32 seconds.
- In 1994 a total of 38 million persons lived in poverty, including 14.6 million children.
- In 1994 44% of families with a female householder, no husband present, and children 18 years of age and under had incomes below the poverty level.
- Almost two thirds of both black children and Hispanic children who live with a single mother live below the federal poverty level.

HOMELESSNESS IS GROWING[f]

- By the mid-1980s the number of homeless people had surpassed anything seen since the Great Depression.
- On any given night up to 600,000 Americans are literally homeless.
- Homeless families with children, over 80% of whom are headed by a single mother, make up about one fifth of homeless persons.
- A significant number of vulnerable persons on public housing waiting lists and involuntarily doubled up with friends and relatives are on the edge of homelessness.

DISPARITIES IN HEALTH CARE ACCESS[e]

- In 1993 it was estimated that 39.7 million Americans, or 15.3%, were without health insurance.
- In 1993 20.5% of blacks and 31.6% of Hispanics were uninsured.
- In 1993 almost 30% of uninsured women 25 to 64 years of age, regardless of poverty status, had no regular source of medical care, compared with less than 10% of women who were insured.

INEFFECTIVE STRESS MANAGEMENT[b,c,d]

- In 1994 over 1 million children were victims of substantial or indicated child abuse and neglect.
- Between 21% and 30% of all women in the United States are estimated to have been beaten by a partner at least once.
- Substance abuse is estimated to be the actual cause of some 120,000 deaths per year.
- An estimated 41.4 million adults have had a mental disorder at some time in their lives.

Data from [a]Institute of Medicine. *The best intentions: unintended pregnancy and the well-being of children and families*, Washington, D.C., 1995, National Academy of Sciences; [b]Maternal and Child Health Bureau. *Child health USA '95*, Washington, D.C., 1996, U.S. Government Printing Office; [c]USDHHS: *Healthy people 2000: national health promotion and disease prevention objectives, full report, with commentary*, Washington, D.C., 1991, U.S. Government Printing Office; [d]USDHHS: *Healthy people 2000: midcourse review and 1995 revisions*, Washington, D.C., 1995, U.S. Government Printing Office; [e]USDHHS: *Health, United States, 1995*, Hyattsville, Md., 1996, Public Health Service; [f]USDHUD: *Priority: home! The federal plan to break the cycle of homelessness*, Washington, D.C., 1994, USDHUD.

MEASUREMENT OF STRESSOR EVENTS

Research since the early 1960s has documented that significant life changes can adversely affect the health status of individuals (Rahe, 1972). The Life Change Questionnaire (see Appendix 8-1), developed by Holmes, Rahe, Masuda, and others, has been used to demonstrate the relationships between a cluster of events requiring life changes and illness. It has been shown that individuals whose life change units (LCU) are greater than the value of 150 in a year's time are more susceptible to illness than individuals whose life change units are below this value. Studies conducted by Rahe demonstrated that 50% of the individuals whose life change units ranged from 150 to 300 LCU had an illness within the following year. In addition, 70% of those individuals whose LCU values exceeded 300 had an illness the following year (Rahe).

Based on the recognition that the types of life change events that produce stress vary across the life span, research has been conducted to increase the relevance of the life event questionnaire for a particular age group or for specific population groups. For example, Norbeck (1984) modified the life event questionnaire to address the needs of adult females of childbearing age. Norbeck's modified tool deals with significant concerns of women, such as having difficulties with contraception, changing child care arrangements, being the victim of violent acts (e.g., rape and assault), and parenting conflicts.

Barnard's (1988) Difficult Life Circumstance (DLC) scale was designed to ascertain the existence of chronic family problems among high-risk families dealing with pregnancy. The items on the DLC scale address such things as domestic violence, child abuse, long-term illness, and problems with alcohol and drug use. Barnard found that families with a high DLC score (a score reflecting the existence of several difficult life circumstances) had less favorable maternal and family outcomes than families with a low DLC score.

Beall and Schmidt (1984) developed a tool for use with adolescents (see Appendix 8-2). The Youth Adaptation Rating Scale is not designed to be used as a predictor of illness. Rather, it was developed "to measure the causes of adolescent adaptation and stress during the adolescent years" (Beall, Schmidt, p. 197). This tool was tested in a variety of settings and by six ethnic groups. Adolescents were asked to rank each item on the tool using a five-point descriptive scale, with zero indicating that the event was not stressful at all and five reflecting a very stressful event that would require a major change in one's life. No significant differences existed between the ethnic groups or the adolescents from communities of different sizes. It was found, however, that the need for adaptation or the recognition of that need becomes more evident as the adolescent grows older and matures (Beall, Schmidt).

Practitioners as well as researchers use life change questionnaires to identify *individuals* at risk for illness. When they discover individuals who are dealing with significant life changes, they discuss the effect of these changes on one's health status and the importance of not making other major life changes at this time.

Family Life Events and Changes

As previously discussed, "families have a distinctive quality apart from the individuals making up the family" which is known as a "*family perception*" (Boss, 1988). To capture a family's perception of stress, McCubbin, Patterson, and Wilson developed the Family Inventory of Life Events and Changes (FILE). FILE examines a family's perception of a range of normative and nonnormative life events (Figure 8-2) and identifies how many of the specified 71 stressors have occurred within the family unit in the past year. Standardized family weights ranging from 21 to 99 have been assigned to each item on FILE to indicate the relative stressfulness of a life event or family change. These weights are included on the file instrument (McCubbin, Thompson, McCubbin, 1996).

In clinical practice FILE is used to assist practitioners in identifying families who are experiencing a pile up of stressors, which makes families more vulnerable to crisis or negative outcomes (McCubbin, Patterson, 1991). The FILE is either completed by the adult family members together, or separately by each partner. If either or both partners record a *yes* on an item, the family couple score is a yes. A high total family/couple score implies high stress. Low-, moderate-, and high-stress scores vary across the seven stages of the family life cycle (McCubbin, Patterson). Scores considered high by family stage are: couple stage (720+), preschool stage (840+), school-age stage (735+), adolescent stage (850+), launching stage (950+), empty nest stage (690+), and retirement stage (700+). The reader is encouraged to review scoring procedures in McCubbin and Patterson (1991) and McCubbin, Thompson, and McCubbin (1996) before using FILE.

FILE provides a guide for quickly assessing a family's level of stress. Families with high-stress scores are helped to analyze their current family situation and how they can mobilize family resources to reduce the demands in their lives. Although families with moderate stress scores fall within the normal range of stressors, these families are particularly vulnerable to future stressful events. They should be counseled about their vulnerability and helped to identify family capabilities that can help them to eliminate or mediate the impact of demands in their lives (McCubbin, Patterson, 1991; McCubbin, Thompson, McCubbin, 1996).

EFFECTS OF CULTURE ON PERCEPTIONS OF STRESS

Cultural patterns of the family must be considered when assessing client situations during periods of stress. Cultural characteristics of families influence their perceptions about the causes of sickness and stress, the meaning and treatment of illness, appropriate coping behaviors, self-care activities,

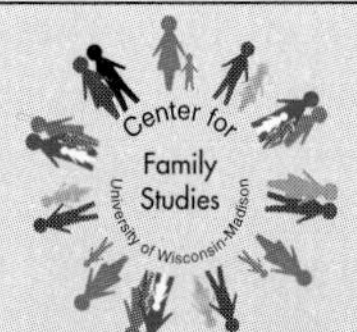

Family Stress, Coping and Health Project
School of Human Ecology
1300 Linden Drive
University of Wisconsin-Madison
Madison, WI 53706

FILE
Family Inventory of Life Events and Changes©

Purpose:

Over their life cycle, all families experience many changes as a result of normal growth and development of members and due to external circumstances. The following list of family life changes can happen in a family at any time. Because family members are connected to each other in some way, a life change for any one member affects all the other persons in the family to some degree.

*"**Family**" means a group of two or more persons living together who are related by blood, marriage or adoption. This includes persons who live with you and to whom you have a long term commitment.*

Directions:

"Did the change happen in your family?"
Please read each family life change and decide whether it happened to any member of your family —**including you** — during the past 12 months and check **Yes** or **No**.

Did the change happen in your family:	During the last 12 months Yes	No	Score
I. Intrafamily Strains			
1. Increase of husband/father's time away from family	○	○	**46**
2. Increase of wife/mother's time away from family	○	○	**51**
3. A member appears to have emotional problems	○	○	**58**
4. A member appears to depend on alcohol or drugs	○	○	**66**
5. Increase in conflict between husband and wife	○	○	**53**
6. Increase in arguments between parent(s) and child(ren)	○	○	**45**
7. Increase in conflict among children in the family	○	○	**48**
8. Increased difficulty in managing teenage child(ren)	○	○	**55**
9. Increased difficulty in managing school age child(ren) (6-12 yrs)	○	○	**39**
10. Increased difficulty in managing preschool age child(ren) (2.5-6 yrs)	○	○	**36**
11. Increased difficulty in managing toddler(s) (1-2.5 yrs.)	○	○	**36**
12. Increased difficulty in managing infant(s) (0-1 yr.)	○	○	**35**
13. Increase in the amount of "outside activities" which the children are involved in	○	○	**25**
14. Increased disagreement about a member's friends or activities	○	○	**35**
15. Increase in the number of problems or issues which don't get resolved	○	○	**45**
16. Increase in the number of tasks or chores which don't get done	○	○	**35**
17. Increased conflict with in-laws or relatives	○	○	**40**

©1983 H. McCubbin

Continued

Figure 8-2 FILE: Family Inventory of Life Events and Changes. *(From McCubbin H, Patterson J, Wilson L: FILE: Family Inventory of Life Events and Changes. In McCubbin HI, Thompson AI, McCubbin MA, eds:* Family assessment: resiliency, coping and adaptation—inventories for research and practice, *Madison, Wi., 1996, University of Wisconsin System, pp. 142-145.)*

Did the change happen in your family:	During the last 12 months Yes	No	Score
II. Marital Strains 18. Spouse/parent was separated or divorced	◯	◯	**79**
19. Spouse/parent had an "affair"	◯	◯	**68**
20. Increased difficulty in resolving issues with a "former" or separated spouse	◯	◯	**47**
21. Increased difficulty with sexual relationship between husband and wife	◯	◯	**58**
III. Pregnancy and Childbearing Strains 22. Spouse had unwanted or difficult pregnancy	◯	◯	**45**
23. An unmarried member became pregnant	◯	◯	**65**
24. A member had an abortion	◯	◯	**50**
25. A member gave birth to or adopted a child	◯	◯	**50**
IV. Finance and Business Strains 26. Took out a loan or refinanced a loan to cover increased expenses	◯	◯	**29**
27. Went on welfare	◯	◯	**55**
28. Change in conditions (economic, political, weather) which hurts the family investments	◯	◯	**41**
29. Change in agriculture market, stock market, or land values which hurts family investments and/or income	◯	◯	**43**
30. A member started a new business	◯	◯	**50**
31. Purchased or built a home	◯	◯	**41**
32. A member purchased a car or other major item	◯	◯	**19**
33. Increased financial debts due to over-use of credit cards	◯	◯	**31**
34. Increased strain on family "money" for medical/dental expenses	◯	◯	**23**
35. Increased strain on family "money" for food, clothing, energy, home care	◯	◯	**21**
36. Increased strain on family "money" for child(ren)'s education	◯	◯	**22**
37. Delay in receiving child support or alimony payments	◯	◯	**41**
V. Work-Family Transitions and Strains 38. A member changed to a new job/career	◯	◯	**40**
39. A member lost or quit a job	◯	◯	**55**
40. A member retired from work	◯	◯	**48**
41. A member started or returned to work	◯	◯	**41**
42. A member stopped working for extended period (e.g., laid off, leave of absence, strike)	◯	◯	**51**
43. Decrease in satisfaction with job/career	◯	◯	**45**
44. A member had increased difficulty with people at work	◯	◯	**32**
45. A member was promoted at work or given more responsibilities	◯	◯	**40**

Continued

Figure **8-2, cont'd**

Did the change happen in your family:	During the last 12 months Yes	No	Score
46. Family moved to a new home/apartment	○	○	43
47. A child/adolescent member changed to a new school	○	○	24
VI. Illness and Family "Care" Strains 48. Parent/spouse became seriously ill or injured	○	○	44
49. Child became seriously ill or injured	○	○	35
50. Close relative or friend of the family became seriously ill	○	○	44
51. A member became physically disabled or chronically ill	○	○	73
52. Increased difficulty in managing a chronically ill or disabled member	○	○	58
53. Member or close relative was committed to an institution or nursing home	○	○	44
54. Increased responsibility to provide direct care or financial help to husband's and/or wife's parents	○	○	47
55. Experienced difficulty in arranging for satisfactory child care	○	○	40
VII. Losses 56. A parent/spouse died	○	○	98
57. A child member died	○	○	99
58. Death of husband's or wife's parent or close relative	○	○	48
59. Close friend of the family died	○	○	47
60. Married son or daughter was separated or divorced	○	○	58
61. A member "broke up" a relationship with a close friend	○	○	35
VIII. Transitions "In and Out" 62. A member was married	○	○	42
63. Young adult member left home	○	○	43
64. Young adult member began college (or post high school training)	○	○	28
65. A member moved back home or a new person moved into the household	○	○	42
66. A parent/spouse started school (or training program) after being away from school for a long time	○	○	38
IX. Family Legal Violations 67. A member went to jail or juvenile detention	○	○	68
68. A member was picked up by police or arrested	○	○	57
69. Physical or sexual abuse or violence in the home	○	○	75
70. A member ran away from home	○	○	61
71. A member dropped out of school or was suspended from school	○	○	38

Figure **8-2, cont'd**

relationships with health care providers and significant others, and expression of stress and discomfort (Ailinger, 1985; Capers, 1985; Davitz, Sameshima, Davitz, 1976; Germain, 1992; Kleinman, Eisenberg, Good, 1978; Lewis, Messner, McDowell, 1985; Ross, 1981; Snow, 1974; Sobralske, 1985; Villarruel, Ortiz de Montellano, 1992).

When considering the effects of culture on perceptions of stress, it is important to understand that scientists and anthropologists have distinguished between the terms *illness* and *disease* to help them explain why health professionals and clients can differ in their views of a hazardous event. Illness does not necessarily correlate with the biomedical interpretation of disease. In Western culture, what an individual/family feels and expresses in terms of stress and discomfort is labeled *illness*. *Disease*, on the other hand, is a physician-diagnosed condition that deviates from clearly defined norms. In terms of these culturally defined definitions, illness can occur in the absence of disease and vice versa (Giger, Davidhizar, 1995; Twaddle, 1981). It is important to differentiate between these concepts because "where only disease is treated, care will be less satisfactory to the patient and less clinically effective than where both disease and illness are treated together" (Kleinman, Eisenberg, Good, 1978).

Kleinman, Eisenberg, and Good (1978, p. 252) believe that illness is culturally shaped in the sense that it is individually perceived—that is, how individuals and families experience and cope with disease is based on their explanations of sickness. In clinical practice it is not uncommon to encounter a wide variation in families' and individuals' explanations of sickness. While community health nurses encounter many clients whose beliefs are consistent with the Western biomedical model, which focuses on scientific explanations for disease and illness occurrence, they also work with many families whose beliefs about health and illness have evolved from the folk medicine system.

Snow (1974), in his classic article on folk medical beliefs, noted that these beliefs promote both natural and unnatural explanations for illness. According to Snow, *natural* explanations emphasize that there is a direct connection between the body and the forces of nature, and that there is safety in harmony and balance and danger in anything that is done to interfere with natural processes. Natural illnesses occur when the individual is inadequately protected against the forces of nature such as cold air and impurities in food, water, and air, or when there is an imbalance between natural forces (Snow). Community health nurses find that families holding these beliefs will take measures to protect themselves against dangerous elements in nature. For example, Chinese families may overdress their infants to prevent cold air from entering their children's bodies (Wong, 1995).

A commonly held natural imbalance supported by the Hispanic, Filipino, and Arab cultures is that which exists between "cold" and "hot," or yin (cold) and yang (hot) in the Chinese culture (Chang, 1995; Wong, 1995). This belief classifies illnesses, foods, areas of the body, and medicines according to intrinsic hot and cold properties (Snow, 1974). These properties can both cause illnesses and treat them and must be kept in balance to maintain health. Persons holding those beliefs will eat yin/cold foods such as honey, vegetables, and fruits when they have a disease with excessive yang/hot forces such as infections, fever, and hypertension (Ludman, Newman, 1984). Crucial to these beliefs are the implications they hold for nursing practice, because community health nurses who respect cultural differences work with families within the context of their cultural perspectives. They may, for instance, assist families in maintaining the harmony of nature by planning a balanced diet with them that avoids hot or cold food at given times.

Not all illnesses have folk explanations involving the disruption of forces in nature. Some result when individuals fall out of favor with the Lord and an evil influence or the devil takes over. Others are caused by witchcraft. "Witchcraft is based on the belief that there are individuals with the ability to mobilize unusual powers for good or evil" (Snow, 1974, p. 85). Snow found that belief in witchcraft as a cause of illness is widespread among Haitians, Trinidadians, Puerto Rican Americans, American blacks, and Mexican-Americans.

Illnesses that result from supernatural evil influences or forces beyond nature have been labeled *unnatural* by Snow (1974). Evil forces can cause all types of physical and mental health stresses that are frightening to families because they cannot be cured by natural remedies or health personnel. A common health belief found among people from Latin American, South Asian, Near Eastern, and some African societies is the belief in the evil eye (Pasquale, 1984). This phenomenon involves the belief that the gaze of the human eye can bring illness and misfortune to people. "Envy is the pivotal emotion that activates people's ability to cause harm and misfortune to others" (Pasquale, p. 32). According to Pasquale, the evil eye phenomenon is a cluster of beliefs that associates people's internal strength-weakness states with the power of the evil eye. When these states are in balance individuals are not likely to cast or fall victim to the evil eye. However, when people have an excess of envy their strength increases and they are capable of casting the evil eye intentionally or unintentionally. Children are particularly vulnerable to the gaze of the evil eye because their internal strength-weakness states are immature. People exposed to the evil eye often have a sudden onset of illness and may have a variety of symptoms such as fever, nausea, diarrhea, and nervousness. Preventive and treatment measures for the evil eye phenomenon usually involve supernatural rituals carried out by the client or approved healers (Pasquale). For example, Hindus paint a spot of lamp-black on children's foreheads as a precautionary measure against the evil eye (Maloney, 1976).

A knowledge of folk health beliefs can assist the community health nurse in understanding clients from the client's perspective and may prevent a client from being labeled noncompliant. This knowledge can also help the nurse to avoid unintentional involvement in spell-casting, such as giving the evil eye when admiring a new baby during a home visit. Lack of understanding can create barriers to therapeutic nursing intervention. When visiting clients from differing cultures it is important to remember that folk explanations for sickness are not limited to the poor and uneducated. Clients from all socioeconomic levels believe in folk explanations for illness (Pasquale, 1984). It is also important to remember that there is significant intracultural variation in relation to health beliefs and practices. As families from different cultures assimilate Western beliefs, some of their traditions are relinquished and others are retained (Louie, 1985). However, folk medical beliefs continue to be documented in the client-health care professional relationship (Eckholm, 1990; Kay, Yoder, 1987).

It should be obvious at this point that similar stressful events can be variously interpreted by clients based on the differing explanatory models of health and illness used by them: a serious infection may be blamed on germs, on evil influences, on impurities in the water, on the entry of cold air into the body of a susceptible individual, or on divine punishment. This in turn affects clients' perceptions about the seriousness of the infection, needed treatment regimens, and acceptance of therapeutic interventions. Illustrative of this are the beliefs held by many Spanish-speaking people. Often they view illness and pain as punishment from God for evil deeds and believe they must accept suffering to atone for their sins. As a result they may refuse pain relievers and nursing care and may engage in various types of penance (Ross, 1981).

Since the meaning of illness and stress is individually perceived within a person's cultural context and self-concept, serious stressful events may or may not evolve into a crisis. Individuals and families who interpret these events as challenges to accomplish significant life goals are often able to develop coping mechanisms to effectively deal with their distress. However, if they perceive stressful events as the will of God, a spirit possession, or events out of their control, a crisis may emerge.

THE CRISIS PHENOMENON

Crisis, like stress, can be identified only by recognizing the manifestations or characteristic signs and symptoms of the crisis state. That is why it is so important for nurses to have a firm understanding of the crisis sequence. Concepts of crisis help the practitioner to quickly recognize clients who need to adjust their coping mechanisms to manage the demands of a stressful event. Boss (1988) defines "family coping to mean the management of a stressful event or situation by the family as a unit with no detrimental effects on any individual in that family" (p. 60).

It is especially critical for community health nurses to be well-grounded in crisis theory because they frequently encounter clients, such as the Slavovi family, in the home environment who are dealing with new, different, or threatening stressful events. Early identification of those clients who are having difficulty coping with these events could prevent an intensified crisis state.

A preventive health philosophy stimulated the development of crisis theory and intervention. Erich Lindemann (1944), in his classic study of grief reactions, identified the need for preventive counseling with clients experiencing loss through death or separation. After investigating the responses of clients who had lost a relative in the famous Coconut Grove fire in Boston, he concluded that appropriate psychiatric intervention with clients who were experiencing grief could prevent prolonged and serious social maladjustment. (Lindemann, p. 147). He further concluded, after observing clients who experienced an "anticipatory grief reaction," that prophylactic counseling could prevent family crisis (p. 148). Anticipatory grief reactions occur when there is a threat of death, such as when soldiers engage in war activities. Clients in these situations go through all the stages of grief. It has been found in some cases that wives of soldiers in the war handled the grief process so effectively that they emancipated themselves from their spouses. This precipitated a crisis if husbands returned from the war, because their wives needed to reestablish marital relationships before they could express feelings of love and caring. Husbands in these situations felt that their wives no longer loved them and frequently asked for a divorce (Lindemann, pp. 147-148).

Crisis reactions such as those described by Lindemann can be predicted and often prevented. Lindemann, Caplan, and other crisis theorists have delineated a sequence of events that occur when a client is experiencing a crisis, as well as factors that intensify the crisis state. They also discovered therapeutic processes that have a positive influence on client functioning during a family crisis. A community health nurse who understands the nature of a crisis and therapeutic crisis intervention can assist families under stress and crisis to adapt and grow.

THE CRISIS SEQUENCE

Gerald Caplan (1961), the founder of preventive psychiatry, describes *crisis* as a state

> provoked when a person faces an obstacle to important life goals that is, for a time, insurmountable through the utilization of customary methods of problem solving. A period of disorganization ensues, a period of upset, during which many different abortive attempts at solution are made. Eventually some kind of adaptation is achieved, which may or may not be in the best interests of that person and his fellows.

When describing the normal sequence of events that occur during a crisis, Caplan (1964) identifies four characteristic phases:

1. An initial phase when an individual's tension rises as he or she uses habitual problem-solving responses to achieve emotional homeostasis.
2. A second stage, in which tension increases and the individual becomes ineffective and upset because normal coping mechanisms were not effective in resolving the state of crisis.
3. A third threshold when tension mounts and stimulates the mobilization of new and emergency problem-solving mechanisms. The problem may be resolved if an individual can redefine the situation in order to cope with it and can adjust to role changes that have occurred.

4. A final phase when tension mounts beyond the limits an individual can tolerate; major disorganization results.

Inherent in Caplan's description of a crisis are several key ideas: (1) change that threatens an individual's ability to meet life goals disrupts the individual's homeostasis; (2) crisis results when an individual's customary methods of adaptation are ineffective in handling change; (3) disorganization occurs during the crisis state; (4) crisis is self-limiting, with a subsequent reduction of emotional tension (adaptation); (5) biopsychosocial homeostasis following a crisis may be at a level the same as, better than, or worse than the precrisis level.

FAMILY CRISIS

From a family perspective, Boss (1988) defines crisis as "(a) a disturbance in the equilibrium that is so overwhelming, (b) a pressure that is so severe, or (c) a change that is so acute that the family system is blocked, immobilized, and incapacitated" (p. 50). During a crisis a family is no longer able to maintain its structural boundaries, is ineffective in carrying out family roles and tasks, and family members have difficulty functioning, physically or psychologically (Boss). Crisis causes disorganization and ineffective functioning within the family unit and among individual family members. Hence the needs of both the family system and individual family members should be assessed when a family is experiencing a crisis.

Family crisis is self-limiting and can promote either growth within the family system or ineffective patterns of family functioning. The goal of crisis intervention is to help the family and individual family members to maintain a level of functioning equal to or better than the precrisis level.

It is not uncommon for community health nurses to work with families who have been unable to return successfully to their precrisis level of functioning after experiencing a crisis. When first encountered by the community health nurse these families often present multiple difficulties, ineffective problem-solving methods, and feelings of helplessness and hopelessness. These families are vulnerable to crises in the future.

Community health nurses also encounter families who not only return to precrisis levels of functioning but, in addition, experience growth during crisis situations. Many families develop new methods of coping that provide alternative ways for them to handle future stresses and crises. Many also develop a cohesive family unity that increases the supportive and nurturing aspects of their family lifestyle and that encourages risk taking. Risk taking may expose individuals and families to other growth-producing opportunities. Characteristics of families who show potential for growth during crisis are delineated in the accompanying box.

Multiple factors affect how well a family handles stress and deals with crises. Community health nurses who understand these variables are better able to help families achieve successful resolution and growth during a crisis state.

NANDA Nursing Diagnosis: Family Coping: Potential for Growth

DEFINITION

Effective management of adaptive tasks involved with the client's health challenge by family member, who now exhibits desire and readiness for enhanced health and growth in regard to self and in relation to the client.

DEFINING CHARACTERISTICS

- Family member is moving in direction of health-promoting and enriching lifestyle that
  1. Supports and monitors maturational processes
  2. Audits and negotiates treatment programs
  3. Generally chooses experiences that optimize wellness
- Individual expresses interest in making contact on a one-to-one basis or on a mutual-aid group basis with another person who has experienced a similar situation
- Family member attempts to describe growth impact of crisis on his or her own values, priorities, goals, or relationships

ETIOLOGICAL OR RELATED FACTORS

- Readiness for seeking goals related to self-actualization

From Gordon M: *Manual of nursing diagnosis, 1997-1998,* St. Louis, 1997, Mosby, p. 453.

FACTORS AFFECTING THE OUTCOME OF STRESS AND CRISIS

It has been well established that there is significant variation in how families and individuals respond to stress and crisis. This variation is influenced by several critical variables that can be categorized under three major headings: *perception of the event, family and individual resources*, and *family and individual coping mechanisms*. These variables affect how clients appraise stressful events and how they mobilize resources to achieve successful adaptation during periods of disequilibrium.

Perception of the Event

Crisis is the emotional reaction that occurs in relation to a new, different, or threatening event, not the event itself. Basically, the extent of this emotional reaction is determined by how the client (individual, family, aggregate) defines his or her particular circumstances (Aguilera, 1994; Boss, 1988; Burr, Klein, Associates, 1994; Caplan, 1964; Glanz, Lewis, Rimer, 1997; Hansen, Hill, 1964; McCubbin, McCubbin, 1993).

Perception of a hazardous event is a multidimensional phenomenon. McCubbin and McCubbin (1993) noted that "the assessments families make include many components of the stressor, such as the intensity, the degree of controllability of the situation, the amount of change expected of the family system, and whether or not the family is capable of responding to the situation" (p. 50). Consistent with this view, Glanz, Lewis, and Rimer (1997) contend that when a person is faced with a stressor he or she "evaluates the potential threat or harm [primary appraisal], as well as his or her ability to alter the situation and manage negative emotional reactions [secondary appraisal]." (p. 116). During the primary appraisal process individuals make judgments about the severity of the threat and their susceptibility to the threat. Additionally, they examine how the stressor impacts on their goals or concerns and the cause of the stressor. During the secondary appraisal process, individuals examine their coping resources and options and assess such things as their perceived ability to change the situation, their perceived ability to manage the emotional reactions to the threat, and expectations about the effectiveness of their coping resources (Glanz, Lewis, Rimer, pp. 118-119).

During the clinical family assessment process it is important to guide the interview to obtain data about the multiple variables that influence how a client perceives a hazardous situation. The accompanying box identifies factors to be considered when assessing a client's response to current stressors. In Chapter 7 information about the structural and process parameters of family functioning was presented. This information helps the practitioner to examine the impact of the stressful situation on the family system. For example, it would be important to assess how the family was handling its division of labor when a family member is ill and unable to carry out his or her normal patterns of functioning. Families experiencing a crisis are no longer able to perform their customary roles and tasks (Boss, 1988).

Even though the responses of individuals and families to hazardous events are highly variable, evidence suggests that distress increases when multiple stressors are encountered (McCubbin, McCubbin, 1993; McCubbin, Patterson, 1983; Rahe, 1974); the stressor or stressors are experienced for a prolonged length of time (Gaynor, 1990; Rowat, Knafe, 1985; Selye, 1976); or the stressful event presents hardship or a threat to life's goals or has serious consequences such as death (Glanz, Lewis, Rimer, 1997; Hill, 1949). Distress also increases if families or their individual family members believe that they have little control over the stressful event (Boss, 1988; McCubbin, McCubbin, 1993).

When distress heightens, clients are more likely to have a distorted view of the current stressor. They may experience feelings such as helplessness, hopelessness, anxiety, fatigue, or depression. It must be emphasized, however, that even when one or more of these factors exist in stressful occurrences, the perceived meaning of occurrences varies from one individual to another. The above factors only place individuals more at risk for developing crisis.

Caplan (1964), in his classic work on crisis, has found that for a stressor to become problematic "it must be perceived as a threat or loss to need satisfaction or as a challenge" (pp. 42-43). He believes that two major variables, personality and sociocultural factors, significantly affect how one perceives life events. These variables determine the type of life experiences one has, prescribe the limits of acceptable behavior when dealing with stress, and influence how one feels about one's abilities to handle changes in life. Case scenarios can best illustrate how the variables of personality and sociocultural influences affect one's perception of an event.

Factors Influencing a Family's Perception of a Stressful Event

- Number of stressors family is experiencing
- Family's past experiences in handling current stressor(s)
- Biopsychosocial status of the client before encountering stressful event(s)
- Duration of exposure to current stressor(s)
- Magnitude or seriousness of current event(s)
- Suddenness of the event
- Family's understanding of the stressor event(s)
- Impact of event on family structure, process, and goals
- Family's perceptions about its ability to manage the demands of the stressful event, including an appraisal of family resources
- Family's perceptions about its ability to change the stressful situation

Case Scenario

Mrs. Farias was 34 years old and left with two sons, 8 and 10 years old, and one daughter, age 14, when her husband was killed in a car accident. The community health nurse had encountered the Farias family before Mr. Farias's death because Carmelina, their 14-year-old daughter, needed orthopedic follow-up for a scoliosis problem discovered through health screening at her high school. During a home visit 8 months after Mr. Farias's death, the community health nurse became concerned about Mrs. Farias's physical and psychological health. She looked uncared for, her home was untidy, and she had no interest in talking about Carmelina's health problems. Weeping, Mrs. Farias shared with the nurse that "nothing was going right lately; the children don't obey, I can't get my husband's life insurance, and my friends haven't visited lately." She became particularly distressed when she talked about how she was going to feed her family in the future. "Our savings are almost gone. I can't get a job. What will I do? I have never worked, because Julio thought that a wife should stay at home. My folks thought that girls should marry and raise a family. I never was good at much except maybe cooking, housekeeping, and loving the kids. My family thinks it is wrong to take money from the welfare department. They say they will help me until I remarry, but I know they don't have anything extra. Besides, I am too old to remarry. Most men I know want their own children, not someone else's. You can't meet men when you are my age."

Another case scenario illustrates different family reactions to the death of its male provider.

CASE *Scenario*

Mrs. Ulisses was a 33-year-old widow with two daughters, 2 and 6 years of age, and two sons, ages 8 and 11. Her husband was killed while hunting. The community health nurse started visiting Mrs. Ulisses after she brought her 2-year-old to the well-baby clinic 6 weeks after her husband's death. At that time she expressed a desire to obtain information about day-care centers. The nurse visited regularly for a year to help Mrs. Ulisses sort out what she would like to do in the future. She and her husband were never able to save much, so Mrs. Ulisses applied for financial assistance from the Department of Social Service. She did not like receiving Temporary Assistance to Needy Families but felt that she needed time to make child care arrangements before she went back to work. Seven and a half months after her husband's death, Mrs. Ulisses enrolled in college. "I know I can find a job, because I have worked off and on since age 15. If I had some training, however, I would be more secure in the future. I am still not sure if I want to get married again, so I better prepare myself to care for my family."

Both Mrs. Farias and Mrs. Ulisses were facing similar situations. They experienced the loss of a significant other who had assumed the provider role in their family system when he was living. Mrs. Farias, however, was more threatened by her circumstances because past and current cultural influences affected her ability to be flexible when role changes were needed. In addition, Mrs. Farias lacked confidence (personality factor) in her abilities to succeed in work and social settings. Her life experiences were focused on preparing her for traditional female roles only.

Mrs. Ulisses, on the other hand, was discouraged at times but was actively involved in planning for a future career. She was better prepared to assume the provider role, having worked off and on since her teenage years, and felt more confident about her abilities to succeed outside the home setting. Her life experiences provided her with a different perception of her female role.

Family and Individual Resources

Families may have both family system resources and social supports that can assist them during periods of stress and crisis. Family system resources such as economic stability, cohesiveness, effective problem-solving abilities and communication patterns, and an adequate knowledge base help families to deal with the harmful health effects of stress and crisis (Boss, 1988; Burr, Klein, associates, 1994; McCubbin, McCubbin, 1993). Chapter 9 expands on family strengths that help families to adjust and adapt during periods of stress and crisis.

Family system resources are the economic, psychological, and physical assets and strengths upon which family members can draw in response to a stressful event or events (Boss, 1988; Burr, Klein, associates, 1994). "Having resources, however, does not imply whether or how a family will use them. For example, a family may use a resource such as money to deal with the event of unemployment in a dysfunctional way (e.g., buy more liquor or a larger television set) or, more functionally, to train for another job" (Boss, 1988, p. 68). During the family assessment process it is important to collect data about how family resources are being used, as well as about the type of resources available to the family. "The greater the breadth, depth, and efficacy of the available personal and family resources, the greater the ease with which the family is able to adapt to the illness situation" (McCubbin, McCubbin, 1993, p. 48).

It has been well established over time that social support can assist families and individuals to cope with the stresses of life (Caplan, Robinson, French Jr et al, 1976; Cassel, 1976; Cobb, 1976; Hamburg, Killilea, 1979; Heaney, Israel, 1997). It has been demonstrated that the presence of social support can play a significant role in buffering the impact of stress and in influencing positive health behaviors, such as the use of health services and adherence to medical regimens. Social support can also stimulate the development of coping strategies and promote mastery or control over one's situation (Cassel, 1976; Cobb, 1976; Hamburg, Killilea, 1979; Pilisuk, Parks, 1983).

Heaney and Israel (1997) distinguish between social networks and social support. They see social networks as the "linkages between people that may (or may not) provide social support and that may serve other functions in addition to that support" (p. 180). In contrast, Heaney and Israel see social support as the aid and assistance exchanged through social relationships and interpersonal transactions that is always intended to be helpful, is consciously provided by the sender, and is provided within an interpersonal context of caring, trust, and respect for each person's right to self-determination (pp. 180-181). Examples of social support are tangible assistance like financial aid and help with daily maintenance activities, the provision of information that helps clients under stress to clarify and address the stressful event, and emotional support that conveys trust, caring, and empathy (House, 1981).

Although it has been shown that social support can positively influence the outcome of a stressful event or crisis, research has also demonstrated that the *nature* of social support is significant to consider when evaluating this variable during the family assessment process (Gottlieb, 1983; Krause, 1986). Thus it is important to ascertain from families their perceptions about the *quality* as well as the *quantity* of support that exists in their environment. Use of a genogram and/or an eco-map (see Chapter 7) often helps the practitioner to assess clients' perceptions about the quality of their internal and external social resources.

During periods of disequilibrium persons need supportive relationships that allow them to verbalize feelings and encourage them to sort out the realities of their situation. Clients also need assistance with problem solving.

In addition, concrete help is frequently needed to facilitate their ability to obtain resources such as financial assistance from their environment (see Chapter 10). Behaviors that support a client's distorted perception of the event are not helpful. A friend, for example, who reinforces a client's blaming behaviors inhibits client growth and successful resolution of a crisis; this type of behavior supports the client's current ineffective coping style, which in turn prevents the client from mobilizing more effective coping mechanisms.

When working with clients who are experiencing a crisis, it is extremely important to remember that their significant others may also be in crisis. Often the practitioner finds that others in a client's social network are experiencing as much or more distress than the client. Thus they are unable to provide the assistance needed by the client to achieve healthy adaptation and may, in fact, be reinforcing maladaptive behaviors. Because of this, significant others are often included in the therapeutic process so that they do not inhibit a client's growth and they themselves receive the help needed to cope with the stressful changes being experienced.

Family and Individual Coping Strategies

The stress-crisis sequence evolves when a family's or an individual's usual coping mechanisms are inadequate to deal with the threatening event(s) being encountered. A major task for a family or an individual who is experiencing stress is to recognize when customary coping mechanisms are ineffective and new patterns for coping must be established. "Coping strategies play a critical role in adaptation" (McCubbin, McCubbin, 1993, p. 57).

Family coping strategies are the active *processes* and *behaviors* families actually try to help them manage, adapt, or deal with stressful events (McCubbin, Dahl, 1985). Examples of specific strategies for managing family stress are gaining useful knowledge about the stressful event, building and enhancing trusting relationships with others, seeking help from relatives, friends, and community agencies, and maintaining family adaptability and flexibility (Burr, Klein, associates, 1994, pp. 134-136).

Coping with stress and crisis is a complex process that may require changes in the basic structure of the famly (e.g., family priorities and beliefs about life) as well as specific patterns of family functioning (e.g., allocations of role responsibilities). For example, as Maria and Angel Slavovi (discussed in the beginning of this chapter) were dealing with the demands of the stressors associated with caring for their child who had disabilities, they changed how the family carried out child care responsibilities and the family's expectations and goals. Mr. Slavovi assumed more responsibility for meeting the basic care needs of his children, and both parents came to realize that their disabled child would never meet the family's educational aspirations. Angel and Maria Slavovi wanted all of their children to go to college so that the children would have a better life than they themselves had. Situations like these are distressing to families because they must compromise or accept a less-than-perfect solution to successfully manage the demands of their stressful event (McCubbin, McCubbin, 1993).

"No (one) coping strategy has been found to be a cure-all" (Burr, Klein, associates, 1994, p. 147). Rather, the literature suggests that families are able to deal with stressors more effectively if they have a rich repertoire of coping strategies (Burr, Klein, associates; McCubbin, McCubbin, 1993). However, Burr, Klein, and associates (1994) stress that "it is important to help families understand that not all coping strategies are helpful for everyone in every situation" (p. 203) and that professional intervention must be individualized to the specific concerns and needs of each family. Their research suggests that the nature of stressors influences family's perceptions about the helpfulness of specific types of coping strategies and that the type of coping strategies used varies by gender. Men appear to use more harmful strategies (e.g., using alcohol or withdrawing) and women tend to reach out to others. Women also tend to use a wider range of coping strategies (Burr, Klein, associates).

Recognizing Inadequate Coping Patterns

Boss (1988) believes that "sometimes it may be better for a family to give up, to let go, to fail to cope even if that precipitates crisis" (p. 63), particularly if maladaptative coping strategies (e.g., social isolation or domestic violence) are used by the family to adapt. These types of coping strategies can cause psychological and physical harm to individual family members and the family unit. The following case scenario illustrates how psychological distress can evolve in a seemingly stable family situation and how maladaptative coping strategies were causing harm to an individual family member.

CASE *Scenario*

Sally Himes called the county health department and requested nursing service for her mother. Without emotion, she stated, "Someone needs to show me how to care for her. I don't know what to do any longer." Sally Himes was a 50-year-old, single woman who lived with her 85-year-old mother. Her mother had a CVA 15 years previously that left her paralyzed and unable to speak. Before her father's death, Ms. Himes had promised him that she would always care for her mother.

When the community health nurse arrived at the Himes home, Sally immediately took her to her mother's bedroom. Although the mother appeared very comfortable and well cared for, Sally insisted that the nurse check her over carefully. "I am doing something that is not right. The doctor needs to visit more frequently to give mother water shots." When the nurse's assessment revealed that the mother's condition was stable, she decided to spend time talking with Sally. Very abruptly in the conversation, Sally replied, "The mailman came today." It took several probing questions like, "Was there something special about the mailman's visit?" before Sally identified that she had received an invitation to her niece's wedding. She was distressed because her mother had not also been invited. "They don't care about her anymore."

Further interviewing revealed that for the past 2 years Sally had isolated herself from family and friends because she felt her mother's condition was deteriorating and that her significant others were too busy to assist her. Sally also shared that she was really discouraged because she wondered if her family cared about her or her mother. "If they cared, they would have invited Mother to Sue's wedding."

Disrupting the status quo when she received an invitation to her niece's wedding was a very positive coping strategy for Sally. "Letting go" and asking for help from others assisted Sally in reevaluating her current situation and seeing that she needed to make changes in her current pattern of functioning. Isolating herself from family and friends and "toughing it out" or keeping feelings to herself resulted in depression and made it more stressful for Sally to care for her mother. Nursing intervention helped Sally to alter her perceptions about her mother's condition, the type of support she needed, and the nature of support her family desired to provide, and helped Sally to realize she was using ineffective coping strategies. One nursing intervention, arranging a conference with the entire family, resulted in a plan in which Sally's brothers and sisters would share responsibility for the care of their mother.

When nurses work with clients who are experiencing stress, they often find that a *triggering event* (e.g., the invitation to Sue's wedding) stimulates the development of a crisis. This event produces a "pile up" of stress beyond the point where the client is able to adapt. This event frequently appears to be a minor occurrence, which makes it difficult for professionals and significant others to recognize the seriousness of the client's situation. For example, a child who comes sobbing into the health clinic at school because of being shoved by peers on the playground may need just a little extra attention. However, if this child perceives the push to mean that he or she is not liked, the child may need help in evaluating social relationships. It is usually wise for a community health nurse to obtain information about the client's daily functioning, support systems, and recent life changes when she or he believes that an emotional reaction to an event is disproportionate to what one would normally expect.

Having an awareness of behaviors that are commonly observed when individuals and families have developed ineffective coping mechanisms enhances the community health nurse's ability to quickly identify clients who are experiencing distress, crisis, or dysfunctional family dynamics. The North American Nursing Diagnosis Association has identified characteristics of individuals and families who have ineffective coping patterns. These characteristics are displayed in the three following boxes and can assist

NANDA Nursing Diagnosis: Ineffective Coping (Individual)

DEFINITION

Impairment of adaptive behaviors and problem-solving abilities for meeting life's demands and roles. Methods of handling stressful life situations are insufficient to prevent/control anxiety, fear, or anger. (Specify stressor[s]—e.g., situational crisis, maturational crisis, event, change.)

DEFINING CHARACTERISTICS

Diagnostic Cues

- Reports presence of life stress/problems (specify)
- Inability to meet role expectations and/or inability to meet basic needs
- Reports feeling anxious, apprehensive, fearful, and/or depressed, angry
- Inappropriate/ineffective use of defense mechanisms

Supporting Cues

- Expresses inability to cope
- Low self-esteem (perceived low self-competency to handle situation)
- Sleep pattern disturbance
- Reports fatigue
- Excess food intake, alcohol consumption; smoking
- Drug abuse
- Digestive, bowel, appetite disturbance; chronic fatigue or sleep pattern disturbance
- High rate of accidents
- Irritability, tension
- Inability to ask for help
- Inability to solve problem effectively
- Destructive behavior toward self and others
- Verbal manipulation
- Alteration in societal participation
- Change in usual communication patterns

ETIOLOGICAL OR RELATED FACTORS

- Ineffective problem-solving strategies/skills*
- Inappropriate/ineffective use of defense mechanisms
- Personal vulnerability
- Knowledge deficit (specify area)

HIGH-RISK POPULATIONS

- Complex disease management
- Overwhelming crisis situations
- Developmental transitions (e.g., adolescence, retirement)

From Gordon M: *Manual of nursing diagnosis, 1997-1998*, St. Louis, 1997, Mosby, pp. 436, 437.

*Ineffective problem-solving strategies/skills had the highest rating in two studies of ineffective coping. Yet it is frequently viewed as a reason for ineffective coping rather than a diagnostic cue to ineffective coping.

NANDA Nursing Diagnosis: Compromised Family Coping

DEFINITION

Usually supportive primary person (family member or close friend) providing insufficient, ineffective, or compromised support, comfort, assistance, or encouragement, which may be needed by client to manage or master adaptive tasks related to health challenge.

DEFINING CHARACTERISTICS

Diagnostic Cues

- Client or another person expresses concern or complaint about significant other's response to client's health problem and one or more of the following:
- Significant person displays protective behavior disproportionate (too little or too much) to client's abilities or need for autonomy
- Significant person describes preoccupation with personal reactions (e.g., fear, guilt, anticipatory grief, anxiety) to client's illness, disability, or other situational or developmental crises
- Significant person describes or confirms inadequate understanding of knowledge base that interferes with effective assistive or supportive behaviors (specify)
- Significant person withdraws or enters into limited or temporary personal communication with client at time of need
- Significant person attempts assistive or supportive behaviors with less than satisfactory results

ETIOLOGICAL OR RELATED FACTORS

- Knowledge deficit (specify area)
- Emotional conflicts (specify)
- Exhaustion of supportive capacity
- Role changes (family)
- Temporary family disorganization
- Developmental or situational crises (specify)

HIGH-RISK POPULATIONS

- 24-hour home care
- Home care with periodic health crises
- History of family life stresses

From Gordon M: *Manual of nursing diagnosis, 1997-1998*, St. Louis, 1997, Mosby.

NANDA Nursing Diagnosis: Disabling Family Coping

DEFINITION

Behavior of significant person (family member or primary person) disables his/her own capacities and client's capacities to effectively address tasks essential to either person's adaptation to the health challenge.

DEFINING CHARACTERISTICS

Diagnostic Cues

- Neglectful care of client in regard to basic human needs and/or illness treatment and one or more of the following:
- Distortion of reality regarding client's health problem, including extreme denial about existence or severity
- Intolerance
- Rejection
- Abandonment
- Desertion
- Carrying on usual routines, disregarding client's needs
- Psychosomaticism
- Taking on illness signs of the client
- Decisions and actions by family that are detrimental to economic or social well-being
- Agitation, depression, aggression, hostility
- Impaired restructuring of a meaningful life for self, impaired individuation, prolonged overconcern for client
- Neglectful relationships with other family members
- Client's development of helpless, inactive dependence

ETIOLOGICAL OR RELATED FACTORS

- Chronically unexpressed guilt/anxiety/hostility by significant other
- Dissonant discrepancy of coping styles (for dealing with adaptive tasks by the significant person and client or among significant people)
- Highly ambivalent family relationships
- Arbitrary handling of family's resistance to treatment (tends to solidify defensiveness as it fails to deal adequately with underlying anxiety)

HIGH-RISK POPULATIONS

- 24-hour home care
- History of family life stresses
- Home care with periodic health crises

From Gordon M: *Manual of nursing diagnosis, 1997-1998*, St. Louis, 1997, Mosby, pp. 459, 461.

community health nurses in determining when individuals and families are having difficulty handling stress. The ineffective behaviors presented in the family coping boxes are primarily identified in terms of how a family relates to a client with an identified problem. During times of distress and crisis families may also develop dysfunctional patterns of functioning that affect the entire family unit. Deceptive, confused, or secretive communication; inability to meet basic needs of family life (e.g., impaired home management); inappropriate or lack of decision making and problem solving; and family interactions characterized by constant conflict are a few examples of such patterns. Others are shared in Chapter 7.

When community health nurses work with families, particularly those who tend to perceive all difficulties as crisis, they often find that problems from the past are reactivated during the crisis state. This occurs because these families have previously used inadequate coping strategies when dealing with stressful situations (Caplan, 1964). Although the resurfacing of old issues can compound the impact of current stressors, it can also provide an opportunity for client growth. Clients can be helped to resolve old as well as new problems during times of crisis and to learn effective ways to address stressful events. Even families who experience extreme types of stress can successfully find new levels of satisfaction and fulfillment in their family lives (Burr, Klein, associates, 1994, p. 204).

SUPPORTIVE FAMILY SERVICES AND INTERVENTIONS

The type of services and interventions needed by families to address stressful situations vary based on the nature of the stressor(s) encountered and the level of family functioning. The Children's Defense Fund (1992) believes that most families can change when offered the right kind of help and that most families in crisis want to be helped to better provide for their family members. This organization advocates for a pyramid (Figure 8-3) of family-focused services in every community that matches the pyramid of family needs and a holistic approach to family stress management that honors cultural variations and is respectful of families (see the accompanying box). Supportive family services and interventions build on family strengths, emphasize prevention, and help families through difficult times (Children's Defense Fund).

Families are especially amenable to outside assistance during periods of disequilibrium or crisis (Caplan, 1964). Caplan found that intervention at this time can be the critical balancing factor in helping clients to achieve positive outcomes during crisis states. Most families in crisis need only some extra support or specialized assistance. For example, refer once again to the Slavovi family discussed in the beginning of this chapter. This family was successful in adapting its family functioning to address the needs of all family members, with supportive assistance from the community health nurse and specialized early intervention workers from the public school system. The community health nurse helped the parents to express their feelings about their child's disabilities, assisted the parents in learning about the nature of their child's health condition (cerebral palsy and mental retardation), and helped the parents to identify appropriate community resources (e.g., early intervention program in the school system). Additionally, the nurse helped the family to establish a pattern of functioning that addressed the needs of all family members. The early intervention workers aided the parents in promoting their child's growth and development and in identifying effective ways to care for their child's needs.

NURSING INTERVENTION STRATEGIES

Community health nurses use a variety of intervention approaches to facilitate adaptation during times of stress and to enhance successful resolution of crisis. Some of these approaches will be briefly summarized under three major categories: *supportive*, *educative*, and *problem-solving*. Separating strategies into categories is an artificial technique that is used here only to focus discussion about ways to effect client change. In reality community health nurses find that often they must integrate several intervention approaches to effectively assist clients under stress.

Establishing rapport and collecting adequate data to identify the task to be accomplished are the essential first steps in any intervention process. These steps are discussed in Chapters 7 and 9 and are not repeated here. They should, however, be kept in mind when selecting a particular intervention approach.

Supportive Approach

The multiple symptoms that clients experience when dealing with stressful events and/or crises were previously discussed in this chapter. These symptoms can be very unpleasant and can create considerable discomfort. Clients can fear that something is seriously wrong with them, and this tends to increase their anxieties and fears.

Often clients who are experiencing symptoms of distress need to reduce their level of stress before they can actively engage in activities that will lead to problem resolution. Supportive intervention by significant others (family, friends, and professionals) can assist clients in stress reduction. Three types of support are especially helpful: (1) providing an opportunity for the client to share feelings with persons who are accepting and nonjudgmental; (2) assisting the client with concrete daily tasks, such as home management and keeping health appointments; and (3) support system enhancement. Community health nurses frequently

Effective Approaches for Working with Families Under Stress

- Emphasize the family unit instead of focusing narrowly on an individual child or other family member.
- Build on family strengths instead of emphasizing deficits.
- Offer preventive services to avert crises instead of merely reacting to emergencies.
- Address family needs comprehensively instead of merely reacting to emergencies.
- Treat families with respect and honor cultural differences.
- Offer flexible, responsive services instead of rigid, single-purpose services.

From Children's Defense Fund (CDF): *The state of America's children 1992*, Washington, D.C., 1992, CDF, p. 65.

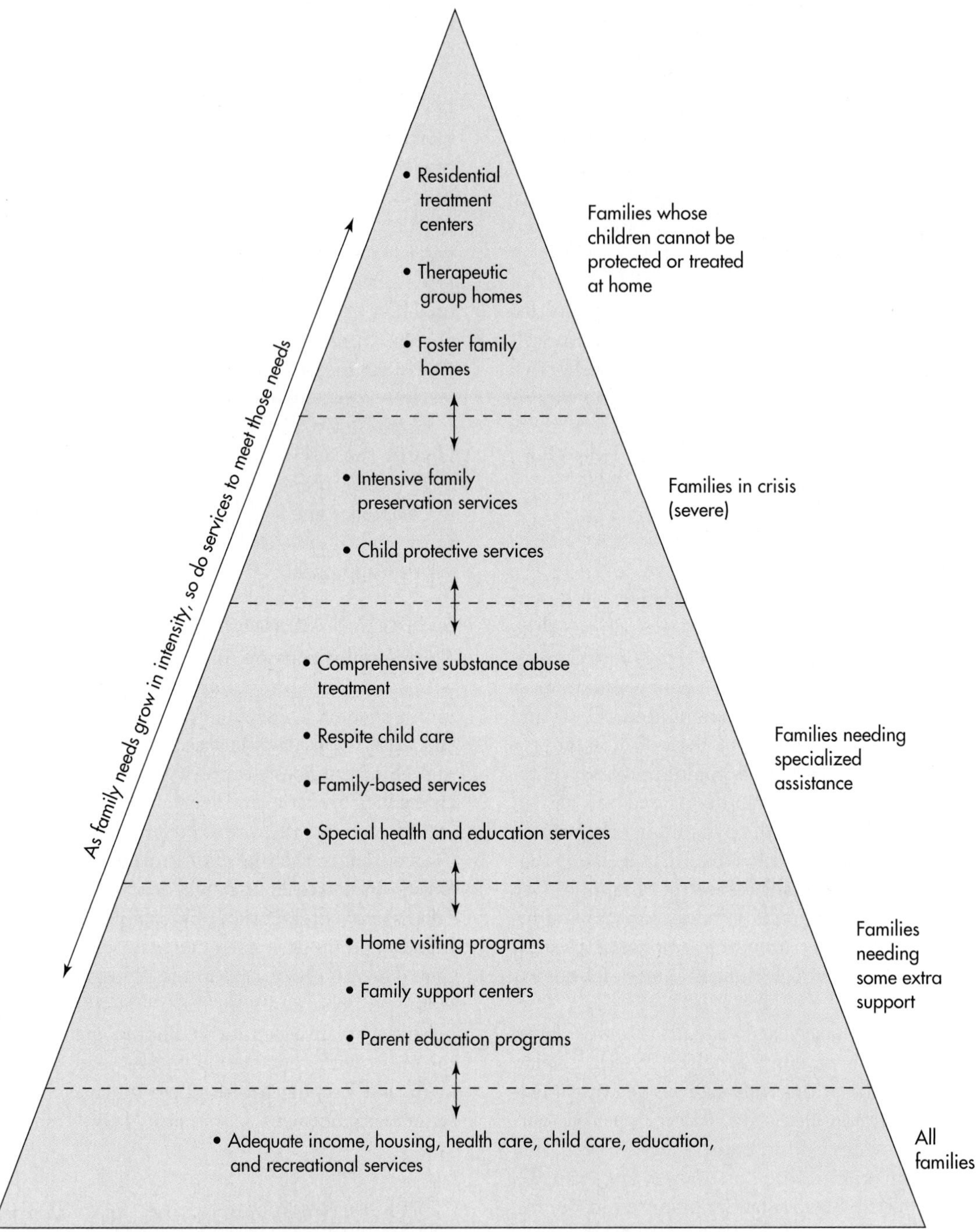

Figure 8-3 Building a pyramid of family-focused services. *(From Children's Defense Fund [CDF]:* The state of America's children 1992, *Washington, D.C., 1992, CDF, p. 68.)*

help clients who are experiencing crisis with concrete tasks by making referrals for homemakers or home health aides or by helping the client to mobilize family resources. At times they also provide this assistance themselves during home visits. They may, for example, feed an infant while talking to a distressed mother.

It is important to remember that clients who are experiencing high levels of stress often need time to deal

NIC Nursing Intervention: Support System Enhancement

DEFINITION

Facilitation of support to patient by family, friends, and community

ACTIVITIES

Assess psychological response to situation and availability of support system
Determine adequacy of existing social networks
Identify degree of family support
Identify degree of family financial support
Determine support systems currently used
Determine barriers to using support systems
Monitor current family situation
Encourage the patient to participate in social and community activities
Encourage relationships with persons who have common interests and goals
Refer to a self-help group, as appropriate
Assess community resource adequacy to identify strengths and weaknesses
Refer to a community-based promotion/prevention/treatment/rehabilitation program, as appropriate
Provide services in a caring and supportive manner
Involve family/significant others/friends in the care and planning
Explain to concerned others how they can help

From McCloskey JC, Bulechek GM, eds: *Nursing interventions classification (NIC)*, ed 2, St. Louis, 1996, Mosby, p. 531.

with their feelings and to reevaluate their perceptions of the stressful event before they can actively engage in problem solving and in learning new knowledge. Ignoring the feeling levels of clients during these times can disrupt the therapeutic relationship and may result in the client withdrawing. Following the principles of crisis intervention discussed in this chapter helps to develop a caring, trusting, professional relationship with clients in crisis.

Families with a limited support system may need assistance in expanding their support base. Nursing interventions that help to enhance family support are displayed in the accompanying box. One strategy important to all social network intervention is to increase awareness among members of the client group of the health-enhancing qualities of social relationships (Heaney, Israel, 1997). "Someone who fully appreciates the importance of social relationships to good health is more likely to be motivated to engage in the processes of providing and receiving support (Heaney, Israel, p. 191).

Educative Approach

Health education has traditionally been a function of the community health nurse. Lillian Wald cared for the sick in the home and also provided instruction so that families were better equipped to assist their ill members. Lina Rodgers taught personal hygiene to school-age children and their families and as a result the spread of disease was reduced and wellness was promoted. Funds were made available through Federal Maternal and Child Health Grants in the 1920s and 1930s so that community health nurses could be hired to provide health teaching in relation to child care, nutrition, and family-life education. Monies were also allocated at this time for preventive, community-wide health teaching services aimed at combating communicable diseases such as tuberculosis and childhood illnesses.

The educative function of nurses in the community setting has remained viable over the years. It is still a major focus of all community health nurses, regardless of the setting in which they practice. Nurses in the community setting use the educative approach to promote health among aggregates at risk and the community as a whole as well as among individuals and families. Chapter 14 addresses how community organization and health planning processes are used to promote health at the community and population level of service. These processes are designed to promote community-wide commitment to healthy living and to deliver health education and other health services to populations in need.

"The central concern of health promotion and health education is health behavior" (Glanz, Lewis, Rimer, 1997, p. 9). Health education activities are designed to identify and address environmental (e.g., political, economic, and social factors) and individual determinants of health that impede or facilitate clients' movement toward a healthy lifestyle.

Although the emphasis of health education in the community health setting is on health promotion and disease prevention, community health nurses use the educative approach to address client needs at all levels of prevention. For example, nurses in the community use this approach to help clients prepare for normative events that produce stress, develop lifestyle patterns that foster optimal health, detect undiagnosed disease and chronic health problems, and handle their rehabilitation needs. Community health nurses use the educative approach with clients across the life span and in a variety of community settings.

THE EDUCATIVE PROCESS The educative intervention approach is a complex process that involves more than instructional activities. It encompasses focused activities aimed at identifying client needs, learner readiness or motivation, and client specific interventions and evaluation criteria that are consistent with client needs. The educative or teaching-learning process as depicted by Redman (1997) is shown in Figure 8-4.

The steps in the teaching-learning or educative process parallel the steps of the nursing process (Table 8-1). Each have a phase that addresses assessment, analysis (diagnosis formulation), planning (goal setting), implementation (intervention), and evaluation (Redman, 1997). However, these processes differ in their focus. The nursing process is designed to address a broad range of client needs, one of which may be an educational need. In contrast, the teaching-learning process focuses on obtaining a more refined assessment of educational needs and client readiness to learn.

The community health nurse uses the educative process to help clients gain an increased understanding of health events and healthy lifestyle functioning through the acquisition of knowledge, and to assist clients in applying newly acquired health information. Need to learn and readiness of the learner must be assessed and established before educational strategies can be successfully implemented. Assumptions should not be made about the client's level of knowledge. For example, a mother may have a clear understanding of the nutritional standards for children but has not applied that information because of financial and time constraints. This mother does not have a need to learn about nutritional guidelines for children. Rather, she may need assistance in obtaining resources (e.g., food stamps or WIC) that expand her food purchasing capabilities or in using low-cost nutritional foods effectively and efficiently. Incomplete assessment of client's learning needs can result in the professional either establishing inappropriate learning goals or neglecting important areas of needs. Assessment of learner needs helps the professional to actively engage the client in the learning process. Accurate assessment of the client's readiness to learn also helps the professional to obtain active client participation.

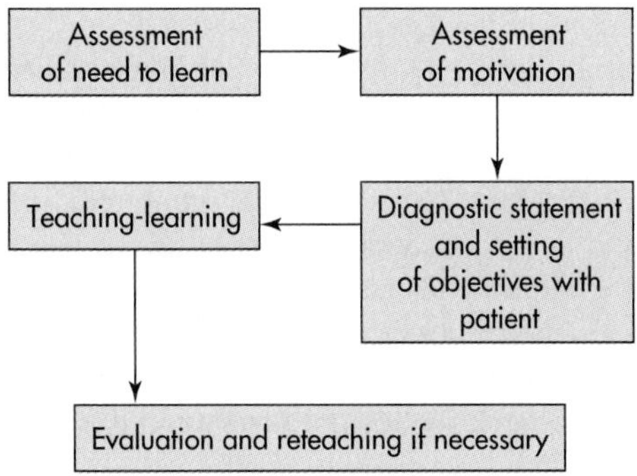

Figure 8-4 The educative, or teaching-learning, process. *(From Redman BK: The practice of patient education, ed 8, St. Louis, 1997, Mosby, p. 4)*

LEARNER READINESS The concept of learner readiness or motivation is a complex, multidimensional phenomenon. It involves the interaction between multiple interrelated variables such as clients' perceptions of health and illness, family patterns of health care, and availability and accessibility of resources. Various models have been proposed by social scientists and nurses to explain why individuals are or are not motivated to engage in health behaviors (Cox, 1982; Fishbein, Ajzen, 1975; Kulbok, 1985; Pender, 1996; Rosenstock, 1966; Rotter, 1966; Strecher, Rosenstock, 1997). One of the most widely used models, the *Health Belief Model*, examines why individuals engage in diagnostic and other disease-prevention activities (Strecher, Rosenstock).

In the mid-1960s Rosenstock stimulated significant interest among health professionals in the use of the Health Belief Model when he examined in the literature why people use health services (Rosenstock, 1966). This model, developed by a group of social scientists, advances the idea that readiness to take health action is dependent on several variables including (1) perceived susceptibility to a specific condition; (2) perceived seriousness of a given health problem; (3) perceived benefits and barriers to taking action; (4) cues to action such as knowledge that someone else has become affected by the condition; and (5) self-efficacy or judgment of one's abilities to take action (Strecher, Rosenstock, 1997). The Health Belief Model emphasizes that the beliefs that define readiness have both cognitive and emotional components and the motivational variables that promote disease-oriented, preventive health action are individually defined (Rosenstock, 1966).

The Health Belief Model is useful in explaining health-promoting behaviors that are triggered by an interest in preventing disease occurrence. Other conceptual models have

table 8-1 Relationship of Teaching Process to Nursing Process

Assessment	Diagnosis	Goals	Intervention	Evaluation
NURSING PROCESS				
General screening questions to detect patient's need to learn; if positive, use teaching process	One of the problem statements may be a need to learn or a nursing diagnosis	Learning goals are a subset of the goals	Teaching intervention may be delivered with other intervention	Evaluating whether the nursing care outcome was met
TEACHING PROCESS				
Refined assessment of need to learn and readiness	Learning diagnosis	Setting of learning goals	Teaching	Evaluating learning

From Redman BK: *The practice of patient education*, ed 8, St. Louis, 1997, Mosby, p. 5.

been developed to examine health-promoting behaviors that are wellness-oriented rather than disease-focused. An example of such a model is the Health Promotion Model developed by Pender (1996).

In Pender's Health Promotion Model behavior-specific cognitions and affect are considered to be the major motivational determinants of behavioral outcome and are identified as (1) perceived benefits of action; (2) perceived barriers to action; (3) perceived self-efficacy; (4) activity-related effect or negative and positive feeling states about a particular behavior; (5) interpersonal influences such as family, peers, providers, and norms; and (6) situational influences, including perceptions of options available, demand characteristics, and aesthetic features of the environment. Personal biological, psychological, and sociocultural characteristics and prior related behavior are hypothesized as influencing health behaviors through behavior-specific cognitive and affect processes. Although health-promoting behavior is the action outcome in Pender's Health Promotion Model, this behavior is ultimately directed toward attaining positive health outcomes for the client (Pender, 1996, pp. 66-73). An in-depth discussion of this model can be found in Pender's book *Health Promotion in Nursing Practice* (1996).

Health behavior models have focused on the individual as client. Loveland-Cherry (1996, p. 27) has proposed a preliminary model for family health promotion (Figure 8-5) based on Pender's revised model for health-promoting behavior, family theory, and research. As illustrated in Figure 8-5, this model identifies general, health-related, and behavioral-specific influences from a family perspective that affect health promotion outcomes.

Health behavior models emphasize the importance of assessing more than cognitive understanding or knowledge when determining learner readiness. Often underlying psychosocial factors are the key variables that influence why people do or do not engage in positive health action. These factors must be addressed before the health professional initiates cognitive teaching strategies.

Use of the nursing process (see Chapter 9), combined with an understanding of the concepts of health behavior and the principles of teaching and learning, aids the community health nurse in assessing learner readiness. These factors also help to individualize educational plans based on

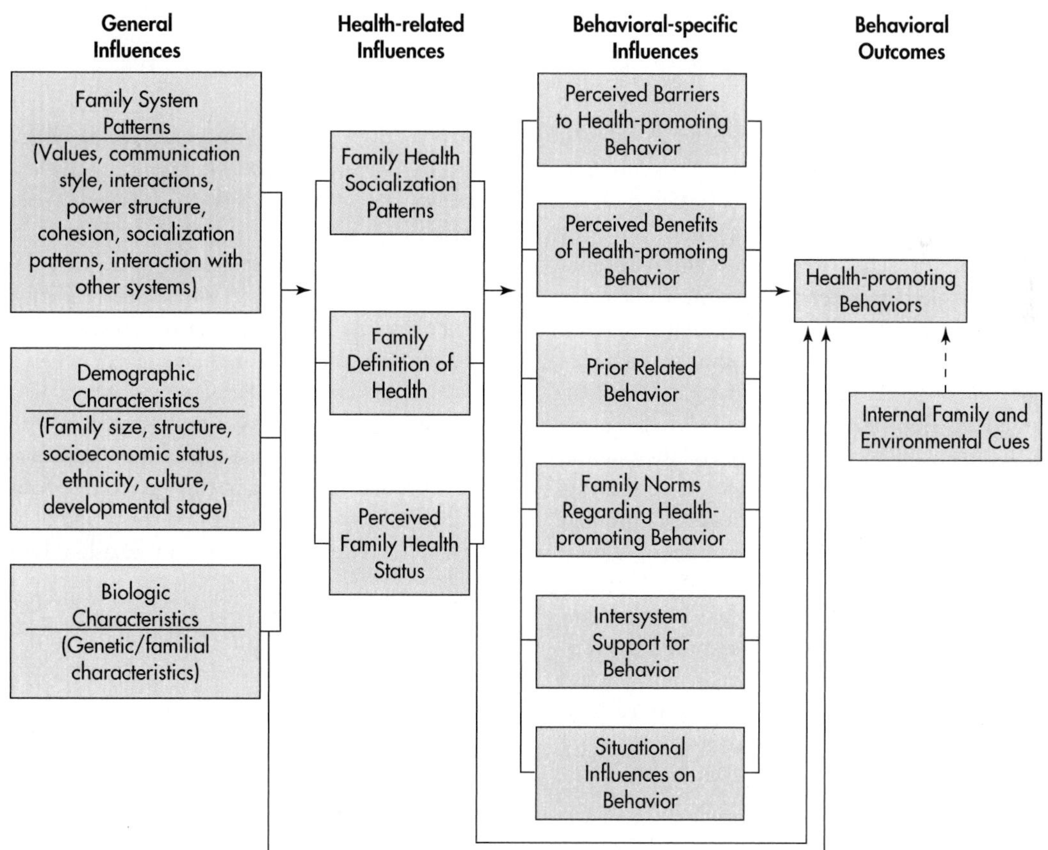

Figure 8-5 **Family health promotion model.** *(Modified from Loveland-Cherry CJ: Family health promotion and health protection. In Bomar PJ:* Nurses and family health promotion: concepts, assessment, and interventions, *ed 2, Philadelphia, 1996, Saunders, p. 27.)*

client needs and circumstances. Writings by Babcock and Miller (1994) and Redman (1997) are valuable resources if one wants to review or expand knowledge in relation to the principles of teaching and learning.

TEACHING/LEARNING PLANS After community health nurses establish learner readiness, they and their clients mutually develop teaching and learning goals. Together they also select from a variety of alternative intervention options a teaching strategy that best fits the client's needs and circumstances. Frequently a combination of two or more teaching methods is used. For example, a community health nurse might combine discussion, demonstration, and use of pamphlets to teach new parents how to bathe a baby. Or the nurse might use group process, audiovisual aids, self-instructional materials, and a baby bath demonstration to teach this same procedure. Whatever techniques are selected, the learner should have the opportunity to obtain new knowledge and to apply the knowledge gained. For instance, understanding how to bathe a baby does not always increase a new parent's level of comfort when doing so. Being allowed to demonstrate what has been learned when assistance is available is more likely to promote ease with such a procedure.

Developing specific, measurable, client-centered goals for the teaching and learning process is essential for several reasons. Specific goals help to determine what content or information is needed by the client. Goals also aid in developing and implementing teaching techniques relevant to the client's needs. In addition, they facilitate evaluation of the learning process because they define what the client desires to learn. A global goal such as "learning about growth and development" does none of these things. It does not define what information parents need in order to handle the developmental needs of their child more effectively. A goal which states that "the parents will verbally identify the developmental characteristics of a 1-year-old" is much clearer. It provides direction for establishing evaluation criteria. One criterion for evaluating the achievement of this goal might be "the parents can articulate the gross motor activities of a 12-month-old child." Using evaluation criteria to assess teaching and learning outcomes is an essential step in the educative process.

Individualizing teaching and learning plans is crucial because client needs vary even when different people encounter similar situations. Some parents understand normal growth-and-development processes very well but have difficulty handling the physical aspects of child care. Others are at ease with feeding, bathing, and clothing their infant but become frustrated when the child does not achieve developmental tasks, even if it is too soon for him or her to accomplish them. Differences such as these are not uncommon among clients who are experiencing similar situations.

When individualizing teaching and learning plans, it is important to take into consideration client characteristics that influence the learning process. Having knowledge of a client's socioeconomic characteristics, including age, educational level, economic and employment status, gender, marital status, cultural background, and place of residence is useful in guiding the tailoring of instructional strategies and educational materials. Printed educational materials need to be tailored to the reading levels of the client and reflect an appreciation of the client's cultural characteristics (Glanz, Lewis, Rimer, 1997, p. 12). They should also be age appropriate. It is important to remember that a client's reading ability and level of educational achievement may not be identical. "The reading levels of many individuals may be up to five grades below the grade they report they completed" (Redman, 1997, p. 45).

STAGES OF CHANGE It is not uncommon in the practice setting to find that clients do not readily change long-established unhealthy lifestyle patterns (e.g., smoking and excessive alcohol use). Prochaska and Di Clemente (1983) propose that for clients to alter these types of behaviors they must move through five discrete stages of change over time. These stages are (1) *precontemplation*, in which individuals have no intention of taking action in the next 6 months; (2) *contemplation*, in which individuals intend to change within the next 6 months; (3) *preparation*, in which individuals seriously intend to take action within the next month and have taken some behavioral steps toward action; (4) *action*, in which individuals have made overt behavior modification within the past 6 months; and (5) *maintenance*, in which individuals work to prevent relapse after successfully changing their behavior for more than 6 months (Prochaska, Redding, Evers, 1997, pp. 61-63).

Movement through these stages is often slow, and many individuals relapse several times before firmly establishing new behaviors. Hence evaluation should occur during each stage of change. Different change processes (e.g., consciousness raising, environmental reevaluation, or contingency management) and intervention strategies are used at each stage. An in-depth discussion of these processes and strategies is beyond the scope of this book. The reader is encouraged to review the writings of the original authors (Prochaska, Di Clemente, 1983; Prochaska, Redding, Evers, 1997).

Problem-Solving Approach

In the community health setting nurses encounter clients who are having difficulty making decisions about a variety of personal life events. Specifically, community health nurses help clients to make decisions about such things as career choices, maintaining or establishing intimate relationships with others, when and where to obtain preventive and curative health care services, how to deal with family conflicts, how to handle financial crisis, or how to provide needed care for aging family members. Clients dealing with situations such as these may have difficulty identifying why they cannot make a decision about what to do.

At times a family's or an individual's problem-solving capabilities are ineffective in addressing the demands of the stressors encountered. "Problem solving refers to the family's ability to organize a stressor into manageable components, to identify alternative courses of action to deal with each component, to initiate steps to resolve the discrete issues, as well as the interpersonal issues, and to develop and cultivate patterns of problem-solving communication needed to bring about family problem-solving efforts" (McCubbin, McCubbin, 1993, p. 30).

A variety of internal and external factors influence why clients are unable to identify and develop solutions which resolve their stress effectively. The following case scenarios identify select factors that influence problem-solving capabilities of families and individuals under stress.

CASE *Scenarios*

Client Has Not Identified the Nature of the Problem

Barb Lehi, a 28-year-old wife and the mother of two children, returned to work when her youngest child entered school. Her family adjusted well to her role change because joint decision-making occurred before Barb's employment. Barb was enjoying what she was doing but began to have tension headaches 2 months after she started her new job. She felt her headaches were related to the adjustments she had to make in her daily routine and assumed that they would go away shortly. They did not, however, until she was able to identify that she was having guilt feelings about being a working mother and its effect on her family.

Client Reaps Benefits from Illness Behavior

Mrs. Jackson, a 68-year-old widow living by herself, kept finding reasons why she should not see a physician after she started having "fainting spells." Her family became frustrated and worried and asked the community health nurse to visit. Referral for medical evaluation was successfully implemented only when Mrs. Jackson was able to verbalize that being ill was the only way she could get attention from her family. Her family visited very sporadically when she was well but daily when she was ill.

Client Is Using Disabling Coping Strategies

Gail Hayes, a 31-year-old mother and wife, provided no stimulation for her 2-year-old daughter who was disabled as a result of rubella exposure in utero. The community health nurse became involved after hearing from a neighbor that Gail left her daughter alone in the house when she visited friends and neighbors. After several home visits, the nurse discovered that Gail did so because, "I can't stand to be with her. She is such a fussy child and wants attention all of the time. I hate seeing her so deformed and feel guilty because if I hadn't gotten measles while pregnant she would be all right." Gail had never before acknowledged these feelings. When she did, she was able to use the help offered by others and to relate more effectively to her daughter.

Client Avoids Accountability for Feelings

Bob Woodrow, a 40-year-old construction worker, was referred to the health department for rehabilitative services after a myocardial infarction. Because of the strenuous nature of construction work it was recommended that he seek other employment. He verbalized an interest in obtaining job training through the Division of Vocational Rehabilitation but took no action. When the community health nurse questioned why, he responded by placing the blame on others. "My wife thinks it is too soon and nags me about not going back to work. I am not sure if my physician thinks I should, because he is always so vague about what is happening with my heart. My car needs fixing before I can use it regularly, and we don't have the money to get it fixed." It took several months for Bob to see that he was not taking action because of his own fears about having another heart attack and about not being able to succeed in a new line of work.

Client Perceptions of Stress Are Distorted

Carol Strang, a 17-year-old junior, repeatedly visited the school nurse for minor physical concerns. Assessments made by the nurse revealed that this occurred when Carol felt that she was not performing well academically. In reality Carol was very successful in her schoolwork, ranking in the top 5% of her class. In addition, she had several close friends who provided praise for her academic achievements. Carol, however, perceived that she was achieving satisfactorily only when she received straight As. When she received anything less than an A, she expressed feelings associated with failure.

Client Lacks Problem-Solving Experience

Mrs. Raabe, a 71-year-old widow, became confused and severely upset after her husband's death. All her life she had been cared for by others. Her parents and her brothers anticipated her needs because she was the "baby" of the family and "helpless." Because her husband assumed the same role as her family, Mrs. Raabe felt lost when he died. She found managing her finances particularly stressful since she had never taken care of the family budget. She needed help with such basics as writing a check, depositing money in the bank, and balancing her income and expenses.

Client Energy Is Depleted Because of Undetected Health Problems

Mrs. La Rosa, a 37-year-old divorced mother of six children, was referred to the health department by her caseworker from the Department of Social Service. Her caseworker believed that Mrs. La Rosa was neglecting her children and felt that environmental conditions were dangerous to the family's health. Mrs. La Rosa told the community health nurse that "I know I should keep my home more tidy, but I am just too tired to keep up with things that need to be done around the house. Sometimes all I want to do is sleep." The community health nurse assisted her in obtaining a medical evaluation. It was found during this evaluation that Mrs. La Rosa had hypertension and diabetes. When both of these conditions were under control, home management and child care skills improved.

Client Has Knowledge and Skill Deficits

Mr. and Mrs. Lueck were extremely upset when their 10-year-old disabled son was sent home from camp because he could not handle activities of daily living such as bathing and toileting. "Tommie always does these things at home. They just don't know how to work with retarded kids." Upon talking with the Luecks, the community health nurse discovered Tommie did wash himself when bathing at home, but that family members helped him with most of the activities necessary for completing a bath. For example, the family ran his bath water for him; assembled the materials he needed to take a bath, including soap, washcloth, and towel; and selected the clothing he would wear afterward. It was obvious to the nurse but not the parents that Tommie had missed essential steps in skill development. He had skill in washing body parts, but lacked decision-making skill about how and when to carry out these activities.

Client Is Unable to Generate or Fears Consequences of Alternative Options

Amy Schmidt, wife and mother of two preschoolers, was physically abused by her husband regularly and expressed a desire to leave him. She found it difficult to take this action because she thought that it was impossible for her to do so. She felt trapped because she had no job skills and her family and friends were unable to assist her financially. In addition, she felt that the abuse would not stop even if she left home because her husband could always find her. The community health nurse assisted Mrs. Schmidt in identifying ways to obtain financial aid and legal assistance to control her husband's behavior. Mrs. Schmidt was also helped to see that living alone could be less frightening for her and her children than being physically abused.

A community health nurse has two major goals when using the problem-solving approach: (1) to assist the client in solving immediate problem(s) and (2) to help the client increase independent problem-solving abilities. Implicit in these goals is the belief that clients can learn skills that will help them to make decisions wisely and to alter behavior accordingly. A community health nurse who has difficulty internalizing this belief will find it hard to move a client toward independence. This nurse is more likely *to do for* the client than *to work with* the client.

A variety of nursing interventions can be used to help a client enhance his or her problem-solving abilities, including such things as individual counseling, group work, role modeling, referral to community resources, client contracting, and behavioral modification. When using any one of these techniques the community health nurse should focus on helping the client to identify the nature of the problem(s), to discover alternative options for problem solving, to make decisions about which option is most appropriate, and to take action to resolve the problem(s). The community health nurse should not assume that the client will take action after making a decision about the most appropriate option and prematurely close the family to service. Taking action is often the most difficult step in the problem-solving process because it is at this point that the client is giving up the secure familiar for the threatening unknown. Clients may need supportive intervention to maintain their commitment to action.

When clients are experiencing crisis, they may express a desire to be rescued and request that others make decisions for them. *Rescue behavior* only temporarily reduces client stress and can prevent the client from developing new ways of coping with threatening events. Adhering to the principles of crisis intervention (see the box on the next page) assists the community health nurse in avoiding rescue activities and providing constructive aid to the family.

Problem-solving takes time. Both the client and the community health nurse must guard against expecting change too rapidly. When progress is slow a client may question if the nurse can really help, and the nurse often begins to wonder whether or not the client really wants to change. At times both of these feelings are justified. More frequently, however, the need is for the client and nurse to recognize that well-established patterns of behavior cannot be changed immediately.

Community health nurses cannot help all clients to learn to make decisions wisely. Some situations are beyond their competence and must be referred to others who are better qualified. Because competence varies from one community health nurse to another as a result of differences in academic preparation and work experiences, nurses must learn how to discriminate between situations that they can and cannot handle. Peer and supervisory conferences will assist a new nurse to objectively evaluate her or his skills.

Underestimating one's ability to help a client, rather than overestimating competency, is often more of a problem when nurses begin practice in the community health setting. Most clients experiencing stress and crisis do not need psychotherapy. Instead, they need someone who cares and who will provide supportive guidance and positive reinforcement for the strength they have. Families

Principles of Crisis Intervention

- *Help the client confront the crisis* by supporting expression of feelings and emotions such as fear, guilt, and crying.
- *Help the client confront the crisis in manageable doses* without dampening the impact of the crisis to a point where the client no longer recognizes the need to alter coping mechanisms. Drugs and diversional activities are helpful when they are used to decrease unmanageable stress. They are harmful when they prevent the client from looking at the realities of his or her situation.
- *Help the client to find the facts* because truth is less frightening than the unknown. Clients may need frequent visits during periods of crisis because they may not have the energy to analyze all the stresses they are experiencing during one home visit.
- *Do not give client false reassurance* because this leads to mistrust and maladaptive coping behaviors. To succeed in resolving a crisis, a client needs reassurance that supports his or her ability to handle the crisis situation.
- *Do not encourage the client to blame others* because blaming only reduces the tension momentarily and can help the client to suppress feelings. This can result in maladaptive behaviors that decrease the client's level of functioning after crisis resolution.
- *Help the client to accept help* because some clients avoid confronting a crisis by denying that they need help and that a problem exists. If the client does not face the crisis, he or she will not mobilize coping mechanisms that will enhance growth.
- *Help the client with everyday tasks* in a manner that reflects kindness and thoughtfulness rather than one that gives a message that the client is weak or incompetent. Clients need help with everyday tasks because it takes considerable energy to resolve a crisis; thus clients often lack sufficient energy to handle daily activities as well.

From Cadden V: Crisis in the family. In Caplan G, ed: *Principles of preventive psychiatry*, New York, 1964, Basic Books, pp. 293-296.

and individuals have tremendous capabilities for "weathering the storms of stress" (Burr, Klein, associates, 1994).

Summary

The community health nurse is often the primary source of assistance when an individual or a family is experiencing stress. Stress is a normal human phenomenon necessary for survival and growth. It triggers the general adaptation syndrome that helps people adapt to the demands and pressures of life. Although stress is essential for survival and growth, individuals and families have limits beyond which stress is no longer tolerated. Prolonged and intensified stress results in crisis, especially when an individual's coping mechanisms are inadequate to reduce disequilibrium.

Families and individuals in crisis experiences disorganization and heightened stress. Crisis is self-limiting but biopsychosocial homeostasis following a crisis may be at a level equal to, better than, or lower than the precrisis level. Timely supportive intervention may be the critical factor that determines if an individual or family has a positive or negative outcome during periods of crisis.

Millions of American families are under stress. Environmental conditions and lifestyle patterns are placing them at risk for situations such as domestic violence, criminal victimization, and economic distress. To address the needs of families from a holistic perspective, every community needs to provide a range of family-focused supportive services and interventions. Most families under stress and crisis want to be helped and can achieve new levels of functioning. The community health nurse plays a key role in helping families to prevent a crisis situation and to adapt when crisis occurs.

Critical *Thinking Exercise*

You are the community health nurse visiting the Slavovi family described on page 197 of this chapter. Shortly after arriving at their home for your first home visit, it becomes obvious that Mr. and Mrs. Slavovi want you to tell them "the right way to do things with Stephanie" and that they are hoping to find someone who can "cure her." (Hospital personnel had shared with the family that Stephanie has cerebral palsy and mental retardation and needs long-term health and educational follow-up.) Considering the factors that influence the outcome of a crisis, discuss with a peer the type of assessment data you would collect on your first home visit and how you would apply the principles of crisis intervention in this situation. Additionally, identify at least three resources in your local community that could assist this family in dealing with its current situation.

References

Ailinger RL: Beliefs about treatment of hypertension among Hispanic older persons, *TCN* 7:26-31, 1985.

Aguilera DC: *Crisis intervention: theory and methodology*, ed 7, St. Louis, 1994, Mosby.

Babcock DE, Miller MA: *Client education: theory and practice*, St. Louis, 1994, Mosby.

Barnard KE: Difficult life circumstances (DLC). In Krentz LG, ed: *Nursing and the promotion/protection of family health: workshop proceedings*, Portland, Or., 1988, Oregon Health Sciences University.

Beall S, Schmidt G: Development of a youth adaptation rating scale, *J School Health* 54(5):197-200, 1984.

Boss PG: Family stress. In Sussman M, Steinmetz S, eds: *Handbook on marriage and the family*, New York, 1987, Plenum, pp. 445-450.

Boss P: *Family stress management*, Newburg Park, Ca., 1988, Sage.

Burr WR, Klein SR, associates: *Reexamining family stress: new theory and research*, Thousand Oaks, Ca., 1994, Sage.

Cadden V: Crisis in the family. In Caplan G, ed: *Principles of preventive psychiatry*, New York, 1964, Basic Books, pp. 228-296.

Capers CF: Nursing and the Afro-American client, *ICN* 7:11-17, 1985.

Caplan G: *An approach to community mental health*, New York, 1961, Grune and Stratton.

Caplan G: *Principles of preventive psychiatry*, New York, 1964, Basic Books.

Caplan RD, Robinson EAR, French JRP Jr. et al: *Adhering to medical regimens: pilot experiments in patient education and social support*, Ann Arbor, 1976, University of Michigan, Institute for Social Research.

Cassel JC: The contribution of the social environment to host resistance, *Am J Epidemiol* 104:107-128, 1976.

Chang K: Chinese Americans. In Giger JN, Davidhizar RE: *Transcultural nursing: assessment and intervention*, St. Louis, 1995, Mosby, pp. 395-416.

Children's Defense Fund (CDF): *The state of America's children 1992*, Washington, D.C., 1992, CDF.

Cobb S: Social support as a moderator of life stress, *Psychosomatic Medicine* 38:300-314, 1976.

Cox C: An interaction model of client health behavior: theoretical prescription for nursing, *Adv Nurs Sci* 5:41-56, 1982.

Davitz LJ, Sameshima Y, Davitz J: Suffering as viewed in six different cultures, *AJN* 76:1296-1297, 1976.

Eckholm E: AIDS and folk healing, a Zimbabwe encounter, *New York Times*, October 5, 1990, 1-2.

Fishbein M, Ajzen I: *Belief, attitude, intention and behavior: an introduction to theory research*, Reading, Ma., 1975, Addison-Wesley.

Gaynor SE: The long haul: the effects of home care on caregivers, *Image J Nurs Sch* 22:208-212, 1990.

Germain CP: Cultural care: a bridge between sickness, illness, and disease, *Holistic Nurse Pract* 6:1-9, 1992.

Giger JN, Davidhizar RE: *Transcultural nursing: assessment and intervention*, St. Louis, 1995, Mosby.

Glanz K, Lewis FM, Rimer BK, eds: *Health behavior and health education: theory, research and practice*, ed 2, San Francisco, 1997, Jossey-Bass.

Gordon M: *Manual of nursing diagnosis, 1997-1998*, St. Louis, 1997, Mosby.

Gottlieb BH: *Social support strategies: guidelines for mental health practice*, Beverly Hills, Ca., 1983, Sage.

Hamburg A, Killilea M: Relation of social support, stress, illness, and use of health services. In Hamburg D, ed: *Healthy people: the Surgeon General's report on health promotion and disease prevention*, DHEW PHS Pub. No. 79-55071A, Washington, D.C., 1979, U.S. Department of Health, Education, and Welfare.

Hansen DA, Hill R: Families under stress. In Christensen HT, ed: *Handbook of marriage and the family*, Chicago, 1964, Rand McNally, pp. 783-819.

Heaney CA, Israel BA: Social networks and social support. In Glanz K, Lewis FM, and Rimer BK, eds: *Health behavior and health education: theory, research, and practice*, ed 2, San Francisco, 1997, Jossey-Bass.

Hill R: *Families under stress: adjustment to the crises of war separation and reunion*, New York, 1949, Harper.

Hill R: Generic features of families under stress. In Parad HJ, ed: *Crisis intervention: selected readings*, New York, 1965, Family Service Association of America, pp. 32-74.

House JS: *Work stress and social support*, Reading, Ma., 1981, Addison-Wesley.

Institute of Medicine: *The best intentions: unintended pregnancy and the well-being of children and families*, Washington, D.C., 1995, National Academy of Sciences.

Kay M, Yoder M: Hot and cold in women's ethnotherapeutics: the American Mexican west, *Soc Sci Med* 25:347-355, 1987.

Kleinman A, Eisenberg L, Good B: Culture, illness, and care: clinical lessons from anthropologic and cross-cultural research, *Ann Intern Med* 88:251-258, 1978.

Krause N: Social support, stress and well-being among older adults, *J Gerontol* 41:512-519, 1986.

Kulbok PP: Social resources, health resources, and preventive health behavior: patterns and predictions, *Public Health Nurs* 2:67-81, 1985.

Lazarus RS: *Psychological stress and the coping process*, New York, 1966, McGraw-Hill.

Lazarus RS, Folkman S: *Stress, appraisal and coping*, New York, 1984, Springer.

Lewis S, Messner R, McDowell WA: An unchanging culture, *J Gerontol Nurs* 11:21-26, 1985.

Lindemann E: Symptomatology and management of acute grief, *Am J Psychiatry* 101:141-148, 1944.

Louie KB: Providing health care to Chinese clients, *ICN* 7:18-25, 1985.

Loveland-Cherry CJ: Family health promotion and health protection. In Bomar PJ: *Nurses and family health promotion: concepts, assessment, and interventions*, ed 2, Philadelphia, 1996, Saunders, pp. 22-35.

Ludman EK, Newman JM: The health-related food practices of three Chinese groups, *J Nutr Educ* 16:4, 1984.

Maloney C: Don't say "pretty baby" lest you zap it with your eye—the evil eye in South Asia. In Maloney C, ed: *The evil eye*, New York, 1976, Columbia University Press, pp. 102-248.

Maternal and Child Health Bureau: *Child health USA '95*, Washington, D.C., 1996, U.S. Government Printing Office.

McCloskey JC, Bulechek GM, eds: *Nursing interventions classification (NIC)*, ed 2, St. Louis, 1996, Mosby.

McCubbin H, Dahl B: *Marriage and family: individuals and life cycles*, New York, 1985, John Wiley.

McCubbin MA, McCubbin HI: Family stress theory and assessment: the T-Double ABCX model of family adjustment and adaptation. In McCubbin HI, Thompson A, eds: *Family assessment inventories for research and practice*, Madison, Wi., 1987, University of Wisconsin-Madison, pp. 3-32.

McCubbin HI, McCubbin MA: Family system assessment in health care. In McCubbin HI, Thompson AI, eds: *Family assessment inventories for research and practice*, Madison, Wi., 1991, University of Wisconsin-Madison, pp. 53-81.

McCubbin MA, McCubbin HI: Families coping with illness: the resiliency model of family stress, adjustment, and adaptation. In Danielson CB, Hamel-Bissell BP, Winstead-Fry P, eds: *Families, health, and illness: perspectives on coping and interventions*, St. Louis, 1993, Mosby, pp. 21-63.

McCubbin HI, Patterson JM: Family stress adaptation to crises: a double ABCX model of family behavior. In Olson DH, Miller BC, eds: *Family studies review year book vol 1*, Beverly Hills, Ca., 1983, Sage, pp. 87-106.

McCubbin HI, Patterson JM: FILE: Family Inventory of Life Events and Changes. In McCubbin HI, Thompson AI, eds: *Family assessment inventories for research and practice*, Madison, Wi., 1991, University of Wisconsin-Madison, pp. 77-98.

McCubbin H, Patterson J, Wilson L: FILE: Family Inventory of Life Events and Changes. In McCubbin HI, Thompson AI, McCubbin MA, eds: *Family assessment: resiliency, coping and adaptation—inventories for research and practice*, Madison, Wi., 1996, University of Wisconsin System.

McCubbin HI, Thompson AI, McCubbin MA: *Family assessment: resiliency, coping and adaptation—inventories for research and practice*, Madison, Wi., 1996, University of Wisconsin System.

Norbeck J: Modification of life event questionnaires for use with female respondents, *Res Nurs Health* 7:61-71, 1984.

Pasquale EA: The evil eye phenomenon: its implications for community health nursing, *Home Health Nurse* 2:32-37, 1984.

Pender N: *Health promotion in nursing practice*, ed 3, Stamford, Ct., 1996, Appleton and Lange.

Pilisuk M, Parks S: Social support and family stress. In McCubbin H, Sussman M, Patterson J, eds: *Social stress and the family: advances and developments in family stress theory and research*, New York, 1983, Haworth, pp. 137-156.

Prochaska JO, Di Clemente CC: Stages and processes of self-change of smoking: toward an integrative model of change, *J Consulting Clin Psych* 51:390-395, 1983.

Prochaska JO, Redding CA, Evers KE: The transtheoretical model and stages of change. In Glanz K, Lewis FM, Rimer DK: *Health behavior and health education: theory, research, and practice*, ed 2, Jossey-Bass, 1997, pp. 60-84.

Rahe RH: Subjects' recent life changes and their near-future illness reports, *Ann Clin Res* 4:250-265, 1972.

Rahe RH: The pathway between subjects' recent life changes and their near-future illness reports: representative results and methodological issues. In Dohrenwend BS, Dohrenwend BP, eds: *Stressful life events*, New York, 1974, Wiley.

Redman BK: *The practice of patient education*, ed 8, St. Louis, 1997, Mosby.

Rosenstock IM: Why people use health services, *Millbank Q* 44:94-127, 1966.

Ross HM: Societal/cultural views regarding death and dying, *TCN* 3:1-15, 1981.

Rotter JB: Generalized expectancies for internal versus external control of reinforcement, *Psychol Monogr* 80(1):1-28, 1966.

Rowat KM, Knafe KA: Living with chronic pain: the spouse's perspective, *Pain* 3:259-271, 1985.

Selye H: *The stress of life*, New York, 1976, McGraw-Hill.

Snow LF: Folk medical beliefs and their implications for care of patients: a review based on studies among Black Americans, *Ann Intern Med* 81:82-96, 1974.

Sobralske MC: Perceptions of health: Navajo Indians, *ICN* 7:32-39, 1985.

Strecher UJ, Rosenstock IM: The Health Belief Model. In Glanz K, Lewis FM, Rimer BK, eds: *Health behavior and health education: theory, research and practice*, ed 2, San Francisco, 1997, Jossey-Bass, pp. 41-59.

Twaddle AC: Sickness and the sickness career: some implications. In Eisenberg L, Kleinman A, eds: *The relevance of social science for medicine*, Dordrecht, Holland, 1981, D. Reidel.

U.S. Department of Health and Human Services (USDHHS): *Health, United States, 1995*, Hyattsville, Md., 1996, Public Health Services.

U.S. Department of Health and Human Services (USDHHS): *Healthy people 2000: midcourse review and 1995 revisions*, Washington, D.C., 1995, U.S. Government Printing Office.

U.S. Department of Health and Human Services (USDHHS): *Healthy people 2000: national health promotion and disease prevention objectives, full report, with commentary*, Washington, D.C., 1991, U.S. Government Printing Office.

U.S. Department of Housing and Urban Development (USDHUD): *Priority: home! The federal plan to break the cycle of homelessness*, Washington, D.C., 1994, USDHUD.

Villarruel AM, Ortiz de Montellano B: Culture and pain: a Mesoamerican perspective, *Adv Nurs Sci* 15:21-32, 1992.

Wong DL: *Whaley and Wong's nursing care of infants and children*, St. Louis, 1995, Mosby.

SELECTED BIBLIOGRAPHY

Antonousky A: *Health, stress, and coping*, San Francisco, 1979, Jossey-Bass.

Barnfather JS, Lyon BL, eds: *Stress and coping: state of the science and implications for nursing theory, research and practice*, Indianapolis, 1994, Sigma Theta Tau International.

Boss PG, Doherty VJ, LaRossa R et al, eds: *Sourcebook of family theories and methods*, New York, 1993, Plenum.

Children's Defense Fund (CDF): *The state of America's children 1995*, Washington, D.C., 1996, CDF.

Craft MJ, Willadsen JA: Interventions related to family, *Nurs Clin North Am* 27:371-396, 1992.

Feetham SL, Meiser SB, Bell JM, Gillis CL, eds: *The nursing of families: theory, research, education, and practice*, Newbury Park, Ca., 1993, Sage.

Fink SV: The influence of family resources and family demands on the strains and well-being of caregiving families, *Nurs Res* 44(3):139-146, 1995.

Frisch NC, Kelley J: *Healing life's crises: a guide for nurses*, Albany, N.Y., 1996, Delmar.

Krentz LG, ed: *Nursing and the promotion/protection of family health: workshop proceedings*, Portland, Or., 1988, Oregon Health Sciences University.

Laffrey SC, Loveland-Cherry CJ, Winkler SJ: Health behavior: evolution of two paradigms, *Public Health Nurs* 3:92-100, 1986.

Mealey AR, Richardson H, Dimico G: Family stress management. In Bomar PJ, ed: *Nurses and family health promotion: concepts, assessment, and interventions*, ed 2, Philadelphia, 1996, Saunders, pp. 227-244.

Murata JM: Family stress, mother's social support, depression and son's behavior problems: modeling nursing interventions for low-income inner-city families, *J Fam Nurs* 1(1):41-62, 1995.

Olson SL, Banyard V: "Stop the world so I can get off for a while": sources of daily stress in the lives of low-income single mothers of young children, *Fam Relations* 42:50-56, 1993.

Rakel BA: Interventions related to patient teaching, *Nurs Clin North Am* 27:397-424, 1992.

Roth P: Family social support. In Bomar PJ, ed: *Nurses and family health promotion: concepts, assessment, and interventions*, ed 2, Philadelphia, 1996, Saunders, pp. 107-120.

Wright LM, Leahey M: *Nurses and families*, ed 2, Philadelphia, 1994, F.A. Davis.

9

Use of Family-Centered Nursing Process with Culturally Diverse Clients

Objectives

Upon completion of this chapter, the reader should be able to:

1. Understand the interrelationship between the phases of the family-centered nursing process.
2. Use the nursing process to plan family-centered nursing care.
3. Articulate the influence of cultural phenomena on client functioning and clinical decision making.
4. Analyze the concept of family health from a holistic perspective.
5. Understand nursing responsibilities and client rights in a provider/client relationship.
6. Understand the significance of using a theoretical base for guiding practice.

> For a green plant to survive, it must reach sunlight. So nature provides that if the plant's growth is blocked in one direction, it can grow in another.
>
> CONOCO OIL COMPANY

People, like green plants, can grow in multiple directions. Stumbling blocks along the way do not necessarily stop growth (Figure 9-1). Caring, support, and assistance from significant others can help humanity to change the course of its development when barriers are inhibiting the growth process. A significant support system for many individuals is the family. Persons can grow, change, and develop within the family unit (Whall, 1991, p. 321). However, at times families need guidance in identifying behaviors that support family growth.

Community health nurses often facilitate the family growth process. They work to develop trusting, supportive relationships so that clients can reach out and use their help when it is needed. Some clients will not seek assistance from community health nurses because they have found other support systems more relevant to them. However, when a client does accept the help offered by community health nurses, it is important for nurses to recognize that their role is to work *with* the client in determining which pathways will promote family health. Nurses who encourage families to make decisions about life choices are more likely to facilitate growth than those who impose on others their beliefs about appropriate life pathways.

Increasingly, health care professionals are encouraging active family involvement in health care decision making. They have identified that doing *for* clients instead of working *with* them can result in client dependence, often limiting client health action. Health care professionals can influence family change, but only families can alter their behavior. Clients must perceive the need for change before they will alter their actions.

To function effectively in the community setting, a nurse must accept the fact that clients are responsible for their health behavior, even when they choose a plan of action that the nurse would not choose. Nurse-defined goals for clients are seldom achieved. Goals defined by the client are more frequently accomplished. The nurse who attempts to take over for clients quickly becomes frustrated with the lack of client response and may "burn out."

The nursing process helps the community health nurse facilitate client goal setting. This therapeutic process is used by nurses in all settings. However, it is labeled the *family-centered nursing process* in the community health setting because community health nurses use it to analyze family functioning and to extend services to the family as a whole. This focus is based on the belief that the family is the basic unit for nursing service: family functioning affects the health of all family members by inhibiting or facilitating the growth process, by influencing when family mem-

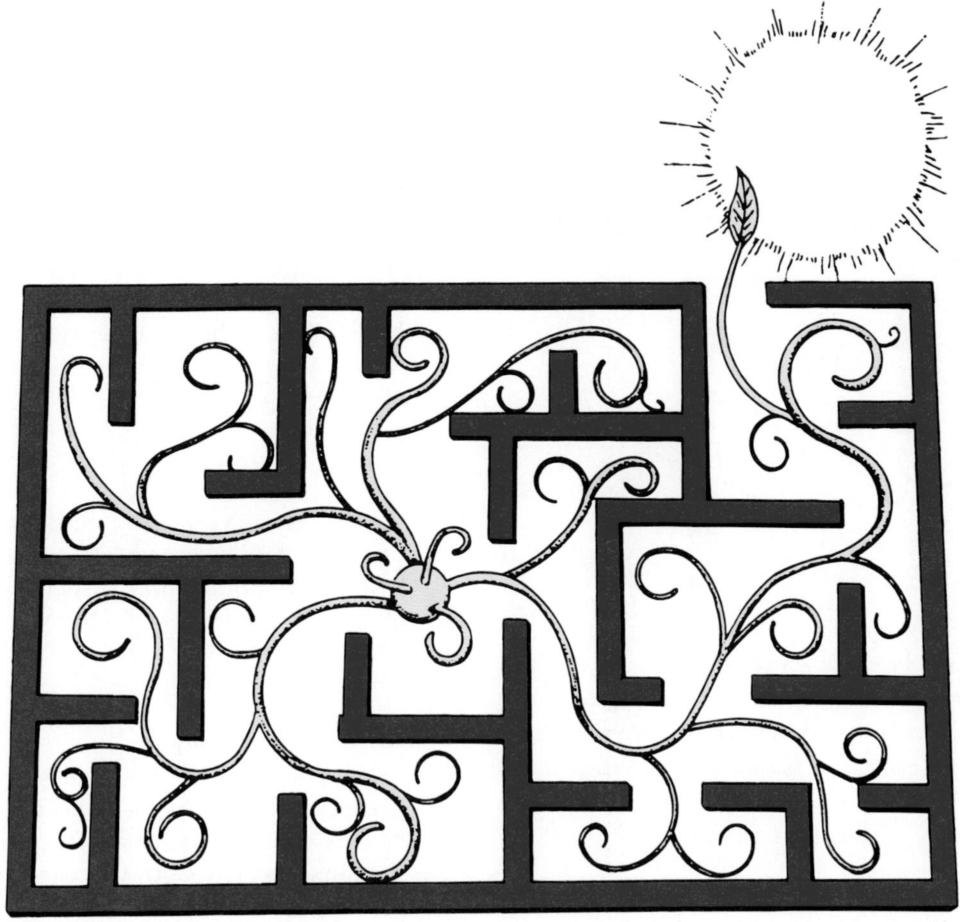

Figure 9-1 Nature doesn't explore just one path to reach a goal. Neither should people. *(Courtesy Conoco Oil Company.)*

bers will accept help from community systems, and by establishing values, attitudes, and beliefs about health practices (Figure 9-2).

THE FAMILY-CENTERED NURSING PROCESS DEFINED

The family-centered nursing process is a systematic approach to scientific problem solving, involving a series of circular dynamic actions—assessing, analyzing, planning, implementing, evaluating, and terminating—for the purpose of facilitating optimum client functioning. This definition has four key elements:

- *Systematic approach*. This process enables the community health nurse to function in an orderly, logical manner. The nurse plans her or his actions to achieve specific goals and recognizes that time and efforts are often wasted if a "hit-or-miss" approach is used.
- *Scientific problem solving*. Decisions made about client needs and appropriate nursing interventions are based on scientific principles. The problem-solving approach is used in everyday life. The nursing process differs from simple problem solving: scientific knowledge gained from advanced study assists the nurse in refining the data analysis process in relation to health, illness, and prevention, and in expanding intervention options that aid clients in maximizing their self-care capabilities. McCain (1965, p. 82), in her classic article on the nursing process, stressed that this process helps nurses function in a deliberative rather than an intuitive way. This notion has been supported in recent literature (Carpenito, 1989; Gordon, 1997, 1993; Weber, 1991).
- *Series of circular, dynamic actions*. No one action alone helps the community health nurse to enhance client growth. All phases of the nursing process must be carried out in order for sound decision making and effective nursing intervention to occur. *Dynamic* implies that care plans are revised when assessment and evaluation data reflect needed change. The nursing process is circular in nature because each phase provides data that either validate or alter original nursing diagnoses, goals, and plans.

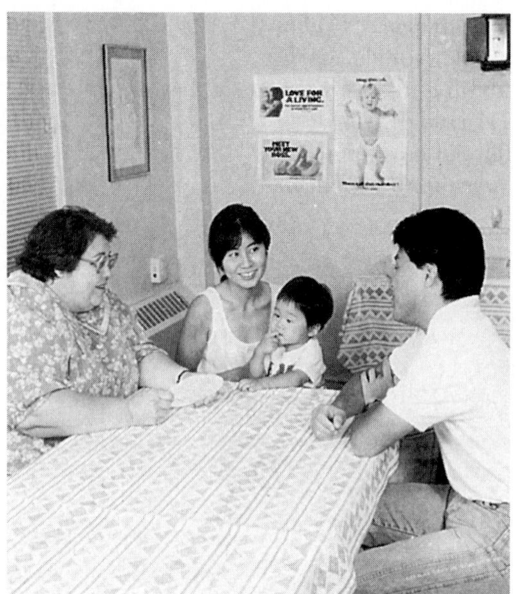

Figure 9-2 The family-centered approach to nursing care focuses on the family as the unit of service. When using the nursing process in the community setting, nurses assess family dynamics as well as individual functioning and establish client-centered goals relevant to the needs of the entire family unit. *(From Barkauskas VH, Stoltenberg-Allen C, Baumann LC, Darling-Fisher C:* Health and physical assessment, *St. Louis, 1994, Mosby.)*

- *Purpose of facilitating optimum client functioning.* Nursing interventions should help the client resolve his or her health care needs and achieve specific, client-defined goals and expected outcomes. A helping, interactive process whereby the client and the nurse share data for the purpose of identifying ways to make things less difficult for the client facilitates this process. To effectively facilitate client functioning, the nurse must individualize nursing actions, since clients define optimum functioning differently.

An effective community health nurse learns that, by using a systematic process, more positive outcomes can be achieved. The nurse understands that it is necessary to base his or her practice on scientific knowledge consistent with the standards of the profession. Standards of community health nursing practice emphasize the need for the nurse to use theoretical concepts from intradisciplinary and interdisciplinary sources, including nursing, public health, social and behavioral sciences, and physical sciences (ANA, 1986, p. 5).

To achieve desired outcomes in a family situation, the nurse must recognize that having knowledge only about a disease process is insufficient to adequately address the impact of illness on the family system. Illustrative of this are the factors nurses take into consideration when they work with a family who has a child with insulin-dependent diabetes. Based on scientific knowledge from the biological sciences, the nurse knows that this child requires an appropriate diet, proper hygiene, insulin injections, regular blood glucose testing, and adequate exercise. However, teaching about these needs may be ineffective unless the nurse applies knowledge from the behavioral and social sciences to gain an understanding of how environmental, lifestyle, and family factors are influencing the child's health behaviors. This is illustrated in the following case scenario:

CASE *Scenario*

One community health nurse intensively visited the family of a 6-year-old child who had an unstable diabetic condition. The child did not follow her prescribed diabetic regimen and one consequence was frequent hospitalization for treatment of diabetic coma. When the nurse discussed with the parents their perceptions of their child's health condition, she learned that they were not ready to accept the diagnosis as permanent. Denying the diagnosis was their way of coping with it. The parents needed assistance in dealing with their feelings of guilt and anger before they could address appropriate treatment plans for their child.

THEORY GUIDES PRACTICE

The ANA (1986) standards of community health nursing practice specify that "the nurse applies theoretical concepts as a basis for decisions in practice. Theoretical concepts define the context within which the community health nurse understands phenomena and their interrelationships, thereby providing a framework for assessment, intervention, and evaluation" (p. 5).

To function effectively in community health, the nurse must use skills and knowledge relevant to both nursing and public health (ANA, 1986; APHA, 1996). Public health knowledge includes concepts from epidemiology, biostatistics, environmental health, social sciences, and public health administration. Core concepts from the epidemiological model (host, agent, and environment) and levels of prevention (primary, secondary, and tertiary) guide public health practice. These concepts are discussed in Chapter 11.

Concepts from epidemiology help the nurse to identify at-risk clients (individuals, families, and aggregates) for the purposes of promoting health and preventing disease. During the assessment phase of the family-centered nursing process, nurses complete a family health risk appraisal. A health risk appraisal is a process whereby data are collected and analyzed to identify characteristics that may make clients vulnerable to illness, premature death, or unhealthy conditions. Examples of such characteristics are unhealthy family patterns that may result in child or elder abuse; lifestyle patterns such as smoking or a high-cholesterol diet that increase the potential for disease occurrence; and hereditary links to disease such as sickle cell anemia. When a health risk is identified, the community health nurse suggests interventions that could reduce this risk. For example, family counseling and caregiver support might decrease the potential for child or elder abuse.

table 9-1 EXAMPLES OF NURSING THEORY BASES APPLICABLE TO COMMUNITY HEALTH NURSING

APPLICABLE CONTENT	NAME OF NURSING THEORY BASE	PRIMARY AUTHOR	NURSING EXAMPLES
Client's self-care ability changing with state of health	Self-Care Framework	Orem, 1971, 1980, 1985, 1991; Orem, Taylor, 1986	Blazek, McCaellen, 1983; Bliss-Holtz, 1988; Campbell, 1986; Chang, Uman, Linn, et al, 1985; Galli, 1984; Hanchett, 1988; Harper, 1984; Hartweg, 1993; Jopp, Carroll, Waters, 1993; Kearney, Fleisher, 1979; Kruger, Shawver, Jones, 1980; Maunz, Woods, 1988; Michael, Sewall, 1980; Nunn, Marriner-Tomey, 1989; Pridham, 1971; Walborn, 1980
Maintaining stressors within client's adaptation Interdependence and role function modes of person in family	Adaptation Model	Roy, 1970, 1976, 1983, 1984, 1987, 1988; Roy, Roberts, 1981; Roy, Andrews, 1991	Fawcett, 1981, 1990; Hanchett, 1988; Kehoe, 1981; Limandri, 1986; Schmitz, 1980; Vicenzi, Thiel, 1992; Wagner, 1976
Primary, secondary, tertiary prevention Lines of defense	Health Care Systems Model	Neuman, 1972, 1980, 1982, 1989, 1990, 1995	Beitler, Tkachuck, Aamodt, 1980; Benedict, Sproles, 1982; Bigbee, 1984; Blank, Clark, Longman, Atwood, 1989; Buchanan, 1987; Hoch, 1987; Pinkerton, 1974; Reed, 1993; Story, Ross, 1986; West, 1984
Holistic health Time perception	Science of Unitary Human Beings	Rogers, 1970, 1980, 1983, 1986, 1989, 1990, 1992, 1994	Boyd, 1985; Fawcett, 1977; Hanchett, 1979, 1988; Laffrey, 1985; Levine, 1976; Rawnsley, 1977; Whall, 1981; Wood, Kekahbah, 1985

Developed by Jan R. Atwood, PhD, MPH, RN, FAAN, Associate Director, Cancer Prevention and Control, University of Nebraska Medical Center/Eppley Cancer Center, and Professor, Colleges of Nursing and Medicine.

Nursing conceptualizations focus on four essential concepts—*person*, *environment*, *health*, and *nursing* (Fawcett, 1984; Flaskerudt, Halloran, 1980; Whall, Fawcett, 1991). Nursing models specify the nursing perspective related to these concepts and their interrelatedness. A nursing "conceptual model comprises abstract, general concepts, and statements that describe and link the concepts. Each conceptual model of nursing represents a particular frame of reference within which patients (persons/ clients), their environments and health states, and nursing activities are viewed, and thus it presents a comprehensive holistic view of nursing care" (Fawcett, Carino, 1989, p. 2).

Several nursing models have been developed in an attempt to capture a comprehensive, holistic view of nursing care. They have met with varying degrees of success. Examples of such models include Johnson's Behavioral System Model, King's Conceptual Framework of Nursing, Neuman's Health Care Systems, Orem's Self-Care Framework, Rogers' Science of Unitary Human Beings, Roy's Adaptation Model, White's Model for Public Health Nursing Practice and Anderson's Community as Client Model. Although most of the nursing models focus on the individual as the unit of analysis, rather than the family and the community, some concepts being advanced by nurse theorists can be applied in the community health nursing arena (Table 9-1). Recent work has begun to provide an understanding of conceptual nursing models as they relate to the community as client (Hanchett, 1988) and the family as client (Chin, 1985; Clements, Roberts, 1983; Gonot, 1986; Hanson, 1984; Johnston, 1986; Riehl-Sisca, 1985; Whall, 1981, 1986; Whall, Fawcett, 1991). Friedemann (1989a, 1989b) is concentrating her scholarly efforts on developing a new conceptual model of nursing that focuses exclusively on the family.

Consistent with the nursing content presented in Table 9-1, community health nursing focuses on the three levels of prevention (primary, secondary, and tertiary), values the holistic nature of humankind, and recognizes the importance of increasing a client's self-care capabilities to promote independence. Community health nurses use a variety of assessment strategies to obtain a holistic perspective about an individual's health status and family dynamics, including a family's role functions and interdependence behaviors (see Chapter 7). Based on assessment data, community health nurses implement intervention strategies that assist clients in maintaining stress at a functional level (within a client's adaptation zone or lines of defense). For example, they coordinate resources for

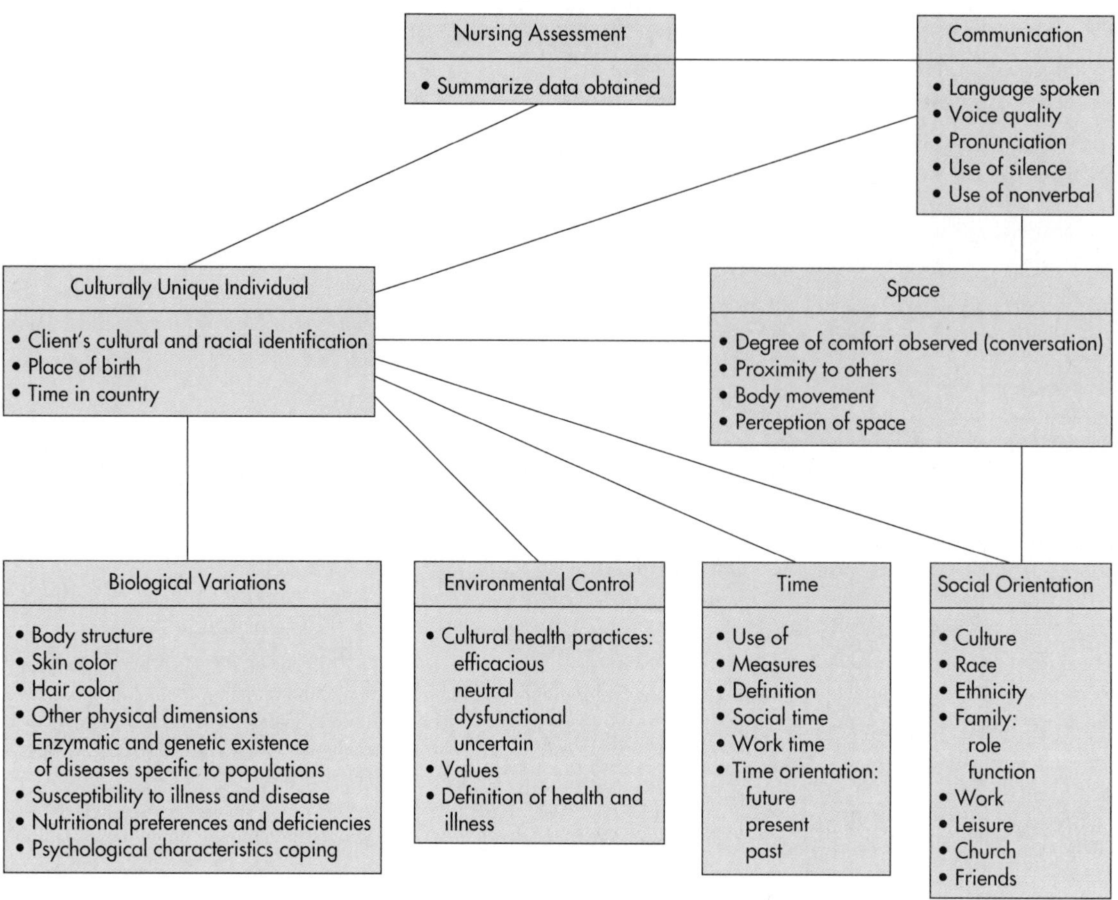

Figure 9-3 Giger and Davidhizar's transcultural assessment model. *(Modified from Giger JN, Davidhizar RE:* Transcultural nursing: assessment and intervention, *ed 2, St. Louis, 1995, Mosby, p. 10.)*

clients who are experiencing stress to decrease the input clients must handle.

Since a comprehensive discussion about nursing theory is beyond the scope of this text, the reader is encouraged to examine writings by the primary author to obtain an accurate understanding of the theoretical and conceptual bases of each nursing model. Examining how others have discussed the application of these models in practice, research, and education can also be beneficial. Table 9-1 provides nursing examples related to community health nursing practice that have applied nursing theory.

CULTURAL FACTORS INFLUENCE PRACTICE

As significant demographic changes have altered the ethnic and racial composition of our nation's population (see Chapter 7), an increased appreciation for cultural diversity has emerged. "The concept of the melting pot, now outmoded, has been replaced by the recognition that this diversity lends strength and uniqueness to the fabric of our society . . . and that greater efforts at understanding and valuing our differences as well as our similarities are needed" (Randall-David, 1989, p. 1). Using an assimilation model that views all clients from the nurse's own cultural perspective negates the value of cultural differences and leads to ineffective nursing practice. It has been well documented that clients bring to the helping relationship values, attitudes, beliefs, and priorities that have developed over generations and that influence health beliefs and practices. Cultural patterning influences families' decisions about when to obtain care and whom they should consult when care is needed. It also influences lifestyle patterns on a daily basis.

Nurses in the community health setting are privileged to enter the homes and lives of culturally diverse families in very intimate ways. They show respect for this privilege by seeking information that increases their awareness of a family's situation from its perspective. The effective community health nurse takes into account cultural factors throughout the helping process. Giger and Davidhizar (1995) have identified cultural phenomena (Figure 9-3) "that vary with application and use, yet are evident in all cultural groups" (p. 8). These phenomena, discussed briefly in the accompanying box, are explored in depth in Giger and Davidhizar's book, *Transcultural Nursing: Assessment and Intervention.*

Cultural Phenomena to Be Considered Throughout the Nursing Process

COMMUNICATION

Communication includes all verbal and nonverbal behavior between people, including things such as vocabulary, grammatical structure, silence, touch, facial expressions, eye and body movements, and expression of warmth and humor.

SPACE

Providing culturally competent care involves examining how families use and control their interpersonal space, including objects in the environment and spatial behavior. Families control their environment to protect themselves from harm, to maintain privacy, to control what occurs in their interpersonal space, and to promote self-identity.

SOCIAL ORGANIZATION

A variety of social organizations (e.g., family, religious groups, ethnic and racial groups, kinship groups, and special interest groups) in a client's environment influences the patterning of cultural behaviors. All of these organizations develop structural and process characteristics that promote specific values, attitudes, beliefs, and norms about growth and development processes, health practices, life goals, and family functioning (refer to Chapter 7).

TIME

Both clock time (an interval of time) and social time influence family behavior. Clock time directs regularity in our lives. Social time refers to patterns and orientations (e.g., past, present, future) that relate to social processes and to the conceptualization and ordering of social life.

ENVIRONMENTAL CONTROL

This term refers to the ability of a family from a particular cultural group to plan activities that control nature or to direct factors in the environment. Health practices and actions taken by families when a family member is ill are affected by how the environment is viewed. Families' views about the environment are influenced by things such as their beliefs about locus of control (internal or external), causes of health and illness (natural or unnatural), and people-to-nature orientation (dominate nature, live in harmony with nature, or subjugate to nature). Views about the environment are also influenced by families' relationships with systems in their environment (e.g., folk medicine or religious system).

BIOLOGICAL VARIATIONS

This phenomena involves examining norms for different cultural/ethnic groups in relation to anatomical characteristics, skin and hair physiology, growth and development patterns, susceptibility and resistance to disease, variations in body systems, and nutritional preferences and deficiencies.

Modified from Giger JN, Davidhizar RE: *Transcultural nursing: assessment and intervention*, ed 2, St. Louis, 1995, Mosby.

The phenomena described by Giger and Davidhizar influence family health factors such as how clients interact with health care providers and others in their environment, clients' beliefs about health and illness and their susceptibility to disease, nutritional preferences and deficiencies, role relationships and communication patterns within a family unit, and time management.

Table 9-2 provides specific examples of how cultural phenomena vary across cultures. These variations influence the use of the nursing process throughout all of its stages. For example, ethnic differences have been found in how members of a specific culture communicate symptoms and how they respond to these symptoms. The Navajo Indians, for instance, have very few words for describing the nature of pain, and their value system supports bearing pain in silence (Simons, 1985). This can lead to an inaccurate assessment and diagnosis regarding the severity of a client's pain, which in turn can influence the nature of interventions (e.g., amount of pain medication given) and evaluation (e.g., relief of pain) of the client's status.

It is important for community health nurses to remember that people are influenced by their culture and that differences among cultures can adversely affect the therapeutic process. For example, it is not unusual for health care providers and clients to have different time perceptions (future-oriented versus present-oriented perceptions) and for the professional to label the client irresponsible when he or she does not keep or is late for appointments. However, "present-oriented individuals do not necessarily adhere strictly to a time-structured schedule" (Giger, Davidhizar, 1995, p. 105). This does not reflect a disregard for others. Rather, it reflects differences in lifestyle patterns that have not been addressed during the therapeutic process.

The box on page 231 describes other situations that illustrate how disparity in health beliefs can adversely affect the therapeutic process. In these situations Eliason (1993) identifies how *ethnocentrism*, "an individual's belief that his or her own cultural group's beliefs and values are the best or the only acceptable beliefs" (p. 226), can adversely influence clients' acceptance of the health care professional and health teaching. Eliason has also identified ethnorelative solutions for reducing cultural barriers to the therapeutic process in the case examples shared in this box. "*Ethnorelativity* is the ability to conceive of alternative viewpoints and to respect the beliefs of another culture even though they are different from one's own" (Eliason, p. 226).

Even though specific incidents can be provided that illustrate how cultural patterning differs across ethnic and racial groups, *it is critically important to mention again that intracultural variations exist and that an individualized assessment*

Table 9-2 Cross-Cultural Examples of Cultural Phenomena Affecting Nursing Care

Nations of Origin	Communication	Space	Time Orientation	Social Organization	Environmental Control	Biological Variations
ASIAN China Hawaii Philippines Korea Japan Southeast Asia (Laos, Cambodia, Vietnam)	National language preference Dialects, written characters Use of silence Nonverbal and contextual cuing	Noncontact people	Present	Family: hierarchial structure, loyalty Devotion to tradition Many religions, including Taoism, Buddhism, Islam, and Christianity Community social organizations	Traditional health and illness beliefs Use of traditional medicines Traditional practitioners: Chinese doctors and herbalists	Liver cancer Stomach cancer Coccidioidomycosis Hypertension Lactose intolerance
AFRICAN West Coast (as slaves) Many African countries West Indian Islands Dominican Republic Haiti Jamaica	National languages Dialect: Pidgin, Creole, Spanish, and French	Close personal space	Present over future	Family: many female, single parent Large, extended family networks Strong church affiliation within community Community social organizations	Traditional health and illness beliefs Folk medicine tradition Traditional healer: root-worker	Sickle cell anemia Hypertension Cancer of the esophagus Stomach cancer Coccidioidomycosis Lactose intolerance
EUROPE Germany England Italy Ireland Other European countries	National languages Many learn English immediately	Noncontact people Aloof Distant Southern countries: closer contact and touch	Future over present	Nuclear families Extended families Judeo-Christian religions Community social organizations	Primary reliance on modern health care system Traditional health and illness beliefs Some remaining folk medicine traditions	Breast cancer Heart disease Diabetes mellitus Thalassemia
NATIVE AMERICAN 170 Native American tribes Aleuts Eskimos	Tribal languages Use of silence and body language	Space very important and has no boundaries	Present	Extremely family oriented Biological and extended families Children taught to respect traditions Community social organizations	Traditional health and illness beliefs Folk medicine tradition Traditional healer: medicine man	Accidents Heart disease Cirrhosis of the liver Diabetes mellitus
HISPANIC COUNTRIES Spain Cuba Mexico Central and South America	Spanish or Portuguese primary language	Tactile relationships Touch Handshakes Embracing Value physical presence	Present	Nuclear family Extended families *Compadrazzo:* godparents Community social organizations	Traditional health and illness beliefs Folk medicine tradition Traditional healers: *Curandero, Espiritista, Partera, Senora*	Diabetes mellitus Parasites Coccidioidomycosis Lactose intolerance

Compiled by Rachel Spector, RN, Ph.D. Modifed from Potter PA, Perry AG: *Fundamentals of nursing: concepts, process, and practice*, ed 4, St. Louis, 1997, Mosby, p. 356.

Examples of Disparity in Health Beliefs

EXAMPLE #1

Carlos is a 15-year-old from a poor urban area where drugs proliferate and many young men trade sex for drugs or money. You are fairly certain that Carlos does not use IV drugs, but know that he often has sex with men for money. Carlos believes that only homosexual men are at risk for AIDS. Because he considers his prostitution a job, not a sexual identity, he does not think of himself as being at risk for AIDS.

Ethnocentric Solutions

1. Convince Carlos that he is gay because he has sex with men; therefore he is at risk for AIDS.
2. Diagnose Carlos as "noncompliant" because he does not alter his behavior after you inform him of the risks.

Ethnorelative Solutions

3. Respect Carlos's beliefs and try to teach him about risky behaviors without discussing sexual identities or applying a label to his behavior.

EXAMPLE #2

Harold and Sarah are expecting their first child. Sarah comes to a prenatal clinic for her first visit. The nurse notes that Sarah is 26 years old, well educated, and healthy. Sarah is informed that she has no unusual risks for her pregnancy. The baby is born healthy, but 10 months later the clinic is being sued because the baby has Tay-Sachs disease and Harold and Sarah were not told that they, as Ashkenazi Jews, were at risk.

Ethnocentric Solutions

1. Blame Sarah for not informing the clinic, because she did not "look Jewish."
2. Blame the clinic administrators, who did not include "Jewish" as a racial identity as well as a religion.

Ethnorelative Solutions

3. Alter clinic health assessment records to ensure reporting of racial/ethnic identity. Educate staff on health and risk for illness factors that differ by race or ethnicity.

EXAMPLE #3

June, a 35-year-old surgical nurse, grew up in a fundamentalist religion, although she rarely attends church now. June admits a middle-aged female patient who is to undergo major surgery the next day. The patient, Barbara, insists that her companion, Alicia, be present for the preop teaching and any discussions of her health. June explains that only spouses or biological family members will be allowed to visit Barbara in the recovery room or the ICU after surgery. When Barbara explains that she considers Alicia her spouse, June leaves the room. Later she comments to coworkers; "It wouldn't be so bad if she didn't throw her homosexuality in my face like that! It really bothers me when those people flaunt their sexuality!" She avoids Barbara's room for the rest of the shift.

Ethnocentric Solutions

1. Uphold hospital policy and do not allow Alicia to visit or make decisions with Barbara.
2. Refuse to care for Barbara, or, if giving her care, avoid any discussion of her sexual identity.

Ethnorelative Solutions

3. Reconsider hospital policies. Must "significant others" be so narrowly defined? What are the purposes of the restrictions?
4. Examine personal beliefs. How did June come to be so negative about lesbians? Does her religious background—much of which she has already rejected—affect her current views?
5. Find out more information about the health care needs of lesbians. Ask Barbara about her wishes and include Alicia in her care.

EXAMPLE #4

Tammi is a 75-year-old woman who was born in China and immigrated to the United States when she was 40. She lives in a predominantly Chinese neighborhood and maintains her traditional values and customs. Although the nurse introduced himself as Tony several times and has asked Tammi to call him by his first name, she continues to call him "doctor." Whenever Tony calls her Tammi, she looks away, but does not say anything about it. Tony is finding it increasingly difficult to communicate with Tammi. Later Tony learns from Tammi's daughter that it is not proper to call strangers by their first name, and it is disrespectful for 25-year-old Tony to call an elder by her first name. It is also not considered polite to make demands upon authority figures, but to take what they offer.

Ethnocentric Solutions

1. Diagnose an alteration in communication or lack of assertiveness because Tammi failed to inform Tony of her wishes.
2. Tell Tammi that in this country, we call people by their first names.

Ethnorelative Solutions

3. Ask her how she would like to be addressed. Offer your whole name and let her choose how to address you.
4. Offer her choices instead of asking open-ended questions.

EXAMPLE #5

Clara is an 82-year-old African-American woman from a small rural community. She has arthritis and congestive heart failure. She has experienced considerable knee pain recently, and Ruth is following up on her prescription for an anti-inflammatory. Ruth, a community health nurse, discovers that Clara never filled the prescription, but is using a "mustard plaster" made of various greens from her garden. She states that the pain is gone and she has no need for expensive pills.

Ethnocentric Solutions

1. Label her as "noncompliant" and encourage her to fill the prescription.
2. Try to persuade her that the greens have no therapeutic value. She should use "real" medicine.

Ethnorelative Solutions

3. Try to determine whether there are other reasons for her rejecting the medication, such as not being able to afford the prescription.
4. Believe her when she says she has no pain and encourage her to continue the mustard plaster treatments.

Modified from Eliason MS: Ethics and transcultural nursing care, *Nurs Outlook* 41(5):227-228, 1993.

is necessary to identify family values, attitudes, beliefs, and norms. However, having an awareness of cultural differences provides a framework for nursing assessment, intervention, and evaluation.

PHASES OF THE FAMILY-CENTERED NURSING PROCESS

The family-centered nursing process has six phases: assessing, analyzing, planning, implementing, evaluating, and terminating. Although each phase is discussed separately, they interrelate and overlap. The interdependent nature of these phases, along with nursing activities during each phase, is presented in Table 9-3. A comprehensive family assessment evaluates multiple components of family health (Figure 9-4). The family is the central focus throughout the nursing process, and assessment data are always validated with the family. The family should be active participants in planning, implementing, and evaluating interventions that are designed to promote family growth. The family-centered nursing process is a client-oriented, not a nurse-oriented, process. This process focuses on strengthening the family's self-care capacities.

Assessing

The assessment phase involves a systematic data collection process that provides the foundation for making nursing diagnoses. During this phase the community health nurse places emphasis on collecting specific data about client (family) functioning so that objective conclusions regarding the client's health status can be made. Inferences about a client's level of functioning should be made only after a sufficient database has been obtained.

The primary responsibilities of the community health nurse during the assessment phase are three-fold: (1) developing a trusting, therapeutic relationship; (2) using a variety of data collection methods to obtain client information from all available resources; and (3) assessing all parameters of family health, including family dynamics, family resources, health status of individual family members, and environmental factors that influence family health. Careful attention given to all three of these activities helps the community health nurse to clearly delineate client needs and goals and interventions that may enhance client growth.

FIRST HOME VISITS Home visiting is a long-established method for promoting family health at all levels of prevention (GAO, 1990; Weiss, 1993). Despite a recent trend emphasizing aggregate-based interventions such as group-work and clinic or school services, home visiting continues to be a significant component of community health nursing practice. In the home health care setting, it is the principal means by which community health nurses provide services for clients and their families. Recent laws, in particular those dealing with Medicaid prenatal care expansions and services to developmentally delayed and at-risk infants and toddlers and their families, include provisions that provide a new impetus for home visiting (GAO, 1990, p. 24).

Making first home visits to families can initially be stressful, especially for a nurse entering an unknown environment controlled by the client rather than the health care professional. First home visits can also be challenging, particularly if the nurse recognizes that he or she is providing a valuable service. In general families are receptive and interested in the services community health nurses have to offer. There may be times, however, when a family prefers to handle its health care needs within the family unit without assistance from "outsiders." If this is the preferred family pattern of functioning, the community health nurse must accept the family's decision and not view this as a personal failure. Sometimes families do not appear interested in home visits because they are unaware of how a community health nurse may assist them.

Educating a family about community health nursing services may provide the family with the information needed to make an informed decision regarding continued visits. When supplying these data the nurse should focus on issues pertinent to the family. For example, when a community health nurse receives antepartum referrals for families having difficulty paying for prenatal care, he or she frequently helps these families to identify community resources that would be helpful to them. Or if the community health nurse receives a referral for an elderly family needing home health care, the nurse would focus attention on home care services relevant to the family's needs, including where to obtain supplies and equipment, the role of the home health aide, and resources in the community that will deliver meals or help with family home maintenance activities.

FIRST HOME VISITS: NURSING RESPONSIBILITIES First home visits can influence families' receptivity to future home visits. Carefully planned first visits can facilitate relationship building and assist nurses in demonstrating the contributions they can make in helping families to deal with current health needs. Table 9-4 outlines how to prepare for a first home visit, tasks to initiate during the visit, and postvisit activities. The goals for the first visit should be to establish a positive client/nurse working relationship, obtain baseline data on the family situation, and address the immediate concerns of the family. The extent to which the nurse carries out the tasks identified in Table 9-4 during the initial visit will vary depending on the family's circumstances. Some tasks will not be done at all because they are not appropriate for the client's situation. For example, doctor's orders are not required for families receiving only health promotion services. On the other hand, nurses do not provide home health or care of the sick services without a doctor's order. It is critical to remember that the assessment phase of the nursing process is ongoing and should extend throughout the length of the nurse/client relationship. *It is not feasible or appropriate to obtain all needed data during the initial contact.*

table 9-3 Relationships Among the Phases of the Family-Centered Nursing Process

Assessing ⟶ / ⟵	Analyzing ⟶ / ⟵	Planning ⟶ / ⟵	Implementing ⟶ / ⟵	Evaluating ⟶ / ⟵	Terminating ⟵
Process for obtaining a data base	A critical thinking process that results in the identification of nursing diagnoses	Formulation of desired family outcomes (goals) and identification of actions (intervention strategies) to achieve goals	A systematic approach to action used by the family and nurse to achieve desired family outcomes	A continuous, concurrent process used to critique each component of the nursing process	A therapeutic process that helps the client and the nurse to end their relationship
Assessing	**Analyzing**	**Planning**	**Implementing**	**Evaluating**	**Terminating**
1. Develop a trusting relationship: a. Explain purpose of community health nursing visit b. Describe what community health nurse has to offer c. Facilitate the sharing of thoughts, feelings, and data d. Set time parameters for evaluation and frequency and length of visits 2. Collect data in variety of ways: a. Observation b. Interview c. Inspection d. Physical assessment e. Contact with secondary sources f. Review of records 3. Assess all parameters of family functioning: a. Family dynamics b. Health status: family and individual members c. Physiological data d. Psychosocial data	1. Make differential conclusions about family needs by: a. Using theoretical knowledge to identify significant signs and symptoms b. Grouping data to show relationships between assessment categories and to identify *patterns* of behavior c. Relating family data to relevant clinical and research findings d. Comparing nursing diagnoses with diagnoses of other health professionals	1. Formulate client-centered goals and expected outcomes: a. Establish realistic goals consistent with the database and nursing diagnoses b. State goals and outcomes in measurable terms c. Develop family and individual goals and expected outcomes in collaboration with the family. 2. Identify intervention strategies: a. Identify direct and indirect care interventions consistent with client needs b. Determine activities that the client, the nurse, and other health care professionals might carry out to achieve expected outcomes	1. Base nursing actions on client needs, lifestyle patterns, level of knowledge, and motivation a. Determine client readiness b. Demonstrate awareness of proper timing for nursing activities c. Adapt or alter nursing interventions if client situation changes d. Modify nursing activities to accommodate lifestyle patterns, level of knowledge 2. Address barriers (e.g., cultural or financial) to client action a. Explore with family reasons for progress or lack of it	1. Elicit ongoing feedback from client to determine if goals, plans, and interventions are appropriate 2. Identify the results of intervention activities taken by: a. Client b. Community health nurse c. Other health care professionals 3. Determine why intervention activities have been ineffective, if warranted 4. Modify the management plan when appropriate	1. Deal with feelings associated with termination 2. Review client achievements 3. Discuss what the therapeutic process has meant 4. Plan carefully the termination of visits 5. Share with client how to reestablish contact if needed 6. Discuss with client self-care requirements upon discharge

Continued

table 9-3 Relationships Among the Phases of the Family-Centered Nursing Process—cont'd

Assessing	Analyzing	Planning	Implementing	Evaluating	Terminating
e. Sociocultural data f. Environmental data g. Preventive health practices 4. Obtain data from multiple sources: a. Client, family b. Health team members c. Community agencies d. Significant others e. Relevant records 5. Use standards of care to focus the interviewing process	2. Formulate specific nursing diagnoses: a. Base diagnoses on a strong data base b. Identify the functional aspects of a client's current health status c. Determine various levels of family functioning (1) Strengths (2) Needs (3) Anticipatory guidance warranted d. Identify when data are insufficient to make a nursing diagnosis	c. Assist the client in identifying the pros and cons of each intervention and in making decisions about the appropriate course of action 3. Identify priority needs, goals, and interventions: a. Use theory to differentiate between problems that need immediate action and those that can wait b. Identify potential crisis situations c. Consider client safety 4. Identify evaluation criteria	b. Assist family in overcoming barriers to action 3. Carry through with planned interventions a. Keep appointments with the family b. Carry out nursing activities in a timely manner c. Discuss with the family the need for altering interventions if necessary d. Assist the family in carrying out planned interventions 4. Base intervention activities on scientific knowledge a. Review scientific literature b. Use acceptable standards (e.g., growth and development or nutritional) c. Consult with peers, supervisors, and other health care providers	5. Use a variety of methods to evaluate: a. Obtain feedback from client b. Consult with peers, supervisors, and other health care professionals c. Summarize records d. Conduct nursing audits	

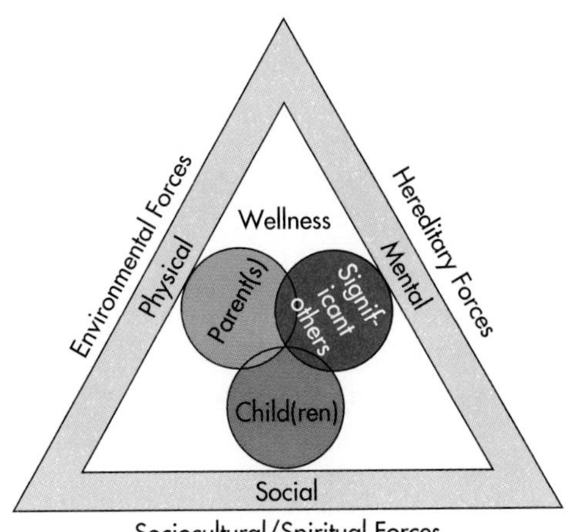

Figure 9-4 Triangle of family health.

Community health nurses encounter a variety of situations on first home visits, such as families who want parenting education or elderly couples who have requested assistance with care of an ill family member. While the major focus on these visits may vary from care of the sick to health teaching, the provision of primary prevention services is a major component of all community health nursing visits. Primary prevention interventions should not be neglected during care of the sick visits. Examples of these types of interventions are teaching to increase the client's self-care capabilities, environmental assessment to prevent home accidents, and referral for respite services to prevent caregiver burnout.

SAFETY IN THE COMMUNITY As in any situation, it is important to consider issues of environmental safety when visiting an unfamiliar area. Statistical data reflect that crime is on the rise in all socioeconomic neighborhoods and in a variety of health and welfare organizations. Although reports of crime involving community health nurses are unusual, take precautions to avoid unsafe or potentially unsafe situations.

It is important to carefully observe environmental conditions and to leave a home or neighborhood if you "sense" that it could be unsafe. Experienced nurses watch for such things as an unusually large number of people congregating in the neighborhood, violent exchanges between family members or individuals in the community, people who appear to be abusing alcohol or drugs, and individuals suspiciously hanging around cars or doorways.

Most community health agencies have safety guidelines to follow, including refusing rides from strangers, dressing professionally, not wearing expensive jewelry and suggestive clothing, planning ahead to avoid appearing lost, leaving an established visit plan in the agency, and not entering an environment where safety is questionable. Families being visited may also provide the nurse with safety guidelines such as where to park one's car in the neighborhood and best times during the day to visit. The nurse may consult with a family by phone if she has questions about environmental conditions.

Some nurses find that they have fears about all aspects of the environment because they are in surroundings entirely different from those they have previously experienced. If this is the case, the nurse will find it helpful to discuss her or his fears with a colleague who can help the nurse to objectively analyze the situation. On the whole nurses have found that the community is an exciting and challenging environment that is open to caring professionals.

RELATIONSHIP BUILDING The type of relationship established during the assessment phase can be the critical factor in helping the client determine whether to accept the assistance offered by the community health nurse. It is natural for clients to evaluate their interactions with community health nurses during the assessment phase. Most people take time to assess how others respond to them before they develop a trusting relationship that allows disclosure of personal thoughts, feelings, and problems.

Explaining the purpose of community health nursing visits, describing services the community health nurse can provide, and fostering a nonthreatening atmosphere that allows the client to share data at his or her own pace are some ways to build trust between the nurse and the client. Clarifying why the community health nurse is visiting is essential. When clients do not understand the purpose of nursing visits it is hard for them to become involved in the therapeutic process. Lack of clarity in the therapeutic relationship can result in frustration and mistrust and inhibit the expression of thoughts, feelings, and data. Clients usually do not share information freely until they understand why the information is needed.

Sharing with clients their rights and responsibilities and agency obligations can help to clarify the purpose of home visits. All clients have the right to be active participants in the care process, including continuity of care decisions, and to have their privacy and property respected. They also have the right to voice complaints without fear of reprisal. Table 9-5 delineates specific client rights and responsibilities and related agency obligations as defined by the Health Care Financing Administration (HCFA, 1991; 1994).

FAMILY INTERVIEWS. Working with families presents special interviewing challenges for the community health nurse, because families are composed of unique individuals who have varying needs, concerns, and communication styles. Since the goal of community health nursing is to enhance the well-being of the family unit (Bomar, McNeely, 1996), as well as to help individual family members, it is important to determine whether the family is successfully executing activities to meet family and individual needs. It is also important to examine at the same time if the family is satisfying societal expectations (Danielson, Hamel-Bissell, Winstead-Fry, 1993, p. 201). For example, when nurses work with a family that is dealing with an unexpected stressful event, such as the birth of a premature in-

table 9-4 First Home Visits: Responsibilities and Tasks

Responsibility	Tasks
I. Previsit preparation	Review available family data including referral information and previous family records. Clarify data with others if unclear (e.g., contact family physician and/or other referral sources or talk with intake nurse). Establish a plan for the visit. Consider appropriate community resources. Review theory related to identified family problems. Prepare for a safe visit (e.g., identify exact location of home, consider safety issues in relation to the neighborhood being visited, and request escort or shared visit services if needed).
II. Establish contact with family	Contact family via phone, if available. Identify self, including name and agency you are representing. Explain who referred family to agency and purpose of referral. Discuss briefly services CHN can provide, such as sharing data about available community resources. Identify family's need for CHN services and willingness to have nurse visits. Schedule home visit at a time convenient for family.
III. Home visit intervention	
A. Relationship-building period	Introduce self and role. Introduce agency, agency obligations, and programs and services. Explain purpose of home visit. Build a nurse/client relationship. Discuss client rights and responsibilities. Assess safety of care plan: is a primary caregiver present and available if needed? Consider safety issues for the health care provider (e.g., park near the home, don't enter the house if the client is not home, and dress professionally, avoiding expensive jewelry and suggestive clothing).
B. Intervention period	Carry out an *initial* client assessment.* Carry out an *initial* family assessment.* Carry out an *initial* environmental assessment,* especially in relation to client safety and health needs. Elicit family's perceptions of how a CHN can assist. Assess doctor's orders and need for changes if appropriate. Assess appropriateness of stated third-party reimbursement. Assess need for other services such as physical therapy or referral to a community agency for parenting classes. Assess need for equipment and supplies. Confirm medication orders, dosages, and client knowledge of medications. Identify client's knowledge base related to identified problems (e.g., disease process or care of infant). Discuss estimated length of service, including limits set by third-party payors, if appropriate.
C. Closing period	Summarize visit activities with family. Together decide what the client/family will be doing between now and the next visit. Inform client/family how to reach nurse between visits. Set time for next visit.
IV. Postvisit activities	Begin the nursing care plan. Document visit. Make contacts on behalf of client/family if needed (e.g., initiate other services, contact physician regarding needed change in order, or inform vendors about needed equipment and supplies). Complete agency reporting forms and paperwork for third-party reimbursement. Evaluate visit progress.

*On the first home visit it is not feasible to complete a comprehensive family assessment. Priority should be given to assessing the family's major concerns and factors that influence these concerns. Referral data can assist a nurse in focusing the initial family assessment.

table 9-5 CLIENT RIGHTS AND RESPONSIBILITIES AND RELATED AGENCY OBLIGATIONS

RIGHTS/OBLIGATIONS	CLIENT RIGHTS	AGENCY OBLIGATIONS
Notice of rights	To be fully informed of all his or her rights and responsibilities	Provide client with a written notice of rights in advance of initiating care Obtain signed verification from client or client's caregiver that they have received written notice of rights
Exercise of rights and respect for property and person	To have property treated with respect To voice grievances and suggest change in service without fear of reprisal or discrimination To have family or guardian voice grievances when judged incompetent To have privacy respected	Investigate complaints made by client or client's family or guardian Document existence of complaint and resolution of complaint
To be informed and to participate in planning care and treatment	To receive appropriate and professional care related to physician orders To choose care provided To receive information necessary to give informed consent before the start of any care To know how to reach agency staff 24 hours a day, 7 days a week, and what to do in an emergency To refuse treatment within the confines of the law and be informed of the consequences of this action To reasonable continuity of care To be informed in reasonable time of anticipated termination of service and plans for transfer to another agency	Admit client for service only if the agency has the ability to provide safe professional care at the level of intensity needed Share with client physician orders Advise client in advance of care, the disciplines that will furnish care, and the frequency of visits Advise client in advance of any changes in care Involve client in the planning of care Inform client of agency policies and procedures
Confidentiality of medical record	To have agency maintain confidentiality of the clinical records	Advise client of agency's policies and procedures regarding disclosure of information in clinical records
Liability for payment	To receive information regarding charges for services, the client's potential liability for these charges, and client's eligibility for third-party reimbursements To referral if service denied solely on the inability to pay for service	Inform client orally and in writing and in advance of care the extent to which third party reimbursement may pay for care and charges client may have to pay Notify client orally and in writing of changes in eligibility for services from third-party reimbursement
Home health hotline	To know about the availability of a toll-free home health hotline in the state to voice complaints about agency services or to have questions answered about home care	Inform client in writing how to reach the home health hotline

Data from Health Care Financing Administration (HCFA): *Conditions of participation: home health agencies*, 42 CFR Part 484, Section 484.10 through 484.52, Washington, D.C., October, 1994, HCFA, Section 484.10.

fant or a diagnosis of cancer, it is crucial to explore how well the family unit is carrying out its role responsibilities (e.g., maintaining work and school schedules and nurturing all family members). During times of stress it is not uncommon for the family to neglect these responsibilities, which can significantly alter family functioning. If this were the situation, the community health nurse would problem-solve with the family to determine ways to achieve a balance in family dynamics (see Chapter 8 for interventions that enhance family problem-solving abilities during times of stress).

When a nurse is allowed to cross the family boundaries and is accepted by the family system, the influences the nurse has on that system must be examined carefully. The nurse needs to watch closely her or his own interactions between individual family members and avoid establishing alliances during the family decision-making process. For example, a nurse who firmly believes that all women need a career outside the home may strongly support a female client's desires to work without allowing her husband or significant other to verbalize his concerns. In situations like these the nurse needs to help the family evaluate the pros

Guidelines for Relating to Clients from Different Cultures

1. **Assess your personal beliefs surrounding persons from different cultures.**
   - Review your personal beliefs and past experiences
   - Set aside any values, biases, ideas, and attitudes that are judgmental and may negatively affect care
2. **Assess communication variables from a cultural perspective.**
   - Determine the ethnic identity of the client, including generation in America
   - Use the client as a source of information when possible
   - Assess cultural factors that may affect your relationship with the client and respond appropriately
3. **Plan care based on the communicated needs and cultural background.**
   - Learn as much as possible about the client's cultural customs and beliefs
   - Encourage the client to reveal cultural interpretation of health, illness, and health care
   - Be sensitive to the uniqueness of the client
   - Identify sources of discrepancy between the client's and your own concepts of health and illness
   - Communicate at the client's personal level of functioning
   - Evaluate effectiveness of nursing actions and modify the nursing care plan when necessary
4. **Modify communication approaches to meet cultural needs.**
   - Be attentive to signs of fear, anxiety, and confusion in the client
   - Respond in a reassuring manner in keeping with the client's cultural orientation
   - Be aware that in some cultural groups discussion concerning the client with others may be offensive and may impede the nursing process
5. **Understand that respect for the client and communicated needs is central to the therapeutic relationship.**
   - Communicate respect by using a kind and attentive approach
   - Learn how listening is communicated in the client's culture
   - Use appropriate active listening techniques
   - Adopt an attitude of flexibility, respect, and interest to help bridge barriers imposed by culture
6. **Communicate in a nonthreatening manner.**
   - Conduct the interview in an unhurried manner
   - Follow acceptable social and cultural amenities
   - Ask general questions during the information-gathering stage
   - Be patient with a respondent who gives information that may seem unrelated to the client's health problem
   - Develop a trusting relationship by listening carefully, allowing time, and giving the client your full attention
7. **Use validating techniques in communication.**
   - Be alert for feedback that the client is not understanding
   - Do not assume meaning is interpreted without distortion
8. **Be considerate of reluctance to talk when the subject involves sexual matters.**
   - Be aware that in some cultures sexual matters are not discussed freely with members of the opposite sex
9. **Adopt special approaches when the client speaks a different language.**
   - Use a caring tone of voice and facial expression to help alleviate the client's fears
   - Speak slowly and distinctly, but not loudly
   - Use gestures, pictures, and play acting to help the client understand
   - Repeat the message in different ways if necessary
   - Be alert to words the client seems to understand and use them frequently
   - Keep messages simple and repeat them frequently
   - Avoid using medical terms and abbreviations that the client may not understand
   - Use an appropriate language dictionary
10. **Use interpreters to improve communication.**
    - Ask the interpreter to translate the message, not just the individual words
    - Obtain feedback to confirm understanding
    - Use an interpreter who is culturally sensitive

Modified from Giger JN, Davidhizar RE: *Transcultural nursing: assessment and intervention*, ed 2, St. Louis, 1995, Mosby, p. 38.

and cons of taking a certain action, and then encourage joint decision making between the couple.

It is particularly easy for community health nurses to support one family member's view over another because they are not always able to see the entire family unit at one time. Remembering that establishing an alliance with an individual family member is not therapeutic and that it can lead to or reinforce ineffective family patterns can help a nurse take action that supports effective communication within the family unit.

The values, attitudes, and beliefs held by the community health nurse can also disrupt the nurse/family interview. Professionals bring to the therapeutic process cultural patterning that influences thinking about variables such as how roles should be implemented, how a home should be managed, and how children should be raised. The nurse may unconsciously label family behavior as ineffective if it is not consistent with her or his beliefs. Use of peer collaboration and supervision helps the professional nurse to identify when personal beliefs are affecting the therapeutic process.

The guidelines presented in the box above can assist the nurse in avoiding barriers to therapeutic communication and in establishing an effective client/nurse relationship in varying cultural situations. A skillful interviewer avoids barriers to communication such as false reassurance, advice giving, excessive talking, and the showing of approval or disapproval. For example, even when asked, "What would you do if you were me?", an empathic interviewer would avoid advice-giving while responding to the family's feelings of distress. A skillful interviewer also adjusts his or her interviewing approach to meet client needs. This involves determining such things as when to be directive or nondirective, when and how to approach sensitive topics, and acceptable social and cultural amenities.

SOURCES AND METHODS FOR COLLECTING DATA During the assessment phase both primary and secondary data are collected from all available sources to determine how well the family is coping with encountered stressors. Primary data are those data which the community health nurse actually obtains from the client or sees, hears, feels, or smells in the client's environment. An astute community health nurse carefully notes observations and verbal information received from the client. Significant clues about a client's level of functioning can be obtained by observing how the client interacts within the environment. It is not unusual for the community health nurse to discern a child discipline problem by repeatedly watching parents interact with their children during home visits. When a nurse observes client functioning, it is important to remember that inferences about client problems should be based on *patterns of behavior* rather than isolated incidents. Labeling behavior ineffective after one observation is a dangerous practice and can adversely affect the nurse-family relationship.

In the community health setting, secondary data are obtained from a variety of sources such as significant others, personnel from health and social agencies, the family's physician, spiritual leaders, and health records. When these data are recorded the source of the information should also be indicated. Generally the community health nurse receives either verbal or written permission from the client before making contact with secondary sources of data outside the family system. This practice not only protects the client's right of privacy but also promotes honesty and trust in the therapeutic relationship. In addition, seeking a client's permission to obtain information from others demonstrates to the client that the nurse respects the client's right of self-determination.

When using secondary data the nurse must recognize that it may not accurately reflect clients' perceptions of themselves or their needs. Instead, secondary data may reflect what others perceive about clients' situations. This point is particularly significant for a community health nurse to keep in mind, because frequently secondary data about the problems of family members are obtained when these individuals are not present. When this occurs the community health nurse often finds it necessary to make arrangements to interview all family members. For example, she or he may visit a child in school or schedule a home visit after school hours in order to identify how the child is reacting to a newly diagnosed health problem. Or the community health nurse may make arrangements to meet with the entire family.

Various assessment methodologies should be used to collect primary and secondary data. Interview, observation, direct examination (auscultation, percussion, palpation, inspection, and measurement), contact with secondary sources of data, and review of relevant records are methods used by the community health nurse to obtain an accurate and complete profile of a family's situation. These methods are used to identify client strengths as well as client needs.

The significance of using a variety of methods to collect data about family functioning cannot be overstated. No one data collection method provides the community health nurse with all the information needed to formulate accurate nursing diagnoses. The Daniels family case scenario that follows illustrates this fact by showing the contrast between the type of data one nurse obtained from interview and from direct observation.

CASE *Scenario*

Following hospitalization of Mr. Daniels for an acute exacerbation episode of multiple sclerosis, the Daniels family was referred to the health department for health supervision follow-up. Ms. Garitt, hospital social worker, requested that a community health nurse assess this family's needs in relation to its understanding of multiple sclerosis, its ability to handle activities of daily living, its knowledge of community resources, and the impact of Mr. Daniels' illness on family functioning. While Jane Mathews, CHN, was interviewing the family and collecting data on the entire family situation, she asked Mr. and Mrs. Daniels how they were managing Mr. Daniels' exercises. Both related that they were doing them regularly. Mrs. Daniels accurately described how the exercises should be done and verbalized that she felt comfortable handling them since she was instructed how to do so by hospital staff. While Mrs. Daniels was demonstrating what she had learned it was found that she did have an understanding about the proper exercises for her husband. However, her body mechanics were inappropriate, and this caused severe backache that she failed to mention during the interviewing process. In addition to Mrs. Daniels' poor body mechanics, the nurse also discovered that Mr. Daniels was very demanding of his wife, expecting her to do exercises for him that he could do independently. Further exploration revealed that Mr. Daniels was doing very little for himself. Before his illness he had been the "man of the house. Now I can't do anything." Through demonstration and return demonstration the nurse showed Mr. Daniels that he was not helpless and assisted Mrs. Daniels in learning how to position herself appropriately when helping her husband. The nurse also helped the family identify family patterns that were fostering dependency.

If the community health nurse in this situation had not observed Mr. and Mrs. Daniels's functioning, it could have taken her a considerable length of time to collect the data

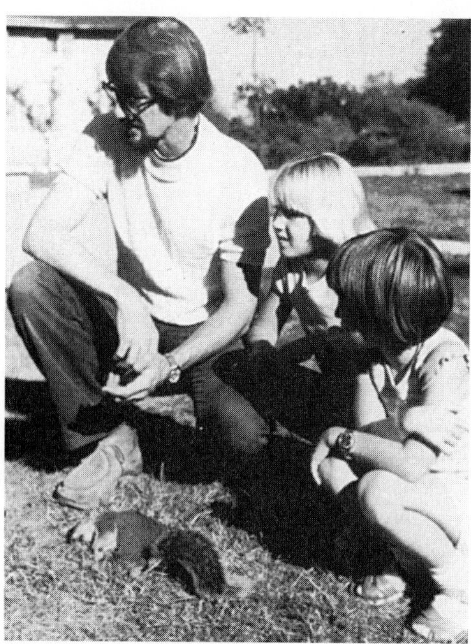

Figure 9-5 Family dynamics influence how well individual family members handle critical life events. The ability to provide support and security during times of stress (exposure to death) is a family strength that should be reinforced.

needed to accurately identify the real concerns in this family situation. Observing family interactions provided this nurse with data about family functioning that were not obtained through interview.

ASSESSING ALL PARAMETERS OF FAMILY HEALTH The family-centered approach to nursing care focuses on the family as a unit rather than a collection of individual family members. This implies that the family is viewed as a system in which the actions and health status of one family member always affect the behavior and health status of all other family members. Thus when community health nurses assess family health they not only examine the health status of individual family members but look at family dynamics as well (Figure 9-5). Chapter 7 presents guidelines for examining family dynamics and includes a family assessment guide (see Appendix 7-2) that facilitates data collection for the purpose of evaluating a family's health status. Hanson and Mischke (1996) have identified a range of family assessment and measurement instruments that have been developed by nonnurses and nurses. Several of these instruments are discussed more extensively in Berkey and Hanson's *Pocket Guide to Family Assessment and Intervention* (1991).

FAMILY HEALTH STATUS. As previously discussed, a major goal of nurses working with families in the community is to enhance the well-being of the family unit. Inherent in this goal is the belief that it is important for families to maintain the integrity of the family unit while meeting the needs of individual family members. It is crucial for both families and nurses to recognize that if the health status of the family unit is neglected, it will be difficult for families to assist individual family members, particularly during periods of stress.

"Family health is the family's quality of life from a holistic perspective as it is affected by such variables as spirituality, nutrition, stress, environment, recreation and exercise, sleep, and sexuality" (Bomar, 1996, p. ix). During the assessment phase of the nursing process, the community health nurse evaluates the health status of the family unit from a holistic perspective to identify both family strengths and needs. Table 9-6 delineates criteria to consider when assessing family strengths. Several themes emerge when reviewing the literature that addresses characteristics of healthy families (Beavers, 1977; Curran, 1983; Lewis, Beavers, Gossett, Phillips, 1976; Otto, 1963; and Pratt, 1976). Healthy families have flexible role patterns, maintain growth-producing relationships within the family unit and between the family and the broader community, have active problem-solving mechanisms, have an ability to accept help, and are responsive to the needs of individual members. Healthy families also have effective communication patterns, provide a warm, caring atmosphere, and have a strong sense of family in which rituals and traditions are shared. "Overall, a well-functioning family is a flexible one that can shift roles, levels of responsibilities, and patterns of interaction as it passes through periods of varying stressful life changes" (Danielson, Hamel-Bissell, Winstead-Fry, 1993, p. 201).

Community health nurses encounter families with varying states of health. Most families visited by nurses in the community setting are dealing with some type of stressor such as the birth of a child, a newly diagnosed health problem, or inadequate resources to meet the family's basic needs. Danielson, Hamel-Bissell, and Winstead-Fry (1993) use a multifaceted framework (Figure 9-6) to assess whether family behavior during these periods of stress is bonadaptive or maladaptive. Bonadaptation is "the ability of the family to stabilize with instituted patterns in place, promote the individual development of its members, and achieve a sense of coherence and congruency even when stressors and substantive changes threaten established patterns of family functioning" (Danielson, Hamel-Bissell, Winstead-Fry, p. 413). Maladaptation occurs when a family is unable to achieve a balance in family functioning during periods of stress (see Chapter 8). Danielson, Hamel-Bissell, and Winstead-Fry's multifaceted assessment framework assists the community health nurse in evaluating the health of the family from three perspectives: "the result of the interaction between individual members and the family unit, between the family unit and the larger social system, and between sociocultural subsystems and individual members" (Danielson, Hamel-Bissell, Winstead-Fry, p. 201).

Since culture affects how a person perceives health and illness and the manner in which clients seek health care,

table 9-6 Criteria to Consider When Assessing Family Strengths: Three Authors' Viewpoints

Assessment Parameters	Authors		
	Otto (1963): Family Strengths	Pratt (1976): Family Structure and Health Behavior Characterizing the Energized Family	Curran (1983): Traits of a Healthy Family
Adaptive abilities	The ability to provide for the physical, emotional, and spiritual needs of a family The ability to use a crisis or seemingly injurious experience as a means of growth The ability for self-help, and ability to accept help when appropriate An ability to perform family roles flexibly The ability to communicate effectively	Combined health behaviors of all family members are energized; all family members tend to care for their health Actively and energetically attempt to cope with life's problems and issues Flexible division of tasks and activities	The healthy family admits to and seeks help with problems The healthy family communicates and listens
Atmosphere and affect	The ability to be sensitive to the needs of family members The ability to provide support, security, and encouragement	Responsive to the particular interests and needs of individual family members Regular and varied interaction among family members	The healthy family teaches respect for others The healthy family has a sense of play and humor The healthy family shares leisure time The healthy family fosters table time and conversation
Individual autonomy and integrity of family system	Mutual respect for the individuality of family members A concern for family unity, loyalty, and interfamily cooperation	Egalitarian distribution of power Provide autonomy for individual family members	The healthy family respects the privacy of individual members The healthy family affirms and supports individual members The healthy family maintains a balance of interaction among members The healthy family has a strong sense of family in which rituals and traditions abound The healthy family exhibits a sense of shared responsibility The healthy family develops a sense of trust The healthy family has a shared religious core
Relationships with others	The ability to initiate and maintain growth-producing relationships and experiences within and without the family The capacity to maintain and create constructive and responsible relationships in the neighborhood, school, town, and local and state government	Provide regular links with the broader community through active participation in community activities	The healthy family values service to others The healthy family teaches a sense of right and wrong

Modified from Otto H: Criteria for assessing family strength, *Family Process* 2:333-336, 1963; Pratt L: *Family structure and effective health behavior: the energized family*, Boston, 1976, Houghton Mifflin, pp. 84-92; Curran D: *Traits of a healthy family*, copyright by Doris Curran, Minneapolis, Mn., 1983, Winston Press, pp. 23-24.

Questions
• Is family flexible in regard to roles?
• How high is anxiety?
• Are individual members' needs being met?
• Is family as a unit participating?
• What is the family type and pattern of functioning?
Individual family members interactions
+
Questions
• Does family have ties to community?
• What are the existing family resources?
• Are there community resources that may be helpful?
Family and larger social system
+
Sociocultural subsystems and individual family members
+
Questions
• Does family self-identify with an ethnic group?
• Do all members perceive themselves as members of the ethnic group?
• What is the family appraisal and values related to the situations?

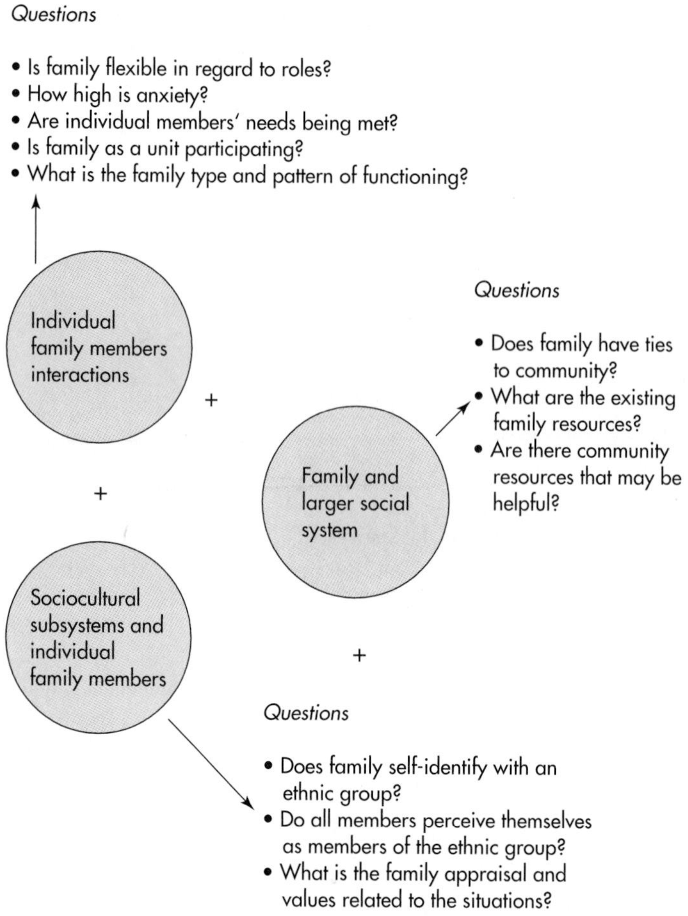

Figure 9-6 Multifaceted family assessment framework. (*From Danielson CB, Hamel-Bissell B, Winstead-Fry P:* Families, health and illness: perspectives on coping and intervention, *St. Louis, 1993, Mosby, p. 202.)*

it is important to examine the family's cultural beliefs, values, and practices when assessing a family's health status. "Cultural assessments are performed to identify patterns that may assist or interfere with a nursing intervention or treatment regimen" (Tripp-Reimer, Brink, Saunders, 1984, p. 81). Cultural assessments help the community health nurse to individualize the nursing care plan for each family. Appendix 7-1 provides guidelines for completing a cultural assessment.

HEALTH STATUS OF FAMILY MEMBERS. The purpose of a family health assessment is to obtain pertinent data about the functioning of individual family members as well as the family system. In keeping with the view of family health just presented, family members are viewed from an integrated, holistic, individual perspective. Biological, psychological, sociocultural, spiritual, developmental, and environmental parameters of functioning are assessed to determine the client's perception of his or her health status. Select cultural and biopsychosocial characteristics to consider when completing an individual health assessment are presented in the box on the next page.

In general, clients do not think systematically about all of the variables that affect their health. A major role of the community health nurse when completing an individual health assessment is to increase the client's awareness of all the factors that influence healthy functioning. A health assessment should be purposeful, meaningful, and goal directed, and should provide the client with an opportunity to identify both personal strengths and needs in relation to the individual's current level of functioning. Data about preventive health practices and healthy aspects of coping, along with information about ways in which the client handles illness, should be elicited.

The vehicles used for organizing an individual functional assessment are the health history and the physical examination. Exploring the techniques of physical appraisal is beyond the scope of this text. Barkauskas, Stoltenberg-Allen, Baumann, and Darling-Fisher (1998) extensively discuss the physical examination process. It is essential for community health nurses to have skill in completing a gross physical appraisal, since clients may lack a regular source of medical care even though they have health problems. Community health nurses must have the ability to distinguish between *abnormal* and *normal* health findings. Price and Wilson (1996) provide a theoretical basis for analyzing health assessment findings. In addition, community health nurses need skill in the use of the referral process (see Chapter 10) in order to help clients obtain needed health care services when abnormal findings are identified.

Select Cultural and Biopsychosocial Characteristics of an Individual

PHYSICAL APPEARANCE (BODY)
Age and developmental stage
Sex and gender identity
Size, height, weight
Skin color
Hair color, configuration, presence/absence
Race (self-identified, perceived by others)
Posture, facial expression
Grooming, personal hygiene
Dress: style, condition
Presence of physical disability
Other characteristics not listed above

MENTAL CHARACTERISTICS, PSYCHOLOGICAL ORIENTATION (MIND)
Cognitive ability, intelligence
Level of consciousness
Emotional disposition, temperament
Aptitude, ability
Sensory acuity (visual, auditory)
Personal traits
Mental health
Other characteristics not listed above

EXTERNAL INFLUENCES (SOCIAL AND PHYSICAL ENVIRONMENT)
Family history, ancestry, geographical origin
Strength of family unit, lines of authority
Role in family, birth order
Languages, communication patterns
Expectations and behavioral norms for age, sex, role
Format (rituals) for major life events (birth, marriage, illness, death)
Economic and work opportunities, access to resources
Housing, living arrangements
Dominant religion, other religions
Theories of disease causation
Availability, quality, variety of health care services
Political, governmental structure
Dietary customs, access to food
Community resources in education, art, music, recreation
Geographical and climatic features
Other influences not listed above

INTERNAL SYNTHESIS OF BODY, MIND, AND ENVIRONMENT (SELF)
Self-concept, self-perception, expectations of self
Beliefs, values, spirituality, religious affiliation
Affect, mood, congruity between words and affect
Attitudes toward health and self care: health history, use of health services
Personal goals, short- and long-term
Work role, economic contribution to self, others
Areas of accomplishment, achievement, sources of pride
Knowledge base, use of educational opportunities
Response to stress, coping strategies, ability to adapt
Language usage: formal, slang, dialect
Food preferences, dietary restrictions
Interests in applied and fine arts, crafts, hobbies, music, literature
Reading ability and preferences
Other characteristics not listed above

Modified from Sibley BJ: Cultural influences on health and illness. In Long BC, Phipps WJ, Cassmeyer VL: *Medical-surgical nursing*, ed 3, St. Louis, 1992, Mosby, p. 32.

Health history. In the community setting, the health history is an important vehicle for assessing the health status of individual family members from a holistic perspective. It has long been recognized that a health assessment from a nursing perspective differs from the health assessment conducted by other disciplines. For example, "a nursing health history differs from a medical health history in that it focuses on the meaning of illness and hospitalization [health care] to the patient [client] and his family as a basis for planning nursing care. The medical history is taken to determine whether pathology is present as a basis for planning medical care" (McPhetridge, 1968, p. 68). When completing a health history, the community health nurse explores carefully the client's perceptions of his or her health status and how current stressors are affecting functioning; emphasis is placed on identifying the client as a unique individual rather than as a person who has a specific disease process.

Components included in a health history vary slightly from one author to another. Basically the goal of a health history is to determine how well the client is meeting health needs and how activities of daily living have been altered to meet these needs. A comprehensive review of the client's past and current health status is elicited to identify an accurate and complete composite of the client's health functioning. With this information the client and the nurse can explore ways for increasing the client's self-care capabilities.

The health history framework developed by Mahoney, Verdisco, and Shortridge (1982) is commonly used in the practice setting. These authors identified seven components of an individual health history, which are presented in Table 9-7.

A commonly used framework for organizing a health status assessment is Gordon's (1997) Functional Health Patterns Typology. Gordon (1987) contends that "all human beings have in common certain functional patterns that contribute to their health, quality of life, and achievement of human potential" and that "these common patterns are the focus of nursing assessment" (p. 92). Table 9-8 provides abbreviated definitions for Gordon's functional health pat-

table 9-7 Seven Components of an Individual Health History

Component	Data Collected
Reason for contact	Why the client is seeking help at this time
Biographical data	Structural variables common to all clients such as name, age, sex, marital status, religious preference, ethnic background, educational level, occupational status, health insurance, and social security information
Current health status	The client's perceptions of his or her health with a specific delineation of current complaints and activities of daily living
Past health history	Data relative to the previous health or illness state of the client and contact with health care professionals, including a description of developmental accomplishments, health practices, known illnesses, allergies, restorative treatment, and social activities, such as foreign travel, that might be related to the client's current health status
Family history	A description of the current health status of each family member, relationships among family members, and a genetic history in relation to health and illness
Social history	An accounting of intrapersonal and interpersonal factors that influence the client's social adjustment, including environmental stressors that may be increasing or decreasing the client's vulnerability to crisis during times of stress
Review of systems*	A systematic assessment of biological functioning from head to toe

From Mahoney EA, Verdisco L, Shortridge L: *How to collect and record a health history*, ed 2, Philadelphia, 1982, Lippincott, pp. 6-7.
*Gordon's (1997) Functional Health Patterns Typology is a commonly used method for examining biological functioning, as well as other aspects of a client's health status.

table 9-8 Gordon's Functional Health Patterns Typology: Abbreviated Definitions for the Eleven Health Patterns

Health Pattern	Abbreviated Definition
Health perception–health management pattern	Describes the client's perceived pattern of health and well-being and how health is managed.
Nutritional-metabolic pattern	Describes pattern of food and fluid consumption relative to metabolic need and pattern indicators of local nutrient supply.
Elimination pattern	Describes patterns of excretory function (bowel, bladder, and skin).
Activity-exercise pattern	Describes pattern of exercise, activity, leisure, and recreation.
Sleep-rest pattern	Describes patterns of sleep, rest, and relaxation.
Cognitive-perceptual pattern	Describes sensory-perceptual and cognitive pattern.
Self-perception–self-concept pattern	Describes self-concept pattern and perceptions of self.
Role-relationship pattern	Describes pattern of role engagements and relationships.
Sexuality-reproductive pattern	Describes patterns of satisfaction or dissatisfaction with sexuality; describes reproductive pattern.
Coping–stress tolerance pattern	Describes general coping pattern and effectiveness of the pattern in terms of stress tolerance.
Value-belief pattern	Describes patterns of values, goals, or beliefs (including spiritual) that guide choices or decisions.

Modified from Gordon M: *Manual of nursing diagnosis, 1997-1998*, St. Louis, 1997, Mosby, pp. 2-5.

terns. Expanded definitions of these functional health patterns can be found in Gordon's (1997) *Manual of Nursing Diagnoses, 1997-1998*.

When completing a health history it is important to elicit the client's expectations of the health care provider. If the client's and the professional's expectations are inconsistent, frustration results for all parties involved. For instance, a client who has diabetes and is expecting a cure will likely have difficulty working with a health care professional whose goal is to help the client live a normal life within the limitations of his or her condition. If the discrepancy between these two goals is not resolved, neither of these goals will be reached.

Every nurse must decide on a format which will facilitate data collection. Although formats may vary, it is crucial to collect data in an orderly fashion on all parameters of client functioning before a nursing care plan is developed. There are times when a crisis situation warrants dealing with the immediate concerns of the client before all data are collected. However, to intervene effectively during times of crisis, the health care professional needs an adequate database. Without this database it is impossible to help the client to make appropriate choices about solutions for resolving current health stress.

Assessment guides can help the community health nurse collect health data in an orderly fashion. Assessment tools designed to collect information about the health status of individual family members should help the nurse to examine multiple aspects of a client's functioning. Appendices 9-1 and 9-2 are examples of assessment forms that help community health nurses organize this beginning phase of the nursing process. These tools aid the nurse in identifying psychosocial as well as physical components of a client's health status. In addition, they help a nurse to integrate individual and family functioning data by raising issues pertinent to the needs of all family members. Other examples of assessment guides, based on the 11 functional health pattern areas, can be found in Gordon's (1997) *Manual of Nursing Diagnosis, 1997-1998*.

Assessment tools have limitations and must be used only as guides to focus a nurse's attention on significant parameters to assess during the health interview and the physical examination process. Spontaneous interchange between the nurse and the client must always be allowed so that the client can fully express needs and can determine priorities that relate to her or his lifestyle. A barrage of questions from an assessment form stifles communication.

Analyzing

Once individual and family data are collected, the analysis phase of the nursing process begins. This phase encompasses a critical thinking process, which results in the formation of *nursing diagnoses*. A nursing diagnosis is "a clinical judgment about an individual, family, or community response to actual or potential health problems/life processes. Nursing diagnoses provide the basis for selection of nursing interventions to achieve outcomes for which the nurse is accountable" (NANDA, 1994, p. 7).

FORMULATING NURSING DIAGNOSES Nursing diagnoses are based on *patterns* reflected in assessment data and identify actual or potential client problems amenable to nursing interventions (Gordon, 1989). They also delineate client strengths that should be reinforced when the nurse is helping the client to enhance his or her self-care capabilities. In the community health setting, nursing diagnoses examine the needs and strengths of family units in addition to the needs and strengths of individual clients. If the identified needs of a family or individual clients are not amenable to nursing intervention, the community health nurse makes a referral to an appropriate care provider (see Chapter 10).

To formulate nursing diagnoses the community health nurse groups data so that relationships between assessment categories can be analyzed and patterns of behavior can be identified. Establishing relationships between assessment categories involves looking at all parameters of individual and family functioning. It requires a synthesis of data to determine the unique combination of biological, psychosocial, developmental, spiritual, and environmental factors that are making an impact on a specific family unit. It is important to synthesize data collected from a family, as client needs vary even when clients are experiencing similar situations. The following case scenarios illustrate this situation:

CASE *Scenario*

One community health nurse was visiting two different families, both of whom were concerned about a child's leaving for school. In one family situation the nurse's diagnosis of this behavior was "anticipatory anxiety related to the family's inability to address the father's health status with all family members." This nursing diagnosis was derived from the following assessment data:

- Susie had enjoyed school until her father had a heart attack;
- Susie's father had his heart attack while she was at school;
- Susie had been asking lately if her father was going to die; and
- The family believed it important to assure the children that everything was fine with the father even though he was unable to work or participate in strenuous family activities at this time.

In the other family situation, the nursing diagnosis in relation to the child's difficulty in leaving for school was quite different. Based on the following assessment data, the nursing diagnosis was "altered growth and development, social skills, related to the family's inability to adjust to normative developmental transitions":

- Bonnie started school a year late because she was "immature" for her developmental age;
- Bonnie has never enjoyed school;
- Bonnie spends most of her free time with her mother, even when children her own age are around; and
- Bonnie clings to her mother when babysitters come to the home.

Nursing diagnoses are derived from assessment data (ANA, 1991) that have been validated by the client and synthesized. Formulating diagnoses without adequate information, or in relation to fragmented pieces of data, leads to invalid diagnoses and inappropriate client goals and nursing interventions. For example, a nursing diagnosis that is based only on environmental observations (fragmented data) and that focuses on "unsafe housekeeping practices" provides very little direction for client and nursing intervention. Unsafe housekeeping practices can result from several factors, including lack of home management skill, energy depletion resulting from normative and nonnormative situational crises, and differing values about environmental safety. How a community health nurse would intervene when unsafe housekeeping practices are encountered is greatly influenced by the database obtained and the nursing diagnosis developed. For instance, an educative strategy is used when a client lacks home management skill, whereas a crisis intervention approach is initiated when a family's energies are depleted because of crisis.

Use of scientific knowledge such as Maslow's hierarchy of needs, theories of growth and development, family theories, and concepts of stress and crisis enhances a community health nurse's ability to synthesize data and to formulate an appropriate nursing diagnosis. Scientific knowledge helps a nurse to identify significant signs and symptoms of distress and to organize collected data into a meaningful whole. Grouping the symptoms presented by a client and then comparing them to clinical and research findings such as those presented in Chapter 8 aids the nurse in determining when a client may be in a state of crisis or vulnerable to stress and crisis.

When comparing collected data with relevant clinical and research findings, it is important to identify nursing diagnoses in relation to client strengths as well as client needs. Discerning client strengths helps the community health nurse to reinforce self-sufficiency skills, which in turn aids the nurse in avoiding dependency-building nursing activities. In the community health nurse setting, special emphasis is also placed on identifying nursing diagnoses that relate to situations or potential problems that warrant anticipatory guidance counseling. This emphasis is based on the belief that primary prevention should be a major focus in community health nursing practice. Situations throughout the life span that warrant anticipatory guidance are covered in Chapters 15 through 21.

NURSING CLASSIFICATION SYSTEMS Using a nursing classification system can help practitioners to refine their diagnostic skills and to document the effectiveness of nursing interventions. In addition, these systems facilitate the collection of assessment data and assist in organizing these data. Two such systems, one developed by The North American Nursing Diagnosis Association and the other by the Visiting Nurse Association of Omaha, Nebraska, are commonly used in the community setting.

NANDA'S NURSING DIAGNOSES CLASSIFICATION The North American Nursing Diagnosis Association was established in St. Louis, Missouri in 1973 for the purpose of developing a standard nomenclature for describing health problems amenable to treatment by nurses (Kim, Moritz, 1982, p. xvii). Since its inception, this association has sponsored several National Nursing Diagnosis Conferences, which have resulted in the identification of appropriate *nursing* diagnostic categories for practitioners. In 1996 over 155 nursing diagnoses had been accepted for clinical testing by the North American Nursing Diagnosis Association (NANDA) and endorsed by the American Nurses Association. Gordon (1997) has grouped these diagnoses under the 11 functional health patterns to facilitate the linking of assessment data and nursing diagnoses (see Appendix 9-3). Gordon's *Manual of Nursing Diagnosis, 1997-1998* explicates in more detail how to use the Functional Health Patterns Typology to facilitate nursing assessments and the identification of nursing diagnoses.

NANDA's nursing diagnoses taxonomy, known as Taxonomy I Revised, is in the process of development. "It is expected that nurses will modify, delete, and add to the currently accepted classifications. Nurses are encouraged to submit refinements of diagnoses to the North American Nursing Diagnosis Association, 1211 Locust Street, Philadelphia, Pennsylvania 19107" (Gordon, 1997, p. x). Further work is needed in the development of family and health promotion nursing diagnoses. Donnelly (1990) noted that only seven of the NANDA diagnostic categories described family-focused needs and only one of these seven addressed the family from a health promotion perspective. Leninger (1990) believes that the NANDA diagnostic taxonomy needs to be refocused to adequately address the health and well-being of people from varying cultures.

THE OMAHA CLASSIFICATION SYSTEM The classification system developed by the Visiting Nurse Association of Omaha was designed to provide an organizing framework for client problems diagnosed by nurses in the community health setting. This classification system, based upon the ANA definition of community health nursing, addresses the needs of families as well as individuals. This system has three major components: Problem Classification Scheme, Intervention Scheme, and Problem Rating Scale for Outcomes (Martin, Scheet, 1992). The Problem Classification Scheme is a taxonomy of nursing diagnoses that is structured at four levels: domains, problems, modifiers, and signs/symptoms. The 40 client problems are grouped into four major domains: environmental, psychosocial, physiological, and health behaviors (Martin, 1994). Definitions for each of these domains are displayed in Table 9-9. Within each of these domains are the names of identified problems that are referenced by two sets of modifiers: each problem is referenced as health promotion, potential (deficit/impairment) or actual (deficit/impairment), as well as family or individual. "When an actual problem modifier is used, a cluster of problem-specific signs and symptoms provides the diagnostic clues to problem identification" (Martin, p. 41). Table 9-10 provides examples of how the Omaha Problem Classification Scheme is organized according to domain, problem label, modifier, and sign or symptom.

Directly related to the problem classification scheme and the nursing process is a Likert-type problem-rating scale that helps nurses to evaluate client outcomes at regular intervals and a nursing intervention scheme consisting

table 9-9 The Omaha System: Definitions of Domains

Domain	Definitions
Environmental	Refers to the material resources and physical surroundings both internal and external to the client, home, neighborhood, and broader community.
Psychosocial	Refers to patterns of behavior, communications, relationships, and development.
Physiological	Refers to the functional status of processes that maintain life.
Health Related Behaviors	Refers to activities that maintain or promote wellness, promote recovery, or maximize rehabilitation.

From Martin K, Scheet N: *The Omaha System: a pocket guide for community health nursing*, Philadelphia, 1992, Saunders, pp. 18-19, 24, 30.

of nursing activities aimed at addressing specific nursing problems. Four nursing intervention categories are delineated in the Omaha System: health teaching, guidance, and counseling; treatments and procedures; case management; and surveillance. Definitions of these categories are presented in Table 9-11. Martin and Scheet's (1992) book, *The Omaha System: A Pocket Guide For Community Health Nursing*, discusses the Omaha System in depth, including how to individualize nursing interventions to client needs, how to use the problem-rating scale, and how to link nursing diagnoses, interventions, and client outcomes.

Planning

After nursing diagnoses are established and validated with the client, the community health nurse and the client move into the planning phase of the nursing process. Three major activities occur during this phase: (1) client-centered goals and expected outcomes for evaluating goal attainment are formulated; (2) interventions and evaluation criteria are identified; and (3) goals, outcomes, and interventions are prioritized. A *goal* is a broad desired outcome toward which behavior is directed, such as "the family will

table 9-10 The Omaha System: Organization of Classification Scheme for Client Problems, Select Examples

Domain	Problem Label	Modifiers	Sign or Symptom*
Environmental	Income	Deficit, family	Low/no income Uninsured medical expenses Inadequate money management Able to buy only necessities Difficulty buying necessities Other (specify)
Psychosocial	Communication with community resources	Impairment, family	Unfamiliar with options/procedures for obtaining services Difficulty understanding roles/regulations of service provider Unable to communicate concerns to service provider Dissatisfaction with services Language barrier Inadequate/unavailable resources Other (specify)
Physiological	Hearing	Impairment, individual	Difficulty hearing normal speech tones Absent/abnormal response to sound Abnormal results of hearing screening test Other (specify)
Health-related behaviors	Health care supervision	Impairment, family	Fails to obtain routine medical/dental evaluation Fails to seek care for symptoms requiring medical/dental evaluation Fails to return as requested to physician/dentist Inability to coordinate multiple appointments/regimens Inconsistent source of medical/dental care Inadequate prescribed mental/dental regimen Other (specify)

From Martin K, Scheet N: *The Omaha System: a pocket guide for community health nursing*, Philadelphia, 1992, Saunders, pp. 18, 20, 24, 32.
*Only those signs or symptoms that apply to the family situation are referenced in the client's record.

table 9-11 THE OMAHA SYSTEM: DEFINITIONS OF THE INTERVENTION CATEGORIES

CATEGORIES	DEFINITIONS
I. Health teaching, guidance, and counseling	Health teaching, guidance, and counseling are nursing activities that include giving information, anticipating client problems, encouraging client action and responsibility for self-care and coping, and assisting with decision making and problem solving. The overlapping concepts occur on a continuum with the variation due to the client's self-direction capabilities.
II. Treatments and procedures	Treatments and procedures are technical nursing activities directed toward preventing signs and symptoms, identifying risk factors and early signs and symptoms, and decreasing or alleviating signs and symptoms.
III. Case management	Case management includes nursing activities of coordination, advocacy, and referral. These activities involve facilitating service delivery on behalf of the client, communicating with health and human service providers, promoting assertive client communication, and guiding the client toward use of appropriate community resources.
IV. Surveillance	Surveillance includes nursing activities of detection, measurement, critical analysis, and monitoring to indicate client status in relation to a given condition or phenomenon.

From Martin K, Scheet N: *The Omaha System: a pocket guide for community health nursing*, Philadelphia, 1992, Saunders, p. 48.

value preventive health care services." An *expected outcome* or behavioral objective delineates client behaviors that reflect when a goal has been reached. "The family will obtain a regular source of care for preventive medical and dental services by September" might be one outcome established to determine if the above goal has been accomplished. *Interventions* are activities that may be implemented by the client, the nurse, and other health care professionals to help the client to achieve the desired goals. For example, in relation to this expected outcome, the nurse might discuss with the family its beliefs about health care, the services of all the available health care resources in the community, and barriers to health care utilization. If barriers to health care utilization exist, the nurse would identify with the family strategies for reducing these barriers (see Chapter 10 for a discussion of these strategies).

All goals and expected outcomes should be stated in specific and realistic terms and linked to the nursing diagnoses that have been established. They should not include expectations that are beyond the professional's or client's resources or capabilities. A goal of a severely retarded child achieving normal growth and development is extremely unrealistic. It is very appropriate to state that the family will work toward maximizing this child's potential, but inappropriate to expect that this child will reach normal growth and development parameters. Expecting that the family of this child will continue to function exactly as they did before the child's birth is also unrealistic. During times of stress and crisis change is necessary and unavoidable. A goal statement that focuses on the family demonstrating constructive behavior to reduce stressors related to the care of their developmentally disabled child is more appropriate.

Goal statements and expected outcomes that are written in positive terms provide direction for nursing interventions more effectively than those that have a negative orientation. Negative goal statements such as "parents will not use harsh disciplinary measures with their children" tend to focus on family weaknesses rather than on family strengths, which can be mobilized to reduce current stresses. Positive goal statements, such as "parents will talk with their children when the children act out," lead to the development of more positive interventions for achieving goals.

The nurse may find that, after client-centered goals are developed, the client finds it impossible to work on all of them immediately. When this happens the nurse and the client should work together to differentiate between problems that require immediate action and those that are of less concern to the client. When establishing priorities in relation to client goals the nurse must keep in mind that the client has the right to make the final decision about goals on which to focus. The nurse does have a responsibility to share concerns when she or he believes that client actions are unsafe or are precipitating a crisis situation.

After client-centered, positively stated goals have been established and priorities determined, expected outcomes that can be measured should be written. The importance of formulating specific outcomes for evaluating goal attainment must be stressed. Broad, general goals do not provide sufficient direction for planning intervention strategies. "Maximizing the potential" of a child who has a developmental lag, for example, does not specifically identify needed areas of improvement. Expected outcomes such as those listed below more appropriately facilitate the identification of intervention strategies because they

Nursing Interventions Classification (NIC) Intervention: Family Integrity Promotion

DEFINITION

Promotion of family cohesion and unity

ACTIVITIES

Be a listener for the family members
Establish trusting relationship with family members
Determine family understanding of causes of illness
Determine guilt family may feel
Assist family to resolve feelings of guilt
Determine typical family relationships
Monitor current family relationships
Identify typical family coping mechanisms
Identify conflicting priorities among family members
Assist family with conflict resolution
Counsel family members on additional effective coping skills for their own use
Respect privacy of individual family members
Provide for family privacy
Tell family members it is safe and acceptable to use typical expressions of affection
Facilitate a tone of togetherness within/among the family
Provide family members with information about the patient's condition regularly, according to patient preference
Collaborate with family in problem solving
Assist family to maintain positive relationships
Facilitate open communications among family members
Provide for care of patient by family members, as appropriate
Provide for family visitation
Refer family to support group of other families dealing with similar problems
Refer for family therapy, as indicated

From McCloskey JC, Bulechek GM, eds: *Nursing interventions classification (NIC)*, ed 2, St. Louis, 1996, Mosby, p. 274.

focus on specific developmental needs of the child and the family.

- Joel's family will help him to achieve daytime bladder and bowel control by December.
- Joel's family will help him to learn how to eat solid foods by October.
- Joel's family will share their feelings about Joel's condition.
- Joel's family will verbally identify how their feelings about Joel's condition positively or negatively affect his growth and development.
- Joel's family will identify strategies to reduce the stress associated with his care.
- Joel's parents will share ways to maintain a healthy spouse relationship.

Interventions, like expected outcomes, should be specific and based on sound scientific knowledge. "Teaching about growth and development" or "provide support to the family" are not specifically stated interventions. They are extremely global and do not take into account the individual needs of a particular family. A community health nurse might better prepare for family visits if the interventions were stated as follows: "implement a urinary habit training program" and "teach caregiver stress management techniques" (McCloskey, Bulechek, 1996, pp. 161, 583).

A research team at the University of Iowa has developed the Nursing Interventions Classification that outlines "the first comprehensive standardized language used to describe the treatments that nurses perform" (McCloskey, Bulechek, 1996, p. ix). This classification identifies 433 nursing interventions and a series of activities for each intervention that help nurses benefit clients. "Each intervention has a label name, a definition, a list of activities that a nurse does to carry out the intervention, and a short list of background readings" (McCloskey, Bulechek, p. ix). The above box presents a sample intervention and illustrates the format for each intervention. "Nursing interventions include both direct and indirect care; both nurse-initiated, physician-initiated, and other provider-initiated treatments" (McCloskey, Bulechek). The definitions for these different types of nursing interventions and nursing activities are presented in the box on the next page.

When delineating a plan for intervention both family and nurse activities should be identified. If only nursing actions are established, the client cannot be an active participant in the therapeutic process. Family resources are frequently overlooked when intervention strategies are developed. For instance, plans are too often made to involve community resources in the client's care even though friends or family members are available and would be more than willing to assist the client in achieving goals.

GUIDING PRINCIPLES OF THE THERAPEUTIC PROCESS

Several key principles must be taken into consideration during all phases of the nursing process. These are (1) individualization of client care, (2) respect of diverse values, (3) active family participation, (4) the family's right of self-determination, (5) confidentiality, and (6) maintenance of therapeutic focus. Adherence to these principles is basic to a trusting nurse-client relationship and reflects a respect for the worth and dignity of human beings.

The family-centered nursing process is a scientific process designed to meet the needs of *clients*. Inherent in

Nursing Interventions Classification (NIC): Definitions of Nursing Intervention and Nursing Activities

NURSING INTERVENTION

Any treatment, based upon clinical judgment and knowledge, that a nurse performs to enhance patient/client outcomes. Nursing interventions include both direct and indirect care; both nurse-initiated, physician-initiated, and other provider-initiated treatments.

A *direct care intervention* is a treatment performed through interaction with the patient(s). Direct care interventions include both physiological and psychosocial nursing actions; both the "laying on of hands" actions and those that are more supportive and counseling in nature.

An *indirect care intervention* is a treatment performed away from the patient but on behalf of a patient or group of patients. Indirect care interventions include nursing actions aimed at management of the patient care environment and interdisciplinary collaboration. These actions support the effectiveness of the direct care interventions.

A *nurse-initiated treatment* is an intervention initiated by the nurse in response to a nursing diagnosis; an autonomous action based on scientific rationale that is executed to benefit the client in a predicted way related to the nursing diagnosis and projected outcomes. Such actions would include those treatments initiated by advanced nurse practitioners.

A *physician-initiated treatment* is an intervention initiated by a physician in response to a medical diagnosis but carried out by a nurse in response to a "doctor's order." Nurses may also carry out treatments initiated by other providers, such as pharmacists, respiratory therapists, or physician assistants.

NURSING ACTIVITIES

The specific behaviors or actions that nurses do to implement an intervention and which assist patients/clients to move toward a desired outcome. Nursing activities are at the concrete level of action. A series of activities is necessary to implement an intervention.

From McCloskey JC, Bulechek GM, eds: *Nursing interventions classification (NIC)*, ed 2, St. Louis, 1996, Mosby, p. xvii.

this concept is the belief that clients have unique needs, values, and ways of functioning that should be determined before diagnoses, goals, expected outcomes, and interventions are established. Actively involving the client in the therapeutic process helps community health nurses to discover the uniqueness of the families they are serving. Active client participation in all phases of the nursing process also promotes client commitment to goal attainment and decreases resistance to change.

Individualizing client care does not negate the value of using standardized assessment tools and nursing diagnoses and intervention classification systems. Rather, this principle focuses on the need to use sound clinical judgment when tools for facilitating data collection and the planning of client care are utilized. McCloskey and Bulechek (1994) believe that "the use of standardized language will allow nurses more time and opportunity to focus on the unique aspects of each patient's care" (p. 59). They see the Nursing Intervention Classification as "a tool that makes it easier to select interventions for a particular patient" (p. 60), but stress that selecting an intervention and carrying out that intervention needs to be tailored for each client. Actively involving the client in the planning process helps the nurse to appropriately select and implement interventions.

When intervention strategies are discussed, the nurse may find that referral to other health care professionals can best help the client to meet his or her needs. In these instances, community health nurses discuss with the family what essential data about their situation can be shared with others. The family's permission should be obtained before releasing information to other health care agencies. The client has the right to determine what data, shared in confidence with the nurse, should or should not be shared with others. Indiscriminate exchange of client information among professionals violates the client's right to confidentiality and promotes mistrust and resistance to professional intervention. The principle of confidentiality is most often violated when goals are not mutually established and the nurse shares or seeks data to validate nurse-focused goals. Interdisciplinary collaboration is appropriate and often essential, but the family must support the need for such an approach before it can be fully successful.

For clients to fully participate in the therapeutic process, they must have the right to refuse any course of action they deem inappropriate. Community health nurses can help a client to examine the pros and cons of certain health actions or the consequences of continuing a particular pattern of functioning, but they also recognize that a client's right of self-determination must be respected when decisions are made. The nurse should not make decisions for the client or expect the client to make decisions in the way the nurse would make them. A community health nurse may intervene without a client's consent if the client is a threat to others (e.g., child abuse, spread of communicable disease) or to herself or himself (suicidal). Even in these situations, the community health nurse works with the client, if possible, to help reduce the distress being experienced and to develop new patterns of coping.

To effectively develop a therapeutic relationship with families, nurses must consistently clarify how their personal attitudes, beliefs, motivations, and conditioning are influencing their professional relationships. Personal biases can subtly influence how professionals interact with clients and can affect the planning and implementation of care. For example, one community health nurse found it difficult to maintain a therapeutic relationship with families when the adult male in the family had a "drinking problem." She would develop an alliance with the female in the family and neglect to help this woman analyze how she might be reinforcing her significant other's ineffective behavior. The nurse recognized the need to discuss this situation with her nursing supervisor and was able to verbalize that she believed her sister died prematurely as a result of stress associated with her husband's drinking problem. When the nurse was conscious of her feelings she was able to deal with them and to better assist clients in these situations.

PROFESSIONAL CONTRACTING Contracting is an intervention designed to promote active client participation in decision making. A *contract*—a mutual agreement between two or more persons for a specific purpose—provides a framework for establishing a facilitative client approach that supports and enhances a client's self-care capabilities. Basic to contracting is a philosophical belief that professional intervention should focus on assisting clients to act effectively on their own behalf. The professional using the contracting method of intervention must feel comfortable with the philosophy that clients have the potential for growth and that they are capable of effective decision making.

Contracting actively engages the client in the therapeutic process for the purpose of developing mutually acceptable goals, expected outcomes, and therapeutic interventions. Simply stated, a professional contract may be defined as a mutually agreed-upon working understanding that relates to the terms of treatment and is continuously negotiable between the nurse and the family (Boehm, 1989; Maluccio, Marlow, 1974; Seabury, 1976). The community health nurse guides the client through the process by facilitating informed decision making, assessing client needs, exploring alternatives for need resolution, assisting clients in carrying out actions that support need resolution, and evaluating expected outcomes.

CONTRACTING PROCESS The community health nurse who believes in contracting involves the client in all aspects of care. She or he makes an agreement with the client that spells out explicitly, mutually defined, client-centered goals. The quality of explicitness implies that terms of intervention are known to both the client and the nurse. When contracting occurs, all involved parties have a mutual understanding about the following:

1. The purpose of client-nurse interactions
2. Nursing diagnoses
3. Desired outcomes (goals) toward which behavior is directed
4. Priority needs in relation to client goals
5. Methods of intervention
6. Specific activities each party will carry out to achieve stated goals
7. Established time parameters for evaluation and the frequency and length of visits

Contracting is a dynamic, complex process that gradually evolves as the therapeutic relationship is strengthened. It should not be viewed as a simple procedure, involving only a discussion about goals, intervention strategies, and time limits. To successfully engage a family in the contracting process, the community health nurse must help the family to gain a clear understanding of its needs and the nature of a therapeutic relationship.

Initially a contract may be very general and include only an agreement to explore the nature of the client's needs. The terms of a contract become more inclusive as the therapeutic relationship evolves and specific data are obtained. Asking clients questions about what they feel they need, what they have been doing to resolve their needs, and how they would like their current situation to change, can elicit specific data that help the client and the nurse structure the therapeutic relationship. Establishing time parameters is important even when a general contract is developed, because these parameters emphasize the need for reviewing progress made in relation to goal attainment.

Contracting increases the clarity in nurse-client interactions. Specific commitments are made orally so that each party is aware of its role in the therapeutic process. Increased clarity often enhances the therapeutic relationship. This is especially true when clients have multiple problems or are unable to identify the nature of their problems. A case scenario can best illustrate this point.

CASE *Scenario*

The Beech family, two parents with five children, had been visited by community health nurses for years. The family folder reflected many problems: marital stress, financial difficulties, poor nutrition, lack of preventive health care for family members, irregular school attendance, and frequent childhood infections were the primary problems with which the family was dealing. Infrequent visits were made by the community health nurse because the family continually failed to deal actively with health care needs. Because they moved frequently, the Beech family never had consistent contact with one nurse for any length of time. Finally the community health nurse decided to talk with Mrs. Beech about terminating nursing service because she believed that the family did not desire assistance. To her surprise, Mrs. Beech verbalized that her family did need help and that she really wanted the nurse to continue visiting. She further shared that she had difficulty concentrating on anything because the family had so many problems to handle. The nurse agreed with Mrs. Beech that it was an impossible task to solve all the family problems at once. She proposed that it might be helpful if the family and the nurse could work together to resolve the one health problem Mrs. Beech felt was most distressing at that time. Mrs. Beech had trouble focusing on one particular concern because she had never before attempted to do so. Because she spent a considerable amount of time talking about Mary, her 10-year-old who had recently failed a hearing test at school, the nurse asked if Mrs. Beech might want to explore ways to resolve this health care problem. The nurse also suggested that it might be helpful to order the family's health problems from most significant to least significant. Since these suggestions were acceptable to Mrs. Beech, the following contract was established:

- *Purpose of client-nurse interactions:* The community health nurse will help the family to establish priorities in relation to their health problems and to handle their problems in manageable doses.
- *Priority need:* Mary's failure of hearing test at school.
- *Mutual goal:* Mary's hearing problem will be evaluated by a physician.
- *Method of intervention:* Family will take Mary to the hearing specialist she had seen before. (This decision was made after the nurse discussed all the possible resources where Mary could obtain care and Mrs. Beech shared that Mary had had hearing problems in the past.)
- *Responsibilities of family:* (1) Make appointment with the doctor; (2) arrange for child care for the two preschoolers for the afternoon of the appointment; (3) arrange for transportation; and (4) together with the nurse, make list of questions to ask the doctor during the visit.
- *Responsibilities of nurse:* Contact the physician to share the results of Mary's hearing test and Mrs. Beech's fears about health care professionals. (Mrs. Beech had been frequently criticized by health care professionals in the past for waiting too long before she sought medical help.) Visit weekly to evaluate how plans for Mary's care are progressing and to help the family establish priorities for health care action.
- *Time limits:* Mary to see the physician by the end of the month.

Mary saw the physician within the appropriate time frame; it was determined that she would need ear surgery. Since the contracting method of intervention helped Mrs. Beech to achieve her first goal, Mrs. Beech and the nurse agreed to renegotiate for follow-up based on the doctor's recommendation. Many other contracts were made before this family case record was closed. Accomplishing resolution of one problem helped family members to see that their situation was not hopeless. Setting priorities in relation to goal attainment decreased the family's anxiety about all the problems they had to handle.

When thinking about contracting with clients, it is important to remember that clients may not know about all the resources available to them. They also may not know why they are experiencing distress at this time. For example, an elderly woman may recognize that she is concerned about the physical aspects of caring for her ill husband, but she may not realize that some of her stress is related to role changes as a result of her caregiver responsibilities.

Contracting is one effective way to involve families in their own health care. However, contracting can reinforce ineffective family patterns if the nurse does not analyze carefully family dynamics. When a contract supports unhealthy family functioning it is labeled a *corrupt contract* (Beall, 1972, p. 77). A corrupt contract might evolve, for instance, when a community health nurse is working with a family who would like their aging parents to move to a nursing home. Sometimes families push for nursing home placement to meet their own needs rather than the needs of their elderly family members. If the community health nurse supports the family's decision and encourages the parents to move without talking to them about their needs and desires, he or she is violating the rights of these family members and the principles of contracting.

During the contracting process a community health nurse may identify problems, such as lack of protection against communicable diseases or inadequate dental care, that do not seem to be of concern to the family. In these situations a nurse-centered goal rather than a client-centered goal is formulated. A nurse-centered goal should be stated as such and should not emphasize family action like "the family will make an appointment at the immunization clinic." Instead it should focus on increasing the family's awareness of the problem and be stated in such terms as "the family will verbalize an understanding of immunizations." Distinguishing carefully between nurse goals and family goals helps the community health nurse to prevent imposing personal values on clients and helps the nurse to focus on the problems and goals important to the family. Generally, families do not explore problems identified by the nurse that they do not see as problems until they have achieved their own client-centered goals.

Implementing

The implementation phase of the nursing process deals specifically with how activities are carried out to achieve client goals. Together the client and the nurse select and test intervention strategies to determine their appropriateness in helping the client move toward need resolution. Priorities concerning when actions will be taken are established so that the client can deal with his or her needs in manageable doses. If needed, other resources are mobilized to help the client handle the change process.

Because change is often threatening, a warm, caring, supportive atmosphere that reinforces client accomplishments should be fostered. Focusing on what remains to be accomplished rather than emphasizing positive results that have already occurred serves only to discourage the client. Honest, positive feedback can be the motivating factor that promotes client involvement in the therapeutic process. Positive feedback can also help to increase clients' self-esteem and confidence in their ability to assume responsibility for maintaining and promoting their health status.

The community health nurse uses a variety of intervention strategies to help clients alter those aspects of life they desire to change. Some of these are discussed in Chapter 8, where the supportive, educative, and problem-solving strategies are explored. Nursing actions should be based on sound scientific principles and knowledge. For example, if a planned intervention is nutritional counseling, the activities the nurse carries out to implement this intervention should reflect knowledge of acceptable nutritional standards and appropriate application of the principles of teaching and learning. Since one principle of teaching and learning is to provide for individual differences (Redman, 1997), effective nursing activities reflect that the nurse took into consideration client characteristics that influence nutritional habits such as cultural preferences in relation to food likes and dislikes, financial resources, and the demands on the homemaker's time.

All other phases of the nursing process are usually carried out during the implementation phase. While clients are actively participating in the intervention process they share data verbally or nonverbally through action taken or not taken. The community health nurse must analyze these new data carefully to determine if care plans need to be revised. Nursing care plans should never be static. Rather, they should be continuously open to renegotiation as the client's situation changes or new data are discovered.

The community health nurse must be flexible when implementing nursing activities, since new data are often generated that alter original nursing diagnoses and client goals. Some clients are unable to identify the nature of their problems until they attempt to change their behavior and find that change does not resolve their need. This was illustrated in Chapter 8, when Mrs. Lehi discovered that her headaches were related to guilt feelings about being a working mother rather than to excessive demands on her time. In this situation the nurse and Mrs. Lehi revised their original goal, "Mrs. Lehi will discover ways to adjust her daily schedule to reduce stress," to "Mrs. Lehi will identify ways to achieve her self-fulfillment needs and maintain the integrity of the family unit without distress." Intervention strategies were altered accordingly. Instead of discussing Mrs. Lehi's daily activities and support systems, the nurse and Mrs. Lehi explored issues such as Mrs. Lehi's feelings about motherhood, the needs of school-age children, an individual's need for self-fulfillment, how a family can grow as its subsystems grow, and ways to reduce Mrs. Lehi's guilt feelings.

During the implementation phase it is not unusual to discover that clients do not wish to pursue a particular goal, even though they previously expressed a desire to work on that goal. Sometimes clients verbalize an *awareness* that a problem exists but are not ready to change their behavior in the way necessary to resolve that problem. Clients may not recognize the difference between awareness and readiness until concrete plans have been made to alter their current situation. If this happens, it can be difficult for these clients to verbally convey to the nurse that they are not ready for change. Frequently they share this message nonverbally by not taking action. That is why it is so important for the community health nurse to find out why clients are not meeting commitments that had been mutually agreed upon. Goals and plans should be modified if clients are not ready to alter their behavior.

Some clients are resistant to change because all their alternatives for change have negative consequences. A woman, for example, who has limited financial resources, no preparation for a job, and few support systems may be very hesitant to divorce her husband even though their marital relationship is destructive to her emotional health. The fear of not being able to support herself and being alone might be far more stressful to her than the emotional pain she is experiencing in the marital relationship. When community health nurses encounter such a situation, they must remain empathic and guard against feeling that the woman has no options. Community health nurses find it difficult to handle situations when all the alternatives for change have some negative consequences. However, clients in these situations can be assisted by helping them to identify their strengths, obtain needed resources to achieve their goals, and recognize that they can achieve control over their lives.

DOCUMENTATION For a variety of reasons, the nurse clearly documents relevant data on the agency record throughout all phases of the nursing process. Accurate record keeping provides direction for the planning, implementation, and evaluation of client care, assists the health care team in coordinating services provided, and helps practitioners to substantiate the quality of care rendered for reimbursement, legal, and certification purposes (Della-Monica, 1994). Accurate record keeping also helps agency administrators to analyze the characteristics of clients served by the agency, including a demographic profile and a profile of client health care needs and service requirements. Having this knowledge assists an agency in analyzing community needs, planning appropriate staffing patterns, and identifying staff competencies needed to provide care to clients served by the agency.

Accurate record keeping is an essential responsibility of the community health nurse. It demonstrates professional accountability and assists the nurse in providing individualized, quality care. To successfully carry out that responsibility, the nurse must have a clear understanding of the agency's documentation policy and the nursing process. A quality client service record reflects appropriate implementation of the nursing process.

Evaluating

Evaluation is the continuous critiquing of each aspect of the nursing process. Although it is discussed as a separate phase, it must take place concurrently with all phases of the nursing process. Ongoing feedback should be elicited from the client to determine whether goals, plans, and intervention strategies are appropriately focused. When expected outcomes are established, defining how they will be evaluated is a necessity. A well-written expected outcome will contain the potential for evaluation. For example, "John will learn how to give his own insulin injection by the end of the month" is a concise statement that can be used to determine whether John has achieved a desired goal.

Evaluation criteria, which help the family and the nurse to determine if expected client outcomes are being reached, should be established very early in the nurse-client relationship. Developing evaluation criteria early in the helping relationship validates the importance of evaluation and provides direction for client and nurse actions. Presented in Table 9-12 is a care plan for the Lopez family (see the ac-

table 9-12 Lopez Family: Initial Care Plan

Assessment Data	Nursing Diagnoses	Expected Client Outcomes	Nursing Interventions	Evaluation Criteria
Children behind in school achievement because of frequent family moves. Family moved north so "children could have a better education."	Family coping, potential for growth as evidenced by family's desire to obtain a better education and life for their children.	Children will succeed in the educational system.	1. Verbally, positively reinforce the family's decision to obtain an education for its children. 2. Identify barriers to successful school achievement. 3. Provide family with information about school policies and procedures.	1. All children will attend school regularly. 2. Children will report satisfying school experiences. 3. Children will obtain passing grades in school.
Family has no regular source of medical care. Family cannot afford to go to the doctor. Family members have obvious health needs. Difficult for family to obtain medical care during daytime hours. Family expresses a desire to follow up on the children's health needs.	Health maintenance, altered, due to limited financial resources and access problems.	Family will obtain the resources needed to follow up on family members' health needs. Family will obtain a regular source of medical and preventive health care.	1. Discuss family's beliefs about health, illness, and health care. 2. Share with family resources in community to assist them in meeting their health needs (e.g., Lions' Club and MSS). 3. Discuss barriers to the use of the referral process. 4. Discern family's interest in obtaining a regular source of care. 5. Advocate for the family if needed. 6. Provide opportunities for breadwinner to meet work responsibilities while obtaining health care for the family.	1. Family members' health needs will be corrected: a. Mr. Lopez will obtain dentures. b. Mrs. Lopez will obtain prenatal care. c. Juanita will obtain an eye examination. d. Francesca will obtain medical care for her ear infection. e. All of the children will obtain dental care. f. All family members' immunization will be up-to-date.
Only grandmother has health insurance. Children have limited clothing for school. Total family income is $465/month.	Income deficit as evidenced by uninsured medical needs and difficulty buying necessities.	Family will be able to obtain the necessities of life.	1. Discuss with the family expectations regarding their needs. 2. Share with family community resources that could help to expand the family income (e.g., food stamps, health department immunization clinic, and clothing closet). 3. Provide assistance in meeting basic family needs.	1. Family will have adequate food and clothing. 2. Family will obtain needed medical care. 3. Family is able to maintain its home.

companying case scenario) that illustrates how one community health nurse initially established evaluation criteria to determine whether expected outcomes were achieved. When reviewing these criteria, note how they relate to each stage of the nursing process.

CASE Scenario

The Lopez family consists of Juan, age 35, Elena, his 30-year-old wife, five children, and Mr. Lopez's mother, Teresa. The family is second-generation Mexican-American from Texas, representative of a stream of Spanish-speaking families who yearly migrate north to harvest a variety of crops. Six months ago the family decided to stay in a northern midwest community when Mr. Lopez was offered a permanent job as a farmhand, because they felt the children could have a better education and life than the parents had experienced. Spanish is spoken in the home. Mr. Lopez speaks some English but is unable to read or write it. Mrs. Lopez has limited comprehension of English and has had no education beyond the fourth grade. Mr. Lopez's mother speaks only Spanish. The children speak English but are behind in school achievement as a result of frequent family moves.

The family lives in a five-room house that is on the farm property. Although housekeeping practices are adequate, the home is in poor condition, in need of paint and repairs. It has running water, the source of which is a well. A septic system is used for sewage disposal. There is electricity for lighting and heating, and bottled gas is used for cooking.

The family lives rent-free in the house, which is provided by the owner of the farm; utilities are also provided by the owner. Family income is limited to Mr. Lopez's income of $100 per week and his mother's income of $65 per month from SSI. Only Grandmother Lopez has health insurance, on the basis of SSI. The tenant farm on which the family lives is 10 miles from the nearest town. Mr. Lopez has a pickup truck that the family uses for transportation when necessary. However, Mr. Lopez finds it difficult to get off work during daytime hours to take the family in for medical care.

table 9-12 Lopez Family: Initial Care Plan—cont'd

Assessment Data	Nursing Diagnoses	Expected Client Outcomes	Nursing Interventions	Evaluation Criteria
Mr. Lopez speaks some English but is unable to read or write it. Mrs. Lopez has limited comprehension of English, as does the grandmother.	Communication with community systems impaired, related to an insufficient number of care providers who speak Spanish.	Family will be able to communicate basic needs with care providers in the community.	1. Use culturally appropriate visual aids to facilitate family understanding. 2. Seek a translator to discuss critical health issues. 3. Show respect for the family's cultural differences (e.g., seek information about family customs, traditions, and health beliefs). 4. Keep language simple and talk slowly. 5. Involve the father in the conversation. 6. Show respect to all family members. 7. Use nonverbal communication (e.g., pictures, drawings, or gestures) to clarify situations with the family.	1. Family will obtain adequate food and clothing. 2. Family will express satisfaction with their encounters in the community.
Home in need of repairs and lead paint removal. Nitrates in well water potentially harmful to a new infant.	Environment impaired, due to presence of lead paint in home and nitrates in well water.	Lead paint will be removed from the environment. Family will use a safe alternative source of water for the new infant.	1. Elicit the family's understanding of lead poisoning and its effects. 2. Assist family in obtaining community resources for repair of home if desired. 3. Help the family to obtain testing to discern safety of water for all family members.	1. Well water is tested. 2. Family verbalizes an understanding of lead poisoning. 3. Family takes action to protect children from lead poisoning.

Health problems are evident in the family. Mr. Lopez is in need of dentures, and all of the school-age children are in need of dental care, as reported by their teachers. Juanita, age 7, was recently referred for ophthalmological examination following vision screening at school. Francesca, age 3, is in need of medical care for a draining ear. All of the children are behind in their immunizations; the adults in the family do not know which "shots" they have had. Mrs. Lopez is in her seventh month of pregnancy and has had no medical care. The family expresses a desire to obtain care for their children but "we have no extra money to pay a doctor. We can hardly afford to buy food and clothing for the kids."

Although evaluation is one of the most significant aspects of the nursing process, it is the one most frequently neglected or haphazardly done. When developing the nursing care plan, intervals should be established for the systematic review of all aspects of the nursing process. Some community health agencies have a policy stating that all records should be summarized and analyzed after a given number of visits have been made or when the family case is being transferred to another nurse. A well-written summary helps the community health nurse synthesize data and vividly identify what has or has not been accomplished in a specified period of time. Consulting with peers, supervisors, and other health care professionals can also help a community health nurse review progress or lack of progress in family situations. Evaluation is absolutely essential and it must be carefully planned. Lack of evaluation often prolongs the therapeutic process.

EVALUATING OUTCOMES When evaluating the effectiveness of interventions implemented by the client, the nurse, and other health care professionals, it is not sufficient to only analyze whether the family is participating in the therapeutic process. The *outcome* of actions taken by the family and health care professionals must also be examined. Noting only that the family has kept an appointment at a clinic provides very little data about the effectiveness of this client behavior. Identifying what happened when the family went to the clinic and what motivated them to do so is far more significant. These types of data provide the key for future interventions. Finding out, for instance, if the family was satisfied with the care they received or if the family understood the recommendations for follow-up can help the nurse to identify barriers to the utilization of health care services. Data obtained from these types of questions can also assist the nurse in planning interventions specific to the current needs of the family.

When evaluating the effectiveness of interventions, the nurse may find that clients are not reaching their expected outcomes. This happens for a variety of reasons that are not always obvious to either the client or the nurse. Outlined in the accompanying box are some factors for the nurse to consider as guidelines when examining why client outcomes have not been reached.

The coordination of services among all professionals is crucial. It should not be assumed that particular services will be provided by an agency when a client is referred to that agency. When multiple agencies are working with a family, clearly defined mechanisms for deciding who will do what and for evaluating the quality of the care being delivered by the health team should be established. The client must be involved in determining how interdisciplinary collaboration and coordination will evolve.

When an interdisciplinary approach is used to provide services for clients, the community health nurse must carefully evaluate when nursing services are and are not needed. Referring a client to another community agency does not necessarily mean that all of the client's needs will be met by that agency. The community health nurse still has a responsibility to evaluate the outcome of the referrals that have been made (see Chapter 10) and to discern if the client has other needs that are amenable to nursing interventions. After the referral has been implemented successfully, it may be found that nursing services are no longer needed. The client is then prepared for termination, and the family case is closed to service.

CLINICAL PATHWAYS Clinical pathways are used in some community health agencies to monitor the achieve-

Common Reasons for Lack of Outcome Achievement

- Database inadequate to identify the *actual* needs of the family.
- Goals and expected outcomes too broad and not tailored to the needs of the family.
- Goals and expected outcomes not mutually established; nurse's goals being imposed on the family.
- Family priorities in relation to goals and expected outcomes not ascertained.
- Family energies not focused on priority family needs; family attempting to deal with all needs at once.
- Family energies depleted as a result of normative and non-normative crises.
- Barriers to care not identified because follow-up on client and nurse actions is neglected.
- Nursing diagnoses, goals, and expected outcomes not revised as the family situation changes.
- Interventions not tailored to the needs of the family.
- Family lacks the support it needs to reduce anxiety during the change process.
- Coordination of care among all health professionals is neglected; family is receiving inconsistent messages about appropriate interventions, or gaps in services exist.

ment of clinical outcomes. A clinical pathway identifies key activities that must occur in a time-sequenced order to achieve specified client goals (Maturen, Zander, 1993). Zander (1988) views the clinical pathway as a unique version of the nursing care plan. Clinical pathways resemble standardized care plans, but in addition to identifying client needs, expected outcomes and interventions, pathways identify very specific timelines for implementing care activities and outcome achievement. They also include a variance record which identifies "any difference between what was planned and what actually occurred" (Marrelli, Hilliard, 1996, p. 27). Variance records portray whether goals are met in a specified time frame and within a cost limit allocation.

Clinical pathways are managed care tools "designed to streamline [client] care, emphasize the achievement of predetermined expected outcomes, minimize length of stay, and control costs while maintaining acceptable quality" (Marrelli, Hilliard, 1996, p. xi). Clinical pathways are standardized care plans that address the needs and service requirements of homogenous, high-volume client case types. For example, a home health care agency might develop a clinical pathway to sequence health care provider activities for clients that have diabetes or hypertension, because these diagnoses are common among home health care clients. In contrast, staff in a public health agency would be more likely to develop clinical pathways for their high-volume maternal child health families or clients that have a communicable disease such as tuberculosis.

A sample clinical pathway is displayed in Appendix 9-4. Agencies using this pathway establish a timeline for interventions and expected outcomes based on the characteristics of the clients served by the agency. For example, if 90% of their diabetic clients required 8 weeks of service, the time frame used would be 8 weeks. Like other types of standardized care plans, clinical pathways are individualized to meet the unique needs of clients. Additional care activities and expected outcomes are added to their pathway based on data obtained during the assessment phase of the nursing process. The reader is referred to Marrelli and Hilliard's (1996) book for a comprehensive discussion of how agencies develop clinical pathways and how pathways are individualized to meet client needs. Clinical pathways can assist the health care team in determining when to prepare clients for termination based on identified client needs.

Terminating

Terminating is seldom identified as a separate phase in the nursing process. It is alluded to during the evaluation phase, but little attention is devoted to discussing the effect termination has on the nurse and the client in the community health setting. Frequently, feelings associated with the separation process are not handled by the client or the nurse. The inability to deal with these feelings can stifle the development of close, caring professional relationships. For this reason terminating is labeled as a separate phase in the family-centered nursing process in this text.

Terminating is the period when the client and nurse deal with feelings associated with separation and when they distance themselves (Kelly, 1969, p. 2381). Ending a meaningful relationship with a client should be carefully planned. Clients, as well as nurses, need time to deal with the strong emotions that are often evoked by separation. Anger, sadness, denial, withdrawal, and regression are some normal reactions associated with termination. The type of reaction that occurs depends, to a great extent, on how the nurse and the client have dealt with separation in the past.

In the community health setting the nurse frequently encounters termination issues. Some clients are seen on a short-term basis, in three or four visits, whereas long-term relationships are established with other clients who have multiple problems to resolve. It is not uncommon to have a client move abruptly or to have a staff nurse's district changed. Clients who have experienced frequent changes in the nurse assigned to their case may have difficulty becoming involved in the therapeutic process. Talking about what these changes mean to the client and the nurse can be a growing process for both.

THE TERMINATION PROCESS The family should be adequately prepared for termination. The family's readiness for ending the therapeutic relationship should be ascertained. Factors the nurse considers when assessing readiness include the family's desire to terminate, progress made in goal achievement, the family's ability to identify personal health care needs and to take action to resolve these needs, and the family's ability to identify and access needed family resources.

The family should be involved in making the decision about how and when the therapeutic relationship will end. Some families find a gradual process, where the nurse decreases the frequency of visits but continues to maintain contact with the family, the most helpful way to terminate. Other families decide when it is time to terminate nursing services and establish a specific time for ending the relationship.

From a realistic perspective, the nurse may find that, because of financial constraints, the number of visits that can be made is limited. When agencies have contracts with managed care companies to provide nursing services, the company decides when termination will occur. The number of visits should be clearly identified during the nurse's initial visit to the client's home. The nurse may need to advocate for additional nursing services when the specified number of visits does not meet client needs, or may need to assist the client to access additional resources in the community.

It is not uncommon for clients, particularly clients who have chronic health problems or who are dealing with multiple family issues, to attempt to prolong the therapeutic relationship even when they agree that it is time to terminate. For example, one 40-year-old client who had multiple sclerosis abruptly stopped doing her exercises after discussing termination with the nurse. She finally verbalized that although the family had adequate resources to handle its needs at this time, she was afraid she would have difficulty obtaining help in the future when her condition deteriorated. The nurse helped this client handle termination by addressing the family's strengths in caring for its family members, addressing the client's fears, and reinforcing how to access services in the future.

When ending a therapeutic relationship, the nurse assists the client in analyzing what has been accomplished and the client's strengths in handling his or her health care needs. The nurse also assists the client in determining how to access nursing services or other community resources in the future.

SUMMARY

The family-centered nursing process is a systematic approach to scientific problem solving, involving a series of circular, dynamic actions—assessing, analyzing, planning, implementing, evaluating, and terminating—for the purpose of facilitating optimum client functioning. Nurses in all settings use this process in order to practice in an orderly, logical manner. It enables the nurse to individualize care for clients. In the community health setting, emphasis is on analyzing the needs of the family unit, as well as the needs of individual family members.

The principles of individualization, active participation, self-determination, confidentiality, and values clarification must be applied in all phases of the nursing process. Contracting is used with clients to promote active client participation in the therapeutic process and to support the client's right of self-determination. *Contracting* is a term used to denote a process that involves the establishment of mutually defined goals and intervention strategies. It is a working agreement between client and nurse, explicitly stated, in which all parties involved are working together to achieve a common goal.

Use of the family-centered nursing process is rewarding and challenging. The family-centered nursing process assists the nurse in helping clients from diverse cultural and ethnic backgrounds to mobilize personal strengths that will enhance their self-care capabilities. It provides the nurse with a framework for facilitating client decision making about health care matters. It also enables the nurse to become truly involved with other human beings in a supportive, therapeutic way.

CRITICAL *Thinking Exercise*

Based on the data provided below, develop an initial care plan for the Athen family, using the following format:

Assessment Data	Nursing Diagnoses	Expected Outcomes/ Goals	Nursing Interventions/ Actions	Evaluation Criteria

THE ATHEN FAMILY

You are the public health nurse from the Pottsville County Health Department and are visiting Mr. and Mrs. Athen, an elderly couple (89 and 85 respectively) who were referred by their family physician for monitoring of a wound on Mrs. Athen's right arm. Mr. Athen dresses this wound twice a day but is concerned because it is healing slowly. Mr. Athen wears glasses and a hearing aid but is in good health considering his age. He does admit that he "tires faster these days." Mr. Athen is the primary caregiver for his wife and caretaker of the household. Mrs. Athen has left-sided hemiplegia from a cerebrovascular accident 3 years ago. She uses a wheelchair for mobility and a guard rail for walking and range-of-motion exercises. The family lives in a well-kept home that is wheelchair accessible. Their daughter and her husband live 30 miles away and are available for emergency help and specific projects. However, they do not visit often because of caregiver responsibilities for their 40-year-old son, who is severely disabled from cerebral palsy. The Athens are devoted to each other and will do everything they can to stay out of a nursing home. They are concerned about what will happen to their grandson should his parents die or become unable to care for him.

REFERENCES

American Nurses Association (ANA): *Standards of community health nursing practice*, Kansas City, Mo., 1986, The Association.

American Nurses Association (ANA): *Standards of clinical nursing practice*, Kansas City, Mo., 1991, ANA.

American Public Health Association (APHA): *The definition and role of public health nursing: a statement of APHA Public Health Nursing Section*, Washington, D.C., 1996, APHA.

Barkauskas VH, Stoltenberg-Allen C, Baumann LC, Darling-Fisher C: *Health and physical assessment*, St. Louis, 1994, Mosby.

Barkauskas VH, Stoltenberg-Allen C, Baumann LC, Darling-Fisher C: *Health and physical assessment*, ed 2, St. Louis, 1998, Mosby.

Beall L: The corrupt contract: problems in conjoint therapy with parents and children, *Am J Orthopsychiatry* 42(1):77-81, 1972.

Beavers WR: *Psychotherapy and growth: a family systems perspective*, New York, 1977, Brunner/Mazel.

Beitler B, Tkachuck B, Aamodt D: The Neuman model applied to mental health, community health, and medical-surgical nursing. In Riehl JP, Roy C, eds: *Conceptual models for nursing practice*, ed 2, New York, 1980, Appleton-Century-Crofts.

Benedict MB, Sproles JB: Application of the Neuman model to public health nursing practice. In Neuman B, ed: *The Neuman systems model: application to nursing education and practice*, New York, 1982, Appleton-Century-Crofts, pp. 223-240.

Berkey KM, Hanson SMH: *Pocket guide to family assessment and intervention*, St. Louis, 1991, Mosby.

Bigbee J: The changing role of rural women: nursing and health implications, *Health Care Women Int* 5:307-322, 1984.

Blank JJ, Clark L, Longman AJ, Atwood J: Perceived homecare needs of cancer patients and their caregivers, *Cancer Nurs* 12:78-84, 1989.

Blazek B, McCaellen M: The effects of self-care instruction on locus of control in children, *J Sch Health* 53:554-556, 1983.

Bliss-Holtz UJ: Primiparas' prenatal concern for learning infant care, *Nurs Res* 37:20-24, 1988.

Boehm S: Patient contracting. In Fitzpatrick JJ, Taunton RL, Benoliel JQ, eds: *Annu Rev Nurs Res*, vol 7, New York, 1989, Springer, pp. 143-153.

Bomar PJ: *Nurses and family health promotion: concepts, assessment, and interventions*, ed 2, Philadelphia, 1996, Saunders.

Bomar PJ, McNeely G: Family health nursing role: past, present, and future. In Bomar PJ: *Nurses and family health promotion: concepts, assessment, and interventions*, ed 2, Philadelphia, 1996, Saunders, pp. 2-21.

Boyd C: Toward an understanding of mother-daughter identification using concept analysis, *Adv Nurs Sci* 7(3):78-86, 1985.

Buchanan BF: Human-environment interaction: a modification of Neuman Systems Model for aggregates, families, and the community, *Public Health Nurs* 4:52-64, 1987.

Campbell JC: Nursing assessment for risk of homicide with battered women, *Adv Nurs Sci* 8(4):36-51, 1986.

Carpenito LJ: *Nursing diagnosis: application to clinical practice*, Philadelphia, 1989, Lippincott.

Chang BL, Uman GC, Linn LS, et al: Adherence to health care regimens among elderly women, *Nurs Res* 34(1):27-31, 1985.

Chin S: Can self-care theory be applied to families? In Riehl-Sisca J, ed: *The science and art of self-care*, Norwalk, Ct., 1985, Appleton-Century-Crofts, pp. 56-62.

Clements IW, Roberts FB, eds: *Family health: a theoretical approach to nursing care*, New York, 1983, Wiley.

Curran D: *Traits of a healthy family*, Minneapolis, Mn., 1983, Winston Press.

Danielson CB, Hamel-Bissell B, Winstead-Fry P: *Families, health and illness: perspectives on coping and intervention*, St. Louis, 1993, Mosby.

Della Monica E: Home health care documentation and record keeping. In Harris MD: *Handbook of home health care administration*, Gaithersburg, Md., 1994, Aspen, pp. 117-142.

Donnelly E: Health promotion, families, and the diagnostic process, *Fam Comm Health* 12:12-20, 1990.

Eliason MS: Ethics and transcultural nursing care, *Nurs Outlook* 41(5):225-228, 1993.

Fawcett J: The relationship between identification and patterns of change in spouses' body images during and after pregnancy, *Int J Nurs Stud* 14:199-213, 1977.

Fawcett J: Needs of Caesarean birthparents, *J Obstet Gynecol Neonat Nurs* 10:371-376, 1981.

Fawcett J: The metaparadigm of nursing: present status and future refinements, *Image J Nurs Sch* 16(3):84-87, 1984.

Fawcett J: Preparation for caesarean childbirth: derivation of a nursing intervention from the Roy Adaptation Model, *J Adv Nurs* 15:1418-1425, 1990.

Fawcett J, Carino C: Hallmarks of success in nursing practice, *Adv Nurs Sci* 11(4):1-8, 1989.

Flaskerudt JH, Halloran EJ: Areas of agreement in nursing theory development, *Adv Nurs Sci* 3:31-42, 1980.

Friedemann ML: Closing the gap between grand theory and mental health practice with families, Part 1: the framework of systemic organization for nursing of families and family members, *Arch Psychiatr Nurs* 3:10-19, 1989a.

Friedemann ML: Closing the gap between grand theory and mental health practice with families. Part 2: the control-congruence model for mental health nursing of families, *Arch Psychiatr Nurs* 3:20-28, 1989b.

Galli M: Promoting self-care in hypertensive clients through patient education, *Home Healthc Nurse*, March-April: 43-45, 1984.

General Accounting Office (GAO): *Home visiting: a promising early intervention strategy for at-risk families*, GAO/HRD-90-83, Washington, D.C., 1990, GAO.

Giger JN, Davidhizar RE: *Transcultural nursing: assessment and intervention*, ed 2, St. Louis, 1995, Mosby.

Gonot PW: Family therapy as derived from King's conceptual model. In Whall AL, ed: *Family therapy for nursing: four approaches*, Norwalk, Ct., 1986, Appleton-Century-Crofts. pp. 33-48.

Gordon M: *Manual of nursing diagnosis, 1988-1989*, St. Louis, 1989, Mosby.

Gordon M: *Manual of nursing diagnosis, 1993-1994*, St. Louis, 1993, Mosby.

Gordon M: *Nursing diagnosis: process and application*, ed 2, New York, 1987, McGraw-Hill.

Gordon M: *Manual of nursing diagnosis, 1997-1998*, St. Louis, 1997, Mosby.

Hanchett ES: *Community health assessment: a conceptual tool kit*, New York, 1979, Wiley.

Hanchett ES: *Nursing frameworks and community as client: bridging the gap*, Norwalk, Ct., 1988, Appleton-Lange.

Hanson J: The family. In Roy C, ed: *Introduction to nursing: an adaptation model*, ed 2, Englewood Cliffs, N.J., 1984, Prentice-Hall, pp. 519-533.

Hanson SMH, Mischke KB: Family health assessment and intervention. In Bomar PJ: *Nurses and family health promotion: concepts, assessment, and interventions*, ed 2, Philadelphia, 1996, Saunders, pp. 165-202.

Harper DC: Application of Orem's theoretical constructs to self-care medication behaviors in the elderly, *Adv Nurs Sci* 6(3):29-46, 1984.

Hartweg DL: Self-care actions of healthy middle-aged women to promote well-being, *Nurs Res* 42:221-227, 1993.

Health Care Financing Administration (HCFA): Medicare Program: home health agencies—conditions of participation, *Federal Register* 56:32967-32975, July 18, 1991.

Health Care Financing Administration (HCFA): *Conditions of participation: home health agencies*, 42CFR Part 484, Section 484.10 through 484.52, Washington, D.C., October 1994, HCFA.

Hoch CC: Assessing delivery of nursing care, *J Gerontol Nurs* 13:10-17, 1987.

Johnston RL: Approaching family intervention through Rogers' conceptual model. In Whall AL, ed: *Family therapy theory for nursing: four approaches*, Norwalk, Ct., 1986, Appleton-Century-Crofts, pp. 11-32.

Jopp M, Carroll MC, Waters L: Using self-care theory to guide nursing management of the older adult after hospitalization, *Rehabil Nurs* 18:91-94, 1993.

Kearney BY, Fleisher BJ: Development of an instrument to measure exercise of self-care agency, *Res Nurs Health* 2:25-34, 1979.

Kehoe CF: Identifying the nursing needs of the postpartum Caesarean mother. In Kehoe CF, ed: *The caesarean experience: theoretical and clinical perspectives for nurses*, New York, 1981, Appleton-Century-Crofts.

Kelly HS: The sense of an ending, *Am J Nurs* 69:2378-2381, 1969.

Kim MJ, Moritz DA: *Classification of nursing diagnoses: proceedings of the third and fourth national conferences*, New York, 1982, McGraw-Hill.

Kruger S, Shawver M, Jones L: Reactions of families to the child with cystic fibrosis, *Image J Nurs Sch* 12:67-72, 1980.

Laffrey SC: Health behavior choice as related to self-actualization and health conception, *West J Nurs Res* 7:279-295, 1985.

Leninger M: Issues, questions, and concerns related to the nursing diagnoses cultural movement from a transcultural nursing perspective, *J Transcult Nurs* 2:23-32, 1990.

Levine NH: A conceptual model for obstetric nursing, *J Obstet Gynecol Neonat Nurs* 5(2):9-15, 1976.

Lewis J, Beavers R, Gossett JT, Phillips UA: *No single thread: psychological health in family systems*, New York, 1976, Brunner/Mazel.

Limandri BJ: Research and practice with abused women: use of the Roy adaptation model as an explanatory framework, *Adv Nurs Sci* 8(4):52-61, 1986.

Mahoney EA, Verdisco L, Shortridge L: *How to collect and record a health history*, ed 2, Philadelphia, 1982, Lippincott.

Maluccio AN, Marlow W: The case for the contract, *Soc Work* 19:28-36, 1974.

Marrelli TM, Hilliard LS: *Home care and clinical paths: effective care planning across the continuum*, St. Louis, 1996, Mosby.

Martin K: The Omaha System: a data base for ambulatory and home care. In Mills MEC, Romano CA, Heller BR: *Information management in nursing and health care*, Springhouse, Pa., 1994, Springhouse, pp. 39-44.

Martin KS, Scheet NJ: *The Omaha System: a pocket guide for community health nursing*, Philadelphia, 1992, Saunders.

Maturen VL, Zander K: Outcome management in a prospective pay system, *Caring* 12:46-53, 1993.

Maunz ER, Woods NF: Self-care practices among young adult women: influences of symptoms, employment and sex-role orientation, *Health Care Women Int* 9:29-41, 1988.

McCain F: Nursing by assessment—not intuition, *Am J Nurs* 65:82-84, 1965.

McCloskey JC, Bulechek GM: Standardizing the language for nursing treatments; an overview of the issues, *Nurs Outlook* 42:56-63, 1994.

McCloskey JC, Bulechek GM, eds: *Nursing interventions classification (NIC)*, ed 2, St. Louis, 1996, Mosby.

McPhetridge LM: Nursing history: one means to personalize care, *Am J Nurs* 68:68-75, 1968.

Michael MM, Sewall KS: Use of the adolescent peer group to increase the self-care agency of adolescent alcohol abusers, *Nurs Clin North Am* 15(1);157-176, 1980.

Neuman B: The Betty Neuman model: a total person approach to viewing patient problems, *Nurs Res* 21(3):264-269, 1972.

Neuman B: The Betty Neuman health-care systems model: a total person approach to patient problems. In Riehl J, Roy C, eds: *Conceptual models for nursing practice*, ed 2, New York, 1980, Appleton-Century-Crofts.

Neuman B, ed: *The Neuman systems model*, New York, 1982, Appleton-Century-Crofts.

Neuman B: *The Neuman systems model, application to education and practice*, ed 2, Norwalk, Ct., 1989, Appleton-Lange.

Neuman B: Health as a continuum based on the Neuman systems model, *Nurs Sci Q* 3:129-135, 1990.

Neuman B: The Neuman systems model. In Neuman B, ed: *The Neuman systems model*, ed 3, Norwalk, Ct., 1995, Appleton and Lange.

North American Nursing Diagnosis Association (NANDA): *Nursing diagnoses: definitions and classification*, Philadelphia, 1994, The Association.

Nunn D, Marriner-Tomey A: Applying Orem's model in nursing administration. In Henry B, Arndt O, Di Vincenti M, Marriner-Tomey A, eds: *Dimensions of nursing administration: theory, research, education, practice*, Boston, 1989, Blackwell Scientific, pp. 63-67.

Orem DE: *Nursing: concepts of practice*, New York, 1971, McGraw-Hill.

Orem DE: *Nursing: concepts of practice*, ed 2, New York, 1980, McGraw-Hill.

Orem DE: *Nursing: concepts of practice*, ed 3, New York, 1985, McGraw-Hill.

Orem DE: *Nursing: concepts of practice*, ed 4, St. Louis, 1991, Mosby.

Orem DE, Taylor SG: Orem's general theory of nursing. In Winstead-Fry P, ed: *Case studies in nursing*, New York, 1986, National League for Nursing, pp. 37-71.

Otto H: Criteria for assessing family strength, *Family Process* 2:329-338, 1963.

Pinkerton A: Use of the Neuman model in a home health-care agency. In Riehl JP, Roy C, eds: *Conceptual models for nursing practice*, New York, 1974, Appleton-Century-Crofts.

Potter PA, Perry AG: *Fundamentals of nursing: concepts, process, and practice*, ed 3, St. Louis, 1993, Mosby.

Pratt L: *Family structure and effective health behavior: the energized family*, Boston, 1976, Houghton Mifflin.

Price S, Wilson L: *Pathophysiology: clinical concepts of disease processes*, ed 5, St. Louis, 1996, Mosby.

Pridham KF: Instruction of a school-age child with chronic illness for increased responsibility in self-care, using diabetes mellitus as an example, *Int J Nurs Stud* 8:237-246, 1971.

Randall-David E: *Strategies for working with culturally diverse communities and clients*, Bethesda, Md., 1989, The Association for the Care of Children's Health.

Rawnsley MM: *Perceptions of the speed of time in aging and in dying: an empirical investigation of the holistic theory of nursing proposed by Martha Rogers*, doctoral dissertation, Boston, 1977, Boston University.

Redman EK: *The process of patient education*, St. Louis, 1997, Mosby.

Reed KS: Adapting the Neuman systems model for family nursing, *Nurs Sci Q* 6:93-97, 1993.

Riehl-Sisca J, ed: *The science and art of self-care*, Norwalk, Ct., 1985, Appleton-Century-Crofts.

Rogers ME: *An introduction to the theoretical basis of nursing*, Philadelphia, 1970, F.A. Davis.

Rogers ME: Nursing: a science of unitary man. In Riehl JP, Roy C, eds: *Conceptual models for nursing practice*, ed 2, New York, 1980, Appleton-Century-Crofts, pp. 329-337.

Rogers ME: Science of unitary human beings: a paradigm for nursing. In Clements JW, Roberts FB, eds: *Family health: a theoretical approach to nursing care*, New York, 1983, Wiley, pp. 219-228.

Rogers ME: Science of unitary human beings. In Malinski UM, ed: *Explorations on Martha Rogers' science of unitary human beings*, Norwalk, Ct., 1986, Appleton-Century-Crofts, pp. 3-8.

Rogers ME: Rogers' science of unitary human beings. In Parse RR, ed: *Nursing science: major metaparadigms, theories, and critique*, Philadelphia, 1989, Saunders, pp. 139-146.

Rogers ME: Nursing science of unitary, irreducible, human beings; update, 1990. In Barrett EAM: *Visions of Rogers' science-based nursing*, New York, 1990, National League for Nursing, pp. 5-11.

Rogers ME: Nursing science and the space age, *Nurs Sci Q* 5:27-34, 1992.

Rogers ME: The science of unitary human beings current perspectives, *Nurs Sci Q* 7:33-35, 1994.

Roy C: Adaptation: a conceptual framework for nursing, *Nurs Outlook* 18(3):42-45, 1970.

Roy C: *Introduction to nursing: an adaptation model*, Englewood Cliffs, N.J., 1976, Prentice-Hall.

Roy C: Family in primary care: analysis and application of the Roy adaptation model. In Clements IW, Roberts FB, eds: *Family health: a theoretical approach to nursing care*, New York, 1983, Wiley, pp. 375-378.

Roy C: *Introduction to nursing: an adaptation model*, ed 2, Englewood Cliffs, N.J., 1984, Prentice-Hall.

Roy C: Roy adaptation model. In Parse RR, ed: *Nursing science: major metaparadigms, theories and critique*, Philadelphia, 1987, Saunders, pp. 35-44.

Roy C: An explication of the philosophical assumptions of the Roy adaptation model, *Nurs Sci Q* 1(1):26-34, 1988.

Roy C, Roberts SL: *Theory construction in nursing: an adaptation model*, Englewood Cliffs, N.J., 1981, Prentice Hall.

Roy SC, Andrews HA: *The Roy adaptation model: a definitive statement,* Norwalk, Ct., 1991, Appleton & Lange.

Schmitz M: The Roy adaptation model: application in a community setting. In Riehl JP, Roy C, eds: *Conceptual models for nursing practice,* ed 2, New York, 1980, Appleton-Century-Crofts.

Seabury BA: The contract: uses, abuses and limitations, *Soc Work* 21(8):39-45, 1976.

Sibley BJ: Cultural influences on health and illness. In Long BC, Phipps WJ, Cassmeyer VL: *Medical-surgical nursing,* ed 3, St. Louis, 1992, Mosby, p. 32.

Simons RC: *Understanding human behavior in health and illness,* ed 3, Baltimore, 1985, Williams and Wilkins.

Story EL, Ross MM: Family centered community health nursing and the Betty Neuman systems model, *Nurs Papers* 18(2):77-88, 1986.

Tripp-Reimer T, Brink PJ, Saunders JN: Cultural assessment: content and process, *Nurs Outlook* 32:78-82, 1984.

Vicenzi HE, Thiel R: AIDS education on the college campus: Roy's adaptation model directs inquiry, *Public Health Nurs* 9:270-276, 1992.

Wagner P: Testing the adaptation model in practice, *Nurs Outlook* 24:682-685, 1976.

Walborn KA: A nursing model for the hospice: hospice primary and self care nursing, *Nurs Clin North Am* 15(1):205-217, 1980.

Weber G: Making nursing diagnosis work for you and your client, *Nurs Health Care* 12:424-430, 1991.

Weiss HB: Home visits necessary but not sufficient, *Future of Children* 3(3):113-128, 1993.

West M: *Patterns of health in mothers of developmentally disabled children,* unpublished master's thesis, University Park, 1984, Pennsylvania State university.

Whall AL: Nursing theory and the assessment of families, *J Psychiatr Nurs Mental Health Serv* 19(1):30-36, 1981.

Whall AL, ed: *Family therapy theory for nursing: four approaches,* Norwalk, Ct., 1986, Appleton-Century-Crofts.

Whall AL: Family system theory; relationship to nursing conceptual models. In Whall AL, Fawcett J: *Family theory development in nursing: state of the science and art,* Philadelphia, 1991, F.A. Davis, pp. 317-342.

Whall AL, Fawcett J: *Family theory development in nursing: state of the science and art,* Philadelphia, 1991, F.A. Davis.

Wood R, Kekahbah J, eds: *Examining the cultural implications of Martha E. Rogers; science of unitary human beings,* Lecompton, Ks., 1985, Wood-Kekahbah Associates.

World Health Organization: Constitution of the World Health Organization, *WHO Chron* 1:29-43, 1947.

Zander K: Nursing case management: strategic management of cost and quality outcomes, *J Nurs Adm* 18:23-30, 1988.

SELECTED BIBLIOGRAPHY

Barnum BJS: *Nursing theory; analysis, application, evaluation,* ed 4, Philadelphia, 1994, Lippincott.

Berg CL, Helgeson DM: That first home visit, *Community Health Nurs* 1:207-216, 1984.

Brink P: Value orientations as an assessment tool in cultural diversity, *Nurs Res* 33:198-203, 1983.

Burr WR, Klein SR, et al: *Reexamining family stress: new theory and research,* Thousand Oaks, Ca., 1994, Sage.

Carey R: How values affect the mutual goal setting process, *Community Health Nurs* 6:7-14, 1989.

Coenen A, Marek KD, Lundeen SP: Using nursing diagnoses to explain utilization in a community nursing center, *Res Nurs Health* 19:441-445, 1996.

Fawcett J: *Analysis and evaluation of conceptual models of nursing,* ed 3, Philadelphia, 1995, F.A. Davis.

Fitzpatrick JJ, Whall AL: *Conceptual models of nursing: analysis and application,* ed 3, Stamford, Ct., 1996, Appleton & Lange.

Gulino C, LaMonica G: Public health nursing: a study of role implementation, *Public Health Nurs* 3:80-91, 1986.

Helgeson DM, Berg CL: Contracting: a method of health promotion, *J Community Health Nurs* 2:199-207, 1985.

Kirschling JM, Gilliss CL, Krentz L, et al: Success in family nursing: experts describe phenomena, *Nurs Health Care* 15:186-189, 1994.

Marek KM: Nursing diagnoses and home care nursing utilization, *Public Health Nurs* 13:195-200, 1996.

Martin ME, Henry M: Cultural relativity and poverty, *Public Health Nurs* 6:28-34, 1989.

McKenry PC, Price SJ, eds: *Families and change: coping with stressful events,* Thousand Oaks, Ca., 1994, Sage.

Muecke MA: Community health diagnosis in nursing, *Public Health Nurs* 1:23-35, 1984.

Porter EJ: Critical analysis of NANDA nursing diagnosis taxonomy I, *Image J Nurs Sch* 13:136-139, 1986.

Radwin LE: Knowing the patient: a process model for individualized interventions, *Nurs Res* 44:364-370, 1995.

Rakel BA: Interventions related to patient teaching. *Nurs Clin North Am* 27:397-423, 1992.

Reed P: A treatise on nursing knowledge development for the twenty-first century: beyond post modernism, *Advances Nurs Sci* 17:70-84, 1995.

Selby-Harrington ML, Tesh AS, Donat PL, Quade D: Diversity in the rural poor: differences between households with and without telephones, *Public Health Nurs* 12:386-392, 1995.

Tadych R: Nursing in multiperson units: the family. In Riehl-Sisca J, ed: *The science and art of self-care,* Norwalk, Ct., 1985, Appleton-Century-Crofts, pp. 49-55.

Wright LM, Leahey M: *Nurses and families: a guide to family assessment and intervention,* Philadelphia, 1994, F.A. Davis.

Wuest J: Removing the shackles: a feminist critique of noncompliance, *Nurs Outlook* 41:217-224, 1993.

10

Continuity of Care through Care Management and the Referral Process

Objectives

Upon completion of this chapter, the reader should be able to:

1. Discuss the concept of continuity of care.
2. Discuss the process of care management.
3. Understand the nurse's role in the discharge planning process.
4. Summarize the basic principles that should be considered when making a referral.
5. Analyze the steps of the referral process.
6. Discuss the nurse's role in the referral process.
7. Distinguish between the levels of nursing intervention in the referral process.
8. Discuss barriers to the use of the referral process.

Continuity of care is a process through which a client's ongoing health care needs are assessed, planned for, coordinated, and met. The process provides for appropriate, uninterrupted care along the health continuum (ANA, 1986a, p. 14) and facilitates the client's transition to different settings and levels of health care.

The significant role of the community health nurse in this process was emphasized by the American Nurses Association (ANA) in both its *Standards of Community Health Nursing Practice* (1986b) and *Standards of Home Health Nursing Practice* (1986a) (see Chapters 21 and 24). In *Standards of Home Health Nursing Practice* the ANA identified a separate standard for continuity of care that charged the nurse with providing for uninterrupted client care through the use of care management, discharge planning, and coordination of community resources (ANA, 1986a, p. 14). The process demands client and family participation, multidisciplinary planning and intervention, and ongoing evaluation.

When continuity of care is not part of a client's care, the results can be disastrous to the client and costly to the health care system. An example of such a situation is given later, illustrating how an ineffectively planned hospital discharge for a ventilator-dependent child resulted in family stress, hospital readmission, and additional health care costs.

Every client should have the opportunity to reach his or her optimum potential for health and recovery; planning for continuity of care helps to ensure that this occurs and helps to assure quality care. Integral components of continuity of care are *care management* and the *referral* process.

CARE MANAGEMENT

The concept of care management is becoming the predominant theme in the evolving managed care system. Managed care is both a structure and a process (Table 10-1). Managed care structures such as HMOs, PPOs, and POSs are discussed in Chapter 4. The process component of managed care, "care management," has historically been a part of community health nursing. More recently care management has been associated with managed care organizations (Girard, 1994, p. 403).

As both a structure and a process managed care heavily emphasizes primary prevention activities, effective utilization of health care services, and high quality health care. As a structure managed care is highly oriented to cost containment. Managed care as a process is client focused and stresses working collaboratively with clients and client satisfaction with services rendered.

The literature on care management does not consistently use or define the term; definitions of the term tend to vary by setting. Care management for the community health nurse is presented in the box on the next page. The care management process follows the steps of the nursing process (see the box on p. 264). Effective care management enhances individual health and the nation's health (Masso, 1995, p. 51).

table 10-1 Managed Care: Structure and Process

	Managed Care Structure	Managed Care Process
Emphasis	Primary prevention (aggregate focused as a cost containment mechanism) Condition focused Cost savings Specialized Match health problem to cheapest intervention	Primary prevention (individualized to meet client needs) Client focused Quality Holistic Match health problem to appropriate intervention
Clients	Those insured by the organization	All in need of services
Funding	Prepaid/capitation	Variable
Locus of Control	Agency guided (external to client)	More internal to perceived needs of client (client is part of decision making)
Outcome Measure(s)	Quality of care Money saved	Quality of care Client satisfaction

Managed care organizations include HMOs, PPOs, and POSs. See Chapter 4 for a discussion of these organizations.

Care Management for the Community Health Nurse*

Care management is a systematic, client-centered process that promotes holistic, comprehensive, continuous care. It focuses on primary prevention, "keeping people healthy," and strives to provide quality care, enhance client outcomes, and efficiently use health care resources (including using the most appropriate level of care). It is designed to reduce fragmentation of health care services and encourages interdisciplinary collaboration. It helps to ensure that health care needs do not go unmet, that health care is coordinated or "seamless," and that clients progress smoothly along the health care continuum. A care manager has caregiving, educative, advocacy, and gatekeeper roles and:

- Utilizes the steps of the nursing process.
- Strives to be culturally sensitive.
- Is client centered and incorporates the client and family in the planning, implementation, and evaluation of care.
- Utilizes the referral process to link clients with appropriate community agencies.
- Utilizes health education interventions to promote health and healthy lifestyles, and teach clients about community resources.
- Strives to optimize client satisfaction with the health care process.
- Strives to promote self-care and independence.

*Case management is part of the care management process.

Community health nurses are involved in care management activities on a daily basis. They build on teaching that was begun in the physician's office or hospital, gather information on community resources, refer clients to appropriate community health agencies, coordinate efforts between community health agencies, assist clients in planning for ongoing health care needs, advocate for health care services, develop holistic plans of care, and take part in discharge planning efforts.

As a holistic, client-centered process, care management includes the client, family, and caregivers in planning health care activities and facilitates continuous, "seamless" care. It consolidates the gains made at one level or setting while arranging for the resources and services necessary to meet the needs of another level or setting. Intervention strategies need to be carefully planned to build on gains made by the client, maximize client strengths, and link the client to appropriate community resources. The process uses anticipatory guidance to assist individuals, families, and communities in planning for health care and making decisions about health.

Care management activities need to be documented. Agencies often have developed standardized forms for tracking care management decisions, activities, and referrals. Such standardized forms may include information on the client's diagnosis, treatment, and level of functioning; health care follow-up needs (including home adaptation and health education needs); support systems available; and community resources that are recommended or already being used.

THE NURSE AND CARE MANAGEMENT

Community health nurses can be proud of the important role they have played in care management efforts. Even before legislation mandated such activities community health nurses recognized the need for care management to facilitate continuity of care.

Historically, community health nurses from local health departments often worked in cooperation with hospitals as *home care coordinators* and *hospital liaisons* to assess client's home care needs and to implement discharge planning activities. Nurses have expanded on these early roles, and

Care Management and the Nursing Process

NURSING ASSESSMENT, DIAGNOSIS, AND PLANNING

A comprehensive nursing assessment of client needs begins the process and is the core of effective care management. The nurse assesses the client's health, including functional status (including ability to carry out activities of daily living) and use of community resources. It is important to assess psychosocial variables such as the client's living situation, level of education, financial resources (including source of payment for health care), social support systems, health values and attitudes, cultural and ethnic background, perceptions of the situation, barriers to care, and care preferences. It is crucial that the nursing assessment be culturally sensitive.

Following assessment the nurse works collaboratively with the client to establish health care needs. Realistic, measurable goals and objectives are formulated with the client.

NURSING INTERVENTIONS

As a caregiver, nursing interventions may be educative, therapeutic, or rehabilitative in nature and frequently the nurse may be placed in an advocacy role. Interventions focus on matching the level of care needed with appropriate community resources and support services. They should assist clients in achieving their maximum level of functioning. Interventions include health education, referrals to appropriate community agencies, and home adaptation strategies.

Nursing interventions frequently involve providing direct care, sharing community resource information with clients, coordinating multidisciplinary care management and discharge planning efforts, and alleviating client and family anxiety about continuing care needs. The nurse needs to be sensitive to the client's and family's readiness to assume care responsibilities and use community resources. Clients and families may find it difficult to consider continuing care needs when they are dealing with an acute care episode.

NURSING EVALUATION

As with all parts of the nursing process, care management efforts need to be evaluated. Evaluation is ongoing and assesses the effectiveness and outcomes of the process including client satisfaction. When evaluating, the nurse elicits information from referral agencies and from the client to determine if continuing care needs were met. Results of evaluation help to revise and shape the care process. In evaluating the discharge planning process the nurse should remember that, whatever the discharge planning needs, efforts focus on facilitating continuity of care, family adaptation and growth, and matching the client with appropriate community resources.

today they are key members of multidisciplinary care management teams.

The nurse involved in care management efforts must realize that not all nurses and clients have a complete or adequate understanding of the process. A major role of the nurse is to "educate" caregivers and clients about care management and community health resources. The nurse develops collaborative relationships to enhance care management efforts. A role that the nurse may assume in care management is that of a case manager. As case managers nurses use the *discharge planning* and the *referral process*.

Nurses as Case Managers

Nurses have historically been involved in case management. Today many nurses work in the contemporary role of a "case manager." As a case manager the nurse assists the client in assessing and planning for health care services, facilitates implementation of services, links clients with community resources, and monitors the care process. As a case manager the nurse is concerned with providing continuous, comprehensive, quality care. Case management *individualizes the care management process*.

Nurses are uniquely qualified to be case managers. Their knowledge of clinical care, interpersonal relationships, and community resources and their readiness to advocate on behalf of clients are all invaluable to case management (Girard, 1994, p. 404). As a health professional the nurse brings a holistic approach to case management and is concerned with the psychosocial aspects of care as well as the medical condition(s) (Girard, p. 404; Hicks, Stallmeyer, Coleman, 1993, p. 43). Nurses are familiar with the services of other health care providers and support an interdisciplinary team approach.

The roles of the nurse as a case manager will vary based on the setting and the individual needs of the client (Girard, 1994, p. 404). Two roles frequently assumed by nurses as case managers are that of advocate and "gatekeeper." When these two roles are carried out simultaneously they can be in conflict with one another and ethical dilemmas can be created (Browdie, 1992, p. 87; Kane, 1992, p. 78). An example of this is when the nurse is employed by a managed care organization and, as a gatekeeper, realizes that the health care organization prefers using the least expensive service. If the least expensive service is inappropriate for the client, as an advocate the nurse would recommend using multiple services, a more costly service, or referring the client to another agency.

As a case manager the nurse needs to ensure that care is client focused (Masso, 1995, p. 50), that the client's right to participate in care decisions is maintained, and that care is of high quality. The nurse can help "to bring coherence to a chaotic and fragmented system of care" (McCloskey, Grace, 1990, p. 166). Some activities of nurses as case managers are given in the box on page 267. One activity that the nurse is involved in as a case manager is discharge planning.

Nurses and Discharge Planning

A forerunner of today's care management process was the discharge planning done by nurses. The box on page 268

A View from the Field: The Child at Home with a Chronic Illness

I am Donnie's mother. I am here to present the parents' view. I will describe the implications of a child's chronic illness on the family, the financial issues, and the complex problems encountered by my family. In addition, I will compare experiences reported by other parents in our parents' group.

Donnie, my sixth child, was born with defects that involved the left side of his body including his left lung, which later on had to be removed. At the time of his birth, we were told that Donnie had to undergo immediate surgery because of what is called an omphalocele, which means that his navel and stomach had evolved outside his abdomen. Within 4 hours of birth, he was transported from Joliet Hospital to Children's Memorial Hospital in Chicago, where the first stage of surgery was performed immediately.

For us as parents, the first shock in the delivery room was knowing that our child had multiple birth defects. We were overpowered by fear of losing our child. Later, the fear was intensified by observing our child in the ICU, when his heart stopped 18 times and he had to be resuscitated. Only because of the prompt response from health care personnel, Donnie survived all this without brain damage.

During his first 3 years in an acute intensive care unit, Donnie underwent a total of 20 operations. Most of the time he was breathing with the help of a machine—a ventilator—receiving numerous intravenous infusions and treatments while we were watching as helpless bystanders. We often did not understand what was done, the reason why, and we had no knowledge of the alternatives.

Our main social contacts were other parents of critically ill children in the ICU waiting area who, over a period of months, became like close friends to us. Some were the unlucky ones; their children died. We grieved with them, always thinking that we could be next. After years of this, we shut ourselves off and avoided contacts with those parents—even to the point of being abrupt.

We did not receive professional help to deal with the psychological stress we were under. My husband dealt with it by talking constantly about it, while I tried not to think or talk about it, which caused great problems between us. We lost a lot of our friends. They did not know what to say, so it was easier for them not to see us. Besides, we were no fun to be with, because we were constantly talking about our problem.

During his years in the ICU, attempts were made to wean Donnie off the ventilator. A pediatrician forcefully suggested that we take Donnie home, that is, to die. We took Donnie home. He had a tracheostomy; that is, a hole in his trachea. He was breathing poorly by himself; we thought he would not live much longer. We were not prepared to properly take care of him at home. We did not even know how to regulate oxygen flow. He was home for two months, only to return to the Children's Memorial ICU because of pneumonia and failure to thrive. By then, we had lived through two months of a nightmare with no help, no medical caregivers, no sleep—only worry. We were exhausted and burned out.

We shared this experience years later with other parents who at the time were sent home unprepared, with a child who could not breathe by himself without a mechanical aid. This couple had ventilated their child by hand 24 hours a day, taking turns day and night for months, until the decision was made that the child needed a mechanical ventilator at home.

Our home is in Joliet, Illinois, 60 miles from Children's Memorial Hospital in Chicago. Rather than spend 2 to 4 hours on the road a day, we chose to move into the waiting rooms at Children's Memorial Hospital, where we lived for over a year. We slept on the couch, showered in the basement locker rooms, ate hospital food, and paid parking fees. Our 5 children, ranging in age from 17 to 12 years, were left unattended most of the time. They learned to take care of themselves. After about a year, my husband and I decided that one of us had to stay at home in Joliet because our other children were beginning to feel the effects of our absence. I went to Joliet, returning to the hospital occasionally, and my husband stayed with Donnie. Consequently, he lost his business and to live we had to borrow money from family members. Besides dealing with this stress, there was no money or time to go on vacations with the other children. We haven't had a family vacation for 10 years!

Our insurance covered $100,000 of Donnie's care. After a few months, we were told to apply for financial assistance to Illinois Public Aid and the Division of Services for Crippled Children. Children's Memorial Hospital was very helpful in helping us apply. We qualified because Donnie was born with multiple deformities.

Why is it much easier to get aid if a child is born with defects than if some illness or accident causes defects at a later date? Others in our parent-group had children who had problems getting financial help. One parent was called into the hospital billing department and was presented with an astronomical hospital bill and was asked, "How are you going to pay for this?" Some parents were advised to go on unemployment, go on public aid, and even get a divorce.

Modified from USDHHS: *Report of the Surgeon General's Workshop on children with handicaps and their families*, DHHS Publication No. PHS 83-50194, Washington, D.C., 1982b, U.S. Government Printing Office, pp. 27-30.

Continued

A View from the Field THE CHILD AT HOME WITH A CHRONIC ILLNESS—cont'd

After spending the better part of 3 years in an Acute ICU, Donnie was transferred into an intermediate care unit for his long-term care. Repeated attempts to wean him from his breathing machine caused him to be lethargic, puffy, and turn blue. He ceased to grow. The only time he was well was when he was on his ventilator. Then he became a very active, happy child. His many arrests had apparently not damaged his brain. He had become a very precocious child, even inventing his own sign language!

Even though we were at his bedside as much as possible, many of the functions of a parent were taken over by nurses and other health caretakers. Correcting bad behavior or eating habits is hard to accomplish outside of a family setting.

Since Donnie was confined to this unit by being on the ventilator, he lacked opportunity for an education appropriate for a 4-year-old. At this time, he got an hour of tutoring a day. Children's Memorial Hospital, being an acute care hospital, was unable to provide additional education for a chronically disabled child.

Then a new idea was presented to us by a new staff physician. Give Donnie optimal ventilation so he can grow. Prepare him to go home safely with his ventilator. With our memories of the past experience, the idea horrified us. But after meeting with qualified medical personnel, we were assured that we would be trained and would have medical help to support us. Donnie needed to go home in order not to become socially handicapped. Once while I was talking to him on the phone, I told him I was sitting at the kitchen table. After he hung up, he asked his nurse, "What is a kitchen table?" My other children were delighted when we told them that Donnie could come home, and they were anxiously awaiting his arrival.

At that time no money was allocated by Federal or State law to care for ventilator-dependent children at home. The State would pay the high costs of intensive care but had no experience in providing funding for less expensive care at home. A long period of negotiation took place. The State officials finally paid for the less expensive care at home. We were luckier than others in the parents' group who were faced with the spend-down money (money to be paid according to income by the family to the state).

Some parents in our group had private insurance. The insurance company refused to change their reimbursement policy for home care. The insurance company was willing to pay everything in hospital, but refused payment for home care. As a result, the insurance company rapidly spent the $500,000 in the hospital. This money could have lasted for years at home. They had no incentive to change. Therefore, public funds were needed sooner, because the private insurance money was gone so quickly while the patient remained in the ICU. So the burden was transferred to the State and ultimately to the taxpayer.

TRANSITION

It took nine months from the time the decision was made to send Donnie home before it really happened. During that time we built a specially adapted addition to our house. Regular meetings with the health care team were held. These meetings clearly defined goals acceptable to all, and provided clear objectives and specific plans for action. Each team member had accountability. The home discharge team included the dedicated clinical staff who had cared for Donnie over the years. The coordinator was his nurse; the educator was his respiratory therapist. Both were caregivers who had received him in the ICU shortly after his birth. The team also involved physical and child-life therapists, special service staff, social workers, etc. Initially, several members had to overcome their own fear and negative thinking, but the more educated they became, the more they were able to overcome this barrier.

My husband and I were trained to handle Donnie's ventilator equipment by both classroom teaching and "hands-on" experience. We passed a test and were certified. Nurses we recruited, selected, and hired to provide 24-hour home care were trained with us at the hospital, in the classroom, and at the bedside. Community support services, including a primary physician and emergency room staff in Joliet, were well-informed about their responsibility prior to their consent. Nursing, physical therapy, and respiratory therapy plans and exact procedures were clearly written, and local suppliers of medical equipment were found, motivated, and well-prepared. Funding was finally approved because of highly motivated and responsible actions of the leaders and staff of the Division of Services for Crippled Children, the Illinois Department of Public Health and SSI Disabled Children's Program.

The team work of all these individuals made the home program a reality.

HOME

It finally happened, our son came home to stay. It has been a difficult task. We are dealing with a lack of privacy, the ventilator breaking down, lack of service for equipment, and difficulties in getting medical supplies.

However, the benefits of having Donnie at home far outweigh the difficulties.

We are now a normal family, maybe different in some ways, but we are all together, sharing all the experiences of

A View from the Field — THE CHILD AT HOME WITH A CHRONIC ILLNESS—cont'd

life. We no longer divide our time among our children. Donnie's health has improved; he has grown several inches. His oxygen need has decreased. His social life is no longer limited to the ICU where he never knew the difference between day and night. He is now getting an education, doing average-to-above-average work. He no longer has to regard cardiac arrests in the bed next to him as his only occasion for "social-get-together." Instead he goes to weddings; he was a ring bearer at his brother's wedding where he never missed a dance. Donnie is a joy to be with. He loves his religion. He celebrated his Holy Communion last month. He tolerates being off the ventilator with oxygen longer. He races his race car (recently he placed first in competition), climbs trees, and he even fell and broke his arm at a birthday party. Donnie worries right now whether he will get married one day. He is concerned that it is not much fun to go trick or treating, because no matter how he dresses up, everybody recognizes him by his tracheostomy. His nightly prayer includes: "Dear God, if you are listening, please get rid of my trach so I can play football."

We know we can go back to Children's Memorial Hospital any time we have any problems with Donnie. He will be well taken care of by loving people who know him and care for him and us.

We are deeply grateful to the staff of Children's Memorial Hospital. They never gave up hope. And thank God nobody pulled the plug in the ICU. Thank you.

THE NURSE AS A CASE MANAGER

The right service, in the right setting, at the right time, by the right provider

- Performs casefinding
- Is knowledgeable about community resources
- Does a comprehensive assessment of the biopsychosocial needs of the client and family
- Develops a plan of care in conjunction with the client and family
- Acts as a resource in identifying and linking the client with the most appropriate resource
- Coordinates care
- Facilitates client access to health care
- Provides direct patient care as appropriate
- Provides client education
- Monitors and evaluates client and program outcomes
- Advocates for necessary and appropriate health care services
- Ensures that high-quality client care is provided
- Ensures that care is patient focused

gives the history of these efforts, how federal legislation still mandates discharge planning for Medicaid and Medicare patients, and how the process remains an integral part of care management. Community health nurses continue to play a major role in discharge planning efforts.

Like other aspects of care management, discharge planning is client focused, interdisciplinary, uses community resources, takes into consideration the setting in which the client is going, and makes revisions as necessary. It strives to provide comprehensive, continuous care and links clients with community resources. The adequacy and timeliness of discharge planning is an important part of care management and meeting client health care needs (Hicks, Stallmeyer, Coleman, 1993, p. 763).

Discharge planning has historically focused on clients who are leaving acute care settings such as hospitals and returning to the community (the referral process is discussed later in this chapter). More recently discharge planning has been used with clients being discharged from health care settings such as nursing homes (Murtagh, 1994) and moving from one level of care to another. As clients leave health care settings "quicker and sicker" their discharge planning needs increase.

The discharge planning process follows the steps of the nursing process. A thorough nursing assessment of client needs begins the process and facilitates planning efforts. Some areas for the nurse to assess in discharge planning are identified in Figure 10-1, page 269, and Appendix 10-1. An example of how a nurse assessed discharge planning needs is presented in Figure 10-2, page 270. Discharge planning makes a difference in client care and has been successful in reducing morbidity and mortality (e.g., using the discharge planning process for premature infants and infants with congenital anomalies) (Mbweza, 1996, p. 53).

The success of discharge planning activities is largely dependent on how accurately discharge needs are assessed and diagnosed, the extent to which the client and family participate in the planning process, and the availability of community resources to meet discharge planning needs.

Discharge planning efforts need to address activities that clients and families will be expected to implement at home, such as administering injections and treatments, using complicated support and assistive devices, and carrying out activities of daily living. In implementing discharge planning activities the client is often referred to community agencies (the referral process is discussed later in this chapter).

History of Discharge Planning

Historically, discharge planning focused on a single event—the referral of a client to community services or facilities upon discharge from a hospital. Being familiar with community resources, community health nurses frequently worked as *hospital liaisons* and *home care coordinators* to make referrals, coordinate care, and "bridge the gap" as the client moved from the hospital to the community.

There is evidence of discharge planning in the late 1800s and early 1900s (O'Hare, Terry, 1988, p. 6; Shamansky, Boase, Horn, 1984, p. 15). Lillian Wald was one of the first to recognize the need for such planning. In 1906 Bellevue Hospital in New York City referred to a nurse whose entire time and care was given to befriending those about to be discharged (O'Hare, Terry, 1988, p. 6).

The 1960s saw the first official use of the term *discharge planning* (Shamansky, Boase, Horn, 1984, p. 16). Discharge planning became a part of many hospital programs, and Edith Wensley's (1963) *Nursing Service Without Walls* urged hospitals to emphasize planning for home care services and referral to community services upon discharge. The National League for Nursing urged hospitals, nursing homes, and home nursing care agencies to have a designated staff person to develop plans for the next stage of nursing care, to implement continuity of care activities, and to develop well-defined, clearly written procedures for client referral (O'Hare, Terry, 1988, p. 7). The passage of Medicaid and Medicare legislation in 1965 placed new emphasis on discharge planning efforts since the home care benefits of these two programs allowed clients to leave hospitals sooner.

In the 1970s discharge planning became inextricably linked with quality assurance. This occurred largely as a result of Medicaid and Medicare legislation in 1972 (Public Law 92-603), which mandated that skilled nursing facilities and hospitals receiving these monies maintain centralized, coordinated programs to ensure that each client had a planned program of continuing care that met post-discharge needs.

In the 1980s federal legislation again shaped the course of discharge planning. A prospective payment system (PPS), aimed at reducing the length of stay in acute care facilities, was enacted for Medicare in 1982. This legislation was instrumental in the development of discharge planning activities across the nation because it gave hospitals a financial incentive to discharge clients as early as possible. Thus discharge planning became a method of cost containment (Willihnganz, 1984).

During the 1980s discharge planning became a hospital priority. The American Hospital Association (AHA) developed guidelines for discharge planning that included early identification of clients likely to need posthospital care; client and family education, assessment, and counseling; discharge plan development, coordination, and implementation; and postdischarge follow-up (AHA, 1984; Corkery, 1989, p. 19). In 1986 Medicare legislation mandated the development of a standardized, uniform needs assessment instrument to evaluate the posthospital "discharge" needs of Medicare patients (Burlenski, 1989, p. 2; McBroom, 1989, p. 1), and required that hospitals receiving Medicare reimbursement notify patients of their right to discharge planning services (Blaylock, Cason, 1992, p. 5; Corkery, 1989, p. 19). Discharge planning is still an important part of care management.

Although discharge planning is an important part of care management, it does not replace the need for ongoing management of client care and does not ensure that client's home care needs are met (Mamon, Steinwachs, Fahey et al, 1994, p. 172-173). Evaluation and follow-up of discharge planning efforts is essential. This follow-up can be in the form of home visiting, written or telephone contacts with clients, and in today's computer age even computer communication linkages. In studies by Garland (1992) and North, Neeusen, and Hollinsworth (1991), cost-effective and time-efficient telephone calls were placed after discharge to follow up on discharge planning efforts. Both studies addressed client and family satisfaction with discharge preparation, identified actual problems after discharge, and obtained information useful for staff to improve discharge planning efforts.

When discharge planning efforts are unsuccessful clients can become discouraged and their confidence is shaken (Glover, King, Green, Shults, 1993, p. 40). Community health nurses frequently work with clients to revise discharge planning efforts. The case of 76-year-old Mrs. Flowers returning home after breaking a hip is an example.

CASE Scenario

Mrs. Flowers was hospitalized for a broken left hip after a fall in her home. From the day of admission her discharge planning needs were assessed and she was involved in establishing and implementing her discharge plan of care. Mrs. Flowers lives alone but has a son and daughter-in-law who live nearby and friends who are willing to help her with grocery shopping and other errands.

As part of discharge planning efforts, options to assist her, such as homemaker services, friendly visitors, Meals-on-Wheels, the local Visiting Nurse Association, and a more supervised living situation, were discussed with her. Assistive devices she would need at home were also considered. Additionally her support systems, financial resources, and goals for care were considered.

A mutually agreeable discharge plan was established for Mrs. Flowers. The necessary assistive devices were ordered. It was decided that she would have a visiting nurse and homemaker services for housework, and her son would help with transportation and groceries. Mrs. Flowers indicated she would like to take care of her own meal preparation.

After a short period at home Mrs. Flowers told the community health nurse/case manager that meal preparation was very difficult. She could prepare some simple meals for herself, but total meal preparation was not working out. The nurse worked with Mrs. Flowers to find an acceptable solution to the situation. The combined efforts of family members and a local Meals-on-Wheels program were utilized, and Mrs. Flowers began to feel more confident in her ability to be independent and care for herself at home.

Rorden and Taft (1990, pp. 24-27) have described the discharge planning process as occurring in three phases: acute, transitional, and continuing care. According to Rorden and Taft, in the acute phase medical attention dominates discharge planning efforts, whereas in the transitional phase the need for acute care is still present but its urgency is reduced and clients can begin to address and plan for future health care needs. In the continuing care phase the client is able to plan and implement continuing care activities. A schema for these phases is given in Figure 10-3.

Nurses and Critical Paths

The term *critical path* is a relatively recent addition to the managed care literature (see Chapter 9 for further discussion of critical paths). It is a form of care management and is primarily used in acute care settings. More recently, critical paths have been used in settings such as home health care agencies (Gartner, Twardon, 1995). They take into consideration the optimal sequencing of health care interventions (Spath, 1995) and function as a map and a time line for interventions and anticipated outcomes (Corbett, Androwich, 1995; Gartner, Twardon, 1995).

Critical paths are based on standards of care for a specified client population and include a client care plan with a time-specific path, identify activities critical to care, and involve case consultation and care collaboration (Girard, 1994, p. 408). They are an interdisciplinary approach to care and attempt to control costs through coordination of services. As with other aspects of care management, critical pathways link clients with community resources that can meet client needs and provide continuity of care. Clients are linked with community agencies by the referral process.

THE REFERRAL PROCESS

The *referral process* is a systematic problem-solving approach involving a series of actions that help clients use resources for the purpose of resolving needs. Clients may be either individuals or groups who require assistance from others in order to achieve their maximum level of func-

Circle all that apply and total.
Refer to the risk factor index.*

Age
- 0 = 55 years or less
- 1 = 56 to 64 years
- 2 = 65 to 79 years
- 3 = 80+ years

Living situation/social support
- 0 = lives only with spouse
- 1 = lives with family
- 2 = lives alone with family support
- 3 = lives alone with friends' support
- 4 = lives alone with no support
- 5 = nursing home/ residential care

Functional status
- 0 = independent in activities of daily living and instrumental activities of daily living

Dependent in:
- 1 = eating/feeding
- 1 = bathing/grooming
- 1 = toileting
- 1 = transferring
- 1 = incontinent of bowel function
- 1 = incontinent of bladder function
- 1 = meal preparation
- 1 = responsible for own medication administration
- 1 = handling own finances
- 1 = grocery shopping
- 1 = transportation

Cognition
- 0 = oriented
- 1 = disoriented to some spheres† some of the time
- 2 = disoriented to some spheres all of the time
- 3 = disoriented to all spheres some of the time
- 4 = disoriented to all spheres all of the time
- 5 = comatose

Behavior pattern
- 0 = appropriate
- 1 = wandering
- 1 = agitated
- 1 = confused
- 1 = other

Mobility
- 0 = ambulatory
- 1 = ambulatory with mechanical assistance
- 2 = ambulatory with human assistance
- 3 = nonambulatory

Sensory deficits
- 0 = none
- 1 = visual or hearing deficits
- 2 = visual and hearing deficits

Number of previous admissions/emergency room visits
- 0 = none in the last 3 months
- 1 = one in the last 3 months
- 2 = two in the last 3 months
- 3 = more than two in the last 3 months

Number of active medical problems
- 0 = three medical problems
- 1 = three to five medical problems
- 2 = more than five medical problems

Number of drugs
- 0 = fewer than three drugs
- 1 = three to five drugs
- 2 = more than five drugs

Total score:

*Risk factor index: score of 10 = at risk for home care resources; score of 11 to 19 = at risk for extended discharge planning; score greater than 20 = at risk for placement other than home. If the patient's score is 10 or greater, refer the patient to the discharge planning coordinator or discharge planning team.
†Spheres = person, place, time, and self.

Copyright 1991 Ann Blaylock

Figure 10-1 Blaylock Discharge Planning Risk Assessment Screen. *(From Blaylock A, Cason CL: Discharge planning predicting patients' needs,* J Gerontol Nurs *18(7):8, 1992.)*

Goals: Successful transition of client to home/community setting; healthy growth and development of mother and infant; successful adjustment to parenting

Psychosocial Factors	Health Status	Functional Status	Assessed Discharge Planning Needs
17-year-old unmarried primipara Resides with mother No means of financial support Unfamiliar with community resources No means of transportation 11th grade education—plans to return to school Has never cared for an infant and requesting help with infant care Bonding well with infant No recent contact with infant's father Requesting home follow-up	Uneventful postpartum period No known medical/health problems Breastfeeding infant No source of regular medical follow-up Infant healthy, Apgar 9	Independent in activities of daily living	Lack of knowledge of infant care Lack of knowledge of community resources Potential lack of social/emotional support systems Need for regular medical follow-up Disruption in normal growth and development processes (e.g., education and other normal developmental tasks)

↓

Incorporation of Client/Family into Planning Process

↓

Multidisciplinary Planning

↓

Possible Community Resources/Referrals

Family — Friends — Work — Neighbors — School — Church

Other

(Local Health Department: Nurses, WIC, Clinics; LaLeche League; Young Mothers Support Group; DHHS: TANF, Medicaid; Child and Family Services; Mom's Day Out Programs; Dial-A-Ride)

Figure 10-2 The nurse as a discharge planner: assessing discharge planning needs. *(Modified from Siegel H: Nurses improve hospital efficiency through a risk assessment model at admission,* Nurs Manage *19(10):42, 1988.)*

tioning. The referral process is an integral part of discharge planning (Glover, King, Green, Shults, 1993, p. 40) and care management.

The referral process is an important part of nursing care. Nurses are frequently called on to refer clients to resources in the community. However, there is little in the nursing literature on referral. Existing studies frequently quantify referrals in terms of numbers sent and received or discuss referral as part of care management. Other studies have looked at referral compliance following public screening initiatives (Maiman, Hildreth, Cox, Greenland, 1992). One study, a qualitative research study by Luker and Chalmers (1989), looked at various aspects of the process and found that the primary purpose of referring clients to other resources was to provide the client with additional expertise or services.

The community health nurse's major goals for initiating a referral are to promote high-level wellness and enhance self-care capabilities and quality of care. As clients move from one care setting and one level of care to another, the referral process is frequently used. Referral criteria are helpful in assisting nurses to identify clients who need referrals to community resources (Nash, 1993, p. 707; Townsend, Edwards, Nadon, 1992, p. 203).

To be implemented effectively, the referral process demands knowledge, skill, and experience. It demands knowledge of community resources and an ability to solve problems, set priorities, coordinate, and collaborate. It is an integral part of comprehensive, continuous client care and is essential to community health nursing practice (Luker, Chalmers, 1989, p. 173).

The community health nurse will make referrals to and receive referrals from health care resources. Referrals can be categorized according to referral initiator, the extent of client contact made with the resource, the level of difficulty of the process, and the source of the referral. Working

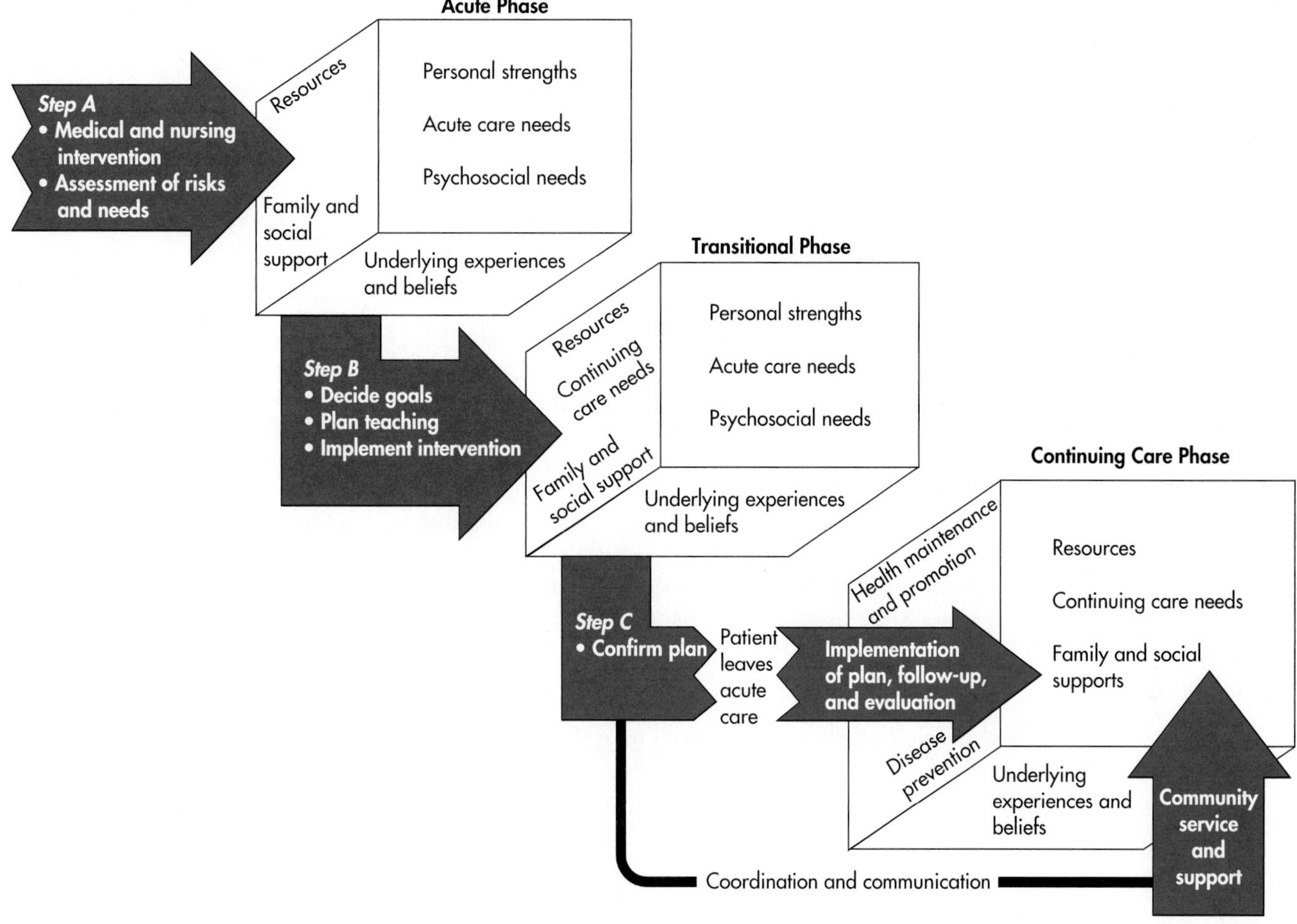

Figure 10-3 Phases of the discharge planning process. *(Redrawn from Rorden JW, Taft E: Discharge planning guide for nurses, Philadelphia, 1990, Saunders, p. 26.)*

through the referral process with a client can be an enriching and rewarding experience. Table 10-2 is a chart illustrating different types of referral. Completing a form or telling a client to contact a community agency is only one small aspect of this process.

Basic Principles of Referral

Wolff's (1962) classic article on referral delineated basic principles to take into consideration when helping clients to use the referral process. Others (Combs, 1976; USDHHS, 1982a; Wheeler-Lachowycz, 1983) have reinforced the value of these principles and have expanded on them. These principles are listed here.

There should be merit in the referral. The referral should meet the needs and objectives of the client and should be necessary and appropriate. Before referring the client to community resources it is important to assess what resources are available in the client's own environment. Often family, friends, and neighbors can do as much as formal community health resources. If a referral is not necessary or appropriate it should not be made.

The referral should be practical. The client should be able to use the referral in an efficient, effective manner. The referral should not be a waste of time, money, and effort on behalf of the client, the resource, or the referral facilitator.

The referral should be individualized to the client. A referral that meets the needs of one client may not meet the needs of another. It is essential to assess the individual needs and concerns of clients before decisions about the appropriateness of a referral are made. For example, some clients can learn very well in a group setting, whereas others cannot.

The referral should be timely. It should come at a time when the client is ready to work on the health care need and when it is the appropriate time to work on the need.

The referral should be coordinated with other activities. The referral should be congruent with other health care activities that are occurring. This aids in maximizing health care interventions, preventing duplication of service and carrying out contradictory intervention strategies.

table 10-2 Types of Referral by Initiator, Extent of Contact with Resource, Level of Difficulty, and Source

	Type of Referral	Example
Initiator	*Primary:* Referral initiated by client, often readily	Client suggesting marriage counseling
	Secondary: Referral initiated by someone other than client	Community health nurse suggesting marriage counseling
Extent of contact with resource	*Formal:* Contact made with a resource on behalf of a client; contact can be made by the client or someone on the client's behalf; contact generally made with client's permission; these referrals are often processed through a system of standardized forms and procedures	Client contacting a local department of social service (DSS) about obtaining food stamps or
	Informal: Discussion of a resource between two or more persons without contact being made with the resource; often the initial step toward a formal referral	Client and community health nurse discussing available DSS services (e.g., food stamps, general assistance, Temporary Assistance to Needy Families, Medicaid)
Level of difficulty	*Simple:* Referral reaches need resolution on the initial attempt	On initial attempt, client goes to DSS and obtains food stamps
	Complex: Referral does not meet need resolution on the initial attempt; process needs to be reworked (see Figure 10-6 for steps in process)	Client goes to DSS seeking food stamps and finds out that she or he is not eligible, but the need for assistance with food budgeting still exists. Other community resources such as the Nutritional Extension Service may be more appropriate
Source	*Interresource:* Referrals made from one resource to another	Community health nurse referring client from the local health department to a neighborhood health clinic
	Intraresource: Referrals made within the resource itself	Community health nurse referring client to local health department sanitarian for water sampling
	Self: Client refers himself to a resource for service; some agencies will not accept these referrals	Client calls local health department to arrange for community health nursing visits

The referral should incorporate the client and family into planning and implementation. It has already been stressed that it is critical for the client and family to be involved in health planning and intervention; without this involvement interventions are likely to fail.

The client should have the right to say no to the referral. This principle acknowledges the client's right to self-determination. A competent client has the right to make decisions about health care (ANA, 1986b). The client has the right to refuse a referral unless legal authority dictates otherwise. Cases of law are the exception and will vary from state to state. An example of a law that requires the community health nurse to refer a client without his or her consent is a child abuse law that mandates reporting suspected child abuse and neglect cases.

To protect this right of self-determination, the client must be aware of the referral. Referrals are sometimes made for clients without their consent, but this is not good referral practice. In following up on a referral the nurse may find that the client was unaware of the referral and does not want it. In such cases the nurse should explain the reason for the referral, the services the nurse can provide, and apologize for any inconvenience to the client. Such interventions may help the client to see why the referral was made and even to accept the referral.

At times individuals are referred without their knowledge or consent because the referring agency considers them a threat to their own safety or the safety of others. The client still has the right to refuse a referral unless legal authority dictates otherwise.

The refusal of a referral may be difficult for the nurse to accept, especially if the referral appears to be helpful to the client. However, the client's right to say no must be respected.

Confidentiality and Referral

Confidentiality of client information is an important professional ethical responsibility. As with self-determination, confidentiality is violated only if laws intervene and mandate that the health care professional must share information. Nurses must receive the client's permission to share personal data; information to be shared should be carefully evaluated. This action should always be in the client's best interest and for purposes of facilitating optimum care. Many agencies have release-of-information forms for sending and

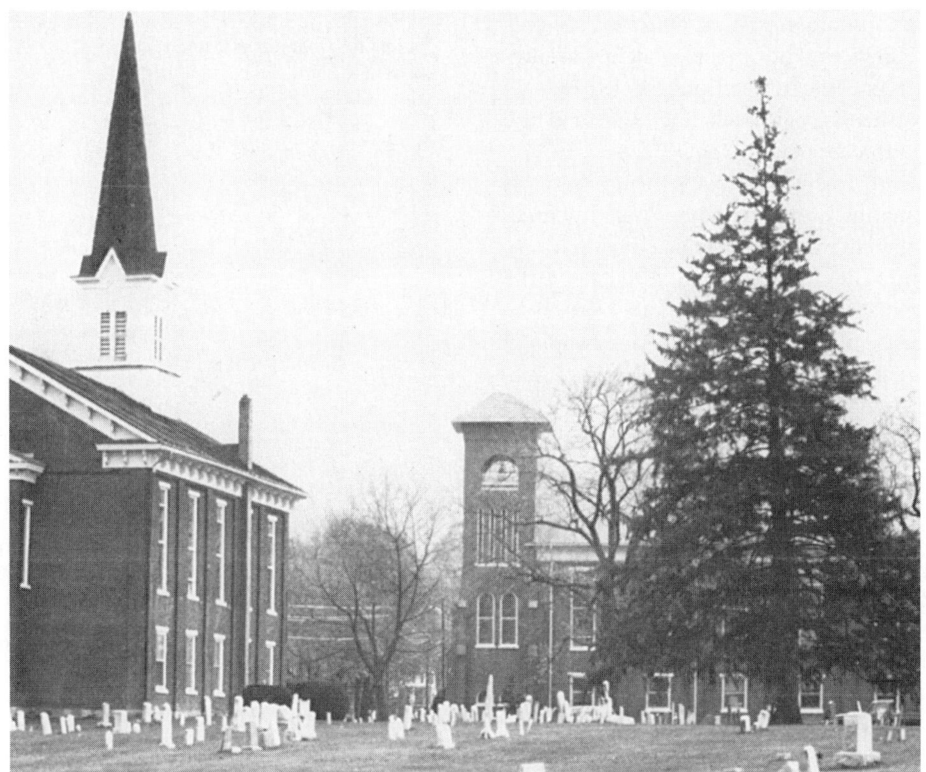

Figure 10-4 Churches are extremely valuable community resources that should not be overlooked by health care professionals. Many churches provide community services, including temporary food, shelter, and clothing; home visiting to ill and disabled persons; home repair services for the needy; and monies to assist families who lack essentials of daily living. Community health nurses frequently find that churches help to fill "gaps" in the resource delivery system and provide services that would not otherwise be available. *(Courtesy Henry Parks, photographer.)*

receiving data about clients. It is preferable to obtain written permission to share data.

Developing a Referral System

Before referral activities occur a referral system needs to be in place. Developing a referral system involves determining the types of resources necessary to carry out health care activities, locating these resources in the community, collecting information on the resources, developing a referral list, developing a referral protocol, developing a follow-up system, training people to make referrals, and periodically updating the referral and resource information (USDHHS, 1982a, p. 27). In developing a system, criteria for both sending and receiving referrals would be established.

Answering a Referral

Answering referrals is an important part of the referral process and helps to maintain effective and ongoing communication between the client, staff, and resources. If referrals are not answered or are answered incompletely or tardily, the referral source may become discouraged and not send further referrals. Interagency communication can be damaged. Prompt, complete, and courteous answering of a referral helps to establish and maintain good working relationships and facilitates follow-up and continuity of client care.

In the written response to the referring agency the nurse should include the following information: the original needs that initiated the referral, current assessment data, nursing diagnoses, and future actions and plans. If nursing service is to be continued, it is often helpful to let the referring agency know this fact. Be sure to thank the referring agency for the referral.

REFERRAL RESOURCES

Once the need for a referral has been established, the appropriate resources must be located in the community. The community health nurse needs to collect information on community resources and be familiar with them (Figure 10-4).

A resource is defined as an agency, group, or individual that assists a client to meet a need. Resources provide multiple services and have varying requirements for usage. The community health nurse needs to be knowledgeable about community resources, increase client awareness of resources, and assist the client in resource use. Health care resources can be described as formal and informal.

Formal health care resources exist primarily for the provision of health care services. They include, but are not limited to, hospitals, extended-care facilities, skilled nursing homes, health departments, outpatient facilities, and the offices of private health care practitioners.

Informal health care resources provide health services but do not exist primarily for this purpose. These resources can be relatives in the client's home, service organizations, and self-help groups. They are scattered throughout the community, are minimally coordinated, and are often more difficult to recognize than formal resources. An example of an informal health care resource is the local Lion's Club, which provides free ophthalmological examinations and eyeglasses to children who could not otherwise obtain them. The Lion's Club provides a health care service, but its primary function is not health-related. Many such resources within the community are important to the provision of community health services.

Local health departments are excellent sources of information on community health resources. Frequently, compilations of local resources are done by groups such as United Way Community Services, chambers of commerce, departments of social service, offices on aging, and health departments. Major service organizations, such as associations for retarded citizens, will compile resources specific to the groups they represent. City offices and planning commissions will also have local resource information. Developing a resource "network" can assist the nurse in finding resource information and facilitating client care. Ideally, the nurse should independently explore the resource before referring clients.

National Foundation March of Dimes
Payne County Office
Address: 20100 Maplewood, Mio, MI 47236
Phone: 811-2110 (Area 516)
Person in charge: Mrs. Nellie Scott, Director

Purpose and services:	Through referral and direct aid, assistance is provided in the areas of prenatal care, genetic counseling, diagnosis, and treatment. Offers prevention and treatment services for clients who have congenital malformations or birth defects through research, direct client services, and public education. Sponsors scholarships in related health fields.
Eligibility:	No restrictions.
Application procedure:	Referrals by private physicians, public health clinics, or health departments. Individuals are encouraged to contact the office for further information.
Fees:	None
Office hours:	9 AM to 3 PM, Tuesday-Saturday
Geographical area served:	Payne County Compiled 12/96
Client satisfaction:	Responds immediately to clients' calls. Especially good at obtaining adaptive equipment.

Figure 10-5 Resource information.

Collecting Information on Referral Resources

When collecting information on referral resources the nurse needs to develop a systematic way of recording resource information (USDHHS, 1982a, p. 28). Creating an ongoing file with a standard format, such as the one shown in Figure 10-5, can be helpful. Such a file should list resources both alphabetically and by service and should note if the resource has available publications and materials explaining its services. Resources that are frequently used, or used with success, may be color-coded or tabbed for easy accessibility. It is necessary that resource information be clear, accurate, and concise.

The following essential information about a resource is readily kept on file cards, in a loose-leaf notebook, or computerized: (1) name of resource (include address, phone number, name and title of person in charge or contact person); (2) purpose and services; (3) eligibility (who may use the resource, including special requirements such as age and income); (4) application procedure; (5) fees; (6) office hours and days; and (7) geographical area served. Resource files should be dated to aid in updating. Data about clients' response to use of the resource is valuable as well.

The nurse should also be aware of specific information that a resource requests of a client when it provides service. Information frequently requested by resources includes the following:

1. Name, address, and telephone number of the client
2. Client age, sex, and marital status
3. Names and birthdates of family members and others living in the household
4. Source of medical care and health history
5. Financial status and records
6. Resources with whom the client is presently working
7. Reason for seeking referral

A grid showing frequently used resources can be a helpful reference when one is visiting clients in the community setting. A grid that includes service areas and specific resources is especially helpful. An example of such a grid is presented in Table 10-3. It is not all inclusive, and resources will vary from area to area, but it does illustrate how a service resource grid can be organized.

STEPS OF THE REFERRAL PROCESS

The referral process is systematic and circular. That is, as data are obtained in one step, other steps may need to be re-table 10-3 RESOURCE GRID

SERVICE NEEDED	TYPES	RESOURCE
Food	1. Emergency	1. Department of Social Services, Salvation Army, local churches, American Red Cross, Goodfellows
	2. Low-cost or free foods	2. Food stamps, food coops, school lunch programs, WIC
	3. Counseling	3. Expanded nutrition program, Health Department
Financial assistance	1. Emergency and short-term	1. Department of Social Services, Salvation Army, Goodfellows, Lion's Club, Traveler's Aid, Volunteers of America, Kiwanis
	2. Long-term	2. Department of Social Service, Social Security Administration, Veterans Administration
Housing	1. Emergency	1. Catholic Social Services, Jewish Action League, United Way Community Service, Department of Social Service, American Red Cross, Salvation Army, local churches, domestic violence facilities
	2. Public (low-cost)	2. Housing Commission, Department of Social Service

Modified from the University of Michigan, School of Nursing, Family and Community Health Nursing: *Resource grid*, Ann Arbor, undated, University of Michigan, School of Nursing.

peated, and as the process stops for one referral, another referral may be initiated. These steps are interconnected and interrelated. The steps involved in the referral process are depicted in Figure 10-6.

The following are the basic steps of the referral process:

1. Establish a working relationship with the client
2. Establish the need for a referral
3. Set objectives for the referral
4. Explore resource availability
5. Client decides to use or not use referral
6. Make referral to resource
7. Facilitate referral
8. Evaluate and follow up

Client participation throughout the process is essential. The community health nurse guides the client through the process by facilitating informed decision making, assessing client needs and objectives, exploring alternatives for need resolution, assisting the client in using resources, and evaluating the results of the entire process. The client is encouraged to be independent whenever possible.

Establish a Working Relationship with the Client

The referral process usually evolves after a working relationship with the client has been established. This involves the formation of trust between the nurse and the client; encouraged by nurses when they show respect, empathy, and genuine concern for the client (Rorden, Taft, 1990, p. 46). As a means of building this relationship the nurse focuses on clients' feelings and perceptions of their situations and starts "where clients are at." The nurse needs to be willing to look at the situation from the client's frame of reference and take into consideration cultural variations regarding health practices, resource use, and perceptions of events.

Trust may develop almost immediately, but more often it evolves over a period of time. While establishing the trust relationship the nurse is able to assess the situation and gather the data necessary for helping the client to make health decisions. A relationship of trust facilitates communication and cooperation in the nurse-client relationship.

In many cases the referral process will commence as this relationship develops to its potential. If referrals are necessitated early in the relationship, the nurse proceeds with caution to be sure that sufficient data have been collected to determine if the referral is appropriate.

Establish the Need for a Referral

The community health nurse and client ought to thoroughly assess the need for referral. Unnecessary or unwanted referrals are costly and time consuming, frustrating for clients, may strain relationships between referring agencies, and can adversely affect nurse-client relationships.

It is important to discriminate between problems the community health nurse can and cannot handle. For example, some budgeting problems can be dealt with by a community health nurse and others cannot. A community health nurse can help a family analyze how they can obtain the most for their food dollars by using meal planning, low-cost meals, and inexpensive sources of protein. On the other hand, if the family is having difficulty with creditors and money management, a credit-counseling resource would be more appropriate.

There may be situations in which the nurse finds it difficult to accept clients' decisions about the need for a referral. People have values, attitudes, and beliefs that may differ from those of the nurse and thus affect resource use. For example, clients may use folk remedies instead of seeking formal health care, may not understand or value the need for preventive health practices such as immunizations for children, and may be unwilling to accept assistance programs. Asking clients questions about the type of services needed, results they hope to achieve from service use, what

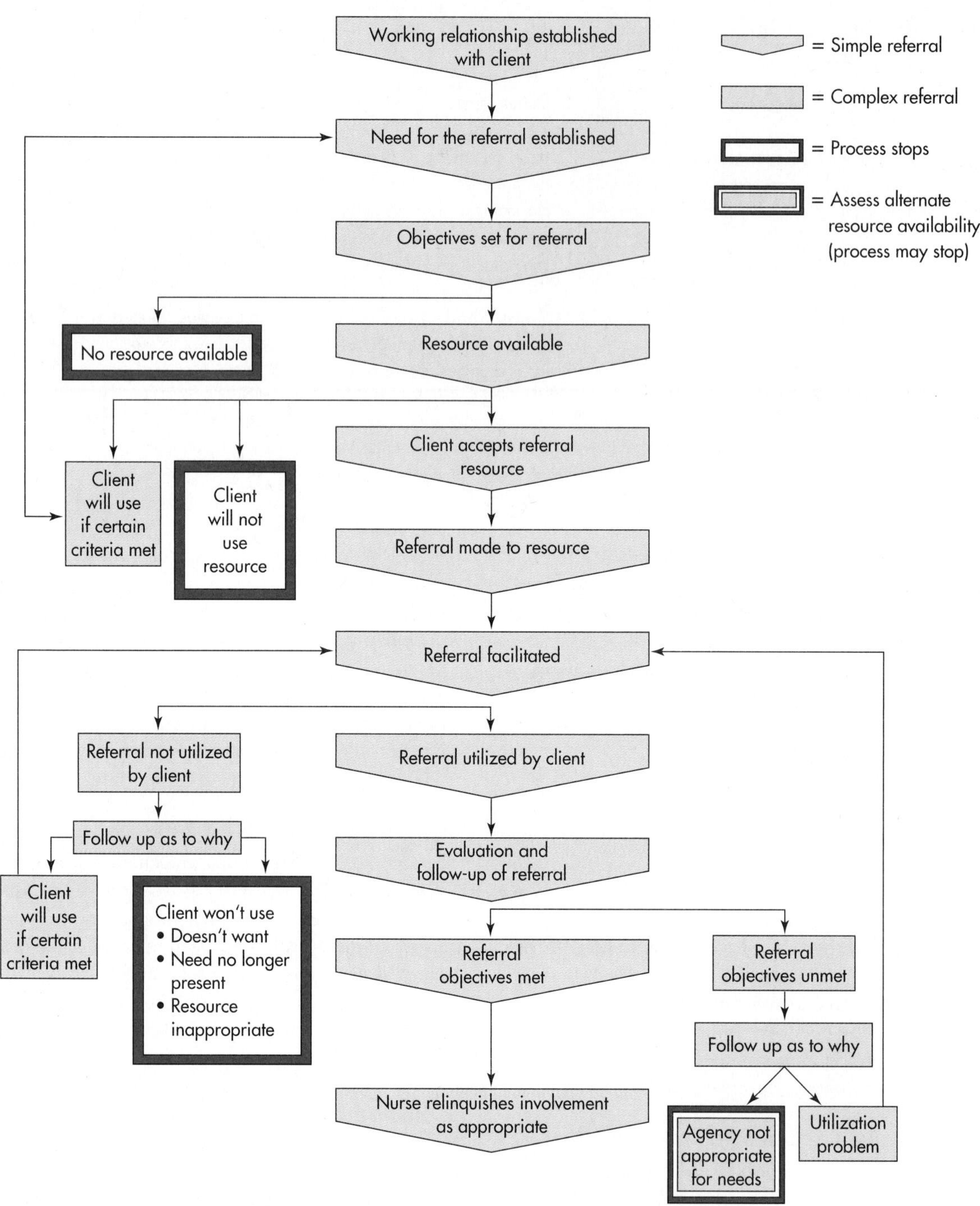

Figure 10-6 The referral process.

they think caused their health problem(s), what they have been doing for their health problems, and what they have been doing to promote health can elicit valuable cultural data. These data assist the nurse in seeing why clients may or may not accept a referral.

When clients are using denial as a coping mechanism it can be difficult to have them realistically assess existing health care needs and the need for a referral. Denial of concerns such as disease conditions, marital crises, and budgeting and childrearing problems can affect the client's perceived health care needs. The nurse can help the client to realistically assess the situation, share professional observations and concerns, and discuss appropriate community resources with the client. Such discussions can help the client to view the situation from a different perspective and motivate the client to take action. This is particularly true when a trust relationship has been established between the client and the nurse and the client realizes that the nurse is acting in his or her best interests. Once the need for a referral has been established, the nurse and client should establish objectives for the services required and look at which resources in the community can best meet the client's needs.

Set Objectives for the Referral

What the client would like to see accomplished, tempered with what is realistically feasible, combine to determine the objectives for the referral. The nurse can help the client to be realistic in resource expectations, but the decision about specific objectives to be achieved should be made by the client. It is often helpful to write out objectives with the client in behavioral terms, such as "Mrs. Armstrong will contact the Department of Social Services about obtaining food stamps by March 30." An integral part of setting objectives for the referral is deciding what services are necessary from the referral source, as well as what time frame to use in obtaining these services.

In this phase of the referral process the nurse may find that the client has unrealistic expectations for the referral. For example, Mrs. Quinn, a single mother, requested counseling for her 16-year-old daughter, who planned to drop out of school and marry her 21-year-old boyfriend. Mrs. Quinn thought a counseling agency could "talk some sense into her." The community health nurse helped Mrs. Quinn to see that a counseling agency would assist the family in working through situations but would most likely not get involved in making family decisions. The nurse helped to arrange joint counseling sessions through the local Family and Neighborhood Counseling Center. These sessions helped both mother and daughter to communicate more effectively and understand each other's concerns and needs. They also helped the family to develop skills in problem solving and decision making.

Explore Resource Availability

A source of aid must be available before a referral can be made. An appropriate resource is one that can meet the client's needs and objectives and is available, acceptable, and accessible to the client. If more than one appropriate resource exists, the client makes the choice about which one to use. If no resource is available, the referral objectives may need to be redefined or a resource developed. Many times resources in the community will reconsider the services they provide to clients, especially if the community health nurse acts as an advocate for certain services.

Client Decides to Use or Not Use Referral

The client can say *yes*, *no*, or *maybe* when deciding to use a referral resource. If the client says *yes*, the referral process continues. If the client says *no* or *maybe*, the nurse should explore with the client the reasons why. If the client does not want the referral under any condition, the right to self-determination must be respected unless legal issues intervene.

In some instances, when clients would use a referral if certain criteria were met, the nurse may be able to assist the client in meeting these criteria. For example, a client might say that she would use a referral to the health department immunization clinic for her 2-year-old if transportation to the clinic could be arranged. The nurse may be able to help this client obtain transportation services from other community resources. However, if a client continues to place conditions on referral use the nurse and client may want to take a close look at the reasons behind these conditions. It is possible that the client really does not want the referral but fears saying *no*.

Sometimes clients do not want to use one resource to meet a health care need but are willing to use another resource. An example of this is Mrs. Morris.

CASE *Scenario*

Mrs. Morris was an elderly client who was eligible for food stamps but would not apply for them. She viewed food stamps as charity and stated, "I do not accept welfare." The community health nurse was frustrated because Mrs. Morris's diet was inadequate, largely for financial reasons. Discussing the food stamp program with Mrs. Morris did not change her mind about using it. The nurse explored alternatives with Mrs. Morris and found that, because she wanted to eat better, she was receptive to learning about how to prepare low-cost, nutritious meals at home and was also interested in applying for a reduced-cost, Meals-on-Wheels program—where she would "pay" for her meals. Mrs. Morris had refused a referral for food stamps, but she and the nurse were able to use other intervention alternatives that helped to meet her nutritional needs.

Make Referral to Resource

The referral should be specific, yet informative enough to reflect the client's objectives for the referral. As the demand for community-based care has increased agencies are developing referral protocols to make the transition from the acute care setting to the community as smooth as possible (Glover, King, Green, Shults, 1993, p. 40). The appropriate forms should be filled out and protocols followed (including a release of information form). Clients usually do not hesitate to sign an authorization for information to be released once they have decided that they need a referral. The client should be encouraged to be as independent as possible in contacting the resource and to make an appointment with the agency if one is necessary.

Timing influences how the client responds to the referral. Studies have shown that a referral should occur as soon as possible after detecting a need; a rapid, well-handled referral often reinforces the importance of taking positive health action to the client (USDHHS, 1982a, p. 27).

Many referrals can be made by telephone and such referrals may be faster and more informative—a written referral

Oakland County Department of Health

1200 North Telegraph Road
Pontiac, Michigan 48053
Telephone 858-1280

27725 Greenfield
Southfield, Michigan 48075
Telephone 424-7000

Referral Form

To: ______________________ From: ______________________

Address: ______________________ ☐ Pontiac Office

______________________ ☐ Southfield Office

Attention: ______________________ Telephone: ____________ Date: ____________

Regarding: ______________________ Aware of referral? ☐ Yes ☐ No

Address: ______________________ Telephone: ____________

Family Roster (Names, birthdates, relationship)

Reason for Referral

Situation

(over)

Known Medical, Agency, Community Resources

Reply Requested: ☐ No ☐ Yes (see back)

Figure 10-7 Sample referral form. *(Courtesy Nursing Division, Oakland County Health Department, Pontiac, Mich.)*

can always follow. If the referral is written it will include information such as client and family awareness of the diagnosis and prognosis; complete and detailed orders for medications and treatments; people living with the client; the client's religion, spoken language, and diet; address and phone number; titles such as Doctor, Mrs., Mr.; goals for and estimated length of service; nursing diagnoses; and method of health care financing (Wheeler-Lachowycz, 1983).

An example of a referral form used by one local health department to refer clients to another resource is presented in Figure 10-7. This form includes essential referral information, such as data about the person making the referral, the individual or family being referred, the reason for the referral, summary of the client's situation, resources being used by the client, a statement on whether or not the client is aware of the referral, and a place for the receiving resource to share information with the referral agency to facilitate follow-up and evaluation.

Often resources request that clients bring specific information with them to their first appointment. If clients are

Continuation of situation:

Agency reply to Oakland County Health Department:

(Signature)

Date:

Figure 10-7, cont'd

not aware of this requirement they may have to return to the resource with the information or be denied service. Returning to a resource takes additional time, effort, and money and may present a barrier to the client using the referral.

Facilitate the Referral

Facilitating a referral involves a number of nursing interventions, including preparing the client for the use of community services and identifying and overcoming barriers to the use of these services. It is important to remember that client motivation is critical; if the client is not motivated to make the referral work, the referral process probably will not be successful. Barriers that decrease client motivation are discussed later in this chapter.

Evaluate and Follow Up

As with all aspects of the nursing process, referrals need to be evaluated. Ongoing evaluation and follow-up are probably of most importance in the referral process. Throughout the process the community health nurse evaluates the client's responses to the referral to determine if changes need to be made.

Some clients need support and encouragement during the process, especially if their problems are not resolved immediately. The case of Mr. Connant is an example.

CASE *Scenario*

Mr. Connant decided that he was not going back to the community mental health center for counseling after his first visit because his counselor "did nothing but talk." In evaluating this situation, the nurse realized that she needed to discuss more specifically with Mr. Connant his expectations of counseling. She talked to him about his feelings about the session, encouraged him to share his feelings with the counselor, and encouraged him to go back "at least one more time." This interaction with the nurse facilitated Mr. Connant's return to the mental health center, and at a later visit he expressed his gratitude to the nurse because counseling was helping him to work through many issues that had been troubling him.

The nurse may notice that a client is evidencing the same problem repeatedly, for example, experiencing the need for frequent emergency food orders. The nurse and client would want to discuss the situation and assess what is happening (e.g., too limited an income, problem with budgeting), use anticipatory guidance, and explore other options.

During evaluation the client's ability to use the process should be assessed and the client should be encouraged to use the process as independently as possible in the future. Probably the hardest part of evaluation is realizing when it is time for the nurse to relinquish involvement with the client (e.g., the client can use the process independently, expected outcomes have been achieved). This can be an especially difficult task when the client and nurse have developed a strong working relationship.

Effective evaluation of the referral process encompasses reviewing how well client needs are being met. Evaluation looks at referral outcomes and enhances the nurse's competency in using the process. When evaluating, the nurse must realize that there are times when a referral was not appropriate or effective.

A goal of the nurse in using the referral process is to assist the client to use the process independently. Usually clients are ready to function independently when they can identify personal health care needs, take initiative to contact health care resources, and take action to resolve health care problems.

BARRIERS TO USE OF THE REFERRAL PROCESS

For each resource and each client, the nurse must identify the barriers that adversely affect the use of referral services. Barriers involve individual and resource components. For example, an agency may have high fees for services (a resource barrier) that the client is unable to afford (a client barrier). In this case fees are both a resource barrier and a client barrier. Some common resource and client barriers are briefly described.

Resource Barriers

ATTITUDES OF HEALTH CARE PROFESSIONALS The attitudes of health care professionals affect client use of resources. Clients are quick to sense the attitudes of health care personnel, and if they are not treated with respect and courtesy they are hesitant to return. Abrupt answers to a client's questions, minimal communication with the client, use of confusing health care jargon, and conveying frustration when clients ask questions are a few examples of behaviors that impede use of resources. Although the values and attitudes of the nurse may differ from the client's, the nurse must be open to the opinions of others and maintain a nonjudgmental attitude. A good rule of thumb is for the nurse to treat clients the way he or she would like to be treated.

An attitude that became a barrier to the use of a health care resource is shown in the following example.

CASE *Scenario*

The nurse in charge of an antepartal clinic for low-income mothers refused to make appointments for clinic clients because "these people wouldn't keep appointments anyway." As a result, the clinic operated on a first-come-first-served basis. Clients frequently traveled by bus to get to the clinic. Since no appointments were available they had to arrive very early to sign in and there were usually long waits to be seen. It was common for clients to leave the clinic before they were seen because of transportation or child-care problems. Many clients became discouraged with the system and did not seek further prenatal care.

Attitudes and practices such as these do not facilitate clients' use of health care services or promote preventive health action.

PHYSICAL ACCESSIBILITY OF RESOURCE Clients are less likely to use resources that are not readily accessible. Once a resource is beyond walking distance, other means of transportation must be found. Public transportation is scarce in this country, and even if a family has a car it may not be available at the time of the appointment, or the family may not have money for gas. The problem is greatly magnified if the resource is at such a distance that the client must make arrangements for overnight stays in order to use its services. Overnight stays often necessitate making arrangements for the care of small children or other members of the family, and they can be very costly to the client.

COST OF RESOURCE SERVICES How much a client can or is willing to pay for a health service is an individual matter. Even the smallest cost may be more than clients can pay if their income is at or below the poverty level. If the service is not absolutely necessary or critical to the client's activities of daily living, the cost may be viewed as prohibitive. On the other hand, if the client places a high priority on receiving a given service, he or she may make concessions in order to pay the fees—such as not paying other bills, not buying needed medications, and not eating well.

Client Barriers

PRIORITIES If the need is not of high priority for the client, he or she may not become actively involved in using the referral services. If other needs are considered to be of higher priority, the nurse should assist the client in meeting these needs first. It may be more important for the family to care for an ill family member than to take a child to the well-baby clinic for immunizations; or if the family is having difficulty meeting its basic needs of food, clothing, and shelter, preventive health care services may not be viewed as a priority.

MOTIVATION If the client is not highly motivated to work on a need, it is not likely that much will be done by the client toward meeting that need. An integral part of client motivation is the concept of *awareness versus readiness*. The fact that the client is aware of a need does not mean that he or she is ready to act on the need. If a differentiation is not made between awareness and readiness, the nurse may feel responsible for the failure of the client to follow through on a referral. Once it is established that the client is not ready to act on a need, the nurse needs to assist the client in prioritizing the needs on which he or she is ready to act. A good example of awareness versus readiness is a client who acknowledges that the house needs to be cleaned but after numerous nursing visits, much discussion, and ample time, still has not cleaned the house. The client is aware of the need but is not ready to act on it.

PREVIOUS EXPERIENCE WITH RESOURCES If a client has not had a positive experience in using a resource in the past, she or he may be hesitant to use this resource again or to use other community resources. *Complaints about resources can be entirely justified*. However, part of a negative experience can be related to the client in terms of perceptions, readiness to make changes, and follow-through. Clients may also have a negative view of the resource because their problems were not resolved. Whatever the reason, it is important to acknowledge the client's feelings and explore ways to make further contacts with community services more meaningful.

LACK OF KNOWLEDGE ABOUT AVAILABLE RESOURCES Clients need to know about resources before they will use them. Lack of knowledge about resources is a major barrier to the use of health care services. A key role of the community health nurse is to educate clients about health care services in the community.

LACK OF UNDERSTANDING REGARDING NEED FOR REFERRAL Clients who do not understand the need for a referral frequently do not take action to obtain referral services. This is often true of families who neglect to have their children immunized. Many people know that children need "baby shots" but do not understand why. Clients will be more likely to follow through in obtaining immunizations on a consistent basis if they know the purpose for receiving immunizations and the consequences of not obtaining adequate protection against communicable diseases.

CLIENT SELF-IMAGE If clients have a negative self-image, they may be hesitant to seek care and may view themselves as unworthy of such care. The nurse should acknowledge these feelings and develop intervention strategies that will help clients to increase self-esteem.

CULTURAL FACTORS Cultural differences can be a barrier to effective use of the referral process. Language is one of the most obvious cultural barriers. In our health care system, clients who do not speak English can have a difficult time using resources and obtaining appropriate health care.

Every culture has beliefs regarding health care practices. Cultural beliefs about the cause of illness, nutrition, preventive health care, and death and dying vary greatly. The norms and values of a culture also affect health care practices. For example, in traditional Arab culture women are generally not allowed to leave their homes or immediate neighborhoods without a male escort, and health care services are better used if they are located in a neighborhood facility.

In some cultural groups where preventive health services are not routinely sought the nurse may have a difficult time gaining compliance on referrals for immunizations and routine physical examinations. Ethnic and cultural values and attitudes pervade a person's life, and it is important that the nurse identify them in relation to health care practices (Rorden, Taft, 1990, p. 97). However, an effective nurse does *not* use racial, cultural, or ethnic stereotypes in anticipating client preferences and providing client care (Rorden, Taft, p. 98).

FINANCES Health care in the United States is expensive. Many clients do not use health care services because they cannot afford them. Chapter 4 discussed methods of health care financing in the United States and the cost of health care. The near-poor client, who does not qualify for welfare assistance but may be medically indigent, frequently has difficulty paying for health care. The same is true for families who are uninsured or underinsured. It is a challenge for the nurse to find resources that will assist such clients. Church groups, private foundations, and voluntary organizations are a few examples of resources that frequently assist these families.

ACCESSIBILITY Access, as a barrier to service, has become a national health care concern and is a major barrier to the use of health care services (Institute of Medicine, 1993; USDHHS, 1991). In many communities necessary health care services are not readily available. This is becoming increasingly evident in rural communities where hospitals and other acute care facilities are closing or cutting back on services at an alarming rate (see Chapter 3). Service access is especially difficult for disadvantaged populations, the disabled, and the elderly (see Chapters 12, 19, and 20).

Lack of access to services because of limited or no transportation is a major barrier to the use of health care services. It has been well documented that clients frequently do not seek health care because they have problems with transportation to health care facilities. If low-cost public transportation is not available, car pooling, the use of volunteer transportation services, or establishing outreach clinic services in the neighborhood may help to reduce transportation barriers. Frequently local churches and departments of human or social services have programs to assist people with transportation needs. Local offices on aging and senior centers frequently have transportation services available for the elderly.

Although lack of resources can limit service utilization, it is crucial for professionals to examine other concerns when considering the concept of access. "Having insurance or nearby health care providers is no guarantee that people who need services will receive them" (Institute of Medicine, 1993, p. 4). Access is a complex concept that involves structural, personal, and economic issues. Families or aggregates having difficulty accessing services often have a complex set of problems that "require organizational solutions that include continuity of care, integration of services, and other subtle characteristics" (Institute of Medicine, p. 18). For example, people who are homeless or victims of domestic violence require an interlinked array of personal, social, and public health services that address psychosocial and economic concerns. Chapter 12 discusses these concerns and interventions needed to facilitate need resolution.

LEVELS OF NURSING INTERVENTION WITH REFERRAL

Clients have varying levels of ability to assume independent functioning when using health care resources, which necessitates different levels of professional intervention by the community health nurse. Identifying the level at which the client is functioning helps community health nurses to focus intervention strategies when they use the referral process. Levels of nursing intervention are presented here.

Level I: At this level the client is largely dependent on the nurse and will need assistance with all aspects of the referral process. Frequently these clients have not had life experiences that have prepared them to deal adequately with systems external to their family unit, or their energies are depleted by crisis. These clients need considerable support and encouragement and, often, concrete help from the community health nurse before they can follow through on a needed referral.

Frequently they assume a passive role. They may sincerely want assistance from others but fail to take action because they lack the energy or knowledge to do so and basically feel inadequate to handle the referral by themselves. Community health nursing intervention with these clients involves health teaching and counseling so that they can identify health needs that necessitate referral. In addition, supportive assistance is necessary while they are learning how to use health care resources.

A major goal at this level is to help clients become more actively involved in taking responsibility for meeting their own health needs. Sometimes it is easier to do for the client than to work with him or her, especially if the client follows through when the nurse makes all the necessary arrangements and decisions. It is important for the community health nurse to work toward helping clients use health resources independently.

Level II: At this level mutual participation is evident. The client does not wait for the community health nurse to initiate discussion about health care needs. Rather, the client actively seeks information to determine what health actions are needed to resolve current health problems or to enhance wellness in the future. Clients at this level may need health teaching to understand the value of preventive health practices, to locate community resources that they can afford, or to learn about community services such as low-cost or free transportation that will help them to use needed resources. They are more likely, however, to raise challenging questions and to identify when health care resources are inappropriate to meet their needs. At times it may be difficult to recognize when these clients need assistance because they are functioning so well in most aspects of their lives.

Level III: At this level the client can use the referral process independently. The nurse may be used as a resource person but otherwise assumes a passive participant role. Reaching this level is a goal for the community health nurse.

SUMMARY

Clients are moving increasingly "quicker and sicker" from one care setting and level of care to another. Community health nurses help to provide client-focused, interdisciplinary, continuous, comprehensive care through care management and the referral processes. Several key concepts are inherent in these processes: (1) clients have the basic responsibility for maintaining their health; (2) clients have the right to accept or refuse health care services; (3) planned intervention by professionals can promote use of resources by clients; (4) interdisciplinary collaboration and coordination are essential to ensure continuity of care; and (5) clients can learn to use health care services independently. Effective use of care management and the referral process helps many clients to resolve their current health needs and provides anticipatory guidance about how to handle future health needs. The historical role of the nurse in discharge planning and care management is expanding. There are limitless opportunities for the community health nurse to facilitate continuity of care through care management and the referral process.

CRITICAL *Thinking Exercise*

You are a health department nurse who has been assigned to work with a local hospital's discharge planning team. You are trying to familiarize yourself with community resources and the nursing role in the discharge planning process. How would you begin to gather data about community resources? What types of information would you want to obtain about your role with the discharge planning team? What type of criteria would you use to identify clients in need of continuing care upon hospital discharge?

REFERENCES

American Hospital Association (AHA): *Guidelines: discharge planning*, Chicago, 1984, AHA.

American Nurses Association (ANA): *Standards of home health nursing practice*, Kansas City, Mo., 1986a, ANA.

American Nurses Association (ANA): *Standards of community health nursing practice*, Kansas City, Mo., 1986b, ANA.

Blaylock A, Cason CL: Discharge planning predicting patients' needs, *J Gerontol Nurs* 18(7):5-10, 1992.

Browdie R: Ethical issues in case management from a political and systems perspective, *J Case Manage* 1(3):87-89, 1992.

Burlenski M: President's message, *Access* 7(1):2, 4, 1989.

Combs PA: A study of the effectiveness of nursing referrals, *Public Health Rep* 91:122-126, 1976.

Corbett CF, Androwich IM: Critical paths: implications for improving practice, *Home Healthc Nurse* 12(6):27-34, 1995.

Corkery E: Discharge planning and home health care: what every staff nurse should know, *Orthop Nurs* 8(6):18-27, 1989.

Garland M: Discharge follow-up by telephone, *Rehabil Nurs* 17(6):339-341, 1992.

Gartner MB, Twardon CA: Care guidelines: journey through the managed care maze, *J WOCN* 22(3):118-121, 1995.

Girard N: The case management model of patient care delivery, *AORN J* 60(3):403-415, 1994.

Glover D, King M, Green C, Shults A: The patient care team advantage, *Caring* 12(10):40-42, 1993.

Hicks LL, Stallmeyer JM, Coleman JR: *Role of the nurse in managed care*, Washington, D.C., 1993, American Nurses Publishing.

Institute of Medicine: *Access to health care in America*, Washington, D.C., 1993, National Academy Press.

Kane RA: Case management in long-term care: it can be ethical and efficacious, *J Case Manage* 1(3):76-81, 1992.

Luker KA, Chalmers KI: The referral process in health visiting, *Int J Nurs Stud* 26(2):173-185, 1989.

Maiman LA, Hildreth NG, Cox C, Greenland P: Improving referral compliance after public cholesterol screening, *Am J Public Health* 82(6):804-809, 1992.

Mamon J, Steinwachs DM, Fahey M et al: Impact of hospital discharge planning on meeting patient needs after returning home, *Health Services Res* 27(2):155-175, 1994.

Masso AR: Managed care and alternative-site health care delivery, *J Care Manage* 1(1):45-51, 1995.

Mbweza E: Bridging the gap between hospital and home for premature infants in Malawi, *Int Nurs Rev* 43(2):53-57, 1996.

McBroom A: Uniform needs assessment instrument nearing completion, *Access* 7(1):1, 3-4, 1989.

McCloskey JC, Grace HK: *Current issues in nursing*, St. Louis, 1990, Mosby.

Murtagh CM: Discharge planning in nursing homes, *Health Services Res* 28(6):751-769, 1994.

Nash A: Reasons for referral to a pallative nursing team, *J Adv Nurs* 18:707-713, 1993.

North M, Neeusen M, Hollinsworth P: Discharge planning: increasing client and nurse satisfaction, *Rehabil Nurs* 16(6):327-329, 1991.

Oakland County Health Department, Nursing Division: Referral form, Pontiac, Mi., undated, Oakland County Health Department.

O'Hare P, Terry M: *Discharge planning: strategies for assuring continuity of care*, Rockville, Md., 1988, Aspen.

Rorden JW, Taft E: *Discharge planning guide for nurses*, Philadelphia, 1990, Saunders.

Shamansky SL, Boase JC, Horn BM: Discharge planning yesterday, today and tomorrow, *Home Healthc Nurse* 2(13):14-21, 1984.

Siegel H: Nurses improve hospital efficiency through a risk assessment model at admission, *Nurs Manage* 19(10):38-40, 42, 44-45, 1988.

Spath PL: Critical paths: maximizing patient care coordination. *Today's OR Nurse* 17(2):13-20, 34-35, 1995.

Stone M: Discharge planning guide, *Am J Nurs* 79:1445-1447, 1979.

Townsend EI, Edwards NC, Nadon C: The hospital liaison process: identifying risk factors in postnatal multiparas, *Can J Public Health* 83(3):203-207, 1992.

United States Department of Health and Human Services (USDHHS): *Source book for health education materials and community resources*, Washington, D.C., 1982a, U.S. Government Printing Office.

United States Department of Health and Human Services (USDHHS): *Report of the Surgeon General's Workshop on children with handicaps and their families*, DHHS Publication No. PHS 83-50194, Washington, D.C., 1982b, U.S. Government Printing Office.

United States Department of Health and Human Services (USDHHS): *Healthy people 2000: promoting health and preventing diseases. Objectives for the nation, full report, with commentary*, Washington, D.C., 1991, USDHHS.

University of Michigan, School of Nursing, Family and Community Health Nursing: *Resource grid*, Ann Arbor, undated, University of Michigan, School of Nursing.

Wensley E: *Nursing service without walls*, New York, 1963, National League for Nursing.

Wheeler-Lachowycz J: How to use your VNA, *Am J Nurs* 83:1164-1167, 1983.

Willihnganz G: The next step: pre-admission planning for discharge needs, *Coordinator* 3:20-21, 1984.

Wolff I: Referral—a process and a skill, *Nurs Outlook* 10:253-256, 1962.

SELECTED BIBLIOGRAPHY

Boyce R: The referral process as an integrated information system and quality assurance tool, *Aust Clin Rev* 10:22-26, 1990.

Bristow O, Stickney C, Thompson S: *Discharge planning for continuity of care*, New York, 1976, National League for Nursing.

Bryant MR: Cabinet on research. Critical pathways: what they are and what they are not . . . optimal care paths, *Tar Heel Nurse* 57(5):18-19, 1995.

Coleman JR: HMOs and individual case management, *Case Manager* 1(3):55-61, 1990.

Coleman JR, Hagen E: Collaborative practice: case managers and home care agency nurses, *Case Manager* 2(4):64-72, 1991.

Courts NF: Steps to a patient satisfaction survey, *Nurs Manage* 26(9):6400-6401, 1995.

Hale C: Case management and managed care, *Nurs Standard* 9(19):33-35, 1995.

Hartigan EG, Brown J: *Discharge planning for continuity of care*, New York, 1985, National League for Nursing.

Janken JK: Cabinet on research. Critical pathways: what they are and what they are not . . . what critical pathways are not, *Tar Heel Nurse* 57(6):36-37, 1995.

Knollmeuller RN: Case management: what's in a name? *Nurs Manage* 20(10):38-42, 1989.

Kromminga DK, Ostwald SK: The public health nurse as a discharge planner: patient's perceptions of the process, *Public Health Nurs* 4:224-229, 1987.

Mackey JF: Lack of referral networks: a parent's perspective, *Birth Defects* 26(2):105-108, 1990.

Managed care and nursing: a view from the front lines, *Mass Nurse* 65(9):4, 10-11, 1995.

McKeehan KM: *Continuing care: a multidisciplinary approach for discharge planning*, St. Louis, 1981, Mosby.

Meisenhelder JB: Networking and nursing, *Image: J Nurs Sch* 14:77-80, 1982.

Newman B: Enhancing patient care: case management and critical pathways, *Aust J Adv Nurs* 13(1):16-24, 1995.

Packard-Helie MT, Lancaster DB: A vital link in continuity of care, *Nurs Manage* 20(8):32-34, 1989.

Petryshen RP, Petryshen PM: The case management model: an innovative approach to the delivery of patient care, *J Adv Nurs* 17:1188-1194, 1992.

Schull DE, Tosch P, Wood M: Clinical nurse specialists as collaborative case managers, *Nurs Manage* 23(3):30-33, 1992.

Shindul-Rothschild J: The economics of managed care, *Mass Nurse* 65(9):4, 6, 1995.

Weilitz PB, Potter PA: A managed care system: financial and clinical evaluation, *J Nurs Admin* 23(5):1-7, 1993.

PART TWO

Planning Health Services for Aggregates at Risk

The uniqueness of community health nursing practice lies in the nurse's ability to assess the health needs of a community, to identify aggregates at risk, and to plan, implement, and evaluate interventions that promote community wellness. A variety of approaches can be used to analyze the health of a community. Because community health nurses work with individuals, families, and populations across the life span, a developmental, age-correlated approach to determining aggregates at risk can be extremely useful. The increasing number of clients across the life span who have long-term care needs is a growing concern of all health care professionals.

Community health nurses use knowledge from nursing, social, and public health sciences to fulfill their responsibility to the population as a whole. Part Two explores how knowledge from these fields of practice is synthesized by nurses in the community when they plan health programs. Emphasis is on analyzing how nurses use epidemiology, community diagnoses, health planning, management, quality improvement, and nursing principles to deliver high-quality services in various community settings. Achieving the *Healthy People 2000* objectives is a major focus in Part Two.

As we approach the year 2000, the impact of *health care reform* is in the forefront of the public mind and is bringing with it many opportunities and challenges for community health nursing. To deal with these challenges nurses must become politically active and advocate for all people in need. They must also understand the urgency of keeping pace with changes in the evolving health care system.

11

Concepts of Epidemiology: Infectious and Chronic Conditions

Objectives

Upon completion of this chapter, the reader should be able to:

1. Define the term *epidemiology* and discuss how its scope has expanded over time.
2. Understand how host, agent, and environmental factors influence the natural life history of a disease.
3. Describe how preventive intervention can alter the natural life history of a disease.
4. Characterize the distribution of health and disease by person, place, and time.
5. Discuss the dynamics of infectious disease transmission.
6. Illustrate the use of epidemiologic measures and methods in the investigation of infectious disease outbreaks and chronic disease occurrence.
7. Understand how public health surveillance influences the control of disease.
8. Summarize barriers to the epidemiological control of infectious and noninfectious disease.
9. Discuss the use of epidemiological concepts in community health nursing practice.

> A hound it was, an enormous coal black hound, but not such a hound as mortal eyes have ever seen. Fire burst from its open mouth, its eyes glowed with a smoldering glare, its muzzle and hackles and dewlap were outlined in flickering flames.
>
> SIR ARTHUR CONAN DOYLE

The quote above is a description of the Hound of the Baskervilles, the object of Sir Arthur Conan Doyle's story based on an actual Devonshire legend and considered the greatest of all Holmesian tales. Sherlock Holmes used his brilliant powers of deduction and keen insight to find out why the demonic howl of this hound had brought fear to the Baskerville family. He was able, with his unique problem-solving abilities, to deduce that the howling of the hound was calculated to cause the death of the rightful heirs of the Baskerville fortune. The inheritance would thus fall into the hand of the bastard son of the villainous Hugo Baskerville.

Professionals in community health function very much like the great detective Sherlock Holmes to promote and protect the health of the community. They use an investigative problem-solving process to study the determinants of health and disease frequencies in populations and to plan and implement health promotion and disease control programs. These persons use knowledge, concepts, and methods of epidemiology to relate causative events (howl of the hound) to given occurrences (death) in order to identify at-risk aggregates (Baskerville heirs).

EPIDEMIOLOGY DEFINED

The word *epidemiology* derives from the Greek word *epidemic*. Literally translated, this means *epi*, "upon," *demos*, "people" (collectively). Historically the major focus of the epidemiologist was on analyzing major disease outbreaks (epidemics) so that ways to control and prevent disease occurrence in populations (people, collectively) could be determined. Today the definition of epidemiology has been expanded to include the study of variables that affect health, as well as those that influence disease and condition occurrence.

There are many variations in the definition of the term *epidemiology*, but most focus on studying determinants of health and disease states among populations. Throughout this chapter the following definition, adapted from MacMahon and Pugh's (1970, p. 1) classic writings, is used:

> Epidemiology is the systematic, scientific study of the distribution patterns and determinants of health, disease, and condition

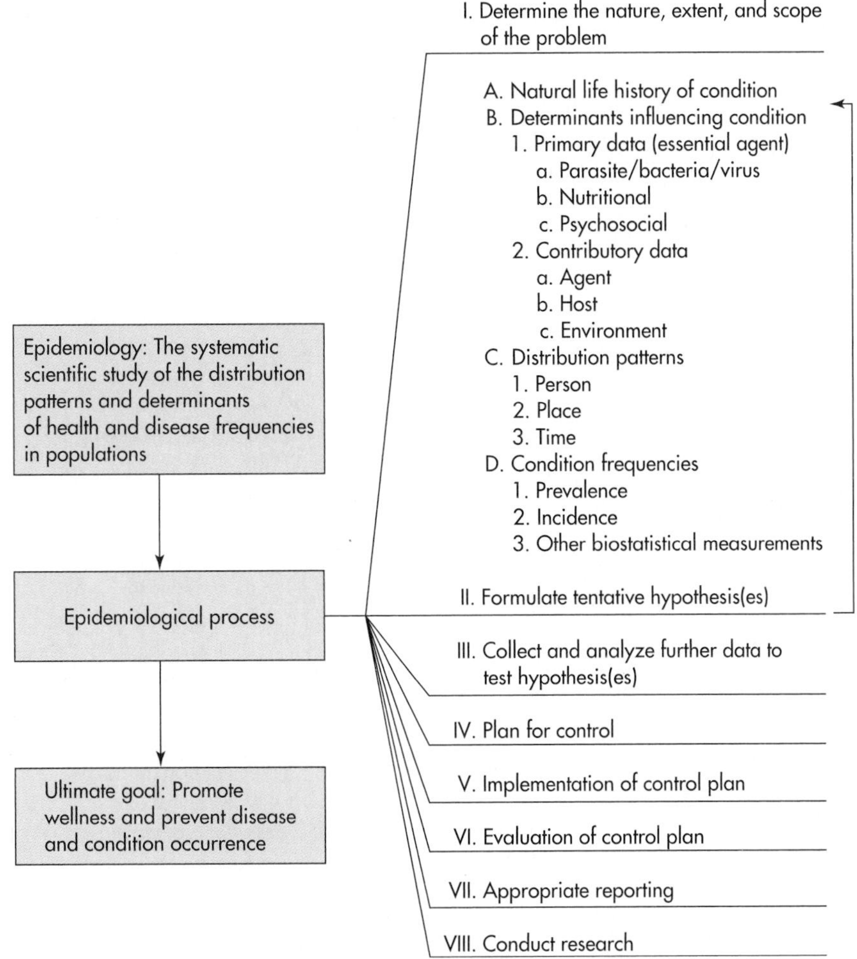

Figure 11-1 Graphical explanation of epidemiology.

frequencies in populations for the purpose of promoting wellness and preventing disease/conditions.

Implicit in this definition are two basic assumptions. The first is that patterns and frequencies of health, disease, and conditions in populations can be identified. The second is that factors determining or contributing to the occurrence of health, disease, or conditions can be discovered through systematic investigation.

Community health nurses use the epidemiological process to carry out their systematic investigation of health, disease, and conditions in populations. This process is graphically depicted in Figure 11-1 and is discussed in detail later in this chapter. Note that the epidemiological process shown in Figure 11-1 is similar to the nursing process. The steps are labeled differently but, in essence, they both involve a series of circular, dynamic problem-solving actions. Table 11-1 illustrates this point. Learning the language of epidemiology gives one a distinct advantage, however, because the terminology of epidemiology is used by all community health professionals; the terminology of the nursing process is not.

History and Scope of Epidemiology

Originally the major focus and scope of epidemiology and public health involved the control of epidemics caused by infectious diseases such as smallpox, plague, diphtheria, whooping cough, cholera, and scarlet fever. The primary goal was to limit the spread of disease and to prevent its recurrence. Although the scope of epidemiology has changed dramatically over time, infectious disease control remains a major priority worldwide. Infectious diseases are still not conquered. In recent years, new ones such as AIDS and Ebola-Marburg viral diseases have emerged, and the incidence of others including cholera, tuberculosis, malaria, and pertussis has increased significantly (CDC, 1994a).

Some of the most dramatic examples of infectious disease occurrence in epidemiological history happened when people who had not acquired natural or passive immunity came in contact with the disease. For example, scholars and scientists believe that the small band of Spaniards who conquered the Aztecs would not have been able to do so without the help of smallpox, which, when introduced into the Aztec community, reduced the community's ability to

table 11-1 Comparison of the Nursing Process and the Epidemiological Process

Nursing Process	Epidemiological Process
Assessing (data collection to determine nature of client problems)	I. Determine the nature, extent, and scope of the problem
	A. Natural life history of condition
	B. Determinants influencing condition
	1. Primary data (essential agent)
	a. Parasite/bacterium/virus
	b. Nutritional
	c. Psychosocial
	2. Contributory data
	a. Agent
	b. Host
	c. Environment
	C. Distribution patterns
	1. Person
	2. Place
	3. Time
	D. Condition frequencies
	1. Prevalence
	2. Incidence
	3. Other biostatistical measurements
Analyzing (formulation of nursing diagnosis or hypothesis)	II. Formulate tentative hypothesis(es)
	III. Collect and analyze further data to test hypothesis(es)
Planning	IV. Plan for control
Implementing	V. Implement control plan
Evaluating	VI. Evaluate control plan
Revising or terminating	VII. Make appropriate report
Research	VIII. Conduct research

defend itself during war; that Captain Cook was able to make his Hawaiian conquests through the accidental transmission of measles; and that the introduction of diseases such as smallpox, scarlet fever, and tuberculosis made Native Americans vulnerable to conquest. The "Lost Colony," the Roanoke Island settlement founded in 1587 by Sir Walter Raleigh, mysteriously disappeared; many historians believe it succumbed to communicable disease. Lost in the mysterious disappearance was Virginia Dare, the first English child born in North America (Prescott, 1936; Woodward, 1932).

The 19th century brought about innovations that helped control infectious diseases, such as the discoveries of Joseph Lister, a British surgeon who pioneered antiseptic surgery; Louis Pasteur, a French microbiologist who originated the germ theory of disease and developed pasteurization; and Robert Koch, a German medical scientist recognized as the father of microbiology. Koch developed pure cultures and discovered the tuberculosis, anthrax, and cholera bacilli.

During the early period in the history of the United States, isolation of the ill and quarantine of travelers were the major control measures used to protect the public against epidemics. These two control measures became quite common by the eighteenth century, and innoculation with material from smallpox scabs was also accepted as an effective control measure. A critical change during this time was the increasing recognition that disease could be controlled through public action (Institute of Medicine, 1988, p. 57).

The work of John Snow during this period helped to establish modern epidemiological methods and emphasized the importance of sanitary measures to control infectious diseases. In his classic study on cholera, Snow demonstrated that this disease could be transmitted by contaminated water and that a simple sanitary control measure could halt an epidemic. During the 1866 London cholera epidemic Snow went door to door to identify victims of this disease and the potential source of infection. He showed, through contact interviews and the use of a spot map that identified where the homes of cholera victims lived, that a public water pump in London was the source of infection. Removal of the pump handle stopped the outbreak of cholera (Jaret, 1991, p. 116).

The "great sanitary awakening" (Winslow, 1923) of the nineteenth century has influenced epidemiology practice throughout the twentieth century (Institute of Medicine, 1988). Knowledge gained during this early period is assisting contemporary epidemiologists to track disease occurrence

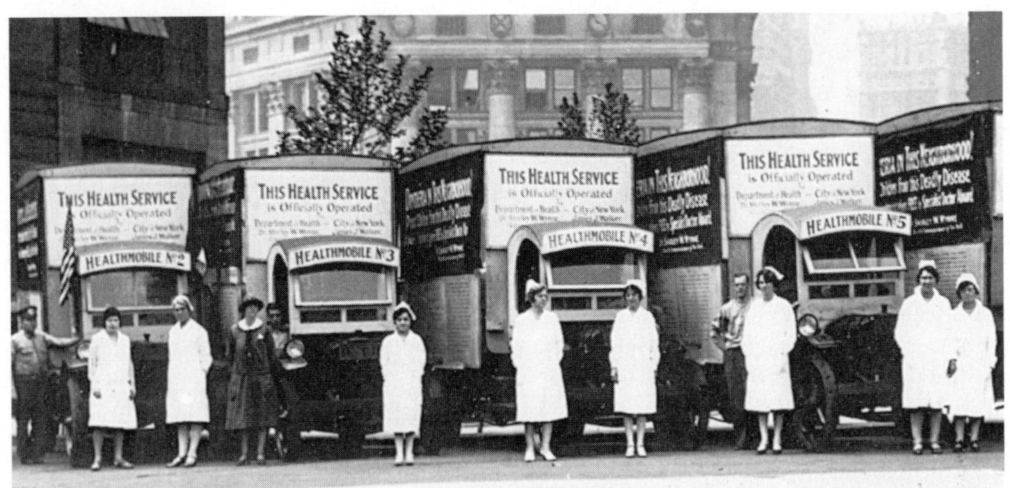

Figure **11-2** Death to diphtheria! Together with the able help of the visiting nurses, Mayor Jimmy Walker and Health Commissioner Hirley T. Wynne waged war on one of America's most dreaded diseases. This 1926 fleet of "healthmobiles" brought trained diptheria detection teams to every hidden pocket of the city. *(Courtesy: Visiting Nurse Service of New York.)*

and to implement effective environmental control measures. Like Snow, epidemiologists currently go door to door to investigate outbreaks of disease such as cholera, Lyme disease, and botulism, and are demonstrating that simple sanitary measures, including basic hand washing, can control infectious disease occurrence (Jaret, 1991).

In the twentieth century, the development of elaborate health care technology, along with the discovery of sulfa drugs, penicillin, and vaccines, has done much to aid in the prevention, control, and treatment of infectious disease. However, most of these advances have not reached the world's 250 million indigenous or "first peoples" living on tribal lands in countries around the world. A significant number of tribal first people exist in developing countries such as Brazil, Guatemala, Papua New Guinea, Thailand, India, and Africa. Tribal first people also live in industrialized nations including Australia (aborigines), Canada (Canadian Indians), and the United States (Native Americans). As the lands of these indigenous people are invaded by outsiders, the world may once again experience massive human destruction such as occurred in our early history. Tribal people are at risk for extinction if infectious diseases are introduced into their communities because they lack natural and acquired immunity against these diseases (McKenna, 1993).

The success of infectious disease control in developed countries brought with it new challenges and expanded the scope of epidemiology. The advances of the twentieth century have dramatically increased life expectancy. However, as longevity increases the prevalence of chronic disease also increases. Today the leading causes of death are chronic conditions, and epidemiologists are focusing attention on early detection and prevention of these conditions. In 1928 New York City sent out "healthmobiles" to rid the city of one of its most dreaded diseases—diphtheria (Figure 11-2). Today healthmobiles are still used in many U.S. cities, but they are currently sent out to screen people for chronic conditions such as hypertension, glaucoma, cancer, and diabetes rather than for infectious disease. This type of screening, as well as longitudinal study of chronic conditions, has helped public health professionals to identify aggregates at risk for chronic disease.

Contemporary epidemiologists examine variables that keep people healthy. They analyze the etiology of chronic conditions, accidents, and other health-related phenomena such as child abuse, abortion, domestic violence, and communicable diseases, including hepatitis B and AIDS. Epidemiologists are emphasizing the importance of studying *social,* as well as physical, factors that affect distributions of disease. Social epidemiologists investigate ways in which social conditions influence the likelihood that disease will develop. They focus attention on studying diseases and conditions—such as ulcers, heart disease, and alcoholism—that are influenced by social variables.

As we approach the twenty-first century, "epidemiology is in transition from a science that identifies risk factors for diseases to one that analyzes the systems that generate patterns of disease in populations" (Koopman, 1996, p. 630). This transition does not negate the importance of addressing factors that place individuals and populations at risk for disease occurrence. Rather, it reflects a shift in thinking about the role the environment plays in promoting health and preventing disease. In recent years community health professions have increasingly recognized that, in addition to lifestyle changes, needed environmental changes must be addressed to resolve many of our contemporary health issues.

EPIDEMIOLOGY AND THE COMMUNITY HEALTH NURSE

Effective implementation of the epidemiological process requires a multidisciplinary approach. Nurses, environmental engineers, physicians, laboratory technicians, statisticians, health officers, social workers, laypersons, and others all carry out necessary and essential roles in the investigation and control of disease and the promotion of wellness. Any health professional can and should function as a member of the epidemiological team.

Community health nurses participate on the epidemiological team in a variety of ways. Their contacts with families in the home and with groups in various settings (clinics, schools, and industry) put them in a unique position to carry out many epidemiological activities. They regularly become involved in case finding, health teaching, counseling, and follow-up essential to the prevention of infectious diseases, chronic conditions, and other health-related phenomena. The actions taken by the community health nurse in the following case scenario illustrate how nurses work to prevent the spread of a streptococcal infection and the occurrence of chronic complications.

CASE Scenario

While visiting the Wills family, the community health nurse learned that Bobbie had a severe sore throat. Because Bobbie's symptoms were indicative of a streptococcal infection, the nurse stressed the significance of a proper medical evaluation to rule out or confirm a diagnosis of strep throat. The family followed through immediately. Bobbie's throat culture came back positive for streptococcal disease, and he was treated with penicillin. The community health nurse, on a follow-up visit, taught the parents about the necessity of continuing the medication for 10 days even if Bobbie had no symptoms; she knew that a 10-day course of penicillin was needed to eliminate the streptococcal organisms. She also knew from theory and experience that if the organisms were not eliminated Bobbie could have serious chronic complications. By using her epidemiological knowledge, this nurse was able to effectively abort rheumatic fever, which can lead to a chronic heart condition or other chronic problems such as kidney disease.

Community health nurses also use concepts from epidemiology to address noninfectious health problems. Their work with children who have elevated blood lead levels (BLL) reflects this type of activity.

CASE Scenario

During a routine health screening for children at a local migrant camp, the community health nurse identified that Eduardo, a 2-year-old child, had a blood lead level of 28 μg/dL. An environmental investigation revealed higher than normal paint lead levels in the homes of the migrants, even though they had just recently been painted. The soil around the migrants' homes also had lead levels above the acceptable norm. Because the family had migrated north for the crop season only recently, the community health nurse questioned the parents about environmental conditions in their home community. The parents stated that they did not use traditional ethnic remedies, because they heard that children got sick from them. However, they had remodeled their older home in one of the Southern states about a year ago. Based on this information and the child's blood lead level, the community health nurse made a referral to the public health department in the family's local home community, requesting medical follow-up for Eduardo and an environmental investigation of the family's home. The community health nurse also shared information about lead poisoning in young children and explained environmental, nutritional, and follow-up interventions needed while the family was at the migrant camp. The importance of follow-up upon their return home was emphasized. The nurse's follow-up was completed when she received notification that Eduardo's family was being visited by a community health nurse in their local home community.

In addition to the activities just described, community health nurses also use epidemiological concepts to carry out research in the community setting. A research team may carry out a study to survey major community needs (see Chapter 13) or to identify gaps in knowledge relative to disease causation, prevention, and control. A community health nurse's ongoing, comprehensive contact with the community and its resources allows her or him to make key contributions during these types of studies.

A community health nurse must apply the principles of epidemiology to provide preventive health services to aggregates in the community. The nurse must understand the significance of expanding epidemiological study to investigate health and disease in populations, as well as in individuals. Only in this way will the community health nurse effectively meet the health needs of the community as a whole.

BASIC CONCEPTS OF EPIDEMIOLOGY

To use the epidemiological process effectively, community health nurses need to have an understanding of the basic concepts, tools, and terms of epidemiology. Since epidemiology is operationally defined in terms of disease measurements, an understanding of the biostatistical concepts is essential. Biostatistics helps to describe the extent and distribution of health, illness, and conditions in the community and aids in the identification of specific health problems and community strengths. Biostatistics also facilitates the setting of priorities for program planning.

In addition to biostatistics, several basic concepts guide epidemiological study. These are aggregates at risk, the natural life history of a disease, levels of prevention, host-agent-environment relationships, multiple causation, and person-place-time relationships. In general these concepts provide a foundation for explaining how disease develops and how health is maintained, who is most susceptible to disease, and how disease can be prevented and health promoted.

Study of Aggregates at Risk

A key concept of epidemiology is that the study of disease in populations is more significant than the study of individual cases of disease. Epidemiological research has demonstrated that using large sampling groups is essential for formulating valid conclusions about the distribution patterns and determinants of health, disease, and condition frequencies in populations. It is by observing large groups that commonalities and differences among people who have or do not have a particular disease or condition can be identified.

The identification of commonalities and differences among groups focuses attention on the essential or contributory factors that produce illness or promote health. For example, it has been found repeatedly, through sampling of large groups, that people who smoke are more likely to develop coronary disease than people who do not smoke. This fact may never have been established if only individual cases had been examined, because many people who develop coronary disease do not smoke.

A preventive health philosophy has led professionals in community health to emphasize the study of groups. The goal of epidemiological study is to identify *aggregates at risk*, so that preventive health measures such as those presented in Table 11-2 can be used to stop the progression of disease or health-related phenomena. As previously defined in Chapter 2, aggregates at high risk are those who engage in certain activities or who have certain characteristics that increase their potential for contracting an illness, injury, or a health problem. For example, parents who were abused as children are at risk for abusing their own children. These activities or characteristics are known as *risk factors*.

RISK FACTORS Risk factors are determined by a risk estimate process. Risk estimates are derived by contrasting the frequency of a disease or health condition in persons *exposed* to a specific trait or risk factor and the frequency in another

table 11-2 Epidemiology in Action: Health Measures Needed to Improve the Health of At-Risk Groups at Each Life Stage

Infants	Children	Adolescents and Young Adults	Adults	Elderly
Education for parenthood Genetic counseling Good prenatal care Sound prenatal nutritional guidance and services Counseling services to decrease adverse maternal habits that affect fetal development (e.g., smoking, drinking, drugs, exposure to radiation) Amniocentesis Breast feeding Regular comprehensive care Immunizations Social services including financial assistance, day care, improved foster and adoption programs, and counseling for families under stress Newborn screening and follow-up	Early comprehensive childhood development programs Special support services to aid families under stress (e.g., child abuse, low income, etc.) Injury reduction education Comprehensive pediatric care Immunizations Lead poisoning screening Fluoridation of water supplies Dental care Nutritional and exercise guidance Education to prevent and eliminate dysfunctional health habits (smoking, alcohol use, drug use, unprotected sexual activity, poor dietary and exercise patterns)	Comprehensive injury prevention programs, including roadway safety Educational programs about smoking, alcohol, and drug use Nutrition and exercise guidance Family planning services Sexually transmissible disease services including education, screening, and treatment Immunizations Mental health Actions to reduce the availability of firearms Comprehensive violence prevention programs	Public education about smoking, alcohol, good nutrition, and adequate exercise, including how poor health habits increase risk of disease Protection from environmental health habits Worksite health and safety programs Hypertension prevention, screening, and control programs Pap smears Regular breast self-examination Education about cancer signs Mental health services Dental care Comprehensive violence prevention programs	Work and social activity for retired persons Education about adequate exercise and nutrition Preventive multiphasic screening programs Education about proper use of medications Immunizations for influenza Home safety programs Community and home services that facilitate independent living

Data from Surgeon General: *Healthy people: the Surgeon General's report on health promotion and disease prevention*, vol II, Washington, D.C., 1979, U.S. Government Printing Office, pp. 149-155; USDHHS: *Healthy people 2000: national health promotion and disease prevention objectives, full report with commentary*, Washington, D.C., 1991, U.S. Government Printing Office, pp. 9-28.

group *not exposed* to a risk factor (Jekel, Elmore, Katz, 1996). Risk factors fall under three major categories: (1) behavioral or lifestyle patterns; (2) environmental factors; and (3) inborn or inherited characteristics (Last, 1995). These risk factors increase one's susceptibility to death, disease, injury, or psychosocial conditions. For example, inherited characteristics may predispose individuals to genetic diseases such as hemophilia or sickle cell anemia and a range of other health problems like cancer, cardiac disease, diabetes, and mental illness.

Although heredity can increase the risk for the occurrence of disease or adverse health conditions, health problems usually result from multiple interacting factors. When these multiple risk factors come together they form an interrelated web of forces that increases their potential for causing harm.

It is increasingly recognized that *environmental factors* and *lifestyle patterns* are crucial variables in the development of disease and adverse conditions. The emphasis on studying these variables began during the 1970s when several major health documents, including the *Lalonde Report on the Health of Canadians* (Lalonde, 1974), the *World Health Assembly Declaration of Commitment to Health For All* (WHO, 1978), and the *United States' Healthy People Mandate* (Surgeon General, 1979), declared that the health care system was not the most important factor in determining health (Pederson, O'Neill, Rootman, 1994). These documents articulated the link between individuals and their social and physical environment (Scherl, Noren, Osterweis, 1992). The *Healthy People* document declared that many of the leading causes of death could be substantially reduced if persons at risk improved their lifestyle patterns of diet, smoking, exercise, alcohol consumption, and use of antihypertensive medication. It was also noted at that time that approximately 20% of all premature deaths could be eliminated if environmental hazards were controlled (Surgeon General, 1979, vol. I).

McGinnis and Foege (1993) reinforced the significance of addressing lifestyle and environmental determinants of health when the root causes of death in the United States were examined. They proposed that the "actual" causes of death were not the pathological disease conditions (e.g., cardiac disease or cancer) existing at the time of death. Rather, the actual causes were external factors such as smoking, diet, and firearms (see the box, above right). The *Behavioral Risk Factor Surveillance System* administered by state health departments in cooperation with the Centers for Disease Control and Prevention collects data related to the leading "actual" causes of death (Michigan Department of Public Health, 1995).

Chapters 15 through 20 discuss many health problems related to lifestyle patterns and environmental factors such as accidents, child abuse, suicide, domestic violence, alcoholism, and sexually transmitted diseases (STDs). Anticipatory guidance at each stage across the life span assists individuals, families, and aggregates in developing lifestyle patterns that promote health and reduce the risk of disease and adverse health conditions. Table 11-2 summarizes the measures which help clients at various life stages to improve their quality of life. Recent U.S. "estimates of years of healthy life years show a decline in health-related quality of life despite increases in life expectancy" (USDHHS, 1995a, p. 6). Self-reported health status and activity limitation data are used to estimate healthy life years (USDHHS, 1995a). Both lifestyle patterns and environmental conditions influence quality of life measures. It has been shown that "health disparities between poor people and those with higher incomes are almost universal for all dimensions of health. Poverty reduces a person's prospects for a long life by increasing the chances of infant death, chronic disease, and traumatic death. Poverty is also associated with significant developmental limitations" (USDHHS, 1991a, pp. 29-30).

Actual Causes of Death

- Tobacco
- Diet/activity
- Alcohol
- Certain infections
- Toxic agents
- Firearms
- Sexual behavior
- Motor vehicles
- Illicit drug use

From McGinnis MJ, Foege WH: Actual causes of death in the United States, *JAMA* 270:2207-2212, 1993, p. 2208.

Natural Life History of Disease

In the search for commonalities that may produce disease and health-related phenomena in specific aggregates, epidemiological study focuses on determining the natural life history of these conditions. Observing the natural life history of disease and health-related phenomena aids in identifying agent-host-environmental factors that influence their development, characteristic signs and symptoms during their different periods of progression, and approaches to preventing and controlling their effects on humans.

The natural life history of disease is defined as "the course of a disease from onset (inception) to resolution. Many diseases have certain well-defined stages that, taken all together, are referred to as the "natural history of the disease in question" (Last, 1995, p. 110). In their classic textbook, Leavell and Clark (1965) identified two distinct periods in the natural history of a disease: *prepathogenesis* and *pathogenesis*.

In the *prepathogenesis* period disease has not developed but interactions are occurring between the host, agent, and environment that produce disease stimulus and increase the host's potential for disease. The combination of high serum

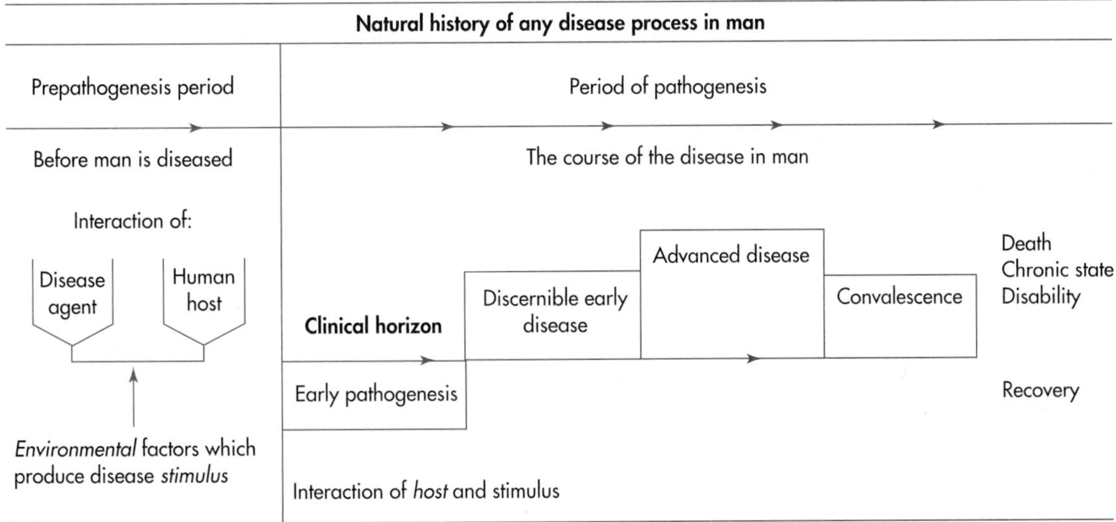

Figure 11-3 Prepathogenesis and pathogenesis periods in the natural history of disease. *(From Leavell HR and Clark EG: Preventive medicine for the doctor in his community: an epidemiologic approach, New York, 1965, McGraw-Hill, p. 18.)*

cholesterol levels and smoking, for example, increases the host's potential for developing coronary heart disease.

The *pathogenesis* period in the natural life history of disease begins when disease-producing stimuli (smoking or elevated serum cholesterol levels) start to produce changes in the tissues of humans (arteriosclerosis in the coronary vessels). Figure 11-3 shows the interrelationship between the prepathogenesis period and the pathogenesis period and how the latter progresses from the presymptomatic stage to advanced, clinical disease. It also shows that disease occurs as a result of processes that happen in the *environment*—prepathogenesis—and processes that happen in *humans*—pathogenesis (Leavell, Clark, 1965, p. 18). Preventive interventions can alter the natural life history of many diseases, especially cardiovascular disease and cancer (Last, 1995).

Levels of Prevention

The study of the natural life history of disease facilitates the achievement of the ultimate goal of epidemiology—the development of effective methods for preventing and controlling disease or conditions in populations. By identifying significant host-agent-environment relationships that influence the progression of the natural life history of a condition, the epidemiologist can identify aggregates at risk and develop ways to prevent disease occurrence among them.

A continuum of preventive activities is essential for the promotion of health in any community. As previously discussed in Chapter 2, preventive activities can be grouped under three levels: *primary* (health promotion and specific protection), *secondary* (early diagnosis, prompt treatment, and disability limitation), and *tertiary* (rehabilitation). Figure 11-4 identifies preventive activities at all three levels that can alter the natural history of disease. The degree to which preventive activities can be implemented will vary depending on the completeness of knowledge one has about the disease or health problem in question, the complexity of these conditions, and the behavioral and environmental factors influencing the natural life history of the disease (Leavell, Clark, 1965).

Host-Agent-Environment Relationships

When epidemiologists analyze the natural life history of a disease or a condition for the purpose of identifying preventive measures to eliminate or halt the disease or condition in question, they study the relationships among three variables: *host*, *agent*, and *environment*. These variables are defined in Table 11-3.

The interactions between the host-agent-environment variables are frequently referred to as the epidemiological triangle (Figure 11-5). These interactions (depicted by arrows in Figure 11-5) influence the level of health in a community. Health is maintained when the host-agent-environment variables are in a state of equilibrium. Pathology occurs when there is a disruption in the balance among those three variables.

Agents are biological, chemical, or physical and include bacteria, viruses, fungi, pesticides, food additives, ionizing radiation, and speeding objects. The normal habitat in which an infectious (biological) agent lives, multiples, and/or grows is called a *reservoir*. These habitats include humans, animals, and the environment and are discussed in a later section of this chapter.

A wide variety of characteristics are classified as host factors. Examples of these factors are age, sex, ethnic group,

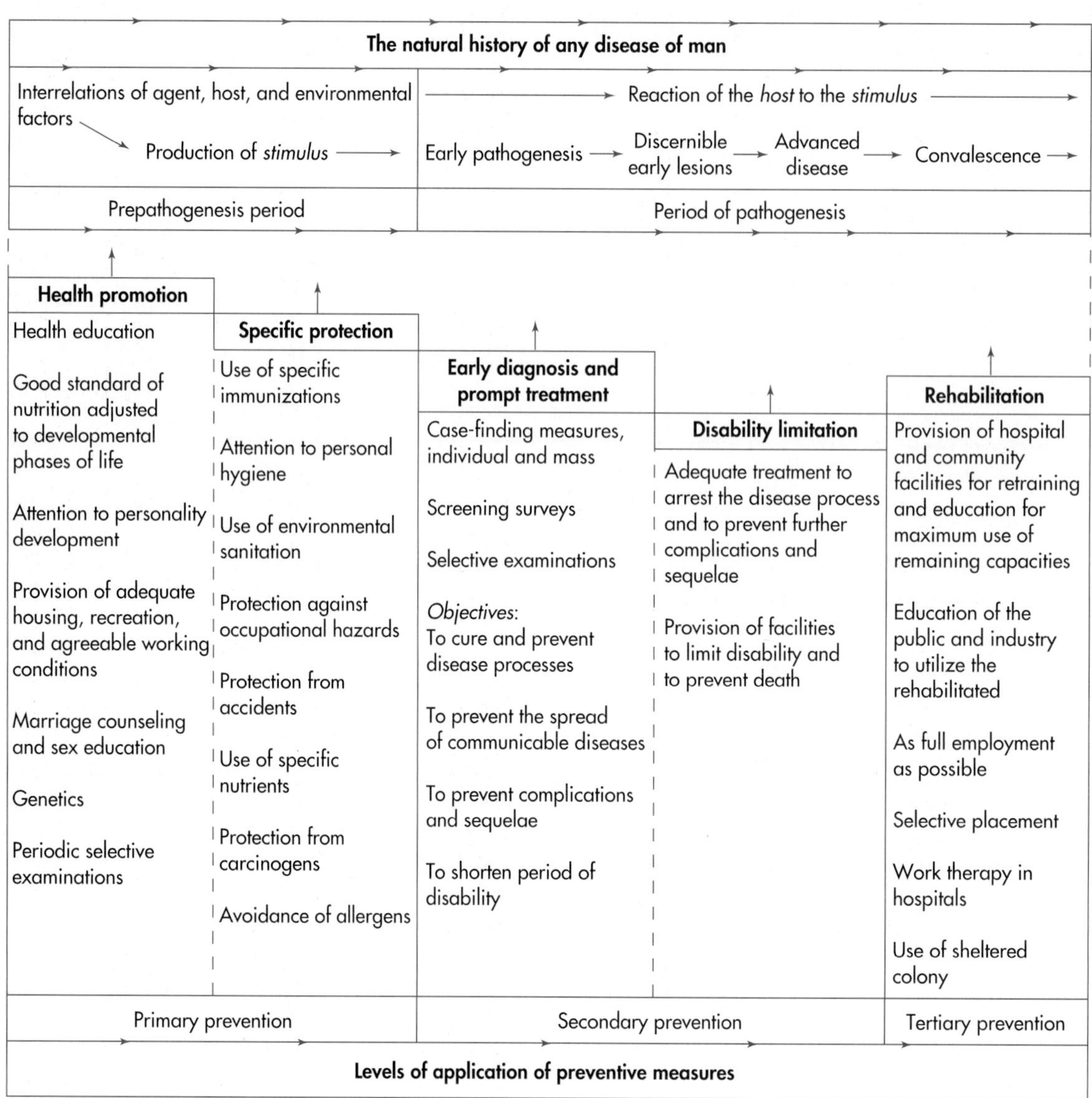

Figure 11-4 Levels of application of preventive measures in the natural history of disease. *(From Leavell HR, Clark EG: Preventive medicine for the doctor in his community: an epidemiologic approach, New York, 1965, McGraw-Hill, p. 21.)*

socioeconomic status, lifestyle, and heredity (CDC, 1987a, p. 5). Four types of environmental factors—physical, social, economic, and family—are discussed in Chapter 6. The dynamic interactions between host-agent-environmental factors, as well as further characteristics of each, are discussed later in this chapter.

Multiple Causation

The theory of multiple causation of disease illustrates and confirms that it is the interactions and relationships between host-agent-environment that actually cause a disease or condition—*not* host, agent, or environmental factors alone. The theory of multiple causation is critical to epidemiology. It is only natural to assume that the introduction of a disease agent (e.g., influenza virus) into a community is enough to cause illness among its members. However, in addition to this causative agent there must be a susceptible host and an environment conducive to the interaction of agent and host. Factors such as the level of immunity in the population, individual susceptibility, availability of vectors, and the amount of contact between members of the population will affect disease/condition occurrence. The following example of an influenza outbreak illustrates how these factors influence disease outbreaks.

An influenza outbreak that occurred in the United States demonstrates the concept of multiple causation. The agent, the influenza virus A/USSR, was introduced into the population. Outbreaks of this disease occurred in groups of young adults and children in environments of close contact: schools, colleges, and military training camps. Attack rates in these

table 11-3 Epidemiology Variables: Host, Agent, and Environment

Variable	Definition
HOST	Living species (humans or other animals) capable of being infected or affected by an agent.
Primary host	Host in which sexual maturation occurs (e.g., in malaria, the mosquito).
Secondary host	Host in which asexual forms of the parasite develops (e.g., in malaria, a human or other vertebrate mammal or bird).
Transport host	Carrier in which the organism remains alive but does not undergo development.
AGENT	Factor, such as a microorganism, chemical substance, or form of radiation, whose presence, excessive presence, or (in deficiency diseases) relative absence is essential for the occurrence of a disease.
ENVIRONMENT	All that which is external to the individual human host. Can be divided into physical, biological, social, cultural, etc., any or all of which can influence health status of populations.

Data from Benenson AS: *Control of communicable diseases manual*, ed 16, Washington, D.C., 1995, APHA, p. 537; Last JM: *A dictionary of epidemiology*, ed 3, New York, 1995, Oxford University Press, pp. 5, 53 and 79.

areas were high, ranging from 40% to 70% in most cases. The disease did not usually appear in adults over 25 years of age.

An analysis of this situation illustrates that the proper combination of multiple factors is necessary before disease will result. Outbreaks occurred in young adults and children because there was a virulent agent, susceptible hosts who lacked immunity, and crowded environmental conditions that supported the spread of the agent. The disease usually did not occur in those over 25 because they had been exposed to this virus earlier and had developed acquired immunity to the organism. This acquired immunity allowed them to maintain a balance in host-agent-environment factors and to escape the disease. If only one variable, such as a virulent agent, was necessary to cause illness, individuals 25 years and older would also have had high attack rates.

The concept of multiple causation becomes even more apparent when one studies the natural life history of noninfectious diseases, chronic conditions, and health-related phenomena. Friedman's (1974, p. 5) classic diagram of the web of causation for myocardial infarction (Figure 11-6) clearly demonstrates that it is the interplay between multiple host-agent-environment characteristics that causes a chronic condition.

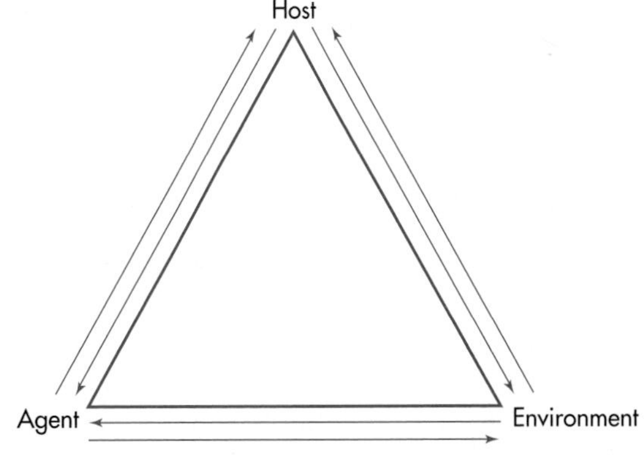

Figure 11-5 Epidemiological triangle.

Person-Place-Time Relationships

The study of relationships is necessary for the community health professional to formulate valid hypotheses about disease or condition causation. Identification of measurable variables that can facilitate rapid and efficient data collection is essential to this study. In epidemiological study the variables found to be most useful are *person* (who is affected), *place* (where affected), and *time* (when affected). Some of the most frequently analyzed characteristics of these variables are presented in Table 11-4.

Timing is a critical factor in disease diagnosis and control. Immediate reporting of a disease outbreak is crucial, since the validity of data is often directly proportional to the time lapse incurred in obtaining the information. If a significant amount of time is lost in reporting, the ability to formulate valid hypotheses is decreased.

When monitoring incidence of infectious disease, the following terms are used to distinguish relative frequency in time and space:

Sporadic: Presence of occasional cases of the event apparently unrelated in time or space

Endemic: Constant long-term presence of an event at about the frequency expected from the past history of the community

Epidemic: Presence of the event at a much higher frequency than expected from the past history of the community, usually over a short period of time (for example, one case of cholera would be labeled epidemic in a U.S. community; on the other hand, in some foreign countries, several cases of cholera would be considered an endemic occurrence).

Pandemic: Presence of an event in epidemic proportions, involving many communities and countries in a relatively short period of time.

THE DYNAMICS OF INFECTIOUS DISEASE TRANSMISSION

Complex interactions between the host, agent, and environment occur before the clinical signs and symptoms of disease are observed. The chain of disease transmission (Figure 11-7) involves a series of events that allows a pathogenic

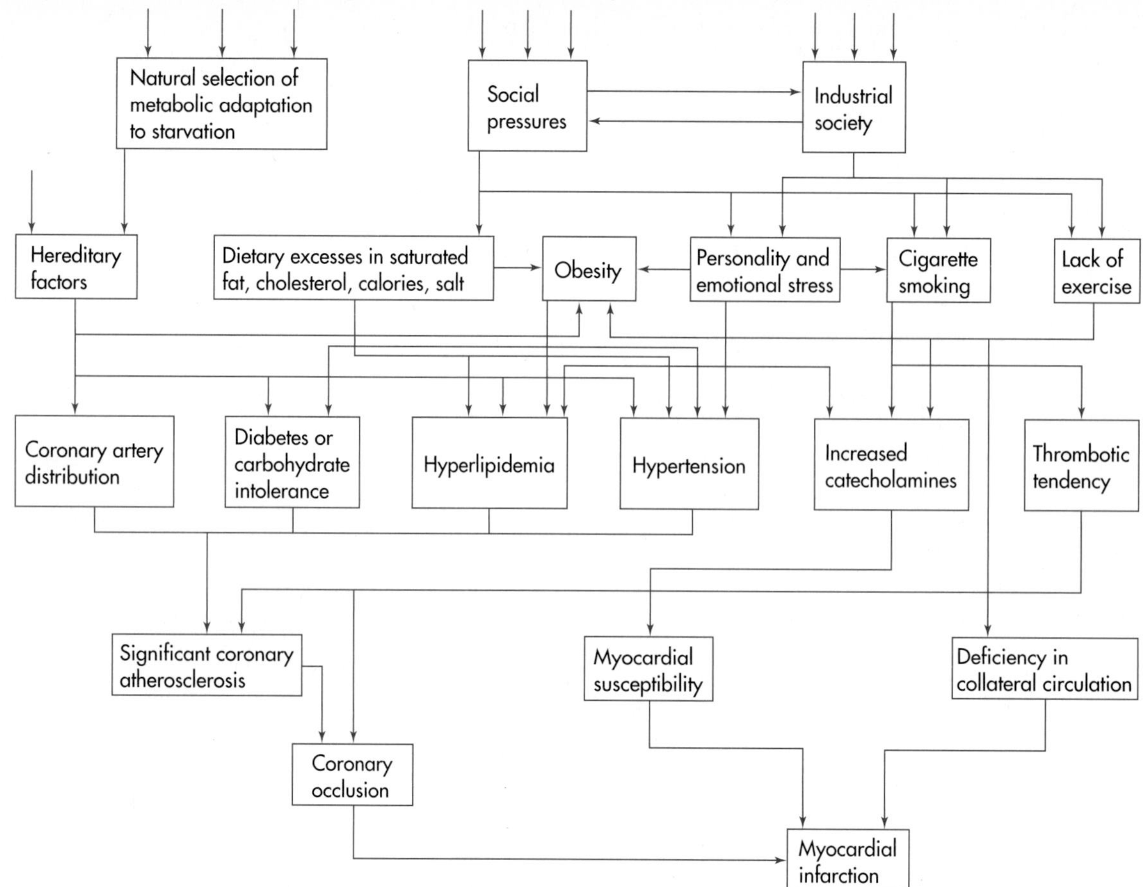

Figure **11-6** The web of causation for myocardial infarction. *(From Friedman GE:* Primer of epidemiology, *New York, 1974, McGraw-Hill, p. 5.)*

table 11-4 Epidemiological Variables

Variable		Characteristics
Person:	delineation of group involved	• Age, sex, race distribution • Socioeconomic status, occupation, education • Health habits and behaviors or lifestyle • Acquired resistance and susceptibility • Health history – natural resistance, hereditary characteristics
Place:	geographical distribution in subdivisions of the area affected	• *Physical environment:* weather; climate; geography; radiation; vibration; noise; pressure; animal reservoirs; pollutants; housing facilities; workplace hazards; and sources of air, water, and food contamination • *Social environment:* population density and mobility; community groups; occupations and other roles; beliefs and attitudes; technological developments; transportation; educational practices; and health care delivery system • *Economic environment:* source of income; income level; employment status; job frustrations; and income for nutrition, housing, and other basic needs • *Family environment:* family history; family dynamics; strategies used to handle stress; type, number, and timing of major life changes; home atmosphere; and family health and cultural patterns (see Chapters 7 and 8)
Time:	chronological distribution of onsets of cases by days, weeks, months	• *Incubation period:* determine life cycle; factors affecting multiplication and virulence of organism • Seasonal trends • Onset of event • Duration of event

Data from MacMahon B, Pugh T: *Epidemiology principles and methods*, Boston, 1970, Little, Brown, pp. 31-32; Surgeon General: *Healthy people: the Surgeon General's report on health promotion and disease prevention*, vol I, Washington, D.C., 1979, U.S. Government Printing Office, pp. 13-14; Centers for Disease Control, Training and Laboratory Program Office: *Principles of epidemiology: agent, host, environment* (self-study course 3030-G, manual 1), Atlanta, 1987a, CDC, pp. 12-30.

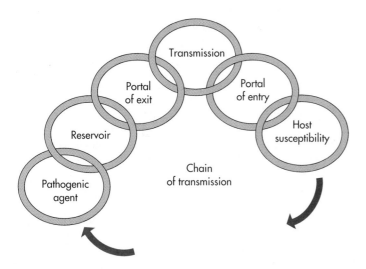

Figure 11-7 Chain of transmission for infection. The chain must be intact for an infection to be transmitted to another host. Transmission can be controlled by breaking any link in the chain. *(From Grimes DE:* Infectious diseases, *St. Louis, 1991, Mosby, p. 21.)*

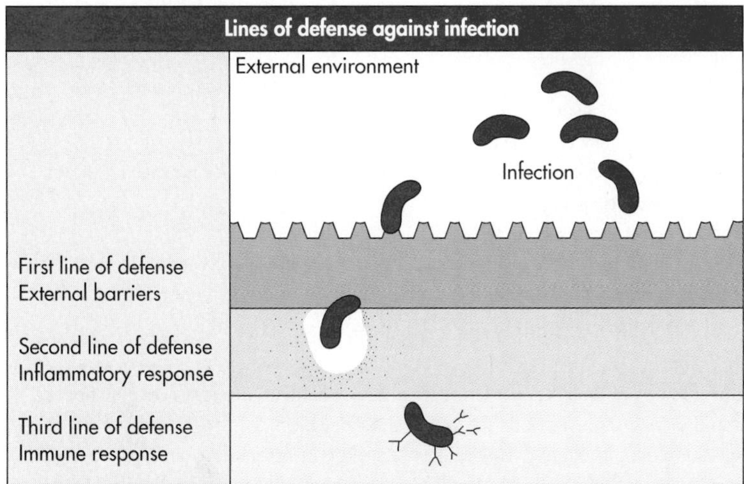

Figure 11-8 Lines of defense against infection. *(From Grimes DE:* Infectious diseases, *St. Louis, 1991, Mosby, p. 4.)*

microorganism to come in contact with a host and to invade, multiply, and elicit a physiologic response in this host. For infection and subsequent disease to occur, the chain of transmission must remain intact. This requires the presence of a pathogenic agent, an appropriate reservoir, a susceptible host with portals of entry and exit, and favorable environmental conditions that support transmission of the agent. Table 11-5 defines select host, agent, and environmental factors that influence disease transmission and progression.

Host Characteristics

Host factors affect the ease of contact between the host and agent and the capability of the host to resist the disease evoking powers of an agent. Lifestyle patterns can significantly influence the host-agent transmission process. Biological characteristics and the host's lines of defense affect how well the host can protect itself against host invasion and dissemination.

A person's (host's) lines of defense (Figure 11-8) can produce inflammatory or immune responses that prevent or contain an infection or destroy the infectious agent. Immunity or protection from infectious disease occurs when an individual's immune response stimulates production of agent-specific antibodies and memory cells (*active immunity*) or when agent-specific antibodies are transferred from one host to another (*passive immunity*). "Active immunity is most desirable" (Atkinson, Furphy, Gantt, Mayfield, 1995, p. 18).

Both passive and active immunity can be acquired either naturally or artificially (Table 11-6). Vaccines produce artificial immunity. Live attenuated (weakened) and inactivated vaccines are used to produce an immune response in a host. "The more similar a vaccine is to the natural disease, the better the immune response to the vaccine. The immune response to a live attenuated vaccine is virtually identical to that produced by a natural infection . . . In contrast, the immune response to an inactivated vaccine is mostly humoral. Little or no cellular immunity results" (Atkinson, Furphy, Gantt, Mayfield, 1995, pp. 15-17). Table 11-7 identifies the available vaccines by type. Having knowledge of the vaccine type helps to predict adverse events, contraindications, and immunization schedule. For example, live attenuated vaccines generally produce long-lasting immunity with a single

table 11-5 Factors Influencing Infectious Disease Transmission and Progression

Term	Definition
HOST CHARACTERISTICS	
Lifestyle factors	Factors (e.g., sanitation practices, sexual habits, food storage and cooking practices) that facilitate or inhibit agent-host contact.
Biological factors	Factors that decrease or increase a host's resistance to infection (e.g., general health status, nutritional intake, immune response).
General defense mechanisms	External barriers (e.g., skin, nose, and digestive system) that prevent the agent from invading the internal organs of the host and the nonspecific inflammatory response that fights and destroys pathogens.
Specific defense mechanisms	An immune response that creates host immunity to a specific infectious agent.
Immunity	Protection from infectious disease associated with the presence of antibodies or cells having a *specific* action on the pathogens that carry a particular infectious disease.
Passive immunity (temporary, short-duration immunity)	Antibody protection *transferred from another person* either naturally by transplacental transfer from the mother or artificially by inoculation of specific protective antibodies.
Active immunity (permanent, or long-lasting, immunity)	Antibody and cell protection *produced by the person's own immune system* either naturally by infection with or without clinical manifestations or artificially by inoculation of the agent itself in a killed, modified, or variant form.
Herd immunity	Resistance of a group or community to invasion and spread of an infectious agent, based on the agent-specific immunity of a high proportion of the population.
AGENT CHARACTERISTICS	
Infectivity	The capability of an infectious agent to evade, survive, and multiply in the host.
Pathogenicity	The power of the agent to produce clinical disease.
Virulence	The degree of pathogenicity of an infectious agent indicated by the *severity* of disease manifestations (e.g., case-fatality rates and tissue damage).
Invasiveness	The capability of an infectious agent to spread and disseminate in the host.
Toxigenicity	The capability of an infectious agent to produce poisonous products such as exotoxins.
Antigenicity	The capability of an infectious agent to stimulate the host to produce an immune response (e.g., production of antibodies or antitoxins).
ENVIRONMENTAL CHARACTERISTICS	
Reservoir	Any person, animal, arthropod, plant, soil, or substance in which an infectious agent lives, multiplies, and reproduces itself in a manner that supports survival and transmission.
Mode of transmission	Any mechanism by which an infectious agent is spread from a source or reservoir to another host.
Direct transmission	Direct *contact* transmission to a portal of entry, as a result of a host physically touching an infected reservoir, transplacental transfer, or transmission of projected airborne droplet spray.
Indirect transmission	Transmission through an *intermediate,* contaminated vehicle or vector or an infective vector.

Data from Benenson AS: *Control of communicable diseases manual*, ed 16, Washington, D.C., 1995, APHA, pp. 536-537, 544-545; Grimes DE: *Infectious diseases*, St. Louis, 1991, Mosby, pp. 2-3, 20-21; Last JM: *A dictionary of epidemiology*, ed 3, New York, 1995, Oxford University Press, pp. 85, 167-168, 172-174.

dose, and adverse reactions to the vaccine are usually similar to those produced by a mild form of the natural illness (e.g., fever and rash). Inactivated vaccines always require multiple doses, often require periodic boosting to maintain immunity, and generally produce mostly localized adverse events (e.g., pain at the injection site) with or without fever (Atkinson, Furphy, Gantt, Mayfield).

Agent Characteristics

Agent characteristics influence the likelihood that infection and disease will occur and affect the nature of the disease process. A microorganism that is capable of producing an infection or an infectious disease is commonly referred to as a pathogenic agent. "Infection is not synonymous with infectious disease; the result may be inapparent or manifest" (Last, 1995, p. 85).

When a pathogenic agent invades a host and multiplies, an inapparent infection occurs. An infection goes through several stages before it produces clinical disease (Figure 11-9). The duration and potential outcomes of each stage vary considerably, depending on agent and host characteristics (Grimes, 1991). Benenson (1995) summarizes significant information about the stages of infection for the major communicable diseases in his book *Control of Communicable Diseases Manual*. This book is a valuable reference for any nurse's library.

The concepts that describe the disease-provoking powers of an agent are *infectivity, pathogenicity, virulence, invasiveness, toxigenicity,* and *antigenicity*. These concepts are defined in Table 11-5. Disease-provoking powers of an agent influence a pathogenic agent's ability to evade, multiply, and survive in a host (infectivity) and to produce clinical disease (pathogencity). They also influence the severity of

table 11-6 Types of Acquired Immunity

Type of Immunity	How Acquired	Length of Resistance
NATURAL		
Active	Natural contact and infection with the antigen	May be temporary or permanent
Passive	Natural contact with antibody transplacentally or through colostrum and breast milk	Temporary
ARTIFICIAL		
Active	Inoculation of antigen	May be temporary or permanent
Passive	Inoculation of antibody or antitoxin	Temporary

From Grimes DE: *Infectious diseases*, St. Louis, 1991, Mosby, p. 18.

table 11-7 Available Vaccines by Type

LIVE ATTENUATED VACCINES	
• Viral	Measles, mumps, rubella, polio, yellow fever, vaccinia, varicella
• Bacterial	BCG
• Recombinant	Typhoid
INACTIVATED VACCINES	
• Viral	Influenza, polio, rabies, hepatitis A
• Bacterial	Pertussis, typhoid, cholera, plague
• Subunit	Hepatitis B, influenza, acellular pertussis
• Toxoid	Diphtheria, tetanus
• Recombinant	Hepatitis B
• Polysaccharide	Pneumococcal, meningococcal, and *Haemophilus* influenzae type b

From Atkinson W, Furphy L, Gantt J, Mayfield M, eds: *Epidemiology and prevention of vaccine-preventable diseases*, Atlanta, 1995, CDC, pp. 15-17.
Note: Subunit vaccines are composed of partial bacteria or viruses; toxoids are composed of fractions of bacterial toxins; polysaccharide vaccines are composed of fractions of bacterial cell wall; recombinant vaccines are antigens created by genetic engineering.

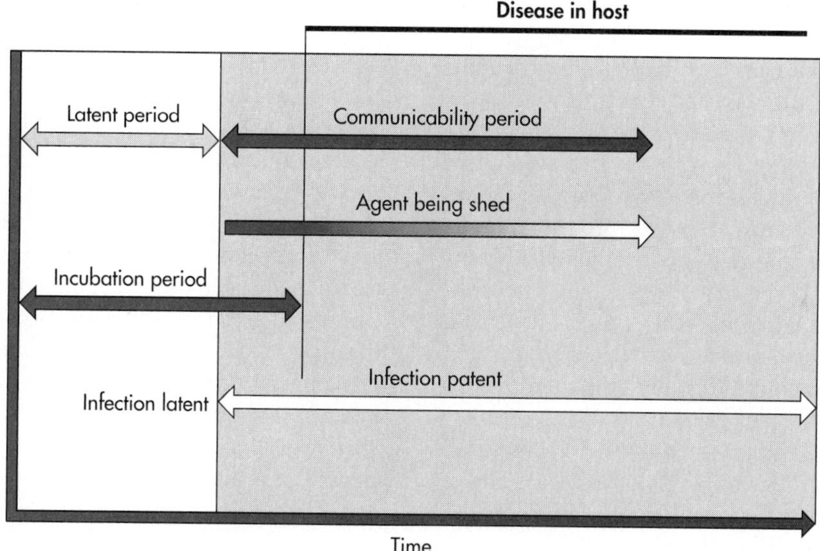

Figure 11-9 Stages of infection. Infection in the host proceeds in identifiable stages: the length of each stage varies with the pathogenic agent and host factors. The *latent period* begins with pathogenic invasion of the body and ends when the agent can be shed (communicability period). The *incubation period* begins with invasion of the agent, during which the organism reproduces, and ends when the disease process begins. The *communicability period* begins when the latent period ends and continues as long as the agent is present. The *disease period* follows the incubation period and ends at variable times. This stage may be subclinical or produce overt symptoms, and it may resolve completely or become latent. (*From Grimes DE:* Infectious diseases, *St. Louis, 1991, Mosby, p. 19.*)

disease (virulence, invasiveness, and toxigenicity). Agents that lack antigenic properties (antigencity) have a greater chance of surviving in a host than those agents that possess these properties.

The disease-provoking capabilities of an agent vary considerably. While many host-agent relationships result in varying degrees of disease, many others result in inapparent or subclinical infection. From a control perspective, it is important to study asymptomatic individuals exposed to an infectious agent as well as those with visible clinical disease. Individuals with inapparent infection can harbor a specific infectious agent without discernible clinical disease and serve as potential sources of infection. These individuals are *carriers* of disease. Carriers of disease present considerable danger to other hosts because they often do not recognize the need to take action to prevent disease transmission. An example of this is a female client who has asymptomatic gonorrhea. She may transmit gonorrhea for a considerable length of time before she knows that she has the disease.

Environmental Characteristics

Environmental factors influence agent survival and transmission processes. These factors can determine what type of agents are present in a region and may provide reservoirs and favorable conditions for the spread of disease. For example, malaria is prevalent in tropical and subtropical areas because environmental conditions support the breeding habits of the Anopheles mosquito, the vector that transmits the disease to human hosts. Human reservoirs are also prevalent in these areas and frequently are carriers of the disease. A *reservoir* is any person, animal, arthropod, plant, soil, or substance in which an infectious agent lives, multiplies, and reproduces itself in a manner that supports survival and transmission (Benenson, 1995). "The human reservoir may be clinically ill, have a subclinical infection, or be a carrier" (Grimes, 1991, p. 20).

Environmental factors support or inhibit direct or indirect transmission of the pathogenic agent from a reservoir to a susceptible host. *Direct* transmission can occur by actual physical contact with an infected reservoir, by transplacental transfer, or by host inhalation of projected airborne droplet spray. *Indirect* transmission occurs through an intermediate vehicle or vector. A *vehicle* is a contaminated inanimate object or material such as food, water, air, blood, feces, soiled linens, or equipment from a diseased person. Objects contaminated by a diseased individual are referred to as *fomites*. A *vector* is an arthropod or other noninvertebrates. Vectors may be simple mechanical carriers (flies) or infected nonvertebrate hosts (mosquitos). Vectorborne transmissions have been responsible for major epidemics of disease (e.g., malaria and yellow fever) and have caused extensive morbidity and mortality (Benenson, 1995).

As discussed earlier in this chapter, a balance between host, agent, and environmental factors must be maintained to prevent disease outbreaks. Altering this balance even slightly can cause significant spread of disease. For example, a daycare worker who neglects to wash his or her hands one time after changing an infant's diaper can transmit bacterial diseases such as salmonellosis. Astute community health professionals have been instrumental in preventing bacterial and other types of disease by carefully observing for environmental and host factors that facilitate disease transmission.

MEASUREMENT OF EPIDEMIOLOGICAL EVENTS

As discussed earlier in this chapter, it is important to monitor the relative *frequency* of an event in time and space to determine health and disease patterns in a community. A variety of methods are used to collect data about these patterns and to identify aggregates at risk in a population. These methods are discussed in Chapter 13 and include such interventions as analyzing all available statistics, carrying out surveys, and interviewing key community informants. Basic statistical concepts used in epidemiology and sources of statistical data are discussed in this chapter.

Types and Sources of Health Statistics

Statistical data aid health professionals in making comparisons over time and between populations. In community health practice, several terms are used to describe health or health-related data. These are biostatistics, vital statistics, morbidity and mortality statistics, and demographic statistics. *Biostatistics* is the overall broad term used to identify any data that delineate health or population events.

Health statistics that describe birth, adoption, death, marriage, divorce, separation, and annulment patterns are labeled *vital statistics*. The National Center for Health Statistics collects and publishes vital statistics from each state. Despite limitations, these data can assist health professionals in examining trends over time and in establishing health improvement plans.

Vital statistics related to the analysis of death trends are classified as *mortality* statistics. Death certificates are used to obtain demographic information about the deceased as well as the frequency of death, the leading causes of death, and premature mortality. This type of information provides a foundation for assessing the level of wellness in the community. For example, infant and maternal death rates have traditionally been used in community health to make judgments about the health status of a community. Deaths in these two population groups are premature, are considered preventable, and are often associated with poor environmental conditions and inadequate health care. Thus they may reflect not only unmet health needs but also deficiencies in the health care delivery system that need to be corrected.

Morbidity statistics are also used to assess the health status of the community. *Morbidity data* describe the extent and distribution of illness and disability in the community, circumstances that affect quality of life as well as productivity. Morbidity in a community is more difficult to evaluate because there is no comprehensive surveillance system that monitors the incidence (new cases) of all conditions contributing to morbidity. Hospital discharge records, cancer registry data, and communicable disease surveillance data are used to obtain select information about the extent and distribution of important health problems (Greenlee, Smith, 1994). Health surveys are selectively conducted to expand the database related to the level of morbidity in a community. As illustrated in the following case scenario, morbidity data can assist the nurse in setting priorities for program planning.

CASE *Scenario*

One midwestern community used morbidity statistics to support the need for a neighborhood health clinic in one of their inner-city districts. A comprehensive analysis of these statistics revealed that 52% of all new tuberculosis cases, 61% of all new syphilis cases, 72% of all new gonorrhea cases, and 37% of all accidental poisoning cases occurred in one particular section of the city in a given period. It was evident from these data that the health needs in this district were much greater than in other sections of the city. Special funds were allocated to determine if a new approach to delivering health services could alter the morbidity trends; significant positive changes were noted after 3 years. Because morbidity statistics were collected before (known as a baseline for comparison) and during the time the clinic was in existence, city officials responded favorably to a request for additional funds to keep the clinic open. Health professionals in this situation had documented the need for, and the effectiveness of, their pilot-health clinic. The use of statistics assisted these health professionals in establishing a neighborhood health center and in keeping the center functioning after the trial period.

Demographic statistics also provide information about significant characteristics of a population which influence community needs and the delivery of health care services. Demographic data describe the number, characteristics, and distribution of people in a given area and socioeconomic changes in the population over time. These data are collected by censuses, special surveys, and registration systems (Duncan, 1988).

Census data provide a wealth of information about a community's population characteristics, such as the size and age structure, educational level, economic status, and household composition. These data provide a baseline for analyzing demographic trends over time. Census tracts and census blocks have been established and maintained throughout the country so that social and economic changes can be easily identified from one census to another.

Census tracts are small areas in large cities that have a population between 3000 and 6000 persons with fairly homogeneous ethnic and socioeconomic characteristics. *Census blocks* are similar to census tracts but are located almost exclusively in nonmetropolitan areas (Robey, 1989). Census data are analyzed because a significant relationship has been documented between educational background, economic status, and living conditions and the frequency of health needs in specified populations (USDHHS, 1991a).

Further sources of health data are shared in Chapter 13. It is important to remember that all data collection systems are subject to error and have limitations. For example, some data collection systems have comprehensive information about a small subset in the population (e.g., cancer registries), whereas others have very selective information on 100% of the population (e.g., census). However, both cancer registries and the census are limited by the amount of information respondents remember and are willing to share. They can also be limited by respondents' interpretations of questions and recording procedures. Users of data systems need to examine strengths and limitations from the perspectives of sample size, characteristics of the population assessed, type of data obtained, and potential sources of inaccuracy (National Center for Health Statistics, 1996). This information is readily available from standardized data sets.

Use of Relative Numbers

When practitioners analyze the *frequency* of health events in populations, they express absolute numbers or actual counts in terms of relative numbers. Using relative numbers makes it easier to compare results in populations of differing sizes or to visualize what proportion of a given population is affected by the event of interest. A relative number is one that shows a relationship between two absolute numbers; this relationship is expressed in terms of a multiplier or a round number. A percentage is an example of a relative number.

The value of using relative numbers becomes clearer when the nurse actually works with raw data. Raw data from populations of differing sizes cannot be compared unless absolute numbers are converted to relative numbers. For example, knowing the number of students who received free lunches in 1996 in each school in the county becomes relevant only when one summarizes the percentage of children in each school who received free lunches. The following figures illustrate how deceptive absolute numbers can be when making comparisons from one population to another; even though the number of children (250 vs. 75) receiving free lunches is much higher in the Burns Park High School, the proportion of children needing free lunches in Kent Elementary School is two times greater than the proportion of children needing free lunches in Burns Park High School:

$$\frac{75}{150} \times 100 = 50\%$$ of the children in Kent Elementary School received free lunches in 1996

$$\frac{250}{1000} \times 100 = 25\%$$ of the children in Burns Park High School received free lunches in 1996

Measures of Central Tendency

At times there is a need to use descriptive measures, such as averages, to organize and characterize health data. This is the situation when a series of measurements or quantitative data are being analyzed. Generally, in any series of data characteristic values tend to cluster near the center of the distribution. Thus averages are often labeled measures of central tendency. The most commonly used averages in community health nursing practice are the arithmetic mean, the median, and the mode.

The *mean* is the arithmetic average of a set of observations. It is the value in a series of data equivalent to the sum of the measurements divided by the number of measurements. The formula for calculating the mean is:

$$\text{Arithmetic mean} = \frac{\text{sum of measurements}}{\text{no. of measurements}}$$

Knowing the mean, or "average," value of a series of measurements helps the community health nurse to identify quickly persons who may have health needs or who are at risk for health problems in the future. Persons who fall far below or far above the average should be comprehensively assessed to determine why this is happening. For example, if the mean weight of children in a second-grade classroom is 51 pounds, a community health nurse would examine why one of these children, who weighs 70 pounds, was deviating so far from the norm.

The *median* is the "middle" value in a series of quantitative data that divides the measurements into two equal parts. That is, 50% of the measurements are less than and 50% are greater than the median value. To calculate the median, the measurements in the distribution must be arranged in order of size.

The median is usually computed when there are very high or very low extremes in a series of measurements, because the mean is distorted by very high or low values but the median is not. For example, when census tract data are reported, median income is usually given because there is such a great variation in family income, ranging from below poverty level to over $50,000.

The *mode* is the measurement that appears most frequently in a series of quantitative data. It is identified by counting the number of times a particular value appears. The measurements do not have to be ordered. The mode is helpful when one wants to identify an average value very quickly. It is only an estimate, however, and not too reliable; other measurements of central tendency should be used when refining data analysis. The mean is the most frequently used measure of central tendency in community health practice because it is the most stable.

Rates and Ratios

In addition to percentages and measures of central tendency, rates and ratios are commonly used to analyze the frequency of health events in a community. A *ratio* is a fraction that expresses the size of one number (numerator) in relation to another number (denominator). It is a general term of which a rate, percentage, and proportion are subsets (Last, 1995). The number of females to males (sex ratio) and per capita expenditure for health care in a given state are examples of ratios. Per capita ratios are obtained by dividing the amount of money spent for health care (event) by the population in a given state.

A *proportion* is a ratio where the numerator is included in the denominator, which means that the population affected is a subset of the total population at risk. A *rate* is also a ratio with the additional features of expressing what has happened in terms of a defined time period and the population at risk for a given event. Some rates are proportions (Last, 1995). Rates delineate the relationship between the number of times an event has occurred to the size of the population at risk. In demographic and epidemiological study, the unit of time for a rate is usually a *year* unless otherwise stated.

A rate is calculated by dividing the number of measured events (numerator) in a specified period by the size of the population at risk (denominator). To adjust for population changes over the year, the estimated midyear population is used as the denominator. A multiplier or a standard base population size is usually used to convert the rate from an awkward fraction or decimal to a whole number: The multiplier is one that makes the rate above the value of 1. For example, if an event such as polio occurs infrequently within a large population at risk, the multiplier used would be "per 100,000 population." On the other hand, when an event such as death occurs frequently within a population at risk, the multiplier used would be "per 1000 population." The relationships between the components of a rate are displayed in the following equation:

$$\text{Rate} = \frac{\text{Number of events in specified period}}{\text{Population at risk during the specified period}} \times \text{multiplier}$$

Frequently used rates and ratios in community health nursing practice are displayed in Table 11-8. It is important to note that some of these rates are restricted by a particular characteristic of interest (e.g., age-specific or cause-specific), whereas others include the total population without reference to any characteristics of the individuals in this population. Rates that restrict the dimensions of the numerator and denominator are known as *specific rates*. Rates that include the total population are known as *general* or *crude rates* (Jekel, Elmore, Katz, 1996). At times a specific rate uses the total population as the denominator because the total population is at risk for a specified event (e.g., cause-specific death rate).

Crude death rates must be standardized or adjusted before comparing them across populations because these rates do not take into consideration the profound impact that age has on death rates (National Center for Health Statistics, 1994). *Standardized rates* or *adjusted rates* are crude rates that have been modified to control for the effects of age or other characteristics and thereby allow for valid comparisons of rates (Jekel, Elmore, Katz, 1996, p. 28).

Morbidity and Mortality Statistics

In epidemiological study morbidity and mortality data are used to provide a foundation for examining the level of health in a community. Crude, or general, death rates assist a community in identifying leading health problems in the

table 11-8 Frequently Used Rates and Ratios in Community Health Nursing Practice

Rate or Ratio	Formula	Commonly Used Multiplier
MORTALITY STATISTICS		
Crude death rate	Number of deaths from all causes during a given year ÷ population estimated at midyear	× 1000 population
Age-specific death rate	Number of deaths for a specified age group during a given year ÷ population estimated at midyear for the specified age group	× 1000 population
Cause-specific death rate	Number of deaths from a specific condition during a given year ÷ population estimated at midyear	× 100,000 population
Maternal mortality rate	Number of deaths from puerperal complications during a given year ÷ number of live births during the same year	× 100,000 live births
Infant mortality rate	Number of deaths under 1 year of age during a given year ÷ number of live births during the same year	× 1000 live births
Neonatal mortality rate	Number of deaths under 28 days of age during a given year ÷ number of live births during the same year	× 1000 live births
Fetal mortality rate	Number of fetal deaths 20 weeks gestation or more during a given year ÷ number of live births and fetal deaths during the same year	× 1000 live births and fetal deaths
Birth-death ratio	Number of live births in a specified population ÷ number of deaths in a specified population	× 100
Case fatality ratio	Number of deaths from specified disease or condition ÷ number of reported cases of the specified disease or condition	× 100
MORBIDITY STATISTICS		
Incidence rate	Number of "new" cases of a specified disease or condition occurring during a given time period ÷ population at risk during the same time period	× 100,000 population
Prevalence rate (ratio)	Number of "old" and "new" cases of specified disease or condition existing at a point ÷ total population at a point	× 100,000 population
VITAL AND DEMOGRAPHIC STATISTICS OTHER THAN MORTALITY		
Crude birth rate	Number of live births during a given year ÷ population estimated at midyear	× 1000 population
General fertility rate	Number of live births during a given year ÷ population estimated at midyear for females ages 15-44 during the same year	× 1000 female population (15-44 years old)
General marriage rate	Number of marriages during a given year ÷ number of persons 15 years of age and over in the population in the same year	× 1000 persons 15 years of age and over
General divorce rate	Number of divorces during a given year ÷ persons 15 years of age and over in the population in the same year	× 1000 persons 15 years of age and over
Dependency ratio	Persons under 20 years of age and persons 65 years and over ÷ total population ages 20-64	× 100

total population. Specific death rates (e.g., age-specific) help a community to target health resources for populations at risk. For example, hypertensive screening and educational programs often target black Americans because the heart disease mortality rate is higher among blacks than among the total population. Formulas for calculating crude and specific death rates are identified in Table 11-8.

A major goal in epidemiology is to prevent premature mortality. The impact of premature death is often described in terms of *Years of Potential Life Lost* (YPLL). The YPLL rate is an age-adjusted measure of premature mortality (death before age 65 years) in a population (Johnson, 1995). Major causes of death that primarily affect younger people, such as infant mortality, homicide, and HIV infections, significantly influence YPLL rates. Significant health disparities among Americans in terms of YPLL continue to be substantiated (USDHHS, 1995a). These disparities are discussed in Chapter 12.

Significant health disparities among Americans in terms of morbidity (disease) also exist. The concepts of incidence and prevalence are used to identify these disparities as well as to track the frequency of disease occurrence. *Incidence* is the number of *new* cases of a disease in a population over a specified period of time. It is often expressed as a rate that is calculated using the following formula:

Incidence Rate =

$$\frac{\text{Number of "new" cases in a specified period}}{\text{Population at risk during the same period}} \times \text{multiplier}$$

Bay City, January through December 1996, 25 new cases of diabetes in a population of 50,000.

$$\text{Incidence rate} = \frac{25}{50,000} \times 100,000 = 50$$

Incidence rate for diabetes in Bay City, 1996: 50 new cases of diabetes per 100,000 population.

Incidence assists community health professionals in examining the rate of increase or decrease of morbidity during a defined time period.

Prevalence examines the extent of morbidity in a community. *Prevalence* is the number of cases (new and old) of a specified disease or condition existing at a given time. Prevalence is often expressed as a rate (National Center for Health Statistics, 1995), which is calculated using the following formula:

Prevalence rate (ratio) = number of "new and old" cases of a specified disease or condition existing at a given point ÷ total population estimated at midyear × a multiplier

Bay City, December 1996, 1200 cases of diabetes in a population of 50,000.

$$\text{Prevalence rate (ratio)} = \frac{600}{50,000} \times 100,000 = 1200$$

Prevalence rate (ratio) for diabetes in Bay City, December 1996: 1200 cases of diabetes per 100,000 population.

Prevalence is also expressed as a percentage (e.g., 1.2% of the population has diabetes in Bay City in December 1996).

The prevalence of disease and conditions in a community is influenced by many factors such as the rate of new cases, the number of existing cases, cause-specific mortality trends, population mobility patterns, and an array of factors that promote disease occurrence. Figure 11-10 illustrates the relationship between incidence and prevalence. Monitoring prevalence and incidence of morbidity assists community planners in developing interventions that prevent disease and promote health.

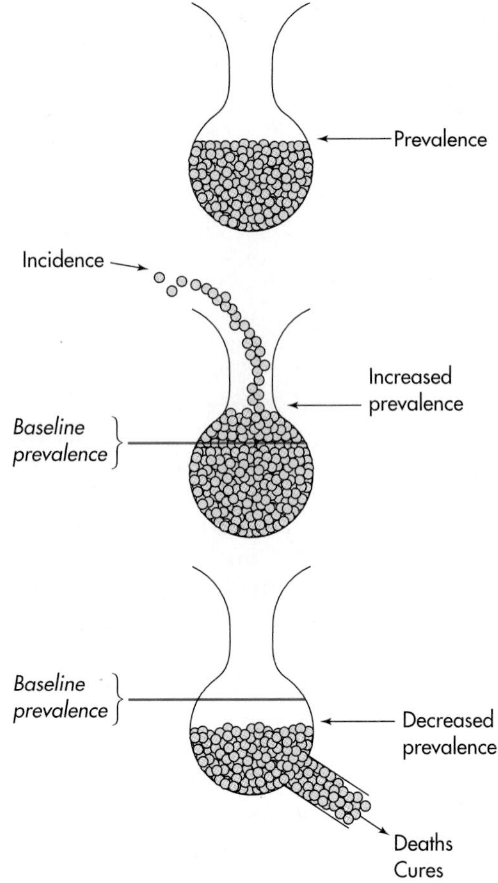

Figure 11-10 Relationship between incidence and prevalence. *(Modified from Gordis L: Epidemiology, Philadelphia, 1996, Saunders, p. 33.)*

EPIDEMIOLOGICAL PROCESS AND INVESTIGATION

Basic concepts in epidemiology have been discussed to lay a foundation for epidemiological investigation of community health problems. These concepts aid in identifying variables that public health professionals consider when they describe the distribution patterns and determinants of health, disease, and condition frequencies in populations. They help to analyze causal relationships in disease or condition outbreaks. To establish these causal relationships, health professionals use a scientific process known as the *epidemiological process*.

The epidemiological process is a systematic course of action taken to identify (1) who is affected (persons); (2) where the affected persons reside (place); (3) when the persons were affected (time); (4) causal factors of health and disease occurrence (host-agent-environment determinants); (5) prevalence and incidence of health and disease (frequencies); and (6) prevention and control measures (levels of prevention) in relation to the natural life history of a disease or a condition.

The epidemiological process has eight basic steps, which are graphically illustrated in Figure 11-1. Although each step is discussed separately, it is important to remember that these steps may overlap and may not always follow a sequential pattern. They are interrelated and dependent on each other. For example, data collected in the initial step provide a foundation for all subsequent steps.

Step I: Determine the Nature, Extent, and Possible Significance of the Problem

The primary responsibilities during this initial step are twofold: (1) to verify the diagnosis by data collection from multiple sources, and (2) to determine the extent and possible significance of the verified problem. Data gathering begins when an index case is reported or when there is a noticeable change in the incidence rate for a particular disease or condition. The *index case* is the case that brings a household or other group to the attention of community health personnel. Once this case is known to health professionals, data are collected from a variety of sources to determine if a problem really exists.

Clinical observations, laboratory studies, and lay reporting assist the epidemiological team in confirming the homogeneity of the current events. If, for instance, four hospital emergency rooms have reported that several individuals were treated for food poisoning in the last 24 hours, health personnel would want to immediately take the following actions:

1. Interview the affected persons to determine the nature of their symptoms and to identify loci of origin according to person, place, and time.
2. Review laboratory studies to confirm a common causative organism. This process could establish that several events are occurring at the same time.
3. Interview friends, relatives, and lay acquaintances to discern their description of the events that led up to the reported illness and to determine if other individuals have symptoms.

It is important to remember that timely, accurate, and thorough data collection are critical factors in Step I. Significant data may be destroyed if the data collection process is too slow. In addition, if only the "tip of the iceberg," or the most obvious events, are observed, the extent of the problem will not be identified. The health professional needs to be like a detective, beginning by interviewing the affected individual and then branching out into this individual's environment to track down the host-agent-environment factors that influence disease occurrence. As previously discussed, the measurable variables that facilitate rapid and efficient data collection about host-agent-environment factors are person, place, and time.

Analyzing data in terms of person, place, and time helps to establish the magnitude of the problem. Data tell the health professional the proportion of the people affected, the seriousness of the effects on the host and the community, improvement or regression over time, and geographical distribution of the disease or condition. They also help in identifying potential sources of infection and causal relationships.

The use of spot maps (see "Analysis of All Available Data" in Chapter 13) facilitates pinpointing the exact geographical location of the disease or condition. This type of map vividly and visually portrays an epidemiological problem very rapidly. If it is used on a regular basis, health personnel can compare current prevalence and incidence with the expected rates and can identify significant departures from normal.

When comparing prevalence and incidence rates, a word of caution is necessary. If there is a distinct departure from normal, it must be ascertained that a problem really exists. It may be that there is only an improvement in reporting, not an actual increase in disease occurrence.

If there has been an actual increase in the incidence of a particular disease or condition, the health professional makes an educated guess as to the nature of the causative agent, based upon the data collected. This formulation of a tentative diagnosis or hypothesis is done to enhance further data collection.

Step II: Formulate Tentative Hypothesis(es)

When dealing with infectious diseases a rapid preliminary analysis of data is imperative. This is essential because infectious diseases can spread quickly, can affect a large number of people in a short period of time, and can have great ranges in severity. Usually this analysis results in the formulation of several hypotheses. Explanation of the most probable source of infection is made in terms of (1) the agent causing the problem; (2) the source of infection, including the chain of events leading to the outbreak of the problem; and (3) environmental conditions that allowed it to occur. Tentative hypotheses must be tested and may be found to be inappropriate. Laboratory tests are invaluable in validating hypotheses. An example of how tentative hypotheses are established is provided in the following scenario. This scenario reflects a commonly occurring community health problem.

CASE Scenario

From September 5-8, the "World's Largest American Indian Fair" was held near Gallup, New Mexico (Horwitz, Pollard, Merson, Martin, 1977, pp. 1071-1076). An estimated 80,000 persons attended the fair. Beginning on September 6th, and during the next few days, several hundred people with gastrointestinal symptoms sought attention at two hospitals near Gallup. Over 130 of them had stool cultures positive for a *Salmonella* group C organism, *Salmonella newport*. The hospitals immediately reported the apparent outbreak to the health department. Preliminary tentative hypotheses indicated that either the community water supply of the area or food served at a free barbeque that attracted thousands on September 5th was the vehicle of transmission for the agent *Salmonella newport*. Evidence favoring a water source included a broken water pipe at the fair grounds in an area soiled with animal feces. The barbeque was suspected because food preparation practices were reportedly improper and those who attended the barbeque appeared to have a high illness attack rate.

Since two possible sources of infection were favored in this situation, health personnel took immediate steps to correct both problem situations and collected and analyzed further data to determine the exact cause of the *Salmonella* outbreak.

Waiting until all data are collected before instituting control measures can amplify the magnitude of the problem. A health professional must be willing to take risks while carrying out an epidemiological investigation.

Step III: Collect and Analyze Further Data to Test Hypothesis(es)

A basic starting point in this step is to identify the group selected for attack by the disease or problem under investigation. Individual epidemiological health histories should be done to classify persons according to their exposure to suspected or causative agents and to identify the clinical data and bacteriological findings needed to substantiate the diagnosis. Significant variation of incidence in contrasted population groups should then be noted. These variations can be identified through study of attack rates.

An *attack rate* is an incidence rate that identifies the number of people at risk who became ill. In studying an outbreak of foodborne disease such as the one at the American Indian Fair, the attack rate for persons who ate certain foods would be compared with the attack rate for persons who did not eat certain foods. This is done in an attempt to identify which food was infected by the causative agent.

Attack rates are calculated in the following manner:

$$\frac{\text{No. of persons affected}}{\text{No. of persons eating food item}} \times 100$$

$$\frac{\text{No. of persons affected}}{\text{No. of persons } \textit{not} \text{ eating food item}} \times 100$$

Table 11-9 illustrates how attack rates are graphically summarized. The attack rates in this table were calculated when people became ill after a banquet. They show that one food item, custard, was probably the infected food (note the differences between the two attack rate percentages). Generally the vulnerable food that shows the greatest differences between the two attack rate percentages is the infected food.

It is essential to remember that attack rates do not positively confirm an infective food. Last (1986, pp. 35-36) has identified the following five reasons why the association of illness with a particular food is often difficult:

1. Some individuals are resistant to the agent and do not become ill even though they are exposed.
2. The definition of an ill person employed may include some who have unrelated illnesses, unless there is a specific test; and even then, if the illness is one that is prevalent, the ill subjects may include some cases not caused by the ingestion of the common vehicle.
3. Contamination of one food by traces of another may take place before or during serving.
4. Errors in history-taking may occur. These may be unbiased errors, caused by memory lapses or misunderstanding, or they may be caused by biases, either on the part of the questioner or the subject. Several kinds of biases are possible; the questioner may have a preconceived notion of what food was responsible and press his questions more vigorously with respect to that food in the case of ill persons than non-ill persons; or the subject may have preconceived notions leading to the same result. The subject may have reasons for wishing to either claim or disclaim illness. Biases may affect the accuracy either of food histories or illness histories and produce spurious association.
5. Finally, biased sampling may also lead to spurious results.

All of these factors can affect the validity of an attack rate and thereby the choice of the appropriate infective food. Laboratory studies are necessary to identify the etiological agent and its vehicle or vector. However, identifying the causative agent is not the only step in preventing further spread of disease. Knowing the agent assists in treating ill individuals who seek medical care but does not tell how the disease is being transmitted. The chain of transmission must be broken to stop the spread of disease.

Since one factor alone never causes a disease or condition, it is not sufficient to identify only a causative agent and the infective food. After the possible agents and the attack group have been identified, the common source(s) to which affected individuals were exposed should be investigated. With foodborne disease the origin, method, and preparation of suspected foods would be primary factors to examine. Concurrently, environmental conditions should be evaluated. These conditions would include such things

table 11-9 Attack Rate Table

	Persons Who Did Eat Vulnerable Food				Persons Who Did Not Eat Vulnerable Food			
Vulnerable Food	Sick	Well	Total	Attack Rate (%)	Sick	Well	Total	Attack Rate (%)
Baked ham	19	56	75	25	30	5	35	86
Custard	45	15	60	**75**	4	46	50	**8**
Jello	20	35	55	36	29	26	55	53
Cole slaw	48	58	106	45	1	3	4	25
Baked beans	45	55	100	45	4	6	10	40
Potato salad	25	45	70	36	24	16	40	60

From Communicable Disease Center: *Food-borne disease investigation: analysis of field data*, Atlanta, 1964, U.S. Public Health Service, p. 8.

as the sanitary status of the restaurant, the area where food was served, and the water and dairy supply. Appendix 11-1 depicts the type of data that one state collects when enteric infections such as *Salmonella newport* are suspected. Community health nurses are frequently responsible for collecting these data during an epidemiological investigation. In some health departments nurses are also responsible for collecting specimens for laboratory analysis. The epidemiological division of the state or local health department will provide information on how to properly collect, preserve, and ship specimens for epidemiological analysis.

Completing an epidemiological case history form provides an opportunity for health teaching and casefinding. Often the community health nurse identifies new cases during this process and helps clients to learn about the nature of the disease and how to prevent its spread.

It is important to use a variety of data-collection methods in determining the extent and source of an epidemiological problem because individuals who have only minor symptoms of illness often do not seek treatment. In the Gallup, New Mexico, outbreak, the extent of the problem was determined by a large questionnaire survey conducted from September 19-25. Using recently made maps of dwellings in the area, 500 dwellings housing 2000 persons were randomly selected for a visit by an interviewer who completed a questionnaire. The interviewer inquired about the occurrence and characteristics of diarrheal illnesses, the types and location of the household water supply, the amount of water consumed at the fair, the time of eating at the barbeque, and the types of food eaten. This survey revealed that attendance at the barbeque was highly associated with illness and confirmed laboratory studies that eliminated water as a vehicle of transmission. It also showed that eating potato salad at the barbeque was strongly associated with illness (Horwitz, Pollard, Merson, Martin, 1977, pp. 1072, 1074).

Often food is strongly associated with gastrointestinal illness, especially when the illness occurs among a large number of people who have attended a social gathering. As was previously discussed, eating custard at a banquet (see Table 11-9) was associated with illness.

Tentative hypothesis(es) must be tested. The survey conducted at Gallup, New Mexico helped to confirm one of the original hypotheses on the source of contamination, the food served at the barbeque, and eliminated another, the contaminated water. At times, however, none of the original hypotheses is appropriate.

Testing hypothesis(es) helps to determine if the initial control measures were sufficient to resolve the current outbreak. It also aids in identifying the natural life history of the disease and where further action is needed.

Step IV: Plan for Control

When planning for control, it is essential to identify preventive activities based on the knowledge of the natural history of the disease in question, which can be used to control the further spread of disease occurrence. Host-agent-environment factors should be analyzed to determine the following:

1. Populations at risk
2. Primary, secondary, and tertiary preventive measures available that would
   a. Alter the behavior or susceptibility of the host (e.g., health education, casefinding, immunization, treatment, or rehabilitation)
   b. Destroy the agent (e.g., heat, drug treatment, or spraying with insecticides)
   c. Eliminate the transmission of the agent (e.g., changes in host's health habits or environmental conditions)
3. Feasibility of implementing the control plan, considering such factors as available community resources, time required, cost of control versus partial or no control, facilities, supplies, and personnel needed
4. Priorities in relation to legal mandates, significance of the problem relative to other community needs, and the feasibility of implementing the control plan

PUBLIC OPINION Public opinion can have a significant impact on the effectiveness of any control plan. In the Gallup outbreak of salmonellosis, one control measure could have been to ban future food preparation and consumption for groups of persons numbering over 100 so that careful attention could be given to details. It is highly unlikely that this plan would be well received, since fairs are a major form of recreation on the Navajo Nation Indian Reservation and people travel considerable distances to attend them. Clearly stating regulations for food preparation, with the mandatory attendance of one environmentalist per 1000 persons to oversee food preparation, would probably be a more realistic control measure for this situation.

BREAKING THE CHAIN OF TRANSMISSION Control measures are generally directed toward breaking the chain of transmission (see Figure 11-7). This includes destroying or treating the reservoir of infection, interrupting the transmission of the agent from the reservoir to the new host, and decreasing the ability of the agent to adapt and multiply within the host. When attempting to break the chain of transmission, the concept of multiple causation must be applied.

Referring again to the Gallup outbreak, the major cause of the disease was error in food preparation. There was prolonged storage of precooked ingredients for potato salad within the 44° to 114° F range in which *Salmonella* have been demonstrated to multiply. The initial source of the *Salmonella* is unknown (Horwitz, Pollard, Merson, Martin, 1977, p. 1074). As is often the case, the food handlers at this large gathering were laypersons and their work was unsupervised. Large gatherings of people at which food is served should be considered high-risk settings for foodborne disease outbreak. It is advisable to have an epidemiologically trained person monitoring food preparation, storage, and serving at such occasions.

HERD IMMUNITY When one is dealing with infectious diseases and establishing a control plan, the concept of herd immunity is also important to consider. *Herd immunity* is the immunity level of a specific group. Immunity is "that resistance usually associated with possession of antibodies that have an inhibitory effect on a specific microorganism, or its toxin, that causes a particular infectious disease" (CDC, 1987a, p. 42). Characteristics of the different types of immunity are presented in Table 11-6.

If 100% of a given group had received measles vaccine, the herd immunity would be 100%. If 80% had received measles vaccine, the herd immunity would be at least 80%. Some people in the group have natural immunity, raising the percentage higher.

Herd immunity does not have to be 100% to prevent an epidemic or to control a disease, but it is not known just what percentage is safe. Communities usually strive to achieve at least a 90% to 95% herd immunity level. A national goal is to increase basic immunization levels among children under age 2 to at least 90% and among children in child care facilities and kindergarten through postsecondary education institutions to at least 95% (USDHHS, 1991a, p. 521).

It is important to realize that as herd immunity decreases, the chances for epidemics rise. In the United States a major concern is that many school-age children are not receiving immunizations for communicable disease. Immunization coverage levels vary substantially by state and large urban areas (CDC, 1996c). This greatly decreases the level of herd immunity and is a major barrier to maintaining community health.

Community health nurses are instrumental in helping the public to see the need for effective control of disease by active immunization. This will continue to be a major function of the community health nurse, because immunizing populations at risk is the most effective way to control many childhood communicable diseases (see Chapter 15 for immunization schedules).

CASEFINDING Casefinding is a major function of epidemiologists and community health nurses. This process focuses on early diagnosis and treatment by discovery of new cases of a disease or condition. It may evolve through clinical observation or laboratory tests and may involve mass or individual testing. Casefinding may also evolve through door-to-door surveying, as in the Gallup, New Mexico situation discussed previously. Opportunities for casefinding are limitless and come through home visits, clinic nursing, school visits, and prenatal classes, to name only a few. Community health nurses in these settings can pick up casefinding clues such as a tired young mother who seems unable to handle her three preschool children, possible scoliosis in a preadolescent girl, or a developmental delay in a toddler. By being alert to such clues many situations will be identified in which nursing skills can be used to prevent disease and promote health. In some instances of casefinding, such as child abuse, a perceptive nurse may observe tendencies of abusive behavior in a parent and be able to assist the parent in working through these tendencies. This could prevent the abuse.

Step V: Implement Control Plan

An active effort should be made to elicit and coordinate the cooperation of the lay public, as well as private and official agencies, when putting control measures into operation. A control program that takes into consideration the beliefs, attitudes, and customs of the community is more likely to be accepted by the public than one that ignores community norms. Health education programs can help to "sell" a control program in the community, especially if they deal with current community attitudes and beliefs.

To evaluate the effectiveness of a control program, broad goals and specific objectives for the program must be identified before the program begins. Defining broad goals and specific outcome objectives such as the ones below makes it easier to determine if control efforts are successful.

Broad Goal: To increase the herd immunity level for DTP to 95% in Centerville.

Objectives: To increase the herd immunity level for DTP in census tracts 4 and 5 by 25% in 4 months by immunizing kindergarten and first-, fifth-, and tenth-grade students.

To increase the herd immunity level for DTP in census tracts 8 and 9 by 17% in 4 months by immunizing kindergarten and first-, fifth-, and tenth-grade students.

Control measures involve primary, secondary, and/or tertiary preventive activities. They include things such as disease reporting, quarantine, environmental control, human carrier control, health education, activities to decrease host susceptibility (e.g., immunizations), and technological advances.

BARRIERS TO CONTROL PROGRAMS There are many barriers to the successful implementation of a control program for both infectious disease and noncommunicable conditions. Barriers to control involve factors such as unknown etiology, no known treatment, unavailable community resources, multifactorial etiology, long latency periods, and lack of reporting.

Low levels of immunity in an exposed population group increase the likelihood of disease occurrence. Mass and individual immunization programs are effective in raising immunity levels for some diseases. For many diseases, however, there are no specific prophylactic immunizations. Examples of such diseases are impetigo and STDs.

Individuals without overt disease symptoms but who harbor the disease organism can be a major vehicle in disease transmission. These individuals are known as *carriers*. Typhoid and salmonellosis are examples of diseases that are often transmitted by carriers.

With any disease and for a variety of reasons, some individuals will delay or not seek treatment. Whatever the reason, a delay in confirmation and treatment of the disease can enhance its spread and continuation and impede control plan implementation.

Individuals for whom the diagnosis is not suspected or confirmed are also barriers to the control of disease. Disease may not be confirmed for several reasons. Some people will evidence atypical symptoms of the disease in question. If clinical symptoms do not fit a disease model the disease may be missed completely or misdiagnosed. Other individuals are seen too early or too late in the course of the disease process to either suspect or confirm the disease. In these situations laboratory tests may be falsely negative, or they may not be done at all because the clinical symptoms do not reflect a need. At other times a diagnosis cannot be confirmed because specimens (stools, emesis, or sputum) have inadvertently been destroyed or handled improperly. When working in the home or in other health care settings it is vitally important to recognize that laboratory tests are needed to confirm most infectious disease diagnoses.

Lack of reporting, often reflecting nonacceptance of a diagnosis, is one of the key barriers in a control program. This can result from clerical error, indifference, fear, shame, or any of a number of variables. In some instances professionals may not want to get involved or do not feel it appropriate to become involved. This is especially true when a social problem such as gonorrhea or child abuse is the disease or condition in question.

Community health nurses need to be acutely aware of these barriers because they are frequently in a position to help individuals, families, or health care professionals overcome them. Through the use of the referral process, knowledge of community resources, interviewing skills, and the ability to understand both health and disease processes, the community health nurse is uniquely able to assist in resolving these barriers.

Step VI: Evaluate Control Plan

An important part of the epidemiological process is evaluation. This ensures that a process can be improved the next time it is repeated. It also ensures, through the problem-solving approach, that all elements of a problem have been reviewed. The first step in evaluation is to determine how well the objectives of the process were met. This implies that, before carrying out the process, objectives were clearly and behaviorally written. The next question to be answered is how the current situation compares to the situation before the investigation. Finally, the practicality of the control measures should be determined. Feasibility and cost in terms of money, time, staff, facilities, and community support should be analyzed.

Step VII: Make Appropriate Report

Prompt, accurate, and concise epidemiological reporting will provide a basis for future investigations and control measures. Appropriate reporting demonstrates to the community the health professionals' accountability and clarifies the epidemiological situation. Reporting should include what was involved in the epidemiological process: diagnosis, factors leading to the epidemic, control measures, process evaluation, and recommendations for preventing similar situations.

Underreporting of many epidemiological investigations occurs. This happens for many reasons. Completion of necessary forms can be tedious and time consuming and, therefore, neglected. Frequently there is no one person assigned the responsibility for seeing that reports are completed, so the responsibility is overlooked. Usually more effective reporting occurs when one person is designated to coordinate the reporting activities of others.

Societal and individual values and attitudes also contribute to underreporting. At times, conditions such as STDs, alcoholism, or mental illness are not discussed or reported because health care professionals are afraid to disturb the status quo in the community.

Accurate reporting is essential for the identification of major community health problems and preventive health action that would correct these problems. Treating only individuals with overt symptoms, rather than collecting and reporting data on populations at risk, does very little to prevent future health problems.

Step VIII: Conduct Research

If health services to populations are to be improved, epidemiological research is essential. Health professionals must be prepared to collect and analyze data systematically so that the gaps in knowledge relative to disease causation, prevention, and control are eliminated. The ultimate goal of epidemiology—the prevention and control of infectious diseases, chronic conditions, and other health-related phenomena in populations—is far from being realized. Infectious diseases such as gonorrhea, syphilis, hepatitis, enteric disorders, and tuberculosis are still major health problems. In spite of scientific advances in the development of immunizations that prevent communicable diseases, epidemic outbreaks of childhood conditions, especially measles and diphtheria, continue to occur. Noninfectious conditions such as accidents and substance abuse, and chronic diseases including cancer and heart conditions, are fast-growing problems. Because of their complex nature, very little is known regarding their etiology or ways to prevent and control them. It is unfortunate that research in the practice setting is often lacking. Research can be exciting and challenging, especially when one discovers significant data that will aid a community to better its health status.

PUBLIC HEALTH SURVEILLANCE

Epidemiologic surveillance is an essential public health function at all levels of government. "Epidemiologic surveillance is the ongoing and systematic collection, analysis, and interpretation of health data in the process of describing and monitoring a health event. This information is used for planning, implementing, and evaluating public health interventions and programs. Surveillance data are used both to determine the need for public health action and to assess the effectiveness of programs" (CDC, 1988b, p. 1).

Public health surveillance activities date back more than three centuries. In the United States these activities were formalized by Congress in 1878 when Congress authorized the U.S. Marine Hospital Service (the forerunner of today's Public Health Service) to collect morbidity reports from U.S. consuls overseas (CDC, 1996d). Consistent with the development of epidemiology, public health surveillance was traditionally limited to the monitoring of infectious diseases. Today public health surveillance systems monitor a variety of issues, including the incidence and prevalence of infectious and noninfectious diseases, the impact associated with these conditions, health risk behaviors in the overall population, components of population growth, and health services, resources, and policy trends. There is a wide range of surveillance data collection systems in the United States. Some of these are discussed in Appendix 13-2).

On a national level, the Centers for Disease Control and Prevention (CDC) is the major agency responsible for public health surveillance. It maintains a national morbidity reporting system that collects, compiles, and publishes demographic, clinical, and laboratory data on many infectious and chronic diseases and conditions from each state. Each state has a department or departments responsible for morbidity reporting to the CDC. Figure 11-11 shows the reporting relationships between local, state, and federal agencies. These relationships extend internationally. The CDC provides an annual summary of disease reports from states to the World Health Organization (WHO) and promptly notifies WHO of any reported cases of the internationally quarantinable diseases (CDC, 1996d).

Because reporting can be mandated only at the state level, reporting to CDC by the states is *voluntary* (CDC, 1996d). State health departments maintain a morbidity reporting system based on regulations adopted by the state board of health. The state board of health derives its authority to issue regulations from acts of the state legislature.

The Council of State and Territorial Epidemiologists is now the CDC's primary collaborator for determining what diseases and conditions are nationally reported (CDC, 1996d). "A notifiable disease is one for which regular, frequent, and timely information on individual cases is considered necessary for the prevention and control of the disease" (CDC, 1994b, p. 800). As of June 1996, 52 infectious diseases were notifiable nationally. In addition, three noninfectious conditions (elevated blood lead levels, silicosis, and acute pesticide poisoning/injuries) and one health risk behavior (prevalence of cigarette smoking) were included in the list of conditions designated as reportable by states to CDC. A listing of notifiable diseases and conditions is provided in Appendix 11-2. This listing changes regularly. Elevated blood lead levels was the first noninfectious condition

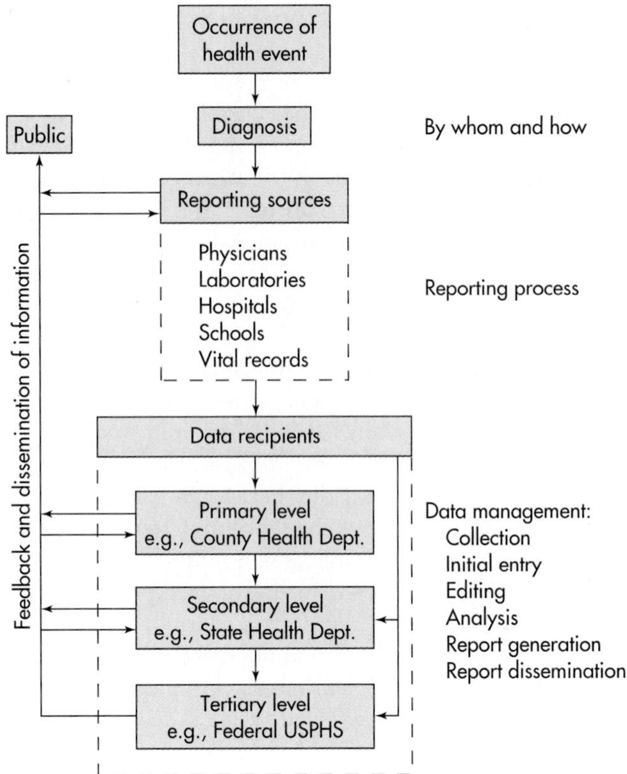

Figure 11-11 United States surveillance system flow chart. *(From Centers for Disease Control (CDC): Guidelines for evaluating surveillance systems,* MMWR *37[Suppl No. S-5]:1-18, 1988, p. 17.)*

added to the list of nationally notifiable diseases. It was included in 1995. The addition of a health risk behavior to the list in 1996 also marked a first (CDC, 1996d). These firsts reflect current trends in epidemiological study.

EPIDEMIOLOGICAL CHALLENGES OF THE FUTURE

Many contemporary challenges for epidemiologists exist. These challenges include the control of infectious and chronic diseases as well as selected psychosocial health phenomena. A major challenge on the epidemiological frontier is the control of acquired immunodeficiency syndrome (AIDS), which is at epidemic proportions in the United States today. AIDS is discussed extensively in Chapter 12.

Infectious Disease: A Neglected Public Health Mandate

The Institute of Medicine's Committee for the Study of the Future of Public Health (1988) alerted the nation in the late 1980s that the control and prevention of infectious disease has become a neglected mandate in the U.S. public health system. The Committee believed that the past strides made in infectious disease control and eradication in the United States have come to be taken for granted

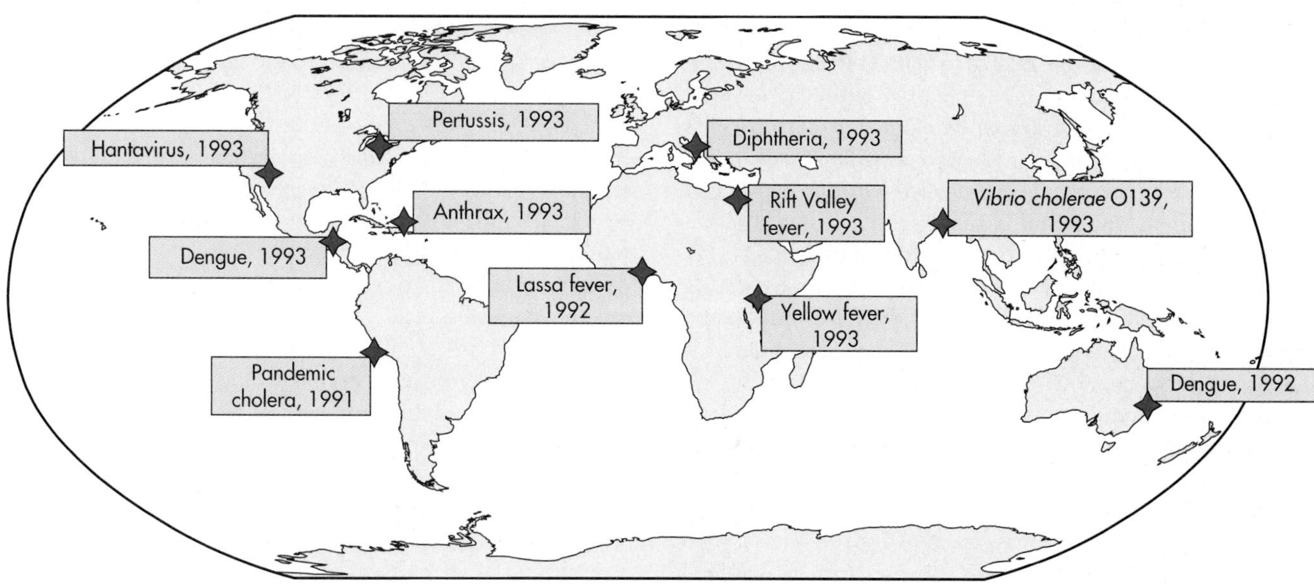

Figure **11-12** Examples of emerging and resurgent infectious diseases in the 1990s. *(From Centers for Disease Control and Prevention (CDC):* Addressing emerging infectious disease threats: a prevention strategy for the United States, *Atlanta, 1994, National Center for Infectious Diseases, p. 8.)*

and that the nation has become increasingly lax in many of its infectious disease practices. Although the CDC achieved notable success in the 1970s and 1980s in tracking new and mysterious disease outbreaks, such as legionnaires' disease and toxic-shock syndrome, and played a key role in the eradication of smallpox (CDC, 1996a), goals such as the eradication of measles by 1977 were not achieved.

Major epidemics of infectious diseases continue to occur in the United States. Influenza is still claiming thousands of lives each year and major *foodborne* (CDC, 1993d; 1993e; 1993f; 1996e), *waterborne* (CDC, 1994a; 1996f), and *vectorborne* (CDC, 1994c) disease outbreaks have been documented in the 1990s. "In the spring of 1993, contamination of a municipal water supply with the intestinal parasite *Cryptosporidium* caused the largest recognized outbreak of waterborne illness in the history of the United States; an estimated 403,000 persons in Milwaukee, Wisconsin, had prolonged diarrhea, and approximately 4400 persons required hospitalization" (CDC, 1994a, p. 2).

Emerging infectious diseases are posing a major threat in the United States and worldwide (Figure 11-12 and the box at right). "Emerging infectious diseases are diseases of infectious origin whose incidence in humans has increased within the past two decades or threatens to increase in the near future" (Institute of Medicine, 1992). Major host, agent, and environmental changes worldwide are significantly influencing this trend. Examples of these changes are disruptions in environmental habitats, microbial adaptation, economic impoverishment, increased international travel, unsafe sexual habits, and the increased frequency of environmental disasters (CDC, 1994a).

Examples of Emerging Infectious Diseases

UNITED STATES

- *E. coli* 0157:H7 disease
- Cryptosporidiosis
- Coccidioidomycosis
- Multidrug-resistant pneumococcal disease
- Vancomycin-resistant enterococcal infections
- Influenza A/Beijing/32/92
- Hantavirus infections

OUTSIDE THE UNITED STATES

- Cholera in Latin America
- Yellow fever in Kenya
- *Vibrio cholerae* 0139 in Asia
- *E. coli* 0157:H7 in South Africa and Swaziland
- Rift Valley fever in Egypt
- Multidrug-resistant *Shigella dysenteriae* in Burundi
- Dengue in Costa Rica
- Diphtheria in Russia

From CDC: *Addressing emerging infectious disease threats: a prevention strategy for the United States*, Atlanta, 1994a, National Center for Infectious Diseases, p. 2.

A GLOBAL PERSPECTIVE The world is facing a global crisis in infectious disease prevention and control. Annually almost half of the 50 million deaths worldwide are directly related to an infectious or parasitic disease; among children, 4.1 million deaths are related to respiratory infections,

3 million each are related to diarrheal disease and tuberculosis, and 1 million each are related to malaria and measles. Additionally, almost half of the population of the world is exposed to malaria to some degree, over one third of the world's population is now infected with *Mycobacterium* tuberculosis, more than 2 billion people are infected with the hepatitis B virus, and more than 16 million adults and 1 million children have acquired HIV infection since the start of the HIV/AIDS pandemic (WHO, 1995, pp. 192-195). These statistics dramatically reflect the magnitude of the infectious disease prevention and control problem. They also reflect a need for a global perspective when infectious disease concerns are addressed. Current international relationships make the United States particularly vulnerable to emerging disease occurrence; international travel, the United States' immigration patterns, and worldwide economic relationships increase the likelihood of disease transmission.

"Global control of infectious diseases can be realized" (Stoeckle, Douglas, 1996). Experiences with the eradication of smallpox and the control of paralytic poliomyelitis have demonstrated that concerted international efforts can produce remarkable results. However, as the population deals with the "emerging killers" such as AIDS, tuberculosis, Hantavirus infections, and Ebola virus hemorrhagic fever, control efforts designed to address common infectious diseases must not be neglected. These diseases can cause significant mortality and morbidity. Appendix 11-3 presents epidemiological information about select common communicable diseases. Chapter 12 addresses the epidemiology of commonly acquired sexually transmitted diseases, including AIDS.

UNIVERSAL PRECAUTIONS—AN ESSENTIAL BUT NOT SUFFICIENT CONTROL MEASURE Primary prevention is the most cost-effective and humane approach to the control of infectious diseases. While the costs of care associated with the treatment of these diseases are tremendous, they do not take into consideration quality of life issues. The burdens of infectious diseases are significant for both society and clients who have acquired them.

Preventing and controlling infectious disease requires that persons at risk for transmitting or acquiring infections change their behaviors (CDC, 1993c). Behavioral aspects of infectious disease control are a leading factor in allowing these diseases to spread. Persons at risk include health care providers as well as clients. It is well documented that lack of adherence to infection control procedures, such as universal precautions, has caused infectious disease among health care workers and clients.

Adherence to universal precautions is essential. This method of infection control was developed by CDC in the mid-1980s to highlight the need to maintain safeguards for protecting workers who are at risk of exposure to bloodborne pathogens, such as the human immunodeficiency (HIV) and hepatitis B (HBV) viruses, and other potentially infectious materials (CDC, 1987c). The importance of maintaining universal precautions was reinforced in 1992 when the Occupational Safety and Health Administration's (OSHA) regulation of bloodborne pathogens was passed (OSHA, 1992).

Based on CDC's universal precautions recommendation, OSHA's bloodborne pathogens standard *requires* that all employers and employees "assume that *all* human blood and specified human body fluids are infectious for HIV, HBV, and other bloodborne pathogens. Where differentiation of types of body fluids is difficult or impossible, *all* body fluids *are* to be considered as potentially *infectious*" (OSHA, 1992). All clinical sites should have a copy of OSHA's Bloodborne Pathogens Standards, which reinforces the need to use sound infection control techniques in the clinical setting, such as handwashing, use of protective equipment, and proper care of needles.

Implementation of universal precautions does not eliminate the need for other category or disease-specific isolation precautions such as those for infectious diarrhea or pulmonary tuberculosis. Special precautions are strongly recommended for oral examinations and treatments in the dental setting and during phlebotomy. In addition to universal precautions, detailed precautions have been developed for procedures and/or settings in which prolonged or intensive exposures to blood occur, such as invasive procedures, dentistry, autopsies or morticians' services, dialysis, and the clinical laboratory.

TUBERCULOSIS: A REEMERGING KILLER Tuberculosis (TB) has been a major killer throughout recorded history. Worldwide it continues to rank among the leading causes of mortality and morbidity. Despite unparalleled biomedical achievement of effective prophylaxis and chemotherapy, it is estimated that the annual incidence of new cases of tuberculosis is about 8 million and that this disease causes almost 3 million deaths annually worldwide (WHO, 1995). In the United States a steady three-decade decline in TB came to a halt in 1984. Beginning in 1985, substantial increases appeared in high-risk populations (Table 11-10). This upward trend continued through 1992 and resulted in over 51,000 more TB cases than expected by the CDC, given earlier decreases (GAO, 1995, p. 8). Despite a recent downward trend, TB remains a major problem in the United States. Although the prevalence of TB varies significantly among different segments of the U.S. population, there is major concern about the potential spread of TB to the general population. During the 1990s there has been documented evidence that transmission of TB to the general population has been associated with air travel and with contact with peers in high school settings (CDC, 1995; GAO, 1995). Additionally, recent outbreaks of TB in health care settings indicate a substantial risk for TB among health care workers in some geographical areas (CDC, 1996g, p. 4).

"At no time in recent history has tuberculosis been as great a concern as it is today" (CDC, 1992a). In addition to the increase of reported cases, recent outbreaks of multidrug-resistant tuberculosis (MDR-TB) have posed a threat to the public's health. Factors contributing to the recent epidemic

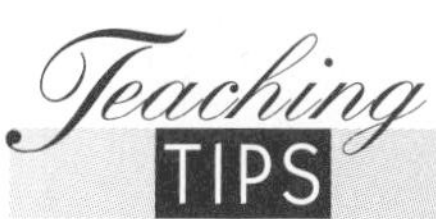

Client Education for Infection Control

Client education is a major focus of community health nurses when providing care. Community health nurses should instruct the client and caregiver about infectious disease, mechanisms of transmission, and specific infection control procedures such as proper techniques in handwashing and needle disposal.

Although community health nurses should use sterile technique when performing all procedural care, clean technique can be taught to the client and caregiver when managing illness at home. Information must be imparted so that the client and caregiver can safely manage infectious disease in the home. The home itself becomes another variable in client management. With this in mind, the following guidelines are recommended.

Bathroom

- When others must share a bathroom with a client whose disease is spread by stool, request that the client cover the faucet and handles with tissue paper before touching them.
- The client should also use a separate toothbrush and drinking glass.
- The person cleaning the bathroom should wear rubber gloves; the gloves should be disinfected with a 10% bleach solution after use; and cracked or torn rubber gloves should be discarded.
- Damp towels and wash cloths should be removed as quickly as possible.
- Recommend that the family use a liquid soap. If the client has an outdoor toilet, 3 to 4 cups of lime should be placed in the toilet weekly.
- The room should be aired out, if possible.

Personal Hygiene

- Clients should be taught to wash their hands in soap and water before and after evacuating bowels or bladder and before handling food. They should cover their mouth when coughing or sneezing and then wash their hands.
- Paper or tissues used by a client experiencing a productive cough need to be discarded into a plastic garbage bag.
- Caregivers should wash their hands before and after delivery of client care.
- The client's body should be kept clean with soap and water baths.
- Gloves should be worn whenever there is a possibility of touching a client's blood or body substances.

Pets

- Pets sometimes harbor organisms (in excreta or hair) that may pose a threat of serious illness to someone with a compromised immune system.
- AIDS clients in particular should not be responsible for cleaning the bird cage, cat litter box, or fish tank.

Other

- Soiled bedpans and commodes should be cleaned with bleach or household detergent and hot water.
- Disposable supplies used during client care should be placed in a separate plastic bag from the rest of the family trash and sealed.
- Sharp containers should be stored in an area that is inaccessible to children or to others who may be injured by them.
- Both plastic bags and needle containers should be disposed of in compliance with local public health department and community waste disposal regulations. Usually, the regular trash disposal system can be used, but local authorities should be consulted if there are any questions.

Kitchen

- Instruct the family to keep the refrigerator clean and set the temperature at 45° F.
- Weekly cleaning of the inside of the refrigerator with regular household cleaning agents will help control microbial growth.
- There is no need to prepare the client's food with separate cooking utensils, but clients should be discouraged from sharing the food off their plate with other members of the household.
- The client's utensils and dishes do not necessarily need to be isolated from those used by other household members if they are washed thoroughly with hot, soapy water. However, the use of common or unclean eating utensils should be avoided. Instruct household members to wash the client's dishes last and then disinfect the sink with a 10% bleach solution.

Laundry

- Soiled linen should be handled as little as possible and should be bagged at the location where it was used.
- Caregivers should be instructed to store infected linen in a separate, leakproof plastic bag and to keep the bag tied shut.
- Hands should be washed immediately after handling soiled laundry to prevent spread of infection.
- Contaminated linens should be washed separately from household laundry in extremely hot water (160° F for 5 minutes). One cup of household bleach in addition to the detergent should be added to each load of laundry. The wash cycle should be run through twice, and then the laundry should be dried.
- To clean the washer, the caregiver should run the empty machine through a complete cycle using a commercial disinfectant or 1 cup of full-strength bleach.
- Rubber gloves should be worn when handwashing soiled laundry and then disinfected with a 10% bleach solution.

Client's Room

- Encourage daily cleaning of the room.
- Items such as toys, books, and games may be cleaned with soap and water or wiped down with alcohol.
- Trash containers should be washed with soap and water and sprayed with commercial disinfectant.
- Floors and furniture should be washed with germicidal solution.

From *Mosby's home health nursing pocket consultant*, St Louis, 1995, Mosby, pp. 160-162.

table 11-10 Tuberculosis: At-Risk Aggregates

Aggregate	Selected Risk Data
Medically underserved low-income populations (e.g., minorities)	In 1995 almost 73% of all TB cases occurred among racial/ethnic minorities. In 1992 Los Angeles estimated that about 12% of their TB cases occurred among homeless persons.
Foreign-born persons entering the United States	In 1995 35.7% of all TB cases in the United States occurred among foreign-born persons. From 1986 through 1992 legal immigrants accounted for 60% of the rise in TB cases. In Los Angeles, foreign-born individuals currently make up about 66% of new TB cases.
HIV-infected persons	HIV-infected persons are at a greatly increased risk of developing active TB once infected because HIV and AIDS weaken the immune system. National data on the number of individuals coinfected with HIV and TB are incomplete, but the estimates from some communities reflect that the number of coinfected persons is very high (e.g., Fulton County, Georgia has reported that 40% of its TB cases are also HIV positive).
Individuals who abuse substances (e.g., alcohol and drugs)	The CDC estimates that substance abuse is a factor in almost 14% of TB cases. Individuals who abuse substances are at a higher risk of developing TB once infected because they often have health problems or unstable living conditions.
Residents in institutions (e.g., nursing homes, prisons, long-term care facilities)	Nursing home residents have an incidence of tuberculosis from two to seven times higher than demographically similar persons living in other settings. Institutional settings are high-risk environments because persons with infectious tuberculosis are likely to live in these settings, the environmental characteristics are conducive to transmission, and large numbers of susceptible persons may be located in these settings. The incidence of TB among inmates of correctional institutions is more than three times higher than that for nonincarcerated adults aged 15 to 64 years.
Persons with medical risk factors that increase the risk of diseases	Medical risk factors that substantially increase the risk of tuberculosis are silicosis; gastrectomy; jejunoileal bypass; weight of 10% or more below ideal body weight; chronic renal failure; diabetes mellitus; conditions requiring prolonged high-dose corticosteroid therapy and other immunosuppressive therapy; some hematological disorders such as leukemia; and other malignancies.
Contacts of infectious cases	Persons in contact with infectious persons are at extremely high risk for developing infection and disease. Most cases of tuberculosis occur in people who are already infected with tubercle bacilli. Individuals in this population who are at highest risk of developing disease are those who have been recently infected and those who are exposed to a variety of stressors.

Data from Centers for Disease Control (CDC): Prevention and control of tuberculosis in correctional institutions: recommendations of the Advisory Committee for the Elimination of Tuberculosis, *MMWR* 38:313-320, 1989b; CDC: Screening for tuberculosis and tuberculosis infection in high-risk populations, *MMWR* 39 (No. RR-8):1-7, 1990b; CDC: Tuberculosis among foreign-born persons entering the United States: recommendations of the Advisory Committee for the Elimination of Tuberculosis, *MMWR* 39 (No. RR-18):1-21, 1990c; CDC: Prevention and control of tuberculosis in U.S. communities with at-risk minority populations, recommendations of the Advisory Committee for the Elimination of Tuberculosis, *MMWR* 41 (No. RR-5):1-11, 1992c; CDC: Prevention and control of tuberculosis among homeless persons, *MMWR* 41 (No. RR-5):18-21, 1992b; GAO: *Tuberculosis: costly and preventable cases continue in five cities*, Washington, D.C., 1995, GAO; CDC: Tuberculosis morbidity—United States, 1995, *MMWR* 45(18):365-370, 1996h.

of tuberculosis in the United States include, but are not limited to, the recent AIDS epidemic, social circumstances such as homelessness and poverty, the migration of refugees and immigrants to this country, and the deteriorating public health infrastructure with a resulting lack of funding for tuberculosis surveillance and control activities. Figure 11-13 depicts the amplifying effect of HIV infection on tuberculosis morbidity and transmission.

Select epidemiological characteristics of tuberculosis are included in Appendix 11-3. Aggregates at high risk for developing the disease are presented in Table 11-10. Reducing tuberculosis to an incidence of no more than 3.5 cases per 100,000 people (baseline: 9.1 per 100,000 in 1988) is a national health objective (USDHHS, 1991a, p. 516). Preventive therapy for the control of tuberculosis infection among high-risk populations is essential. The key strategies of the national action plan for eliminating tuberculosis focus on (1) identification and treatment of infectious cases so that they do not continue to transmit infection and (2) identification and treatment of infected people before they develop the infectious form of the disease (USDHHS, 1991a, p. 517). The major components in the United States'

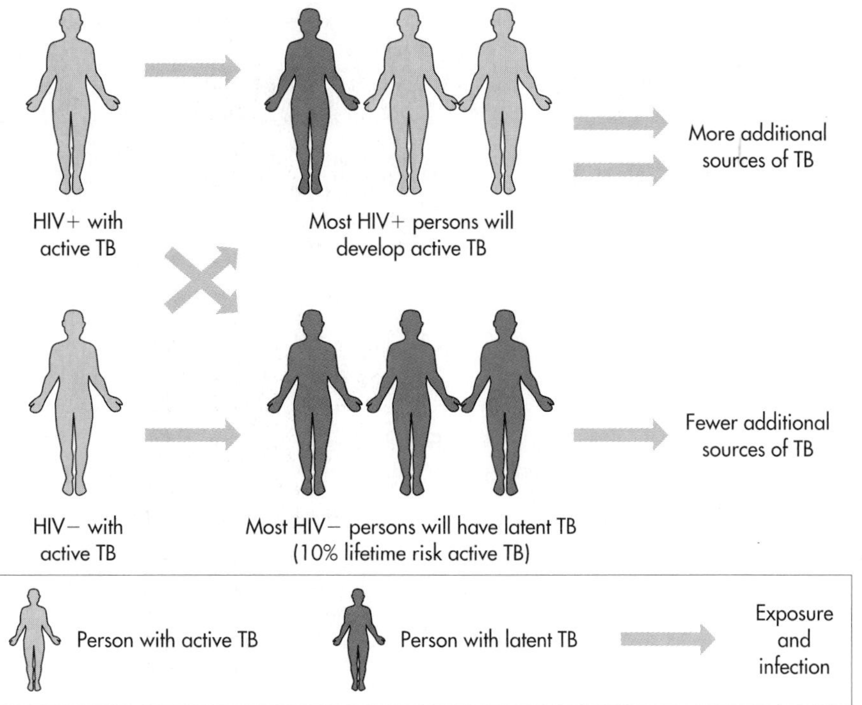

Figure **11-13** The amplifying effect of HIV infection on TB morbidity and transmission. *(From Centers for Disease Control and Prevention [CDC]:* CDC HIV/AIDS prevention: fact book, 1993, *Atlanta, 1993b, CDC, p. 18.)*

action plan to combat multidrug-resistant tuberculosis are presented in the box at right.

Tuberculosis is now "the other epidemic" (Allen, Ownby, 1991) that needs to be addressed by all health care professionals across the nation. Large-scale, epidemic transmission of tuberculosis is a major threat to all health care providers and patients (CDC, 1996g). Community health nurses have and will continue to play a role in the prevention and treatment of tuberculosis. Taking precautions to prevent the transmission of multidrug-resistant tuberculosis in all settings is a major challenge for nurses in the coming decade.

Chronic Disease and Conditions: An Increasing Challenge

Chapter 19 deals with chronic and disabling conditions. Chronic disease and conditions are of great concern to health professionals because they are long term and often limit a person's ability to carry out major activities of daily living. Major activity refers to ability to work, keep house, or engage in school or preschool activities (National Center for Health Statistics, 1996). Chronic diseases and conditions have been studied extensively in the United States since the late 1940s. The prevalence of these diseases and conditions is increasing worldwide. Individuals experiencing chronic health problems require ongoing and comprehensive community health nursing and other health services.

U.S. National Action Plan to Combat Multidrug-Resistant Tuberculosis (MDR-TB)

Surveillance and epidemiology: determine the magnitude and nature of the problem

Laboratory diagnosis: improve the rapidity, sensitivity, and reliability of diagnostic methods for MDR-TB

Patient management: effectively managing patients who have MDR-TB and preventing patients with drug-susceptible TB from developing drug-resistant disease

Screening and preventive therapy: identifying persons who are infected with or at risk of developing MDR-TB and preventing them from developing clinically active TB

Infection control: minimizing the risk of transmission of MDR-TB to patients, workers, and others in institutional settings

Outbreak control: facilitate collaboration of various officials and organizations in controlling MDR-TB outbreaks

Program evaluation: ensuring that TB programs are effective in managing patients and preventing MDR-TB

Information dissemination/training and education: develop a cadre of health-care professionals with expertise in the management of TB, including MDR-TB

Research: identify better methods for combating MDR-TB

From Centers for Disease Control and Prevention (CDC): National action plan to combat multidrug-resistant tuberculosis, *MMWR* 41(No. RR-11):5-48, 1992a.

Number of Selected Reported Chronic Conditions by Age Group, 1993
(Noninstitutionalized Population, Numbers in Thousands)

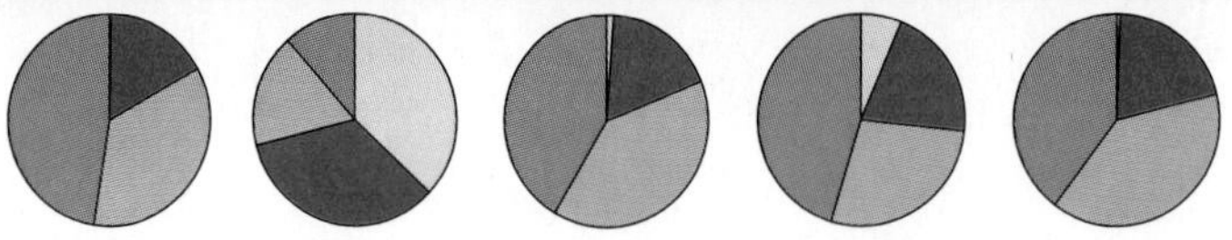

By Age	Arthritis	Asthma	Diabetes	Heart Disease	High Blood Pressure
<18	154*	4,830	104	1,367	212*
18-44	5,439	4,495	1,389	4,353	5,630
45-64	11,627	2,242	3,081	5,926	10,808
65+	15,422	1,506	3,238	9,609	10,899

*proportionally, this number is too small to chart

Some chronic conditions, such as arthritis, affect the elderly predominantly. Others, such as asthma, affect persons of all ages.

Figure **11-14** Selected chronic conditions by age group (From The Institute for Health and Aging, University of California, San Francisco: *Chronic care in America: a 21st century challenge,* Princeton, N.J., 1996, The Robert Wood Johnson Foundation, p. 24.) *Sources: (1) Hoffman, C, Rice, DP: Estimates based on the 1987 National Medical Expenditure Survey. University of California, San Francisco—Institute for Health & Aging, 1995. 2) National Center for Health Statistics:* Current estimates from the National Health Interview Survey, 1993, *Vital & Health Statistics, Series 10 (No. 190), Table 62, December 1994.*

The Commission on Chronic Illness, a national voluntary group, examined the extent of chronic disease and illness in the United States from 1949 to 1956. This commission defined chronic diseases as impairments or deviations from normal that have at least one of the following characteristics: permanency, residual disability, irreversible pathological causation and alteration, need for special rehabilitation training, and need for a long period of supervision, observation, or care (Commission on Chronic Illness, 1957, p. 4). These concepts still guide practice related to chronic disease prevention and control.

Currently, data about the prevalence of selected chronic conditions are collected regularly by the National Center for Health Statistics by means of the National Health Interview Survey. In this survey a condition is considered chronic if (1) the condition is described by the respondent as having been first noticed more than 3 months before the week of the interview, or (2) it is one of the conditions always classified as chronic regardless of time of onset. Examples of conditions always viewed as chronic are ulcers, emphysema, diabetes, arthritis, neoplasms, all congenital anomalies, and psychoses and other mental disorders (National Center for Health Statistics, 1996). The National Health Interview Survey also examines the concepts of impairment and disability related to chronic disease and conditions. These concepts are discussed in Chapter 19.

People of any age can evidence chronic conditions; these conditions are not synonymous with old age. It should be remembered that aging is the normal process of biological, psychological, and sociological change over time. However, because aging involves a gradual lessening in levels of efficiency and functioning in the various body systems, elderly people are more likely than young people to have chronic conditions. They also are likely to have more of them.

THE SCOPE OF CHRONIC CONDITIONS Approximately 100 million persons residing in the community have one or more chronic conditions. It is projected that by the year 2020 the number of individuals with chronic conditions will increase by almost 35 million. "Chronic conditions affect people of all ages and all strata of society, from newborns to octogenarians, and from the very wealthy to the impoverished" (The Institute for Health and Aging, 1996, p. 22). As illustrated in Figure 11-14, some chronic conditions predominantly affect the elderly, whereas others affect persons of all ages. Nearly 40 million Americans have a *comorbidity*, or more than one chronic condition. This varies by age and gender: women and the elderly have more comorbidities (The Institute for Health and Aging).

Chronic conditions cause significant stress for families, individuals, and society. Roughly 41 million Americans had some degree of activity limitation in 1995, of which 12 million were unable to carry out a major life activity. Chronic conditions are the major cause of illness, disability, and death: collectively, chronic conditions account for three out of every four deaths in the United States (The Institute for Health and Aging, 1996, pp. 4, 8).

The economic burden associated with chronic conditions is staggering (Figure 11-15). In addition to the $470 billion (in 1990 dollars) spent on direct medical services in 1995, chronic conditions cost the economy more than $230 billion in lost productivity. These costs do not take into account the lost productivity of caregivers or costs of non-

**The Numbers of Americans with Chronic Conditions Are Increasing...
As Are the Costs of Their Care**

Estimated Number of Persons with Chronic Conditions and Direct Medical Costs for Persons with Chronic Conditions, Selected Years, 1995-2050

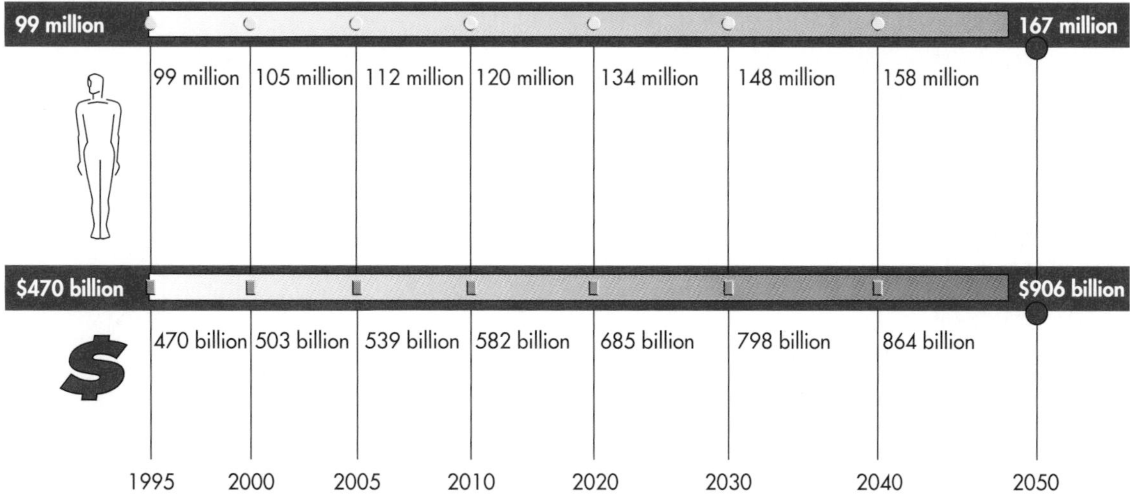

Notes: Chronic conditions is a general term that includes chronic illnesses and impairments. Chronic illness: The presence of long-term disease or symptoms. (A common definition of "long-term" in population surveys is a duration of 3 or more months.) Impairment: A physiological, psychological, or anatomical abnormality of bodily structure or function; includes all losses or abnormalities, not just those attributable to active pathology.

This estimate is of persons in the United States with chronic conditions characterized by persistent and recurring health consequences lasting for periods of years. Costs are in 1990 dollars, estimated by applying the rates of chronic conditions and the per capita costs in 1990 dollars to the estimated projected population with chronic conditions by gender and age.

Figure **11-15** Estimated number of persons with chronic conditions and direct medical costs for persons with chronic conditions, selected years, 1995-2050. *(From The Institute for Health and Aging, University of California, San Francisco:* Chronic care in America: a 21st century challenge, *Princeton, N.J., 1996, The Robert Wood Johnson Foundation, p. 9.) Source: Hoffman C, Rice DP: Estimates based on the 1987 National Medical Expenditure Survey, University of California, San Francisco—Institute for Health & Aging, 1995.*

medical services (e.g., adequate housing and personal care services). Persons with chronic conditions require a host of chronic care services that they frequently find difficult to use, unacceptable because of quality, or unavailable (Figure 11-16). Chronic conditions limit access to private insurance, force reliance on public funds, and drain both public and individual resources (The Institute for Health and Aging, 1996, pp. 9-10, 48-49).

The risks and burdens associated with chronic conditions vary by age, race, the nature of the condition, and socioeconomic status. Chapters 15 through 20 discuss these variations. However, it is important to remember that many chronic conditions found in later life have their roots in childhood or young adulthood and continue throughout the life span. Since life expectancy is increasing for people with chronic conditions, as well as for the general population, a major concern is emerging about the nation's ability to provide for chronic care services for all who need them. The emphasis in health care spending must be on preventing chronic conditions in childhood and young adulthood.

LEVELS OF PREVENTION FOR CHRONIC DISEASE The first of a four-volume series based on the work of the Commission on Chronic Illness was appropriately titled *Prevention of Chronic Illness*. Prevention must be the underlying approach to chronic conditions or these problems will only increase with time. Prevention on all three levels—primary, secondary, and tertiary—is essential for effective management and control of chronic conditions.

Primary prevention of many serious chronic illnesses is frequently impossible because health professionals are unable to determine the exact point in time when a condition begins. When, for example, does schizophrenia or asbestosis begin? Each of these diseases goes through a long latent period before symptoms are seen. They may stem from such variables as hereditary characteristics, occupational conditions, environmental stresses, or nutritional factors. Some chronic conditions can be prevented. Primary preventive efforts that control communicable disease, reduce accidents, emphasize adequate care during pregnancy, and suggest ways to cope with emotional stress all contribute to the prevention of certain chronic conditions. Primary prevention is an important task of the community health nurse.

Detection and treatment of chronic conditions (secondary prevention) are often possible. For many conditions such as diabetes, hypertension, breast cancer, and glaucoma, large-scale national programs for early detection represent a profitable and economical approach to secondary prevention. Early diagnosis plays a significant role in the control of chronic disease and conditions.

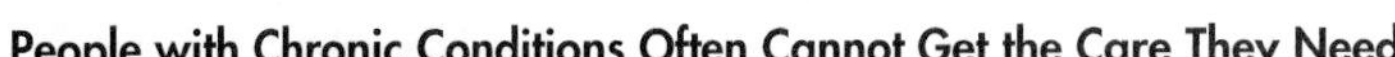

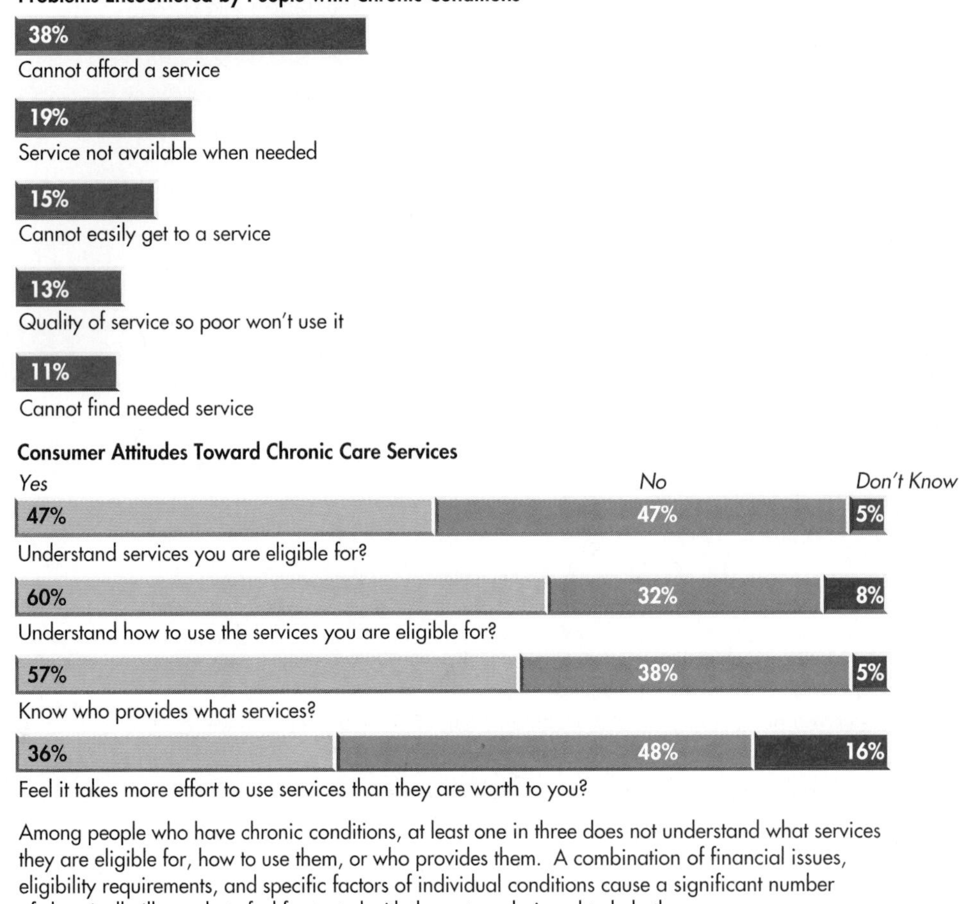

Figure 11-16 Consumer attitudes toward and problems encountered with chronic care services: results from the 1992 Gallup Poll of People with Chronic Illness. *(From The Institute for Health and Aging, University of California, San Francisco:* Chronic care in America: a 21st century challenge, *Princeton, N.J., 1996, The Robert Wood Johnson Foundaion, p. 10.) Source: Kabcenell, AI, et al.* People with disabling chronic conditions report on their service system. *Unpublished data from the Poll of People with Chronic Illness by The Gallup Organization, 1992.*

A major secondary prevention effort relative to chronic illness occurred in the United States when the National Health Survey was authorized and conducted in 1956 to secure information about health conditions in the general population. This survey was enacted under the National Health Survey Act, which was proposed in 1955 by the U.S. Department of Health, Education, and Welfare (USDHEW). Under this act the Surgeon General of the Public Health Service was authorized to conduct a survey in order to produce uniform national statistics on disease, injury, impairment, disability, and related topics.

In 1972 a new survey mechanism initiated by USDHEW, the Health and Nutrition Examination Survey (HANES), began. Persons 1 to 74 years of age were examined, with emphasis on their nutritional status. Statistical data were collected on health records, fertility patterns, morbidity, and mortality. Today HANES is the primary source of nationwide data on illnesses, disabilities, and physiological measurements.

Tertiary prevention activities, as well as primary and secondary ones, should be planned when working with people who have chronic conditions. Tertiary prevention involves rehabilitation, with the ultimate goal being cure or full restoration of the client's level of functioning. For some chronic conditions this may be impossible; hence the ideal goal must be replaced by more limited objectives such as maximizing remaining functional potential or minimizing further deterioration. Another option would be to learn to live within the limitations that the chronic disease has imposed. A more detailed discussion of the concept of rehabilitation is presented in Chapter 19.

APPROACHES TO THE STUDY OF CHRONIC CONDITIONS Two basic approaches to the study of chronic conditions and other diseases are retrospective and prospective studies. Retrospective and prospective studies are designed to determine if there is a relationship between a factor and a disease, as well as the intensity of that relationship. Mausner and Kramer (1985, pp. 159-174) discuss the principles involved in these types of studies. Since only a brief summary of their thoughts is presented below, the reader should refer to Mausner and Kramer's text to obtain a better understanding of these approaches.

Retrospective studies look at people who are diagnosed as having a disease and compare them with those who do not have disease. The persons who do not have the disease are called *controls*. The controls come from the same general population segment as the individuals who have the condition and have the same characteristics as the study group except for the disease condition. A retrospective study examines factors in the person's past experience. One of the disadvantages of retrospective studies is that detailed information may not be available or accurate. The greatest problem, however, is finding a control group that is alike in all respects except for the condition under study. The advantages of this type of study are cost and the number of subjects needed. Retrospective studies are relatively inexpensive and require a small sampling size because cases are identified at the onset.

Prospective studies start with a group of people—a *cohort*—all presumed to be free from a condition but who differ in their exposure to a supposedly harmful factor. This cohort is followed over a period to discover differences in the rate at which disease develops in relation to exposure to the harmful factor. A major advantage of this type of study is that the cohort is chosen for study before the disease develops. The cohort is therefore not influenced by knowledge that disease exists, as in retrospective studies.

Prospective studies allow calculation of incidence rates among those exposed and those not exposed. Thus absolute difference in incidence rates and the true relative risk can be measured. The major disadvantage is that a prospective study is a long, expensive project. A large cohort must be used, especially if the disease has low incidence. Also, the larger the number of factors to be studied, the larger the cohort must be. The loss of people from the cohort as a result of death, lack of interest, or job mobility is a major problem when a study lasts over an extended period. Changes in diagnostic criteria, administrative problems, loss of staff or funding, and the high cost of record keeping can all contribute to make this a study that should not be undertaken without careful planning.

Retrospective and prospective studies assist in identifying causes of disease and effective disease control mechanisms. It is not intended that this brief description of retrospective and prospective studies will prepare community health nurses to do them. The purpose is to familiarize readers with the basic concepts involved in the study of chronic conditions.

The community health nurse does, however, play an active role in the control of chronic conditions. Casefinding through screening programs is a significant aspect of this part of the community health nurse's role.

SCREENING AS A METHOD FOR DETECTION AND CONTROL OF CHRONIC CONDITIONS Screening programs can be an efficient way to identify individuals in a community who may unknowingly have a chronic condition in addition to an infectious disease.

There are two types of screening programs whereby chronic and infectious disease is sought in apparently healthy individuals: the *single screening test*, where only one condition is being identified, such as giving a group of teachers a TB tine test, and the *multiphasic screening test*, where a battery of tests is used at one time to detect several disease conditions. Doing height and weight measurements, audiometry, and vision screening of all persons at a county fair is an example of multiphasic screening.

Screening tests do not provide a conclusive diagnosis of a disease but rather are used to identify asymptomatic individuals who may unknowingly have a problem. Anyone who evidences symptoms of a disease through a screening program should have further medical diagnostic testing. This is essential, since early diagnosis and treatment are the primary goals of a screening program. Early diagnosis and treatment are particularly beneficial for conditions—such as hypertension and cancer—for which treatment measures are available to prevent progression of the condition.

Advantages of screening programs are that often they are relatively inexpensive, take little time, need few professionals to administer them, provide opportunity for prevention, early diagnosis, and treatment, and present statistics on the prevalence of disease when there is adequate follow-up. Major disadvantages of screening programs are that people tend to substitute them for medical examination, findings of screening programs are presumptive and further testing should be done to confirm a diagnosis, screening programs often do not reach vulnerable groups of people, and conditions may be missed during screening, resulting in persons receiving a false impression of their health status.

Not all chronic conditions lend themselves to screening. Many authors have discussed criteria to consider when establishing screening programs. The following principles are seen as essential to good screening practices (Mausner, Kramer, 1985; Wilson, Jungner, 1968).

1. The condition sought should be an important health problem (affect a significant percentage of people).

2. There should be an accepted treatment for clients with recognized disease.
3. Facilities for diagnosis and treatment should be available.
4. There should be a recognizable latent or early symptomatic stage.
5. There should be a suitable test or examination that is able to detect the disease earlier than without screening.
6. The test should be acceptable to the population.
7. The natural history of the condition, including development from latent to declared disease, should be adequately understood.
8. The cost of casefinding (including diagnosis and treatment) should be economically balanced in relation to possible expenditure for medical care as a whole.
9. Casefinding should be thought of as a continuing process and not a "once and for all" project.

It should be clear from reviewing these principles that although screening can be one method for early discovery of asymptomatic disease, it should be used judiciously and discriminately. Screening results need to be thoroughly evaluated, and the conditions found must be treated.

An especially valuable reference in helping one to evaluate the effectiveness of screening tests and procedures is the *Guide to Clinical Preventive Services* (1996) by the U.S. Preventive Services Task Force. The importance of the above principles of screening are reinforced in this textbook.

Summary

The epidemiological process helps community health nurses to identify the health status of the community in which they are working and to prevent disease, chronic conditions, and other health-related phenomena such as child abuse, mental illness, and domestic violence. This process places emphasis on analyzing the needs of aggregates rather than the needs of individual clients. Like the nursing process it is a scientific, systematic problem-solving approach to the study of health needs.

Several key concepts are inherent in the understanding and utilization of the epidemiological process. These are study of aggregates at risk, natural life history of the disease, levels of prevention, host-agent-environment relationships, multiple causation of disease, and person-place-time relationships. These concepts provide a foundation for understanding the dynamics of disease transmission and occurrence and aggregate-focused preventive interventions. In addition to these concepts, a community health nurse must understand biostatistics to effectively use the epidemiological process.

By applying the concepts and methods of epidemiology, community health nurses play a vital role in the prevention of disease, injuries, and social problems in a community. Through their contacts in a variety of settings they are in a key position to do casefinding, to eliminate barriers to the control of disease, and to promote health through teaching and counseling.

CRITICAL *Thinking Exercise*

Select a contemporary health problem of interest (e.g., elder abuse, teenage pregnancy, suicide, drug abuse, AIDS, tuberculosis, or homelessness) and discuss agent, host, and environmental factors that have contributed to the occurrence of this problem and have presented barriers to control. Identify primary, secondary, and tertiary preventive activities designed to reduce the condition occurrence and the role of nursing in implementing these activities.

REFERENCES

Allen MA, Ownby KK: Tuberculosis: the other epidemic, *JANAC* 2:9-24, 1991.

Atkinson W, Furphy L, Gantt J, Mayfield M, eds: *Epidemiology and prevention of vaccine-preventable diseases*, Atlanta, 1995, CDC.

Benenson AS: *Control of communicable diseases manual*, ed 16, Washington, D.C., 1995, APHA.

Benson V, Marano MA: *Current estimates from the National Health Interview Survey*, National Center for Health Statistics, Vital Health Stat 10(189), 1994.

Centers for Disease Control (CDC), Training and Laboratory Program Office: *Principles of epidemiology: agent, host, environment* (self-study course 3030-G, manual 1), Atlanta, 1987a, CDC.

Centers for Disease Control (CDC), Training and Laboratory Program Office: *Principles of epidemiology: disease surveillance* (self-study course 3030-G, manual 5), Atlanta, 1987b, CDC.

Centers for Disease Control (CDC): Recommendations for prevention of HIV transmission in health care settings, *MMWR* 36(Suppl S-2), August 21, 1987c.

Centers for Disease Control (CDC): Guidelines for evaluating surveillance systems, *MMWR* 37(Suppl No.S-5):1-18, 1988b.

Centers for Disease Control (CDC): Prevention and control of tuberculosis in correctional institutions: recommendations of the Advisory Committee for the Elimination of Tuberculosis, *MMWR* 38:313-320, 1989b.

Centers for Disease Control (CDC): Screening for tuberculosis and tuberculous infection in high-risk populations, *MMWR* 39(No. RR-8):1-7, 1990b.

Centers for Disease Control (CDC): Tuberculosis among foreign-born persons entering the United States: recommendations of the Advisory Committee for the Elimination of Tuberculosis, *MMWR* 39 (No. RR-18): 1-21, 1990c.

Centers for Disease Control and Prevention (CDC): National action plan to combat multidrug-resistant tuberculosis, *MMWR* 41(No. RR-11): 5-48, 1992a.

Centers for Disease Control and Prevention (CDC): Prevention and control of tuberculosis among homeless persons, *MMWR* 41(No. RR-5): 18-21, 1992b.

Centers for Disease Control and Prevention (CDC): Prevention and control of tuberculosis in U.S. communities with at-risk minority populations, recommendations of the Advisory Committee for the Elimination of Tuberculosis, *MMWR* 41(No. RR-5):1-11, 1992c.

Centers for Disease Control and Prevention (CDC): Summary of notifiable diseases, United States, 1992, *MMWR* 41:3, 1993a.

Centers for Disease Control and Prevention (CDC): *CDC HIV/AIDS prevention: fact book, 1993*, Atlanta, 1993b, CDC.

Centers for Disease Control and Prevention (CDC): 1993 sexually transmitted diseases treatment guidelines, *MMWR* 42(No. RR-14):3-59, 1993c.

Centers for Disease Control and Prevention (CDC): Update: Multistate outbreak of *Escherichia coli* 0157:H7 infections from hamburgers—western United States, 1992-1993, *MMWR* 42:258-263, 1993d.

Centers for Disease Control and Prevention (CDC): Multistate outbreak of viral gastroenteritis related to consumption of oysters—Louisiana, Maryland, Mississippi, and North Carolina, *MMWR* 42:945-948, 1993e.

Centers for Disease Control and Prevention (CDC): Salmonella serotype Tennessee in powdered milk products and infant formula—Canada and the United States, 1993, *MMWR*, 42:516-517, 1993f.

Centers for Disease Control and Prevention (CDC): *Addressing emerging infectious disease threats: a prevention strategy for the United States*, Atlanta, 1994a, National Center for Infectious Diseases.

Centers for Disease Control and Prevention (CDC): National notifiable disease reporting, 1994, *MMWR* 43:800, 1994b.

Centers for Disease Control and Prevention (CDC): Hantavirus pulmonary syndrome—United States, 1993, *MMWR* 43:45-48, 1994c.

Centers for Disease Control and Prevention (CDC): Exposure of passengers and flight crew to Mycobacterium tuberculosis on commercial aircraft, 1992-1995, *MMWR* 44:137-140, 1995.

Centers for Disease Control and Prevention (CDC): CDC's 50th Anniversary—July 1, 1996, *MMWR* 45:525-530, 1996a.

Centers for Disease Control and Prevention (CDC): Infectious diseases designated as notifiable at the national level—United States, 1996, *MMWR* 25(3):42, 1996b.

Centers for Disease Control and Prevention (CDC): National, state, and urban area vaccination coverage levels among children aged 19-35 months—United States, April 1994-March 1995, *MMWR* 45:145-150, 1996c.

Centers for Disease Control and Prevention (CDC): Notifiable disease surveillance and notifiable disease statistics—United States, June 1946 and June 1996, *MMWR* 25(45):531-537, 1996d.

Centers for Disease Control and Prevention (CDC): Outbreak of trichinellosis associated with eating cougar jerky—Idaho, 1995, *MMWR* 45:205-207, 1996e.

Centers for Disease Control and Prevention (CDC): Shigella sonnei outbreak associated with contaminated drinking water—Island Park, Idaho, August 1995, *MMWR* 45:229-231, 1996f.

Centers for Disease Control and Prevention (CDC): The role of BCG vaccine in the prevention and control of tuberculosis in the United States: a joint statement by the Advisory Council for the Elimination of Tuberculosis and the Advisory Committee on Immunization Practices, *MMWR* 45(No. RR-4):1-18, 1996g.

Centers for Disease Control and Prevention (CDC): Tuberculosis morbidity—United States, 1995, *MMWR* 45(18):365-370, 1996h.

Collins JG: *Prevalence of selected chronic conditions: United States, 1986-88*, National Center for Health Statistics, Vital Health Stat 10(182), 1993.

Commission on Chronic Illness: *Chronic illness in the United States, vol I: prevention of chronic illness*, Cambridge, Ma., 1957, Harvard University Press.

Communicable Disease Center: *Food-borne disease investigation: analysis of field data*, Atlanta, 1964, U.S. Public Health Service.

Doyle, AC: *The hound of the Baskervilles*, New York, 1971, Berkley.

Duncan DF: *Epidemiology: basis for disease prevention and health promotion*, New York, 1988, Macmillan.

Friedman GE: *Primer of epidemiology*, New York, 1974, McGraw-Hill.

General Accounting Office (GAO): *Tuberculosis: costly and preventable cases continue in five cities*, Washington, D.C., 1995, GAO.

Gordis L: *Epidemiology*, Philadelphia, 1996, Saunders.

Greenlee R, Smith U: *Community health profile, Kent County, Michigan: a guide for the Healthy Kent 2000 Committee based on the format of APEXPH*, Grand Rapids, Mich., 1994, Kent County Health Department.

Grimes DE: *Infectious diseases*, St. Louis, 1991, Mosby.

Horwitz M, Pollard R, Merson M, Martin SA: A large outbreak of foodborne salmonellosis on the Navajo Nation Indian Reservation: epidemiology and transmission, *AJPH* 67:1071-1076, 1977.

Institute of Medicine—Committee for the Study of the Future of Public Health: *The future of public health*, Washington, D.C., 1988, National Academy Press.

Institute of Medicine: *Emerging infections: microbial threats to health in the United States*, Washington, D.C., 1992, National Academy Press.

Iseman MD: A leap of faith: What can we do to curtail intrainstitutional transmission of tuberculosis? *Ann of Intern Med* 117: 251-253, 1992.

Jaret P: Stalking the world's epidemics: the disease detectives, *National Geographic* 179:116-190, 1991.

Jekel JF, Elmore JG, Katz DL: *Epidemiology, biostatistics, and preventive medicine*, Philadelphia, 1996, Saunders.

Johnson NE: *Health profiles of Michigan populations of color*, Lansing, Mi., 1995, Michigan Department of Public Health.

Koopman JS: Comment: emerging objectives and methods in epidemiology, *AJPH* 86:630-632, 1996.

Lalonde M: *A new perspective on the health of Canadians*, Ottawa, 1974, Information, Canada.

Last JM, ed: *Maxcy-Rosenau public health and preventive medicine*, ed 12, Norwalk, Ct., 1986, Appleton-Century-Crofts.

Last JM: *A dictionary of epidemiology*, ed 3, New York, 1995, Oxford University Press.

Leavell HR, Clark EG: *Preventive medicine for the doctor in his community: an epidemiologic approach*, New York, 1965, McGraw-Hill.

MacMahon B, Pugh T: *Epidemiology principles and methods*, Boston, 1970, Little, Brown.

Mausner JS, Kramer S: *Mausner and Bahn epidemiology: an introductory text*, ed 2, Philadelphia, 1985, Saunders.

McGinnis MJ, Foege WH: Actual causes of death in the United States, *JAMA* 270:2207-2212, 1993.

McKenna N: A disaster waiting to happen, *World AIDS* 27:5-9, 1993.

Michigan Department of Community Health: *Michigan Critical Health Indicators 1996*, Lansing, Mi., 1996, The Department.

Michigan Department of Public Health, Division of Epidemiology: *Enteric infections case history*, Lansing, Mi., undated, MDPH.

Michigan Department of Public Health: *Health risk behaviors 1993*, Lansing, Mi., 1995, The Department.

Mosby's home health nursing packet consultant, St Louis, 1995, Mosby.

National Center for Health Statistics: *Health, United States, 1993*, Washington, D.C., 1994, U.S. Government Printing Office.

National Center for Health Statistics: *Health, United States, 1994*, Hyattsville, Md., 1995, Public Health Service.

National Center for Health Statistics: *Health, United States, 1995*, Hyattsville, Md., 1996, Public Health Service.

Occupational Safety and Health Administration (OSHA): *Occupational exposure to bloodborne pathogens*, Washington, D.C., 1992, OSHA.

Pederson A, O'Neill M, Rootman I: *Health promotion in Canada: provincial, national, and international perspectives*, Toronto, 1994, Saunders, Canada.

Prescott WH: *History of the conquest of Mexico*, New York, 1936, Random House.

Robey B: Two hundred years and counting: the 1990 census, *Pop Bull* 44(1), Washington, D.C., 1989, Population Reference Bureau.

Scherl D, Noren J, Osterweis M (eds): *Promoting health and preventing disease*, Washington, D.C., 1992, Association of Academic Health Centers.

Stoeckle MY, Douglas RG: Infectious diseases, *JAMA* 275:1816-1817, 1996.

Surgeon General: *Healthy people: the Surgeon General's report on health promotion and disease prevention*, vol I & II, Washington, D.C., 1979, U.S. Government Printing Office.

Tennessee Department of Health and Environment: *Protect them from harm*, Murfreesboro, Tn., 1983, Lancer.

The Institute for Health and Aging, University of California, San Francisco: *Chronic care in America: a 21st century challenge*, Princeton, N.J., 1996, The Robert Wood Johnson Foundation.

Trupin L, Rice DP: Health status, medical care use, and number of disabling conditions in the United States, *Disability Statistics Abstract* 9:1-4, 1995.

U.S. Bureau of the Census: *Statistical abstract of the United States*, ed 116, Washington, D.C., 1995, The Bureau.

U.S. Department of Health and Human Services (USDHHS): *Healthy people 2000: national health promotion and disease prevention objectives, full report, with commentary*, Washington, D.C., 1991a, U.S. Government Printing Office.

U.S. Department of Health and Human Services (USDHHS): *Healthy People 2000: midcourse review and 1995 revisions*, Washington, D.C., 1995a, U.S. Government Printing Office.

U.S. Department of Health and Human Services (USDHHS): *Health status of minorities and low-income groups*, ed 3, Washington, D.C., 1991b, U.S. Government Printing Office.

U.S. Department of Health and Human Services (USDHHS): *Health United States, 1994*, Washington, D.C., 1995b, U.S. Government Printing Office.

U.S. Preventive Services Task Force: *Guide to clinical preventive services*, Baltimore, 1996, Williams and Wilkins.

Valanis B: *Epidemiology in nursing and healthcare*, Norwalk, Ct., 1992, Appleton and Lange.

Vaughan G: *Mummy, I don't feel well*, London, 1970, Causton and Sons, Ltd.

Wilson JMG, Jungner F: Principles and practice of screening for disease, *Public Health Papers No* 34, Geneva, 1968, WHO.

Winslow CE-A: The evolution and significance of the modern public health campaign, *J Public Health Policy*, South Burlington, Vt., 1923.

Woodward SB: The story of smallpox in Massachusetts, *N Engl J Med* 206:1181, 1932.

World Health Organization (WHO): *Alma-Ata 1978: primary health care: report of the International Conference on Primary Health Care, Alma-Ata, USSR*, Geneva, 1978, WHO.

World Health Organization (WHO): Health Status, *World Health Statistical Q* 48:189-199, 1995.

SELECTED BIBLIOGRAPHY

AARP: *Living in the community with a disability: demographic characteristics of the population under age 65*, Washington, D.C., 1995, AARP.

Bayer R, Dupuis L: Tuberculosis, public health, and civil liberties, *Annu Rev Public Health* 16:307-326, 1995.

Bellenir K, Dresser PD, eds: *Food and animal borne diseases sourcebook*, Detroit, Mi., 1995, Ommigraphics Inc.

Bowden KM, McDiarmid MA: Occupationally acquired tuberculosis: what's known, *J Occupational Medicine* 36:320-325, 1994.

Centers for Disease Control and Prevention (CDC): *Manual of procedures for the reporting of nationally notifiable diseases to CDC*, Atlanta, 1995, CDC.

Clever LH, LeGuyader Y: Infectious risks for health care workers, *Annu Rev Public Health* 16:141-164, 1995.

DeHovitz JA: Directly observed therapy initiative: a 1990s tuberculosis treatment imperative, *J Public Health Manag Pract* 1:vi-vii, 1995.

Forstar J, Wolfson M: Is the message the medium? Perception, social position, and health. A commentary on "the importance of social interaction: a new perspective on social epidemiology, social risk factors, and health," *Health Education Q* 21:465-469, 1994.

Krieger N: Epidemiology and the web of causation: has anyone seen the spider? *Soc Sci Med* 39:887-903, 1994.

LeDuc J: World Health Organization strategy for emerging infectious diseases, *JAMA* 275:318-320, 1996.

Mandell GL, Bennett JE, Dolin R: *Principles and practice of infectious diseases*, ed 4 (vol 1 and vol 2), New York, 1995, Churchill Livingstone.

Morton RF, Hebel JR, McCarter RJ: *A study guide to epidemiology and biostatistics*, ed 4, Gaithersburg, Md., 1996, Aspen.

Pinner RW, Teutsch SM, Sinorsen L, et al: Trends in infectious disease mortality in the United States, *JAMA* 275:189-193, 1996.

Subedi J, Gallagher EB: *Society, health and disease: transcultural perspectives*, Upper Saddle River, NJ, 1996, Prentice-Hall.

Verbrugge LM, Patrick DL: Seven chronic conditions: their impact on U.S. adult's activity levels and use of medical services, *AJPH* 85:173-182, 1995.

Walker H, ed: *Global infectious diseases, prevention, control, and eradication*, New York, 1992, Springer-Verlag.

Winkelstein W: A new perspective on John Snow's communicable disease theory, *Am Epidemiol* 142:53-59, 1995.

Winkelstein W: Editorial: eras, paradigms, and the future of epidemiology, *AJPH* 86:621-622, 1996.

12

Aggregate-Focused Contemporary Community Health Issues

Ella Mae Brooks, RN, PhD

OBJECTIVES

Upon completion of this chapter, the reader should be able to:

1. Discuss select aggregate-focused contemporary community health issues.
2. Discuss minority health and health risks.
3. Apply roles of the community health nurse in addressing select aggregate-focused contemporary health problems.
4. Apply the levels of prevention when intervening to resolve select contemporary community health problems.
5. Understand health risks associated with selected contemporary community health issues.
6. Discuss critical variables influencing contemporary community health issues.
7. Discuss community-focused interventions for addressing selected contemporary community health issues.

Numerous health issues face the nation. Although some health issues may be more salient in one community and less in another, most communities are affected by contemporary health issues. Geographically, health issues vary and community health nurses must keep abreast of health concerns in their respective communities. As a result of the ease of geographical mobility and spread of disease, no community can ever live in ignorance, thinking, "This will not happen here, and I don't need to know about this." It is imperative that community health nurses be aware of contemporary community health issues throughout the nation and the world. Frequently contemporary health problems are multifaceted and individuals are caught up in a web of social problems. Figure 12-1 illustrates the web of social problems that influence the development of many health problems.

As discussed previously, *Healthy People 2000* has established three major goals to improve the quality of life among all Americans (see Chapter 5). To achieve these goals our nation must address health-related threats to individuals across the life span, health risks for disadvantaged populations, and specific issues involving population groups at risk for poor health. Additionally, contemporary community-based health issues must be examined to determine critical variables influencing the occurrence of these problems and interventions to resolve them. Chapters 15 through 21 discuss the health profiles of specific developmental age groups and aggregates at risk among these groups. This chapter will focus on "universal" contemporary health issues that reach across the life span, affect multiple aggregates, and span developmental stages. Using *Healthy People 2000* goals and objectives, the needs of select populations will be addressed. Specifically, these select populations include minorities, persons with low incomes, those who abuse alcohol and drugs, persons who are homeless, those who are at risk for sexually transmitted diseases including HIV/AIDS, and persons who are affected by violence. Issues facing these populations create challenges and opportunities for community health nurses.

A comprehensive, multifaceted intervention approach is needed to address the web of problems experienced by aggregates at risk in contemporary society. As community health nurses deal with these aggregates they must be prepared to assess and intervene both collaboratively and individually to meet the multifaceted needs. The role of the nurse in primary, secondary, and tertiary prevention of these issues will be discussed. Emphasis will be placed on primary preventive interventions.

MINORITY HEALTH

After the publication of *Healthy People 2000* the Office of Minority Health (OMH) was established as part of the U.S. Department of Health and Human Services (USDHHS). The primary focus of the OMH was to develop, coordinate, and monitor a national strategy to improve minority health. The office has helped to make the health of minority Americans a public concern. With the publication of *Healthy People 2000* a goal to reduce health disparities among Americans and numerous objectives in relation to improving

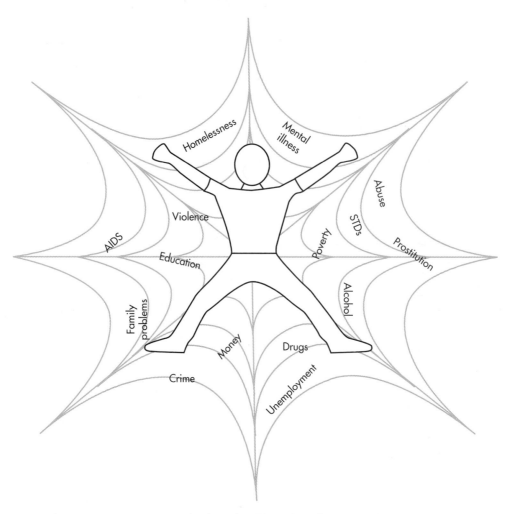

Figure 12-1 Aggregates experiencing a web of social problems that influence the development of many health problems. *(Modified from Massaro J, Pepper B: The relationship of addiction to crime, health and other social problems. In Crowe AH, Reeves RR:* Treatment for alcohol and other drug abuse: opportunities for coordination, *DHHS Pub No. (SMA)94-2075, Rockville, Md., 1994, U.S. Government Printing Office, p. 14.)*

minority health were established. These objectives address disparities across the life span.

In the past decade the size of U.S. minority populations has increased dramatically, and the United States has become more culturally diverse. In 1976 the federal government began to classify individuals into the following racial groups: black, white, Asian or Pacific Islander, and American Indian or Alaskan Native. Hispanics were classified among "other" populations (National Center for Health Statistics, 1996, p. 108). The first year that Hispanics were classified as an ethnic group in population data was 1980 (USDHHS, 1991b, p. 11). The black and Hispanic populations are growing faster than the white population, and between these two groups the number of Hispanics is increasing more rapidly. In 1993 about 10% of the estimated 258 million persons in the United States were Hispanic (National Center for Health Statistics, 1996, p. 4).

The predominant categories of minorities addressed in *Healthy People 2000* are blacks, Hispanics, Asian and Pacific Islanders, and American and Alaskan Indians (these categories do not have absolute boundaries and many subgroups exist within each category) (USDHHS, 1995). For example, the Hispanic subgroups include Mexican-Americans and Puerto Ricans, and some Asian and Pacific Islander subgroups include Chinese, Japanese, and Filipinos.

Figure 12-2 depicts the total U.S. population by race and by growth of population groups from 1980 through 1993. It is interesting to note that the number of Hispanics has almost doubled between 1980 and 1993, while the number of Asian/Pacific Islanders has more than doubled.

Minority Populations and Health Disparities

There are notable health disparities among Americans (USDHHS, 1995). From a survey of almost 4000 minority

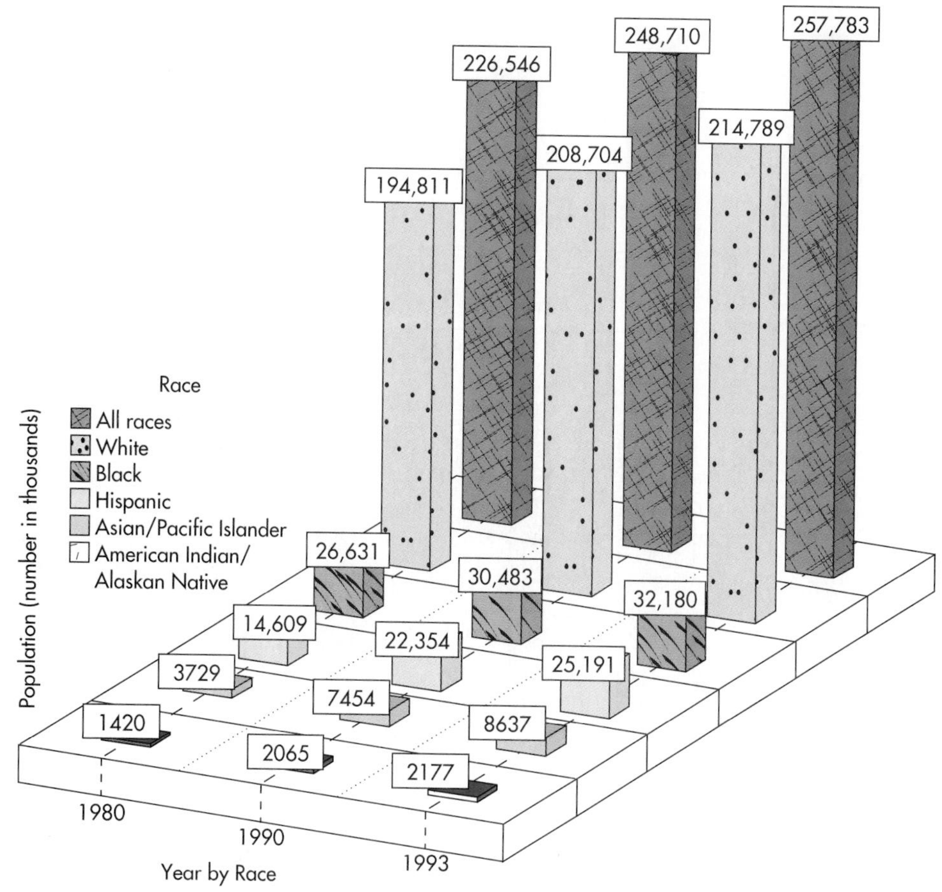

Figure 12-2 U.S. total population (all races) and population by race, 1980-1993. *(Modified from National Center for Health Statistics:* Health, United States, 1995, chartbook, *Pub No. (PHS)96-1232, Hyattsville, Md., 1996, U.S. Government Printing Office, pp. 78-89.)*

adults, the Commonwealth Fund reported disparity in health opportunities between minority Americans and white Americans (Commonwealth Fund, 1995). The report noted that minorities were more likely to lack health insurance, have difficulty accessing health care, have little or no choice in care, and have difficulty obtaining specialty care as a result of low income and less than, or lack of, adequate insurance coverage (Commonwealth Fund). Additionally, the survey reported that minority groups experience more health problems than their white counterparts; minorities experience more stress and violence, are less likely to maintain a healthy diet and exercise regularly, have lower incomes, are more likely to live in substandard housing, and are more likely to have incomplete education. These problems all contribute to a poorer quality of life. The gap between minority and majority health is most dramatic when mortality is measured in "excess deaths."

Minority Populations and Excess Deaths

Excess deaths are defined as deaths that would not have occurred if minorities had the same age and sex-specific death rate as the majority population (OMH—Resource Center, 1989, p. 1). Over 80% of minority excess deaths fall into the six categories of heart disease, stroke, cancer, infant deaths, homicide/accidents, and chemical dependency (USDHHS, 1991a). Even when the socioeconomic effects (e.g., poverty, education, social class) are accounted for, health and survival disparities still exist for minorities (USDHHS, 1991b, p. 32). This was further exemplified in a national longitudinal mortality study (Sorlie, Backlund, Keller, 1995) involving 530,000 subjects, which reported significantly higher mortality in blacks than whites after adjusting for socioeconomic variables. An understanding of the extent and causes of mortality variations between the minority and majority populations provides a foundation for targeting services and designing interventions to reduce these variations (Blane, 1995).

Figure 12-3 depicts death rates by race in the United States and displays the disparity in deaths between whites and minorities. Deaths among minorities exceed those among whites in all age groups except those 15 to 19 and those 85 and over. The life expectancy has been consistently

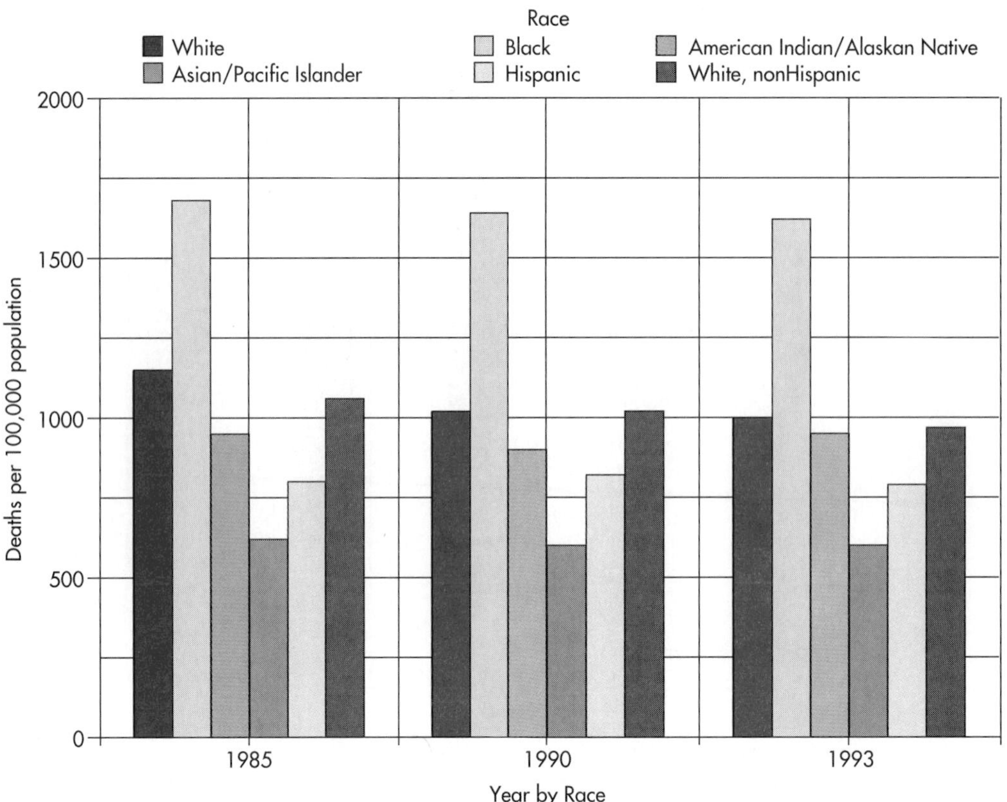

Figure 12-3 Death rates for all causes by race, for all ages, age adjusted 1985-1993. *(Modified from National Center for Health Statistics:* Health, United States, 1995, chartbook, *Pub No. (PHS)96-1232, Hyattsville, Md., 1996, U.S. Government Printing Office.)*

lower among the minority populations than the white majority.

Nursing and Health of Minority Populations

As discussed in Chapter 1, Lillian Wald and the Henry Street Settlement nurses worked to improve the health of immigrants in the United States and strove to provide culturally sensitive care (Wald, 1915). This concern with the health of minority and disadvantaged populations has continued into contemporary community health nursing practice. Nursing organizations across the nation are working with diverse minority populations to achieve "health for all."

Nurses' Commitments to Health of Minority Populations

Consistent with *Healthy People 2000*, the American Nurses Association (ANA) has made a legislative commitment in the 104th Congress to encourage unified efforts of health care providers and educators to meet the health care needs of minority groups (ANA, 1995, p. 23). According to this legislative commitment, "ANA will lobby for expansion of health care programs to ensure quality health care for all populations . . . [and ANA] will pursue educational funding for health care workers to increase the number of ethnically and culturally competent professionals" (ANA, p. 23). ANA's commitment to minorities includes both programming to target minority health and the education and development of culturally competent health care providers. Currently minority groups report more negative experiences with the health care system than do white adults (Commonwealth Fund, 1995).

Nurses and Cultural Competence

Chapters 7 and 9 elaborate on the concepts of culturally sensitive and culturally competent care. To provide competent care to culturally diverse minority populations, nurses must have an understanding of the health needs of the minority population being considered. They must also "possess specific knowledge and information about the particular cultural groups they are working with" (Randall-David, 1994, p. 3).

ANA's (1996c) Position Statement on Cultural Diversity provides an operational definition for cultural diversity to guide nurses in their practice with minority groups. "Cultural diversity refers to the differences between people based on a shared ideology and valued set of beliefs, norms, customs, and meanings evidenced in a way of life" (ANA, p. 90). In practice this is known as *cultural sensitivity,* meaning that nurses must be sensitive to the values, beliefs, traditions, and health practices of various cultures that may affect nursing interventions designed to meet the needs of members of these groups (Spector, 1993).

Community Empowerment

Using the health education strategy to mobilize communities to make decisions regarding their own health care needs and solutions (as discussed in Chapters 3 and 13) is one intervention that can help to reduce the disparities in the health status of minority populations. "Health education can empower [mobilize] individuals to take control of their lives, empower communities to influence public policies, and raise awareness among health service providers about their crucial health promotion role" (McDermott, 1995). Mobilizing communities means getting individuals and aggregates involved and enthused about taking responsibility for their own health destiny. There is no doubt that community involvement is crucial to reducing health disparities. As budgets are cut, government and private agencies "are increasingly turning their support to community empowerment initiatives" (Eisen, 1994). Community health nurses must be involved in developing initiatives in their respective communities.

Key Considerations for Providing Culturally Competent Care to a Target Minority Population

- Identify the culture.
- Describe its demographics, health beliefs, health practices, health attitudes, and values.
- Describe its communication patterns, religious beliefs, rituals, and symbols.
- Identify one's own personal culture, health values, health beliefs and practices, rituals, and symbols that affect communication with targeted population.
- Identify cultural differences between oneself and the targeted population.
- Determine whether personal cultural values and beliefs or an understanding of the targeted population's values is guiding communication and health planning with the targeted population.
- Establish collaborative relationships with key community leaders.
- Involve the client in all aspects of the planning process.
- Develop health planning and intervention strategies based on the targeted population's values, needs, and characteristics.

Facilitating Community Empowerment

Effective community health nurses facilitate community empowerment when they work with minorities. To effectively facilitate empowerment and deliver culturally competent care the nurse must be culturally sensitive. It is important that health intervention programs be specific to group needs because many health promoting behaviors are group specific (Marin, Burhansstipanov, Connell et al, 1995). For example, in developing a cancer prevention program for a black minority group one must consider that "perceptions and beliefs are known to play an integral part in cancer prevention" (Underwood, 1994, p. 20). Many blacks recognize the severity of cancer but "tend to believe that little can be done to prevent it" (Underwood, p. 20). For a prevention program to effectively mobilize the targeted aggregate, these beliefs must be *incorporated* in planning the interventions. The box above right provides some key considerations for delivering culturally competent care to a target minority population.

Community health nurses can be instrumental in getting health education materials and programs to minority aggregates, ensuring that these materials are culturally sensitive, improving accessibility to services, and serving as advocates for minority health and research. Strategies for reaching minority aggregates are discussed in Chapter 14.

Although minority populations have increased and continue to increase, they make up a small percentage of registered nurses and professional school enrollments (Eisen, 1994; Waters, 1996). Nurses at all levels can encourage minorities to become health care professionals and ultimately leaders and advocates for their communities. One community intervention could be to target select minority populations in local private and public schools and health systems and work with career counselors to deliver culturally/community-specific career opportunity programs. It is advantageous to seek out minority professionals to participate in these programs to enhance cultural competence.

Since lifestyles vary according to culture, lifestyle assessments are a key component in meeting health care needs of the culturally diverse (Pender, 1996, pp. 132-135). Prevention efforts that are not culturally sensitive will be ineffective because they will not be understood by targeted individuals, groups, and populations (Bayer, 1994, p. 895). A health promotion program with characteristics appropriate to a targeted Hispanic population may not necessarily be appropriate to the needs of an American Indian population in the same community. Health education programs must be culturally congruent. Lack of cultural sensitivity will impede or inhibit implementing health promotion interventions.

Chapter 7 provides characteristics about specific cultures that may influence health practices and should be taken into consideration during health programming. However, a culturally competent practitioner "understands that diversity *within* cultures is as important as diversity *between* cultures" (Randall-David, 1994, p. 3). Working with key community leaders helps practitioners to identify this diversity (see Chapter 13).

Grossman (1994, p. 62) described seven steps to help nurses develop cultural competence:

1. Know yourself.
2. Keep an open mind.

3. Respect differences in people.
4. Be willing to learn.
5. Learn to communicate effectively.
6. Don't judge.
7. Be resourceful and creative.

Chapter 9 provides guidelines for establishing a therapeutic relationship with clients of other cultures. Two key factors to consider when working with aggregates are "involving community members in every step of the process and networking with community-based organizations that already have good working relationships with the target population" (Randall-David, 1994, p. 23).

Transcultural Resources

Numerous nursing research studies and publications have addressed transcultural issues. The Transcultural Nursing Society is an international organization that addresses cultural care and diversity in nursing. The nurse can also obtain current information on local, state, and federal minority health programs, resources, publications, and statistics by calling the Office of Minority Health's Resource Center 1-800-444-MHRC.

POVERTY

The correlation between socioeconomic status and health care status has been well established (Benjamin, 1996). Low socioeconomic status is the basis of many health problems experienced by Americans, particularly minority blacks, Hispanics, Asian and Pacific Islanders, American Indians, and Alaskan Natives (USDHHS, 1991a). Nearly 1 of every 7 Americans lives in a family with an income below the federal poverty level (USDHHS, 1995, p. 65). Table 12-1 gives information on poverty level and race that dramatically illustrates that people of color are disproportionally experiencing poverty. It is significant to note that the percentage of blacks and Hispanics living in poverty is almost three times greater than the percentage of whites living in poverty.

As was discussed in Chapter 4, poverty and health has been the focus of numerous legislation throughout the years. Most recently the 104th Congress has proposed new legislation to address poverty in America. Poverty was a major issue in the 1996 election campaigns with every indication that it will continue to be a prominent concern in the 105th Congress and thereafter, with emphasis shifting from federal welfare solutions to state, grassroots, and community solutions (Evers-Williams, 1996; Gingrich, 1996; Woodson, 1996). However, health care professionals and advocates for people living in poverty are concerned that massive cuts in federal aid could spell disaster for families and neighborhoods "teetering on the edge of survival and stability" (Children's Defense Fund, 1996, p. xxviii). A major role for community health nurses in the future will be the political advocate role. The health of every disadvantaged group must be safeguarded during all state and federal legislative sessions.

Poverty and Health Risk Factors

Poverty coexists with many risk factors that influence health. Poor academic achievement, cognitive and developmental delays, decreased productivity in adulthood, high infant mortality, inadequate housing, unaffordable and inaccessible health care, poor nutrition, decreased mental well-being, and unemployment are some of the poverty risks that influence a community's health status (Benjamin, 1996; Garbarino, 1996; Grimes, 1996; Hartmann, Spalter-Roth, Chu, 1996). Increasingly the importance of the interrelationships between environmental or societal forces and the health status of aggregates is being recognized. Forces such as the economy of the nation, state, and local community; the availability of affordable health care services; and health policies greatly affect health programming and outcome.

A dynamic relationship also exists between low socioeconomic status and health risks such as lifestyle behaviors including smoking, drug use, exercise, and diet (Link, 1996). Death rates of people below the poverty level are much higher than those who are above it (Benjamin, 1996; USDHHS, 1991b). This is not surprising because health risks increase significantly in lower-income families. Low income has been identified as the key factor in almost all of the chronic illnesses in the United States (USDHHS, 1991a, p. 29). For example, infectious diseases and death rates from heart disease and cancer are significantly higher in low-income groups than their counterparts above the poverty level; low socioeconomic status is also associated with higher risks of accidents and homicides and has been associated with academic and developmental delays in children (USDHHS, 1991a, pp. 29-30). Additionally, low income has been a factor contributing to a higher incidence of low birth weight infants because low-income mothers are less likely to have early and adequate prenatal care (National Center for Health Statistics, 1996, p. 4). Chapter 15 elaborates on health risks of children living in poverty.

Clearly community efforts are needed throughout this country to increase educational and socioeconomic opportunities that would decrease risks of mortality in the less fortunate. For example, "working welfare mothers with a high-school education and job training are more likely to escape poverty" (Hartmann, Spalter-Roth, Chu, 1996) than those who drop out of school and remain uneducated and untrained. Changes in income and educational attainment can positively influence the health status of populations. This was illustrated in a longitudinal study that, after adjusting for various socioeconomic and demographic factors, demonstrated a decrease in mortality in both men and women under 65 years of age as income and educational level increased (Sorlie, Backlund, Keller, 1995). Hence community efforts to encourage education to help decrease socioeconomic disparities and ultimately develop healthy communities must be continually reiterated.

table 12-1 Persons and Families Below Poverty Level, According to Selected Characteristics, Race, and Hispanic Origin: United States, Selected Years 1973-1994

Selected Characteristics, Race, and Hispanic Origin	1973	1980[1]	1985	1988	1989	1990	1991	1992	1993	1994
					PERCENT BELOW POVERTY					
ALL PERSONS										
All races	11.1	13.0	14.0	13.0	12.8	13.5	14.2	14.8	15.1	14.5
White	8.4	10.2	11.4	10.1	10.0	10.7	11.3	11.9	12.2	11.7
Black	31.4	32.5	31.3	31.3	30.7	31.9	32.7	33.4	33.1	30.6
Hispanic	21.9	25.7	29.0	26.7	26.2	28.1	28.7	29.6	30.6	30.7
Mexican American			28.8	28.5	28.4	28.1	29.5	30.1	31.6	32.3
Puerto Rican			43.3	33.7	33.0	40.6	39.4	36.5	38.4	36.0
RELATED CHILDREN UNDER 18 YEARS OF AGE IN FAMILIES										
All races	14.2	17.9	20.1	19.0	19.0	19.9	21.1	21.6	22.0	21.2
White	9.7	13.4	15.6	14.0	14.1	15.1	16.1	16.5	17.0	16.3
Black	40.6	42.1	43.1	42.8	43.2	44.2	45.6	46.3	45.9	43.3
Hispanic	27.8	33.0	39.6	37.3	35.5	37.7	39.8	39.0	39.9	41.1
Mexican American			37.4	37.5	36.3	35.5	38.9	38.2	39.5	41.8
Puerto Rican			58.6	49.1	48.0	56.7	57.7	52.2	53.8	50.5
FAMILIES WITH FEMALE HOUSEHOLDER, NO HUSBAND PRESENT, AND CHILDREN UNDER 18 YEARS OF AGE[2]										
All races	43.2	42.9	45.4	44.7	42.8	44.5	47.1	46.2	46.1	44.0
White	35.2	35.9	38.7	38.2	36.1	37.9	39.6	39.6	39.6	38.3
Black	58.8	56.0	58.9	56.2	53.9	56.1	60.5	57.4	57.7	53.9
Hispanic		57.3	64.0	59.2	57.9	58.2	60.1	57.7	60.5	59.2
					NUMBER BELOW POVERTY IN THOUSANDS					
ALL PERSONS										
All races	22,973	29,272	33,064	31,745	31,528	33,585	35,708	38,014	39,265	38,059
White	15,142	19,699	22,860	20,715	20,785	22,326	23,747	25,259	26,226	25,379
Black	7,388	8,579	8,926	9,356	9,302	9,837	10,242	10,827	10,877	10,196
Hispanic	2,366	3,491	5,236	5,357	5,430	6,006	6,339	7,592	8,126	8,416
Mexican American			3,220	3,584	3,777	3,764	4,149	4,404	5,373	5,781
Puerto Rican			1,011	785	720	966	924	874	1,061	981
RELATED CHILDREN UNDER 18 YEARS OF AGE IN FAMILIES										
All races	9,453	11,114	12,483	11,935	12,001	12,715	13,658	14,521	14,961	14,610
White	5,462	6,817	7,838	7,095	7,164	7,696	8,316	8,752	9,123	8,826
Black	3,822	3,906	4,057	4,148	4,257	4,412	4,637	5,015	5,030	4,787
Hispanic	1,364	1,718	2,512	2,576	2,496	2,750	2,977	3,440	3,666	3,956
Mexican American			1,589	1,819	1,785	1,733	2,004	2,019	2,520	2,805
Puerto Rican			535	389	354	490	475	457	537	485
FAMILIES WITH FEMALE HOUSEHOLDER, NO HUSBAND PRESENT, AND CHILDREN UNDER 18 YEARS OF AGE[2]										
All races	1,987	2,703	3,131	3,294	3,190	3,426	3,767	3,867	4,034	3,816
White	1,053	1,433	1,730	1,740	1,671	1,814	1,969	2,021	2,123	2,064
Black	905	1,217	1,336	1,452	1,415	1,513	1,676	1,706	1,780	1,591
Hispanic		288	493	510	491	536	584	598	706	700

From National Center for Health Statistics: *Health, United States, 1995, Chartbook*, Pub No. (PHS) 96-1232, Hyattsville, Md., 1996, U.S. Government Printing Office, p. 81.

[1]Data for Hispanic families with female householder, no husband present, and children under 18 years are for 1979.

[2]Data not available for Mexican American and Puerto Rican families.

Notes: The race groups, white and black, include persons of both Hispanic and non-Hispanic origin. Conversely, persons of Hispanic origin may be of any race. Some numbers in this table have been revised and differ from previous editions of *Health, United States*.

A midcourse review of the *Healthy People 2000* goal to reduce health service disparities among Americans showed that significant disparities still existed between low-income Americans and other minority population groups (USDHHS, 1995, p. 6). Like minority Americans, Americans with low income have difficulty affording and gaining access to health care and preventive services. Lack of appropriate health care places individuals at high risk for development of acute and chronic illnesses. To reduce health disparities among low-income Americans, national, state, and community efforts must be made to increase access to health care and decrease the number of people living in poverty.

Where Is Poverty?

Poverty spans all ages, exists in rural America as well as inner city America, and exists in white populations as well as minority populations (Flynt, 1996). Poverty exists at some level in every geographical community. Young families and one-parent families have had dramatic rises in poverty rates in recent years (Burg, 1994, p. 125). For example, "single-mother families are more likely to experience poverty than almost any other group" (Hartmann, Spalter-Roth, Chu, 1996, p. 24).

Although minority groups experience a disproportionate amount of poverty, the majority of Americans living in poverty are white and reside in rural or suburban areas. Additionally, the majority of poor families with children work. In 1994 poor families with children received twice as much income from work as from governmental assistance (Children's Defense Fund, 1996, p. 2).

Nursing and Poverty

Historically, community health nurses have served low-income families. At the Henry Street Settlement Lillian Wald saw and responded to the health care needs of the poor in the community. Concerns such as poor nutrition and sanitation, poor infant health, child labor, lack of recreational facilities, school absences caused by sickness, and lack of access to appropriate health services became areas to be addressed by the Henry Street nurses. At the Frontier Nursing Service Mary Breckenridge worked with poor, rural Appalachian families to promote health.

Today's community health nurses provide numerous services to low-income populations. Nurses need to be sensitive to the needs and concerns of these populations and be familiar with community resources that can assist them. Examples of resources that can assist low-income families and children are Medicaid, Temporary Assistance to Needy Families, WIC, and Food Stamps.

Poverty and Nursing Interventions

Working with low-income populations provides many challenges and opportunities for community health nurses. Managed-care models, neighborhood health clinics, and community-based nursing centers are some ways of meeting the challenges of providing effective, culturally sensitive care to these aggregates (Craig, 1996; McCreary, 1996; Murphy, 1995). Community health nurses need to be innovative in developing interventions to promote the health of those living in poverty.

How can nurses intervene? As budgets are cut, financial resources become more and more difficult to obtain, and as responsibility for developing solutions shifts from federal programs to states and local communities, health care providers and local community leaders must become resourceful and creative in developing interventions to solve many of the problems associated with poverty. Certainly one cannot expect to eliminate poverty and poverty-related health risks in one step or by a one-provider approach. However, it is possible for nurses to identify at-risk aggregates (e.g., teen parents) that can be targeted for preventive interventions. Nurses can develop collaborative interventions and make great strides toward improving health and reducing the risk of people living in poverty.

Interventions cannot be developed before risks and problems are defined in communities. One way for nurses to identify health risks and problems is to conduct a community assessment of needs within a local community (Chapter 13 elaborates on how to conduct a community health assessment). The box below is an example of how risk identification at a local community level can effectively meet needs of at-risk aggregates. In this example the nurses identified a high-risk aggregate and targeted this population for preventive interventions. Efforts such as these are needed to expand the limited resources available for health programming in local communities.

An Example of Risk Identification at a Community Level: School-Based Tuberculin Testing

A review of tuberculosis surveillance data from a program of school-based tuberculin testing demonstrates the natural evolution of targeted populations. In the 7 years encompassed by this study, the prevalence of tuberculin reactivity ranged from 4.3% to 6.1% in the Amarillo public school populations which were tested. The initial screening was a sampling of all students in the school district. In subsequent years' screening, the targeted populations were increasingly refined to eliminate lower-risk populations. Children enrolled in "English as a Second Language" (ESL) classes were found to have an 8.5% tuberculosis infection rate. The purpose of this study was to alert nurses that culturally sensitive approaches are needed for successful future testing.

From Denison AV, Shum SY: The evolution of targeted populations in a school-based tuberculin testing program, *Image J Nurs Sch* 27(4):263-266, 1995.

Interventions will vary from one community to another based on each respective community's risks and needs. The most effective interventions for aggregate health are those that are population based, that mobilize populations to be enthusiastic about taking personal responsibility for their future health, and that shape the overall health of the community (Eisen, 1994; Woodson, 1996). Interventions that involve collaborative efforts (e.g., health care agencies and key community leaders) are thought to have higher outcomes than non-collaborative interventions (Marin, Burhansstipanov, Connell et al, 1995). Community health nurses play an important role in collaborating with community agencies to improve the health of the impoverished. Clearly the most ideal interventions are those that focus on primary prevention, including health promotion and specific protection. It costs less to prevent than to cure.

As nurses address the health risks of populations in communities, it is helpful to keep in mind the various roles of community health nurses in addressing the health needs of populations. Some examples of key community health nursing roles that may be implemented with the impoverished in a community are that of *health planner, casefinder, advocate, teacher,* and *clinic nurse*. Some typical situations in which these roles emerge are as follows:

- *Health planner:* Collaborate with local community health agencies and educational systems to determine population-specific health needs. The box below provides an example of a community-specific collaborative effort to complete a needs assessment that benefited all involved partners. Collaborative relationships are also being developed to plan innovative health programs. For example, community health nurses in Texas developed a community partnership to plan a health program designed to reduce infant mortality. Volunteer mothers in the community were used for outreach to teach Hispanic women at risk about the importance of early prenatal care in reducing the incidence of low birth weight babies. "Since the beginning of the program in 1989, not one low-birthweight baby has been born to a woman followed by a volunteer mother" (McFarlane, 1996, p. 880). Chapter 14 elaborates on this example and illustrates the health planning role with aggregates at risk.
- *Advocate:* Meet with local health agency personnel to promote development of a mobile health unit to access low-income populations at risk in the community.
- *Casefinder:* Conduct a community assessment to identify at-risk aggregates, such as a population living in a potentially toxic environment.
- *Teacher:* Apply teaching and learning principles to educate a group of single teen mothers about parenting skills that foster healthy child development. Keep in mind that "effective health education interventions should be tailored to a specific population" (Freudenberg, Eng, Flay et al, 1995, p. 297). For example, peer education strategies are often very effective with teen mothers.
- *Clinic nurse:* Focus on all three levels of prevention and use many community health nursing roles in addressing the needs of the less fortunate. For example, as a *casefinder* identify risks (such as nutritional deficiencies, violence, STDs) among the clinic clientele, as a *researcher* document trends (such as nutritional deficits, abuse, STD incidence and prevalence) within the clinic population, and as a *counselor* develop "culturally sensitive," population-specific interventions (e.g., community nutritional education programs to reduce hypertension, a support group for grandparents who are parenting young children, or a survivors' grief support group for families that have experienced violence).

An Example of a Community-Specific Collaborative Effort to Determine Population-Specific Needs

Health care reform can provide opportunities for collaboration between universities and the public at large. An advanced community nursing class within a post-RN program at a university combined resources with a nearby rural community to complete a community health and social needs assessment. The partners in the project included the local hospital, health unit, and the university; funding was secured from the Regional Center for Health Promotion and Community Studies and the two health agency partners also made a financial donation. Community liaisons who were both registered nurses and residents of the community were instrumental in completing tasks and activities related to the project. The students were taught the various data collection methods and participated in class assignments refining the necessary skills required for the actual assessment. This project benefited the community by providing baseline health status and social needs data in an era of dramatic health care reform while simultaneously affording undergraduate nursing students the opportunity to apply theory to practice.

From Kulig JC, Wilde IW: Collaboration between communities and universities: completion of a community needs assessment, *Public Health Nurs* 13(2):112-119, 1996.

HOMELESSNESS

Homeless persons are becoming more and more common in communities across the United States, and the number of Americans who are homeless is increasing dramatically. Factors that have contributed to homelessness include the lack of affordable housing, the deinstitutionalization of psychiatric patients, the economic recession, unemployment, catastrophic illness, mental illness, drug and alcohol abuse, and the reduction of funding for shelter programs. Homelessness has often been thought to exist primarily in urban areas. However, the number of rural families who have become homeless has increased significantly over the past few years (Wagner, Menke, Ciccone, 1995). Like other contemporary health-related problems, few communities are exempt from homeless populations. Community health nurses must be astute in identifying and meeting the needs of the homeless in their respective communities.

Over the past two decades, estimates of the number of homeless persons have ranged between 2 to 3 million or more people at various times (USDHUD, 1994). An accurate estimate is almost impossible to obtain because definitions of homelessness vary, sampling and survey methods differ (Link, Susser, Stueve et al, 1994), and the number of people homeless at any given time differs greatly from the number of people who have ever experienced homelessness in their lifetimes. According to one study, it was estimated that 13.5 million adults have been homeless at some time in their lives (Link, Susser, Stueve et al, p. 1910). Regardless of the precise number of homeless persons, it cannot be disputed that the number is continuing to increase for a variety of reasons.

Young families are the fastest-growing group of homeless people in the United States. Those families most at risk for homelessness are teenage and one-parent families, whose poverty rates have increased dramatically in recent years (Burg, 1994, p. 125). One-parent families, usually headed by women, represent the majority of all homeless families nationwide (Burg, 1994; Mihaly, 1991; Norton, Ridenour, 1995; Wagner, Menke, Ciccone, 1995).

It has been estimated that 60,000 to 500,000 American children go to sleep homeless on various nights (USDHHS, 1996). Mihaly (1991) stated that "the fundamental cause of homelessness among children today is the rapidly growing gap between the incomes of poor, minority, and young families and the cost of available housing" (p. 10).

Homelessness may have a lifelong impact on children that adversely affects them in adulthood. This impact was demonstrated in a Los Angeles County study of 1563 homeless adults, in which the majority reported growing up in poor socioeconomic conditions and over half had experienced some type of housing disruption as children that ranged from subsidized housing, eviction, crowded living conditions, and homelessness (Koegel, Melamid, Burnam, 1995, p. 1647). It is necessary to intervene early to prevent the cycle of homelessness in ongoing generations and to promote the health of children so that they will be healthy, contributing individuals as they move into adulthood.

Health Problems Among the Homeless

Homeless adults have a high prevalence of social, physical, and chronic problems that may have their roots in a homeless childhood. Homeless children have numerous health problems that may contribute to chronic problems in adulthood. Studies have noted that homeless children have incomplete immunizations and immunization delays, putting them at increased risk of serious and disabling communicable disease. For example, in New York City Mihaly (1991) found that homeless children were three times more likely to be behind in their immunizations than their "housed" poor counterparts. Similarly, in Ohio Wagner, Menke, and Ciccone (1995) studied the health of 76 rural homeless families, which included 125 children ranging from 1 month to 12 years of age, and identified several health risks including allergies, bronchitis, incomplete immunizations, and developmental risks. Eighty-five of the children in this study were under 6 years of age, and over half (52%) were found to have developmental delays (based on Denver Developmental Screening Tests), including 20 children who completely failed fine motor testing.

Findings from a study of homeless children in Los Angeles were consistent with findings in the Ohio study by Wagner, Menke, and Ciccone (1995). Zima, Wells, and Freeman (1994) found that homeless children were more likely to be academically delayed and have depressive and social disorders than those not homeless. Another study revealed that homeless children had various chronic physical disorders including asthma, anemia, and malnutrition, and that skin ailments, ear infections, eye disorders, dental problems, upper respiratory infections, and gastrointestinal problems were also common (Berne, Dato, Mason, Rafferty, 1990, p. 8). The mental health of homeless children in this study was profoundly affected. Developmental delays, depression, anxiety, suicidal ideation, sleep problems, shyness, withdrawal, and aggression were evident. Homeless children often do not have regular schooling, lack stable familial support systems, and lack friends. This can be personally and developmentally devastating, which leaves them vulnerable to a variety of health, social, and behavioral problems as they mature to adulthood.

Both adults and children who are homeless often find it difficult to obtain health care services. Riemer, Van-Cleve, and Galbraith (1995) identified common barriers that impede preventive health care for homeless children. These barriers included difficulties in selecting and obtaining health care providers, resource variables such as waiting time for obtaining care and during appointments, attitudes of health care professionals, and transportation costs. Most homeless people do not have health insurance, and the cost of health care services is often prohibitive. The challenge for community health nurses is to find ways to reach out to the homeless populations in their communities. Outreach services are often essential for the homeless.

There is no doubt that homeless children are at risk for health, developmental, and social problems that may extend into adulthood. It is important for community health nurses to assess the childhood experiences of homeless adults, as well as assessing the homeless children themselves when intervening with homeless populations. Homeless adults who were homeless as children may have unidentified health and developmental problems that began in childhood.

The Homeless and Their Environment

Persons who are homeless are exposed to the elements (Figure 12-4) and experience overcrowding and unsanitary conditions. Homelessness is often a cause and effect of multiple social and chronic health problems. It is not surprising that homeless people have a high prevalence of severe and chronic mental disorders and substance abuse; a high risk of becoming victims of rape and violence; an increased incidence of physical problems, such as hypertension and trauma; an increased susceptibility to infectious disease conditions, including tuberculosis, influenza, scabies, lice, and pneumonia; and a variety of nutritional deficiencies.

Murray (1996), from interviews with 150 homeless men who were part of a day treatment program for mentally ill and chemically dependent persons, described two major fears of homeless men: fear of violence and fear of being unable to meet basic needs. A third of the men had suffered some kind of violent assault such as beating (most common), knifing, robbing, or shooting. As a result, the majority feared violence and were fearful of being unable to protect themselves. The homeless also cited frustration with shelter staff and negative reactions of other people. These data reflect the need for nurses to holistically address, and be sensitive to, the needs of the homeless without passing judgment in order to competently intervene. Nurses who work with the homeless visit them in a variety of places, including homeless shelters, shacks, benches in a park, and under bridges.

Homelessness and Legislation

On a national level, the Stewart B. McKinney Homeless Assistance Act (Public Law 100-77) provides assistance to protect and improve the lives and safety of the homeless with special emphasis on the elderly, handicapped persons, and families with children. The Act authorized emergency food and shelter, supportive housing, programs for primary health care, substance abuse services, community mental health care, adult education, education for children and youth, job training, and studies of homelessness. Further information about this Act can be found in Chapter 4.

Homelessness and Isolation

Homeless people are often isolated from the mainstream of society. Families find themselves without the necessary support or resources to cope with even minor problems and difficulties. Kinzel (1991), in research with the homeless, found that a recurring theme among people who are homeless was the need to interact with a caring person. "The feeling that no one cares, a lack of self-worth, and a sense of limited control over their lives may lead to depression, hopelessness, and finally illness. The extent and effectiveness of health-seeking behaviors among this group are limited because of decreased trust, decreased motivation for self-care, and isolation from social and health care systems" (Kinzel, 1991, p. 189).

It is estimated that one third of homeless people have serious mental health and substance abuse problems that have interfered with their own ability to seek health care and

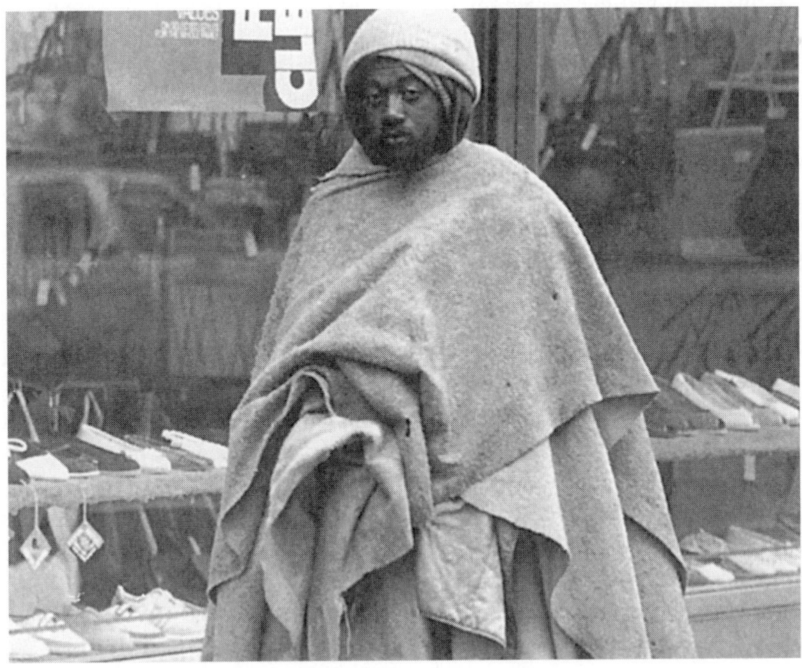

Figure 12-4 Homelessness is often the cause and effect of multiple social and chronic health problems. *(Courtesy Brian Lafferty.)*

provide shelter for themselves (USDHHS, 1994c). In response to this need, five large multisite demonstration projects known as the *Center for Mental Health Services* (CMHS), funded by the *Stewart B. McKinney Homeless Assistance Act*, began in 1990 and targeted the homeless mentally ill in five sites: Boston, Baltimore, San Diego, and two projects in New York (USDHHS, 1994c).

The CMHS projects involved a total of 896 homeless adults who were between 36 and 40 years old and had mental illnesses such as nonaffective psychotic disorder, schizophrenia, and depression. The majority (67%) were single, about 33% were high school dropouts, about 25% were veterans, over 50% had alcohol or drug abuse problems, and less than 33% had any income benefits (USDHHS, 1994c, pp. i-ii). Within this CMHS multisite population 75% were homeless for 1 year or more, 30% for 10 or more years, and 22% before age 18 (USDHHS, 1994c, pp. i-ii). The interim key findings from these longitudinal projects that have implications for the development of community health outreach services are as follows (USDHHS, 1994c, pp. ii-iii):

- *Homeless people with severe mental illnesses will use accessible, relevant community health services.*
- *Appropriate services decrease homelessness.*
- *Advocacy helps increase access to entitlement income.*
- *Formerly homeless persons with severe mental illnesses are an important resource.*
- *Substance abuse is a major factor in homelessness among persons with severe mental illness.*
- *Housing stability, appropriate mental health treatment, and increased income lead to an improved quality of life.*

In addition to the key findings, the CMHS interim report (USDHHS, 1994c, p. iii) identified five policy implications that need to be considered when providing for the health needs of the homeless:

- *Service systems must be integrated at all levels to remove barriers and promote efficient services.*
- *Substance abuse treatment must be an integral part of comprehensive services for persons with severe mental illnesses to prevent recurrent homelessness.*
- *A range of housing options is required to respond to the needs and preferences of the homeless.*
- *Preventive health care and health education are critical components in health planning for the homeless since many are at risk for acute and chronic illnesses.*
- *Longer-term follow-up studies should focus on how to sustain early gains.*

From both the CMHS key findings and policy implications, there is no doubt that interventions with the homeless must be *community-based, population-specific*, and designed to meet the needs of the particular homeless populations in communities throughout the country. Despite the recognized need of outreach programs to access the homeless "there are virtually no health insurance programs that support the efforts of outreach workers" (Wells, 1996). Because of this there is a tremendous need to develop methods to enhance the primary care, mental health, and substance abuse resources available to the homeless.

Nursing Interventions with the Homeless

Community health nurses provide health care to people who are homeless in traditional settings such as health departments and outpatient clinics. Consistent with the changing health care delivery system, community health nurses from traditional and other settings are also demonstrating that innovative community-based approaches to caring for the homeless are effective. Community health nurses are establishing community-based centers and clinics targeting the homeless (McNeal, 1996; Scholler-Jaquish, 1996; Simandl, 1996), providing health promotion and protection activities such as tuberculosis treatment and control in homeless shelters (Kitazawa, 1995; May, Evans, 1994; Mayo, White, Oates, Franklin, 1996), and taking care to the "streets" with on-the-spot mobile units (Berne, Dato, Mason, Rafferty, 1990). Lillian Wald's Henry Street Settlement House in New York provides supportive, 24-hour care to homeless families. In Lexington, Kentucky nurses are addressing the health needs of the homeless through the "Hope Center," a nurse-managed clinic (Ossege, Berry, 1994, p. 22). Wells (1996) emphasized the need for outreach programs to be mobile and to meet the homeless wherever they are, which means going beyond clinics and offices to parks, bridges, and shelters.

Berne, Dato, Mason, Rafferty (1990) described a model program that used comprehensive pediatric mobile units to access children living in homeless shelters and hotels in New York City. A major component of the program included public health nurses on-site at homeless centers to casefind and do initial client assessments and nurse practitioners to diagnose and treat health problems. Clients were referred to community resources such as WIC, the department of social services, and community mental health services. A primary focus in working with the homeless is to mobilize their skills and capacities to become self-sufficient and to break the homeless cycle by building hope and self-esteem. Specific self-esteem enhancement interventions are discussed in Chapter 19. Self-esteem enhancement nursing activities assist clients to increase their personal judgment of self-worth (McCloskey, Bulechek, 1996, p. 492).

Nurses can provide the "caring" aspect that people who are homeless covet in service provision. A recent study with homeless veterans found high levels of depression were linked to low levels of self-esteem, hope, and self-efficacy (Tollett, Thomas, 1996). Through the use of a nursing theory–based intervention Tollett and Thomas were able to "care" for the veterans and make significant changes in their level of hope (p. 87). Specifically, Tollett and Thomas used small-group therapy sessions to assist veterans in identifying reasons for hope, personal strengths, and areas in which they felt pride. The researchers believed that a personal feeling of having hope was an essential first step before the homeless veterans could learn to be self-sufficient. It is vital to intervene whenever possible to increase self-sufficiency and decrease the risk of intergenerational homelessness. "Prevention is the most cost-effective way to address homelessness" (USDHUD, 1994, p. 50). Nurses can help to link people who are homeless to community resources and provide the "caring" aspects of health care.

Like other contemporary problems the most ideal intervention is primary prevention. Prevention should be inherent in every facet of health programming for the homeless. A primary long-term outcome goal should always be directed toward providing the homeless with tools to become self-motivated and self-sufficient in maintaining their own health and shelter. It is evident that the most efficient interventions are those that are community and population specific. Collaborative efforts between a multidisciplinary health care team and the homeless assists communities in developing population-specific interventions. "No single service system can adequately address the many service needs of people recovering from homelessness and mental illnesses" (Wells, 1996, p. 8).

SUBSTANCE ABUSE

Substance abuse undermines health and is a serious problem in the United States. Each year millions of Americans abuse alcohol and other drugs. Substance abuse is estimated to be the actual cause of 120,000 deaths annually in the United States and contributes significantly to injury, suicide, homicide, violent crime, and AIDS transmission (USDHHS, 1995, p. 42). The psychological, familial, and social damage that accompanies substance abuse is devastating. A rising concern is the increased substance abuse among children, with an estimated "11% of 22 million teens using drugs" (Friend, 1996, p. A1). The *Monitoring the Future Project* discussed in Chapter 16 provides data annually on the range of substance abuse among American youth. Smoking is discussed extensively in Chapter 17.

Healthy People 2000 has a separate priority area for substance abuse (alcohol and other drugs) with numerous national health objectives. Both government and private organizations are working to combat substance abuse in the nation. To assist in disseminating treatment and resource information the federal government sponsors the National Alcohol and Drug Abuse Information and Referral Hotline (1-800-662-HELP) as well as a hotline for information on all drugs (1-800-COCAINE). In response to the *Healthy People 2000* objectives that focused on reducing substance abuse, schools and worksites across the nation have implemented drug and alcohol education, treatment, and prevention programs. According to the *Healthy People 2000 Midcourse Review* (USDHHS, 1995, p. 42), great strides in reduction of alcohol use were made. However, while alcohol use declined among teens, drug use increased and continues to rise at an alarming rate (Friend, 1996; Leland, 1996; Schoemer, 1996). Heightened drug awareness programs in schools, as well as increased community-based substance abuse prevention programs, are needed. The rise in drug use and need for prevention was a prime issue in the 1996 presidential campaign (Klaidman, 1996; Nichols, 1996).

Two federal government agencies assist local communities in developing effective programs for addressing substance abuse. The National Clearinghouse on Alcohol and Drug Abuse offers information, educational materials, and referral sources. The National Institute on Alcohol Abuse and Alcoholism strives to increase knowledge and promote effective strategies to deal with the health problems associated with alcoholism. It sponsors research and education programs including youth alcohol awareness programs, education on alcohol and pregnancy, and national drunk driving awareness.

Health Risks of Alcoholism

Alcoholism is the largest drug problem in the United States today. Millions of American adolescents and adults are alcohol abusers (Crowe, Reeves, 1994). Although more men than women abuse alcohol and drugs, the problem among women is substantial. While the annual per capita consumption of alcohol has declined in recent years to 2.3 gallons of alcohol for every U.S. resident above the age of 14 years, it is still above the year 2000 national health objective of 2 gallons annual average (USDHHS, 1995, pp. 42, 183).

Alcoholism contributes to health problems such as nutritional deficiencies, pancreatitis, cirrhosis, and cancer. Cirrhosis is a leading cause of death among adults, and as many as 90% of cases are associated with excessive use of alcohol (USDHHS, 1995). Alcohol is a contributing factor in other causes of death, including accidents, suicides, and homicides. Nearly half of all traffic deaths are alcohol related. Studies show that careless handling of smoking materials by intoxicated persons is dangerous and contributes substantially to burn injuries, death, and property damage.

"The reduction of alcohol-related vehicle deaths is one of the greatest success stories of public health in this decade" (USDHHS, 1995, p. 42). At midcourse review the *Healthy People 2000* objective for alcohol-related motor vehicle crashes was met for the overall population and for people aged 15 to 24 (USDHHS, p. 44). Because targeted outcomes for these groups were achieved, revisions to the *Healthy People 2000* objectives were made to target special population groups. The 1995 revisions included (a) to reduce the number of cirrhosis deaths among all American Indian/Alaskan Native men, not just those living in reservation states; (b) to begin tracking cirrhosis deaths among Hispanics; and (c) to monitor drug-related deaths among blacks and Hispanics (USDHHS, p. 44).

Contradictory to the *Healthy People 2000* midcourse report, and after a 10-year decline in the number of alcohol-related traffic deaths, Johnson and Dowling (1996) reported a rise in the number of alcohol-related traffic deaths in 1995. Johnson and Dowling cited a 4.13% increase over the 1994 alcohol-related traffic deaths (p. A2). Although a reason for this recent rise was unclear, it triggered a national media and law enforcement blitz that targeted drunk drivers and increased state and community awareness efforts to stop drunk driving. The number of alcohol-related traffic deaths will continue to be closely monitored, and evaluation of *Healthy People 2000* objectives is ongoing with annual reporting on the status of outcomes.

Substance abuse is a serious health problem. The effects of substance abuse are devastating to the health of communities (Emblad, 1995, p. 4). The psychosocial consequences of alcoholism are immense. Such consequences include disruption of family life, loss of on-the-job productivity and financial prosperity, lowered self-esteem, and devastating emotional effects for friends and co-workers. The families of alcoholics are victims of alcoholism themselves. Self-help groups such as Alcoholics Anonymous, Children of Alcoholics, and counseling services are available for alcoholics and their families. The National Council on Alcoholism (1-800-NCA-CALL) is a voluntary organization that offers information and referral services. Many employers have employee assistance programs that help employees to obtain help with their drinking problems.

Some rather innovative, and sometimes controversial, methods were recommended by former Surgeon General C. Everett Koop to decrease alcohol use in the United States. These measures included an increase of alcohol-related public service ads to match the number of beer, wine, and spirit ads; an increase in the federal and state taxes on liquor; elimination of "happy hours" and drink discounts; an end to alcohol ads that use celebrities and appear on college campuses; a halt to liquor producers sponsoring sports events, rock concerts, and other programs where the majority of the target audience is under age 21; and a reduction in the legal blood-alcohol level for motorists to 0.04% by the year 2000 (Cox, 1989). Some of these measures were implemented, have contributed to the favorable outcomes related to the *Healthy People* objectives, and have promoted the development of alcohol prevention programs for at-risk groups. For example, numerous substance abuse prevention programs have targeted adolescents and teens; baseline deaths from alcohol-related vehicle accidents dropped from 9.8 deaths per 100,000 in 1987 to 6.8 deaths per 100,000 in 1993; 11 states reduced blood alcohol concentration limits from .10 to .08; and stricter enforcement of laws against driving while intoxicated (DWI) have contributed to some of the *Healthy People* successes (USDHHS, 1995, p. 42).

Fetal Alcohol Syndrome

Fetal Alcohol Syndrome (FAS) consists of a variety of health problems with infants that have been linked to exposure to alcohol in utero. It has been estimated that between one and three infants per 1000 births have FAS (Crowe, Reeves, 1994, pp. 84-85). The adverse effects of alcohol on fetal development has been and continues to be a health concern. The infants of mothers who consume alcohol suffer from low birth weight, birth defects, brain and physical malformations, lower IQs, aggression, mental retardation, and learning, memory, and attention deficits (Crowe, Reeves, pp. 84-85). Studies have shown that both chronic drinking and binge drinking affect pregnancy outcomes.

The public is becoming increasingly aware of conditions such as FAS, but education about this problem is an important element in a FAS prevention program. Women of childbearing years, especially pregnant women, need to know the effects of drinking during pregnancy. Increased programs to help pregnant women prevent FAS by eliminating alcohol and substance use during pregnancy are needed to decrease the health risks to the mother, the fetus, and the infant.

Health Risks of Illegal Drugs

Drug use is a serious health concern among adults as well as children. According to the *Healthy People 2000* midcourse review, alcohol and marijuana use among adolescents declined from 1988 to 1992. However, in 1992 this decline halted as the use of these drugs increased among American teens (USDHHS, 1995, p. 43). Among high school seniors in 1995, 49% had tried an illicit drug (Johnston, O'Malley, Bachman, 1995). Millions of Americans use illicit drugs each year. More recently, rising substance abuse among children has been noted, as in an alarming *USA Today* headline that stated *Teens and Drugs: in classroom of 25, three kids are users* (August 21, 1996). According to Friend (1996), some of the reasons for the increased use of drugs by teens included failure to recognize harmful effects of drugs, peer pressure, unhappy homelife, curiosity, and a reglamorization of drug use by the movie industry. "This nation's secondary school students and young adults show a level of involvement with illicit drugs which is greater than is documented in any other industrialized nation in the world" (Johnston, O'Malley, Bachman, 1995, p. 27). Clearly drug prevention programs must target adolescents and young adults before addiction cycles are established. Drug use is linked to other concerns such as death, violent crime, transmission of HIV, and physical, behavioral, and developmental problems in infants of drug-addicted mothers.

Drug use is a direct or contributing factor in thousands of deaths each year in the United States. Accidental overdose is the most common cause of these deaths. Alcohol, heroin, cocaine, crack, marijuana, stimulants, and tranquilizers are commonly ingested in overdoses (Leland, 1996; Schoemer, 1996). There is a disproportionate number of drug deaths among minorities.

Violent crimes are linked to drug use and the drug trade. According to a survey of state prisons, 28% of inmates who had been convicted of murder and 32% of inmates who had been convicted of rape were under the influence of drugs and/or alcohol at the time the crime was committed (Robert Wood Johnson Foundation, 1991, p. 58). Often crimes are committed in an effort to procure drugs when addicted persons do not have the cash resources to maintain their addiction (Needle, Mills, 1994). Research has shown that there is a relationship between drug use and crime and more than 50% of the individuals in correctional facilities have alcohol and other drug abuse problems (Massaro, Pepper, 1994, p. 11). More than half of the men and women booked for crimes in many of the nation's larger cities have tested positive for illicit drugs at the time of their arrest (Massaro, Pepper, p. 13).

Illicit drug use is related to the HIV epidemic. HIV is prevalent among intravenous drug users. Substance abuse has many other adverse health consequences. Some of these consequences include malnutrition, low birth weight and premature infants, accidental injuries and death, infectious diseases, and mental disorders (Crowe, Reeves, 1994).

The devastating effects of illegal drugs hit hardest among some of the most vulnerable population groups in our country: the poor, women and children, minorities, and those infected with HIV. Drug abuse has killed hundreds of thousands of young adults who will never have the opportunity to contribute their skills to society.

Who Becomes Addicted?

Who becomes addicted? In the largest global study on cocaine use ever undertaken by the World Health Organization (WHO) it was reported that drug abuse has no boundaries. The study concluded "that there is no average cocaine user, there is an enormous variety in the types of people who use cocaine" for a variety of reasons, and cocaine users often use other drugs as well (Cocaine use, 1995, p. 25). This means that drug abuse transcends boundaries of race, culture, religion, communities, economics, and age. No community is exempt from substance users, and community health nurses have a tremendous responsibility to identify populations at risk for substance abuse. Community health nurses can then intervene before addiction occurs.

No one begins to use drugs and alcohol with the intention of becoming addicted (Crowe, Reeves, 1994, p. 2). However, all too frequently what began as an experience to satisfy curiosity leads to a point of no return where addiction has occurred. The process of addiction progresses from experimental, social use to dependency and addiction (Crowe, Reeves, p. 1). Substance abuse is multifaceted, and numerous views have been espoused in relation to causes of substance addiction (Crowe, Reeves, p. 25). Family and environmental factors have been thought to contribute to addiction (see the box on the next page). Additionally, other factors such as genetics, altered brain chemistry, personality traits, social learning, and self-medication have also been thought to be possible risk indicators in addiction (Crowe, Reeves, p. 29).

The Process of Addiction

The process of addiction generally occurs in three stages: experimenting, abuse, and addiction. The first stage involves experimental and social use of alcohol and/or drugs. During this stage drugs/alcohol are used intermittently, and there are periods of abstinence (Crowe, Reeves, 1994, p. 2). Table 12-2 on the process of addiction identifies reasons for drug and alcohol use, the frequency and the effects of use, and the sources of alcohol and drugs.

The second stage in the addiction process is characterized by abuse of alcohol and drugs. The amount and frequency of substance used is increased with frequent intoxication. In this stage some negative consequences start to appear (note the behavior indicators listed in the box on the next page). Users are considered dependent when they stop taking the drugs and experience some physical and psychological distress with drug withdrawal (Crowe, Reeves, 1994, p. 3).

The third stage of the addiction process is that of addiction. With addiction users have no self-control over using the substance. There is a compulsive need to maintain the addiction, and to do so criminal activity, including prostitution, is not uncommon (Crowe, Reeves, 1994, pp. 3-4). The consequences of alcohol and drug use during this stage are profoundly negative.

Substance Abuse and the Role of the Community Health Nurse

Figure 12-5 diagrams the process of addiction through its various stages. As substance users progress through the stages of addiction, various personal, social, and psychological problems occur. When drug users undergo recovery, community health nurses must keep in mind that recovery is not an *end;* instead, recovery is a *process* that is ongoing. Therefore preventive efforts must also include tertiary prevention interventions that focus on how to prevent intermittent relapses. Understanding the process helps health care providers to casefind and develop primary, secondary, and tertiary preventive programs and interventions.

Assessment is the first stage of any treatment or intervention process (Crowe, Reeves, 1994). The community health nurse's role with populations who are substance abusers begins with a comprehensive assessment. Special attention should be placed on assessing for this problem among pregnant women. A comprehensive assessment is essential to design appropriate interventions for appropriate problems (Crowe, Reeves). Often drug users are caught up in a web of personal, social, and cultural problems (see Figure 12-1) and require services from multiple community resources. Therefore a comprehensive assessment must be multifaceted and holistic, with interagency collaboration. A holistic approach will involve a collaborative network of care in treatment and relapse prevention, as depicted in Figure 12-6.

Crowe and Reeves (1994) described five key objectives in conducting a comprehensive substance abuse assessment:

Text continues on p. 341.

Family and Environmental Factors Contributing to Alcohol and Drug Addiction

FAMILY FACTORS

- **Parent and sibling drug use.** Parental and sibling alcoholism and use of illicit drugs increases the risk of alcoholism and drug abuse in offspring. Attitudes and early drinking behaviors appear to be shaped more by parents and relatives than by peers (Hawkins, Lishner, Jenson et al, 1987; Knott, 1986).
- **Poor and inconsistent family practices.** Children from families with lax supervision, excessively severe or inconsistent disciplinary practices, and low communication and involvement between parents and children are at high risk for later delinquency and drug use (Hawkins, Lishner, Jenson et al, 1987). Lack of acceptance, closeness, warmth, and praise for good behavior also are family characteristics associated with adolescent substance abuse (Jaynes, Rugg, 1988).
- **Family conflict.** Children raised in families with high rates of conflict appear at risk for both delinquency and illicit drug use. It is the conflict, rather than the actual family structure (e.g., "broken home" or single parent family), that predicts delinquency and drug use (Hawkins, Lishner, Jenson et al, 1987).
- **Family social and economic deprivation.** Social isolation, poverty, poor living conditions, and low-status occupations are circumstances that appear to elevate the risk of delinquency and drug use (Hawkins, Lishner, Jenson et al, 1987).

SCHOOL-RELATED FACTORS

- **School failure.** School failure is a predictor of delinquency and drug use. Truancy, placement in special classes, and early dropout from school are factors associated with drug abuse (Hawkins, Lishner, Jenson et al, 1987).
- **Low degree of commitment to education and attachment to school.** This factor is sometimes called school bonding. Low commitment to school is related to drug use. Drug users are more likely than nonusers to be absent from school, to cut classes, and to perform poorly. Dropouts tend to have patterns of greater drug use (Hawkins, Lishner, Jenson et al, 1987).

BEHAVIORAL AND ATTITUDINAL FACTORS

- **Early antisocial behavior.** Conduct problems in early elementary grades have been associated with continued delinquency and use of drugs in adolescence. Early delinquent behavior appears to predict early initiation of the use of illicit drugs; and early initiation of drug use increases the risk for regular use and the probability of involvement in crime (Hawkins, Lishner, Jenson et al, 1987).
- **Attitudes and beliefs.** Alienation from the dominant values of society, low religiosity, and rebelliousness are related to drug use. Adolescents who are problem drinkers tend to value independence and autonomy, be more tolerant of deviance, and place more importance on the positive than on the negative functions of drinking. They also tend to have lower expectations of achievement. Individuals with positive attitudes toward drug use are more likely to become substance users. Perceiving substance use as normal and widespread behavior is correlated with engaging in substance use. The initiation into use of any substance is preceded by values favorable to its use (Hawkins, Lishner, Jenson et al, 1987; Knott, 1986; Schinke, Botvin, Orlandi, 1991).

ENVIRONMENTAL FACTORS

- **Neighborhood attachment and community disorganization.** Disorganized communities, such as those with high population density, high neighborhood crime rates, and lack of informal social controls, have less ability to limit drug use among adolescents (Hawkins, Lishner, Jenson et al, 1987).
- **Peer factors.** Drug behavior and drug-related attitudes of peers are among the most potent predictors of drug involvement. Adolescents tend to increase use of drugs due to the influence of friends, and they also tend to choose friends who reinforce their own drug norms and behaviors (Hawkins, Lishner, Jenson et al, 1987). Adolescents who are problem drinkers usually do not feel their peer group and their parents are compatible, are more easily influenced by peers than by parents, and feel more pressure from peers for drinking and drug use (Knott, 1986).
- **Mobility.** Transitions (such as from elementary to middle school and from junior high to senior high school) and residential mobility are associated with high rates of drug initiation and frequency of use (Hawkins, Lishner, Jenson et al, 1987).

CONSTITUTIONAL AND PERSONALITY FACTORS

- **Constitutional factors.** These factors are often present from birth or early childhood and are thought to have neurological or physiological origins. Attention and cognitive deficits, such as low verbal ability and poor language and problem-solving skills, have been associated with delinquent behavior. There also is evidence of a constitutional predisposition toward alcoholism, suggesting that genetic factors may play a role in this area (Hawkins, Lishner, Jenson et al, 1987).
- **Personality factors.** Alienation, low motivation, sensation-seeking, willingness to take risks, and need for stimulation are associated with drug and alcohol use (Hawkins, Lishner, Jenson et al, 1987). Other characteristics associated with substance use include low self-esteem and self-confidence, need for social approval, high anxiety, low assertiveness, rebelliousness, low personal control, and low self-efficacy (Schinke, Botvin, Orlandi, 1991).

PHYSICAL AND SEXUAL ABUSE

- This area of investigation is relatively recent. However, some studies have found a high correlation between physical and/or sexual abuse and drug use and/or other deviant behavior. It is postulated that child maltreatment leads adolescents to become disengaged from conventional norms and behaviors and to initiate patterns of deviant behaviors (Dembo, Williams, Wish et al, 1988). There also appears to be a high correlation between parents' abuse of drugs and alcohol and abuse and neglect of their children. These emotional wounds, in turn, increase the likelihood that youth will use substances to compensate for unmet emotional needs (Nowinski, 1990).

Modified from Crowe AH, Reeves RR: *Treatment for alcohol and other drug abuse: opportunities for coordination*, DHHS Pub No. (SMA)94-2075, Rockville, Md., 1994, U.S. Government Printing Office, p. 27.

table 12-2 The Process of Addiction

Stage	Frequency of Use	Sources	Reasons for Use	Effects	Behavioral Indicators
1: Experimental and Social	Occasional, perhaps a few times monthly. Usually on weekends when at parties or with friends. May use when alone.	Friends/peers primarily. Youth may use parent's alcohol.	To satisfy curiosity. To acquiesce to peer pressure. To obtain social acceptance. To defy parental limits. To take a risk or seek a thrill. To appear grown up. To relieve boredom. To produce pleasurable feelings. To diminish inhibitions in social situations.	At this stage the person will experience euphoria and return to a normal state after using. A small amount may cause intoxication. Feelings sought include: Fun, excitement. Thrill. Belonging. Control.	Little noticeable change. Some may lie about use or whereabouts. Some may experience moderate hangovers. Occasionally there is evidence of use, such as a beer can or marijuana joint.
2: Abuse	Regular, may use several times per week. May begin using during the day. May be using alone rather than with friends.	Friends; begins buying enough to be prepared. May sell drugs to keep a supply for personal use. May begin stealing to have money to buy drugs/alcohol.	To manipulate emotions. To experience the pleasure the substances produce. To cope with stress and uncomfortable feelings such as pain, guilt, anxiety, and sadness. To overcome feelings of inadequacy. Persons who progress to this stage of drug/alcohol involvement often experience depression or other uncomfortable feelings when not using. Substances are used to stay high or at least maintain normal feelings.	Euphoria is the desired feeling; may return to a normal state following use or may experience pain, depression, and general discomfort. Intoxication begins to occur regularly. Feelings sought include: Pleasure. Relief from negative feelings, such as boredom and anxiety. Stress reduction. May being to feel some guilt, fear, and shame. May have suicidal ideations/attempts. Tries to control use, but is unsuccessful. Feels shame and guilt. More of a substance is needed to produce the same effect.	School or work performance and attendance may decline. Mood swings. Changes in personality. Lying and conning. Change in friendships — will have drug-using friends. Decrease in extra curricular activities. Begins adopting drug culture appearance (clothing, grooming, hairstyles, jewelry). Conflict with family members may be exacerbated. Behavior may be more rebellious. All interest is focused on procuring and using drugs/alcohol.
3: Dependancy/ Addiction	Daily use, continous.	Will use any means necessary to obtain and secure needed drugs/alcohol. Will take serious risks. Will often engage in criminal behavior such as shoplifting and burglary.	Drugs/alcohol are needed to avoid pain and depression. Many wish to escape the realities of daily living. Use is out of control.	Person's normal state is pain or discomfort. Drugs/alcohol help person feel normal; when the effects wear off, the person again feels pain. Unlikely to experience euphoria at this stage. May experience suicidal thoughts or attempts. Often feel guilt, shame, and remorse. May experience blackouts. May experience changing emotions such as depression, aggression, irritation, and apathy.	Physical deterioration includes weight loss, health problems. Appearance is poor. May experience memory loss, flashbacks, paranoia, volatile mood swings, and other mental problems. Likely to drop out or be expelled from school or lose jobs. May be absent from home much of the time. Possible overdoses. Lack of concern about being caught — focused only on procuring and using drugs/alcohol.

Data from Beschner, 1986; Institute of Medicine, 1990; Jaynes, Rugg, 1988; Macdonald, 1989; Nowinski, 1990. Modified from Crowe AH, Reeves RR: *Treatment for alcohol and other drug abuse: opportunities for coordination*, DHHS Pub No. (SMA) 94-2075, Rockville, Md., 1994, U.S. Government Printing Offie, pp. 2-4.

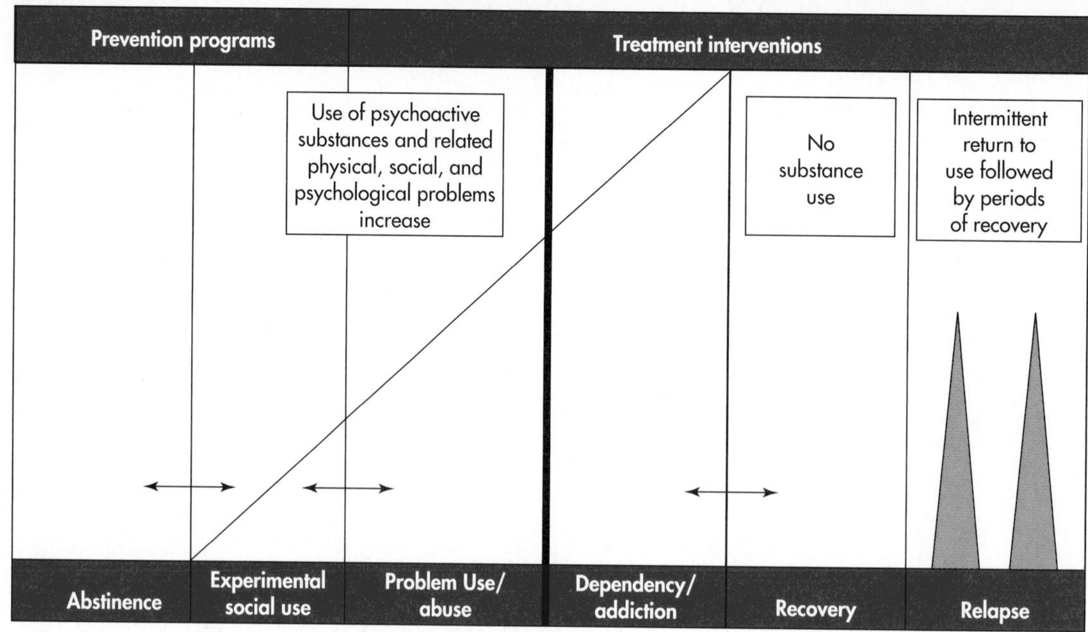

Figure 12-5 The process of addiction. *(From Crowe AH, Reeves RR:* Treatment for alcohol and other drug abuse: opportunities for coordination, *DHHS Pub No. (SMA)94-2075, Rockville, Md., 1994, U.S. Government Printing Office, p. 5. Data from Doweiko, 1990; Institute of Medicine, 1990.)*

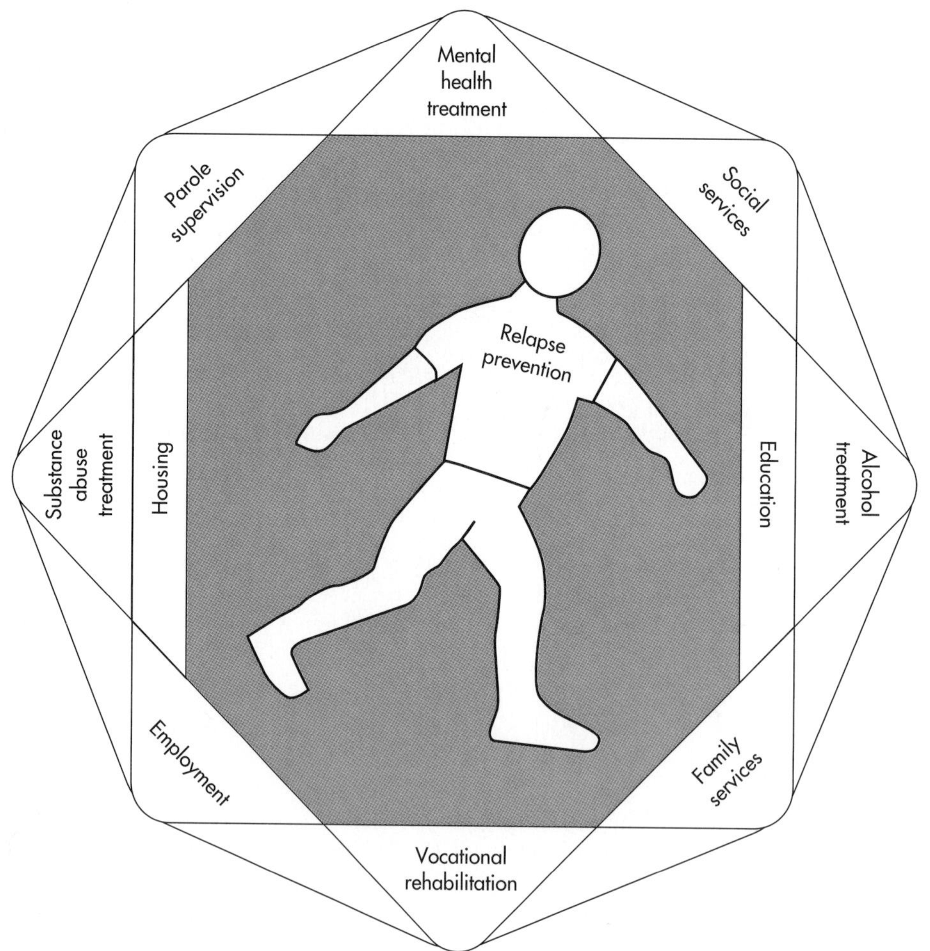

Figure 12-6 Substance abuse populations in a collaborative network of care. *(From Massaro J, Pepper B: The relationship of addiction to crime, health, and other social problems. In Crowe AH, Reeves RR:* Treatment for alcohol and other drug abuse: opportunities for coordination, *DHHS Pub No. (SMA)94-2075, Rockville, Md., 1994, U.S. Government Printing Office, p. 21.)*

- Identify drug abusers and those at risk for drug abuse.
- Assess the full spectrum of problems and risks that may need interventions.
- Plan appropriate interventions.
- Involve appropriate family or significant others in the intervention process.
- Evaluate effectiveness of interventions that have been implemented (p. 48).

The following box provides five key considerations in screening for alcohol and drug abuse. Screening procedures assist health care providers in identifying clients who need a comprehensive substance abuse assessment.

Identifying risk factors is an essential element in a comprehensive assessment. The box on the next page describes areas of assessment and questions to ask to aid in determining substance abuse and risk factors for substance abuse. Most agencies will have an assessment protocol that will guide the nurse in data collection. Every health history should include questions about substance use, including the use of alcohol and illegal and prescription drugs. Community health nurses should be alert to signs of substance abuse. The answer to questions in the comprehensive assessment can help nurses to recognize substance abuse signs. Nurses can also use these questions as a guide when working with other community personnel and families to teach them about early signs and symptoms of substance abuse.

To develop appropriate interventions, community health nurses must be aware of the social supports and resources that are available and needed in their respective communities. Local communities often have substance abuse hotlines, resources, and support groups. The nurse's knowledge about community resources, payment systems, and the referral process (see Chapter 10) can assist the drug abuse population in obtaining treatment services. The intervention plan should identify the interventions to decrease drug involvement and address related psychosocial and financial problems. Interventions may include such things as preventive and primary care, testing for infectious diseases (e.g., AIDS, TB), counseling, support group intervention, periodic drug screening, and relapse prevention (Crowe, Reeves, 1994, p. 56).

The community health nurse can carry out health education activities, actively participate in the treatment program, offer support to the client, remain nonjudgmental, and refer the client to appropriate community resources. Other nursing roles include that of researcher regarding such issues as the most effective treatment modalities and reasons for the upward trends in substance abuse. As an advocate, the community health nurse may have an active role in developing policies and advocating for services at the local, state, and federal levels.

Key Considerations in Screening for Alcohol and Drug Abuse

- Screening should be conducted on persons recognized to be at risk, in a variety of settings, by a range of professionals.
- There should be collaboration among agencies and professionals on screening processes, techniques, and instruments.
- All instruments and processes should be sensitive to racial, cultural, socioeconomic, and gender-related concerns.
- Initial screening procedures should be brief.
- Information should be gathered from various sources.

From Crowe AH, Reeves RR: *Treatment for alcohol and other drug abuse: opportunities for coordination*, DHHS Pub No. (SMA)94-2075, Rockville, Md., 1994, U.S. Government Printing Office, p. 53.

SEXUALLY TRANSMITTED DISEASES

Historically, sexually transmitted diseases (STDs) have been a major community health problem. A sexually transmitted disease is defined as any infection "spread by transfer of organisms from person to person during sexual contact" (USDHHS, 1991a, p. 496). Before the 1980s only five STDs were monitored by the CDC on a regular basis. Since then the number, scope, and spectrum of STDs has grown immensely, and by 1990 more than 50 STD organisms and syndromes were recognized (USDHHS, 1991a, p. 496).

Because of the current epidemic of HIV/AIDS and its devastating effects, and being consistent with *Healthy People 2000* listing STDs and HIV/AIDS as two separate priority areas, STDs and HIV/AIDS will be discussed in two separate categories. However, there is often a reciprocal connection where "STDs and HIV infection are often linked not only by common underlying risk behaviors but also by biological mechanisms" (USDHHS, 1995, p. 116). Because of this reciprocal connection, prevention and treatment efforts for STDs or HIV/AIDS cannot be addressed to the exclusion of the other without considering the dynamics of disease transmission (e.g., underlying health risk behaviors).

The following section addresses STDs and HIV/AIDS in separate categories, discusses health risks for both STDs and HIV/AIDS, and presents nursing's role in prevention and treatment interventions of STDs and HIV/AIDS. The epidemiological control measures for STDs and other infectious diseases are examined in Chapter 11.

STDs

STDs have been, and continue to be, a high priority in public health programming. An estimated 12 million cases of STDs occur every year in the United States (USDHHS, 1995, p. 116). On the federal level, *Healthy People 2000* listed STDs as a separate priority area and had numerous objectives to reduce their incidence and prevalence. The STDs that are specifically addressed in this document are syphilis, gonorrhea, *Chlamydia trachomatis* infections, genital herpes, human papillomavirus, chancroid, genital mycoplasmas, cytomegalovirus, hepatitis B, vaginitis, enteric infections, and ecotoparasitic diseases.

New methods for screening, determining the epidemiology of the disease process, diagnoses, and treatments are emerging. Today some STDs are becoming drug resistant and very difficult to treat. The emergence of HIV in the 1980s as a major STD has brought about a heightened awareness and mass campaign to prevent STDs (USDHHS, 1991a, p. 496). However, because of the overwhelming focus on AIDS, other sexually transmitted diseases are becoming what some consider "a neglected public health priority" (Yankauer, 1994, p. 1895). Neglecting STD control increases the risk of HIV transmission. "It is known that the STDs that cause ulcerative lesions such as syphilis, chancroid, or genital herpes, increase the risk of HIV transmission" (Newmann, Nishimoto, 1996, p. 20). Behavioral risk factors, such as intravenous drug use and unprotected sex, that place individuals at risk for development of STDs are also factors that place individuals at risk for the development of HIV. Hence HIV prevention efforts must also include STD prevention.

Comprehensive Substance Abuse Assessment: Areas of Assessment through Patient and Collateral Interviews

- **Drug history and current patterns of use.** When did alcohol or other drug use begin? What types of alcohol or other drugs does the individual currently use? Does the person use over-the-counter medications, prescription drugs, tobacco, and caffeine? How frequently are the substances used and in what quantity?
- **Substance abuse treatment history.** Has the individual ever received treatment for substance abuse? If so, what type of treatment (inpatient, outpatient, methadone maintenance, twelve-step programs, etc.)? Were these treatment experiences considered successful or unsuccessful and why? Has the person been sober and experienced relapse, or has s/he never attained recovery?
- **Medical history and current status.** What symptoms are currently reported by the patient? Are there indicators of infectious and/or sexually transmitted diseases? Has the individual been tested for HIV and other infectious diseases? Are there indicators of risk for HIV or other diseases for which testing should be done? What kind of health care has been received in the past? The causes and effects of various illnesses and traumas should be explored.
- **Mental status and mental health history.** Is the individual orientated to person, place, and time? Does s/he have the ability to concentrate on the interview process? Are there indicators of impaired cognitive abilities? What is the appropriateness of responses during the interview? Is the person's affect (emotional response) appropriate for the situation? Are there indicators from collateral sources of inappropriate behavior or responses by the person? Is there evidence of extreme mood states, suicidal potential, or possibility of violence? Is the individual able to control impulses? Have there been previous psychological or psychiatric evaluations or treatment?
- **Personal status.** What are this person's critical life events? Who constitutes his/her peer group? Does the individual indicate psychosocial problems that might lead to substance abuse? Does the person demonstrate appropriate social, interpersonal, self-management, and stress management skills? What is the individual's level of self-esteem? What are the person's leisure time interests? What are his/her socioeconomic level and housing and neighborhood situation?
- **Family history and current relationships.** Who does the individual consider his/her family to be; is it a traditional or nontraditional family constellation? What role does the individual play within the family? Are there indicators of a history of physical or sexual abuse or neglect? Do other family members have a history of substance abuse, health problems or chronic illnesses, psychiatric disorders, or criminal behavior? What is the family's cultural, racial, and socioeconomic background? What are the strengths of the family and are they invested in helping the individual? Have there been foster family or other out-of-home placements?
- **Positive support systems.** Does the person have hobbies, interests, and talents? Who are his/her positive peers or family members?
- **Crime or delinquency.** Have there been previous arrests and/or involvement in the criminal or juvenile justice system? Has the person been involved in criminal or delinquent activity but not been apprehended? Is there evidence of gang involvement? Is the person currently under the supervision of the justice system? What is the person's attitude about criminal or delinquent behavior?
- **Education.** How much formal education has the person completed? What is the individual's functional educational level? Is there evidence of a learning disability? Has s/he received any special education services? If currently in school, what is the person's academic performance and attendance pattern?
- **Employment.** What is the individual's current employment status? What employment training has been received? What jobs have been held in the past and why has the person left these jobs? If currently employed, are there problems with performance or attendance?
- **Readiness for treatment.** Does the patient accept or deny a need for treatment? Are there other barriers to treatment?
- **Resources and responsibilities.** What is the individual's socioeconomic status? Is the person receiving services from other agencies, or might s/he be eligible for services?

Data from Doweiko, 1990; McLellan, Dembo, 1992; Tarter, Ott, Mezzich, 1991.
From Crowe AH, Reeves RR: *Treatment for alcohol and other drug abuse: opportunities for coordination*, DHHS Pub No. (SMA)94-2075, Rockville, Md., 1994, U.S. Government Printing Office, p. 55.

STDs affect all people, regardless of gender, race, or socioeconomic status. However, the incidence of STDs is higher in young people than ever before and is continuing to increase in young people and women. "Two-thirds of the STD cases occur among young people under the age of 25" (USDHHS, 1995, p. 116). Overall the incidence is disproportionately represented in the poor and minority groups (USDHHS, p. 116).

Early in 1996 the CDC identified six prominent nationally notifiable STDs that have the highest incidence and prevalence: AIDS, chancroid, chlamydia, gonorrhea, pediatric HIV infection (not notifiable in all states, however), and syphilis (CDC, 1996a). Appendix 12-1 provides information about the most commonly acquired STDs. CDC plays a major role in national disease surveillance. The CDC works collaboratively with states in maintaining a national disease reporting system (Chapter 11 elaborates on the CDC's role in public health surveillance). The primary responsibility for monitoring and controlling STDs rests on surveillance by state and local health departments (LHDs). However, the surveillance activities by these organizations would be incomplete without the assistance of other health care providers and services (USDHHS, 1995, p. 116). Most LHDs have STD clinics that provide diagnostic and treatment services at no cost to the individual.

The midcourse review of the year 2000 health objectives reported that nearly all STDs are declining (USDHHS, 1995, p. 117). However, the review noted that the number of 15- to 17-year-old adolescents engaging in intercourse has increased and is rapidly moving away from the *Healthy People 2000* objective. Although the number of adolescents who report using condoms has increased, adolescents were found to have some of the highest rates of gonorrhea and chlamydia (USDHHS, p. 118). At midcourse review, revisions to the *Healthy People 2000* objectives included new objectives urging health promotion campaigns and activities to focus on reducing gonorrhea, syphilis, and pelvic inflammatory disease (PID).

HIV/AIDS

Human immunodeficiency virus disease (HIV) and acquired immunodeficiency syndrome (AIDS) were first diagnosed in the early 1980s and are now epidemic worldwide. When *Healthy People 2000* was published in 1990 there were 114,500 reported cases of AIDS in the United States (USDHHS, 1995, p. 112). Five years later the number of AIDS cases reported in the United States exceeded a half-million, and at the same time the World Health Organization estimated that there were approximately 4.5 million AIDS cases worldwide (CDC, 1995a, p. 849, 851). At the beginning of this decade the World Health Organization estimated that 15 to 20 million persons will be infected worldwide by the year 2000 (Rice, 1991, p. 300).

By the end of 1995 513,436 AIDS cases in the United States had been reported to the Centers for Disease Control, and over 62% of these cases were fatal (CDC, 1995b, p. 5). AIDS cases are reported to the CDC based on a uniform case definition and a case report form. The case definition of AIDS was changed in 1987 to incorporate a broader range of AIDS indicator diseases and conditions (CDC, 1987). In 1993 the definition was again revised to include "severe immunosuppression, based on CD4 T-lymphocyte cell counts, as well as an expanded set of HIV-associated illnesses" (Aday, 1994, p. 498). These changes in the AIDS definition, the long incubation period between HIV infection and symptoms, and the variation in state HIV surveillance and reporting has made it difficult to accurately predict the number of AIDS cases (USDHHS, 1995, p. 112). These factors have also made it difficult to uniformly gather surveillance data on the progress toward achieving *Healthy People 2000* HIV/AIDS objectives (USDHHS, pp. 112-113). Since there is no systematic screening or reporting of HIV, the number of cases of AIDS does not reflect HIV trends (Hitchcock, 1996). However, as national and international surveillance increases and as the AIDS epidemic continues to rise without an immediate cure or vaccine, it is entirely possible that the number of AIDS cases could even exceed Rice's (1991) World Health Organization year 2000 prediction.

AIDS has become the leading cause of death in people between ages 25 to 44 and the eighth leading cause of death worldwide (USDHHS, 1995, p. 112; CDC, 1995a, p. 850; CDC, 1996e, p. 121). In 1993 AIDS was the fourth leading cause of death among 23- to 44-year-old women and the fifth leading cause of death among 1- to 4-year-old children (CDC, 1995d, p. 2). By 1995 there were more than 58,000 cases among adolescents and adult women, and more than 6948 cases among children who acquired HIV perinatally (Maternal and Child Health Bureau, 1996, p. 30). The highest overall number of deaths have been among minorities (CDC, 1995b, p. 20). The human and economic costs of the AIDS epidemic are astronomical and beyond estimation. By 1993 "more than one million children in the developing world had already been orphaned by AIDS. The World Health Organization estimates that during the 1990s between 10 and 15 million children around the world will lose a mother, father or both parents to AIDS" (Armstrong, 1993, p. 2).

AIDS initially appeared in gay men, and many people still think that it is a disease of this aggregate. Even though "men who have sex with men continue to account for the largest proportion of cases" (CDC, 1995a, p. 851), the number of AIDS cases resulting from heterosexual transmission has drastically risen. As a result women are increasingly developing AIDS. In 1995 19% of adult and adolescent AIDS cases were women, which was the highest percentage ever reported, and the numbers continue to grow (CDC, 1995b, pp. 5-6). Figure 12-7 shows AIDS cases in the United States at time of diagnosis, according to race for persons 13 years of age and over diagnosed through June 1995. Note the

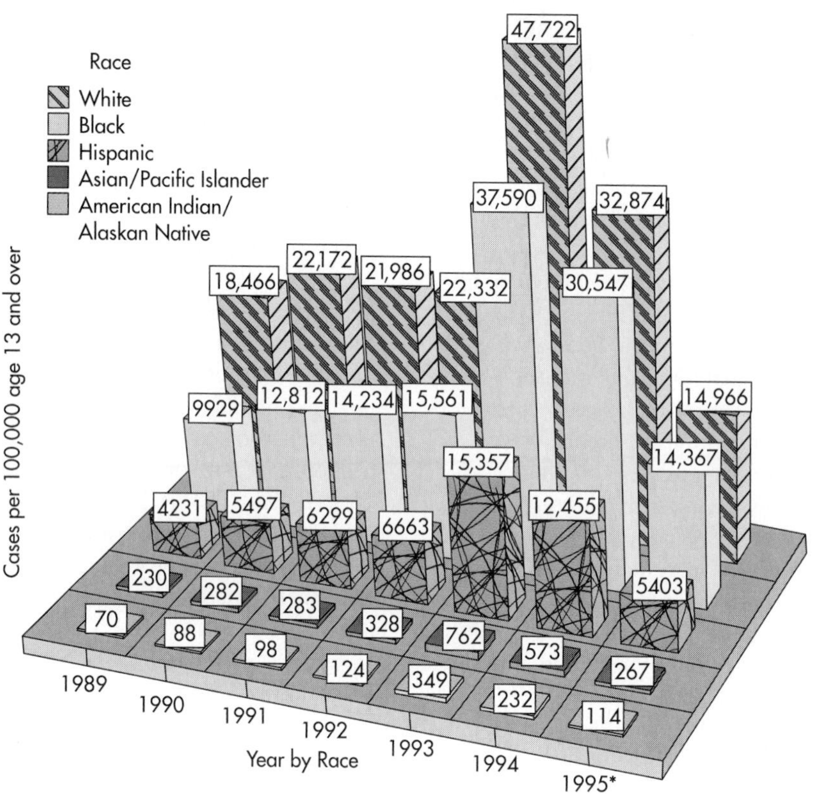

Figure 12-7 AIDS cases in the United States at time of diagnosis, according to race, selected years 1989-1995. *(Modified from National Center for Health Statistics:* Health, United States, 1995, chartbook, *Pub No. (PHS)96-1232, Hyattsville, Md., 1996, U.S. Government Printing Office, p. 165.)*

dramatic increase in 1993 for all races and the decline in 1994. The increase reflects the 1993 revisions in the AIDS case definition rather than a drastic increase in the incidence of AIDS.

Healthy People 2000 has a separate priority area for HIV/AIDS with numerous prevention objectives. These objectives provide direction for state and local health programming efforts. They emphasize increased testing for HIV infection with counseling and follow-up accompanied by public education efforts on the risks and precautions needed to slow the spread of the disease.

Health Risks for STDs and HIV/AIDS

Health risks for STDs and HIV/AIDS will be addressed in two categories. The first discusses health behaviors that increase the risk of acquiring STDs and HIV/AIDS. The second category addresses opportunistic infections that increase the risk of AIDS and AIDS mortality.

HEALTH RISK BEHAVIORS Numerous health behaviors place individuals at risk for developing STDs and HIV/AIDS. According to the *Healthy People 2000* midcourse report nearly all STD rates are on the decline. However, when broken down into special population groups, the decline is not as great. For example, one objective that has regressed from the year 2000 target is the increase in the number of adolescents who are engaging in sexual intercourse (USDHHS, 1995, p. 117). This places the adolescent and young adult population groups at high risk for acquiring STDs and HIV/AIDS.

As discussed in the previous section, tracking progress toward *Healthy People 2000* HIV infection objectives in the population has been difficult. However, to identify progress towards achieving the year 2000 targets risk behaviors for acquiring HIV are monitored. Some of these risk factors include the number of adolescents engaging in sexual intercourse, use of condoms, number of intravenous drug users in treatment and the number of AIDS cases acquired through blood transfusions (USDHHS, 1995, p. 113). According to the *Healthy People 2000* midcourse report, progress has been made toward increasing the use of condoms; increasing the number of drug users who have enrolled in treatment or are using uncontaminated drug paraphernalia; increasing the percentage of HIV-infected persons being tested; and increasing the safety of the nation's blood supply (USDHHS, p. 113). However, like STDs, the objective pertaining to HIV transmission that regressed from the year 2000 target is the increase in the number of adolescents engaging in sexual intercourse (USDHHS, p. 114).

Several reports have noted the increase in sexual activity among adolescents, particularly those 15 to 17 years old (Adams, Schoenborn, Moss et al, 1995; USDHHS, 1995). A national youth risk behavior study in 1994 revealed some startling information regarding unhealthy adolescent behaviors. It was found that about one out of three 14- to 15-year-old youths had engaged in sexual intercourse; almost four out of five had had intercourse by ages 18 to 21; and 12.1% of the 18- to 21-year-old males who participated in the study had reported having their first sexual intercourse by age 12 (Adams, Schoenborn, Moss et al, 1995). Although the number of adolescents having sexual intercourse has increased, there has been an increase in the number of adolescents using condoms (USDHHS, 1995). Clearly STD and HIV prevention efforts must target young adolescents so that they can begin to develop healthy behaviors at an early age to minimize the risk of STDs and HIV. The following box lists unhealthy behaviors that increase the risk of acquiring STDs and HIV/AIDS.

Even though progress has been made in reducing risk behaviors in communities throughout the United States, there are still populations who have not grasped the serious and potentially fatal consequences of engaging in high-risk sexual activities. In a study involving knowledge and behavioral issues with 175 HIV-positive subjects, Sowell, Seals, and Cooper (1996) identified 10 reasons the HIV-infected participants gave for engaging in unprotected sex. These reasons are displayed in the box, below right.

Sowell, Seals, and Cooper found that "being drunk or high" was the most frequently cited reason for engaging in unsafe sexual behavior. This study has tremendous implications for primary prevention. Preventive interventions must be multifaceted and include education about all facets of disease transmission, including various reasons for engaging in unhealthy sexual activities. Sowell, Seals, and Cooper's study suggests that in addition to educating persons about the disease process and risk factors, discussing responsible sexual behavior and the building of trusting intimate relationships is essential. Knowledge alone will not prevent the spread of HIV. Sowell, Seals, and Cooper's study does reflect, however, that there is still lack of knowledge about HIV and its spread. It is imperative that populations fully understand the nature of HIV and the manners in which it may be spread. Education must also increase awareness that the exchange of body fluids between HIV-infected persons "may result in reinfection with HIV or exposure to other harmful pathogens that can cause morbidity" (Sowell, Seals, Cooper, 1996). It is crucial that HIV-infected persons understand that it is not "safe" to engage in unprotected sex regardless of the circumstances (see the Teaching Tips box).

OPPORTUNISTIC INFECTIONS AMONG HIV POPULATIONS

It is important to remember that "HIV is an asymptomatic disease and the host is infectious for many years" (Hitchcock, 1996, p. 83). For this reason many individuals can be infected with HIV before the host carrier is personally aware of being HIV infected. The time between being infected with HIV and developing AIDS varies, but about half of HIV-infected persons develop AIDS within 10 years (USDHHS, 1994b, p. 2). The first realization that the host is infected often occurs with the manifestation of an opportunistic infection.

There are numerous opportunistic infections. HIV-infected persons often develop opportunistic infections that lead to AIDS and that frequently parallel the occurrence of AIDS. The common opportunistic conditions that were included in the 1993 AIDS surveillance case definition for reporting and determining categories of HIV/AIDS progression are shown in the box on page 347.

Risk Behaviors for STDs and HIV/AIDS

- Engaging in unprotected anal, vaginal, or oral sexual activities (both receptive and insertive).
- Having sex with a person known to be HIV-positive.
- Sharing, or having sex with persons who share drug needles, syringes, or other injection equipment that has been used by others.
- Having multiple sex partners.
- Having sex in exchange for drugs, money, or other inducements.
- Using alcohol and drugs with sexual activity.
- Having a history of STDs, especially genital lesions (such as syphilis, chancroid, herpes), and engaging in sexual activity.

Modified from CDC: *HIV counseling, testing, and referral: standards and guidelines*, Atlanta, 1994a, CDC, p. 7.

Reasons for Engaging in Unprotected Sex

- Was drunk or high on alcohol/drugs
- Did not have condom available
- Was turned on and didn't want to stop
- Didn't know at the time that it was risky
- Didn't know reason why
- Knew risk but chose to take it
- Safer sex was not satisfying
- Don't like condoms
- Was not comfortable asking partner
- Both partners HIV-positive and monogamous

From Sowell RL, Seals BF, Cooper JA: HIV transmission knowledge and risk behaviors of persons with HIV infection, *AIDS Patient Care and STDs* 10(2):111-115, 1996, p. 115.

Recent research that tracked patterns of opportunistic infections in 1530 HIV-infected persons has provided evidence that the development of one opportunistic infection significantly increases the risk of developing additional opportunistic infections (Finkelstein, Williams, Molenberghs et al, 1996). Findings from this research also provided support that the risk of developing opportunistic infections can be predicted (and used to begin AIDS prophylaxis that is consistent with CDC 1993 revised recommendations) by monitoring the CD4 T-lymphocyte cell counts in HIV-

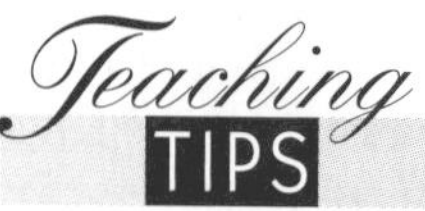

Safer Sex

What Does It Mean to Practice "Safer Sex"?

The term "safer sex" refers to the practice of protecting yourself against sexually transmitted diseases (STDs), sometimes referred to as venereal diesease (VD). There are at least 50 different kinds of these diseases: some of them even life-threatening. You can catch an STD by having sex with someone who is infected.

What If I Have Sex Without Actually Having Intercourse?

You can still get an STD without having vaginal intercourse or penetration. STDs are spread by having vaginal, oral, or anal sex with an infected person. STD-causing germs can pass from one person to another through body fluids such as semen, vaginal fluid, saliva, and blood; genital warts and herpes are STDs that are spread by direct contact with a wart or blister.

No One I Dated Looks to Me as If They Could Have an STD. They Look Really Healthy.

You can't tell if a person has an STD just by appearance. In fact, some people with STDs have no signs at all and may not even know they are infected. Still, some signs to look for in your partner are a heavy discharge, rash, sore, or redness near your partner's sex organs. If you see any of these, don't have sex or be sure to use a condom.

How Can I Tell If I Might Have an STD?

You may have an STD if you experience burning or pain when urinating; sores, bumps, or blisters near the genitals or mouth; swelling around the genitals; fever, chills, night sweats, or swollen glands; or tiredness, vomiting, diarrhea, or sore muscles. In addition, you may have an unusual discharge or smell from the vagina; burning and itching around the vagina; pain in the lower abdomen; vaginal pain during sex; or vaginal bleeding between periods. *But don't forget: you may not have any warning signs at all. Regular medical checkups are essential to your health . . . If you have sex with more than one partner, routine cultures and blood tests may be needed.*

I Think I Have an STD! What Should I Do?

Get help right away. If you don't, you may pass the STD to your partner or, if you're pregnant, to your baby. In fact, without treatment an STD may make it impossible for you to have a baby at all. You may also develop brain damage, blindness, cancer, heart disease, or arthritis. In some cases you can even die. So go to a doctor or clinic right away.

If your health care provider determines that you do have an STD, tell your partner or partners to get tested, too. Take all of your medication; don't stop just because all your symptoms go away. Do not have sex until you have received full treatment. The disease could still be present in your body. Finally, keep all your appointments, and always use a condom and spermicide when you have sex.

What Are the Signs of STDs?

There are many different kinds of STDs, and some of them have similar symptoms. You should never attempt to make a diagnosis on your own. The nurse can give you a list with general descriptions of a few of the most common sexually transmitted diseases.

How Can I Reduce My Chances of Contracting an STD?

Remember, the more sexual partners you have, the greater your risk. Naturally, the best way to reduce your risk is by not having sex or by having sex with one mutually faithful, uninfected partner, or by using a latex condom and spermicide with nonoxynol-9 during sex. Some STDs may be avoided by placing spermicide in the vagina before having sex, because it kills sperm and some STD germs. It helps to urinate and wash after sex (but do not douche, because douching may actually force germs higher up into the body). Avoid having sex with someone who uses intravenous drugs or engages in anal sex. Don't engage in oral, anal, or vaginal sex with an infected person. If you think you may be at risk for AIDS or an STD, seek medical help immediately. Use a new condom each time you have sexual intercourse. *Recent research indicates that the prevention of HIV transmission and developing AIDS may be only 60% to 70% effective when using condoms as a barrier against this infection.*

What If the Condom Breaks? What Should We Do?

If a condom breaks, do not douche. Insert more spermicide into the vagina right away. Men should wash their genitals immediately. Go to a doctor or clinic for an STD examination as soon as possible.

From *Mosby's patient teaching guides*, St. Louis, 1995, Mosby, p. 221.

Opportunistic Conditions Included in the 1993 AIDS Surveillance Case Definition

- Candidiasis of bronchi, trachea, or lungs
- Candidiasis, esophageal
- Cervical cancer, invasive
- Coccidioidomycosis, disseminated or extrapulmonary
- Cryptococcosis, extrapulmonary
- Cryptosporidiosis, chronic intestinal (> 1 month's duration)
- Cytomegalovirus disease (other than liver, spleen, or nodes)
- Cytomegalovirus retinitis (with loss of vision)
- Encephalopathy, HIV-related
- Herpes simplex: chronic ulcer(s) (>1 month's duration); or bronchitis, pneumonitis, or esophagitis
- Histoplasmosis, disseminated or extrapulmonary
- Isosporiasis, chronic intestinal (>1 month's duration)
- Kaposi's sarcoma
- Lymphoma, Burkitt's (or equivalent term)
- Lymphoma, immunoblastic (or equivalent term)
- Lymphoma, primary, of brain
- *Mycobacterium avium* complex or *M. Kansasii,* disseminated or extrapulmonary
- *Mycobacterium tuberculosis,* any site (pulmonary or extrapulmonary)
- *Mycobacterium,* other species or unidentified species, disseminated or extrapulmonary
- *Pneumocystis carinii* pneumonia
- Pneumonia, recurrent
- Progressive multifocal leukoencephalopathy
- *Salmonella septicemia,* recurrent
- Toxoplasmosis of brain
- Wasting syndrome due to HIV

From Centers for Disease Control and Prevention (CDC): 1993 revised classification system for HIV infection and expanded surveillance case definition for AIDS among adolescents and adults, *MMWR* 41(RR-17):15, December 18, 1992.

infected persons (Finkelstein, Williams, Molenberghs et al, 1996). Clearly, with HIV-infected populations, attention must focus on promoting healthy behaviors and lifestyles that would decrease transmission to uninfected persons, decrease the risk of developing opportunistic infections, and prolong the time before the development of AIDS. The rate at which HIV infection progresses to AIDS varies. The CD4 T-lymphocyte counts are used to guide clinicians in placing HIV-infected persons on prophylaxis that protects them against serious opportunistic infections and delays the development of AIDS (CDC, 1992).

CDC provides guidelines for prevention and treatment of opportunistic infections (CDC, 1995c). These guidelines divide the CD4 T-lymphocyte cell markers into three categories according to the number of cells per microliter of blood. Category 1 refers to 500 or more CD4 T-lymphocytes per microliter of blood; category 2 refers to 200 to 499 cells per microliter of blood; and category 3 refers to less than 200 cells per microliter of blood. Adults with a CD4 T-lymphocyte count below 200 are considered to be severely immunosuppressed (CDC, 1995c, p. 1). Depending on the number of CD4 T-lymphocyte cells and the presence or absence of clinical indicators such as opportunistic infections (clinical indicators are divided into asymptomatic, symptomatic, and AIDS indicators), physicians will place the HIV-infected person on some form of chemoprophylaxis. The CD4 T-lymphocyte cell counts and clinical indicators are considered in determining HIV infection and AIDS. For example, for prevention of *Pneumocystis carinii* guidelines recommend beginning chemoprophylaxis if HIV-infected persons have a CD4 T-lymphocyte count of less than 200 cells, unexplained fever that is more than 100° F for 2 or more weeks, or a history of oropharyngeal candidiasis (CDC, 1995c, p. 5). The guidelines also provide recommended drug regimen, as well as behavior activities to prevent exposure to opportunistic infections.

Acquiring opportunistic infections increases the progression of HIV and the onset of AIDS. As discussed in Chapter 11, people who are HIV infected are at high risk for developing active tuberculosis (TB), particularly in settings where cough-inducing procedures (sputum induction and aerosolized pentamidine treatments) are being performed. Persons with HIV have a more rapid conversion to active TB than those who are not HIV infected and have a higher probability of contracting TB on exposure because of the risk factors (Benenson, 1995; Grimes, Grimes, 1995).

TB has a strong epidemiological link with AIDS, with some communities estimating that up to 40% of its TB clients are also HIV positive (GAO, 1995). In the past "assessment of the relation between HIV infection and TB has been limited by incomplete reporting of information" (CDC, 1996d, p. 369) so the prevalence may actually be higher than has been reported. To address this issue, the CDC is collaborating with state and local health departments to make a unified effort to collect this information. These results will be used to develop strategies to more accurately report HIV and TB infection and to improve HIV and TB testing and counseling (CDC, 1996d, p. 369). Because of the increased incidence and prevalence of TB among AIDS populations, community health nurses must think TB, become vigilant in assessing for comorbidity (Grimes, Grimes, 1995, p. 166), and increase TB surveillance along with HIV surveillance (Sbarbaro, 1996, p. 33). This means that any person who is HIV positive should automatically be tested for TB.

A cure or vaccine for AIDS does not seem to be on the near horizon. Presently, vaccine development is uncertain and has been impeded because of the long incubation period of AIDS, as well as the enormous costs for vaccine development (Koopman, Little, 1995). Although there is no cure for AIDS, great strides have been made in drug prophylaxis that decreases the rate of HIV progression to AIDS. Clearly the emphasis with AIDS needs to be on prevention of the disease. The war against AIDS must continue, and all possible avenues of prevention and cure must be considered.

The Nursing Role and STDs

In response to the *Healthy People 2000* objectives, the American Nurses Association (ANA) has made a commitment to support all efforts of disease prevention (ANA, 1995, p. 20). Community health nurses have a unique opportunity to help decrease incidence, prevalence, and complications of STDs through primary, secondary, and tertiary prevention activities. Nurses have access to populations across the life span and have the opportunity to be involved in community education programs that address preventive interventions for all age groups.

The ANA made a legislative commitment in the 104th Congress to fight the AIDS epidemic through research, education, and prevention (ANA, 1995, p. 31) and has articulated Position Statements for sexually transmitted diseases and various HIV-related issues (ANA, 1996b).

The National League for Nursing has also made a commitment to assist nurses in addressing HIV and AIDS issues. It has developed the Caring for Persons with AIDS Test to assist nurses in learning more about AIDS. This test is intended for nurses working in hospitals, long-term care facilities, home health agencies, and schools of nursing to measure the nurse's knowledge and ability to apply basic principles in AIDS patient care (National League for Nursing, 1989, p. 563). To obtain more information about this test, contact the National League for Nursing at 1-800-NOW-1-NLN, or in New York City at 1-212-989-9393.

The National Institute of Nursing Research's (NINR) commitment to AIDS is reflected in its research priorities. NINR has awarded grants to promote research in nursing care of persons with AIDS and continues to fund nursing research in relation to HIV/AIDS. Nursing research is becoming part of the solution to the AIDS epidemic.

To provide competent care, nurses need to be aware of their own attitudes about STDs when working with clients. People with STDs, and especially people with AIDS, are well aware of the prejudices that have surrounded the disease. One study found that nurses' attitudes toward persons with AIDS were significantly different according to the mode in which AIDS was acquired (Cole, Slocumb, 1993). Clients who acquired AIDS through blood transfusions were thought of as innocent victims and were viewed more favorably than those who acquired the disease through homosexual contact or use of drug needles (Cole, Slocumb, p. 116). A goal for all community health nurses should be that clients will never feel that they lack support from their nurses. Nurses have unique skills to help fight this terrible disease and must make every effort to prevent its spread.

Primary, Secondary, and Tertiary Preventive Nursing Interventions

A continuum of preventive services is essential to address problems associated with AIDS and other STDs. The key goal when addressing STDs and HIV/AIDS control is primary prevention. The most successful outcomes will come from comprehensive and collaborative efforts that are community specific. These efforts must address the needs of communities and aggregates and involve clients and a range of community organizations and providers (e.g., health care agencies, nurses, physicians, volunteers, and educators) in providing preventive and treatment services. This means developing community outreach programs that access at-risk populations where they are. Nurses work with local community and school leaders to provide STD/HIV/AIDS awareness education to community members, parents, teachers, school children, adolescents, college students, homeless shelters, family planning clinics, and other community-based clinics such as emergency rooms and 24-hour emergency agencies.

Nurses need to assume a major role in educating people about STDs and HIV/AIDS by providing competent nursing care and linking clients with appropriate community resources. Education is an important asset. Lack of knowledge about STDs/HIV/AIDS can lead to risk-taking behaviors, delays in seeking testing and treatment, exclusion from clinical drug trials, and higher mortality rates. Nurses working with persons who have STDs/AIDS must be able to deal with personal biases to be competent therapeutic agents. Education is a vital component at all levels of prevention. Confidentiality is extremely important with STD populations. Standards and guidelines exist for STDs and HIV that must be adhered to in working with STD populations (CDC, 1993; USDHHS, 1994a).

CDC guidelines for prevention and control of STDs/HIV emphasize four main areas: (1) education to reduce risk or transmission; (2) detection of asymptomatic and symptomatic infected persons; (3) effective diagnosis and treatment of infected persons; and (4) evaluation, treatment, and counseling of sex partners of those who have an STD (CDC, 1993, p. 3). Table 12-3 provides examples of select primary, secondary, and tertiary preventive nursing interventions that address these guidelines.

PRIMARY PREVENTION Primary prevention focuses on active prevention of contracting STDs/HIV. Primary prevention of STDs/HIV is carried out by identifying those at risk for transmitting and acquiring STDs and working with them to change their risky behaviors. Preventive efforts should be population specific and tailored to the particular risks that have been identified in the assessment of that population. For example, it has been found among some

table 12-3 NURSING APPLICATION OF PRIMARY, SECONDARY, AND TERTIARY LEVELS OF PREVENTION FOR STDs AND HIV/AIDS

PREVENTION LEVEL	PRIMARY PREVENTION	SECONDARY PREVENTION	TERTIARY PREVENTION
AREAS TO FOCUS OBJECTIVES	PROMOTE HEALTHY BEHAVIORS ADVOCATE SPECIFIC PROTECTION	EARLY DIAGNOSIS PROMPT TREATMENT	REHABILITATION PREVENT RELAPSE
Examples of Nursing Interventions	• Conduct risk assessments to identify populations at risk for acquiring STDs • Develop community education programs: – STD/AIDS awareness – Involve community residents and agencies such as teachers, parents, health care agencies, community centers, etc. • Provide "safe sex" education such as the proper use of condoms and advocate abstinence and monogomy in high-risk groups • Teach adolescents about risks of acquiring STDs in sexual experimentation associated with alcohol and drug use • Educate groups of parents and teachers on how to recognize risk behaviors (such as alcohol and drug abuse) in their children or students	• Conduct risk assessment to casefind, identify STD-exposed partners, and refer individuals to appropriate community agency for diagnosis and treatment • Conduct TB screening in HIV-infected and refer for prompt treatment • Educate STD/HIV-infected populations that abstaining from sexual activity is the most effective way to prevent disease transmission; additionally educate regarding use of protective methods that prevent exchange of body fluids • Refer drug and alcohol abusers for treatment • Work with HIV populations to eliminate risk behaviors (such as sharing drug syringes and needles) that would spread the disease	• Case manage STD/HIV-infected persons to prevent disease complications • Conduct periodic risk assessments in infected populations to casefind and prevent disease reinfection and development of opportunistic infections • Work with support agencies to keep alcohol and drug populations in treatment to prevent abuse relapse • Provide supportive nursing care, such as adequate nutrition, to improve quality of life and delay progression of HIV infection to AIDS

ethnic and socioeconomic groups that mass media educational efforts do not adequately address the educational needs of these groups (Calvillo, 1992). With these groups a more focused educational experience where the client is would be more beneficial.

Prevention messages must be developmentally appropriate. For example, it is important to understand that sexual inquisitiveness is normal in adolescents as they are beginning to establish their own sexual identities. Therefore prevention messages that take into consideration sexual inquisitiveness must target the young so that they can develop safe and healthy habits at an early age instead of engaging in risky behavior that may lead to acquiring STDs.

The predominant theme in primary prevention should be that *abstinence* is the only sure method of preventing and acquiring an STD. Other methods, such as using condoms, decrease risks of transmitting and acquiring STDs but do not insure absolute safety. Latex condoms provide a strong protection against HIV if properly used. The CDC recommends that prevention messages on the effectiveness and proper use of condoms should be clear and tailored to the population (CDC, 1993, p. 5). It is imperative for the nurse to adequately instruct clients on how to use condoms properly.

In primary prevention of STDs the concern is with promoting healthy behaviors and avoiding or changing risky behaviors, such as unprotected sex or drug and alcohol use. Nursing activities focus on health promotion and specific prevention of STDs.

SECONDARY PREVENTION Secondary prevention focuses on early diagnosis and treatment of STDs and those who are infected with HIV. Secondary prevention stresses early and immediate management of infections, promotion of the practice of healthy habits to prevent transmission of the disease to others, and prevention of opportunistic infections. For example, if partners are HIV positive, the message must include that it is not "safe" to engage in unprotected sex regardless of the circumstances because of the risk of reinfection or the potential of being infected with other STDs or opportunistic infections.

Secondary prevention includes finding those who have been exposed to STDs and notifying partners of STD-infected persons of the need for diagnosis and treatment. Referral for treatment can be by client referral, where the infected person notifies the partner(s), or by provider referral, where the provider (e.g., physician) refers the infected person to the local health department for contact follow-up on partners for early treatment (CDC, 1993, p. 7). Regardless of the type of contact follow-up done, health care providers do report actual cases of STDs and AIDS to the official local reporting agency (see Chapter 11).

Early intervention is intervening before there are symptoms (CDC, 1993, p. 11). Early intervention links people to appropriate community resources for treatment and support. If the population includes drug users, particularly IV drug users, then secondary prevention and treatment is concerned with getting this population into drug treatment programs and preventing the sharing of equipment. Some community health agencies are developing innovative needle exchange programming to prevent the spread of infection.

Collaborative efforts are needed to effectively address the complexity of STD transmission. It is not sufficient to only diagnose and treat the disease. An effective control program must include identifying contributing behaviors (e.g., alcohol and drugs) that enhance the risk for reinfection and transmission. This can be done through risk assessment to determine individualized risks and also by developing an intervention plan that appropriately targets the risk behaviors in aggregates (USDHHS, 1994a, p. 7).

TERTIARY PREVENTION Tertiary prevention for STDs and HIV is concerned with rehabilitation. Nursing activities focus on preventing reinfection, preventing complications from STDs, preventing opportunistic infections to delay HIV progression to AIDS, and providing supportive nursing care. Treatment for STDs or HIV should not be done without assessing other areas of risks, such as IV drug use, that may contribute to reinfection or transmission. Like other contemporary problems a web of cofactors must often be addressed to have successful outcomes. In tertiary prevention the ideal is to prevent unhealthy behaviors that would increase the risk of STD transmission, or reinfection, and progression of HIV infection to AIDS.

Although there is no cure for AIDS, much has been done to delay the progression of HIV infection to AIDS by various drugs that delay development of AIDS. Again, tertiary prevention involves comprehensive and collaborative activities. Tertiary prevention in HIV populations is concerned with strengthening the immune system. This includes pharmacologic drug management as well as promoting healthy behaviors. CDC provides recommended guidelines for pharmacologic management of HIV opportunistic infections and for STDs (CDC, 1995c; CDC, 1993).

VIOLENT AND ABUSIVE BEHAVIOR

Violent behavior refers to behaviors that intentionally inflict injury to self (as in suicide) and to others (Rosenberg, O'Carroll, Powell, 1992). More than two million people are injured by violent assaults each year (USDHHS, 1995, p. 60). Violent and abusive behavior poses enormous threats, with considerable physical costs and emotional consequences, to the health and safety of communities, workplaces, and schools.

When costs are examined in monetary expenditures the amount is staggering. Medical expenses, lost earnings, and the financing of public programs dealing with violent crime is estimated to cost $105 billion annually. When pain, suffering, and reduced quality of life are added to this, the cost is estimated at $450 billion annually, with violent crime accounting for $426 billion and property crime the other $24 billion (Miller, Cohen, Wiersema, 1996). Every effort must be made to eliminate violence.

Why violence is so widespread, often occurring in families where bonds are strongest, is difficult to understand. Hanrahan, Campbell, and Ulrich (1993) have summarized various explanations for violence in our society (see the accompanying box on the next page). Different cultures have varying interpretations about what constitutes violence, and the nurse must consider others' views of violence from economic, kinship, and territoriality perspectives, as well as the influence of spiritual, moral, psychological, and metaphysical issues (Hanrahan, Campbell, Ulrich, p. 30).

Violent and abusive behavior was a major priority area in the *Healthy People 2000* document. The national objectives were directed toward reducing morbidity and mortality associated with violence, including homicides, suicides, and domestic partner and child assault (USDHHS, 1991a). The following section discusses homicide and suicide, addresses domestic violence with a focus on violence against women, and discusses nursing interventions for violent and abusive behaviors. Chapters 15 and 16 discuss violence among children.

Homicide and Suicide

There are more than 50,000 homicide and suicide victims each year (USDHHS, 1995, p. 60). The *Healthy People 2000* midcourse report identified some disturbing trends in violent behavior. There has been an increase in the number of young people, particularly 14- to 17-year-olds, who have become both perpetrators and victims of violence; and there has been an increase in the number of women who are physically and sexually violated by persons (spouses, ex-spouses, and others) known to them (USDHHS, p. 60).

Violent behavior is a complex issue involving a web of cofactors and no single solution. Like other contemporary problems, violent behavior cannot be addressed as a separate entity without examining the societal and socioeconomic cofactors often associated with the violence. For example, alcohol, substance abuse, poverty, drug trafficking, socioeconomic status, adolescent criminal activity, easily accessible weapons, and victims of family violence are some factors that are known to contribute to violent behavior and place aggregates at risk for homicides (Stephenson,

Summaries of Explanations of Violence

- **Biological**
  Aggression is an innate characteristic that is either an instinctual drive (the instinctivist school of thought) or neurologically based (neurophysiological theories). The latter examines how brain functioning and/or hormones influence degrees of aggressive tendencies and/or violent behaviors. Research evidence links increased testosterone levels to increases in aggression, but the studies do not indicate a causal relationship and factors such as mood, sampling difficulties, and environment must be considered as intervening characteristics.
- **Role of alcohol**
  Research indicates that alcohol seems to facilitate aggression because of the negative affect it has on conscious cognitive processing, yet violence occurs as frequently *without* the presence of alcohol. Alcohol is often used as an excuse or a justification for violence.
- **Psychoanalytical viewpoint**
  This position, espoused by Freud and followers, states that violence results from ego weaknesses and the internal need to discharge hostility. Frustration is the stimulus that leads to the expression of aggression. Catharsis or the expression of the aggression results in a decrease of subsequent aggressive behaviors.
- **Social-learning theory**
  Aggression and violence are learned responses and may be considered adaptive or destructive depending on the situation. The family, television, and environmental conditions serve as models for children to learn how to be aggressive and/or violent.
- **Cultural attitudes fostering violence**
  Tacit acceptance of violence as a means to resolve conflict. War and weapons are justified as protection. In everyday language, we jokingly threaten to "kill" people or "beat them up." We accept physical punishment as a way to discipline children under "certain circumstances." Pornographic depictions of women are legal and deemed as erotica.
- **Power and violence**
  Violence or its threat is often used as a method of persuasion, as in rape or incest. Fear of being a victim of violence keeps people, primarily women, in positions of submission.
- **Poverty**
  Being poor is a condition of oppression, and aggression and violence are methods of expressing such oppression. Poverty needs to be considered as a circumstance in which violence occurs rather than as factor causing such behaviors.
- **Subculture of violence**
  There is a theme of violence that permeates the lifestyle values of the individuals who are part of this "cultural group." Violence is a fairly typical method of resolving conflict.

From Hanrahan P, Campbell J, Ulrich Y: Theories of violence. In Campbell J, Humphreys J, eds: *Nursing care of survivors of family violence*, St. Louis, 1993, Mosby, p. 6.

1992, p. 43; USDHHS, 1995, p. 60). Many of the cofactors that increase the risk for homicide also place individuals at risk for suicide. Specifically it has been found that suicide results from an interaction of many cofactors and usually involves a history of psychosocial problems and mental illness that often do not surface until after the suicide has occurred (CDC, 1994b).

The *Healthy People 2000* midcourse report noted some progress toward reducing the suicide rate in the overall population. In the overall population, the number of suicides has remained stable over the last 10 years. However, the suicide rate among young white and minority men has increased. Figure 12-8 illustrates the death rate trends according to race for male suicide since 1989. After 2 years of relative stability in the suicide rates, there is a notable increase in suicides among minorities. The most notable increase between 1992 and 1993 is among American Indians/Alaskan Natives and Asian/Pacific Islanders.

The number of homicides occurring annually demonstrates regression from the *Healthy People 2000* objective for reducing homicides. Nationally the homicide rate has significantly increased, and it is higher among young black men (USDHHS, 1995, p. 61). Blacks generally have a higher homicide rate than whites and other minority populations. This difference is illustrated in Figure 12-9, which depicts the male homicide trends between 1989 and 1993.

The Role of the Nurse with Homicide and Suicide

Community health nurses play an important role in primary prevention of violent and aggressive behavior. Nurses have opportunities to intervene with populations across the life span. They develop collaborative relationships with other health care providers for the purpose of developing comprehensive health programming that targets aggregates at risk for suicide and homicide. Because of the complexity of violent and aggressive behavior, social cofactors must be considered when developing multifaceted community interventions to eliminate violent and abusive behavior in the communities (USDHHS, 1995, p. 61).

Community health nurses are involved in community risk assessment, determining populations at risk for violence and suicide, and developing and implementing interventions to decrease violence in the community (see Chapters 13 and 14 for assessing and planning interventions with communities and aggregates at risk). Solutions to eliminate violence are complex and require multidisciplinary and multifaceted approaches. Like other contemporary problems, the most effective intervention is prevention. Interventions to prevent violent behavior that leads to homicide and suicide must include long-range planning that begins at home, is supported in the schools and communities, and involves state, local, media, religious, and cultural organizations (Wolman, 1995, p. xix). Chapter 16 presents a range of preventive interventions to reduce youth suicide and violence.

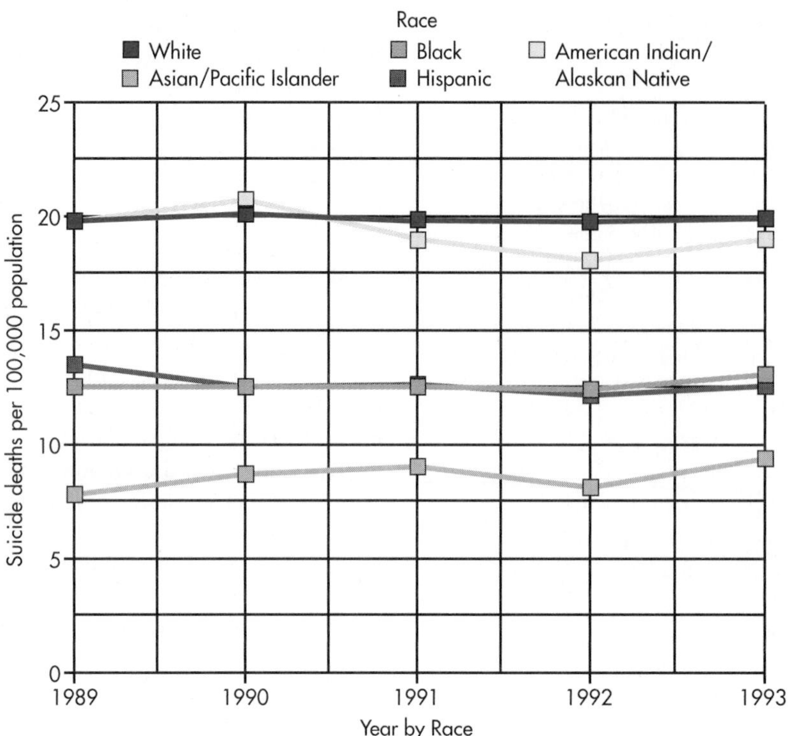

Figure 12-8 Suicide deaths for males of all ages, by race, for 1989-1993, age adjusted. *(Modified from National Center for Health Statistics:* Health, United States, 1995, chartbook, *Pub No. (PHS)96-1232, Hyattsville, Md., 1996, U.S. Government Printing Office, pp. 152-154.)*

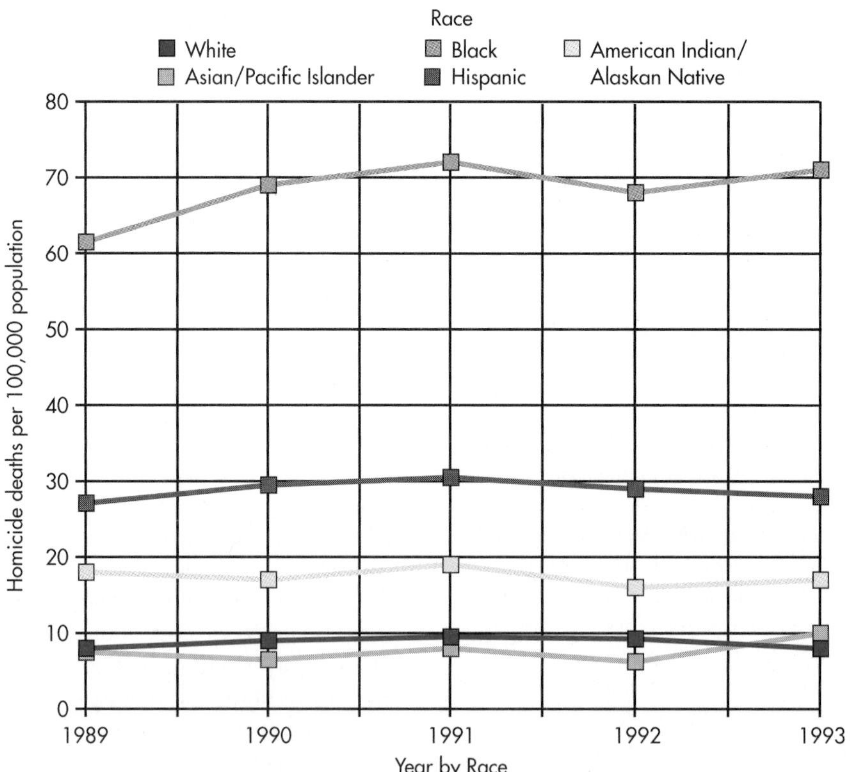

Figure 12-9 Homicide deaths for males of all ages, by race, for 1989-1993, age adjusted. *(Modified from National Center for Health Statistics:* Health, United States, 1995, chartbook, *Pub No. (PHS)96-1232, Hyattsville, Md., 1996, U.S. Government Printing Office, pp. 149-151.)*

Working collaboratively with other disciplines and agencies to identify those at risk and to intervene effectively through prevention is crucial. For example, it is important to ensure that suicide prevention programs are linked to community mental health resources (CDC, 1994b, p. 6). This requires community health nurses to be knowledgeable about the mental health resources available in the community. Knowledge of community resources is necessary for any intervention with community populations, and community health nurses must be able to identify which resources exist and which are needed, and have a strong network with community agencies to develop preventive and treatment measures.

Recognizing populations that are prone to violent behavior is essential. Multiple social, economic, and psychological factors, such as unemployment and societal attitudes about violence and drug abuse, place aggregates at risk for homicides. Like other social problems, this one does not exist in isolation, and there is no single indicator. However, certain characteristics are known to contribute to homicide and suicide. These characteristics are part of a larger web of crime cofactors and are a point from which to begin a risk assessment. A few questions nurses might ask to ascertain the extent and cofactors of violence that may be existing in their communities are listed in the box below.

Answers to these questions can provide a starting point for understanding the potential web of violence in respective communities and can provide a base for developing prevention interventions. This would include such things as public awareness campaigns, supporting law enforcement in arrest, supporting stringent legal sanctions for perpetrators and treatment for the chemically addicted, treating injured victims, advocating for shelter, and advocating for strong protective and treatment policy development.

Community health nurses can intervene at the primary, secondary, and tertiary levels of prevention. The roles of the community health nurse may vary with various interventions. Every aspect of prevention and intervention should have an overall goal to *stop violence*. Table 12-4 shows examples of various nursing interventions and nursing roles involved in eliminating violent behavior.

Domestic Violence

Recently awareness of domestic violence has increased. As a result, many myths concerning domestic abuse have been dispelled, and it has become clear that domestic violence occurs in every community. Domestic violence occurs in every race at all socioeconomic levels, all educational levels, all ages, in both men and women, among the employed and unemployed and celebrities and noncelebrities. In other words, no populations are unaffected by domestic violence. Every reader of this textbook will undoubtedly have heard of, or personally known, someone within his or her community who has been a victim of domestic violence. Domestic violence has serious ramifications for the individual, family, and community. It can result in physical and emotional injury, death, temporary or permanent separation of families, and financial hardship. Intrafamilial violence is more prevalent than is often recognized. As will be shown

Questions to Determine the Extent of Violence and Resources Addressing Violence in the Community

How safe do you feel in the community?
Are the schools in the community safe? What is the incidence of truancy and dropout?
Is there any indication of gang activity?
What is the incidence of stolen property, auto vehicle theft, and breaking and entering homes?
Are the community parks safe? What are the parks used for? Who uses them?
Is there a homeless population in the community?
What is the number of single-parent families?
What is the average socioeconomic status?
What is the poverty rate?
What is the unemployment rate?
What is the illiteracy rate?
Is there evidence of drug dealing? At what ages?
What are the alcohol use, abuse, and/or addiction rates in the community?
What are the number of driving arrests related to intoxication?
What are the drug use, abuse, and/or addiction rates?
What is the incidence of adolescent violence?
What are the homicide and/or attempted homicide statistics?
What are the suicide and/or attempted suicide statistics?
What is the incidence of adolescent suicide and/or attempted suicide?
Is there suicide education that spans all ages?
Is there a high incidence of domestic violence in the community?
What is the incidence of child abuse?
Is there a shelter for domestic abuse victims?
What support groups are active? What peer support groups are needed?
What crisis intervention exists (for suicide, drugs, alcohol, STDs, AIDS, victims of violence, families/friends of suicide/homicide victims)?
What, if any, are the crisis hotline telephone numbers? Where are the centers?
What referral agencies are available?
Are there community partnerships to deal with violence?
How many worksites have employee assistance programs?
How many worksites have developed policies to address alcohol, drugs, and violence?
How does the media address the issue of violence in the community?

table 12-4 NURSING APPLICATION OF PRIMARY, SECONDARY, AND TERTIARY LEVELS OF PREVENTION FOR VIOLENT AND ABUSIVE BEHAVIOR

PREVENTION LEVEL	PRIMARY PREVENTION	SECONDARY PREVENTION	TERTIARY PREVENTION
GOAL	STOP VIOLENCE	STOP VIOLENCE	STOP VIOLENCE
Examples of nursing interventions	• Conduct risk assessment to identify populations at risk for violent behavior • Develop community public awareness programs to alert public of indicators of criminal activity • Involve community members such as teachers, parents, health care agencies, and community centers in prevention • Educate aggregates (e.g., parents, teachers, adolescents) on how to recognize signs of suicidal ideation • Collaborate with community leaders to destroy the base of violence, suicide, and homicide, and provide awareness of domestic abuse shelters and other options for protection • Advocate policy development that limits access to drugs and weapons	• Research the number of suicide attempts in the population, crime statistics, domestic abuse police calls, drug/alcohol-related arrests, and injuries related to violent behavior • Refer victims of violence to support groups and shelters • Support enforcement of legal sanctions for perpetrators • Casefind by screening select populations for depression and refer for counseling/treatment • Work with affected populations to eliminate risk behaviors (such as drug and alcohol abuse) • Facilitate development of peer support groups	• Conduct follow-up risk assessments for relapse • Coordinate follow-up therapy of victims of violence to prevent recurrence and to break the cycle of abuse • Collaborate with community providers to establish community support groups for helping perpetrators stop violent behavior • Advocate enforcement of stringent legal sanctions for perpetrators • Collaborate with support agencies to ensure ongoing treatment for victims and perpetrators • Advocate for development of shelters for victims

here and discussed in Chapters 15, 16, and 20, domestic violence crosses the life span.

Although domestic violence has been prevalent for some time, in recent years more stringent laws have been passed that enable protective action before behaviors escalate into physical injury and death. For example, in the early 1990s antistalking legislation was passed that gives the police power to arrest individuals for this behavior, and currently almost all states and the District of Columbia have passed antistalking legislation (U.S. Department of Justice, 1996b). In 1994 Congress passed the Violence Against Women Act, which, along with the celebrity murders of Nicole Brown-Simpson and Ronald Goldman, has also brought about national campaigns for violence against women. As a result, every state has established a state organization of Violence Against Women. A national hotline (1-800-799-SAFE) has been established, and many states have developed toll-free hotlines as well (U.S. Department of Justice, 1996a).

Domestic violence laws vary from state to state in the types of acts (e.g., stalking, assaults, threats) they cover. How each state defines domestic violence determines what constitutes a crime (Stark, Flitcraft, 1996, p. 160; U.S. Department of Justice, 1996b). A 36-month study by the CDC and the National Institute of Justice that is currently underway will be examining multiple forms of violence against women (U.S. Department of Justice, 1996b). The study is designed to provide in-depth knowledge about the nature of domestic violence, abusive partners, and victims. The findings will be used as a basis to develop more effective programming to prevent and treat domestic violence.

Both men and women are victims of domestic violence, but women are the most frequently and seriously injured victims. Studies suggest that at least 2 million women are physically battered each year by intimate partners, including husbands, former husbands, boyfriends, and lovers, including gay or lesbian partners (Crowell, Burgess, 1996, p. 1). The findings from a national crime victimization survey provided some poignant facts about victims of domestic violence. These facts are shown in the box on the next page.

No segment of the population is free of battered women; they come from all walks of life. However, some characteristics of domestic violence victims that have been observed with consistency include an early exposure to violence as a

Victims of Domestic Violence: Select Facts from a National Crime Victimization Survey

- Women are attacked about six times more often by offenders with whom they had an intimate relationship than are male violence victims.
- Nearly 30% of all female homicide victims are known to have been killed by their husbands, former husbands, or boyfriends.
- In contrast, just over 3% of male homicide victims are known to have been killed by their wives, former wives, or girlfriends.
- Husbands, former husbands, boyfriends, and ex-boyfriends committed more than one million violent acts against women.
- Family members or other people that the victim knew committed more than 2.7 million violent crimes against women.
- Husbands, former husbands, boyfriends, and ex-boyfriends committed 26% of rapes and sexual assaults.
- Forty-five percent of all violent attacks against female victims 12 years old and older by multiple offenders involve offenders they know.
- The rate of intimate-offender attacks on women separated from their husbands was about three times higher than that of divorced women and about 25 times higher than that of married women.
- Women of all races are equally vulnerable to attacks by intimates.
- Female victims of violence are more likely to be injured when attacked by someone they knew than female victims of violence who are attacked by strangers.

Modified from U.S. Department of Justice: *Domestic violence awareness: stop the cycle of violence*, Pub No. U.S.G.P.O.: 1996-405-033/54261, Washington, D.C., 1996a, U.S. Government Printing Office, p. 5.

child, economic dependence on one's partner, lack of awareness of alternatives, poor self-image, and inadequate support systems. Often friends and relatives of the battered woman find it easier to ignore the situation or even sanction the abuse.

The vast majority of domestic homicides are preceded by episodes of violence (USDHHS, 1991a, p. 61). Between 21% and 30% of all women in the United States are estimated to have been beaten by a partner at least once, and more than 1 million women each year seek help for injuries caused by battering. This help is often sought out at emergency rooms where fewer questions may be asked and anonymity may be maintained.

When a victim of domestic abuse presents to the emergency room or clinic, nurses are often the first contact the victim has following the assault. Because of the complexity of the abuse cycle, nurses must be sensitive to the fear experienced by these victims when questioning and intervening. This is especially critical in cases of rape, where nurses are dealing with emotional trauma and may also be gathering forensic evidence that will used if legal charges are filed against the perpetrator (Crowell, Burgess, 1996, p. 109). Domestic violence involves battering (such as pushing, slapping, punching, kicking, knifing, shooting, and throwing objects) and verbal and emotional abuse. Most battering relationships "pass through phases marked by increasing fear, isolation, and control, often accompanied by increasingly complex psychological and psychosocial adaptations" (Stark, Flitcraft, 1996, p. 205).

Within these phases there is often a time of remorse; the perpetrator may feel guilty and remorseful following an episode of abuse, and things may calm down for awhile. However, it does not take much to trigger a new episode. In fact, the abuse cycle is very likely to occur again, and it may become more severe. A violent relationship can easily go on to become a violent system that ultimately leads to death. Nurses must be perceptive and prepared to comprehensively assess, intervene, and refer appropriately when victims present themselves for care.

Domestic violence is different from other forms of violence in that the victim is in close relationship to the perpetrator and the perpetrator has continued access to the victim (Stark, Flitcraft, 1996, p. 161). Domestic violence is often difficult to identify. Travis (1996) has described three predominant indicators to distinguish domestic violence from other forms of violence. First, the victim often knows the perpetrator, and often there have been repeated offenses that have progressively become more violent; second, the victim often lives in a state of terror and powerlessness as the perpetrator exerts physical, psychological, and emotional control over the victim; and last, the violence is often known to the community, where there have been fragmented indicators of abuse in medical records, police records, and school and work records that reflect patterns of absence or visible signs of battering, yet the community has looked the other way and ignored the indicators (Travis, 1996, pp. 24-25). When the violence is finally noted it is often severe and in some cases deadly. It is crucial for community health nurses to be aware of these characteristics to intervene in an efficacious manner.

The battered victim may be kept from contact with others who could provide help. The victim may be depressed and may frequently mention minor somatic complaints when seen by health care personnel; she may or may not show obvious signs of physical injury. Many women who have experienced battering are unrecognized during health care visits (Davidson, 1996, p. 13). Domestic violence is difficult to deal with because of emotional ties between the individuals involved (NIJ, 1996, p. 28).

Shelters and safe homes for battered women exist in many communities throughout the country. As mentioned earlier, there is a national hotline (1-800-799-SAFE) with daily 24-hour coverage by people who respond to requests

table 12-5 Indicators of Potential or Actual Wife Abuse from History

Area of Assessment	At-Risk Responses*
PRIMARY CONCERN/REASON FOR VISIT	
	Unwarranted delay between time of injury and seeking treatment
	Inappropriate spouse reactions (lack of concern, overconcern, threatening demeanor, reluctance to leave wife, etc.)
	Vague information about cause of injury or problem; discrepancy between physical findings and verbal description of cause; obviously incongruous cause of injury given
	Minimizing serious injury
	Seeking emergency room treatment for vague stress-related symptoms and minor injuries
	Suicide attempt; history of previous attempts
FAMILY HEALTH HISTORY	
Family of origin	Traditional values about women's role taught
	Spouse abuse or child abuse (may not be significant for wife but should be noted)
Children	Children abused
	Physical punishment used routinely and severely with children
	Children are hostile toward or fearful of father
	Father perceives children as an additional burden
	Father demands unquestioning obedience from children
Partner	Alcohol or drug abuse
	Holds machismo values
	Experience with violence outside of home, including violence against women in previous relationships
	Low self-esteem; lack of power in workplace or other arenas outside of home
	Uses force or coercion in sexual activities
	Unemployment or underemployment
	Extreme jealousy of female friendships, work, and children, as well as other men; jealousy frequently unfounded
	Stressors such as death in family, moving, change of jobs, trouble at work
	Abused as a child or witnessed father abusing mother
Household	Poverty
	Conflicts solved by aggression or violence
	Isolated from neighbors, relatives; few friends; lack of support systems
PAST HEALTH HISTORY	
	Fractures and trauma injuries
	Depression, anxiety symptoms, substance abuse
	Injuries while pregnant
	Spontaneous abortions
	Psychophysiological complaints
	Previous suicide attempts
Nutrition	Evidence of overeating or anorexia as reactions to stress
	Sudden changes in weight
Personal/social	Low self-esteem; evaluates self poorly in relation to others and ideal self, has trouble listing strengths, makes negative comments about self frequently, doubts own abilities
	Expresses feelings of being trapped, powerlessness, that the situation is hopeless, that it is futile to make future plans
	Chronic fatigue, apathy
	Feels responsible for spouse's behavior
	Holds traditional values about the home, a wife's prescribed role, the husband's prerogatives, strong commitment to marriage
	External locus of control orientation, feels no control over situation, believes fate or other forces determine events
	Major decisions in household made by spouse, indicates far less power than he has in relationship, activities controlled by spouse, money controlled by spouse
	Few support systems, few supportive friends, little outside home activity, outside relationships have been discouraged by spouse or curtailed by self to deal with violent situation
	Physical aggression in courtship

From Campbell J, McKenna LS, Torres S et al: Nursing care of abused women. In Campbell J, Humphreys J, eds: *Nursing care of survivors of family violence*, St. Louis, 1993, Mosby, pp. 255-256.
*At-risk responses are derived from clinical experience and review of the literature.

table 12-5 INDICATORS OF POTENTIAL OR ACTUAL WIFE ABUSE FROM HISTORY—CONT'D

AREA OF ASSESSMENT	AT-RISK RESPONSES
Sleep	Sleep disturbances, insomnia, sleeping more than 10 to 12 hours per day
Elimination	Chronic constipation, diarrhea, or elimination disturbances related to stress
Illness	Frequent psychophysiological illnesses Treatment for mental illness Use of tranquilizers and/or mood elevators and/or antidepressants
Operations/ hospitalizations	Hospitalizations for trauma injuries Suicide attempts Hospitalization for depression Refusals of hospitalization when suggested by physician
Personal safety	Handgun(s) in home History of frequent accidents Does not take safety precautions
Health care utilization	No regular provider Indicates mistrust of health care system
Review of systems	Headaches, undiagnosed gastrointestinal symptoms, palpitations, other possible psychophysiological complaints Sexual difficulties, feels husband is "rough" in sexual activities, lack of sexual desire, pain with intercourse Joint pain and/or other areas of tenderness, especially at the extremities Chronic pain Pelvic inflammatory disease

for information, discuss options, and provide shelter referrals. Individuals who call the hotline can get an immediate crisis intervention referral to agencies in their local communities, including domestic abuse shelters and emergency services. The National Coalition against Domestic Violence in Washington, D.C. (202-638-6388) is an excellent source of information and referral. In response to the Violence Against Women Act, the National Institute of Justice is carrying out extensive research on this problem, and new data and information will be forthcoming in the next few years.

The Role of the Nurse with Domestic Violence

The American Nurses Association has developed a strong position statement on violence against women. The position document defines violence against women as "behavior intended to inflict harm and includes slapping, kicking, choking, punching, pushing, use of objects as weapons, forced sexual activity, and injury or death from a weapon" (ANA, 1996a, p. 203). ANA has made an active commitment to eliminate all forms of domestic violence "through the legislative, regulatory, and health care arena" (ANA, 1995).

Because nurses have the unique opportunity to interact with clients individually as well as in groups, it is important to complete thorough interviews with victims or potential victims to more effectively intervene and to identify the most appropriate referrals. Humphreys (1993) believes that every family should be assessed for family violence. Table 12-5 lists the indicators of potential or actual wife abuse from history. Table 12-6 gives the indicators of wife abuse from physical examination. Indicators for child abuse are identified in Chapter 16.

Davey and Davey (1996) encourage nurses to interview clients when screening for abuse because the victims are more likely to disclose personal information during an interview with a nurse than when responding to a written form. The Teaching Tips box presents a domestic violence assessment tool, and the following box (p. 359) gives a list of guidelines to use when interviewing victims about domestic violence. Community health nurses can use these guides to assess women at risk; assessment data are then used as a basis for developing nursing interventions, including referral to community resources as indicated. Identifying women at risk is essential for intervention at both primary and secondary levels of prevention (Davidson, 1996, p. 13).

An important role of the community health nurse is casefinding. The community health nurse is in a unique position to see the family at home and may be the first to observe an abusive relationship. The nurse must be comfortable in exploring possible abuse issues with clients; this may involve examining personal attitudes and beliefs related to domestic abuse (Dickson, Tutty, 1996). Community health nurses, like other health care providers, are legally responsible for reporting abuse, and it is imperative that nurses do not allow personal issues and biases to interfere with their professional responsibility to clients. Early intervention is necessary to break the cycle of abuse and prevent the escalation of violence. The nurse can help clients to look at

table 12-6 Indicators of Wife Abuse from Physical Examination

Area of Assessment	At-Risk Findings
General appearance	Increased anxiety in presence of spouse Watching spouse for approval of answers to questions Signs of fatigue Inappropriate or anxious nonverbal behavior Nonverbal communication suggesting shame about body Flinches when touched Poor grooming, inappropriate attire
Vital statistics	Overweight or underweight Hypertension
Skin	Bruises, welts, edema, or scars, especially on breasts, upper arms, abdomen, chest, face, and genitalia Burns
Head	Subdural hematoma Clumps of hair missing
Eyes	Swelling Subconjunctival hemorrhage
Genital/urinary	Edema, bruises, tenderness, external bleeding
Rectal	Bruising, bleeding, edema, irritation
Musculoskeletal	Fractures, especially of facial bones, spiral fractures of radius or ulna, ribs Shoulder dislocation Limited motion of an extremity Old fractures in various stages of healing
Abdomen	Abdominal injuries in pregnant women Intra-abdominal injury
Neurological	Hyperactive reflex responses Ear or eye problems secondary to injury Areas of numbness from old injuries Tremors
Mental status examination	Anxiety, fear Depression Suicidal ideation Low self-esteem Memory loss Difficulty concentrating

From Campbell J, McKenna LS, Torres S, et al: Nursing care of abused women. In Campbell J, Humphreys J, eds: *Nursing care of survivors of family violence*, St. Louis, 1993, Mosby, p. 257.

their situation and to seek alternatives to their current lifestyle. This usually involves examining available community resources and agencies for both immediate and long-term assistance. A collaborative approach is necessary for assessment, intervention, and prevention of domestic violence.

Referrals for counseling, shelters for battered women and their children, self-help programs, job training, and financial assistance are a few of the community services available to help domestic violence victims. Community health nurses provide supportive assistance when the client is using these community services. Community health nurses also facilitate, through referral, coordination, and managed-care roles, comprehensive ongoing care that is coordinated with other community groups and agencies. Nurses also refer clients to safe houses and serve as client advocates.

Increasingly, community health nurses are providing valuable services in shelters for battered women and children. Nurses complete health assessments, make referrals to community resources, provide health counseling, conduct group health education sessions, and provide consultation to the shelter staff relative to the health aspects of operating a group home. Community health nurses' knowledge of the community and health issues make them valuable members of a domestic violence team.

In sheltered group settings community health nurses are active members of an interdisciplinary team and provide a unique perspective to the delivery of comprehensive health care. Their focus on preventive, as well as curative, services

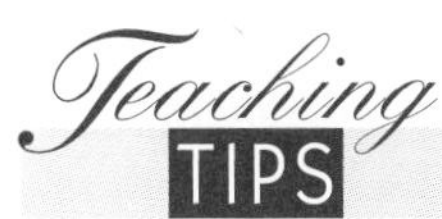

Domestic Violence Guide*

I. Identify Signs and Signals:

A. Physical (any injuries if pregnant, hair missing, edema, limited motion)
B. Emotional (feels depressed, suicidal, or responsible for abuse and for meeting partner's needs)
C. Behavioral (hypervigilant, quiet in partner's presence, victimizes others)
D. Social (isolated from friends and family, few financial or other resources)

II. When Domestic Violence is Suspected:

A. Assess the existence of violence and presence of danger
B. Educate about domestic violence and choices
C. Assist in the development and practice of a safety plan
D. Encourage short- and long-term counseling

III. Assess the Abuser for Increasing Threat:

A. Threatens homicide or suicide
B. Acutely depressed or feeling hopeless
C. Brings gun or other weapon into home
D. Obsessive about partner or family
E. Increases frequency or roughness of battering
F. Uses drugs or alcohol
G. Hurts or kills family pets
H. Rages or fights with other people

IV. Identify Options:

A. Seek legal advice
B. Get protective order
C. Have abuser arrested
D. Leave
E. Stay
F. Develop safety plan

V. Establish a Client-Centered Safety Plan:

A. Determine the effects of violence on the client's children, how to predict imminent danger, how to physically leave situation
B. Hide money, important papers, cards, numbers, clothing, medication for quick, easy access
C. Hide extra keys for house and give extra set to trusted person
D. Set up "code" with family and friends so they'll know when to call police
E. Hide phone number for local shelter, establish contact with social worker
F. Reestablish contact with estranged family and friends
G. Identify places of sanctuary
H. Make current plan more detailed than last "escape" attempt

VI. Organizing Framework for the Clinician:

A. Develop protocol for handling domestic violence, put in Policies and Procedures manual
B. Offer educational sessions for staff
C. Post phone numbers for local domestic violence shelters in prominent place
D. Compile a list of therapists and social workers who specialize in treating victims on an outpatient basis
E. Contact attorney general to learn status of laws about reporting abuse in your state

From Davey PA, Davey DB: Domestic violence: a clinical view, *Home Health Focus* 2(10):78-79, 1996.
*This document is for use by clinicians only and is not to be left in the home.

Guidelines for Interviewing Clients about Domestic Violence

Remember that your client is a survivor.
Talk unhurriedly in a private environment.
Maintain confidentiality.
Use active listening skills.
Maintain eye contact without staring.
Show empathetic concern, not horror.
Don't offer simplistic solutions.
Don't use demonstrative sympathy or anger.
Don't ask "why" questions.
Believe your client, don't disregard or minimize the situation.
Don't make judgments.
Acknowledge injustice.
Give supportive messages.
Respect your client's right of self-determination.
Record without judgments what has been said and observed.

From Davey PA, Davey DB: Domestic violence: a clinical view, *Home Health Focus* 2(10):78-79, 1996.

enhances the care provided to this population group. Because of the complex dynamics related to family violence, confidentiality in regard to the location of shelters for battered victims is maintained by health professionals throughout the community. Crisis hotlines help clients to access services from these shelters. Nurses have been working to strengthen services for victims of domestic violence across the nation.

The Nursing Network on Violence Against Women (NNVAW) was founded in 1985 during the first National Nursing Conference on Violence Against Women held at the University of Massachusetts at Amherst. The ultimate goal of NNVAW is to provide a nursing presence in the struggle to end violence in women's lives. A book written specifically for nurses on family violence is *Nursing Care of Survivors of Family Violence* (1993) by Campbell and Humphreys. The book is an excellent practical resource for clinicians, researchers, and teachers. The authors stress that preventive interventions at both the family and community level are essential to reduce future domestic violence.

Since the passage of the 1994 Violence Against Women Act, publications are becoming available that provide new perspectives and in-depth understanding of the complexity of violence against women and guidance for therapists. For example, *Counseling to End Violence Against Women* (Whalen, 1996) provides a feminist perspective and a counseling model that was derived from research with counselors who were working with domestic and sexual assault victims. This model provides a counseling method, encompassing counseling approaches, that relates to a woman's problems, needs, roles, and relationships. Nursing activities developed by the Iowa Intervention Project to intervene in abuse protection are listed in the box on page 361. As research continues, more publications will become available and, as researcher roles are implemented, community health nurses will make a contribution to nursing's knowledge base for preventing and intervening in violent and abusive situations.

SUMMARY

Aggregate-focused contemporary community health issues are multifaceted and complex. Community health nurses have an important role in assessing populations at risk, identifying health problems, and developing interventions to promote the health of the community. This chapter addressed the issues involving select population groups at risk and discussed the community health nurse's role in primary, secondary, and tertiary prevention of contemporary health issues. Particular emphasis was given to primary prevention and developing community-based interventions.

As responsibility for meeting the needs of disadvantaged populations shifts from the federal government to state and local communities, the need for comprehensive community-based programming is a priority. In community-based programming interventions are tailored specifically to the needs of communities. Examples of such interventions include the use of peer counselors and the use of culturally relevant health education materials.

Community-based programming requires a holistic approach that addresses the multifaceted web of contemporary health problems (poverty, homelessness, substance addiction, STDs, HIV/AIDS, violence, and abusive behavior). Many of the problems do not exist in isolation but are part of a larger web of social, economic, and other related health issues. Because community health nurses have access to the populations at risk and knowledge of the resources in their respective communities, they play an important role when they use the nursing process in intervening with aggregates to assist and diagnose contemporary health issues and to implement and evaluate effective interventions.

Comprehensive programming requires mobilization of community resources to ensure comprehensive intervention. Community resources such as social support services, drug/alcohol abuse treatment centers, mental health professionals, nurses in acute care agencies, school and youth leaders, law enforcement agencies, legal advisors, family planning services, and primary care providers are used. There must also be a willingness to develop community initiatives that mobilize resource providers to address the multifaced problems that interact and threaten the health and safety of the community. Through their knowledge and experience in applying the levels of prevention, community health nurses can make a unique contribution in comprehensive community planning and intervention.

CRITICAL *Thinking Exercise*

Read the following scenario (Berne, Dato, Mason, Rafferty, 1990, p. 11) and then write a paragraph describing your feelings and the course of action you would take in the next week. Do you believe that this situation could ever happen to you or someone that you know?

Imagine You Are Homeless . . .

Imagine you are a 33-year-old woman with three children. Your apartment burned down 6 months ago. You and your children had been living with your sister in her cramped apartment until she had another baby, and now there simply is not enough room for everyone.

You sleep in your car at night. During the day, you walk the streets with your children trying to find an apartment you can afford. Finally, you go to the department of social services to try to find shelter for the night and are told that your children may have to be placed in foster care if a place cannot be found for all of you. Knowing that the foster care system in this city is unreliable and sometimes unsafe, you agree to spend the first night in an overcrowded warehouse-type shelter, where you end up sleeping on the floor.

You and your children have no privacy here. Many of the children and adults have colds, and you hear that tuberculosis

NIC Nursing Intervention: Abuse Protection

Definition

Identification of high-risk, dependent relationships and actions to prevent further infliction of physical or emotional harm

NURSING ACTIVITIES

Identify adult(s) with a history of unhappy childhoods associated with abuse, rejection, excessive criticism, or feelings of being worthless and unloved as children
Identify adult(s) who have difficulty trusting others or feel disliked by others
Identify whether individual feels that asking for help is an indication of personal incompetence
Identify level of social isolation present in family situation
Determine whether family needs periodic relief from care responsibilities
Identify whether adult at risk has close friends or family available to help with children when needed
Determine relationship between husband and wife
Determine whether adults are able to take over for each other when one is too tense, tired, or angry to deal with a dependent family member
Determine whether child/dependent adult is viewed differently by an adult based on gender, appearance, or behavior
Identify crisis situations that may trigger abuse, such as poverty, unemployment, divorce, or death of a loved one
Monitor for signs of neglect in high-risk families
Observe a sick or injured child/dependent adult for signs of abuse
Listen to the explanation on how the illness or injury happened
Identify when the explanation of the cause of the injury is inconsistent among those involved
Encourage admission of child/dependent adult for further observation and investigation as appropriate
Record times and duration of visits during hospitalization
Monitor parent-child interactions and record observations as appropriate
Monitor for underreactions or overreactions on the part of an adult
Monitor child/dependent adult for extreme compliance, such as passive submission to hospital procedures
Monitor child for role reversal, such as comforting the parent, or overactive or aggressive behavior
Listen attentively to adult who begins to talk about own problems
Listen to a pregnant woman's feelings about pregnancy and expectations about the unborn child
Monitor new parent's reactions to infant, observing for feelings of disgust, fear, or unrealistic expectations
Monitor for a parent who holds newborn at arm's length, handles newborn awkwardly, or asks for excessive assistance
Monitor for repeated visits to a clinic, emergency room, or physician's office for minor problems
Monitor for a progressive deterioration in the physical and emotional care provided to a child/dependent adult in the family
Monitor child for signs of failure to thrive, depression, apathy, developmental delay, or malnutrition
Determine expectations adult has for child to determine whether expected behaviors are realistic
Instruct parents on realistic expectations of child based on developmental level
Establish rapport with families who have a history of abuse for long-term evaluation and support
Help families identify coping strategies for stressful situations
Instruct adult family members on signs of abuse
Refer adult(s) at risk to appropriate specialists
Inform the physician of observations indicative of abuse
Report any situations where abuse is suspected to the proper authorities
Refer adult(s) to shelters for abused spouses as appropriate
Refer parents to Parents Anonymous for group support as appropriate

From McCloskey JC, Bulecheck GM, eds: *Nursing interventions classification (NIC)*, ed 2, St. Louis, 1996, Mosby, pp. 71-72.

has been an increasing problem among the homeless. When the opportunity arises, you agree to move into one of the single-room occupancy hotels that the city is using to house homeless families "temporarily." That temporary shelter becomes your home for 13 months.

The temporary shelter consists of one 10 by 10 ft. room. You have no kitchen, no refrigerator, no stove or cooking facilities. There is one bed for you and your three children.

You pull the mattress off the bed at night to make room for all of you to sleep and then pull the sheets off the bed in the day to eat on the floor.

You use running water to keep your baby's milk cool and you do the dishes in the tub where you bathe and store things.

There is no place for your children to play, no place to sit, no place to do homework. When they try to play in the hall, they are approached by drug dealers and sometimes even pimps.

This is what life is like for you and your children. Imagine the gradual dissipation of your own and your children's self-esteem and the isolation and depression that eventually overwhelm you. Imagine having a future without space, without privacy, without hope.

Ella M. Brooks acknowledges the work from previous editions of this text in the development of this chapter.

REFERENCES

Adams PF, Schoenborn CA, Moss AJ et al: *Health risk behaviors among our nations youth: United States, 1992*, National Center for Health Statistics, Vital Health Statistics 10 (192), 1995.

Aday L: Health status of vulnerable populations, *Annu Rev Public Health* 15:487-509, 1994.

American Nurses Association (ANA): *Legislative and regulatory initiatives for the 104th Congress*, American Nurses Association: Department of Governmental Affairs, 1995, ANA.

American Nurses Association (ANA): *American Nurses Association position statement on physical violence against women*, Washington, D.C., 1996a, ANA.

American Nurses Association (ANA): American Nurses Association position statement on tuberculosis and HIV. In *Compendium of American Nurses Association position statements*, Washington, D.C., 1996b, ANA.

American Nurses Association (ANA): *American Nurses Association position statement on cultural diversity in nursing practice*, Washington, D.C., 1996c, ANA.

Armstrong S: The lost generation, *World AIDS* 30:2-5, 1993.

Bayer R: AIDS prevention and cultural sensitivity: are they compatible? *Am J Public Health* 84(6):895-897, 1994.

Benenson A: *Control of communicable diseases manual*, ed 16, Washington, D.C., 1995, APHA.

Benjamin R: Feeling poorly: the troubling verdict on poverty and health care in America, *National Forum* 76(3):39-42, 1996.

Berne AS, Dato C, Mason DJ, Rafferty M: A nursing model for addressing the health needs of homeless families, *Image J Nurs Sch* 22(1):8-13, 1990.

Beschner G: Understanding teenage drug use. In Beschner G, Friedman AS, eds: *Teen drug use*, Lexington, Ma., 1986, D.C. Heath.

Blane D: Editorial: Social determinants of health—socioeconomic status, social class, and ethnicity, *Am J Public Health* 85(7):903-905, 1995.

Burg M: Health problems of sheltered homeless women and their dependent children, *Health Soc Work* 19(2):125-131, 1994.

Calvillo ER: AIDS knowledge and attitudes among Latinas. In Western Institute of Nursing: *Communicating nursing research, silver threads: 25 years of excellence*, vol 25, Boulder, Co., 1992, The Institute.

Campbell JC, Humphreys JC: *Nursing care of survivors of family violence*, St. Louis, 1993, Mosby.

Campbell J, McKenna LS, Torres S et al: Nursing care of abused women. In Campbell J, Humphreys J, eds: *Nursing care of survivors of family violence*, St. Louis, 1993, Mosby.

Centers for Disease Control and Prevention (CDC): Changes in notifiable diseases data presentation, *MMWR* 45(2):41-42, January 19, 1996a.

Centers for Disease Control and Prevention (CDC): *HIV counseling, testing, and referral: standards and guidelines*, Atlanta, 1994a, CDC.

Centers for Disease Control and Prevention (CDC): First 500,000 AIDS cases—United States, 1995, *MMWR* 44:849-853, November 24, 1995a.

Centers for Disease Control and Prevention (CDC): HIV/AIDS education and prevention programs for adults in prisons and jails and juveniles in confinement facilities—United States, 1994, *MMWR* 45(13):268-270, 1996b.

Centers for Disease Control and Prevention (CDC): *HIV/AIDS Surveillance Report*, 7(2):5-39, December 1995b.

Centers for Disease Control (CDC): 1989 sexually transmitted diseases treatment guidelines, *MMWR* 38(No. S-8):4-40, 1989.

Centers for Disease Control and Prevention (CDC): 1993 revised classification system for HIV infection and expanded surveillance case definition for AIDS among adolescents and adults, *MMWR* 41(RR-17):1-15, December 18, 1992.

Centers for Disease Control and Prevention (CDC): 1993 sexually transmitted diseases treatment guidelines, *MMWR* 42(No. RR-14):1-102, 1993.

Centers for Disease Control and Prevention (CDC): Prevention and control of tuberculosis in correctional facilities, *MMWR* 45(RR-8):1-6, June 7, 1996c.

Centers for Disease Control and Prevention (CDC): Programs for the prevention of suicide among adolescents and young adults, *MMWR* 43(RR-6):3-18, April 22, 1994b.

Centers for Disease Control (CDC): Revision of the CDC surveillance case definition for Acquired Immunodeficiency Syndrome, *MMWR* 36(No. 1S):3S-15S, 1987.

Centers for Disease Control and Prevention (CDC): Tuberculosis morbidity—United States, 1995, *MMWR* 45(18):365-370, 1996d.

Centers for Disease Control and Prevention (CDC): Update: Mortality attributable to HIV infection, *MMWR* 16(45):10-125, 1996e.

Centers for Disease Control and Prevention (CDC): USPHS/IDSA guidelines for the prevention of opportunistic infections in persons infected with human immunodeficiency virus: a summary, *MMWR* 44(RR-8), 1995c.

Centers for Disease Control and Prevention (CDC): U.S. Public Health Service recommendations for human immunodeficiency virus counseling and voluntary testing for pregnant women, *MMWR* 44(RR-7):1-15, 1995d.

Children's Defense Fund (CDF): *The state of America's children yearbook 1996*, Washington, D.C., 1996, CDF.

Cocaine use: the largest global study ever undertaken, *World Health* 4(July-August):25, 1995.

Cole F, Slocumb E: Nurses' attitudes toward patients with AIDS, *J Adv Nurs* 83:112-117, 1993.

Commonwealth Fund: *National comparative survey of minority health care*. New York, 1995, The Fund.

Cox J: Koop says up tax, cut liquor ads, *USA Today*, June 1, 1989, A1.

Craig C: Making the most of the nurse-managed clinic, *Nurs Health Care* 17(3):124-126, 1996.

Crowe AH, Reeves RR: *Treatment for alcohol and other drug abuse: opportunities for coordination*, DHHS Pub No. (SMA)94-2075, Rockville, Md., 1994, U.S. Government Printing Office.

Crowell NA, Burgess AW: *Understanding violence against women*, Washington, D.C., 1996, National Academy Press.

Davey PA, Davey DB: Domestic violence: a clinical view, *Home Health Focus* 2(10):78-79, 1996.

Davidson L: Editorial: Preventing injuries from violence toward women, *Am J Public Health* 86(1):12-14, 1996.

Dembo R, Williams L, Wish ED et al: The relationship between physical and sexual abuse and illicit drug use: a replication among a new sample of youths entering a juvenile detention center, *Int J Addict* 23(11):1102-1123, 1988.

Denison AV, Shum SY: The evolution of targeted populations in a school-based tuberculin testing program, *Image J Nurs Sch* 27(4):263-266, 1995.

Dickson F, Tutty LM: The role of public health nurses in responding to abused women, *Public Health Nurs* 13(4):263-268, 1996.

Doweiko HE: *Concepts of chemical dependency*, Pacific Grove, Ca., 1990, Brooks/Cole Publishing.

Eisen A: Survey of neighborhood-based, comprehensive community empowerment initiatives, *Health Educ Q* 21(2):235-252, 1994.

Emblad J: Dispelling the myths, *World Health* 4:4(July-August), 1995.

Evers-Williams M: Ending welfare as we know it, *National Forum* 79(3):12-14, 1996.

Finkelstein DM, Williams PL, Molenberghs G et al: Patterns of opportunistic infections in patients with HIV infection, *J Acquir Immune Defic Syndr Hum Retrovirol* 12:38-45, 1996.

Flynt W: Rural poverty in America, *National Forum* 76(3):32-34, 1996.

Freudenberg N, Eng E, Flay B et al: Strengthening individual and community capacity to prevent disease and promote health: in search of relevant theories and principles, *Health Educ Q* 22(3): 290-306, 1995.

Friend T: Cover story: today's youth just don't see the dangers, *USA Today*, August 21, 1996, A1, A2.

Garbarino J: Children and poverty in America, *National Forum* 76(3):28-31,42, 1996.

General Accounting Office (GAO): *Tuberculosis: costly and preventable cases in five cities*, Washington, D.C., 1995, GAO.

Gingrich N: Rethinking our approach to poverty, *National Forum* 79(3):9-11,19, 1996.

Grimes D, Grimes M: Tuberculosis: what nurses need to know to help control the epidemic, *Nurs Outlook* 43(4):164-173, 1995.

Grimes ML: Forum on education & academics, middle-class morality: Postures toward the poor, *National Forum* 76(3):3-4, 1996.

Grossman D: Enhancing your cultural competence, *Am J Nurs* 94: 58-62, 1994.

Hanrahan P, Campbell J, Ulrich Y: Theories of violence. In Campbell J, Humphreys J, eds: *Nursing care of survivors of family violence*, St. Louis, 1993, Mosby.

Hartmann H, Spalter-Roth R, Chu J: Poverty alleviation and single-mother families, *National Forum* 76(3):24-27, 1996.

Hawkins JD, Lishner DM, Jenson JM, et al: Delinquents and drugs: what the evidence suggests about prevention and treatment programming. In Brown BS, Mills AR, eds: *Youth at high risk for substance abuse*, Rockville, Md., 1987, National Institute on Drug Abuse.

Hitchcock PJ: Adolescents and sexually transmitted diseases, *AIDS Patient Care* 10(2):79-86, 1996.

Humphreys J: Children of battered women. In Campbell J, Humphreys J, eds: *Nursing care of survivors of family violence*, St. Louis, 1993, Mosby.

Institute of Medicine (IOM): *Treating drug problems* (vol 1), Washington, D.C., 1990, National Academy Press.

Jaynes JH, Rugg CA: *Adolescents, alcohol and drugs*, Springfield, Il., 1988, Charles Thomas.

Johnston LD, O'Malley PM, Bachman JG: *National survey results on drug use from the monitoring the future study*, 1975-1994, NIH Pub No. 95-4026, Washington, D.C., 1995, U.S. Government Printing Office.

Johnson KV, Dowling C: After a decade of decline, a deadly statistic rises, *USA Today*, July 2, 1996, A2.

Kinzel D: Self-identified health concerns of two homeless groups, *West J Nurs Res* 13(2):181-194, 1991.

Kitazawa S: Tuberculosis health education needs in homeless shelters, *Public Health Nurs* 12(6):409-416, 1995.

Klaidman D: The politics of drugs: back to war, *Newsweek*, August 25, 1996, 57-58.

Knott DH: *Alcohol problems: diagnosis and treatment*, New York, 1986, Pergamon Press.

Koegel P, Melamid E, Burnam A: Childhood risk factors for homelessness among homeless adults, *Am J Public Health* 85(12):1642-1649, 1995.

Koopman JS, Little RJ: Assessing HIV vaccine effects, *Am J Epidemiol* 142(10):1113-1119, 1995.

Kulig JC, Wilde IW: Collaboration between communities and universities: completion of a community needs assessment, *Public Health Nurs* 13(2):112-119, 1996.

Leland J: The fear of heroin is shooting up: kids on dope are still rare, but parents are right to be scared, *Newsweek*, August 26, 1996, 55-56.

Link B: Editorial: Understanding sociodemographic differences in health—the role of fundamental social causes, *Am J Public Health* 86(4):471-473, 1996.

Link B, Susser E, Stueve A et al: Lifetime and five-year prevalence of homelessness in the United States, *Am J Public Health* 84(12): 1907-1912, 1994.

Macdonald DI: *Drugs, drinking and adolescents*, St Louis, 1989, Mosby.

Marin G, Burhansstipanov L, Connell CM et al: A research agenda for health education among underserved populations, *Health Educ Q* 22(3):346-363, 1995.

Massaro J, Pepper B: The relationship of addiction to crime, health, and other social problems. In Crowe AH, Reeves RR: *Treatment for alcohol and other drug abuse: opportunities for coordination*, DHHS Pub No. (SMA)94-2075, Rockville, Md., 1994, U.S. Government Printing Office.

Maternal and Child Health Bureau: *Child health USA '95*, Washington, D.C., 1996, U.S. Government Printing Office.

May K, Evans G: Health education for homeless populations, *J Community Health Nurs* 11(4):229-237, 1994.

Mayo K, White S, Oates SK, Franklin F: Community collaboration: prevention and control of tuberculosis in a homeless shelter, *Public Health Nurs* 13(2):120-127, 1996.

McCloskey JC, Bulechek GM, eds: *Nursing interventions classification* (NIC), ed 2, St. Louis, 1996, Mosby, pp. 71-72, 492.

McCreary M: Collaboration among communities: NLN's new center for collaborating organizations and community groups introduces exciting plan for health care futures, *NLN Update* 2(2):3, 5, 1996.

McDermott S: The health promotion needs of older people, *Prof Nurse* 10(8):530-533, 1995.

McFarlane J: De Madres a Madras: an access model for primary care, *Am J Public Health* 86:879-880, 1996.

McLellan T, Dembo R: *Screening and assessment of alcohol and other drug (AOD)–abusing adolescents* (Treatment Improvement Protocol 3), Rockville, Md., 1992, Center for Substance Abuse Treatment.

McNeal G: Mobile health care for those at risk, *Nursing and Health Care: Perspectives on Community* 17(3):134-140, 1996.

Mihaly LK: *Homeless families: failed policies and young victims*, Washington, D.C., 1991, Children's Defense Fund.

Miller TR, Cohen MA, Wiersema B: *Victim costs and consequences: a new look*, National Institute of Justice research report, Pub No. NIJ 155282, Washington, D.C., February 1996, U.S. Department of Justice.

Mosby's patient teaching guides, St. Louis, 1995, Mosby.

Murray RB: Stressors and coping strategies of homeless men, *J Psychosoc Nurs* 34(8):16-22, 1996.

Murphy B, ed: *Nursing centers: the time is now*, New York, 1995, National League for Nursing.

National Center for Health Statistics: *Health, United States, 1995, Chartbook*, Pub No. (PHS) 96-1232, Hyattsville, Md., 1996, U.S. Government Printing Office.

National Institute for Justice (NIJ): *The criminalization of domestic violence: promises and limits*. Rockville, Md., 1996, U.S. Department of Justice.

National League for Nursing (NLN): Caring for persons with AIDS test, *Nurs Health Care* 10(10):563, 1989.

Needle RH, Mills AR: *Drug procurement practices of the out-of-treatment chronic drug abuser*, NIH Pub No. 94-3820, Rockville, Md., 1994, National Institutes of Health.

Newmann RE, Nishimoto PW: 1996 Human Immunodeficiency Virus Update for the primary care provider, *Nurse Pract Forum* 7(1):16-22, 1996.

Nichols B: White house GOP spar on drug report, *USA Today*, August 21, 1996, A1.

Norton D, Ridenour N: Homeless women and children: the challenge of health promotion, *Nurse Pract Forum* 6(1):29-33, 1995.

Nowinski J: *Substance abuse in adolescents and young adults: a guide to treatment*, New York, 1990, Norton.

Office of Minority Health—Resource Center (OMH-RC): Cancer hits some minorities hard. In *Cancer and minorities: closing the gap*, Washington, D.C., 1989, Department of Health and Human Resources.

Ossege J, Berry R: Nurse managed care for the homeless in Lexington, *Ky Nurse* 43(4):22, Oct-Dec, 1994.

Pender N: *Assessment of health, health beliefs, and health behaviors. Health promotion in nursing practice*, ed 3, 1996, Appleton and Lange, pp. 115-144.

Randall-David E: *Culturally competent HIV counseling and education*, McLean, Va., 1994, The Maternal and Child Health Clearinghouse.

Rice DP: Health status and national health priorities, *West J Med* 154:294-302, March, 1991.

Riemer J, Van-Cleve L, Galbraith M: Barriers to well child care for homeless children under age 13, *Public Health Nurs* 12(1):61-66, 1995.

Robert Wood Johnson Foundation: *Challenges in health care: a chartbook perspective 1991*, Princeton, N.J., 1991, The Foundation.

Rosenberg ML, O'Carroll PW, Powell KE: Let's be clear, violence is a public health problem, *JAMA* 267(22):3071-3072, 1992.

Sbarbaro J: TB control is indeed an exercise in vigilance, *Public Health Rep* III:32-33, 1996.

Schinke SP, Botvin GJ, Orlandi MA: *Substance abuse in children and adolescents: evaluation and intervention*, Newbury Park, Ca., 1991, Sage.

Schoemer K: Rockers, models and the new allure of heroin, *Newsweek*, August 26, 1996, pp. 50-54.

Scholler-Jaquish A: Walk-in health clinic for the homeless, *Nurs Health Care* 17(3):119-123, 1996.

Simandl G: Nursing students working with the homeless, *Nurse Educ* 21(2):18-22, 1996.

Sorlie P, Backlund E, Keller J: U.S. mortality by economic demographics and social characteristics: the national longitudinal study, *Am J Public Health* 85(7):949-956, 1995.

Sowell RL, Seals BF, Cooper JA: HIV transmission knowledge and risk behaviors of persons with HIV infection, *AIDS Patient Care and STDs* 10(2):111-115, 1996.

Spector R: Sociocultural perspective of prevention. In Knollmueller R, ed: *Prevention across the life span*, Washington, D.C., 1993, American Nurses Publishing, pp. 11-19.

Stark E, Flitcraft A: *Women at risk: domestic violence and women's health*, Thousand Oaks, Ca., 1996, Sage.

Stephenson GM: *Preparedness for crime, the psychology of criminal justice*, Cambridge, Ma., 1992, Blackwell.

Tarter RE, Ott PJ, Mezzich AC: Psychometric assessment. In Frances RJ, Miller SI, eds: *Clinical textbook of addictive disorders*, New York, 1991, Guilford Press.

Tollett JH, Thomas SP: A theory-based nursing intervention to instill hope in homeless veterans, *Adv Nurs Sci* 18(2):76-90, 1996.

Travis J: Violence against women: reflections on NIJ's research agenda, *National Institute of Justice Journal* 2(230):21-25, February 1996.

Underwood SM: Issues and challenges in cancer nursing research: increasing the participation and involvement of African-Americans in cancer programs and trials. In American Cancer Society, ed: *Nursing Research and Underserved Populations*, 1994, The Society.

U.S. Department of Health and Human Services (USDHHS): *Directory of outreach and primary health services for homeless children, draft*, Bethesda, Md., May 1996, Public Health Service Health Resources and Services Administration.

U.S. Department of Health and Human Services (USDHHS): *Healthy People 2000: midcourse review and 1995 revisions*, Washington, D.C., 1995, U.S. Government Printing Office.

U.S. Department of Health and Human Services (USDHHS): *Healthy People 2000: national health promotion and disease prevention objectives, full report, with commentary*, Washington, D.C., 1991a, U.S. Government Printing Office.

U.S. Department of Health and Human Services (USDHHS): *Health status of minorities and low-income groups*, ed 3, Washington, D.C., 1991b, U.S. Government Printing Office.

U.S. Department of Health and Human Services (USDHHS): *HIV counseling, testing and referral standards and guidelines*, Public Health Service, Washington, D.C., 1994a, U.S. Government Printing Office.

U.S. Department of Health and Human Services (USDHHS): *HIV infection and AIDS: are you at risk?* Public Health Service, Washington, D.C., 1994b, U.S. Government Printing Office.

U.S. Department of Health and Human Services (USDHHS): *Making a difference: interim status report of the McKinney Demonstration Program for homeless adults with serious mental illness*, Rockville, Md., 1994c, Center for Mental Health Services, Substance Abuse and Mental Health Services Administration.

U.S. Department of Housing and Urban Development (USDHUD): *Priority: Home! The Federal plan to break the cycle of homelessness*, Pub No. HUD-1454-CPD(1), Washington, D.C., 1994, U.S. Government Printing Office.

U.S. Department of Justice: *Domestic violence awareness: stop the cycle of violence*, Pub No. U.S.G.P.O.:1996-405-033/54261, Washington, D.C., 1996a, U.S. Government Printing Office.

U.S. Department of Justice: *Domestic violence, stalking, and antistalking legislation*, Pub No. 1996-405-037/40024, Washington, D.C., 1996b, U.S. Government Printing Office.

Venereal Disease Action Coalition: *Sexually transmitted diseases: a community information and resource guide*, Detroit, 1983, United Community Services of Metropolitan Detroit.

Wagner JD, Menke EM, Ciccone JK: What is known about the health of rural homeless families? *Public Health Nurs* 12(6):400-408, 1995.

Wald L: *The house on Henry Street*, New York, 1915, Holt.

Waters CM: Professional development in nursing research—a culturally diverse postdoctoral experience, *Image J Nurs Sch* 28(1):47-50, 1996.

Wells SM: Recovering from homelessness and serious mental illness, *Access: information from the National Resource Center on Homelessness and Mental Illness* 8(2):1,3-4,8, 1996.

Whalen M: *Counseling to end violence against women*, Thousand Oaks, Ca., 1996, Sage.

Wolman B: Foreword. In Adler LL, Denmark FL, eds: *Violence and the prevention of violence*, Westport, Ct., 1995, Praeger.

Woodson RL: Welfare reform, *National Forum* 79(3):15-19, 1996.

Yankauer A: Sexually transmitted diseases: a neglected public health priority, *Am J Public Health* 84(12):1894-1897, 1994.

Zima B, Wells K, Freeman H: Emotional and behavioral problems and severe academic delays among sheltered children in Los Angeles County, *Am J Public Health* 84(2):260-264, 1994.

SELECTED BIBLIOGRAPHY

Campbell JC: Violence against women: where policy needs to go, *Nurs Policy Forum* 1(6):10-17, 1995.

Cull V: Exposure to violence and self-care practices of adolescents, *Fam Community Health* 19(1):31-41, 1996.

Dickson F, Tutty LM: The role of public health nurses in responding to abused women, *Public Health Nurs* 13(4):263-268, 1996.

Killion C: Special health care needs of homeless pregnant women, *Adv Nurs Sci* 18(2):44-46, 1995.

Koop CE, Lundberg GD: Violence in America: a public health emergency, *JAMA* 267(22):3075-3076, 1992.

Marzuk PM, Tardiff K, Hirsch CS: The epidemiology of Murder-Suicide, *JAMA* 267(23):3179-3183, 1992.

McFarlane J, Parker B, Soeken K: Abuse during pregnancy: frequency, severity, perpetrator, and risk factors of homicide, *Public Health Nurs* 12(5):284-289, 1996.

Miller RB, Boyle JS: "You don't ask for trouble": women who do sex and drugs, *Fam Community Health* 19(3):35-48, 1996.

Owens DK, Nease RF, Harris RA: Cost-effectiveness of HIV screening in acute care settings, *Arch Intern Med* 156:394-404, 1996.

Purdy LJ: Knife and gun clubs of America, *JAMA* 267(22):3086, 1992.

Rose A: Treatment programs for the homeless: a review of the literature, *J MARC Res* 1(1):65-74, 1993.

Rouse BA, ed: *Substance abuse and mental health statistics sourcebook*, DHHS Pub No. (SMA)95-3064, Washington, D.C., 1996, U.S. Government Printing Office.

Schafran LH: Topics for our times: rape is a major public health issue, *Am J Public Health* 86(1):15-17, 1996.

Shinn M, Weitzman B: Research in homelessness: an introduction, *J Soc Issues* 46(4):1-11, 1990.

Talashek ML, Gerace LM, Starr KL: The substance abuse pandemic, determinants to guide interventions, *Public Health Nurs* 11(2):131-139, 1994.

Whalen M: *Counseling to end violence against women*, Thousand Oaks, Ca., 1996, Sage.

13

Community Assessment and Diagnosis

Objectives

Upon completion of this chapter, the reader should be able to:

1. Describe the relevance of community analysis activities to community health nursing practice
2. Discuss the importance of developing partnerships when assessing a community.
3. Discuss the application of the nursing process to community-oriented practice.
4. Identify parameters for assessing a community's level of functioning.
5. Summarize methods for assessing a community's health status.
6. Explain the relevance of public health statistics to community health nursing practice.
7. Summarize international, federal, state, and local sources for obtaining community data.
8. Formulate guidelines for implementing community analysis activities in the practice setting.

Chapter 2 explored the ANA's and the APHA's definitions of community health nursing practice, which state that the dominant responsibility of nurses in community health is to the community or the population as a whole (ANA, 1986; APHA, 1996). Recently both private foundations (The Pew Charitable Trusts) and nursing organizations (ANA and NLN) confirmed the importance of focusing on the health of the community (ANA, 1991; NLN, 1993; Pew Health Professions Commission, 1995; Shugars, O'Neil, Bader, 1991). These organizations' visions for the future emphasize a consumer-driven, community-based health care system and the need for changes in the education of health professionals to prepare them to deal with current issues in health care delivery. They advocate that health professionals be educated to address health promotion and disease prevention at aggregate and community levels, as well as the personal care level (NLN, 1993). This emphasis is consistent with the *Healthy People 2000* mandate (USDHHS, 1991) that challenges communities to develop local health plans to reduce morbidity and premature mortality through preventive health action.

Preventive health action at the community level requires the implementation of community analysis strategies that allow health providers to work with community residents in identifying a unique community profile. To establish this profile, community health nurses must "see," "smell," and "hear" the community and describe its people, its environment, its health status, and its health resources. Further, they must work with the community to systematically analyze all facets of community dynamics (described in Chapter 3) for the purpose of identifying appropriate community- and aggregate-focused health interventions.

"*Community analysis* is the process of assessing and defining needs, opportunities and resources involved in initiating community health action programs" (Haglund, Weisbrod, Bracht, 1990, p. 91). This process involves a variety of assessment and diagnostic activities that aid the community in setting priorities for health planning. These activities are discussed in a later section of this chapter.

WHY ASSESS THE COMMUNITY?

It is essential for the community health nurse to have an understanding of community dynamics because health action occurs in the community. Every community has *patterns* of functioning or community dynamics that either contribute to or detract from its state of health. The community health nurse must recognize these patterns to anticipate community responses to health action and to facilitate community health planning efforts. Without this knowledge it is difficult to effect change.

Knowledge of community dynamics is obtained through systematic community assessment. Community assessment helps the nurse and other health care professionals to identify cultural differences in relation to consumer interests, strengths, concerns, and motivations. This assessment also assists health care professionals in analyzing processes through which community beliefs, values, and attitudes are transmitted. Having this information allows health professionals to individualize community health planning activities.

It is important for the community health nurse to recognize that, as the traditions and health experiences in each community vary, the type of programs designed to meet consumer needs should also vary. Programs appropriate for one community or for an aggregate within a community may be ineffective in meeting the needs of other community aggregates.

Calvillo (1992) substantiated this fact when she examined AIDS knowledge and attitudes among Latina women in Los Angeles compared to a national sample of Hispanic women in the United States. The Los Angeles sample had lower educational and income levels. These respondents were less knowledgeable about AIDS and held more erroneous misconceptions about the transmission of AIDS than their national counterparts. Calvillo (p. 415) also found that "women in the Los Angeles sample who were more acculturated had significantly higher knowledge scores, fewer erroneous beliefs and greater knowledge of preventive measures." These facts suggested to Calvillo that socioeconomic status, differing levels of acculturation, and ethnicity all affect health programming and that targeted educational efforts are needed to meet the needs of diverse subgroups within communities. Other researchers (Breen, Kessler, 1994; Marin, Burhansstipanov, Connell et al, 1995; Winkleby, Flora, Kraemer, 1994) have also found that community health interventions must take into consideration the unique demographic, socioeconomic, and cultural characteristics of community residents and need to be tailored for differing subgroups to produce *sustained* health behavior change.

Studies such as those conducted by Calvillo reinforce the need to study the characteristics of the community in which one is working. They demonstrate that assumptions cannot be made about community response to health promotion and disease prevention interventions, and they point out the relevance of identifying factors that facilitate or inhibit change in health beliefs. Such studies also provide data that support the need for collaborative relationships between the consumer and the health care provider to enhance the delivery of health care services.

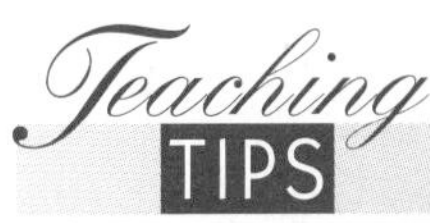

Strategies for Educating the Community About Health Issues

- Elicit the community's perspective of health issues through focus group discussions or community surveys.
- Use the community partnership approach to share community assessment data with culturally diverse segments of the population.
- Conduct a health fair that provides information on major health problems across the age continuum and health promotion activities to prevent these problems.
- Write a health column for the local newspaper or newsletters sent home from schools, churches, and other community organizations.
- Use the mass media (e.g., radio or television) to inform the public about significant community health issues.
- Sponsor special events around national health celebration days (e.g., smoking cessation and healthy heart activities during Healthy Heart month or on the Great American Smokeout day).
- Sponsor a community health awareness symposium.
- Place health information on bulletin boards in local gathering places (e.g., grocery stores, laundromats, churches, or community centers).
- Have a health booth at local community events (e.g., ethnic festivals, county fairs, powwows).

COMMUNITY HEALTH ASSESSMENT: A PARTNERSHIP PROCESS

Within any community setting there are concerned citizens and professionals from many disciplines interested in health action activities that are designed to assess a community's health status for the purpose of identifying unmet need. Since it would be impossible for any one group to handle all the health care needs of a community, efforts by many should be promoted and supported. Developing effective partnerships with clients and other health providers is the key to successful health planning in the future. "Public health, in a reformed health care system, will forge partnerships between communities and all levels of government. Communities and public health agencies—together—will keep the public healthy by assessing the community's health needs fully, developing the best policies to meet those needs, and assuring that all of us have access to high quality health and medical services and the highest attainable level of individual and community health" (APHA, 1993, unnumbered forward).

The importance of forging community health partnerships is emphasized by public health leaders across the nation (Aubel, Samba-Ndure, 1996; Berkowitz, 1995; Children's Defense Fund, 1996; Cleary, 1996; Flynn, Ray, Rider, 1994; Kreuter, 1992; McFarlane, 1996; Oberle, Barker, Magenheim, 1994; Oros, 1995; Sen, 1994). Frequently cited benefits of such partnerships are displayed in the box on the next page. Partnerships are being established to develop *local Healthy People 2000* objectives, to strengthen a community's capacity to respond to health problems, and to revitalize communities. They are also being used to improve access to health care, advocate for underserved populations, increase public awareness about the consequences of

SELECTED POTENTIAL BENEFITS OF COMMUNITY PARTNERSHIPS

- Raise the public's consciousness concerning health status indicators, available community resources, gaps in service delivery, and health behavior interventions
- Promote a shared vision around health goals and outcomes
- Encourage individuals and organizations to use their skills and resources in collective health action
- Activate citizens to participate in health decision making
- Promote a community-wide focus on "health for all"
- Help health care providers to focus on priority concerns of community residents
- Demonstrate respect for cultural diversity and the needs of differing community subgroups
- Expand community health action resources
- Promote commitment to community health improvement efforts
- Facilitate development and implementation of culturally sensitive health interventions

ASSESSMENT FUNCTION

MICHIGAN'S PUBLIC HEALTH NURSES TELL THEIR STORIES. . .

The public health nursing staff at a local health department kept encountering teens in the community who were not only pregnant, but also were living in community environments which were unhealthy for them and their unborn children.

For example, in one case, a 15-year-old female who was 4 months pregnant was living at a local shelter with a man in his 20s. In another situation, a 16-year-old female who was 8 months pregnant was living with older friends in unsanitary conditions. Both of these adolescents had difficulty maintaining prenatal care appointments because of lack of permanent and stable living arrangements and lifestyles. As a result, the nursing staff began working with the community to develop a transitional living program for pregnant and parenting teens.

Modified from Nurse Administrators Forum: *Promoting healthy Michigan communities: the role of public health nursing in health reform*, Lansing, Mi., 1994, Michigan Department of Public Health, p. 9.

unhealthy lifestyles, and establish culturally relevant and age-appropriate health interventions.

A community partnership is a union of people that is focused on collective action for a common endeavor or goal (see Chapter 3). Phrases including *coalition*, *grass-roots movement*, *leadership boards*, *networks*, *consortia*, and *citizen panels* reflect the movement to have people actively participate in community health action efforts. The differences in terminology relate to how partnerships are organized and citizen participation is facilitated (Bracht, Gleason, 1990). For example, the term *coalition* is used when formal community structures (existing organizations and groups) are linked together to address a pressing community issue such as violence. On the other hand, a grass-roots movement uses informal structures (e.g., church groups or parents of disabled children) to mobilize community residents for health action (Bracht, Gleason).

Successful community partnerships promote an active participatory process that encourages individuals and organizations to use their skills and resources in collective action, to understand health problems, and to promote local ownership of health interventions and programs. Although building active community participation in health activities can be challenging at times, it is absolutely crucial to the successful resolution of many community health problems. No community agency can address by itself situational problems such as violence, homelessness, and infant mortality.

THE NURSE'S ROLE IN COMMUNITY ASSESSMENT

Community health nurses at both administrative and staff levels must become involved in community health assessment and development activities to maintain health in the community. Although nursing administrators have the primary responsibility for establishing mechanisms that facilitate community involvement in the health assessment process, staff nurses play a pivotal role in identifying community needs on a daily basis. While working with clients in the community setting, staff nurses assess the characteristics of their work environment (neighborhood, census tract, or district) and the health status of aggregates (e.g., the homeless, elderly residents in a senior citizens' housing project, pregnant teenagers, or Asian refugees) within these work regions. This assessment process aids staff in identifying barriers to service delivery and in determining ways to mobilize community resources to reduce these barriers.

The public health nursing stories in the above box illustrate the advantage of staff nurse involvement in community health assessment activities. The data collected from the two adolescents described in this story assisted the nurses in realizing that community efforts were needed to assure positive pregnancy outcomes for teenagers in their communities. This type of knowledge aids health care organizations and community residents in planning relevant programs and services for aggregates at risk.

"Public (community) health nurses have great opportunities for community development because of their knowledge of and positions in the community" (Clarke, Beddome, Whyte, 1993, p. 309). Their daily contact with families and individuals provide significant linkages with the community as a whole, which allows them to gain knowledge and trust of the community (Conley, 1995). "This trust provides the public (community) health nurse with ready access to client populations that are difficult to engage, to agencies, and to health care providers" (Conley, p. 3). Having access to underserved populations and key community leaders permits community health nurses to gain a qualitative perspective about a community's health status. This type of perspective is not achieved when only statistical health status indicators are analyzed. Qualitative data are needed to identify *determinants* of health and disease (Conley).

In addition to assessing their work environments, community health nurses participate in comprehensive community health status assessment activities. Public health agencies have the responsibility to "regularly and systematically collect, assemble, analyze, and make available information on the health of the community, including statistics on health status, community health needs, and epidemiologic and other studies of health problems" (Institute of Medicine, 1988, p. 9). As discussed above, community partnerships are being formed to fulfill this function. As an active member of this partnership, the community health nurse participates in a variety of data collection efforts such as interviewing key informants and conducting focus groups. These and other data collection approaches are described in a later section of this chapter.

The unique perspective that the community health nurse brings to a community assessment team is a holistic philosophy derived from a synthesis of nursing and public health knowledge. The community health nurse's professional experience, educational preparation, value system, and relationships with consumers provide the skills necessary to integrate biopsychosocial data into a meaningful whole. Since all parameters of human functioning and all aspects of community dynamics have an impact on the client's (community) health status, the whole must be analyzed to determine the real causes of health and illness.

"Public (community) health nurses contribute the human and functional perspectives to community description and assessment" (Conley, 1995, p. 4). They assess the community environment to determine if environmental factors are adversely affecting a client's level of functioning. They also examine lifestyle patterns that affect preventive health practices. Refer again to the public health nursing stories. Those stories reflect the human, functional, and environmental aspects of health behavior.

The community health nurse's primary purpose in assessing the community is to identify strengths and needs in relation to preventive health practices. When needs are identified, community health nurses work with consumers and other health care professionals to improve preventive and health promotion practices. "Only programs that systematically work to promote health and to prevent disease and injury on a community-wide basis can keep people from getting sick. It has always been the mandate of public health to prevent, rather than merely treat, our health problems" (APHA, 1993, p. 1).

DIAGNOSING PREVENTIVE HEALTH NEEDS IN THE COMMUNITY

When participating in community analysis activities the community health nurse uses the nursing process as described in Chapter 9 but shifts emphasis from the family as client to the community as client and partner. Data are collected from multiple sources (*assessing*) and *analyzed* in order to formulate nursing diagnoses about community health problems. Nursing diagnoses about existing health needs, community dynamics that either positively or negatively influence health action, and deficiencies in the existing health care delivery system are generated for the purpose of facilitating community organization and health planning activities. Nursing diagnoses about community strengths are also made, because it is through its strengths that a community is able to resolve its health problems. Some examples of nursing diagnoses that might be made after the community health nurse has analyzed community assessment data are listed here:

- Children in census tracts 10 and 11 are at risk for lead poisoning because most homes were built before 1950, homes are poorly repaired, and housing regulations are inadequately enforced.
- Thirty-five percent of the aging persons in the community are experiencing social isolation because recreational activities and transportation for these persons are lacking.
- Teenagers are at risk for unwanted pregnancies because health care resources in the community refuse to provide birth control information for teenagers without parental consent.
- Community health nursing services need to be increased in census tract 5 because the number of new referrals from this area exceeds the time the current nurse has available for home visiting.
- Local churches within the community readily support health education efforts.
- Service clubs within the community respond very favorably when health care professionals request financial assistance for meeting unresolved health problems.

"A nursing diagnosis is a clinical judgment about an individual, family, or community response to actual or potential health problems/life processes . . . which . . . provides the basis for selection of nursing interventions to achieve outcomes for which the nurse is accountable" (NANDA, 1994, p. 7). Community-focused nursing diagnoses are derived from a synthesis of assessment data, are based on the concepts of risk and health needs (discussed in Chapter 11), and are situations that can be influenced by nursing intervention. Note the sample nursing diagnoses shared above. These diagnoses reflect several aggregates at risk in the community (e.g., children, teenagers, and the elderly) and pertinent functional nursing roles. For example, community health nurses are often in a key position to prevent or diagnose lead poisoning among children. Since many families are unaware of the dangers of this condition and its causes (etiology), community health nurses frequently plan and implement health education programs designed to inform the public about lead poisoning. They also carry out lead poisoning surveillance activities by assessing the environment during home visits and when traveling through their districts. If community health nurses identify that a significant number of homes in their work regions are old and in poor condition, they may also implement screening programs to identify children with lead poisoning. Children at highest risk for lead poisoning live in homes built before 1950, a time when a high dose of lead was included in interior household paint. However, "although the use and manufacture of interior lead-based paint declined during the 1950s and thereafter, exterior lead-based paint and lesser amounts of interior lead-based paint continued to be available until the mid-1970s" (CDC, 1991b, p. 18).

Once nursing diagnoses are established, the community health nurse uses the principles of planning (see Chapter 14) to prioritize health needs, to determine alternative ways to resolve these needs, to develop specific expected outcomes for health programming, and to identify ways to accomplish the stated objectives (*planning*). Following are a few examples of expected outcomes that might be developed when planning a health program to meet the social needs of aging citizens in the community. These expected outcomes reflect the advocacy role of nursing and a recognition that environmental factors significantly influence the psychosocial health of clients in the community setting.

- The county commissioners will appropriate funds for a senior citizens project in census tract 2.
- St. Francis Catholic Church will donate space in their facilities once a week for recreational activities for the aging.
- Community volunteers will plan and implement recreational activities for the aging at St. Francis Church.
- The local chapter of the American Red Cross will provide transporation for aging citizens once a week so that these persons can participate in the social activities planned at St. Francis Church.

These expected outcomes can be met by initiating several intervention strategies (*implementing*). For example, the community health nurse might make all the necessary contacts personally or might mobilize community resources to address these needs. Church groups, service clubs, and social workers from community agencies, for instance, often know of individuals who are interested in volunteering their time and energies for worthy community projects. Community health nurses frequently develop partnerships when planning a health program because they know that active participation by consumers and other professionals promotes long-term support and involvement.

Aggregate-focused nursing interventions must be *evaluated* to determine if the desired outcomes were achieved. During this process, new problems can emerge and may reflect a need for intervention strategies different from those already identified. If this were the case, the community health nurse would revise her or his nursing care plan to address new and existing needs.

Diagnosing community health problems and planning action to correct these problems are often more difficult than was just indicated. However, the community health nurse uses the nursing process—assessing, analyzing, planning, implementing, and evaluating—when intervening in affairs of the population as a whole, as well as when working with individual families. A range of community-focused nursing functions, categorized by the phases of the nursing process, is presented in the box on the next page.

How community health nurses assess the health status of populations and how they analyze community data is further elaborated on in this chapter. An overview of community organization and health planning activities is presented in Chapter 14.

COMMUNITY ASSESSMENT PARAMETERS

A significant component of community assessment is the identification of what needs to be addressed during the process. Establishing assessment guidelines helps a community partnership to organize data collection and to identify significant factors that influence a community's state of wellness.

Figure 13-1 summarizes parameters for community assessment and illustrates that community wellness is a multidimensional concept, influenced by interrelated characteristics including people, the environment, and health resources. If any one of these components changes, the balance of community health is altered. For example, economic depression can reduce funding for health care services and other essential communities activities. It can also affect the physical, mental, and social health status of community residents. When analyzing community needs, it is important to examine all components of wellness and to identify community dynamics that detract from or enhance a community's level of functioning. Chapter 3 presents the knowledge needed to analyze community dynamics.

In addition to delineating assessment parameters, it is important to determine questions that need to be answered during the assessment process. This helps the assessment team to determine the information base and methods needed to make decisions about a community's health status. The extent of the questions to be addressed will vary based on available resources and local health objectives. The box on page 372 displays one state's views about the *minimum* number of questions to be answered by a community health assessment.

The *Healthy People 2000* mandate (USDHHS, 1991) challenges state and local health care professionals to

Community-Focused Nursing Functions

ASSESSMENT

1. Identifies pertinent information about community.
2. Gathers descriptive data about the community.
3. Assesses health-related learning needs of populations.
4. Participates in identifying community health states and health behaviors, including the knowledge, attitudes, and perceptions of groups regarding health and illness.
5. Collects pertinent information about community in a systematic way.
6. Aids in community health surveys.
7. Includes members of the community as partners in the assessment process.
8. Uses basic statistics and demographic methods to collect health data.
9. Collaborates with other health care providers to assess the community.
10. Consults with community leaders to describe the community.

ANALYSIS

11. Identifies common and recurrent health problems that have potential for illness consequences.
12. Identifies health needs of help-seeking and nonseeking populations.
13. Describes health capability of community based on assessment.
14. Applies selected epidemiologic concepts in analyzing assessment data (population-at-risk, incidence, prevalence, for instance).
15. Describes present community health problems in the perspective of time (recognizes trends).
16. Describes and analyzes resources available including patterns of utilization.
17. Analyzes data for relationships and clues to the community's health.
18. Aids/participates in analysis of community health data base.
19. Forms ideas and hypotheses concerning data gathered in community assessment to derive inferences for nursing programs.
20. Includes members of the community in analyzing assessment data.

PLANNING

21. Assists in developing plans to meet needs arising from gaps or deficiencies identified.
22. Develops service priorities and plans for intervention based on analysis, community expectations and accepted practice standards.
23. Participates in planning community health programs.
24. Determines priorities for community health care based on information gathered during assessment.
25. Participates with community leaders in planning to meet identified health needs.
26. Participates with others in developing health plans applicable to the community at large.
27. Develops service objectives of identified community problems.
28. Uses knowledge of change process in planning community programs.
29. Plans for community-wide or age-specific screening programs.
30. Includes members of the community as partners in planning community health programs.

IMPLEMENTATION

31. Mobilizes the community's collective resources to help achieve higher community health goals.
32. Functions as a health advocate for the community.
33. Serves as vital link in the communication network between all kinds of community agencies and clients.
34. Seeks opportunities to participate with other disciplines in projects to bring about changes in the availability, accessibility, and accountability of health care and related systems.
35. Sets up immunization campaigns with community leaders and public health officials.
36. Initiates and monitors disease prevention programs in the community.
37. Educates the community through media regarding health issues.
38. Organizes community groups to work on alleviating community health problems.
39. Acts as a catalyst/potentiator for community change.
40. Sets up ongoing community health education programs with community leaders and public health officials.

EVALUATION

41. Monitors health services for desired quality.
42. Continually validates appropriateness of public health programs (discusses with residents, collects more data, for example).
43. Contributes information for use in evaluation of nursing programs.
44. Evaluates community response to nursing intervention.
45. Ensures necessary community health program evaluation data are collected accurately and systematically.
46. Analyzes results of service in relation to proportion of population served.
47. Promotes systematic evaluation of community resources.
48. Evaluates the impact of nursing activities on the health of the community as a whole.
49. Includes members of the community as partners in evaluating health programs.
50. Analyzes results of service in relation to whether community program objectives were reached.

From Anderson ET: Community focus in public health nursing: whose responsibility? *Nurs Outlook* 31:44-48, 1983, p. 46.
© 1981, E. Anderson.

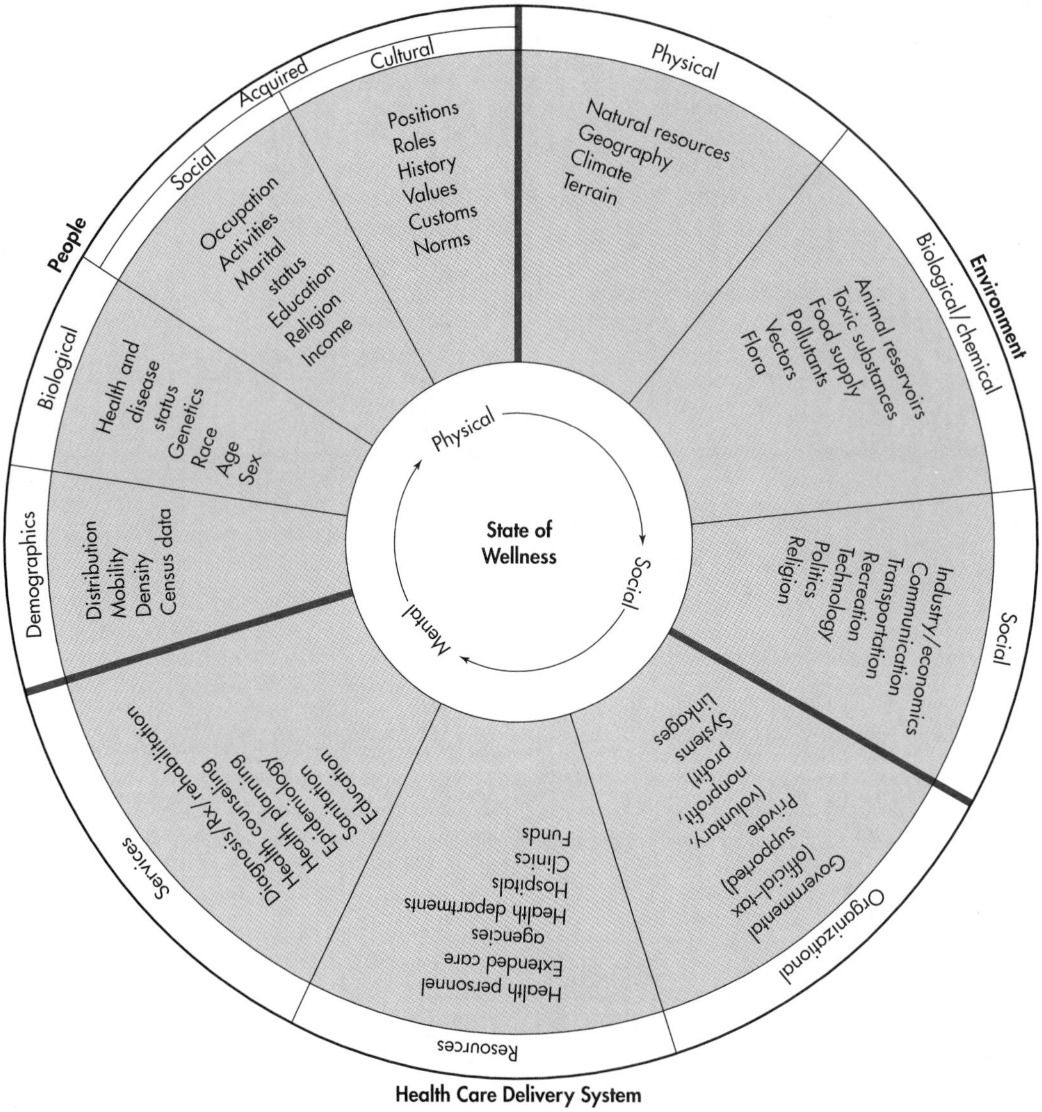

Figure 13-1 The community: its people, its environment, and its health care delivery system.

Community Health Assessment

The questions to be answered by the health assessment include, at a minimum:

1. What are the demographic, social and economic characteristics of the community's population?
2. What is the health status?
3. What are the levels of health risk?
4. What is the utilization pattern for health services?
5. What are the key environmental/occupational health issues?
6. What are the expenditures for health care services?
7. What are the available community health resources?
8. Is the supply of health care providers, (e.g., primary care practitioners) sufficient?
9. Does the population have access to health care?

From Office of Policy, Planning, and Evaluation, Michigan Department of Public Health: *List of national and state databases*, Lansing, Mi., 1995, The Office, p. 2.

compare community health status indicators against the benchmarks delineated in *Healthy People 2000* (Oberle, Baker, Magenheim, 1994). To facilitate national, state, and local comparisons, a committee representing all levels of public health was convened by the Centers for Disease Control to develop a consensus set of 18 health status indicators (see the box on the next page). "Priority in selecting the indicators was given to measures for which data are readily available and that are commonly used in public health" (CDC, 1991a, p. 449). These indicators provide health outcome and risk parameters for persons to consider during a community assessment.

After determining the information needed to establish appropriate diagnoses about the health status of the community and factors influencing a community's level of functioning, the community assessment team uses both qualitative and quantitative data collection methods to obtain

Consensus Set of Indicators* for Assessing Community Health Status and Monitoring Progress Toward the Year 2000 Objectives

INDICATORS OF HEALTH STATUS OUTCOME

1. Race/ethnicity-specific infant mortality, as measured by the rate (per 1000 live births) of deaths among infants <1 year of age

Death rates (per 100,000 population)† for:

2. Motor vehicle crashes
3. Work-related injury
4. Suicide
5. Lung cancer
6. Breast cancer
7. Cardiovascular disease
8. Homicide
9. All causes

Reported incidence (per 100,000 population) of:

10. Acquired immunodeficiency syndrome
11. Measles
12. Tuberculosis
13. Primary and secondary syphilis

INDICATORS OF RISK FACTORS

14. Incidence of low birth weight, as measured by percentage of total number of live-born infants weighing <2500 g at birth
15. Births to adolescents (females age 10-17 years) as a percentage of total live births
16. Prenatal care, as measured by percentage of mothers delivering live infants who did not receive prenatal care during first trimester
17. Childhood poverty, as measured by the proportion of children 15 years of age living in families at or below the poverty level
18. Proportion of persons living in counties exceeding U.S. Environmental Protection Agency standards for air quality during previous year

From Centers for Disease Control: Consensus set of health status indicators for the general assessment of community health status—United States, *MMWR* 40(27):449-451, 1991a, p. 450.
*Position or number of the indicator does not imply priority.
†Age-adjusted to the 1940 standard population.

this information. These methods are discussed in the next section.

METHODS FOR ASSESSING A COMMUNITY'S HEALTH STATUS

A variety of approaches are used to analyze existing community data and to obtain additional information about a community's health status. No one method is sufficient for obtaining a comprehensive view of how a community is functioning. With the increasing recognition that effective health assessment efforts must address factors that influence health and disease occurrence (e.g., environmental influences and lifestyle patterns), as well as health status outcomes and risk indicators, the need for multiple approaches to data collection becomes quite evident.

Regardless of the approach used to obtain needed community information, community analysis efforts should be structured. "Verification that adequate sampling and accurate description and interpretation have taken place is also essential" (Ruffing-Rahal, 1985, p. 135). A structured approach helps to ensure that all assessment parameters are addressed and that an adequate sampling of community perceptions has occurred.

Structure can be provided in a variety of ways during the community assessment process including developing specific goals and expected outcomes for the different phases of the process, establishing focused questions for community interviews, and using survey tools and assessment guides. Focusing data collection efforts helps to ensure that sufficient data for establishing community diagnoses are collected.

Use Assessment Guides

A systematic approach to data collection is needed to obtain a comprehensive profile of a community's level of functioning or competence. Use of a community assessment guide is one way to obtain focused information about community dynamics, including health status data. A community assessment guide developed around critical assessment parameters aids health care professionals and consumers in addressing essential assessment components. This guide can also help to organize data in a meaningful way, which facilitates the development of appropriate diagnoses about community strengths and needs and the identification of effective intervention strategies.

Reference citations for several community assessment guides that assist the practitioner in obtaining community data were presented in Chapter 3. The assessment guide in Appendix 13-1 is systematically organized around the components of a community and community dynamics. This guide aids the practitioner in doing a comprehensive community assessment over an extended period.

When completed, a community assessment guide provides a visual summary of significant community data. However, to use this guide effectively, an assessment team must have an understanding of community dynamics and community health concepts, which describe the qualitative and quantitative aspects of community assessment. Community assessment guides can never replace a need for this theoretical background. When this understanding is lacking, it is easy to miss significant clues about community functioning or not to recognize the importance of critical assessment parameters.

Analyze Available Statistics

Many people immediately associate the term *statistics* with a long list of numbers, boring to read and difficult to use. Data can be exciting and intriguing if used effectively. As illustrated in the case scenario below, statistics can quickly reveal facts about a community, including characteristics of the population being served and clues about why citizens may or may not participate in health activities. This, in turn, can help the nurse to predict health needs and interests and to plan health services accordingly.

CASE *Scenario*

One community health nurse was concerned because parents in one of the schools she serviced were not participating in health activities designed to promote child safety. When this nurse looked at census tract data, she found that 64% of the households in her district were headed by single-parent, working mothers who had marginal incomes. This information suggested to the nurse that to reach these women she would have to plan activities around the mothers' work schedules. It also pointed out to her that she was dealing with families who were at risk for financial, social, and psychological crises. These data stimulated the nurse to design health programs that were relevant to mothers' and children's needs. One program, *How to Meet Your Social Needs While Caring for Small Children*, was particularly well received. This program was planned because the nurse on several home visits heard mothers complain about the lack of time for leisure activities. The expressed concerns of these mothers, coupled with knowledge obtained from census tract data, led the nurse to believe that other mothers in the area had the same concern. Her nursing diagnosis was supported and resulted in a meaningful health program that was well attended. Since this one program was so well received, an ongoing activity and discussion group for these mothers was established, with equally positive results. The processes this nurse used to develop her mothers' group and to maintain it are presented in Chapter 22.

Statistical data often provide the basis for decision making in the face of uncertainty. Community health nurses frequently find that there are several requests for nursing service and that it is necessary to plan time to benefit the greatest number of people. Using census tract data, vital statistics, and health statistics can help community health nurses to determine where to focus their efforts. Take, for instance, the community health nurse who has several requests for the establishment of a well-baby clinic in various locations. If only one clinic can be funded, this nurse may use statistical data to document a need for a clinic in one location rather than another. The concentration of preschool children in a given area, the illness and death rates of these children, and the level of immunization protection can all be obtained from statistical data. These data provide information about where the greatest need exists and can be used to substantiate a decision a nurse might make about clinic location.

The importance of understanding and using statistical data becomes increasingly apparent to the community health nurse when decisions such as those described above must be made. Statistical data help the community health nurse to carry out many daily responsibilities more effectively. These data help the nurse to:

- Identify aggregates at risk
- Document accountability
- Predict health needs of individuals, families, and populations
- Determine priorities when needs are greater than staff time available
- Evaluate the outcomes of nursing services
- Support the need for increased funding for nursing services

Specific types of statistical data were presented in Chapter 11. It is important for health care professionals to analyze a range of available health or health-related data, such as demographic, morbidity, and mortality statistics, to assess community strengths and needs. Comparing local, state, and national statistics is equally important. Analyzing data related to the national consensus health status indicators identified previously in this chapter can facilitate these comparisons. Examining statistical trends over time is also essential. These analyses help a community assessment team to more effectively make decisions about a community's health status and needed health action. For example, if a community's death rate for breast cancer is significantly higher than state and national rates over a 5-year period, this community should seriously consider developing a breast cancer prevention program. However, if this situation was noted only in 1 given year, the community would want to establish an effective monitoring system to determine whether this was an isolated occurrence or the beginning of a trend.

GRAPHICAL PRESENTATION OF DATA Graphical presentation of data is an efficient way to show large numbers of observations at one time. Numerical figures are more easily remembered when presented graphically because data are organized and relationships are demonstrated. Tables, graphs, and charts are some of the instruments used to present statistical information symbolically. Guidelines for presenting data in this form include the following:

- Illustrate only the amount of data that is visually appealing.
- Number a table, graph, or chart if more than one is used (Table 13-1).
- Title each table, graph, or chart, including in the title information identifying *what*, *where*, and *when*.
- Define unclear terms and/or abbreviations in the footnote.
- Label both the horizontal and vertical axes of the graphical presentation.
- Identify the source of the data at the bottom of the chart, including author, title of publication, publisher, data of publication, and reference page number.

table 13-1 Distribution of Reported AIDS Cases by Exposure Category, Age, and Sex in the United States, Cumulative Totals through December 1995

Horizontal Axes

	% of AIDS Cases			
Exposure Category (Risk Group)	Men* (N=434,719)	Women* (N=71,818)	Children <13 yrs (N=6,948)	Total (N=513,487†)
VERTICAL AXES				
Male homosexual contact with HIV	60%	–	–	51%
IV drug users (IVDU)	22%	47%	–	25%
Male homosexual and IVDU	7%	–	–	7%
Heterosexual contact with HIV	3%	37%	–	8%
Transfusion recipient	1%	4%	5%	2%
Mother with HIV	–	–	90%	1%
Hemophiliac	1%	–	3%	1%
Undetermined	6%	12%	2%	6%
Total	100%	100%	100%	101%‡

Modified from Centers for Disease Control and Prevention: *HIV/AIDS surveillance report, year-end edition* 7:1-39, 1995, pp. 10-12.
*Includes adults and adolescents.
†Includes one person whose sex is unknown.
‡Percentage greater then 100% due to rounding of numbers.

When these guidelines are used, a table would look like the example presented in Table 13-1.

Graphical presentation of data has popular appeal and is frequently used to portray quickly a large number of facts. Graphs, charts, and tables can be misused or misunderstood, however, especially if one attempts to relate data that are unrelated. Also, attempting to present too many facts in one table defeats the purpose for using data display methods. When this is done, it confuses rather than clarifies the events being illustrated.

Available data on a community should be used in the most effective way possible to get across the significance of a community's health problems. These data should not, however, be misrepresented on tables, graphs, and charts. If available data are not sufficient to reach decisions about a community's state of health, they should not be displayed. Rather, further data should be collected.

Carry Out Surveys

Surveys are commonly conducted in community health nursing practice because existing health and health-related data are inadequate to substantiate a need for the development of a particular health program. Standard sources of data may show that suicide is one of the leading causes of death for older adolescents. This information is significant in that it focuses attention on a major health problem of this developmental age group. It is not sufficient, however, to identify health action needed in a particular community for reducing adolescent suicide. Other types of information must be collected before initiating a local health program. Data about things such as adolescent use of available mental health resources, attitudes of professionals and consumers about adolescent needs, and reasons for teenage suicide must be ascertained before health planning can be effective. A survey is frequently conducted to obtain this type of information.

A community survey is a systematic study designed to collect data about a community's level of functioning. Data about a specific segment of the population, about a particular component of the health care delivery system, or about health needs of the entire community may be collected during a survey. The scope varies depending on the purpose and the financial and work force resources available. It is important to define specifically the reason for doing a survey because this process can be costly and time-consuming. On the other hand, this process can provide essential data for health programming and may save time and monies if it is carefully planned (Figure 13-2). Conducting a pilot study or a small-scale survey during the planning phase can help to eliminate major problems during the survey process.

A community can survey its needs in a variety of ways. Personal interviews, telephone interviews, or written questionnaires are a few examples of the methods that can be used. It is important to select carefully survey methods and tools to minimize financial costs. Reviewing the literature about what other professionals are discovering in their work is useful.

Surveys should be used to obtain data that are not available from other sources. Generally, accurate data can be obtained about vital events (births, deaths, or marriages), but morbidity data are often incomplete. Disease rates and data about health-related phenomena (alcoholism, mental

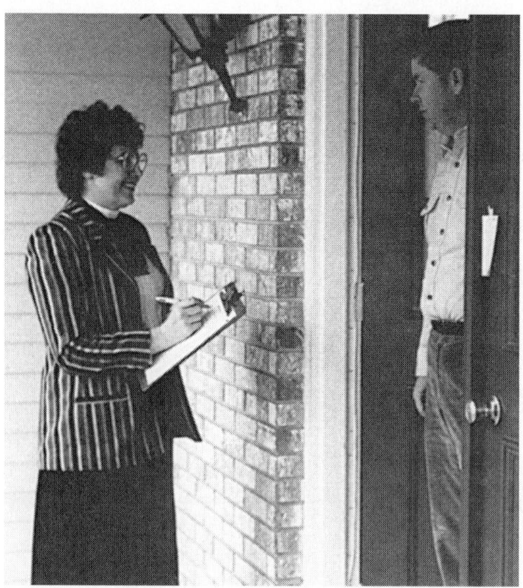

Figure 13-2 House-to-house surveys assist health care professionals in obtaining a comprehensive understanding of their local communities. A well-planned survey can provide data about such things as resource utilization patterns, social concerns, and specific health needs of a subgroup within the community. The public health professional pictured was a member of an epidemiological team that was conducting a city-wide family health study. Higher-than-average infant deaths prompted the local health department to initiate this study. The results of the survey helped the health department to target its maternal-child health (MCH) efforts on high-risk groups. Five years after the survey was completed, this local community no longer qualified for special state MCH funds, because of its low infant mortality rate. *(Courtesy Henry Parks.)*

disorders, child abuse) are usually estimates as a result of underreporting. It is frequently unknown how many individuals are affected by these conditions or whether affected individuals are receiving adequate care. Surveys may be able to elicit such data. In addition, a survey can help to determine comprehensive needs of a particular segment of a population. Routinely collected statistics often do not provide data about functional health problems, social needs, or health care resources.

Data obtained from a survey provide the foundation for more extensive investigation of health needs in a community. Research is frequently conducted after surveys are completed to explore the potential cause-and-effect relationships between community phenomena. Surveys do not provide sufficient evidence to substantiate cause-and-effect conclusions since generally very few controls are built into a survey design (Polit-O'hara, Hungler, 1995). Focus group interviews and community forums can help researchers identify community priorities for health intervention and obtain support for their research efforts.

Conduct Focus Group Interviews

Conducting focus group interviews is another approach for obtaining information about health needs and strengths from a community's perspective. "The focus group interview or discussion is a qualitative approach to learning about population subgroups with respect to conscious, semiconscious and unconscious psychological and sociocultural characteristics and processes" (Basch, 1987, p. 411). The focus group method is useful for obtaining culturally relevant and community-specific assessment data because it aids health care providers in gaining an understanding of a range of community attitudes and beliefs about a problem. It also assists the health professional in obtaining data about peoples' perceived needs and priorities and their preferences regarding health programming (Gonzalez, Gonzalez, Freeman, Howard-Pitney, 1991, p. 19).

The standard focus group format is similar to the processes used with small groups (Basch, 1987; Gearhart-Pucci, Haglund, 1992; Krueger, 1994). The leader or moderator uses a variety of leadership interventions to establish the focus groups, to promote a supportive group atmosphere, and to accomplish specific goals. These interventions are discussed in Chapter 22 and include such things as finding an appropriate and easily accessible setting, creating a nonthreatening climate in which all members feel safe to participate, and facilitating group process by clarifying and highlighting significant issues.

Like other small groups, a focus group usually lasts no more than 1 to 3 hours. A focus group differs from many small groups in that the participants are usually homogenous with respect to characteristics such as age, sex, and social variables. Focus group interviews are structured around a specific set of questions designed to identify community needs and strengths. This structure is established to learn about and assist the community as a whole, rather than individual group participants (Basch, 1987).

A diversity of views is needed to detect patterns and trends in relation to critical health problems, priorities for health programming, and strategies for addressing concerns of multiple aggregates at risk. When using a focus group approach, diversity is achieved by controlling the size of the group and conducting a *series* of group interviews or by interviewing multiple groups with similar participants. The size of the focus group should be small enough to allow all participants to share their insights yet large enough to promote diversity of perceptions. Usually a focus group is composed of 6 to 10 people (Krueger, 1994, p. 17).

As indicated in Chapter 12, the majority of our contemporary health problems affect aggregates across the life span and most ethnic groups. An example of this is the concern about accessibility of preventive health care services. To gain an understanding about the extent of this concern, a local community assessment team would need to ascertain information from multiple groups with similar participants. They may discuss this issue with a group of senior citizens, parents of young children, teenagers, low-income families, and several groups representing the ethnic subgroups in the community. Only with this type of representation can the community assessment team obtain data about perceived need in relation to the community as a whole.

Conduct Community Forums

The community forum approach to data collection is similar to the focus group approach in that it is a qualitative method designed to obtain grass-roots opinions. Both approaches place people in natural, real-life situations that can increase the possibility of spontaneous, candid expression of views. Both approaches also can provide speedy results and cost relatively little (Krueger, 1994).

Although community forums may contain some of the characteristics of a focus group, there are significant differences. A community forum consists of open meetings for all members of the community (Balacki, 1988). This is in contrast to the homogenous, structured focus group. Focus groups are structured to promote public opinion representation from a variety of at-risk groups. The open approach of a community forum may not attract this type of representation. Balacki questions the assumption that the neediest within a community will attend a formal gathering and be a vocal element (p. 305). Further, the number in attendance can influence how well participants would vocalize their needs. Even though community forums do provide a naturalistic environment for discussion, many people find it difficult to express their views in a large group setting.

Community forums, commonly called *town hall meetings*, are used across the nation to elicit public opinion about health care issues (Group takes pulse of public via town hall meetings, 1992; Harris, 1993; Lauter, 1993; Ross, 1993; Toner, 1994; Town meetings air reform issues, 1993). New technology is facilitating citizen participation in forum activities. President Clinton used telecommunication to bring his health care reform messages to residents in local communities. Many communities air their significant political and decision-making meetings (e.g., city council and school boards) on local cable television channels (Snider, 1994). "Electronic town hall meetings" are the wave of the future (Snider).

Like other group intervention strategies, a successful community forum requires careful planning and organization. Chapter 22 discusses factors that nurses take into consideration when planning a group experience for client action. The literature has consistently highlighted the need for a concerted mass media saturation before a forum, strong leadership that can focus participants on forum objectives, and a method for recording consumer input (Balacki, 1988; Group takes pulse of public via town hall meetings, 1992; Warheit, Bell, Schwab, 1974).

Town hall meetings are a creative strategy that actively engages the community in dialogue about community needs and interests (Randall-David, 1994). They can assist practitioners in identifying perceived unmet need as well as factors that inhibit or promote health action. Although community forums may not provide representative views from all segments of the population, they can provide direction for more focused community group experiences.

Conduct Research

Research to document the effectiveness of nursing services and to identify cause-and-effect relationships is critically needed in the community health nursing setting. Funders of health care services are demanding concrete data that support the need for nursing personnel, the need for certain health programs, and the value of using one intervention strategy rather than another. If qualitative data are not available, funders evaluate effectiveness only on the basis of quantitative counts, such as the numbers of home, school, or clinic visits. When this happens the quality of nursing care can suffer.

Research can help the health care professional to document community needs as well as interventions that effectively address these needs. A study conducted by Street Health, a community-based nursing organization in Toronto that operates clinics for women and men who are homeless or underhoused, illustrates the importance of clinical research (Crowe, Hardill, 1993, p. 21). Recognizing that they lacked quantitative data to document both the health problems of their homeless clients and barriers to services—structural and attitudinal—the Street Health nurses established a research survey project to obtain the data needed to strengthen their lobby efforts for homeless people. This survey showed that homeless women and men had health problems similar to the general population but the prevalence of many health problems, such as emphysema, chronic bronchitis, and epilepsy, was significantly greater in the homeless population than in the general public. It also showed that life circumstance had a tremendous impact on homeless persons' abilities to cope with these problems and that a number of barriers were preventing the homeless from receiving appropriate and/or compassionate care (Crowe, Hardill, pp. 22-23). Based on these survey results, Street Health developed over 40 recommendations that target a variety of community health agencies and educational institutions. For example, Street Health has recommended that emergency room staff receive sensitivity training about the community they serve, that the Ministry of Health prohibit all publicly funded health care institutions from refusing care to individuals who do not have their health card, and that Toronto's metro police develop a standing order to address the problem of discriminatory treatment of and violence towards homeless people (Crowe, Hardill, p. 23). The Street Health nurses are currently using these research findings to advocate needed health services for their clients.

Research use is a critical component of professional nursing practice. It is imperative that the community health nurse be familiar with research in the field and integrate research findings into clinical nursing practice. Reading journals and attending professional conferences are important ways to remain clinically current. The *Annual Review of Nursing Research* is a unique nursing research reference that has been published every year since 1983. Each volume has chapters summarizing nursing research in selected areas by experts in the field. A number of areas that have been addressed in the *Review* would be of interest to community health nurses.

"Not all nurses need to conduct research, but all should use it to guide their practice" (Lusk, 1993, p. 153). The ANA has spelled out a research role for nurses at all levels of preparation (ANA, 1989). Research-based knowledge in community health nursing is rapidly evolving and nurse researchers are an integral part of the scientific community, helping to move nursing into the twenty-first century. Practitioners must make time to investigate clinical practice issues and concerns. Only in this way can a profession remain viable.

Contact Key Community Informants

Research and surveys tend to focus on the present. Since a community's current characteristics are an outgrowth of its historical development, it is beneficial to interview consumers and community leaders to identify how community traditions are affecting community functioning. The values, attitudes, and interests of previous community leaders often subtly influence the current direction of health planning. Contact with key community persons, or *informants*, can help community health nurses to understand factors influencing health behavior and identify those with whom they might work to enhance their effectiveness.

Directors of housing projects, clergy, professionals in other health care agencies, local politicians, owners of long-established businesses, and unofficial community spokespersons are some of the individuals a nurse might contact to obtain information about community dynamics. These individuals can help the nurse to gain knowledge about the power relationships within a local area, community values and attitudes, and environmental factors that enhance or detract from a community's state of health. Unofficial spokespersons often provide the most candid opinion of how the consumer views health and the health care delivery system. Clergy, agency clients, and cultural organizations, such as International Neighbors or the Polish club, can frequently assist a community health nurse in identifying these unofficial spokespersons.

A community health nurse should use every opportunity available to relate to community people outside and within the agency. The opportunities are limitless and require only motivation on the part of the nurse and supervisory support to take advantage of them. A visit to the local library can provide very valuable information about a community's history. Talking with people the nurse meets while carrying out regular caseload responsibilities can be just as valuable. Spontaneous dialogue with community residents aids community health nurses in gaining community trust and creating a positive professional image. The ability to relate to others in the community, such as school principals, physicians, administrators in mental health agencies, secretaries, and clergy, is essential if one wants to diagnose community needs accurately.

Observe, Listen, and Analyze

Data about a community can be obtained daily by observing, listening, and analyzing. What the environment looks like when the nurse drives in the district, how families are dressed when they are seen in the clinic setting, and who relates to whom during community meetings all provide the community health nurse with clues about a community's state of health.

Participant observation during significant community events such as community health and political meetings, social gatherings, religious ceremonies, and special celebrations is an important process for community health nurses. This process can assist the health care provider in learning about people's behavior and practices and their differences and similarities. During this process the nurse might notice how business is conducted, how decisions are made, who attends community events, health concerns of community residents, and differences in attitudes about service usage (Gonzalez, Gonzalez, Freeman, Howard-Pitney, 1991; Randall-David, 1989). Participant observations help the community health nurse to identify significant cultural differences in the community and health concerns that need to be addressed. They also assist the nurse in identifying key informants.

Community health nurses who are truly interested in the welfare of their community will take time to analyze what has been observed and heard. They will be alert to environmental conditions that adversely affect the state of a community's health. If, when driving through the district, a nurse finds children playing in the streets and limited recreational facilities, she or he can raise questions about the need for safe playgrounds. An astute nurse can effect change as illustrated in the following case scenario.

CASE *Scenario*

One community health nurse was able to promote environmental changes in her district because she identified that the parents in the area were genuinely concerned about the welfare of their children. Rat-infested vacant lots in the neighborhood presented a serious threat to the children who played in them. This nurse, with the assistance of a minister, was able to mobilize parents' energies so that the garbage from these lots was removed and rats were killed. Maintaining the lots as suitable play areas became a major community project.

A community health nurse who views the community as the unit of service is more likely to meet the needs of individual families than the nurse who focuses only on family health care needs. Family problems are interrelated with community problems and often cannot be resolved until changes occur within community systems or the environment. The case situation above reflects this view.

SOURCES OF COMMUNITY DATA

A community health nurse can contact numerous international, federal, state, and local agencies and individuals to obtain health data. Some have been mentioned previously in this chapter but are summarized here to give a composite picture of the multiple sources of data one can use when diagnosing community needs.

International Sources

The United Nations is the major source of worldwide health and health-related data. Most countries report demographic statistics and health data to this organization, which then compiles the data into two major documents. The *Demographic Year Book* is a comprehensive collection of international demographic statistics. The *World Health Statistics Annual* is a yearly publication of information on vital statistics and causes of death (National Center for Health Statistics, 1995). These documents permit the United States to compare its health status with other developed nations. They also help local communities with high immigration rates to identify among immigrants health problems that are not normally experienced in the United States. Chapter 11 identifies some of these problems.

National Sources

The federal agency specifically established for the collection and dissemination of health data is the Public Health Services' National Center for Health Statistics. This center conducts the National Health Survey, which provides valuable information on the health and illness status of U.S. residents (see Chapter 11). In addition, it provides official information on vital statistics and data about the supply and use of health resources (Office of the Federal Register, 1995).

The U.S. Public Health Service also publishes two documents that provide extensive resource information related to our nation's major health issues. Its *Starting Points for Creating a Healthy Community* document delineates resources which assist communities in establishing "Healthy Cities and Communities" programs and identifies national, state, and local agencies that provide information related to the 22 priority areas in *Healthy People 2000*. Its *Federal Health Information Centers and Clearinghouses* document lists almost 300 centers or organizations that serve as a resource for health information.

Several other federal and national agencies will supply health data on request. The Substance Abuse and Mental Health Services Administration, the National Institutes of Health, the Bureau of the Census, the Alan Guttmacher Institute, and the Public Health Foundation are a few examples of such agencies. The *United States Government Manual*, which can be purchased from the Superintendent of Documents, U.S. Government Printing Office, Washington, D.C., is a valuable reference for identifying other government agencies that disseminate health data. This manual is updated regularly and describes the purposes and programs of most federal agencies. The *Health United States* document, a report on the health status of the nation, is also updated regularly and contains information on both federal and private agencies that provide health information. Selected ongoing national health data collection systems and health surveys are displayed in Appendix 13-2. The national health data collection systems regularly publish major reports on trends. These reports can be obtained in most professional libraries or from the federal agency that assumes responsibility for ongoing data collection.

The importance of obtaining data from the Bureau of the Census on the size, distribution, structure, and change of populations in the United States cannot be overemphasized. These data demonstrate patterns over time and provide general characteristics of a community's total population. Knowing the age structure in a community assists health care professionals located there in predicting the types of health problems and health care services needed. This knowledge, as well as census data about the economic status, housing conditions, and household composition in an area, assists community health nurses in predicting aggregates at risk in segments of the population. The previously discussed case situation about the needs of a high concentration of single working mothers in a nurse's district illustrates the importance of using census tract data.

Population or disease/condition-specific organizations on all three levels of governments are significant sources of community data. Examples of such organizations are the American Association of Retired Persons (AARP), the Children's Defense Fund (CDF), National Council on Disability, American Cancer Society, American Diabetes Association, Mothers and Students Against Drunk Drivers (MADD and SADD), and National Coalition Against Domestic Violence. These organizations provide significant demographic, health status and health risk data, as well as information about community resources and major service delivery issues. Many of them provide information that helps a community assessment team to compare local health data with national and state trends. For example, the Public Policy Institute of the American Association of Retired Persons has published on a yearly basis since 1991 the document titled *Reforming the Health Care Systems: State Profiles*. This document provides a profile for each state that includes eight major categories of information: (1) demographics; (2) health status; (3) utilization of services; (4) administration and quality issues; (5) health care expenditures and financing; (6) resources available; (7) health care coverage; and (8) health care reform activities. States can use these profiles to determine how their health needs rank in comparison to the health needs in other states.

Legislators and public officials on all three levels of government are also valuable resources. They are often willing to assist health care professionals in analyzing social and health care legislation. Laws and ordinances related to community health reflect the values and priorities of a community, the state, and the federal government. Every health care professional should be familiar with legislation that influences the health of his or her community. Legislation that influences the delivery of community health services is discussed throughout this text.

State Sources

State health departments are a major source of health data. Vital statistics, morbidity data, health workforce, and resource information are usually collected and disseminated by this agency. Frequently this agency has health information clearing houses and hot lines that quickly provide health information to interested providers and consumers. State health departments often have an extensive listing of health promotion and disease prevention resources.

Legislators and the population or disease/condition-specific organizations identified above are also valuable information resources on the state level. The Department of Education, the Bureau of Mental Health, and the Office of Services to the Aging are some of the state agencies that supply health and health-related information. Obtaining a state directory of health and social service agencies will help each reader to determine which agencies in her or his state furnish information about specific health needs in local communities. These directories often can be obtained from local health councils or at local libraries.

Local Sources

On the local level, some key sources for obtaining community data are the chamber of commerce, city planner's office, health department, county extension office, intermediate school district, libraries, health and welfare professionals, hospital records, clergy, community leaders, and consumers. In addition to providing health statistics and information about major health problems, health, education, and social service agencies can share significant information about service utilization patterns. The city planner's office can provide population mobility data that can assist health providers in predicting service needs. Community residents provide important qualitative data about perceived community needs, the traditions of the community, and informal information resources.

Most cities and counties have directories that provide information on the major health and welfare resources in their community. These directories are often published by local health departments or United Way organizations. Experienced practitioners are valuable resources for new practitioners who are interested in learning about formal community services. Experienced practitioners are also very knowledgeable about informal community resources.

SYNTHESIZE ALL AVAILABLE DATA

Once community data are assembled they should be organized in a meaningful way so that patterns and trends can be ascertained. Many techniques can be used to synthesize community data. Charts, figures, and tables are often used for this purpose. Graphical presentation of population distributions, morbidity data, or vital statistics for several decades can be very effective in pinpointing significant community problems. Growth or lack of growth in a community, for instance, can be identified when population distributions are graphically visualized. Lack of growth in a community can seriously affect the availability of health and social service resources and the economic status of the community.

Mapping is another technique that facilitates data analysis. Dotted scatter maps can be used to determine at a glance such things as high-risk populations, poor environmental conditions, the distribution of illness, disease, and health, and the accessibility of health care services. When this technique is used, school districts or political jurisdictions are usually outlined on a county map. Point symbols or spots are then distributed within these divisions as specified events happen (disease, death, health-related phenomena, or condemned housing), at the exact locations where the events occurred. Figure 13-3, Reported Cases of Hepatitis in Howard County, illustrates the mapping technique. The clustering of hepatitis cases in census tracts 13, 12, and 9 was related to an outbreak of hepatitis that occurred in a trailer camp in census tract 12. Relatives and friends from census tracts 9 and 13 had contact with family and friends in census tract 12 while they were in a communicable state. An epidemiological investigation provided evidence showing that a major outbreak of hepatitis had occurred in these census tracts in a very short time. This investigation also showed that the clustering of hepatitis cases in census tract 6 was a result of drug problems.

Dotted scatter maps can be very impressive and useful, but they can also be misleading if the population base is not analyzed. One geographical area may have far fewer cases than another because far fewer people are in that area. Calculating rates, ratios, and percentages aids in making comparisons between census tracts. These descriptive statistics also help to compare the occurrence of significant events with other communities and with state and national rates.

Comparing community rates with state and national rates is essential. This comparison can highlight specific health problems and community strengths and can help a community to determine priorities for program planning. For example, if a community's infant and maternal mortality rates are much higher than state and national rates, a community would examine carefully its maternal-child health programming. On the other hand, a community may find, when making these comparisons, that

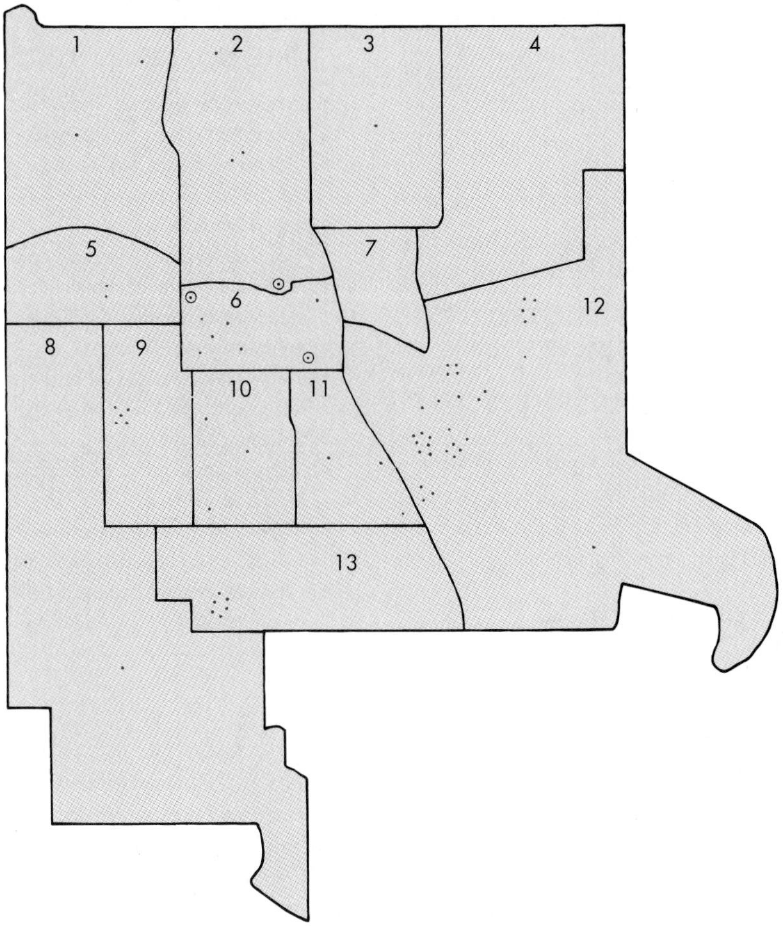

Figure 13-3 The mapping technique: reported cases of hepatitis in Howard County, January through June 1996. • = cases of hepatitis; ⊙ = drug suppliers; 1-13 = census tracts.

its maternal-child health statistics are far superior to those of other areas. This in turn could demonstrate to the community the value of maintaining adequate health programs for these two age groups in the population.

Analysis of data often supports the need for further data collection. This is illustrated in the following case scenario:

CASE *Scenario*

The health department became aware of a maternal-infant health problem in one census tract of a large urban area. This census tract was a residential rental area with basement efficiency apartments renting for $540 or higher per month. The population was 75% students and young working people, referred to as the "yuppies." Of the remaining 25%, 20% were elderly first-generation immigrant merchants, and 5% were young families living in the city housing project. The area had a high reported incidence of mugging, purse snatching, and apartment thefts, with rumors of drug manufacturing, pushing, and usage.

Few referrals were made to the health agencies in the area; casefinding was negligible; records of nursing services showed few home visits to individuals in this district. The explanation given for this situation was that the majority of the population in this census tract was either at school or working and, therefore, inaccessible to agency personnel during the working day. Evening office hours were scheduled by private physicians and several health clinics in the area. The health department became particularly concerned about the lack of referrals from this census tract when they analyzed the infant and maternal death rates for the entire county. It was discovered that only in this census tract did these rates significantly vary from national statistics.

Infant and maternal mortality rates for the specified census tract were:

23.4 infant deaths per 1000 live births
5.2 maternal deaths per 1000 live births

Infant and maternal mortality rates in the United States during the same time period were:

9.1 infant deaths per 1000 live births
3.1 maternal deaths per 1000 live births

It was obvious from the vital statistics that something had to be done to improve the health status of mothers and children in this area. However, more specific data were needed to determine causes of death, health status of area residents, and use of health care services, as well as related health problems, including socioeconomic difficulties, drug use, and attitudes about the "establishment." Personnel from a drug clinic and the student organization at a local college assisted the health department in collecting the data they needed. Lack of transportation, extremely limited incomes, lack of knowledge, inadequate nutrition, and resistance to normal channels of health care were some of the major problems identified. The establishment of a neighborhood health clinic, staffed mostly by college students and area residents, produced positive results. Data analysis at the end of 3 years reflected a significant decrease in both the infant and maternal mortality rates for this area.

This scenario dramatically illustrates the importance of synthesizing data once they are compiled. Community diagnostic activities are carried out so that appropriate decisions about health planning can be made. When data analysis is lacking, significant health issues can be missed.

TIPS FOR IMPLEMENTING COMMUNITY ANALYSIS ACTIVITIES

Community assessment and diagnostic activities are exciting and challenging. It should be apparent, however, that they cannot be left to chance. To effectively implement these activities, time for planning, assessing, and analyzing must be set aside. Equally important is the need to always keep the framework of the "community" in clear perspective when providing nursing care. Community dynamics that adversely affect the health status of individuals, families, and aggregates at risk should not be ignored. Nursing intervention strategies should be planned to resolve community needs, as well as the needs of families and individuals.

New practitioners often experience feelings of frustration and disillusionment when first entering the practice setting as a result of gaps between reality and the ideal. Presented below are suggestions for bridging some of these gaps in community-oriented practice.

Do Preliminary Community Assessment during Orientation Period

It is only natural for newly employed nurses to want immediate involvement in client casework. Reading policy and procedure manuals and attending orientation meetings can be tiring and less than rewarding. It is important, however, to remind yourself that orientation periods are designed to facilitate functioning in all aspects of one's job responsibilities. Do not overplan family visits during this time period. Rather, balance family and community activities so that time is available to learn about community dynamics and population characteristics. Allowing time in one's schedule to engage in community-focused activities during the orientation period will help the nurse to function more effectively in the community health setting. The above box identifies some of these activities.

Most agencies allow new employees to help design their own orientation. The activities in the accompanying box should be planned for, even if similar experiences were available during your course of study in the academic environment. In the educational setting these types of experiences are planned to help students apply theoretical concepts in the practice setting. Educational experiences cannot, however, provide the practitioner with the specific information needed to understand the unique characteristics of the population in the practitioner's work area.

SELECTED COMMUNITY-FOCUSED ORIENTATION ACTIVITIES

- Analyze census tract and vital statistics data to learn about population characteristics in your district.
- Attend case conferences and community meetings (PTA, social service council, citizen group activities) with an experienced employee.
- Conduct a windshield survey of your work area (Figure 13-4).
- Attend a board of health meeting or other policy-focused meetings to identify the values and attitudes of leaders in policy-making positions.
- Identify the locations of health and social service resources, recreational facilities, local churches, school systems, and shopping areas.
- Shop in your district to determine cost of essentials such as food and clothing.
- Make field visits with personnel from other departments in your agency (environmental health, mental health, or nutrition).
- Observe in clinic settings (well-baby, STD, adult screening, or prenatal).

Discuss Community-Focused Activities with Supervisors

In community health nursing practice the practitioner is frequently unable to meet client needs because of deficiencies in the health and welfare systems. Insufficient time may be available to work comprehensively with all the families referred to the nurse. These difficulties should be discussed with the nursing supervisor because the supervisor is in a favorable position for initiating major change in community systems. In addition, the supervisor can provide support and assistance in relation to caseload management activities and give suggestions about innovative intervention strategies for dealing with community problems. For example, it is not uncommon for the nursing supervisor to help the staff develop a new well-baby clinic when child health services

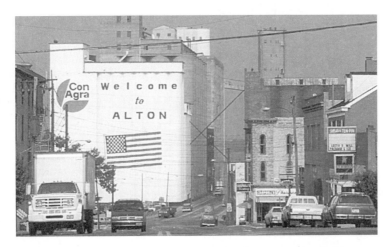

Figure 13-4 Direct observation of a community provides the nurse with valuable assessment data.

are lacking. It is also not uncommon for the nursing supervisor to provide support and assistance when a staff member wants to establish group activities to expand her or his services to a larger number of clients.

Develop Community-Focused Evaluation Criteria

Staff-level community-focused activities are seldom evaluated or rewarded. As a result, very little priority is placed on these types of activities and the focus of service shifts from the community as a whole to individual clients. To alter this pattern the practitioner must take time to revise evaluation tools and procedures so that community activities are assessed during the evaluation process. Only if this is done will time be allocated for community work. Listed below are a few examples of items you might want to include under a community service category on a staff evaluation tool:

- Assesses health needs and strengths of specific populations (school, clinic, industry) in assigned district
- Works with nursing supervisor to discern health action needed for at-risk aggregates in assigned district
- Works with the nursing supervisor to develop intervention strategies (group work, clinic services) for aggregates at risk in assigned district
- Collaborates with other professionals on health planning projects for aggregates at risk in the community

Summary

Meeting the health needs of at-risk aggregates is a major community health nursing function. A nurse must know the community before this responsibility can be effectively carried out. A variety of strategies must be used to assess the health status, the health capability, and the health action potential of the nurse's community. Data must be analyzed, as well as collected, so that target groups for nursing service can be identified. Use of the nursing process facilitates implementation of these activities. Developing community partnerships also facilitates this process.

Numerous professionals and consumers will assist the community health nurse in identifying community health needs and strengths. Interdisciplinary collaboration and consumer participation must be fostered during the community analysis process since no one person alone can appropriately diagnose community needs.

Exploring the community, its organization, and its activities is extremely rewarding. This exploration provides a clearer picture of community health action and a foundation for health planning activities designed to improve the health status of high-risk groups. It further helps the community health nurse to assist individual families more effectively. Often family health problems cannot be resolved until changes occur in community systems. It may be difficult for the community health nurse to integrate community-focused activities into an already busy schedule, but it is essential to do so to meet the needs of individuals, families, and aggregates at risk.

CRITICAL *Thinking Exercise*

You are a community health nurse who works for a local health department that was directed by the city commissioners to develop short- and long-range plans to combat local community violence. The agency's violence task force, of which you are a member, recognizes that it has insufficient data to make decisions about specific community interventions. Thus the committee's first goal is to assess community perceptions regarding this problem and to collect and analyze quantitative data relative to the nature of the problem. Taking into consideration that several types of violence (e.g., child and elder abuse, domestic violence, homicide, and intentional and unintentional injury) occur in a community, identify the key informants who could assist your task force in obtaining the community's perspective about the problem. Additionally, discuss the kinds of quantitative data you would need to document the extent of violence in your community and where and how you might obtain this data. Further, discuss how community attitudes about violence could facilitate or inhibit your data collection process.

REFERENCES

American Nurses Association (ANA), Community Health Nursing Division: *Standards of community health nursing practices* (Pub No. CH-10), Kansas City, Mo., 1986, ANA.

American Nurses Association (ANA): *Education for participation in nursing research*, Kansas City, Mo., 1989, ANA.

American Nurses Association (ANA): *Nursing's agenda for health care reform*, Kansas City, Mo., 1991, ANA.

American Public Health Association (APHA), Public Health Nursing Section: *The definition and role of public health nursing: a statement of APHA public health nursing section*, Washington, D.C., 1986, APHA.

American Public Health Association (APHA): *Public health in a reformed health care system: a vision for the future*, Washington, D.C., 1993, APHA.

Anderson ET: Community focus in public health nursing: whose responsibility? *Nurs Outlook* 31:44-48, 1983.

Aubel J, Samba-Ndure K: Community participation: lessons on sustainability for community health projects, *World Health Forum* 17:52-57, 1996.

Baker EL, Melton RJ, Stange PU et al: Health reform and the health of the public: forging community health partnerships, *JAMA* 272(16):1276-1282, 1994.

Balacki MF: Assessing mental health needs in the rural community: a critique of assessment approaches, *Issues Ment Health Nurs* 9:299-315, 1988.

Basch C: Focus group interview: an underutilized research technique for improving theory and practice in health education, *Health Educ Q* 14:411-448, 1987, Winter.

Berkowitz B: Health system reform: a blueprint for the future of public health, *J Public Health Manage Prac* 1:1-6, 1995.

Bracht N, Gleason J: Strategies and structures for citizen partnerships. In Bracht N, ed: *Health promotion at the community level*, Newbury Park, Ca., 1990, Sage, pp. 109-124.

Breen N, Kessler L: Changes in the use of screening mammography: evidence from the 1987 and 1990 National Health Interview Surveys, *Am J Public Health* 84:62-66, 1994.

Calvillo ER: AIDS knowledge and attitudes among Latinas. In Western Institute of Nursing: *Communicating nursing research, silver threads: 25 years of nursing excellence*, vol 25, Boulder, Co., 1992, The Institute, p. 415.

Centers for Disease Control (CDC): Consensus set of health status indicators for the general assessment of community health status—United States, *MMWR* 40 (27):449-451, 1991a.

Centers for Disease Control (CDC): *Preventing lead poisoning in young children: a statement by the Centers for Disease Control*, Atlanta, 1991b, CDC.

Centers for Disease Control and Prevention (CDC): *HIV/AIDS surveillance report, year-end edition* 7:1-39, 1995.

Children's Defense Fund (CDF): *The state of America's children yearbook 1996*, Washington, D.C., 1996, CDF.

Clark NM, McLeroy KR: Creating capacity through health education: what we know and what we don't, *Health Educ* 22:273-289, 1995.

Clarke HF, Beddome G, Whyte NB: Public health nurses' vision of their future reflects changing paradigms, *Image: J Nurs Sch* 25:305-310, 1993.

Cleary D: Florida goes statewide with alcohol health warning signs, *Am J Public Health* 86:880-881, 1996.

Conley E: Public health nursing within core public health functions: "back to the future," *J Public Health Manage Pract* 1:1-8, 1995.

Crowe C, Hardill K: Nursing research and political change: the Street Health Report, *Can Nurse* 88:21-24, 1993.

Flynn BC, Ray DW, Rider MS: Empowering communities: action research through Healthy Cities, *Health Educ* 21:395-405, 1994.

Gearhart-Pucci L, Haglund BJA: Focus groups: a tool for developing better health education materials and approaches for smoking intervention, *Health Promotion Int* 7:11-15, 1992.

Gonzalez U, Gonzalez J, Freeman U, Howard-Pitney B: *Health promotion in diverse cultural communities*, Palo Alto, Ca., 1991, Health Promotion Resource Center, Stanford Center for Research in Disease Prevention.

Group takes pulse of public via town hall meetings, *Public Relations J* 48:5, 1992.

Haglund B, Weisbrod R, Bracht N: Assessing the community: its services, needs, leadership, and readiness. In Bracht N, ed: *Health promotion at the community level*, Newbury Park, Ca., 1990, Sage, pp. 91-108.

Harris HR: A heavy dose of questions for Clinton's health care plan, *The Washington Post* 116:DCI(Col 1), October 21, 1993.

Institute of Medicine (IOM): *The future of public health*, Washington, D.C., 1988, National Academy Press.

Jamieson MK: Block nursing: practicing autonomous professional nursing in the community, *Nurs Health Care* 11:250-253, 1990.

Kreuter MW: PATCH: its origin, basic concepts, and links to contemporary public health policy, *J Health Educ* 23:135-139, 1992.

Krueger RA: *Focus groups: a practical guide for applied research*, ed. 2, Thousand Oaks, Ca., 1994, Sage.

Lauter D: Town hall health hearing presents few cures, *Los Angeles Times* 112:A21 (col 1), March 13, 1993.

Lusk SL: *Linking practice and research*, *AAOHN J* 41:153-157, 1993.

Marin G, Burhansstipanov L, Connell C et al: A research agenda for health education among underserved populations, *Health Educ Q* 22:346-363, 1995.

McFarlane J: De Madras a Madres: an access model for primary care, *AJPH* 86:879-880, 1996.

National Center for Health Statistics: *Health, United States*, 1994, Hyattsville, Md., 1995, U.S. Government Printing Office.

National League for Nursing (NLN): *A vision for nursing education*, New York, 1993, NLN.

North American Nursing Diagnosis Association (NANDA): *Nursing diagnoses: definitions and classification*, Philadelphia, 1994, NANDA.

Nurse Administrators Forum: *Promoting healthy Michigan communities: the role of public health nursing in health reform*, Lansing, Mi., 1994, Michigan Department of Public Health.

Oberle MW, Baker EL, Magenheim MJ: *Healthy People 2000* and community health planning, *Annu Rev Public Health* 15:259-275, 1994.

Office of the Federal Register: *United States government manual, 1995/1996*, Washington, D.C., 1995, The Office.

Office of Policy, Planning, and Evaluation, Michigan Department of Public Health: *List of national and state databases*, Lansing, Mi., 1995, The Office.

Oros M: Creating a vision for health, *The Enterprise Foundation* 5:3-5, 1995 (Fall).

Overbo B, Ryan M, Jackson K, Hutchinson K: The homeless prenatal program: a model for empowering homeless pregnant women, *Health Educ Q* 21:187-198, 1994.

Pew Health Professions Commission: *Critical challenges: revitalizing the health professions for the twenty-first century*, San Francisco, 1995, UCSF Center for the Health Professions.

Polit-O'hara DF, Hungler BP: *Nursing research: principles and methods*, ed. 3, Philadelphia, 1995, Lippincott.

Rafferty AP, McGee HB, Skarupski KA: *Results from Michigan's Behavioral Risk Factor Survey*, Lansing, Mi., 1995, Michigan's Department of Public Health.

Randall-David E: *Strategies for working with culturally diverse communities and clients*, Bethesda, Md., 1989, The Association for the Care of Children's Health.

Randall-David E: *Culturally competent HIV counseling and education*, McLean, Va., 1994, The Maternal and Child Health Clearinghouse.

Ross M. Health plan takes heat at GOP meetings, *Los Angeles Times* 113:A20 (col 1), December 5, 1993.

Ruffing-Rahal MA: Qualitative methods in community analysis, *Public Health Nurs* 2:130-137, 1985.

Sen R: Building community involvement in health care, *Social Policy* 24:32-43, 1994.

Shugars DA, O'Neil EH, Bader JD, eds: *Healthy America: practitioners for 2005, an agenda for action for U.S. health professional schools*, Durham, N.C., 1991, The Pew Health Professions Commission.

Snider JH: Democracy on-line: tomorrow's electronic electorate, *The Futurist* 28(5):15-19, 1994.

Steckler A, Allegrante JP, Altman D et al: Health education intervention strategies: recommendations for future research, *Health Educ Q* 22:307-328, 1995.

Toner R: Wanting health care help, voters tell of apprehension, *The New York Times* 143(Sec. 1):1 (col 2), April 3, 1994.

Town meetings air reform issues, *Employee Benefit Plan Review* 47:12, 1993.

U.S. Department of Health and Human Services (USDHHS): *Healthy People 2000: national health promotion and disease prevention objectives, full report, with commentary*, Washington, D.C., 1991, U.S. Government Printing Office.

Warheit GJ, Bell RA, Schwab JJ: *Planning for change: needs assessment approaches*, Rockville, Md., 1974 National Institute of Mental Health.

Winkleby MA, Flora JA, Kraemer HC: A community-based heart disease intervention: predictors of change, *Am J Public Health* 84:767-771, 1994.

SELECTED BIBLIOGRAPHY

Courtney R, Ballard E, Fauver S et al: The partnership model: working with individuals, families, and communities toward a new vision of health, *Public Health Nurs* 113:177-186, 1996.

Eisen A: Survey of neighborhood-based, comprehensive community empowerment initiatives, *Health Educ Q* 21:235-252, 1994.

Finnegan L, Ervin NE: An epidemiological approach to community assessment, *Public Health Nurs* 6:147-151, 1989.

Flynn BC: Developing community leadership in healthy cities: the Indiana Model, *Nurs Outlook* 40(3):121-126, 1992.

Freudenberg N, Lee J, Germain LM: Reaching low-income women at risk of AIDS: a case history of a drop-in center for women in the South Bronx, New York City, *Health Educ Res* 9:119-132, 1994.

Goeppinger J: Health promotion for rural populations: partnership interventions, *Fam Community Health* 16:1-10, 1993.

Gordon RL, Baker EL, Roper WL, Omenn GS: Prevention and the reforming U.S. health care system: changing roles and responsibilities for public health, *Annu Rev Public Health* 17:489-509, 1996.

Hamilton P: Community nursing diagnosis, *Adv Nurs Sci* 5(3):21-36, 1983.

Kaufman JE: Personal definitions of health among elderly people: a link to effective health promotion, *Fam Community Health* 19:58-68, 1996.

Labonte R: Health promotion and empowerment: reflections on professional practice, *Health Educ Q* 21:253-268, 1994.

Muecke MA: Community health diagnosis in nursing, *Public Health Nurs* 1:23-35, 1984.

Pearson TA, Spencer M, Jenkins P: Who will provide preventive services? The changing relationships between medical care systems and public health agencies in health care reform, *J Public Health Manage Pract* 1:16-27, 1995.

Schultz PR: When client means more than one: extending the foundational concept of person, *Adv Nurs Sci* 10:71-86, 1987.

Schwab M, Neuhauser L, Morgen S et al: The Wellness guide: towards a new model for community participation in health promotion, *Health Promotion Int* 7:27-36, 1992.

Selby-Harrington ML, Riportella-Muller E: Easing the burden on health departments: a cost-effective method for public health nurses to increase private sector participation in the early and periodic screening, diagnosis and treatment program, *Public Health Nurs* 10:114-121, 1993.

Stevens PE: Focus groups: collecting aggregate-level data to understand community health phenomena, *Public Health Nurs* 13:170-176, 1996.

14

Community Organization and Health Planning for Aggregates at Risk

Objectives

Upon completion of this chapter, the reader should be able to:

1. Discuss the concepts of community organization and health planning.
2. Distinguish between comprehensive health planning and health program planning.
3. Understand the relationships among the concepts inherent in epidemiology, demography, community organization, and health planning.
4. Trace the development of comprehensive health planning activities and legislation in the United States and discuss trends that influenced this development.
5. Analyze the steps of the health program planning process.
6. Describe how to work with communities as partners to solve contemporary health problems.
7. Discuss the use of health planning concepts in community health nursing practice.
8. Discuss barriers to health planning.

Chapter 3 describes how aggregates at risk and the community are the client for the community health nurse. A distinguishing feature of this specialty area is a focus on interventions that protect and promote the health of communities; this chapter describes how nurses put that concept into practice. Problems that contemporary community health nurses frequently encounter include crack-addicted neonates, family violence, child abuse, and drug and alcohol abuse. Further, declining family incomes, lack of access to health care, and growing hunger and homelessness face too many people. These are awesome problems that require interventions different from those developed by nurses working with individual clients and family members. Community health nurses use community-based health promotion efforts that stimulate community organization. They are involved in policy decisions that address the environmental, social, and behavioral variables making an impact on the health of families and populations.

Lillian Wald, the founder of modern community health nursing, was a role model for this behavior. She described how nurses helped to make the community a positive environment that facilitates the self-actualization of individuals through the life span. In describing how nurses from Henry Street Settlement House functioned, she wrote that the nurses are "enlisted in the crusade against disease and for the promotion of right living, beginning even before life itself is brought forth, through infancy, into school life, on through adolescence. . . . The nurse is being socialized, made part of a community plan for the communal health. Her contribution to human welfare, unified and harmonized with those powers which aim at care and prevention, rather than at police power and punishment, forms part of the great policy of bringing human beings to a higher level" (Wald, 1915, p. 60). Wald noted early in her career that working with political leaders to change the social and physical environment was as important as helping individuals modify their health behaviors. This activist changed child labor laws, helped build playgrounds, and established school nursing, all examples of how political and social structures influence the health of communities, aggregates, families, and individuals.

Community organizations using health care planning processes facilitate work with communities as partners, assisting and motivating aggregates to bring about changes. These changes are designed to solve health problems and to create environments that prevent health problems from developing. Using this approach to deal with health concerns means that community health nurses shift from a one-to-one reactive model of care to a multidisciplinary, proactive, community-based model that involves the community in problem identification and resolution.

The need for such an approach is currently endorsed by most *professional* (ANA, 1995; APHA, 1996; Fisher, 1996; NLN, 1993), *private* (Children's Defense Fund, 1996; Pew Health Professions Commission, 1995), and *government* (Berkowitz, 1995; USDHHS, 1995) organizations and local communities around the world (Aubel, Samba-Ndure, 1996; Sen, 1994; USDHHS, 1995). The nation's agenda for health, *Healthy People 2000*, also emphasizes the need for aggregate and community-based comprehensive health planning, guided by a multidisciplinary and lay partnership model for health.

DEFINING HEALTH PLANNING

Health planning is an ongoing process whereby information about the nation, a state, or a local community is systematically collected and *used* to structure a health improvement plan that facilitates client empowerment for health action. "Planning is a method of trying to ensure that the resources now and in the future are used in the most efficient way to obtain explicit objectives" (Green, 1992, p. 3).

The health planning process is a scientific problem-solving approach that helps a community to evaluate and bring about specific changes for the purpose of improving the health status of the community. In community health practice, this approach is used on a community-wide level to develop "healthy public policy" that supports health promotion and disease prevention efforts (Kickbusch, Draper, O'Neill, 1990). "Such policies are articulated not only in laws and regulations that govern the behavior of individuals but also in practice guidelines for health care providers, educational requirements for health professionals, and reimbursement schemes for health care" (Scherl, Noren, Osterweis, 1992, p. 3). Community-wide planning also helps to provide a framework for the development of population-focused interventions and the coordination of client and provider health action efforts. For example, the *Healthy People 2000* documents, which have been developed at all levels of government, provide direction for targeting interventions for aggregates at risk as well as resources to resolve priority health problems.

Community-wide health planning is known as *comprehensive health planning* or *policy planning*. In the community setting planning also occurs at the organizational level to develop strategies for thriving in a competitive environment (*strategic* and *visionary planning*) and to develop health programs and services (*health program planning* or *operational planning*). This chapter expands discussion on comprehensive health planning and health program planning.

COMPREHENSIVE HEALTH PLANNING: HISTORICAL AND CURRENT PERSPECTIVES

Comprehensive health planning began as a *voluntary movement* in the early 1930s with the establishment of area-wide hospital planning councils. These councils were formed to raise and allocate money for hospital construction and modernization. Their membership included lay persons involved in philanthropic and civic affairs and professionals such as hospital administrators (National Academy of Sciences, 1980, p. 13).

Formalized government involvement in health planning became evident in the mid-1930s when a provision of the Social Security Act of 1935 provided aid to states for maternal child health and disease control service programming with the stipulation that states develop plans on how to use this aid (Bergwall, Reeves, Woodside, 1973). Since that time, most federal legislation that provides aid to states for the development of health services or the construction of health facilities has commonly required state planning activities. For example, the Hospital Survey and Construction Act of 1946, commonly referred to as the *Hill-Burton Act*, authorized grants to states for statewide planning for hospitals and public health centers and construction grants for facilities. An annual updated state plan was required to maintain Hill-Burton funding from year to year. The Heart Disease, Cancer, and Stroke Amendments of 1965, known as The Regional Medical Program, also had planning requirements. It involved professionals in health planning for regional centers for treatment of heart disease, cancer, and stroke.

For a long time, health planning was primarily reactive. Only after a health problem affected a large number of people was there an attempt to solve it. However, beginning with some of President Johnson's Great Society Programs in the 1960s, the emphasis in health planning became more comprehensive, with the recognition that all components of the community influenced the health status of the community. Consumer participation in the planning process was also stressed. The National Commission on Community Health Services (1966) summarized these beliefs in its classic report, *Health Is A Community Affair*.

> Action planning for health should be community wide in area, continuous in nature, comprehensive in scope, all-inclusive in design, coordinative in function, and adequately staffed. . . . The Community Action Studies Project (CASP) analysis especially emphasizes the relationship of one aspect of community health to another, and the interrelatedness of health with the total social, educational, and economic enterprise. Action-planning should be all-inclusive in design—a partnership between private, voluntary, and governmental sectors representing all elements of the community, including consumers as well as providers of services, civic leaders, and, importantly, health professionals (pp. 168-169).

Consistent with these beliefs, two types of legislation designed to improve the health status of communities emerged—community development and health service legislation. Through the Economic Opportunity Act of 1964, the federal government supported broad community development initiatives to make a comprehensive attack on poverty. These initiatives had a "healthy cities" focus. They established community action agencies that worked to revitalize distressed communities and to help people in these communities obtain needed education, social services, and housing. Some of them focused on improving the physical environment. Programs under the Economic Opportunity Act found it difficult to significantly influence the practice of community agencies or to improve service delivery because they lacked sufficient authority and political support at the federal and local levels. Although the Office of Economic Opportunity eventually disbanded, local community action agencies continue to operate (GAO, 1995b, p. 7). These agencies are eligible for Community Services Block Grant funding, which is discussed later in this section.

Private sector efforts, especially private foundation support, have advanced community revitalization programs since the early 1960s. Currently at least 2500 private nonprofit Community Development Corporations around the country focus their efforts on improving distressed geographical areas. However, many of them do not offer comprehensive services. It is the hope of planners that the Empowerment Zones and Enterprise Communities Program, adopted in 1992 under the Omnibus Budget Reconciliation Act, will promote comprehensive community revitalization efforts (GAO, 1995b).

Comprehensive health service planning efforts ran parallel to the community revitalization efforts. The Comprehensive Health Planning and Public Health Service Amendment of 1966 was passed to enable states and communities to plan for better use of health resources. This legislation was not effective because of lack of authority, inadequate funding, and political opposition (Reeves, Coile, 1989). Because of these problems, other legislative action was taken in the mid-1970s.

The National Health Planning and Resources Development Act of 1974 consolidated the Hill-Burton Act, Regional Medical Programs, and the Comprehensive Health Planning Programs. This act was passed to facilitate the development of a national health planning policy and to augment state and local health planning. The goals of this act were improved accessibility of health care services, curtailment of rising costs, and monitoring of the quality of care being provided. To accomplish these goals, a network of regulatory local health systems agencies, state health planning and development agencies, and statewide health coordinating councils was established. A new National Council for Health Policy was also created. This legislation emphasized the need for strong local planning and control over the development of services. Additionally, it mandated consumer and third-party payer participation in the planning process.

The antiregulatory philosophy of the Reagan administration advanced the belief that the control of health planning and service development should occur at the local level. The Omnibus Budget Reconciliation Act (OBRA) of 1981 ended the federal mandate for planning under the National Health Planning and Resources Development Act. It also consolidated federal programs and reorganized how federal expenditures were allocated to the states under its *block grant* provision. The Omnibus Budget Reconciliation Act created 9 block grants by consolidating more than 50 categorical grant programs and 3 existing block grants; 4 of the 9 block grants were for health, 3 were for social services, 1 was for education, and 1 was for community development (GAO, 1995a, p. 27). The four areas of health covered by block grants were maternal and child health; preventive health and health services; alcohol, drug abuse, and mental health; and primary care.

A block grant is a funding mechanism through which the federal government supports state and local health programs. In contrast to categorical grants, which specifically designate how the funds are to be spent, the block grant provides a lump sum of money to states and allows states to determine how these monies will be spent. This type of federal aid is designed to provide states greater discretion in the use of federal funds. However, state flexibility was reduced over time as funding constraints were added to the block grants (GAO, 1995a). Currently, as Congress is considering adding new block grants, concerns about the ability of states to adequately fund health and social services are emerging. History has shown that federal aid to states is reduced under the block grant financing mechanism.

By the end of the 1980s it was becoming evident that the focus on cost containment was affecting health planning activities at state and local levels. The Committee for the Study of the Future of Public Health (IOM, 1988) identified that "increases in public health spending were not keeping pace with the growing need for assessment, policy development, and assurance activities demanded by the range of immediate and impending crises and ongoing problems in public health" (p. 80). Once again, health planning was becoming primarily reactive, responding to the issue of the moment rather than benefiting from careful assessment processes (IOM). The IOM Committee challenged the nation to strengthen essential public health activities to improve the health and well-being of the American people.

COMPREHENSIVE HEALTH PLANNING: THE 1990s AND BEYOND

The 1990s produced dramatic changes in health planning activities and legislation. Experience with the abolishment of the national health planning framework, created under the National Health Planning and Resources Development Act, showed that the "free market" of business had not controlled costs nor had it adequately addressed the health problems of the American people (Reeves, Coile, 1989). Major debates about the most effective and cost-efficient way to meet the health needs of all occurred at every level of government and among professional and lay advocacy groups during the 1990s. These debates continue.

The health planning experiences in the 1980s also showed that some form of external oversight and guidance for health planning was essential. During this time, the type and degree of health planning activities at state and local levels became very diverse. Coalitions, appointed state and local health committees, and health task forces increasingly emerged to provide a needed structure for community health planning efforts (Reeves, Coile, 1989).

Health planning experiences during the 1980s and early 1990s highlighted the need to reexamine the nation's health planning efforts. Many of the visions of the 1960s National Commission on Community Health Services are reemerging as central themes in health planning. Currently the emphasis is on comprehensive community health status assessment and action, professional and consumer planning partnerships for health, and community revitalization. The Year 2000 Health Objectives Planning Act of 1990 is facilitating the development of state and local community health plans. Community health partnerships are advancing community development efforts as well as community action. Importantly, planning efforts are focusing on the significant influence that environmental factors have on health. In contrast to the 1960s' emphasis on how changes in health services delivery will resolve community problems, the current emphasis during health planning is on identifying *community health needs* and a range of appropriate interventions for addressing these needs. This change reflects the recognition that client need must be our focus and that a range of interventions must be developed to address contemporary health problems.

As was discussed in Chapter 2, many international and national movements have reoriented health planning and policy toward prevention during the past decade. "Two phrases that capture the essence of a new vision for health care in the 1990s are *promoting health* and *preventing disease* . . . A significant catalyst for action has been *Healthy People 2000: National Health Promotion and Disease Prevention Objectives* (Scherl, Noren, Osterweis, 1992, p. 1).

HEALTHY PEOPLE 2000 MANDATE PROMOTES HEALTH PLANNING

The *Healthy People 2000* mandate, the nation's vision for improving the health status of all citizens, has provided an impetus for government agencies, private organizations and businesses, and local communities to strengthen their community development and health planning efforts. This mandate created a framework for monitoring the nation's changing health status and for guiding public health policy at all levels of government (Stoto, 1992; USDHHS, 1991, 1995). The *Healthy People 2000* mandate specifies national health objectives that must be achieved to improve the health of populations across the life span. These objectives help communities to focus on major health problems. They also help policymakers to promote legislation that addresses major health concerns in the nation.

The *Healthy People 2000* mandate challenges states and local communities to develop their own *Healthy People 2000* objectives and action plans to address these objectives. It is expected that these governmental units will carry out the core public health functions—assessment, policy development, and assurance (IOM, 1988)—to promote healthy community living. To support local communities in fulfilling these functions, several national endeavors have emerged. National funds are being allocated to states under the Year 2000 Health Objectives Planning Act (PL101-582) to assist communities with community analysis and health planning activities (Stoto, 1992). "As of June 1995, 42 states, the District of Columbia, and Guam had developed year 2000 plans. All other states have undertaken assessments related to the year 2000 objectives" (USDHHS, 1995, p. 130).

Major national surveillance and data systems (see Appendix 13-2) are also available to aid states and local communities in their health planning endeavors. These systems are being strengthened to ensure that communities have accurate and timely health data in a useable form. In the *Healthy People 2000* document, "one of its 22 priority areas is devoted to specific objectives for surveillance and data systems" (USDHHS, 1995). These objectives are designed to strengthen public health assessment and planning efforts (Stoto, 1992): "Data represents the single most critical element to successful [health] planning" (IOM, 1990, p. 23). Without data it is difficult to identify the health status of the nation, a state, or a local community. When data is lacking, it is also difficult to determine whether health programs and interventions are effective and how to target resources to the areas of greatest need (USDHHS, 1995, p. 130). Community development and health planning activities focus on effective and efficient targeting of scarce resources.

Healthy People 2000 objectives are increasingly used by local health departments to mobilize communities for health. The objectives assist local agencies to increase awareness and understanding of how problems and activities at the local level reflect national and state community health problems. They also aid local agencies in formulating a clear vision about local community needs, in advocating for budget or resource prioritization, and in building partnerships for health action (Oberle, Baker, Magenheim, 1994). The *Healthy People 2000* objectives help local communities to advance comprehensive community and aggregate-focused health planning efforts.

COMMUNITY DIAGNOSIS

To facilitate the development of *Healthy People 2000* plans, states and local communities complete a population-based community health status assessment. Understanding the concepts presented in Chapter 13 relative to community diagnosis, along with the epidemiological variables of person, place, and time, is essential to answer the key questions that health planners must ask as they assess health planning needs. *Person* involves the "who" of community diagnosis. The cultural, ethnic, psychosocial, spiritual, and biological characteristics of the person variable must be considered when health services are planned. These characteristics influence how persons define health and illness. Since these terms do not have a common meaning to all people, it is crucial to identify how the population being served views them. If, for instance, a population narrowly defines *health* as the absence of disease, this population would probably respond more favorably to the provision of curative care than to the provision of preventive care.

Place describes the setting where services are planned, which may be rural, urban, inner city, or suburbia. When the characteristics of place are examined, the availability, accessibility, and cost of present services should be analyzed. Size is also a factor that needs to be considered. A community with 1000 residents will have different needs than a community with a population of 1 million. The cost to deliver health services, the kinds of personnel and financial resources that are available, and the complexity involved in planning and implementing services are some factors that vary among populations of different sizes.

The basic unit of service in health planning is the population to be served and its distribution. Any planning should take into consideration population size and distribution and population needs as reflected by health statistics. Population size and mortality and morbidity rates for the future should be estimated. Future demands on the health care delivery system are determined in this way.

Time in relation to urgency also needs to be considered during the health planning process. If the problem under consideration, for example, is an emergency such as influenza among aging citizens, immediate action must be taken. Other health problems such as accident prevention may not require immediate action but can necessitate action over time.

Long-term action makes more complex demands on the health planner. When long-term intervention is needed, mechanisms must be established to ensure that evaluation occurs periodically during the intervention phase, that coordination of all persons involved in the process is supported, and that public awareness of the problem and the health program is maintained.

It is important to determine the appropriate time to initiate the health program under consideration. Analyzing community values and attitudes, availability of resources, and cost-benefit factors aids the health planner in determining the appropriate time to begin health-planning intervention.

Examining a community's developmental history is another significant factor to examine when considering timing. An older, inner-city ethnic community might have more established values and attitudes about health and illness than a newer community such as a prospering subdivision. Analyzing how values and attitudes have evolved over time in an older community assists the health planner in identifying key community leaders who can actively participate in developing interventions that would be acceptable to the community.

SETTING PRIORITIES FOR HEALTH PLANNING

Throughout the nation, local communities are using *Healthy People 2000* plans to establish priorities for the effective and efficient use of scarce health resources. This has become an especially difficult task because communities are facing an increasing range of pressing problems that require community-based interventions (CDC, undated).

A review of the literature reveals that a common set of criteria is being used for setting health planning priorities. This set of criteria is labeled either the Hanlon Method or the Basic Priority Rating System (CDC, undated; Pickett, Hanlon, 1990). These criteria as well as potential evaluation parameters for each are presented in Table 14-1. Following is the formula for establishing a numerical

table 14-1 Criteria for Health Planning Priority Setting

Criteria	Potential Evaluation Parameters
Size of problem	Percentage of population with health problem Population to be considered (entire population or a target group)
Seriousness of the problem	*Urgency*—emergent nature of problem; importance relative to the public (epidemic/endemic, community's perception of problem) *Severity*—premature mortality; years of potential life lost; disability; community beliefs about seriousness of the health problem *Economic loss*—to the community (city/county/state); to the individual *Involvement of others*—potential impact on populations (measles) or impact on family groups (child abuse, homicide)
Estimated effectiveness of interventions	Is there an acceptable preventive/treatment intervention? Does the intervention improve the likelihood of favorable health outcomes? What is the potential adverse effect of the interventions (e.g., screening tests)? What proportion of the target population can be reached by the intervention?

From CDC: *A guide for establishing public health priorities*, Atlanta, undated, CDC, p. 4; Pickett GE, Hanlon JJ: *Public health administration and practice*, ed 9, St. Louis, 1990, Mosby, pp. 226-227.

score when these criteria are used (CDC, undated; Pickett, Hanlon, 1990):

Basic Priority Rating = (A + 2B) × C
A = size of the problem
B = seriousness of the problem
C = estimated effectiveness of interventions

This formula reflects that the seriousness of the problem and the effectiveness of interventions receive a higher priority than the size of the problem.

Tables 14-2, 14-3, and 14-4 provide examples of how to obtain a numerical rating when using the Basic Priority Rating (BPR) formula. How to rank problems based on the BPR system is illustrated in Table 14-5. The ranking will vary from one community to another based on community characteristics. One community may rank a health problem a number one, while a neighboring community may rank the same problem a number five. These rankings are based on both quantitative data and qualitative perceptions of the problem. For example, a local community may rank motor vehicle accidents among its youth higher than another community, if the rate of mortality from motor vehicle accidents among people 15 to 24 years has significantly increased over the past year. The local community's ranking might be influenced by the community's emotional reactions to the premature death of its youth, as well as by statistical data (cause-specific and age-specific mortality rates).

After rating the size and seriousness of the problem and intervention effectiveness, a group of factors commonly known as the "PEARL" are examined. These factors—*propriety, economics, acceptability, resources,* and *legality*—do not relate directly to the health problem but significantly influence a community health agency's ability to address the

table 14-2 Criteria for Scoring Size of a Health Problem

Percent of Population with Health Problem	Size of Problem Rating
25% or more	9 or 10
10% through 24.9%	7 or 8
1% through 9.9%	5 or 6
.1% through .9%	3 or 4
.01% through .09%	1 or 2
Less than .01% (1/10,000)	0

From Centers for Disease Control and Prevention (CDC): *A guide for establishing public health priorities*, Atlanta, undated, CDC, p. 3.

table 14-3 Criteria for Scoring Seriousness of a Health Problem

How Serious	"Seriousness" Rating
Very serious (e.g., very high death rate; premature mortality; great impact on others; etc.)	9 or 10
Serious	6, 7, or 8
Moderately serious	3, 4, or 5
Not serious	0, 1, or 2

From Centers for Disease Control and Prevention (CDC): *A guide for establishing public health priorities*, Atlanta, undated, CDC, p. 5.

table 14-4 Criteria for Scoring Effectiveness of Intervention

Effectiveness of Interventions	"Effectiveness" Rating
Very effective 80% to 100% effective (e.g., vaccine)	9 or 10
Relatively effective 60% to 80% effective	7 or 8
Effective 40% to 80% effective (e.g., laser treatment for diabetic retinopathy to prevent blindness)	5 or 6
Moderately effective 20% to 40% effective	3 or 4
Relatively ineffective 5% to 20% effective (e.g., smoking cessation interventions)	1 or 2
Almost entirely ineffective Less than 5% effective	0

From Centers for Disease Control and Prevention (CDC): *A guide for establishing public health priorities*, Atlanta, undated, CDC, p. 6.

table 14-5 Problem Ranking Using the Basic Priority Rating (BPR)

Health Problem	Components A	B	C	BPR Score (A + 2B) × C	Rank
Access to preventive care	6	9	7	168.00	4
Teen pregnancy	5	9	2	46.00	6
Uninsured	6	8	9	198.00	2
Ground water protection	9	9	9	243.00	1
Sexually transmitted diseases	7	8	6	138.00	5
Motor vehicle accidents	6	9	8	192.00	3

From Centers for Disease Control and Prevention (CDC): *A guide for establishing public health priorities*, Atlanta, undated, CDC, p. 7.

table 14-6 PEARL Component of Priority Setting

PEARL Factors	Questions Considered
P = Propriety	Is the problem one that falls within the agency's overall scope of operation?
E = Economic feasibility	Does it make economic sense to address the problem; are there economic consequences if the problem is not addressed?
A = Acceptability	Will the community and/or target population accept a program to address the problem?
R = Resources	Are, or should, resources be available to address the problem?
L = Legality	Do current laws allow the problem to be addressed?

From Centers for Disease Control and Prevention (CDC): *A guide for establishing public health priorities*, Atlanta, undated, CDC, p. 5.

problem (CDC, undated). The questions addressed by the PEARL are presented in Table 14-6. Yes-or-no scoring is used with the PEARL factors. Health problems that receive a *no* answer to any of the PEARL questions are either dropped from consideration for the present or receive further investigation to determine if the PEARL factor can be corrected (CDC).

To effectively use a priority rating method, community health planners must have a qualitative and a quantitative understanding of the community in which they work. Using community assessment data and concepts from epidemiology and establishing collaborative relationships with consumers and other health care providers facilitates this understanding.

THE COMMUNITY HEALTH NURSE AND HEALTH PLANNING

Nurses have played a significant role in advancing action for health. It was a nurse, in cooperation with a local community, that started the Healthy Cities initiative in the United States (Flynn, Ray, Rider, 1994). Nurses are assuming leadership roles at all levels of government in carrying out the core public health functions of assessment, policy development, and assurance (Berkowitz, 1995; Conley, 1995; News, 1992). Nurses are also assuming leadership roles in the new emerging health care structures where they advocate for quality client services.

The community health nurse is particularly well qualified to work with community citizens in carrying out population-based health planning. Each day the nurse sees the needs of aggregates at risk within the community through home visits, clinics, classes, schools, and other nursing activities. She or he is able to obtain a composite picture of the health needs of an aggregate such as lack of prenatal care, family planning services, or public transportation. The nurse's continual, comprehensive contact with the community makes her or him knowledgeable about available resources, gaps in service provision, and unhealthy environmental conditions. The staff nurse should share these assessed health needs with supervisory personnel, and together they can discuss the alternatives to the situation. The agency's philosophy of service, policies, priorities, and staff variables will affect the alternatives offered. By sharing assessed needs with people in an agency who are in a position to assist in implementing change, the nurse is taking a beginning step in health planning for the needs of the community.

Nurses usually see only the "tip of the iceberg" when diagnosing problems common to families in their caseloads. What has been assessed, however, can become the basis for an epidemiological investigation of community needs. Epidemiological studies examine groups of families in an agency's geographical area. They frequently involve investigation of needs in census tracts or specific political boundaries such as cities, towns, or counties (Figure 14-1). "Public health nurses provide a critical linkage between epidemiological data and clinical understanding of health and illness as it is experienced in peoples' lives" (APHA, 1996, p. 3). This linkage assists planners in validating community needs and strengths.

Nurses also provide a critical linkage between providers and consumers. They articulate community needs to health planners and policy makers and advocate for essential health policies and programs (APHA, 1996). Additionally, nurses plan, implement, and evaluate population-focused health services. Planning and implementing health screenings at the worksite, coordinating health fairs in schools or shopping malls, and developing clinic services for the uninsured are a few examples of *health planning interventions* commonly implemented by community health nurses.

Health needs of aggregates can also be addressed by building on research studies and known problems and solutions. How this is done is illustrated by graduate students in community health nursing at the University of Texas who assessed an aggregate at risk, nearby immigrant and refugee Hispanic persons. Evidence showed that this community of approximately 100,000 Central American immigrants fared poorly in terms of both potential and realized access to medical care. The purpose of the assessment was to gather information to document systematically whether expanded public health services were needed in the area, and, if so, what types of services were needed (Rojas-Urruita, Aday, 1991). Bilingual interviewers spoke with 242 people. Questions adapted from an interview survey on access to medical care were part of the interview schedule. The results indicated that 67% of this group sought health care, compared to 87% of the general population for comparable illnesses. One in 10 persons in the study population had been denied access

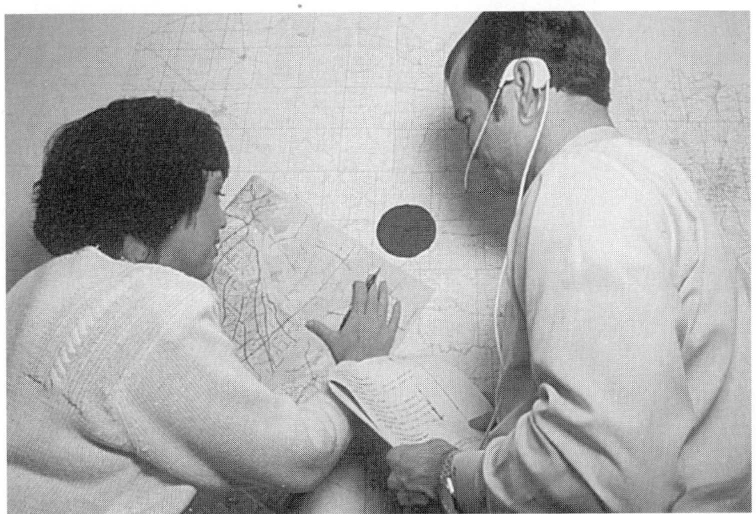

Figure 14-1 Health planners study aggregates within specific geographical and political boundaries and community trends using maps and other tools.

to medical care for some reason. Study findings were given to both local and county health authorities and other area agencies. "The result was a series of meetings with agency personnel and community representatives that resulted in proposals from the city health department, for, in the short run, establishing a storefront public health clinic in the area, and for the long term, developing a multiservice center to provide preventive and treatment-related care . . ." (Rojas-Urruita, Aday, p. 25). The project demonstrated that research can both identify problems and promote the implementations of solutions to reduce community problems.

As we move toward the twenty-first century, the challenges for nurses and other health planners will be extensive and opportunities will be abundant. While safeguarding the health of vulnerable populations, such as those described above, nurses, other health care providers, and consumers will have an opportunity to develop creative service delivery approaches and health interventions. Change and innovation will be the norm. As changes are occurring, exciting role opportunities for nurses and other health care providers are emerging, and innovative service delivery patterns for meeting the nation's critical health needs are evolving.

PROGRAM PLANNING FOR HEALTH*

Program planning for aggregates at risk involves the same steps used in the individual and family-centered nursing process: assessing, analyzing, planning, implementing, and evaluating (Table 14-7). Basic concepts of epidemiology, biostatistics, and demography (see Chapter 11) and management principles (see Chapter 23) are used to refine decision-making and diagnostic skills and to expand intervention options during the program planning process.

The emphasis in the program planning model is on the health of aggregates at risk and the community as a whole, and problems, solutions, and interventions are defined on this level. In contrast, the clinical practice model focuses on the individual as the unit of service. During the program planning process, the community is viewed as the client and a vehicle for social participation and collective action (Checkoway, 1988).

Another distinguishing feature of community and aggregate-based program planning is its focus on the prevention of existing health problems in the population being served, as well as on the promotion of health and well-being. The goals are to have "healthy people in a healthy world" and to "make prevention a way of life, not just an idea" (CDC, 1995, pp. 1, 5). The box on the next page identifies prevention strategies needed to have healthy people in healthy communities. Community planning strategies are addressed in this chapter. Chapters 15 through 21 focus on the health of aggregates from a developmental age perspective, health threats among these aggregates, and specific preventive interventions needed to reduce these threats.

TRENDS AFFECTING HEALTH PROGRAM PLANNING

To assist community residents in identifying priority health needs and in planning programs that meet these needs requires an understanding of the demographic, epidemiological, and health care delivery trends in the United States. Prevailing attitudes, as well as these trends, influence both

*Christine DeGregorio, Ph.D., while a University of Rochester doctoral student in political science, first wrote the phases and steps of the community planning process as outlined here. Much of the content and many of the illustrations in this section reflect her thinking and creativity. It is used with her permission.

table 14-7 Comparison of the Nursing, Epidemiological, and Health Care Planning Processes

Nursing Process	Epidemiological Process	Health Planning Process
Assessing Data collection to determine nature of client problems	I. Determine the nature, extent, and scope of the problem A. Natural life history of condition B. Determinants influencing condition 1. Primary data (essential agent) a. Parasite, bacterium, or virus b. Nutrition c. Psychosocial factor 2. Contributory data a. Agent b. Host c. Environment C. Distribution patterns 1. Person 2. Place 3. Time D. Condition frequencies 1. Prevalence 2. Incidence 3. Other biostatistical measurements	Preplanning Assessment Data collection to determine needs of populations and the community as a whole Assessment of resources
Analyzing	II. Formulate tentative hypothesis(es)	Development of problem statement, goals, expected outcomes
Formulation of nursing diagnoses or hypotheses	III. Collect and analyze further data to test hypothesis(es)	Policy development
Planning	IV. Plan for control	Plan strategies to achieve expected outcomes
Implementing	V. Implement control plan	Implementation
Evaluating	VI. Evaluate control plan	Evaluation
Revising or terminating	VII. Make appropriate report	
	VIII. Conduct research	

An Ounce of Prevention = a World of Cure

Successful implementation of the following strategies will make prevention a way of life:

- Promoting healthy behaviors
- Preventing chronic diseases
- Preventing infectious diseases
- Participating in community planning
- Preventing injuries and disabilities

Modified from Centers for Disease Control and Prevention (CDC): *CDC vision: healthy people in a healthy world through prevention*, Atlanta, 1995, CDC, p. 5.

the services needed and the organization of these services. The box on the next page presents a summary of trends that are influencing health planning efforts; an examination of them makes it clear that the health care delivery system and local communities will be dealing with unprecedented demands that will require creative planning and programming.

THE PROGRAM PLANNING PROCESS

After identifying priority health needs, local agencies will initiate the health planning process to address client needs and gaps in service delivery. As illustrated in Table 14-7, the program planning process is orderly and logical. It is a tool that helps those using it to organize large amounts of community data that describe community problems and strengths, as well as health planning solutions. For purposes of discussion, the program planning process is divided into five phases: *preplanning, assessment, policy development, implementation*, and *evaluation*. Each of these phases is separately described, but in reality they are overlapping and inseparable. For example, in practice, evaluative activities may occur during any phase of the process or goals may be altered when resource implications of different alternatives are discussed, with the realization that original goals were too ambitious or overly cautious (Green, 1992, p. 24).

Trends Affecting Health Care Planning

EPIDEMIOLOGICAL TRENDS

- Conditions of the aging, including cardiovascular disease, cancer, diabetes, osteoarthritis, cognitive impairment, and advancing age, place crucial demands on the health care system. With the number of people growing older, these demands will increase.
- Diseases of lifestyle and behavior, including obesity, trauma, substance abuse, sexually transmitted diseases, teenage pregnancy, occupational and environmental hazards, and homelessness and disability, mean that social policies have to change and that health education should take place in nontraditional forms.
- Diseases and technology have brought about a marked reduction in premature mortality and an overall reduction in morbidity. These changes have also produced social, legal, and ethical dilemmas
- The AIDS epidemic has produced immeasurable human suffering and costs of 2.3 billion dollars annually. In the absence of a cure or vaccine, this epidemic will spread.
- Infant mortality rates place the United States at twenty-second in the world; there are large discrepancies in deaths of infants between whites and African Americans.
- Enhanced understanding of diseases is helping researchers to understand that people do not progress from health to disease but that genetic predisposition interacts with exposure to various physical, chemical, and biological factors. Preventing disease is much more complex than once thought.
- Environmental factors that predispose to and/or cause disease are present. Our industrial age has created conveniences, but at a price. The world will need to choose between convenience and environmental destruction in some cases.

DEMOGRAPHIC TRENDS

- The aging population is dramatically increasing. The population over age 85 will grow steadily to 15.5% by 2010.
- The baby boom generation, those born between 1946 and 1964, reversed a downward trend and added 1.5 million persons each year of the boom. This group is one of the best-educated generations and will place demands on the health care sector over the next 50 years.
- A declining younger population will produce smaller numbers for schools and colleges.
- Racial and ethnic diversity, including growth in the African-American and Hispanic-American populations, will make an impact on all aspects of the health care system, since both groups are currently underserved and underrepresented in health care.
- Changes in the family unit mean that a mother, father, and two children are no longer the norm. Locations and hours of delivery of health care will need to change, as will the traditional set of medical problems focusing on emotional health and well-being.

HEALTH CARE DELIVERY TRENDS

- A system more managed with better integration of services and financing.
- A system more accountable to those who purchase and use health services.
- A system more aware of and responsive to the needs of enrolled populations.
- A system able to use fewer resources more effectively.
- A system more innovative and diverse in how it provides for health.
- A system more inclusive in how it defines health.
- A system less focused on treatment and more concerned with education, prevention, and care management.
- A system more oriented to improving the health of the entire population.
- A system more reliant on outcome data and evidence.

From Shugars DA, O'Neil EH, Bader JD, eds: *Healthy America: practitioners for 2005, an agenda for action for U.S. health professional schools*, Durham, N.C., 1991, The Pew Health Professions Commission, pp. 31-32, 39-40; O'Neil EH: *Health professions education for the future: schools in service to the nation*, San Francisco, Ca., 1993, Pew Health Professions Commission, pp. 6-7. Pew Health Professions Commission: *Critical challenges: revitalizing the health professions for the twenty-first century*, San Francisco, 1995, UCSF Center for the Health Professions, pp. 9-10.

The Preplanning Phase

This phase builds a foundation for the rest of the process. Before developing policies for health planning, it is crucial that planners test their ideas and validate that what they perceive as a problem is also seen by others as a problem severe enough to warrant changes. The planning organization and environment needs to be "tested" to ascertain whether sufficient resources and commitment are available to devote to the work required to bring about the change. Preliminary expectations and skeleton organizational plans need to be outlined. These sound like simple commonsense comments. In reality these very basic parts to the process are often skipped, and positive results are then difficult to achieve.

The preplanning phase has six steps: (1) obtaining community and consumer support and participation, (2) development of a broadly defined problem statement, (3) statement of a goal, (4) delineation of a timetable that accounts for the remaining four phases of the process, (5) assessment of resources for the task that needs to be accomplished, and (6) planning for data collection strategies to be used. Each of these steps helps to build a framework needed for future planning activities.

OBTAINING COMMUNITY AND CONSUMER SUPPORT AND PARTICIPATION Encouraging people to be involved in making decisions and addressing policy issues that affect their quality of life helps to ensure that programs will progress beyond the ideas of the planners. Changes in client behavior and community relationships, as well as in the social environment, are necessary to reduce the morbidity and mortality associated with problems encountered by community health nurses. For example, teenagers can be taught the importance of wearing seat belts, driving the posted speed limits, and not drinking while driving. However, this behavior is enhanced by roads that have adequate shoulders and no hidden curves and by stiff penalties for breaking the traffic laws. Since many traditional health promotion approaches that focused on changing client behavior have failed, a variety of new models to promote consumer participation have been tested.

Phrases including *community participation*, *community organization*, *community empowerment*, and *empowerment education* reflect the movement to have people "buy into" the changes needed for healthy living. Community organization activities are designed to stimulate conditions for change and to mobilize citizens and communities for health action. A major goal during this process is to facilitate community empowerment. As discussed in Chapter 3, to be empowered means that one (community, family, or individual) has the knowledge, skills, and capacity for effective and self-determined action (Courtney, 1995, p. 370; Courtney, Ballard, Fauver et al, 1996, p. 180). Courtney, Ballard, Fauver, Gariota, and Holland and other professionals in the field (APHA, 1996; Flynn, Ray, Rider, 1994; Goeppinger, Lassiter, Wilcox, 1982; Sen, 1994) believe that strengthening a community's capacity to act on its own behalf requires the implementation of partnership relationships that focus on community strengths and active client participation in all aspects of the health planning process. In contrast, the professional clinical model emphasizes client deficiences and often places the client in a passive role. Further differences between the professional model and the partnership model are presented in Table 14-8.

As stated previously, "A partnership process is the negotiated sharing of power between health professionals and individual family and/or community partners. These partners agree to be involved as active participants in the process of

table 14-8 Comparison of Professional Model with Partnership Model

Professional Model	Partnership Model
FOCUS	
The problem or the diagnosis	Fostering the skills and capacity of the partner as a primary focus in the process of improving health and well-being (the initial stimulus may be a problem, but the primary focus will be strengthening/facilitating empowerment of the partner)
HEALTH PROFESSIONAL'S ROLE	
Expert who does "to" or "for," not "with"; the professional serves as decision maker and problem solver	Professional working "with," not "doing to"; facilitator, enabler, resource person who shares leadership and power with partner; services are provided in nonjudgmental, noncontrolling manner
PARTNER'S ROLE	
Often passive recipient of "service" that is defined by professional	Active and willing participant in self-determination of strengths, problems, and solutions
NATURE OF RELATIONSHIP	
Professional is director of the process, instructing or "telling" others what to do; interventions tend to be standardized and are seldom tailored to individual or cultural needs; interventions tend to focus on the problem, not the person	Professional actively facilitates the partner's participation in the relationship; requires ongoing negotiation of goals, roles, and responsibilities; respects individual and cultural differences
GOAL/PLAN	
Determined by the professional; focused totally on the problem	Mutual goal setting; plan of action developed with partner who is involved as active participant
ACTIVITY/SERVICE	
Unilateral action by the professional to diagnose problem, establish intervention, assess progress, and revise intervention as needed	Joint action and assessment of progress that includes ongoing negotiation of roles and responsibilities; implements the partnership process; emphasizes involving natural helpers; families, groups, and/or coalitions as resources
EXPECTED OUTCOME	
The problem is solved or corrected or the patient is considered noncompliant	The partner's capacity to act more effectively on their own behalf is strengthened (i.e., more empowered); the "problem" may or may not be solved, but the partner's capacity is enhanced to prevent future problems or to address them more effectively

From Courtney R, Ballard E, Fauver S et al: The partnership model: working with individuals, families, and communities toward a new vision of health, *Public Health Nurs* 13:177-186, 1996, p. 179.

mutually determining goals and actions that promote health and well-being. The ultimate goal of the partnership process is to enchance the capacity of individual, family, and community partners to act more effectively on their own behalf" (Courtney, Ballard, Fauver et al, 1996, p. 180). Active client participation, mutual goal-setting, and community capacity building are key goals during the health planning process. Although all clients may not wish to engage in a partnership relationship, it is important for the health care professional to develop a therapeutic relationship with clients, which strengthens clients' self-care capabilities.

"Mobilizing community partnerships and action to identify and solve health problems" (CDC, 1995) is viewed as an essential public health service. The process of facilitating community empowerment through a partnership relationship can occur in various ways. Schlaff (1991), in a prize-winning idea for the 1990 Secretary's Award for Innovation in Health Promotion and Disease Prevention, described an ideal scenario in one city: a health center worked with the neighborhood council to deal with health problems; the council was an elected body of residents and activists representing the community. The health center director reported directly to the council, and working with them were lay community health workers who reflected the ethnic and cultural diversity of the community. Community health workers carried out health education in homes; people indigenous to the population of concern also assisted planners in accurately defining problems that needed correction. The program combined the use of community organization activities, efforts to form organizational structures involving members of the community, and the use of lay health workers who lived in the community where they worked.

Another illustration of facilitating community empowerment to change both the health behavior of individuals and their collective health is the Abbotsford Community Nursing Center in Philadelphia. The Center is located in a tenant-managed public housing development and delivers primary health services ranging from prenatal to geriatric care. Need for the services offered was in part based on a resident-administered survey that defined the major health issues in the community. Residents have control of the 12-member board that makes final decisions about program design, hiring of personnel, and policy. Residents of the project are hired to be the outreach workers, drivers, security personnel, and receptionists. Using these indigenous resources puts money directly back into the community being served and also brings information about the community to the Center. The outreach workers visit households in the development on a regular basis, provide information on health education and prevention issues, and follow up on missed appointments and concerns such as prenatal and postnatal difficulties. The Center is *community driven*, which means that the residents have control both over the resources and ownership in the results of the program (Resources for Human Development, Inc., and the Abbottsford Homes Tenant Management Corporation, Project Abstract, undated). This behavior illustrates well the first step of program planning: obtaining community and consumer support and participation.

DEVELOPMENT OF A PROBLEM STATEMENT A problem is a condition that is sufficiently distressing that change to bring relief is desired or sought. An example of a broadly defined problem statement from which policy development could begin might be the following: "Deaths from motor vehicle accidents for people 15 to 24 years of age in Jones County have substantially increased over the past year." This statement has a broad, yet clear, focus. All involved in the planning process would know that the concern is increased motor vehicle accidents for a certain age group in a specific area in a given year. As Table 14-8 reflects, the identification of a community problem is often the initial stimulus for developing a health action partnership.

STATEMENT OF A GOAL A goal is a general statement of intent or purpose that provides guidance for the activities that are to take place. A goal emanating from the above problem statement might be, "Jones County citizens will work toward reducing the rate of fatalities from motor vehicle accidents among people 15 to 24 years of age by 10% in 3 years."

DELINEATION OF A TIMETABLE To develop a realistic timetable that accounts for the remaining four phases of the process, planners must have a general idea of what they plan to accomplish in the months ahead. After a specific goal is delineated, health planners have a preliminary discussion about what needs to be done to achieve the stated goal, and how they can facilitate community participation for action. This discussion focuses on examining the nature of the tasks to be accomplished and what is feasible for community agencies and citizens to do together, considering other priorities.

Table 14-9 presents a sample health planning timetable. As discussed earlier, this table illustrates how the phases overlap and build on one another.

ASSESSMENT OF RESOURCES Resources are needed to effectively carry out the planning process. An assessment of resources is completed to determine whether current resources are adequate to accomplish program planning goals. Resources can be both internal (part of the organization) and external to an organization. Examples of resources include money, enthusiasm for the planning goals, community commitment, space in which to work, time, staff competencies, and experienced workers who have popularity, esteem, charisma, and commitment to the planning project. If resources are inadequate planning goals may need to be altered, or strategies for obtaining sufficient resources will need to be developed.

Resources may be found within the organization or elsewhere. Space and money, for example, may need to be

table 14-9 Timetable for Jones County Health Department's Motor Vehicle Accident Project

	Time in Months											
Phases	Dec	Jan	Feb	Mar	April	May	June	July	Aug	Sept	Oct	Nov
Preplanning	—	—										
Assessment		—	—	—	—							
Policy development				—	—	—	—	—				
Implementation							—	—	—	—	—	
Evaluation									—	—	—	—

obtained from voluntary community agencies and technical expertise requested from a university. Knowing the community in which one works helps the community health nurse to quickly identify valuable resources during the planning process (see Chapter 13).

One of the most valuable health planning resources is a committee that works toward the goal and that has power and authority to make decisions. To be viable the committee must have tasks assigned to it that are crucial to the goal; the committee must also have an audience that expects results. Health planning committee members should be chosen on the basis of their interpersonal skills, their knowledge of the planning process and the community, and their commitment to the goals. Not every committee member will likely have all of these ingredients for successful planning; however, these ingredients must be present in some degree if successful planning is to take place. Inexperienced planners should be part of the group so that learning can take place for future planning activities. The planning committee may need to be trained in the planning process if this is an entirely new activity for committee members. Help with the process may be obtained from a variety of community resources such as the United Way, the county health planning council, and local university faculty members.

An example of how community leaders are organized and trained to deal with health problems is the collaborative effort between the Indiana University School of Nursing Institute of Action Research for Community Health, the Indiana Public Health Association, and six Indiana cities (Flynn, Rider, Bailey, 1992). Healthy Cities Indiana is a community development approach to health promotion and involves a public-private partnership in developing healthier cities. Citizens participate in examining problems and solutions to promote healthy cities. Community leadership development that supports health promotion is fundamental. Central to the process is the local healthy city committee that represents the community. Its members come from various sectors of the city, including arts and culture, business, dentistry, education, employment, environment, finance, health and medical care, local government, media, parks, and other areas such as religion and transportation. The Healthy Cities Indiana program emphasizes experiential learning with these leaders, teaching what people want and need rather than setting goals for them. Emphasis is on strengthening a community's capacity to deal with its own perceived needs.

DEVELOPING DATA COLLECTION STRATEGIES A plan needs to be developed to assess the problem of concern. When developing this plan the planning group focuses on *what* data are needed, from *whom* they need input, *how* they should obtain data, *who* will be responsible for collecting the data, and *when* the data collection process will be completed. For example, the Jones County Health Department planning group would want active participation from parents, teachers, legislators, police officers, and health providers when they examine vehicle fatalities.

The plan for data collection should be written in sufficient detail so that all involved parties are clear about what needs to be accomplished. A worksheet such as the one presented in Table 14-10 facilitates the planning process.

At the conclusion of these five steps, the planning group should have a good grasp of the problem, should be aware of the power and authority they have from the involved community, should know their strengths and weaknesses, and should have delineated the time frame for the process. The group is then ready to move to the next phase of the planning process: *assessment*.

The Assessment Phase

In population-based planning, community health nurses "evaluate health trends and risk factors of population groups and help determine priorities for targeted interventions" (APHA, 1996, p. 3). Examining risk factors as well as health trends broadens the health planner's perspective and reflects a recognition that health problems are influenced by multiple interrelated factors such as those discussed in Chapter 11. Identifying the multiple forces that influence illness aids communities in developing appropriate interventions. "The ultimate aim of a [community] health plan

table 14-10 Jones County Health Department Motor Vehicle Accident Project: Worksheet for Planning Data Collection Strategies

Goal: Reduce the rate of motor vehicle accidents among 15- to 24-year-old youth in Jones County.
Rationale for Goal: The rate of fatal motor vehicle accidents (MVA) among 15- to 24-year-old youth has increased 5% in the past year.

Type of Data	Data Source	Collection Method	Time for Completion	Responsibility of
DATA COLLECTION PLAN FOR ORGANIZATIONAL ASSESSMENT				
Characteristics of accident victims	Clients	Personal interview	April 30, 1996	Staff CHN
Epidemiological data	Accident reports and interview data	Review of reports	April 30, 1996	Planning committee
DATA COLLECTION PLAN FOR COMMUNITY ASSESSMENT				
Causes of accidents	Law enforcement officers	Mail survey	April 30, 1996	Planning committee
Content covered in driver education courses	Driver education staff	Telephone interview	April 30, 1996	Planning committee

is to improve levels of health rather than health services—although the latter may, of course, be an important means to that end" (Green, 1992, p. 167).

In population-based planning, three steps in the assessment phase of the health care planning process are completed. These are (1) conducting a needs assessment, (2) setting priorities upon which the planning committee can focus, and (3) specifying outcomes to which organizational and community resources can be applied. Each of these steps helps planners to become more specific as they progress through the planning process.

CONDUCTING A NEEDS ASSESSMENT During the program planning process, health planners build upon community assessment data and use epidemiological concepts to identify the specific nature of the problem being addressed. When examining the nature and extent of the problem, planners discern trends over a specified period of years and cite the problem's significance, implications, and comparisons with norms or other standards.

Assessing a population's need relative to a circumscribed health problem (e.g., motor vehicle accidents, domestic violence, or teenage pregnancy) is a complex matter that goes beyond defining the population at risk. Needs are relative, and they are based on values, cultures, history, and the experiences of the individual, the family, and the community. Human needs are not easily identified, but are diffuse and related. For example, motor vehicle deaths may be related to poor roads that are the result of a low-level tax base for road repairs, which is due to high unemployment. Human needs often change because the forces that influence need often change. A need today may not be a need next year.

Translating assessed needs into community programs and interventions is greatly influenced by the availability of human and financial resources in addition to the availability of technology. Thus a needs assessment delineates population strengths, such as concerned citizen groups, that can be tapped when developing policies, implementing strategies, and evaluating program outcomes. A *health resource inventory* is also completed to prevent duplication of services and to identify potential partnerships for action. A health resource inventory identifies the type of services community agencies are providing relative to the specified health problems, service utilization patterns and barriers, and perceived community need.

The box on the next page presents a simple needs assessment tool designed to collect data about motor vehicle accidents in Jones County. It can be used as an assessment guide to collect data about other health problems in a community. How and where health planners obtain data for a needs assessment is presented in Chapter 13.

A community will be readier to act if it believes that a given issue is important and if the issue affects a number of people. People in a community will also be readier to act if they have had previous success with community action and if there is a network of organizations to facilitate change (Brown, 1991, p. 442). Communities, classified as anomic, transitory, stepping-stone, or diffuse will likely have more difficulty with community organization and change than

A Sample Needs Assessment Tool: Motor Vehicle Accidents in Jones County

1. Community assessment of factors influencing fatalities from motor vehicle accidents
   a. Mortality data
   b. Morbidity data (incidence and prevalence) trends in recent years
   c. Demographic characteristics associated with mortality and morbidity (at-risk aggregates) in the defined community
   d. Local factors, such as road conditions, thought to influence trends
   e. Lifestyle of population groups
      (1) Environmental characteristics promoting health or illness
      (2) Economic base of population, income, and occupation
      (3) Lifestyle behaviors, such as drinking patterns, that influence health states
   f. Local perception of needs, problems, or priorities
2. Community resources
   a. Health services, strengths, and limitations
   b. Population coverage
   c. Usage rates for health services and barriers to utilization
3. Extent of knowledge related to the problem under consideration
   a. Magnitude of the problem in other populations: national and state data
   b. Etiological factors (*results* of case-control and cohort studies or theories)
   c. Physiological, sociological, and psychological processes related to pathology
   d. Inferences for *primary* prevention and early detection of problems
   e. Treatment potential
      (1) Inferences for therapeutic strategies at the individual, family, or aggregate level
      (2) Inferences for *secondary* and *tertiary* prevention (both of above are based on *results* of clinical trials and other types of evaluative studies or theories)

will parochial or integral communities (see Chapter 3 for a description of these types of communities).

SETTING PRIORITIES During this step in the assessment process, planners make decisions about priorities for a program focus. To determine this focus, health planners examine the factors influencing problem occurrence, as well as gaps in existing services. Based on this exploration, a target population is identified and the nature of the problem is specifically defined. Using the motor vehicle mortality problem in Jones County among youth ages 15 to 24 years as an example, possible target groups could be all youth in the 15- to 24-year-old age span, or high school students ages 15 through 18, or young adults ages 18 through 24. Jones County program developers determined that priority should be placed on addressing the problem among high school students, since the majority of fatal accidents were occurring among this age group. It was further established that addressing drinking and driving should be the program emphasis, since all but one death among high school students was associated with excessive alcohol intake.

Analysis of health statistics aids planners in making decisions about priorities for a program focus. Criteria similar to those previously discussed in this chapter are also used to guide decision making regarding priorities. Green (1992) cautions planners to be aware of the danger of "paralysis by analysis" syndrome, where no action is taken until all data are available. One of the objectives of the program may be to focus on data collection if gaps in data are identified and the problem is considered to be a major health concern.

Whatever method is used by the planning committee to set priorities, the priority chosen will affect the timing and the amount of resources allocated to that priority. Human as well as financial resources are important to consider when establishing resource needs. With the rapidly changing nature of practice in health care organizations, *staff competencies* are a critical factor to assess as well.

SPECIFY OUTCOMES The last step in this assessment phase is to specify outcomes to which organizational and community resources can be applied over a specified period of time. Outcomes are specific, concrete, measurable statements that need to be accomplished in order to eventually reach a broad goal. They are intended to guide the operations of the agency to reach the goal.

Outcomes focus on the what and when. They specify *results*, not strategies for getting results. For example, outcomes that help to reach the goal of reducing the rate of fatalities from motor vehicle accidents might be (1) lower the motor vehicle fatality rate for youth ages 15 to 18 years in Jones County by 3% in the next year; (2) ensure enforcement of the provisions of the Zero Tolerance Bill (no alcohol at school activities) during the 1997-1998 school year; (3) limit teenage access to alcohol by 1998; and (4) design and implement an ongoing alcohol awareness educational program during 1997-1998. These outcomes are designed to provide direction for achieving the goal of the program, "Jones County Citizens will work toward reducing the rate of fatalities from motor vehicle accidents among people 15 to 24 years of age by 10% in 3 years."

When establishing outcomes it is important to take into consideration what can feasibly be accomplished in a specified time frame. Ideally, Jones County would like to reduce fatal motor vehicle accidents among their youth by 5% immediately. However, this is not realistic considering the nature of the problem, the characteristics of the target population, and the resources needed to affect change. Multiple factors influence the motor vehicle accident fatality rate, especially among youth. Teenagers and young adults are known to engage in behaviors (e.g., drinking while driving,

driving without a seat belt, and speeding) that place them at high risk for fatal driving accidents. Comprehensive programming is needed to address all of these factors, which can require extensive resources.

At the conclusion of the three steps of the assessment phase, planners will know the details of the problem under consideration. They will also know the resources available both within and outside the organization and the community that can help deal with the problem. When this information is known, health planners concentrate on the third step in the planning process, *policy development*.

The Policy Development Phase

Policy development involves the determination of strategies to achieve the expected outcomes that emerge as the result of the assessment done in phase two of the planning process. These strategies include methods for allocating resources such as money, personnel, and equipment and interventions directed toward prevention. The strategies also clarify relationships that affect rights, status, and resources. In this phase planners pay attention to social and political parameters: Where are the greatest resources? Where is there resistance to the expected outcomes? What methods or strategies could best achieve the expected outcomes? How can the community be mobilized for health action? Will one of the strategies be a modification of what already exists or will it be a new innovative approach? Will the strategies to meet the expected outcomes involve contracts with other organizations and/or support for these organizations so that they can better meet the expected outcome? Answers to these questions will result in an allocation of resources, the identification of responsibilities, and, finally, the establishment of an action plan that has tasks, responsibilities, interventions, and a time frame clearly delineated.

Policy development is frequently a process of negotiation among the different groups involved in the planning process: consumers, service providers, decision makers, and resource persons. Further, during the policy development phase planners must anticipate expected changes in services, legislation, and general trends, and then must foresee what impact these changes will have on the local community. A balance must be achieved that will most effectively use community resources to meet the needs perceived by ordinary citizens, as well as needs perceived by professionals with expertise.

It is easier to discuss the policy development phase of the planning process by dividing it into four steps: (1) assess various strategies to achieve expected outcomes, (2) match tasks with resources, (3) negotiate new organizational liaisons as needed, and, finally, (4) establish contracts as needed. The result will be an action plan.

GENERATE STRATEGIES TO ACHIEVE EXPECTED OUTCOMES

Generating alternatives to meet the expected outcomes written in phase two is one of the most exhilarating steps in the process. It is a time to be creative and innovative, to exercise a flair for originality.

There are a variety of ways to generate strategies that can be effective in reaching desired outcomes. Reviewing the literature that addresses successful and unsuccessful strategies related to the health problem of concern is one. Talking with communities and/or advocacy groups that are dealing with similar problems is another. *Brainstorming*—throwing caution to the wind and citing any idea that comes to mind—or conducting a *think tank* with people affected by the health problem are two other approaches for generating community-based interventions.

One of the most exciting aspects of this phase of the health planning process is the development of client interventions that will reach the target population. In community health practice, a major challenge is to develop interventions that reach underserved populations. Freudenberg, Eng, Flay et al (1995) have proposed principles to consider when planners mobilize communities for the purpose of addressing the needs of the underserved. These guidelines are presented in the above box and reinforce many of the concepts presented throughout this chapter. Examples of community-based *interventions* used to prevent disease and promote health are peer modeling and education, use of lay health advisors, coalition building for advocacy, educating policy makers and members of community leadership groups (e.g., Tribal Councils and City Councils),

PRINCIPLES FOR BUILDING INDIVIDUAL AND COMMUNITY CAPACITY

- Effective health education interventions should be tailored to a specific population within a particular setting.
- Effective interventions involve the participants in planning, implementation, and evaluation.
- Effective interventions integrate efforts aimed at changing individuals, social and physical environments, communities, and policies.
- Effective interventions link participants' concerns about health to broader life concerns and to a vision of a better society.
- Effective interventions use existing resources within the environment.
- Effective interventions build on the strengths found among participants and their communities.
- Effective interventions advocate for the resources and policy changes needed to achieve the desired health objectives.
- Effective interventions prepare participants to become leaders.
- Effective interventions support the diffusion of innovation to a wider population.
- Effective interventions seek to institutionalize successful components and to replicate them in other settings.

From Freudenberg N, Eng E, Flay B et al: Strengthening individual and community capacity to prevent disease and promote health: in search of relevant theories and principles, *Health Educ Q* 22:290-306, 1995, pp. 297-298.

participating in community events (e.g., health fairs and pow-wows), and using an education format that actively engages the community (e.g., distribution of useful items with imprinted messages such as T-shirts and use of videos, plays, art, or music) (Freudenberg, Eng, Flay et al, 1995; Marin, Burhansstipanov, Connell et al, 1995; Randall-David, 1994).

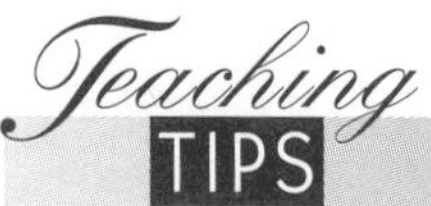

TIPS

Providing Culturally Appropriate Community Educational Messages

- Learn about the learning style of the members in the community. Most audiences relate more when they hear, see, and then do.
- Utilize many different strategies for educating culturally diverse communities.
- Limit the use of lectures and workshops.
- Employ strategies that exist in the community when making group presentations, such as the "call and response" method used in the African American community. With this strategy, the leader/teacher/preacher states a message in an emphatic way and the audience calls back a response.
- Use a *format* that actively engages the community, such as games, dance, street theater, videos, and storytelling.
- Use existing community educational strategies (e.g., church newsletters, announcements at street fairs or tribal gatherings, and neighborhood flyers).
- Identify language (e.g., street vocabulary or vernacular) that is most appropriate to use and rules for communicating.
- Limit the use of brochures, since most people remember only 10% of what they read.
- For imparting the message, choose a *messenger* who is respected by the targeted segment(s) of the community (e.g., spiritual leaders, healers, influential opinion leaders, gang leaders, sports figures, and tenant association leaders).
- Design a *message* that is simple, uncomplicated, and "do-able," that is consistent with the cultural values of the community and encourages community members to take charge.
- Offer education in settings that are familiar, safe, clean, and easily accessible (e.g., natural gathering places such as community centers, playgrounds, soup kitchens, and malls).

Modified from Randall-David E: *Culturally competent HIV counseling and education*, McLean, Va., 1994, The Maternal and Child Health Clearinghouse, pp. 24-26.

MATCH TASKS WITH RESOURCES After several strategies have been chosen for each expected outcome, resources need to be assigned to make certain that the task or strategy is accomplished. This results in an action plan specifying the work activities needed to achieve the expected outcome. It includes what is to be done, who is responsible, and by what date each step should be completed. It should be possible to accomplish action steps in 1 to 12 months; each expected outcome may have many action steps. For example, if one expected outcome is "To limit teenager access to alcohol by 1998," the action plan that matches strategies with resources to achieve this outcome might look like the one presented in Table 14-11.

Step two of the policy development phase results in an action plan that delineates specific action steps with responsible individuals, along with a realistic time frame. This type of plan facilitates the completion of necessary health planning activities.

ESTABLISH ORGANIZATIONAL LIAISONS AND CONTRACTS These steps help planners to complete action steps. For example, if Ms. Alexander is responsible for a monthly newspaper article focused on alcohol awareness issues, she will need to have a firm commitment from the editor that the paper will print it. This may involve a visit by administrative personnel in the health department to the editorial director of the newspaper and a written or verbal agreement that such a plan is feasible. This may also be the situation if support from law enforcement agencies is desired; coalition building with community organizations and concerned citizens interested in causes of motor vehicle accidents among youth and the health department who then, together, ask for changes in enforcement practices is likely to be necessary. These two steps may be the most difficult, and yet the most important aspects needed to achieve positive outcomes from program planning activities.

Table 14-12, showing the planning sequence, summarizes the differences between goals, plans, outcomes, and action steps, as well as the following parameters of each of these: functions, leadership, database, time span, and accountability. Having an awareness of these differences is important, because each level of planning must be com-

table 14-11 JONES COUNTY HEALTH DEPARTMENT: ONE ACTION PLAN FOR THE MOTOR VEHICLE ACCIDENT PROJECT

Expected Outcome: To limit teenager access to alcohol by 1998.

ACTION STEPS	DATE	PERSON RESPONSIBLE
Get support of the 15 Jones County PTAs	March 15, 1997	Eigsti
Get support of all law enforcement agencies	March 15, 1997	Clemen and Jones
Put one article each month of the year in the "Jones County Chronicle"	Monthly	Alexander
Get support of grocery association	August 1, 1997	McGuire

pleted to ensure effective and efficient community health planning.

The Implementation Phase

The fourth phase of the health care planning process is implementation. All the work of the other phases finally leads to achievement of concrete outcomes in the real world. Implementation is, to a great extent, a political process that requires that those seeking to bring about change be very aware of the various forces present in the community. Will these forces help the changes to take place or can they be mobilized to provide support for the changes? Implementation involves incentives for people to change, public hearings, and advocacy for change. This phase calls for trust, rapport, and patience to work out new and different relationships and to respond to the unanticipated ramifications of the change.

In short, implementation is carrying out the plan. It involves organizing, delegating, and managing work so that the action steps prepared in the last phase are completed and outcomes are accomplished within the specified time. These are the questions that planners need to answer in the implementation phase: What is to be done? How will it be done? Who will do it? What are the deadlines for each step? Who will monitor progress? How and when will the solution be evaluated?

A timeline flowchart delineating operational activities to be accomplished to achieve program goals is used throughout the implementation phase. This flowchart visually displays the major program activities and a time frame in which each activity is to take place. One of the first timeline flowcharts to be formalized was the Gantt chart (Timmreck, 1995). Usually only a simple Gantt chart (Figure 14-2) is used at the program planning level in community health practice

On a simple timeline flowchart, only major activities of a project rather than a breakdown of the elements of activities are identified. For example, "train staff" on Figure 14-2 is a major activity. Elements of this activity, such as needs assessment of staff, development of training materials, and implementation and evaluation of training, are not displayed on Figure 14-2. The projected completion time for each major activity is indicated on the chart by a solid line or arrow. The original Gantt chart reflected projected starting time and desired completion time but did not indicate what actually occurred during the specified time frame. Some agencies modify the Gantt chart to include this type of information.

A timeline flowchart helps program directors avoid planning too many tasks for the same time period or tackling less urgent tasks until all essential tasks have been completed. It is important to monitor the implementation plan to make certain that the correct sequence of activities needed to achieve program goals and expected outcomes is being carried out. This monitoring enables the organization to identify successful and unsuccessful strategies and organizational issues related to program implementation. While monitoring the implementation phase, the emphasis among planners is on the next phase of the health planning process—*evaluation*.

table 14-12 The Planning Sequence

Planning Level	Function	Primary Leadership	Database	Time Span	Accountability
Goals	To provide broad purpose and general direction for the organization	Board	Ideology, values, role, mission	Infinite	Everyone
Plans	To provide definitive direction and a plan for the organization	Chief executive Planning chairman Planning committee Adopted by board	Operational Societal (issues & trends) Opinions of community leaders, key internal lay & staff leaders	2-3 years	President, planning chairman, executive director
Outcomes	To provide measurable specification of attainable outcomes within operational goals	Unit executives Unit boards and committees	Operational Clients Community Opinions of key internal lay and staff leaders of operating units	1 year	Executive director, specific staff
Action steps	To provide specification of steps to be taken and activities to be conducted to achieve outcomes; persons responsible; completion dates	Unit Executives Staff	Operational Available resources	1-12 months	Individual staff

Developed by Christine DeGregorio, Ph.D., while a doctoral student in political science, University of Rochester, Rochester, N.Y.

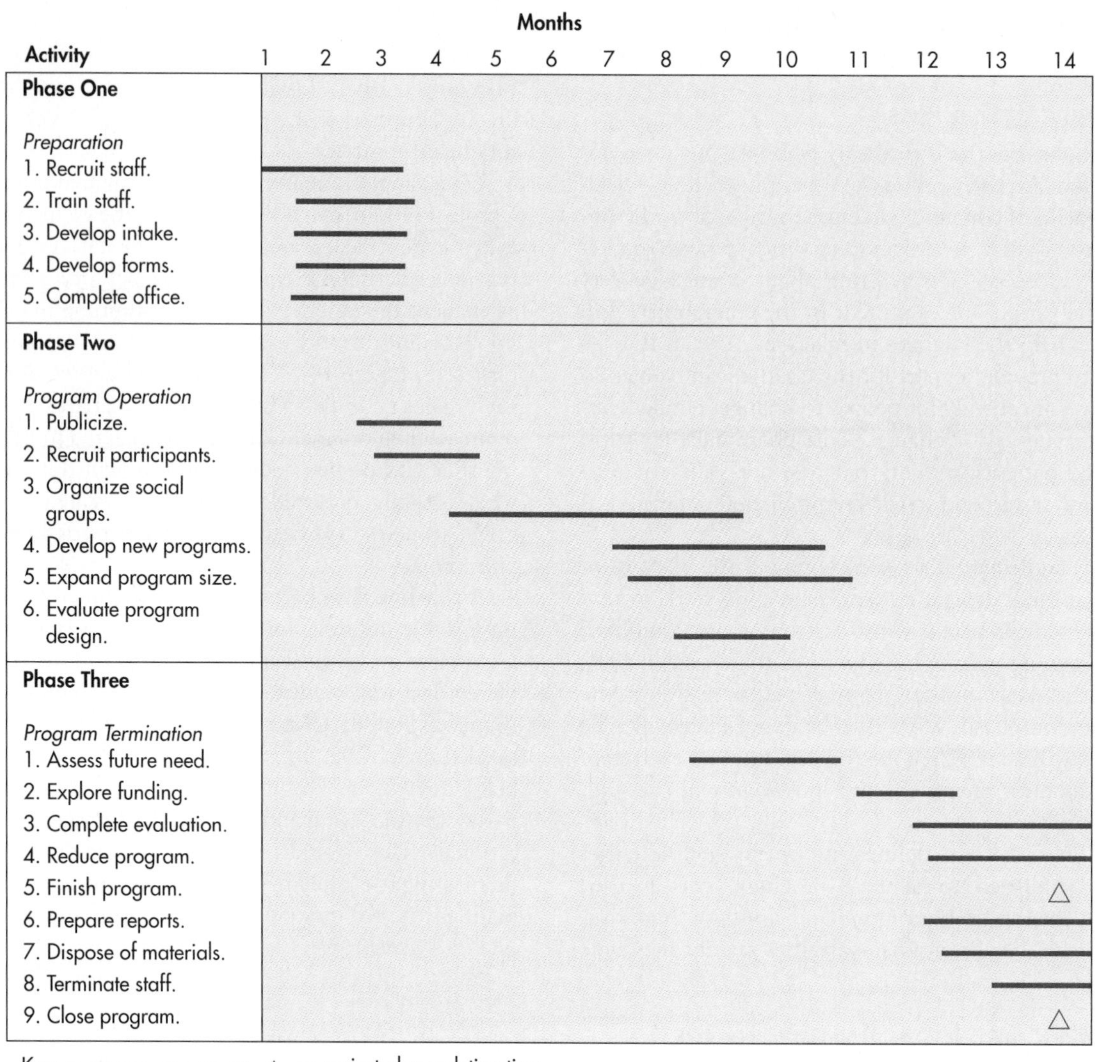

Figure 14-2 Modified Gantt chart. *(Developed by Christine De Gregorio, Ph.D., while a graduate student in political science, University of Rochester, Rochester, N.Y.)*

The Evaluation Phase

The fifth phase of the health care planning process, *evaluation,* is best seen as a continuous feedback process. It looks back on actions to determine their efficiency in order to make decisions regarding future actions. Figure 14-3 illustrates the feedback nature of the evaluation process.

Evaluation is an objective critical assessment of the degree to which entire services or their component parts (e.g., effectiveness and efficiency of a specific intervention or completion of activities within a specified time frame) fulfill stated goals (St. Leger, Schnieden, Walsworth-Bell, 1992, p. 1). Evaluation occurs throughout the health planning process *(formative evaluation)* to document progress in carrying out program activities within the designated time frame and to monitor achievement of intermediate outcomes. Evaluation also occurs as the program ends *(summative evaluation)* to assess program impact or outcome and efficiency. When program impact is evaluated, the relationship between program interventions and outcomes as well as actual program outcomes are examined (Timmreck, 1995). "Program efficiency is used to ascertain if the same outcomes could have been achieved in a more effective manner at a lower cost" (Timmreck, p. 182).

Program evaluation should occur from three perspectives (Donabedian, 1982): *structure* (environment in which program operates), *process* (how well program activities are planned and services delivered), and *outcomes* (program impact and efficiency). Chapter 25 examines these concepts more extensively. In the evolving managed care environment, emphasis is on both program impact (outcomes) and efficiency.

The evaluation phase has three steps: documenting progress, comparing achievements against a performance standard, and preparing for needed modifications. If any one

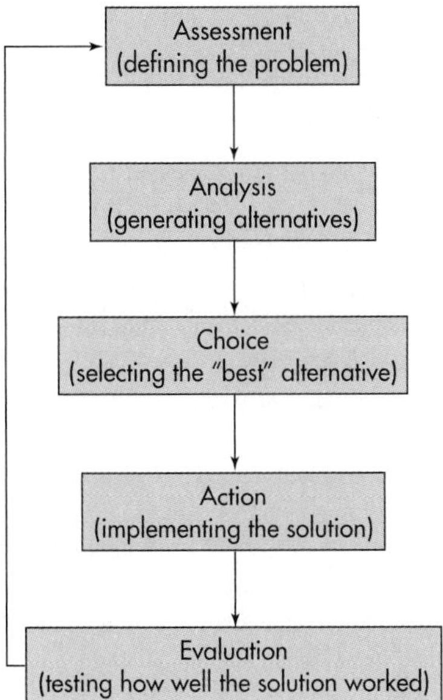

Figure **14-3** Summary of the planning process. *(Developed by Christine De Gregorio, Ph.D., while a graduate student in political science, University of Rochester, Rochester, N.Y.)*

of these steps is ignored, the evaluation process will be incomplete.

DOCUMENT PROGRESS Keeping accurate and complete records of successes and problems in the process is a key activity to a productive evaluation. Examples of the type of questions asked to document progress are identified below:

1. Are problems clearly defined?
2. Are the problems documented?
3. Are the solutions appropriate?
4. Do the solutions have many associated risks?
5. Is the envisioned scope of change satisfactory?
6. What impact will the change have on rights, resources, and structures?
7. Are the risks worth the gains?
8. Are the objectives feasible?
9. Are outcomes being achieved within the specified time frame?
10. Is the evaluation plan appropriate?

With the information obtained by asking these questions, planners can move to the next step in the evaluation phase.

COMPARE ACHIEVEMENTS AGAINST A PERFORMANCE STANDARD Performance standards are based on the expected outcomes that were written in the assessment phase of the process. For each action step written to reach each expected outcome, criteria or indicators should be established before implementation. "An indicator is an objective, measurable, well-defined variable relating to the structure, process, or outcome of care" (SCAHO, 1990, p. 29). For example, if the expected outcome is "to reduce teenager access to alcohol by 1998," and one of the action steps is to get support of the 15 Jones County Parent Teacher Associations, standards to evaluate this action step might be:

1. High achievement—support of all 15 PTAs
2. Adequate achievement—support of 10 PTAs
3. Inadequate progress—support from fewer than 10 PTAs

Indicators for evaluation should be established before implementing action steps. In addition, ways to determine whether the indicators were met should be developed. The method to obtain data about PTA support might involve a verbal report from the coordinating PTA group. This method would be delineated on an action plan as follows:

1. Source of data: verbal report from coordinating PTA group
2. Time: March 1997
3. Responsibility: Mary Cox, CHN

Developing performance indicators that address structure, process, and outcome dimensions of evaluation is challenging in the community setting. Many aggregates at risk, such as the homeless and those dealing with domestic violence, have multiple and complex needs, and only a comprehensive health programming approach is adequate to address the needs experienced by these groups. This type of programming is difficult to evaluate because the range of variables that need to be addressed is extensive and "numerous personal and societal factors outside the clinicians' control may impact the final outcomes for individual clients" (Bureau of Primary Health Care, USDHHS, 1996, p. ii). When planners develop performance standards for comprehensive programming, they *selectively* evaluate those outcomes they are able to influence.

Table 14-13 displays key questions planners might ask to evaluate whether providers are addressing program outcomes for the homeless. These questions examine how well the system (structure and process standards) functions on behalf of homeless people, as well as the impact that interventions have on individual clients (outcome standards). For each of the desired outcomes (e.g., increased level of functioning or improved access to services) performance indicators are developed. For example, if the expected outcome is "to increase the level of functioning of homeless school-age children during the 1997-1998 academic year," a performance indicator that addresses school attendance would be appropriate, since school attendance is a major standard used to assess a child's level of functioning. To measure school attendance, planners might use the following indicators:

- High achievement—less than 5 school days missed (the national average number of days missed per school-age child is 3.8 days.)
- Adequate achievement—less than 10 school days missed
- Inadequate progress—more than 10 school days missed

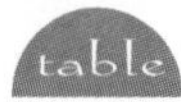 14-13 MEASURING CLIENT-LEVEL AND SYSTEM-LEVEL OUTCOMES KEY QUESTIONS FOR HEALTH CARE FOR THE HOMELESS PROVIDERS

	SELECTED HEALTH CONDITIONS			
OUTCOMES	VIOLENCE AGAINST WOMEN (ADULTS)	OTITIS MEDIA (PEDIATRICS)	MENTAL ILLNESS	SUBSTANCE ABUSE
CLIENT-LEVEL OUTCOMES				
Involvement in treatment	Are women involved in counseling?	Are children receiving antibiotics?	Are clients engaged in treatment?	Are clients engaged in treatment?
Improved health status	Is victimization reduced? Is self-esteem improved?	Do children have fewer recurring infections? Is hearing loss reduced?	Are psychiatric symptoms reduced? Is physical health addressed?	Are co-morbid physical and psychiatric symptoms reduced?
Improved level of functioning	Are physical, psychiatric, and social functioning improved?	Are children missing fewer days of school?	Are physical, psychiatric, and social functioning improved?	Are physical, psychiatric, and social functioning improved?
Disease self-management	Can women avoid risks? Are they involved in self-help groups?	Do children and their parents understand risks and how to avoid them?	Are patients able to manage their symptoms? Are they involved in self-help groups?	Are clients able to reduce their usage? Are they involved in self-help groups?
Improved quality of life	Do women have safe housing? Do they have a support network? Do they have income or work?	Do children have safe housing? Do they have family support? Are they in school?	Are clients housed? Do they have a support network? Do they have income or work?	Are clients housed? Do they have a support network? Do they have income or work?
Client choice	Do women feel they have treatment options?	Do parents (and older children) feel they have treatment options?	Do clients feel they have treatment options?	Do clients feel they have treatment options?
Client satisfaction	Are women satisfied with the services they receive?	Are parents (and older children) satisfied with the services they receive?	Are clients satisfied with the services they receive?	Are clients satisfied with the services they receive?
SYSTEM-LEVEL OUTCOMES				
Access	Do providers screen for violence? Do they conduct outreach?	Do patients receive care for acute symptoms within 24 hours?	Are appointment times convenient? Is crisis care available?	Are detox and residential services available?
Comprehensive services	Are appropriate options available that are attractive to clients?	Are appropriate options available to meet the child's needs?	Are appropriate options available that are attractive to clients?	Are appropriate options available that are attractive to clients?
Continuity of care	Is a referral network available? Are referrals successful?	Do providers offer follow-up care? Do they make specialty referrals?	Do providers offer follow-up care? Do they make specialty referrals?	Do providers offer follow-up care? Do they make specialty referrals?
Systems integration	Do other providers (e.g., housing, employment) make services available to clients?	Are other key systems (e.g., education) involved in the child's care?	Do other providers (e.g., housing, employment) make services available to clients?	Do other providers (e.g., housing, employment) make services available to clients?
Cost-effectiveness	Are emergency room visits and repeat episodes reduced?	Are surgical procedures and emergency room visits reduced?	Are emergency room visits and inpatient care reduced?	Are emergency room visits and inpatient care reduced?
Prevention	Is educational material available? Do providers screen for gun possession?	Is educational material available for parents and patients?	Is educational material available? Are risk factors addressed?	Is educational material available? Are risk factors addressed?
Client involvement	Do patients participate in treatment decisions?	Do parents (and older children) participate in treatment decisions?	Do clients participate in treatment decisions?	Do clients participate in treatment decisions?

From Bureau of Primary Health Care, USDHHS: *The working group on homeless health outcomes, meeting proceedings*, Rockville, Md., June 1996, The Bureau, pp. 14-15.

In this era of cost containment, the importance of objectively measuring program impact and efficiency cannot be overemphasized. Program funders expect health care providers to demonstrate an ability to produce quality, cost-effective outcomes (Bureau of Primary Health Care, USDHHS, 1996).

All five phases of the planning process—preplanning, assessment, policy, development, implementation, and evaluation—are interrelated and are, in reality, not carried out separately in the manner that they have been presented. When the basic elements included in each phase are followed, planners have a much greater likelihood of success than when they are passed over. The health care planning process is a valuable tool for planners who wish to bring about change to solve a difficult problem.

PREPARE FOR NEEDED MODIFICATIONS The information obtained in the final step of the evaluation phase is used by planners to make decisions about the changes that need to be made in the objectives and associated action plans. Questions such as the following need to be asked about the planning process:

1. Have any key informants been left out of the community planning process—citizens, professionals, leaders?
2. Was an adequate decision-making process used?
3. Have responsibilities and tasks been allocated appropriately?
4. Has there been negative feedback or a destructive impact (lost trust or commitment or heightened resistance) thus far?
5. What positive community responses (improved cooperation, trust, problem solving, heightened commitment, or greater resources) have occurred thus far?
6. Are resources adequate to achieve desired outcomes?
7. Are program goals, objectives, and performance indicators appropriate?

OPERATION WITHIN AN INTERDEPENDENT SYSTEM

Numerous voluntary and official agencies at the local, state, and federal level have detailed programs that contribute to successful methods for preventing disease and promoting the health of both aggregates at risk and the community. Much of this text has presented facets of these contributions, beginning with the multiple voluntary organizations such as the American Heart Association and the United Way and the work of health departments at the local, state, and federal levels. Although the most effective point for health promotion and disease prevention is the community (Kreuter, 1992, p. 136), the responsibilities and contributions of all of these organizations to the health of the local community is critical. Thus health care professionals planning health intervention programs need to develop techniques of working within an interdependent system that connects local, state, and federal planning efforts.

One technique, developed in 1983 at the Centers for Disease Control, is PATCH: Planned Approach to Community Health. PATCH is designed to "strengthen state and local health departments' capacities to plan, implement, and evaluate community-based health promotion activities targeted toward priority health problems" (Kreuter, 1992, p. 135). PATCH uses the existing system of official public health agencies, but it nutures leadership to develop intervention programs wherever it can be found. *Horizontal* and *vertical* networks are key to PATCH. At each level of government—local, state, and federal—coalition building, collaboration, and partnership formation activities are required. Further, from the top federal level down to the local health department, leaders are expected to work together to strengthen each other. PATCH builds strongly on the concept of community empowerment discussed earlier in this chapter, but in the process it provides practical skills-based programs of technical assistance where health education leaders in state health agencies can work with people at the local level to establish needed programs. The health care planning process as presented in this chapter is the methodology used to develop programs. Community health professionals can expect to see an increased emphasis on working interdependently to achieve health for all of the citizens of the world. An entire volume of *The Journal of Health Education* (1992, 23:3) explicates the PATCH concept in greater detail.

COLLABORATION FOR INTERDISCIPLINARY FUNCTIONING

Although community health nursing is exciting and challenging, nurses in this specialty area encounter problems that can be overwhelming: pregnant women addicted to crack, aging people living alone with no caretakers, child and spouse abuse, and clients having difficulties obtaining access to care, all accompanied by the terrible conditions of poverty. Nurses cannot solve these crises alone. They need to work competently with other disciplines and professions to begin to solve them. Interdisciplinary functioning and collaboration is a learned skill: individuals working in one group do not automatically come together as a united team. Understanding the definitions of interdisciplinary functioning and collaboration and the factors that facilitate teamwork help the nurse to participate in a setting that includes other professions.

Collaboration is the process of working jointly with others. An interdisciplinary team is a group of people "who have a unified direction, who are committed to achieving common objectives, and who are focused on an integrated outcome . . ." (Mariano, 1989, p. 286). Mariano discusses three factors that affect collaboration: goal and role conflict, decision-making skills, and communication skills. Goals need to be clear to all team members, and the role or the skills that each professional contributes toward that goal must be made clear. Competent professionals know their own strengths, limitations, and contributions and are capable of communicating these to others. The process used in decision making by the team is influenced by these factors and is successful when there is respect for the contributions of everyone (Chapters 16 and 21 discuss the role contributions of various disciplines on the health care team). Data available for making the decisions need to be adequate as well. Synthesizing information from multiple sources such as clients, families, and health records for the purpose of obtaining a comprehensive picture of client situations is another crucial aspect of collaboration. Communication skills, enhanced by respect and knowledge of the goals and roles of team members, succeed with a climate of openness and the guarantee that people can express thoughts freely.

BARRIERS TO HEALTH PLANNING

Each step in the process of health planning goes down neatly on paper. Carrying out the process in "real life" is a different and challenging activity. Several barriers to health planning need to be acknowledged. Some of these, such as unavailability and inaccessibility of resources, inadequate knowledge, and lack of commitment to health planning, were addressed previously. Others are presented in the following section.

A major barrier to effective health planning is a lack of understanding of the term *health*. Health is an elusive state that is difficult to define. What causes health is not easy to enumerate. It is possible to list healthy behaviors, but no one can guarantee health because both health and disease are affected by multiple interrelated variables (multiple causation principle). Epidemiological research has not yet been sufficient to document what these multiple causes are for many conditions or what health actions most effectively promote health and prevent disease. Thus it is difficult for health planners to develop health action strategies for many situations. As more epidemiological research is conducted this barrier should become less acute.

The disease-oriented focus in our present health care delivery system presents another key barrier to health planning. Health promotion and prevention concepts are very often not accepted by laypersons and professionals alike in this system. Skyrocketing health costs have severely disrupted the country's health care system, and thus community health prevention programs have been badly neglected. Basically what has happened is that persons spend so much money curing illness that little money is left for preventive health care.

Lack of sufficient money and personnel is a constant barrier. Health may not be a priority for communities, so that energy and money are spent in other directions. Health planning is often a political rather than a technical or analytical exercise, and it is possible to see an ongoing contest between local, state, and federal organizations for control of planning activities and money.

Noncompliance with health-planning activities is also a barrier. In the United States freedom of choice is a highly prized right. Safety belts save lives, but one chooses whether or not to use them, even when existing laws mandate their use. Healthy behaviors can be presented as options but that is all. Differing values promote different priorities. If an individual is not motivated to seek preventive care, preventive health-planning action will be ineffective.

The health care system in the United States is an enormous industry that has unbelievable growth each year. Health care is a basic part of the American economy. It is inevitable that it does not function perfectly. Efforts are being made, however, to improve the quality of health care in our country.

Health care providers are being confronted with awesome tasks when facing issues such as AIDS and lack of insurance coverage for many Americans. Clearly, health care reform with changes in the health care delivery system demands restructuring of the organizational culture. We will continue to see "changes in leadership orientations, and increasing flexibility to accommodate flattening of organizational authority systems. Incorporated in these changes are needs for the implementation of a more collaborative model of team building for the delivery of public health nursing services. Collaborative models should include the consumers of our services to whom we must listen" (Graham, 1992, p. 73).

The nursing profession's reason for being is caring for others, a revolutionary concept in health policy.

> The challenge to nurses and other health and social activists is one of leadership, of rebuilding communities, of reclaiming spaces and places for humane and caring interactions, and of articulating a compelling vision of another way for society and its people to be. The challenge is ultimately one of transforming such a vision into a reality of rebuilt and reclaimed communities. . . . nursing needs to consider its role in creating new realities that ensure that caring is a core value in both health and social policies. (Moccia, 1990, p. 76)

SUMMARY

Health planning for aggregates at risk is a major function of the community health nurse. In any community setting there are aggregates at risk for specific health problems. The developmental framework helps the community health nurse to identify these groups across the life span.

Health planning occurs at all levels of government and within national, state, and local private organizations. Health planning occurs at a community-wide level (*comprehensive health planning*) to identify the health status of the community and to promote the development of healthy public policy. Health planning also occurs at the operational level (*program planning*) in an organization to develop health programs, services, and interventions. Both types of planning are essential for addressing the health needs of the community and aggregates within the community. The *Healthy People 2000* mandate has provided direction for all types of health planning.

During the health planning process, emphasis is placed on mobilizing the community for health action. Partnership building facilitates the achievement of this goal and supports a community in effective and self-determined action. Innovation in practice is needed to address the complex needs in the nation.

Community health nurses provide unique contributions during the health planning process. Educational experiences prepare nurses to comprehensively analyze needs of families and populations. Clinical practice brings them in touch daily with consumer concerns and helps to identify gaps or duplication in the health care delivery system.

Currently there are obvious deficiencies in the health care delivery system, that warrant health planning action. Health care services are frequently fragmented, extremely costly, and often lacking for specific segments of the population. However, there has been a positive trend evolving that places emphasis on developing new ways to meet the health care needs of all citizens.

Involvement in health planning activities can be exciting and rewarding. Nurses are increasingly recognizing the importance of actively participating on health planning teams and engaging in political activities aimed at changing health policy.

A View *from the* Field

DE MADRES A MADRES: A COMMUNITY PARTNERSHIP FOR HEALTH

Joan Mahon, M.S., R.N., Judith McFarlane, R.N., Dr.P.H., and Katherine Golden, B.S.N., R.N.

Abstract To increase the number of Hispanic women who begin early prenatal care, a community partnership for health was initiated among the general public, businesses, 14 volunteer mothers, and one community health nurse. Volunteer mothers living in the targeted community were taught how to identify Hispanic women at risk for not starting early prenatal care, and how to provide social support and community resource information within a culturally acceptable milieu. At the end of the first year of the partnership, over 2000 women at risk for not starting early prenatal care had been contacted by the volunteer mothers.

As a single teenage mother, I felt alone and frightened when I was pregnant. I asked myself what I was going to do, how I would manage, where I could go for help, and who would help me. Women in my community need information and support during pregnancy.
—19-year-old single parent and volunteer mother in de Madres a Madres

A NATIONAL DISGRACE

Almost 40,000 infants die each year before their first birthday due to low birth weight. The cost of intensive care, special education, and social services for these infants and their families can average $400,000 over the children's life. In comparison, the cost of routine prenatal care is $400 (American Public Health Association, 1989a). The Surgeon General's goal for the nation was that by 1990, 90% of all pregnant women would begin prenatal care within the first three months of pregnancy (USDHHS, 1980). Based on the 1978-1986 rate of progress, however, the nation will not meet this goal until the year 2094, 100 years after the target date (Children's Defense Fund, 1989). As reported by the American Public Health Association (1989b), maternal and infant health has clearly suffered and markedly declined in recent years, as chronicled by 12 key indicators, including prenatal care, rates of low birth weight, and infant mortality.

A WIDENING MINORITY GAP

Compounding the problem are major disparities between the maternal and infant health of white and minority Americans (USDHHS, 1989). Between 1984 and 1985 there was no improvement in the proportion of infants with low birth weight. Among black and nonwhite infants, the frequency of low birth weight increased (Children's Defense Fund, 1989).

Low birth weight, infant mortality, and pregnancy complications are clearly associated with inadequate prenatal care. To improve access to prenatal care, the National Institute of Medicine (1988) set forth a seminal document detailing demographic risk factors associated with insufficient prenatal care, barriers to the use of prenatal care, and recommendations to improve the use of prenatal care. The report profiled Hispanic women as substantially less likely than non-Hispanic white mothers to begin prenatal care early, and 3 times as likely to obtain late or no care. Moreover, Hispanic mothers as a group are more likely than non-Hispanic black mothers to begin prenatal care late or not at all. Clearly, when compared to non-Hispanic white and black women, Hispanic women are at far greater risk to not receiving early prenatal care; many receive no prenatal care. In addition to minority status, age is a major indicator, with teenagers and mothers over age 40 years being at highest risk of receiving late or no prenatal care. Women with less than a high school education are also at

From *Publ Health Nurs* 8(1):15-19. © 1991 Blackwell Scientific Publications, Inc. Reprinted by permission of Blackwell Scientific Publications, Inc.

Address correspondence to Judith McFarlane, R.N., Professor and Director, de Madres a Madres: A Community Partnership for Health, Texas Woman's University, College of Nursing, 1130 M.C. Anderson Boulevard, Houston, TX 77030.
Joan Mahon is the clinical nurse associate with de Madres a Madres and Katherine Golden is research associate. Both are at Texas Woman's University.

This program was aided by grant CHE-255 from the Texas Gulf Coast Chapter, March of Dimes Birth Defects Foundation.

Continued

A View from the Field: de Madres a Madres: A Community Partnership for Health—cont'd

increased risk. Finally, poverty was cited as one of the most important correlates of insufficient prenatal care.

In Houston, the fourth largest city in the nation, the minority health gap is widening. According to the latest figures from the City of Houston Health Department (1988), 68.6% of pregnant women initiate prenatal care during the first trimester; for Hispanic women the figure falls to 60.4%. Stated another way, 40% of the Hispanic women in Houston do not receive early prenatal care. The 1989-1990 Texas State Health Plan designated access to prenatal and maternity care for low-income pregnant women in Texas as the top priority issue. Texas accounts for 8% of all births nationally. Nearly 1 in every 12 infants in this country who died in 1985 was a Texas resident (Texas Department of Health, 1988). Improving birth outcomes in the state would have a major impact on meeting the Surgeon General's goals for the nation.

CULTURALLY RELEVANT SOCIAL SUPPORT AND INFORMATION TO FACILITATE EARLY PRENATAL CARE

With the Hispanic woman at high risk for not receiving early prenatal care, innovative approaches to provide access to care are essential. Barriers were well defined and verified by the National Institute of Medicine (1988) as sociodemographic (age, education, parity), system access (transportation, clinic availability, insurance), and cultural-personal (fear, stress, depression, denial). To mitigate barriers to prenatal care, de Madres a Madres: A Community Partnership for Health was initiated in a Hispanic community. (De Madres a Madres means "from mothers to mothers.")

The program is a collaborative effort among the general public, businesses, and volunteer mothers to identify Hispanic women at risk for not starting early prenatal care. Other objectives are to provide social support and information on community resources within a culturally acceptable framework. The value of social support in promoting a healthy pregnancy is well supported in the literature (Nuckolls, Cassel, & Kaplan, 1972; Norbeck & Tilden, 1983; Omer et al., 1987; Gray, 1987; American Nurses Association, 1987). The use of lay volunteers and paraprofessionals to offer education and support services in the home setting to pregnant women is also widely reported in the literature (National Institute of Medicine, 1988; Heins, Nance, & Ferguson, 1987; Olds et al., 1986). The conceptual basis for the program was drawn directly from a community as client model (Anderson and McFarlane, 1988). An analysis of each community system was completed to yield community strengths and portals for intervention as well as identify community leaders and levers for change. Community as client information was used to strategize planning, implementation, and evaluation of the de Madres a Madres program.

The pregnant women in all cited studies received intensive social support by volunteers or lay professionals after they initiated prenatal care in a clinic setting, which for most was in the second or third trimester. No program has been reported to date that offers targeted support and information to high-risk women before they enter the health care system. De Madres a Madres proposed culturally relevant social support and community resource information to identified at-risk women before they entered the system. The premise was that culturally relevant social support coupled with community resource information would enable pregnant women to transcend barriers to early prenatal care.

The program will be evaluated by the number of women who begin early prenatal care before as compared to after implementation of the program. The percentage of pregnant women who obtain early prenatal care at the neighborhood health clinic, located within the target community and the only provider of public prenatal care, will be evaluated for the two years of the program and compared to a two-year period before the program was initiated. Additional variables include the number of at-risk women visited by the volunteer mothers, and the number of health and social service referrals completed by the volunteer mothers. Finally, structured interviews of at-risk women who are assisted by the volunteer mothers will be used to evaluate the program. Requirements for the volunteer mothers include residence in the community, at least 18 years of age, and completion of an eight-hour training program offered by the community health nurse. Community awareness, involvement, commitment, and ownership are the essential program elements.

Community Awareness and Recruitment of Volunteer Mothers

Begun in 1989 and funded by a two-year community service grant from the local chapter of the March of Dimes, de Madres a Madres employed one master's-prepared community health nurse (CHN). Based on the fact that Houston's Hispanic women are the least likely to obtain early prenatal care, an inner-city Hispanic community was selected by the March of Dimes for program implementation. This community has a population of 13,555, of which 34% are women of childbearing age. Median family income is $12,782, and 19% of the households receive public assistance. The CHN completed a community assessment that identified 31 key community leaders.

The 31 community leaders, many of whom were Hispanic, included school principals, the clergy, civic leaders, attorneys, social service administrators, a state representative, health care providers, elected city council represen-

A View from the Field — DE MADRES A MADRES: A COMMUNITY PARTNERSHIP FOR HEALTH—cont'd

tatives, school board members, and law enforcement officers. Most were visited individually several times. The objectives and purpose of the program were explained during each visit. Each community leader was asked for names of potential volunteer mothers. (Since most community leaders were men, sharing the names of women yielded an endorsement for the program from the male hierarchy.)

Simultaneously, the CHN made formal presentations about the program at scheduled community functions, including school meetings, civic association gatherings, church functions, and crime-prevention meetings. At least 100 people attended most formal meetings and learned about de Madres a Madres. In addition, informal presentations were made by the community health nurse at community health fairs, school-sponsored fiestas, and church-supported bazaars and social events.

The CHN assimilated herself into community activities, and on a typical day might begin by visiting with a cluster of women at the local bakery to learn of their concerns during pregnancy and perceived barriers to care. The next stop might be a discussion with the school nurse regarding how the de Madres a Madres program could be integrated into the nurse's regularly scheduled group meeting with pregnant teens. Then on to churches in the area to meet with lay groups of volunteer women interested in outreach and community service. The evening might consist of making a formal presentation on the program at a neighborhood meeting to prevent crime, followed by informal chats with women interested in becoming volunteer mothers.

The community assessment and establishment of trust between the CHN and residents was the lengthiest phase of the program. It was quickly learned that, although most of the 13,000 residents were considered of Hispanic ethnicity, the residents segregated themselves by nation of birth. For example, second-generation Mexican-Americans would not associate with the newly immigrated Mexicans, and neither group would mingle with Guatemalans, El Salvadorans, or Nicaraguans. Values, beliefs, and health practices were nationality specific. It was necessary to recruit volunteer mothers from each group. In addition to nation of origin, immigration status differed widely and was a definite barrier to prenatal care. Women in the amnesty program were at highest risk of not receiving prenatal care and, like teen mothers, required special efforts on the part of the volunteer mothers and CHN.

Community Commitment and Involvement

At the end of nine months, 14 volunteer mothers had completed the eight-hour training session with the CHN. They ranged in age from 19 to 65 years, had experienced roles from teenage mother to grandmother, and, because of their positions in the community, came into daily contact with women at risk for not starting early prenatal care. The women met in small groups for two hours and were guided through information on the importance of early prenatal care, how to identify women at risk for not starting early care, resources for pregnant women, and effective supportive communication skills. The mothers learned and shared their perceptions of the many barriers to obtaining care during pregnancy. Information was provided on how effective listening and social support can decrease isolation and enable pregnant women to obtain resources and early prenatal care. The volunteer mothers learned how to be advocates for healthy pregnancies. The following is an outline of the curriculum.

A. Role as advocate
   1. Overview of de Madres a Madres: A Community Partnership for Health
   2. Importance of volunteer neighborhood mothers
   3. Volunteer role in the home and the community
B. Resources in the community
   1. Health, food, job training, education, financial aid, transportation, housing
C. Communication/support techniques
   1. Development of trust; use of empathy; verbal skills relating to trust and empathy
   2. Nonverbal skills relating to trust and empathy; use of touch
D. Effective supportive communication skills
   1. Techniques for effective communication; barriers to communication; ways of facilitating communication
E. Aspects of quality prenatal care
   1. Places to receive prenatal care; probable cost; what the visit will entail; outcome of good prenatal care; maternal complications from lack of prenatal care; ambivalence about pregnancy and fears of prenatal care
F. Health resources (detailed description)
   1. Agencies offering prenatal care; eligibility requirements; how agencies coordinate care
G. Low-birth-weight infants, known causes
   1. Prenatal care
   2. Nutrition
   3. Substance abuse
   4. Stress (battering)
H. Family dynamics, interpersonal relationships
   1. Supportive family relationships
   2. Spousal abuse
I. Importance of social support, effects of stress on pregnancy
   1. Methods to decrease stress and increase problem solving skills

Continued

A View from the Field — DE MADRES A MADRES: A COMMUNITY PARTNERSHIP FOR HEALTH—cont'd

2. Effective listening; decreasing isolation; guiding to proper resources; role modeling
3. Increasing mother's self-worth

Strategies for presenting the curriculum varied. Some of the content was taught during a visit to the local hospital's intensive care unit for low-birth-weight infants. Other sessions focused on role playing and group sharing of experiences. Guest speakers discussed how to obtain health and social services programs for pregnant women. Volunteers who completed the training program were given a tote bag with the program name and logo. They proudly carried the bag daily and turned queries about the logo into discussion sessions about the program with colleagues at work as well as the general public.

A great deal of camaraderie developed among the volunteer mothers, who established a strong social support network for each other. Such group support was essential for the successful coping of these volunteers as they assisted women in dire circumstances. The mothers met regularly with the CHN to discuss their experiences and plans for community events, and receive additional and updated information. They also met informally as a group and began to establish an organizational infrastructure with leadership positions.

Because these mothers were of the same culture and spoke the same language as women in their community, information was offered in a culturally acceptable milieu. Methods of providing the information varied. One mother invited women into her home to discuss concerns and community resources for a healthy pregnancy. Others visited women in their homes. Several of them were present at the food pantry in the community where they offered social support and community resource information with 75 to 100 women weekly. Many of the women who frequented the pantry were undocumented residents and unaware of how to obtain care for their pregnancy without fear of reprisal.

Although the fact of pregnancy is frequently obvious, exact status was not solicited. The basic premise of de Madres a Madres is primary prevention. If at-risk women are offered culturally relevant information, they will be able to use it when a pregnancy is confirmed. It also was assumed that mothers would share the information with family and friends, creating a ripple effect of information throughout the community. The volunteer mothers were taught that information is empowering and contact is success. The at-risk women would choose when and how to use the information.

The volunteer mothers planned and implemented several community-wide events to share information, including a de Madres a Madres party for all women in the community and an information booth at community functions. A brochure that included community resources and a video about the program were developed for use by the volunteers. A small purse mirror with community resource numbers was given to all mothers visited by the volunteers.

A COMMUNITY PARTNERSHIP FOR HEALTH

Community ownership follows community awareness, involvement, and commitment. To facilitate community ownership, the second year of the de Madres a Madres program will focus on strengthening involvement of the business community, including financial support for the program. The CHN will assist the community in exploring sources for continuation funding, including the United Way and Hispanic Chamber of Commerce. A community advisory board will be formed, with representatives from business, community leaders, and volunteer mothers. A task of the board will be to assume future direction and support mechanisms for the program.

After the first year of the program, more than 2000 at-risk women had received information from a volunteer mother. The type of woman seen daily is exemplified by Olivia.

Olivia, age 21, was five months pregnant and a recent immigrant to Houston. She did not speak English and had not begun prenatal care. After seeing a notice about a de Madres a Madres event, she walked the one mile to the neighborhood elementary school where the program was being held. At the event, Olivia learned about community resources including the location of the prenatal clinic and health and social service agencies. A volunteer mother arranged to visit her the next day. During the home visit, Olivia stated that she was in need of basic food staples for her family, and that her husband was physically abusive. The volunteer mother offered information about the shelter for battered women, location of neighborhood food pantries, and eligibility requirements for specific health and social services. After contact with the volunteer mother, Olivia initiated prenatal care, enrolled in the Women, Infants, and Children (WIC) program, and received weekly food staples from the neighborhood pantry.

Maternal and child health is essential for a healthy and prosperous community. De Madres a Madres developed a community support network to form a partnership of the general public, businesses, and volunteer mothers to protect and promote the health of pregnant women. When a volunteer mother with two children who works full time was asked why she donated her time, her reply was quick and sure, "Why would I not help these women? This community is my home. I care about these women."

Article References

American Nurses' Association. (1987). *Access to prenatal care: Key to preventing low birthweight*. Kansas City, MO: Author.

A View from the Field: DE MADRES A MADRES: A COMMUNITY PARTNERSHIP FOR HEALTH—cont'd

American Public Health Association. (1989a). The nation's health [editorial] Washington, D.C.: Author.

American Public Health Association. (1989b). *Monitoring children's health: Key indicators*. Washington, D.C.: Author.

Anderson, E., & McFarlane, J. (1988). *Community as client. Application of the nursing process*. Philadelphia: J.B. Lippincott.

Children's Defense Fund. (1989). *The health of American's children. Maternal and child health data book*. New York: Author.

City of Houston Health Department. (1988) *The health of Houston 1984-1986*. Houston: Author.

Gray, L. (1987). A descriptive study on perceived social support among clients assessed by public health nurses. Unpublished thesis, Texas Woman's University, Houston, Texas.

Heins, H.C., Nance, N.W., & Ferguson, J.E. (1987). Social support in improving perinatal outcome: The resource mothers program. *Obstetrics and Gynecology*, 70:263-266.

National Institute of Medicine. (1988). *Prenatal Care: Reaching Mothers, Reaching Infants*. Washington, D.C.: National Academy Press.

Norbeck, J.S.., & Tilden, V.P. (1983). Life stress, social support, and emotional disequilibrium in complications of pregnancy: A prospective multivariate study. *Journal of Health and Social Behavior*, 24, 30-46.

Nuckolls, K.B., Cassel, J., & Kaplan, B.H. (1972). Psychosocial assets, life crises and the prognosis of pregnancy. *American Journal of Epidemiology*, 95, 431-441.

Olds, D.L., Henderson, C.R., Tatelbaum, R., & Chamberlin, R. (1986). Improving the delivery of prenatal care and outcomes of pregnancy: A randomized trial of nurse home visitation. *Pediatrics*, *77*, 16-28.

Omer, H., Elizur,V., Barnea, T., Friedlander, D., & Palti, Z. (1987). Psychological variables and premature labour: A possible solution for some methodological problems. *Journal of Psychosomatic Research*, 30, 559-565.

Texas Department of Health. (1988). *1989-90 Texas state health plan*. Texas Statewide Health Coordinating Council. Austin: Author.

U.S. Department of Health and Human Services. (1980). *Promoting health/preventing disease: Objectives for the nation*. Washington, D.C.: Government Printing Office.

U.S. Department of Health and Human Services. (1989). *Health, United States, 1988*. Washington, D.C.: Government Printing Office.

CRITICAL *Thinking Exercise*

The View From the Field (Mahon J, McFarlane J, Golden K: de Madres a Madres: a community partnership for health, *Public Health Nurs* 8[1]:15-19, 1991) describes how community health nurses used the health care planning process to begin solving the problem of lack of prenatal care in an aggregate at risk. "Since the beginning of the program in 1989, not one low-birthweight baby has been born to a woman followed by a volunteer mother" (McFarlane, 1996, p. 880). Analyze how the concepts of community empowerment and education were used in the program. What changes would you make to increase community involvement in the program?

REFERENCES

American Nurses Association (ANA): *Nursing's social policy statement*, Washington, D.C., 1995, American Nurses Publishing.

American Public Health Association (APHA): *Public health in a reformed health care system: a vision for the future*, Washington, D.C., 1993, APHA.

American Public Health Association (APHA), Public Health Nursing Section: *The definition and role of public health nursing: a statement of APHA Public Health Nursing Section*, Washington, D.C., 1996, APHA.

Aubel J, Samba-Ndure K: Community participation: lessons on sustainability for community health projects, *World Health Forum* 17:52-57, 1996.

Bergwall DF, Reeves PN, Woodside NB: *Introduction to health planning*, Washington, D.C., 1973, Information Resources Press.

Berkowitz B: Health system reform: a blueprint for the future of public health, *J Public Health Management Pract* 1:1-6, 1995.

Brown ER: Community action for health promotion: a strategy to empower individuals and communities, *Int J Health Services* 21(3):441-456, 1991.

Bureau of Primary Health Care, USDHHS: *The working group on homeless health outcomes, meeting proceedings*, Rockville, Md., June 1996, The Bureau.

Centers for Disease Control and Prevention (CDC): *CDC vision: healthy people in a healthy world through prevention*, Atlanta, 1995, CDC.

Centers for Disease Control and Prevention (CDC): *A guide for establishing public health priorities*, Atlanta, undated, CDC.

Checkoway B: Community-based initiatives to improve health of the elderly, *Danish Medical Bulletin*, Special Supplement Series No. 6:30-36, 1988.

Children's Defense Fund (CDF): *The state of America's children year book 1996*, Washington, D.C., 1996, The Author.

Conley E: Public health nursing within core public health functions: "back to the future," *J Public Health Management Pract* 1:1-8, 1995.

Courtney R: Community partnership primary care: a new paradigm for primary care, *Public Health Nurs* 12:366-373, 1995.

Courtney R, Ballard E, Fauver S et al: The partnership model: working with individuals, families, and communities toward a new vision of health, *Public Health Nurs* 13:177-186, 1996.

Donabedian A: *Exploration in quality assessment and monitoring*, vol 2, Ann Arbor, Mich, 1982, Health Administration Press.

Fisher JK: What kind of general practitioner for the twenty-first century? *World Health Forum* 17:178-180, 1996.

Flynn BC, Rider MS, Bailey WW: Developing community leadership in healthy cities: the Indiana model, *Nurs Outlook* 40(3):121-126, 1992.

Flynn BC, Ray DW, Rider MS: Empowering communities: action research through Healthy Cities, *Health Ed* 21:395-405, 1994.

Freudenberg N, Eng E, Flay B et al: Strengthening individual and community capacity to prevent disease and promote health: in search of relevant theories and principles, *Health Educ Q* 22:290-306, 1995.

General Accounting Office (GAO): *Block grants: characteristics, experience, and lessons learned*, Washington, D.C., 1995a, GAO.

General Accounting Office (GAO): *Community development: comprehensive approaches address multiple needs but are challenging to implement*, Washington, D.C., 1995b, GAO.

General Accounting Office (GAO): *Community health centers: challenges in transitioning to prepaid managed care*, Washington, D.C., 1995c, GAO.

Goeppinger J, Lassiter PG, Wilcox B: Community health is community competence, *Nurs Outlook* 30:464-467, 1982.

Graham KY: Health care reform and public health nursing, *Public Health Nurs* 9:6, 73, 1992.

Green A: *An introduction to health planning in developing countries*, New York, 1992, Oxford University Press.

Institute of Medicine (IOM): *The future of public health*, Washington, D.C., 1988, National Academy Press.

Institute of Medicine (IOM): *Healthy People 2000: citizens chart the course*, Washington, D.C., 1990, National Academy Press.

Joint Commission on Accreditation of Healthcare Organizations (JCAHO): *Quality assurance in home care and hospice organizations*, Oakbrook Terrace, Il, 1990, JCAHO.

Kickbusch I, Draper R, O'Neill M: Healthy public policy: a strategy to implement the Health for All philosophy at various governmental levels. In Evers W, Farrant W, Trojan A eds., *Healthy public policy at the local level*, Boulder, Colorado, 1990, Westview Press.

Kreuter MW: PATCH: its origin, basic concepts and links to contemporary public health policy, *J Health Educ* 23(3):135-139, 1992.

Marin G, Burhansstipanov L, Connell C et al: A research agenda for health education among underserved populations, *Health Educ Q* 22:346-363, 1995.

McFarlane J: De Madres a Madres: an access model for primary care, *Am J Public Health* 86:879-880, 1996.

Mahon J, McFarlane J, Golden K: De Madres a Madres: a community partnership for health, *Public Health Nurs* 8(1):15-19, 1991.

Mariano C: The call for interdisciplinary collaboration, *Nurs Outlook* 37(6):285-288, 1989.

Moccia P: Reclaiming our communities, *Nurs Outlook* 38(2):73-76, 1990.

National Academy of Sciences, Institute of Medicine: *Health planning in the United States: issues in guidelines development*, Washington, D.C., 1980, The National Academy.

National Commission on Community Health Services: *Health is a community affair*, Cambridge, Ma., 1966, Harvard University Press.

National League for Nursing (NLN): *A vision for nursing education*, New York, 1993, NLN.

News: In a first, Texas elects a nurse legislator to Congress, *Am J Nurs* 92(12):71, 80, 1992.

Oberle MW, Baker EL, Magenheim MJ: Healthy People 2000 and community health planning, *Annu Rev Publ Health* 15:259-275, 1994.

O'Neil EH: *Health professionals education for the future: schools in service to the nation*, San Francisco, Ca., 1993, Pew Health Professions Commission.

Pew Health Professions Commission: *Critical challenges: revitalizing the health professions for the twenty-first century*, San Francisco, 1995, UCSF Center for the Health Professions.

Pickett GE, Hanlon JJ: *Public health administration and practice*, ed 9, St. Louis, 1990, Mosby.

Randall-David E: *Culturally competent HIV counseling and education*, McLean, Va., 1994, Maternal and Child Health Clearing House.

Reeves PN, Coile RC: *Introduction to health planning*, ed 4, Arlington, Va., 1989, Information Resources Press.

Resources for Human Development, Inc. and Abottsford Homes Tenant Management Corporation: *Project abstract*, Philadelphia, undated, The Corporation.

Rojas-Urruita X, Aday LS: A framework for community assessment: designing and conducting a survey in a Hispanic immigrant and refugee community, *Public Health Nurs* 8(1):20-25, 1991.

Scherl D, Noren J, Osterweis M: *Promoting health and preventing disease*, Washington, D.C., 1992, Association of Academic Health Centers.

Schlaff AL: Boston's Codman Square community partnership for health promotion, *Public Health Reports* 106(2):186-191, 1991.

Sen R: Building community involvement in health care, *Social Policy* 24:32-43, 1994.

Shugars DA, O'Neil EH, Bader JD, eds: *Healthy America: practitioners for 2005, an agenda for action for U.S. health professional schools*, Durham, N.C., 1991, The Pew Health Professions Commission.

St. Leger AS, Schnieden H, Walsworth-Bell JP: *Evaluating health services' effectiveness: a guide for health professionals, service managers and policy makers*, Philadelphia, 1992, Open University Press.

Stoto MA: Public health assessment in the 1990s, *Annu Rev Publ Health* 13:59-78, 1992.

Timmreck T: *Planning, program development, and evaluation: a handbook for health promotion, aging, and health services*, Boston, Ma., 1995, Jones & Bartlett.

U.S. Department of Health and Human Services (USDHHS): *Healthy People 2000: national health promotion and disease prevention objectives, full report, with commentary*, Washington, D.C., 1991, U.S. Government Printing Service.

U.S. Department of Health and Human Services (USDHHS): *Healthy People 2000: midcourse review and 1995 revisions*, Washington, D.C., 1995, U.S. Government Printing Office.

Wald L: *The house on Henry street*, New York, 1915, Henry Holt.

SELECTED BIBLIOGRAPHY

American Nurses Association (ANA): *Community-based nursing services: innovative models*, Kansas City, Mo., 1986, ANA.

Anderson ET, McFarlane J: *Community as partner: theory and practice in nursing*, ed 2, Philadelphia, 1996, Lippincott.

Battista RN, Lawrence RS, eds: *Implementing preventive services*, New York, 1988, Oxford University Press.

Bennett EJ: Health needs assessment of a rural county: impact evaluation of a student project, *Fam Community Health* 16:28-35, 1993.

Burton L: *The ethical dilemmas of the Oregon Health Plan*, *Nurs Pract*, 21:62-72, 1996.

Butterfoss FD, Goodman RM, Wonderman A: Community coalitions for prevention and health promotion: factors predicting satisfaction, participation, and planning, *Health Educ Q* 21:235-252, 1994.

Coast J, Donovan J, Frankel S: *Priority setting: the health care debate*, New York, 1996, John Wiley & Sons.

Ducanis AJ, Golin AK: *The interdisciplinary health care team: a handbook*, Germantown, Md., 1979, Aspen Publishers.

Eisen A: Survey of neighborhood-based, comprehensive community empowerment initiatives, *Health Educ Q* 21:235-252, 1994

Evers A, Farrant W, Trojan A, eds: *Healthy public policy at the local level*, Boulder, 1990, Westview Press.

Halbert TL, Underwood JE, Chambers LW et al: Population-based health promotion: a new agenda for public health nurses, *Can J Public Health* 84:243-249, 1993.

Hale CD, Arnold F, Travis MT: *Planning and evaluating health programs: a primer*, Albany, 1994, Delmar.

McKenzie JF, Smeltzer JL: *Planning, implementing, and evaluating health promotion programs: a primer*, ed 2, Boston, 1997, Allyn & Bacon.

Navarro U: Why some countries have national health insurance, others have national health services, and the United States has neither, *Int J Health Services* 19:384-404, 1989.

Pederson A, O'Neill M, Rootman I: *Health promotion in Canada: provincial, national and international perspectives*, Toronto, 1994, W.B. Saunders Canada.

Pirie PL, Stone EJ, Assaf AR et al: Program evaluation strategies for community-based health promotion programs: perspectives from the cardiovascular disease community research and demonstration studies, *Health Educ Res* 9:23-36, 1994.

Steckler A, Allegrante JP, Altman D et al: Health education intervention strategies: recommendations for future research, *Health Educ Q* 22:307-328, 1995.

Winkelstein W: Determinants of worldwide health, *Am J Publ Health* 82(7):931-932, 1992.

Needs and Services of Children from Birth to 5 Years

Objectives

Upon completion of this chapter, the reader should be able to:

1. Describe U.S. trends in infant and maternal mortality and why health care professionals are concerned about these trends.
2. Discuss the *Healthy People 2000* maternal and infant health objectives.
3. Discuss the leading causes of mortality among infants and children 1 to 5 years of age.
4. Analyze factors associated with high-risk pregnancies and births.
5. Discuss common health risks for infants and children 1 to 5 years of age.
6. Analyze health promotion needs of families with children in the newborn to 5-year-old age group and community health nursing interventions to address these needs.
7. Discuss significant legislation that has influenced maternal and child health care delivery.
8. Describe barriers to the delivery of services to the newborn to 5-year-old population and their parents.
9. Identify the roles assumed by the community health nurse to promote maternal, infant, and child health.

Stand for Children: Leave No Child Behind

CHILDREN'S DEFENSE FUND, 1996, P. IX

On June 1, 1996, parents, grandparents, religious and civic community leaders, advocates for children, and concerned citizens converged upon Washington, D.C. to take a "*Stand For All Children.*" This national mobilization effort was a day of spiritual, family, and community renewal and personal commitment to children. At the Lincoln Memorial, masses of people from communities nationwide stood united in their commitment to help all children have a healthy start, a head start, a fair start, a safe start, and a moral start (Children's Defense Fund, 1996). This national day for children was a day for speaking out against violence, child abuse and neglect, poverty, disparities in health care and health status, and political and socioeconomic forces that contribute to family and community stress and crisis. It was a day for sharing the fact that it is no longer acceptable for even one child to suffer from life's hardships.

INFANT AND MATERNAL HEALTH: A SIGNIFICANT INDICATOR OF A NATION'S HEALTH STATUS

The importance of infant and maternal mortality rates as significant indicators of a nation's health status is well documented in the literature (Hargraves, Thomas, 1993; Maternal and Child Health Bureau, 1996; Singh, Yu, 1995; WHO, 1995). These rates are used worldwide as global indicators of the health status of the population as a whole because they are closely related to socioeconomic and environmental conditions. A nation's maternal and infant mortality rates are a measure of its success in combating poverty, ignorance, and disease (Mason, 1991).

Worldwide, maternal death rates range from approximately 520 per 100,000 live births to less than 10 per 100,000, and infant death rates range from 112 per 1000 live births to 7 per 1000. As would be expected, the highest death rates are in the least developed countries, such as those in Africa and southeast Asia (WHO, 1995).

At the beginning of the century, maternal mortality rates in the United States mirrored those currently seen in developing countries. In 1935, the year when Title V of the Social Security Act was passed to improve the health of all mothers and children in the nation, the maternal mortality rate was 582 deaths per 100,000 live births, and the infant mortality rate was almost 56 deaths per 1000 live births (Maternal and Child Health Bureau, 1996). Statistics such as these motivated concerned individuals to develop community-based maternal and child health programs.

Nurses have assumed a major leadership role in maternal and child programming since the early 1900s (Figure 15-1).

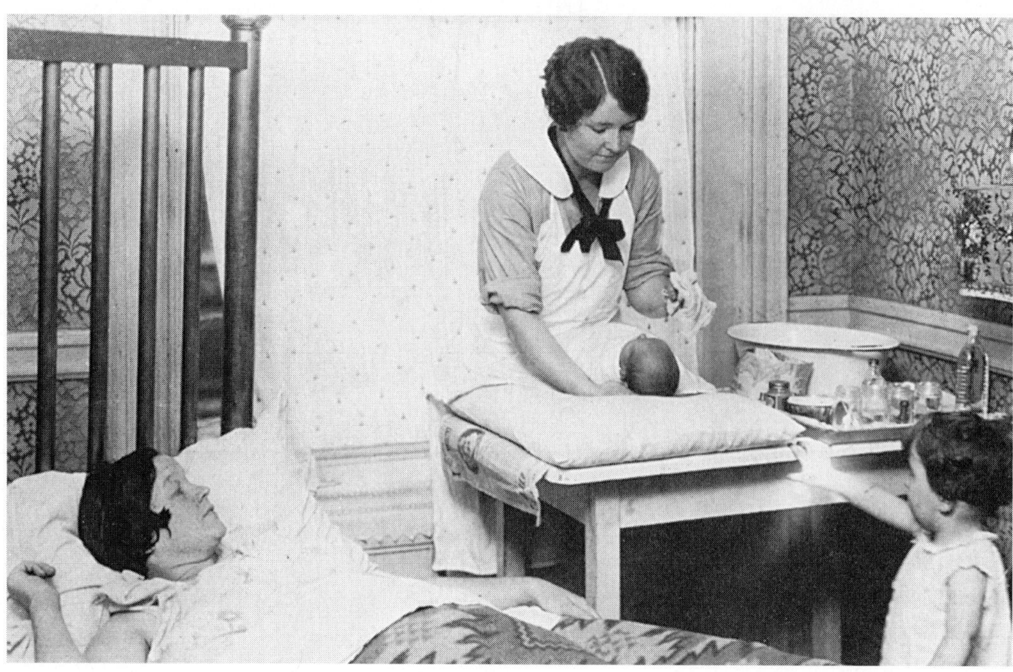

Figure 15-1 A community health nurse from the Visiting Nurse Service of New York City visits a mother with a new baby at home in the early 1930s. *(Courtesy Visiting Nurse Service of New York City.)*

Lillian Wald, the pioneer community health nurse and feminist, helped establish milk stations in 1903 at the Henry Street Settlement House in New York City to ensure the safety of milk for babies. Diarrhea caused by contaminated milk in the summer months was the cause of many deaths. The City of New York followed this example and in 1911 authorized the establishment of 15 milk stations:

> A nurse is attached to each station to follow into the homes and there lay the foundation, through education, for hygienic living. A marked reduction in infant mortality has been brought about and moreover, a realization, on the part of the city, of the immeasurable social and economic value of keeping the babies alive. (Wald, 1915, p. 57)

Traditionally, childbearing women, infants, and children are considered to be the most dependent and vulnerable members in a society. As the society develops there is a trend toward greater concern for this segment of the population. The health of a society's children ensures that society's future, so this concern for infants and children is justified on economic, as well as other grounds.

The vast majority of mothers and children in the United States are healthy, and successful efforts at preventing mortality and morbidity among these populations mean that there will be further improvement in their health. However, the United States cannot take its maternal and child health achievements for granted. Although infant and maternal deaths have decreased significantly over the past 60 years, our nation still has serious maternal and child health issues that need to be addressed. Maternal deaths are of concern because many of these might be preventable if the health system functioned more effectively (Maternal and Child Health Bureau, 1996, p. 11).

When the infant mortality rate for the United States is compared with the same rate in other developed countries, a striking reason is apparent why those who care about the public's health should be concerned: *this nation ranked lower than 21 other industrialized countries in 1992* (Figure 15-2). Japan has had the lowest infant mortality rate in the world since 1980. The risk of a Japanese infant dying in 1992 (the latest available data) was 55% lower than that observed in the United States (Maternal and Child Health Bureau, 1996, p. 23).

The mortality disparities among American infants (Figure 15-3) are particularly distressing to the nation. The 1993 infant mortality rate for black infants was 2.4 times the rate for white infants (Maternal and Child Health Bureau, 1996, p. 24). The proportional discrepancy between black and white rates has remained unchanged throughout the century. This discrepancy is noted in both neonatal and postneonatal mortality. Native Americans and Puerto Ricans also have infant mortality rates substantially higher than the United States average (USDHHS, 1991, 1995a). These data have provided the stimulus for the United States to increase its national efforts in the combat against infant mortality.

In 1986 the National Commission to Prevent Infant Mortality was created by Congress (PL 99-660) to establish

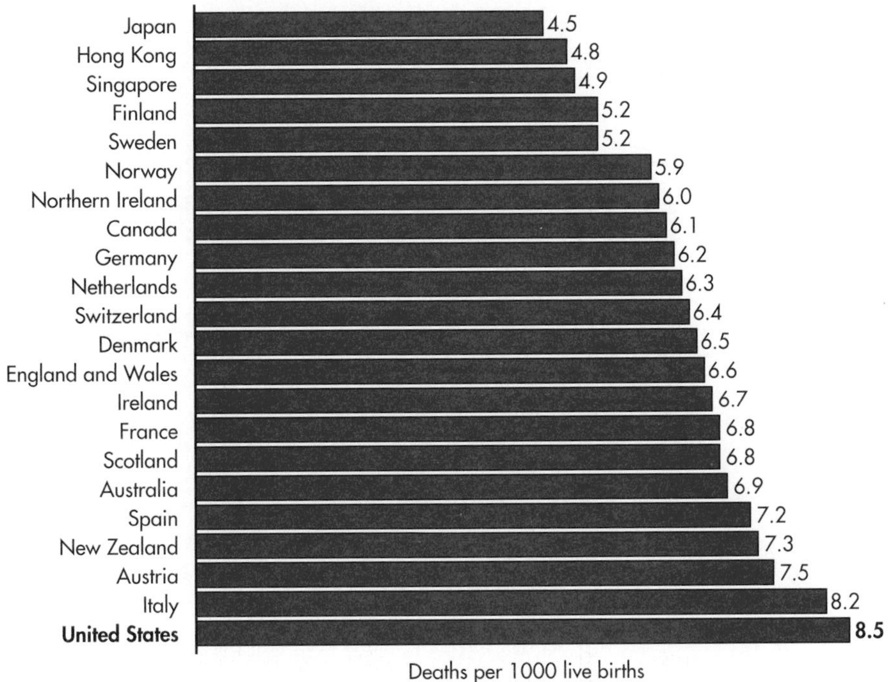

Figure **15-2** Comparison of national infant mortality rates: 1992. *(From Maternal and Child Health Bureau:* Child health USA '95, *Washington, D.C., 1996, U.S. Government Printing Office, p. 23. Source: National Center for Health Statistics.)*

a national strategic plan for reducing infant mortality and morbidity (National Commission to Prevent Infant Mortality, 1988). In its report, *Death Before Life: the Tragedy of Infant Mortality*, the commission focused on practical solutions for improving maternal and child health and identified two major goals: (1) that every pregnant woman and infant receive adequate care, the woman as soon as she knows she is pregnant and the infant from the moment of birth; and (2) that maternal and child health and well-being become a national priority (National Commission to Prevent Infant Mortality). Maternal and child health is one of the 22 priority areas identified in the *Healthy People 2000* document.

HEALTHY PEOPLE 2000: MATERNAL AND CHILD HEALTH OBJECTIVES

The *Healthy People 2000* maternal and child health objectives in the box on page 419 reflect the nation's commitment to reducing infant mortality. These objectives address the major health concerns of infants, including low birth weight, congenital anomalies, sudden infant death syndrome, and respiratory distress syndrome. They include maternal factors associated with these concerns. Special population groups are targeted, including low-income, black, American Indian/Alaskan native and Hispanic women, and black and American Indian/Alaskan native infants. Puerto Ricans were added to the special population targets during the *Healthy People 2000* midcourse review (USDHHS, 1995a).

Progress toward achieving the nation's maternal and child health objectives is mixed. Although infant mortality has reached record low levels, the proportional discrepancy between black and white rates has not changed. Additionally, the infant mortality rates among Puerto Ricans have risen, overall low birth weight and very low birth weight rates have increased, and the number of babies born with fetal alcohol syndrome has increased. Little progress has been made in promoting breast-feeding among women 5 to 6 months postpartum. Objectives moving in the right direction are improving survival for low birth weight infants, decreasing cesarean deliveries, increasing the percentage of pregnant women who abstain from tobacco, and increasing the percentage of women who breast-fed their infants during the early postpartum period. A consistent tracking data source is lacking for several objectives (USDHHS, 1995a, pp. 94-96).

National objectives for improving the health of mothers and children are focused on modifying behaviors and lifestyles that affect birth outcomes and removing financial, educational, social, and logistical barriers to care (USDHHS, 1991). The *Healthy People 2000* mandate challenges states and local communities to develop specific maternal and child health objectives and action plans to address these objectives. Problems among mothers and children will not be resolved until our nation has dedicated commitment from all state and local communities.

MATERNAL AND CHILD HEALTH CONCERNS

Improving the health of mothers, infants, and children under 5 years of age has become a national challenge

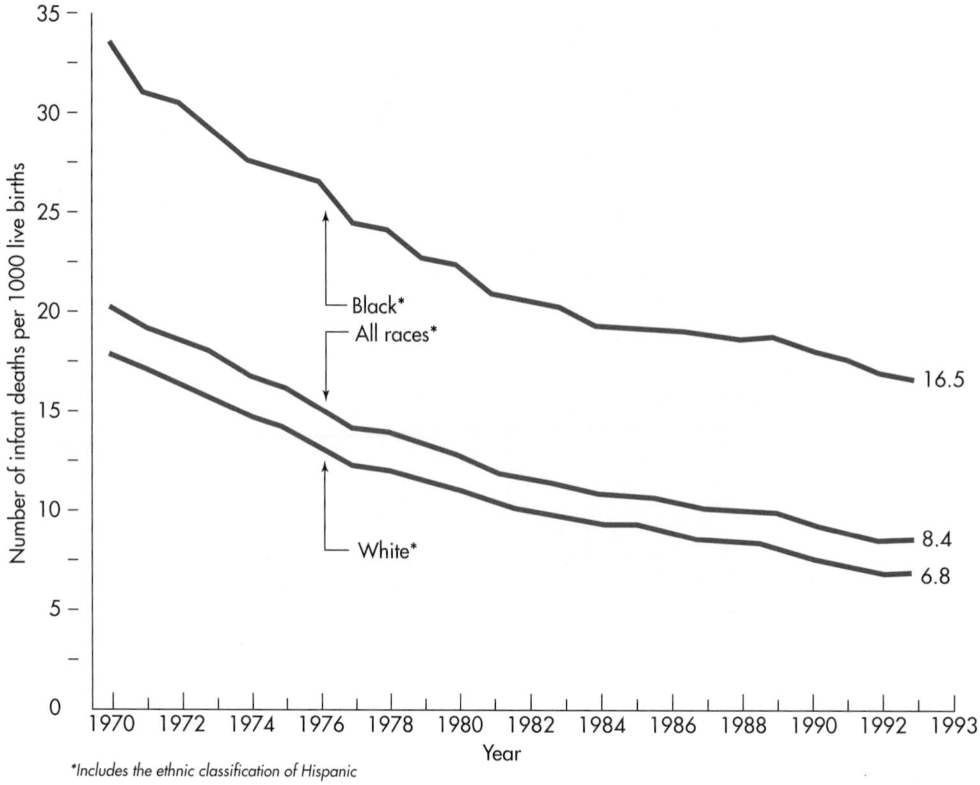

*Includes the ethnic classification of Hispanic

Figure 15-3 U.S. infant mortality rates by race of mother: 1970-1993. *(From Maternal and Child Health Bureau:* Child health USA '95, *Washington, D.C., 1996, U.S. Government Printing Office, p. 24. Source: National Center for Health Statistics.)*

(USDHHS, 1991, p. 366). Although the United States has made tremendous progress in reducing maternal and infant deaths since the turn of the century, the pace of progress in recent years has slowed. The 1995 midcourse review of the progress made toward reaching our maternal and child health goals reflects an urgent need to develop creative strategies for improving pregnancy outcomes for at-risk populations. Poor pregnancy outcomes increase the health risks for mothers as well as for infants and children.

It is clear from the literature that the problems among infants, children, and mothers in the United States are multifaceted, involving numerous complex variables, including demographic, medical, physical, environmental, educational, behavioral, and attitudinal factors, as well as the ability to receive care. It is proposed that the recent slowing of progress in reducing infant mortality is related to maternal lifestyle behaviors (e.g., use of illicit drugs) that place a mother at increased risk for poor pregnancy outcomes, the increasing rate of unintended pregnancy, and the approaching maximization of benefits in advances in neonatal intensive care (USDHHS, 1991, p. 366).

It is estimated that almost 60% of all pregnancies are unintended, either mistimed or unwanted altogether (IOM, 1995). There are several consequences of unintended pregnancy. "A woman with an unintended pregnancy is less likely to seek early prenatal care and is more likely to expose the fetus to harmful substances (such as tobacco or alcohol). The child of an unwanted conception especially (as distinct from a mistimed one) is at greater risk of being born at low birthweight, of dying in its first year of life, of being abused, and of not receiving sufficient resources for healthy development" (IOM, p. 1).

Strategies to improve pregnancy outcomes must include *preventive*, integrated efforts targeted to both the community and the individual. A dedicated national commitment to assuring adequate support to individuals and families is also needed. This support must include protection against poverty and high-quality health care (Hughes, Simpson, 1995, pp. 97-98). Chomitz, Cheung, and Lieberman (1995) believe that "pregnancy and the prospect of pregnancy provide a window of opportunity to improve a woman's health before pregnancy, during pregnancy, and after the birth of her child" (p. 132). A preventive approach to maternal and child health programming can help mothers to modify lifestyle behaviors, before and during pregnancy, that increase the risk for poor pregnancy outcomes.

Health risks to women, such as smoking, drug abuse, and environmental conditions associated with poor health, have been discussed in Chapters 12, 17, and 18. The emphasis in this chapter is on health risks common to infants

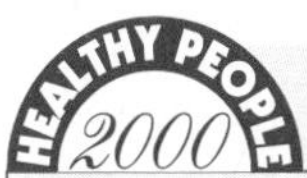

Maternal and Infant Health Objectives

HEALTH STATUS OBJECTIVES

- Reduce the infant mortality rate to no more than 7 per 1000 live births. (Baseline: 10.1 per 1000 live births in 1987)
- Reduce the fetal death rate (20 or more weeks of gestation) to no more than 5 per 1000 live births plus fetal deaths. (Baseline: 7.6 per 1000 live births plus fetal deaths in 1987)
- Reduce the maternal mortality rate to no more than 3.3 per 100,000 live births. (Baseline: 6.6 per 100,000 in 1987)
- Reduce the incidence of fetal alcohol syndrome to no more than 0.12 per 1000 live births. (Baseline: 0.22 per 1000 live births in 1987)
- Reduce low birth weight to an incidence of no more than 5% of live births and very low birth weight to no more than 1% of live births. (Baseline: 6.9% and 1.2%, respectively, in 1987)
- Increase to at least 85% the proportion of mothers who achieve the minimum recommended weight gain during their pregnancies. (Baseline: 67% of married women in 1980)
- Reduce severe complications of pregnancy to no more than 15 per 100 deliveries. (Baseline: 22 hospitalizations before delivery per 100 deliveries in 1987)
- Reduce the cesarean delivery rate to no more than 15 per 100 deliveries. (Baseline: 24.4 per 100 deliveries in 1987)
- Increase to at least 75% the proportion of mothers who breastfeed their babies in the early postpartum period and to at least 50% the proportion who continue breast-feeding until their babies are 5 to 6 months old. (Baseline: 54% during early postpartum and 21% who are still breastfeeding at 5 to 6 months in 1988)
- Increase abstinence from tobacco use by pregnant women to at least 90% and increase abstinence from alcohol, cocaine, and marijuana by pregnant women by at least 20%. (Baseline: 75% of pregnant women abstained from tobacco use in 1985)
- Increase to at least 90% the proportion of all pregnant women who receive prenatal care in the first trimester of pregnancy. (Baseline: 76% of live births in 1987)
- Increase to at least 60% the proportion of primary care providers who provide age-appropriate preconception care and counseling. (Baseline: 18% to 65% in 1992)
- Increase to at least 90% the proportion of women enrolled in prenatal care who are offered screening and counseling on prenatal detection of fetal abnormalities. (Baseline: 29% in 1988)
- Increase to at least 90% the proportion of pregnant women and infants who receive risk-appropriate care. (Baseline data unavailable)
- Increase to at least 95% the proportion of newborns screened by state-sponsored programs for genetic disorders and other disabling conditions and to 90% the proportion of newborns testing positive for disease who receive appropriate treatment. (Baseline: For sickle cell anemia, with 20 states reporting, approximately 33% of live births screened [57% of black infants]; for galactosemia, with 38 states reporting, approximately 70% of live births screened)
- Increase to at least 90% the proportion of babies aged 18 months and younger who receive recommended primary care services at the appropriate intervals. (Baseline data: unavailable)
- Reduce the incidence of spina bifida and other neural tube defects to 3 per 10,000 live births. (Baseline: 6 per 10,000 in 1990)

From USDHHS: *Healthy people 2000: national health promotion and disease prevention objectives, full report, with commentary*, Washington, D.C., 1991, U.S. Government Printing Office, pp. 110-111; USDHHS: *Healthy people 2000: midcourse review and 1995 revisions*, Washington, D.C., 1995a, U.S. Government Printing Office, pp. 226-231.

as well as to children under 5 years of age. Many of the problems among children begin before birth and extend throughout life. It is important to remember, however, that the health concerns of children cannot be examined in isolation. Socioeconomic and environmental factors, including the health status of mothers and families, significantly influence healthy or unhealthy development throughout childhood.

Morbidity and mortality among the newborn to 5-year-old population present a major public health concern. In the process of growing up, children encounter injuries and illnesses that interfere with normal functioning. Jack and Jill's broken crown and Humpty Dumpty's fall off the wall are common experiences known to every child.

There are health problems common to the newborn to 5-year-old age group that can be prevented, as well as problems that necessitate secondary and tertiary prevention. To plan health services for this group, the community health nurse should be familiar with factors that increase children's risk for morbidity and mortality. Having this knowledge facilitates application of the three levels of prevention and casefinding.

INFANT HEALTH RISKS

Figure 15-4 shows the leading causes of death for children less than a year. Almost *three quarters* of all infant deaths occur in the neonatal period—the first 28 days of life (Paneth, 1995). Major causes of neonatal mortality are congenital anomalies, disorders related to short gestation and low birth weight, respiratory distress syndrome, and maternal complications of pregnancy (Maternal and Child Health Bureau, 1996). Infants most at risk during this period are low birth weight (less than 2500 grams, or 5 pounds 8 ounces, at birth) babies, especially very low birth weight (less than 1500 grams, or 3 pounds 5 ounces, at birth) babies, and those born preterm.

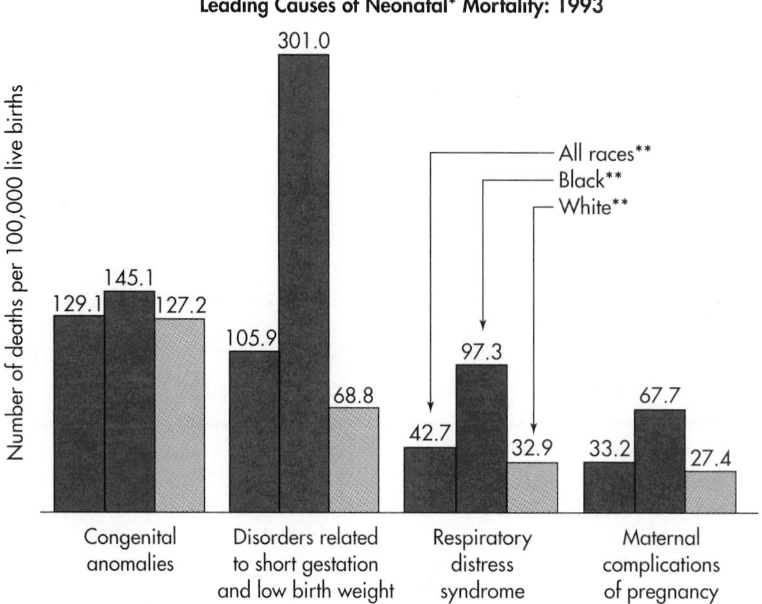

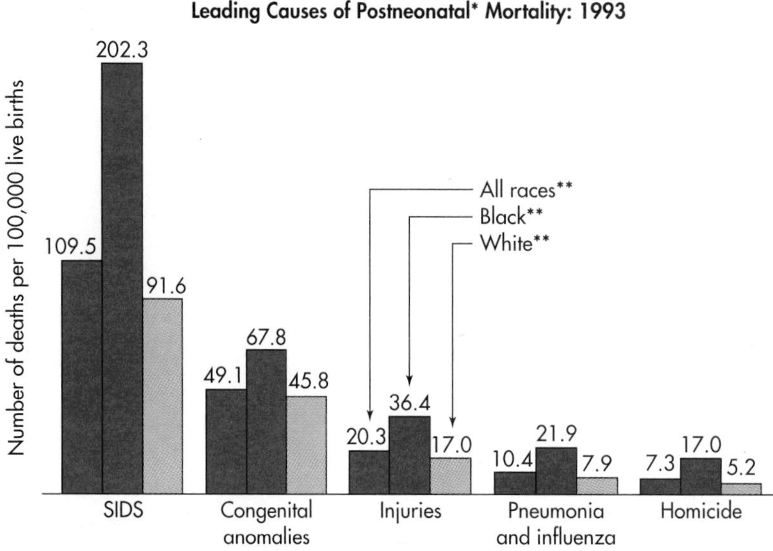

Figure 15-4 Leading causes of neonatal and postneonatal mortality: 1993. *(From Maternal and Child Health Bureau:* Child health USA '95, *Washington, D.C., 1996, U.S. Government Printing Office, p. 25. Source: National Center for Health Statistics.)*

Low birth weight and/or preterm delivery are the major factors that fuel the proportional discrepancy between black and white infant mortality rates in the United States. These factors also account for the United States' high infant mortality ranking among industrialized countries. Figure 15-5 "shows that infant mortality parallels the low birthweight rate and the preterm birth rate quite consistently in international comparisons" (Paneth, 1995, p. 22). In other words, countries that have a high proportion of low birth weight and preterm births have high infant mortality. In 1993 7.2% of all infants in the United States were born too small (Maternal and Child Health Bureau, 1996).

Congenital anomalies cause a significant number of infant deaths during both the neonatal and postneonatal periods. The most important cause of death during the postneonatal period is sudden infant death syndrome (SIDS).

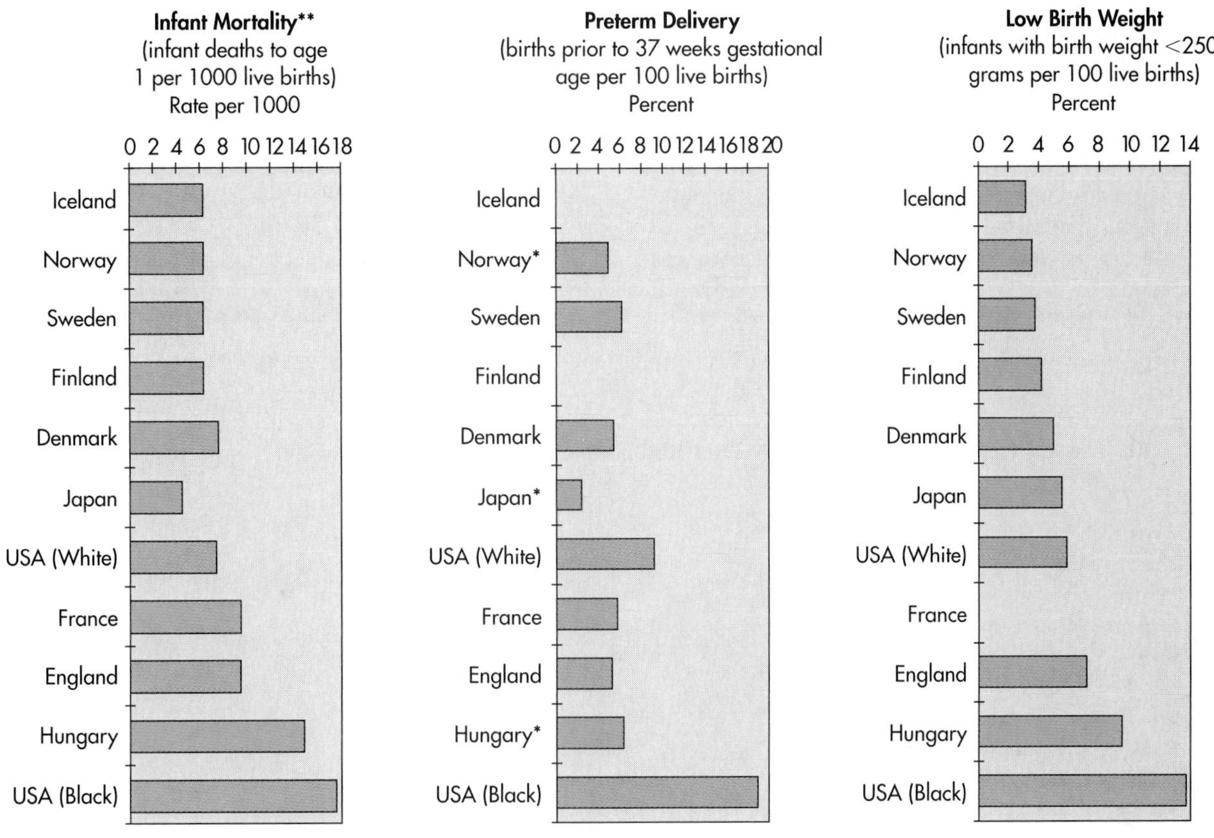

*Prior to 35 completed weeks.
**All infant mortality rates for 1991 except Finland and Hungary (1990).

Figure **15-5** International comparison of birth outcomes. *(From Paneth NS: The problem of low birthweight,* The Future of Children, *5(1):19-34, 1995, p. 23.) (Sources: Proceedings of the international collaborative effort on perinatal and infant mortality; vol III. DHHS/PHS 92-1252. Hyattsville, Md., 1992, National Center for Health Statistics; Kohler L, Jakobsson G: Children's health and well-being in the Nordic countries, London, 1987, Mac Keith; Berkowitz GS, Papiernik E: Epidemiology of preterm birth, Epidemiology Reviews 15:414-43, 1993; World Health Organization: World health statistics annual, 1991, Geneva, 1993, WHO; World Health Organization: United Nations demographic yearbook, 1986. Geneva, 1988, WHO; National Center for Health Statistics: Advance report of final natality statistics, 1991, Monthly Vital Statistics Report, Vol. 42, No. 3, Suppl. Hyattsville, Md., 1993, Public Health Service; National Center for Health Statistics: Advance report of final mortality statistics, 1991, Monthly Vital Statistics Report, Vol. 42, No. 2, Suppl. Hyattsville, Md., 1993, Public Health Service.)*

SIDS claims the lives of about 7000 infants annually (Wong, 1995).

Risks to the Infant Before Birth

Factors associated with high-risk pregnancies are displayed in the box below. These factors are important for nurses to consider during the prenatal period, because they provide the basis for the high mortality and morbidity rates during infancy and contribute to the high maternal mortality rates. They are danger signs signaling threat to the newborn and the mother. Those caring for the pregnant woman can effectively use these risk indicators to identify mothers and infants who have special needs and can benefit from preventive interventions.

Many variables influence intrauterine growth and gestational duration (Table 15-1) and infant survival. "Cigarette smoking during pregnancy, low maternal weight gain, and low prepregnancy weight account for nearly two-thirds of all growth-retarded infants" (Shiono, Behrman, 1995, p. 8). Poverty, low level of educational attainment, and minority status are also associated with risk of low birth weight (Maternal and Child Health Bureau, 1996, p. 27). As previously mentioned, the infant mortality rate for black infants is over two times the rate for white infants. Unraveling the underlying reasons for ethnic variations in pregnancy outcomes is one of the great challenges to public health research (Paneth, 1995).

"Socioeconomic status is one of the most powerful risk factors for poor health outcomes" (Hughes, Simpson, 1995, p. 88). Low socioeconomic status is associated with reduced access to health care, poor nutrition, lower education, and inadequate housing. It is also strongly linked to race, ethnicity, and unhealthy lifestyles (Hughes, Simpson).

Socially and economically deprived persons are more likely than others to have high-risk pregnancies. This is at least partially explained by the lack of adequate prenatal care, which is often unavailable to many population groups, including the inner city and rural poor, teenage mothers, and disadvantaged ethnic groups. "Risk factors for not receiving prenatal care include being less than 18 years of age,

Factors Associated with High-Risk Pregnancy

ECONOMIC

Poverty
Unemployment
Uninsured, underinsured health insurance
Poor access to prenatal care

CULTURAL-BEHAVIORAL

Low educational status
Poor health care attitudes
No care or inadequate prenatal care
Cigarette, alcohol, drug abuse
Age less than 16 or over 35 yr
Unmarried
Short interpregnancy interval
Lack of support group (husband, family, church)
Stress (physical, psychological)
Black race

BIOLOGICAL-GENETIC

Previous low birth weight infant
Low maternal weight at her birth
Low weight for height
Poor weight gain during pregnancy
Short stature
Poor nutrition
Inbreeding (autosomal recessive?)
Intergenerational effects
Hereditary diseases (inborn error of metabolism)

REPRODUCTIVE

Prior cesarean section
Prior infertility
Prolonged gestation
Prolonged labor
Prior infant with cerebral palsy, mental retardation, birth trauma, congenital anomalies
Abnormal lie (breech)
Multiple gestation
Premature rupture of membranes
Infections (systemic, amniotic, extraamniotic, cervical)
Preeclampsia or eclampsia
Uterine bleeding (abruptio placenta, placenta previa)
Parity (0 or more than 5)
Uterine or cervical anomalies
Fetal disease
Abnormal fetal growth
Idiopathic premature labor
Iatrogenic prematurity
High or low levels of maternal serum α-fetoprotein

MEDICAL

Diabetes mellitus
Hypertension
Congenital heart disease
Autoimmune disease
Sickle cell anemia
TORCH infection
Intercurrent surgery or trauma
Sexually transmitted diseases

Modified from Nelson WE, Behrman RE, Kliegman RM, Algin AM (eds): *Nelson textbook of pediatrics*, Philadelphia, 1996, Saunders, p. 440.

unmarried status, low educational attainment, and being in a minority group. Regardless of age, black women (Figure 15-6) are less likely to receive prenatal care than are white women" (Maternal and Child Health Bureau, 1996, p. 60).

Prenatal care provides a number of benefits, including the prevention of maternal deaths; education regarding pregnancy, labor and delivery, and newborn care; the potential for linking disadvantaged women to important social services; and an increased likelihood that newborns will receive needed preventive care (Shiono, Behrman, 1995, p. 13). It also provides an avenue for preventing congenital syphilis in the newborn (Millman, 1993).

"The lowest neonatal mortality rate occurs in infants of mothers who receive adequate prenatal care and who are 20 to 30 years of age" (Nelson, Behrman, Kliegman, Algin, 1996, p. 440). Numerous personal and system barriers limit participation in prenatal care (see the box on p. 425). Economic status and health insurance coverage play large roles in determining whether a woman obtains prenatal care (Brown, 1989). Nevertheless, the number of women of childbearing age without insurance is increasing, while at the same time the cost of maternity care is rising.

Shiono and Behrman (1995) and other health professionals (Alexander, Korenbrot, 1995; Johnson, Primas, Coe, 1994) believe that resources should be concentrated on improving the content and structure of prenatal and obstetric care, with an emphasis on addressing modifiable risks for low birth weight and preterm births. "The most likely known targets for prenatal interventions to prevent low birth weight rates are: (1) smoking, (2) nutrition, and (3) medical care" (Alexander, Korenbrot, 1995, p. 107).

Community-wide, well-coordinated initiatives are needed to address problems related to negative pregnancy outcomes. Since needs vary among different segments of the population, a comprehensive array of programs must be developed (Alan Guttmacher Institute, 1989; Chamberlin, 1988; National Commission to Prevent Infant Mortality, 1989). Coalition- or constituency-building among all sectors of society is a must to enhance service delivery to mothers and children. There is renewed interest in the importance of home visiting to reach geographically isolated and/or other disadvantaged groups (Chamberlin, 1988; National Commission to Prevent Infant Mortality, 1989). Home visiting activities can improve many health outcomes, including increasing attendance in cost-effective prenatal care, encouraging healthy behaviors, and discouraging harmful activities during pregnancy such as smoking and drug use (National Commission to Prevent Infant Mortality).

table 15-1 Factors Assessed for Independent Causal Impact on Intrauterine Growth and Gestational Duration

	Genetic and Constitutional	Demographic and Psychosocial	Obstetric	Nutritional	Maternal Morbidity During Pregnancy
Factors assessed	Infant sex* Racial/ethnic origin* Maternal height* Maternal prepregnancy weights‡	Maternal age†,§ Socioeconomic status†,§ Marital status Maternal psychological factors	Parity* Birth or pregnancy interval Sexual activity Intrauterine growth and gestational duration in prior pregnancies In utero exposure to diethylstilbestrol‡ Prior induced abortion Prior stillbirth or neonatal death Prior infertility Prior spontaneous abortion‡	Gestational weight gain* Vitamin B_6 Caloric intake* Energy expenditure, work, and physical activity Protein intake/status Iron and anemia Folic acid and vitamin B_{12} Calcium, phosphorus, and vitamin D Other vitamins and trace elements Zinc and copper	General morbidity and episodic illness* Malaria* Urinary tract infection Genital tract infection

From Kramer MS: The etiology and prevention of low birthweight: current knowledge and priorities for future research. In Berendes H, Kessel S, Yaffe S, eds: *Advances in the prevention of low birthweight: an international symposium*, Washington, D.C., 1991, National Center for Education in Maternal and Child Health, p. 35.

*Established direct determinants of intrauterine growth include infant sex, racial/ethnic origin, prepregnancy weight, paternal height and weight, maternal height and weight, parity, prior LBW, gestational weight gain, caloric intake, general morbidity, malaria, cigarette smoking, alcohol consumption, and tobacco chewing.

†Established indirect determinants of intrauterine growth include maternal age and socioeconomic status.

‡Factors with well-established direct causal impact on gestational duration include prepregnancy weight, prior prematurity, prior spontaneous abortion, in utero diethylstilbestrol exposure, and cigarette smoking.

§Factors with well-established indirect causal impact on gestational duration include maternal age and socioeconomic status.

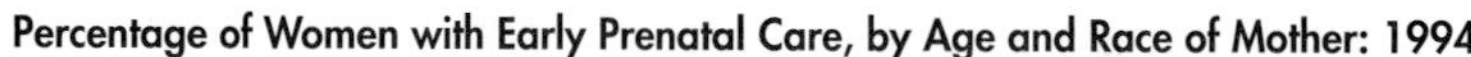

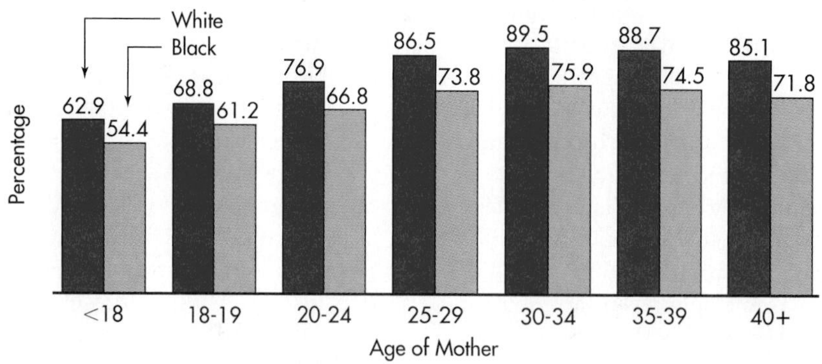

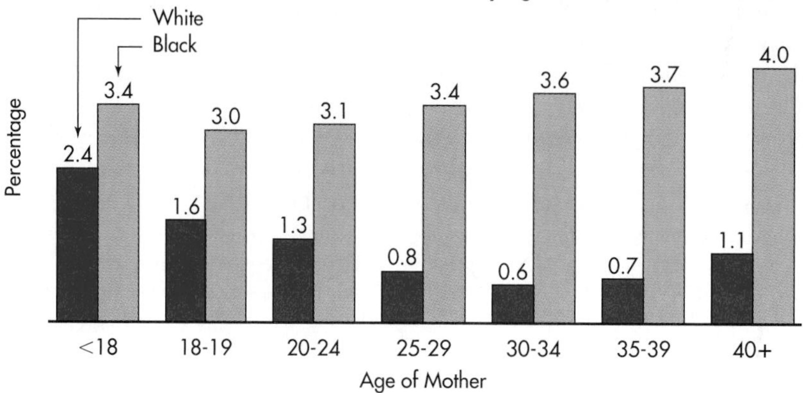

Figure 15-6 Percentage of women with early and no prenatal care, by age and race of mother: 1994. *(From Maternal and Child Health Bureau:* Child health USA '95, *Washington, D.C., 1996, U.S. Government Printing Office, p. 60.) Source: National Center for Health Statistics.*

Risks to the Infant After Birth

As previously discussed, once a baby is born, gestational age, birth weight, congenital anomalies, and the infant's environment are significant factors in the chances for survival. These factors also significantly influence the child's growth and development throughout life. For example, although many low birth weight and preterm infants are healthy, they are more likely than children with a normal birth weight to experience health and developmental problems. Low birth weight infants have a higher incidence of neurological impairments or chronic health conditions (Lewit, Baker, Corman, Shiono, 1995). "A greater incidence of cerebral palsy, attention deficit disorder, visual-motor deficits, and altered intellectual functioning is observed in preterm than in full-term infants" (Wong, 1995, p. 389). Respiratory distress syndrome (RDS) is seen almost exclusively in infants born preterm. This condition causes more infant deaths than any other disease and often results in long-term respiratory and neurological complications (Wong).

Families experience considerable stress when dealing with the needs of a low birth weight infant or an infant with a disability. The costs of caring for these children can be high from both a humanistic and an economic perspective. "Children with chronic conditions spend about 10 times as many days in the hospital as children without activity limitations" (Maternal and Child Health Bureau, 1996, p. 58). Frequent hospitalization of a child is a significant stressor that can result in a family having to change its normal pattern of functioning and its goal expectations.

Problems developing before the infant reaches 1 month of age are usually related to gestational age and birth weight and in utero problems. Problems after 1 month are more often related to environmental factors. Here the community health nurse plays a significant role in prevention, especially in relation to morbidity.

Parent-Infant Bonding (Attachment)

Parent-infant bonding can be adversely affected when an infant is physically separated from its primary caregiver for a period of time. This separation can occur when an infant is premature or otherwise at risk and must have extended health care away from its parents. "When an infant is sick, the necessary physical separation appears to be accompanied by an emotional estrangement on the part of parents that may seriously damage the capacity for parenting their infants" (Wong, 1995, p. 385). Research has indicated that

Barriers to Use of Prenatal Care

I. SOCIODEMOGRAPHIC

Poverty
Residence: inner-city or rural
Minority status
Age: <18 or >39
High parity
Non–English-speaking
Unmarried
Less than high school education

II. SYSTEM-RELATED

Inadequacies in private insurance policies (waiting periods, coverage limitations, coinsurance and deductibles, requirements for up-front payments)
Absence of either Medicaid or private insurance coverage of maternity services
Inadequate or no maternity care providers for Medicaid-enrolled, uninsured, and other low-income women (long wait to get appointment)
Complicated, time-consuming process to enroll in Medicaid
Availability of Medicaid poorly advertised
Inadequate transportation services, long travel time to service sites, or both
Difficulty obtaining child care
Weak links between prenatal services and pregnancy testing
Inadequate coordination among such services as WIC and prenatal care
Inconvenient clinic hours, especially for working women
Long waits to see physician
Language and cultural incompatibility between providers and clients
Poor communication between clients and providers exacerbated by short interactions with providers
Negative attributes of clinics, including rude personnel, uncomfortable surroundings, and complicated registration procedures
Limited information on exactly where to get care (phone numbers and addresses)

III. ATTITUDINAL

Pregnancy unplanned, viewed negatively, or both
Ambivalence
Signs of pregnancy not known or recognized
Prenatal care not valued or understood
Fear of doctors, hospitals, procedures
Fear of parental discovery
Fear of deportation or problems with the Immigration and Naturalization Service
Fear that certain health habits will be discovered and criticized (smoking, eating disorders, drug or alcohol abuse)
Selected lifestyles (drug abuse, homelessness)
Inadequate social supports and personal resources
Excessive stress
Denial or apathy
Concealment

From Brown S: Drawing women into prenatal care, *Family Planning Perspectives* 21(2):75, March/April 1989. © The Alan Guttmacher Institute.

during the period immediately after birth and for a short time after that, parents have a unique ability to bond with their infants (Klaus, Kennell, 1982).

It is important for community health nurses to understand that early parent-infant separation increases the risk for bonding difficulties. It is also significant for community health nurses to understand that bonding difficulties can arise among families who have full-term babies. Early recognition of attachment problems can prevent long-term adverse consequences such as failure to thrive difficulties and behavioral problems. Community health nurses play a significant role in facilitating attachment between infants and parents. The box on the next page provides suggestions for facilitating parent-infant attachment, taking into consideration the needs of economically disadvantaged mothers and ethnic and cultural variations in childbearing practices. Cultural beliefs influence parent-infant interactions, as well as the care of the mother during the postpartum period (see the box on p. 427).

Failure to Thrive (FTT)

Another problem associated with high-risk infants—those who are small or have other physical, familial, and psychological problems—can be their failure to thrive. A child who fails to thrive is one whose weight and sometimes height fall below the *fifth percentile* for the child's age (Wong, 1995, p. 596). Three general categories of failure to thrive have been defined (Wong, p. 596):

- **Organic failure to thrive (OFTT),** which is the result of a physical cause, such as congenital heart defects, neurologic lesions, microcephaly, chronic urinary tract infection, gastroesophageal reflux, renal insufficiency, malabsorption syndrome, endocrine dysfunction, or cystic fibrosis. This category accounts for less than half of all FTT.
- **Nonorganic failure to thrive (NFTT),** which has a definable cause that is unrelated to disease. NFTT is most often the result of psychosocial factors, such as inadequate nutritional information by the parent; deficiency in maternal care or a disturbance in maternal-child attachment; or a disturbance in the child's ability to separate from the parent, leading to food refusal to maintain attention (Chatoor, Dickson, Schaefer, James, 1985). NFTT has been described under a variety of less acceptable names, including maternal deprivation, environmental deprivation, and deprivation dwarfism.

Nursing Considerations to Foster Bonding Among Specific Populations

WOMEN IN ECONOMICALLY DISADVANTAGED SITUATIONS

Low-income mothers may have to contend with stressors that distract them from developing a relationship with their babies. Inability to pay for infant supplies or child care, chaotic home situations, and worry over eligibility for social and health care services deplete these women's psychological energy.

Nurses need to conduct nonjudgmental, individual assessments of resources and social networks to avoid inaccurate and stereotypical assumptions. Nurses can help economically disadvantaged mothers access social services, such as the Women, Infants, and Children (WIC) program and Medicaid. For mothers whose home environments provide little or no support and multiple stressors, early discharge may not be optimal. Nurses can advocate for longer hospital stays for these mothers when the hospital environment is more conducive to bonding.

Economically disadvantaged mothers, especially adolescents, are not as likely to be aware of the benefits of bonding or to be knowledgeable of normal infant behaviors. These women may not be aware of maternity care options, such as rooming-in, or may be less assertive in asking for such options. The nurse needs to be a client educator and advocate, explaining the choices and the potential benefits. The nurse should ensure a supportive, encouraging environment that will help mothers engage in positive interactions with their infants. By use of the Brazelton Neonatal Assessment Scale, the nurse can capture the mother's attention with a mother-infant interactional experience and, at the same time, increase the mother's knowledge of infant behavior. Written material can be provided after the assessment to reinforce the behavioral concepts. Examples, from sections of an individualized handout written as if from the baby, include "My Strengths: great motor maturity—I stretch my arms way up over my head" and "How you can help: swaddle my arms so I can suck on my hands" (Tedder, 1991).

WOMEN OF VARYING ETHNIC AND CULTURAL GROUPS

Childbearing practices and rituals of other cultures may not be congruent with standard practices associated with bonding in the Anglo-American culture. For example, Chinese families traditionally use extended family members to care for the newborn so that the mother can rest and recover, especially after a cesarean birth. Some Native American, Asian, and Hispanic women do not initiate breastfeeding until their breast milk comes in. Haitian families do not name their babies until after the confinement month. Amount of eye contact varies among cultures, too. Yup'ik Eskimo mothers almost always position their babies so that eye contact can be made.

Nurses should become knowledgeable of the childbearing beliefs and practices of diverse cultural and ethnic groups. Because individual cultural variations exist within groups, nurses need to clarify with the client and family members or friends what cultural norms the client follows. Incorrect judgments may be made about mother-infant bonding if nurses do not practice culturally sensitive care.

From Lowdermilk DL, Perry SE, Bobak IM: *Maternity and women's health care*, ed 6, St. Louis, 1997, Mosby, p. 474.
Source: Geissler EM: *Pocket guide to cultural assessment*, St Louis, 1994, Mosby; Symanski ME: Maternal-infant bonding, *J Nurs Midwifery* 37:675, 1992; Tedder JL: Using the Brazelton Neonatal Assessment Scale to facilitate the parent-infant relationship in a primary care setting, *Nurse Pract* 16(3):26, 1991.

- **Idiopathic failure to thrive,** which is unexplained by the usual organic and environmental etiologies but may also be classified as NFTT. Both categories of NFTT account for the majority of cases of FTT.

Causes of failure to thrive include poverty, inadequate nutritional knowledge, health beliefs such as fad diets, family stress, feeding resistance, and insufficient breast milk (Wong, 1995, p. 596). Wong has suggested that nursing care for families who have children that fail to thrive must include support that encourages adaptive mothering behaviors and promotes mother-child attachment. The nursing care should also include teaching specific nurturing techniques, including adequate feeding and interaction with the environment. Assistance to the family in resolving problems that interfere with their ability to provide a nurturing environment is another important element of nursing care. Dealing with families who have a parent-child disturbance can be difficult. Wong discusses this care in depth.

Community health nurses play an important role in preventing FTT, identifying infants at risk for FTT, and assisting families in promoting normal growth and development. It is not unusual for the community health nurse to work with parents who lack adequate resources to purchase formula or parents who lack knowledge about formula preparation. It is also not unusual for the community health nurse to work with families who are experiencing considerable stress, which can interfere with the bonding process.

Child Abuse

Child abuse involves direct harm or intent to injure, including intentionality without physical injury. Different types of child maltreatment occur, including physical and/or psychological abuse and neglect and sexual abuse. In general, *abuse* refers to acts of commission such as beating or excessive chastisement. *Neglect* refers to acts of omission such as failure to provide adequate food, clothing, or emotional care. However, the line separating the two is a very thin one (U.S. Congress, OTA, 1988, p. 167).

The problem of child maltreatment is growing. In 1994 an estimated 2.9 million children nationwide were referred for suspected abuse or neglect, meaning that 45 of every 1000 children were reported. Between 1985 and 1993 there was an approximately 50% increase in the reporting of child abuse and neglect (Lewit, 1994). Forty-three states reported

Some Cultural Beliefs About the Postpartum Period and Contraception

POSTPARTUM CARE

Chinese, Mexican, Korean, and Southeast Asian women may wish to eat only warm foods and drink hot drinks to replace blood lost and to restore the balance of hot and cold in their bodies. These women may also wish to stay warm and avoid bathing in a tub or shower, exercising, and washing their hair for 7 to 30 days after childbirth. Self-care may not be a priority; care by family members is preferred. These women may wear abdominal binders. They may prefer not to give their babies colostrum. Other family members may care for the baby.

Haitian women may ask to take the placenta home to bury or burn it.

Japanese women may request part of the umbilical cord, which they will place in a special box.

Muslim women follow strict religious laws concerning modesty and diet. A Muslim woman must keep her hair, body, arms to the wrist, and legs to the ankles covered at all times. She cannot be alone in the presence of a man other than her husband or a male relative. Observant Muslims will not eat pork or pork products. They are obligated to eat meat slaughtered according to Islamic law (halal meat) but will usually accept kosher meat, seafood, or a vegetarian diet if halal meat is not available.

CONTRACEPTION

Birth control is government mandated in *China*. Most Chinese women have an IUD inserted after the birth of their first child.

Saudi Arabian women usually do not practice birth control.

Mexican women are likely to choose the rhythm method because most are Catholic.

East Indian men are encouraged to undergo voluntary sterilization by vasectomy.

Muslim couples may practice contraception by mutual consent, so long as its use is not harmful to the woman. Acceptable contraceptive methods include foam, condoms, the diaphragm, and natural family planning.

From Lowdermilk DL, Perry SE, Bobak IM: *Maternity and women's health care*, ed 6, St. Louis, 1997, Mosby, p. 458.

that child maltreatment resulted in 1111 deaths in 1994 and 48 states substantiated, upon investigation, that 1,012,000 children were victims of abuse and neglect in that same year. Over half of all reports alleging maltreatment (53%) came from professionals; only one in five reports came from either the victimized child or a family member of the victim (Maternal and Child Health Bureau, 1996, p. 37).

Child abuse or neglect is a cumulative problem since the scars that result from such behavior have long-term effects. The most damaging aspect of child abuse and neglect is on the developmental process and emotional growth of the child. Abused children do not feel safe and are unable to trust others—Erikson's first stage in development. Almost 50% of all victims of child maltreatment in 1994 were under the age of 6 (Maternal and Child Health Bureau, 1996, p. 37).

"The most important parental risk factors for child maltreatment are those related to poverty and unemployment and a history of abuse as a child" (U.S. Congress, OTA, 1988, p. 176). Parents may follow *their* parents' method of child rearing: if it was characterized by abuse and neglect, their child-rearing style may duplicate their own experience. At the same time, it is possible that intergenerational violence could be related in part to the perpetuation of poverty from one generation to the next (U.S. Congress, OTA, p. 175). There are conflicting findings about the relationship between being abused as a child and intergenerational violence (Wong, 1995).

Parents of abused children often do not understand normal growth and development patterns and expect too much of their children. As a result, the child is criticized and physically and emotionally punished. A sense of failure and lack of confidence and faith in one's own abilities often results in abused and neglected children who in turn may abuse and neglect others.

Community health nurses need to be alert to situations where abuse and neglect might occur and intervene before they happen. Marital strain, poverty, isolation, and overwhelmed parents are signals to be heeded. Premature births or having children with developmental disabilities are stressful situations that need to be noted. Parents who expect infants to be responsible for their acts and who respond with physical punishment also bear watching.

Mental retardation, emotional disorders, and learning disorders can be other evidences of a less-than-positive nurturing environment for infants. Organic pathological factors are contributors to these disorders, but psychosocial and other factors also influence the development of these disorders. A summary of physical and behavioral indicators that can assist nurses in identifying child abuse and neglect can be found in Chapter 16.

Presently no states have enough resources and personnel to deal adequately with the increasing number of reported cases of abuse and neglect, not to mention working with families who have already been identified as needing care.

Sudden Infant Death Syndrome

Another sequel to high-risk pregnancy may be the sudden infant death syndrome (SIDS). In the United States, 2 of every 1000 live-born infants die annually from SIDS. It is the number one cause of death in infants between the ages of 1 month and 1 year. Although SIDS was identified as early as in the writings of the New Testament, no single cause for this condition has been discovered. It is suspected that SIDS is caused by a combination of events and some type of biochemical, anatomical, or developmental defect or deficiency (National SIDS Clearinghouse,

1989; Wong, 1995). Risk factors for SIDS are displayed in Table 15-2.

Helping parents handle grief and guilt feelings is the major role of the community health nurse in these situations. The impact of death on siblings is another area where the nurse must intervene. Increasingly, communities are setting up crisis teams to assist families who have experienced a child's death from SIDS. One health department in a northern city employs a pediatric nurse practitioner who works full-time with such families. She facilitates family adjustment as they work through the grief process after death has come to a seemingly healthy infant. Helping families to deal with their feelings about future parenting is very important (Chan, 1987). Since the mourning process takes at least a year for completion of acceptance and social reorganization, nurses should call on the family periodically to evaluate their progress (Wong, 1995, p. 605).

table 15-2 EPIDEMIOLOGY OF SIDS

FACTORS	OCCURRENCE
Incidence	1.4 : 1000 live births
Peak age	2 to 4 months; 95% occur by 6 months
Sex	Higher percentage of males affected
Time of death	During sleep
Time of year	Increased incidence in winter; peak in January
Racial	Greater incidence in Native Americans and blacks, followed by whites, Asians, and Hispanics
Socioeconomic	Increased occurrence in lower socioeconomic class
Birth	Higher incidence in: Premature infants, especially infants of low birth weight Multiple births* Neonates with low Apgar scores Infants with central nervous system disturbances and respiratory disorders such as bronchopulmonary dysplasia Increasing birth order (subsequent siblings as opposed to firstborn child) Infants with a recent history of illness
Sleep habits	Prone position; use of polystyrene-filled cushions; overheating (thermal stress)
Feeding habits	Lower incidence in breast-fed infants
Siblings	May have greater incidence
Maternal	Young age; cigarette smoking, especially during pregnancy; substance abuse (heroin, methadone, cocaine)

From Wong DL: *Whaley and Wong's nursing care of infants and children*, ed 5, St. Louis, 1995, Mosby, p. 603.

*Although a rare event, simultaneous death of twins from SIDS can occur.

Public health professionals have a significant preventive intervention role as well as a therapeutic role when dealing with SIDS. A 7-year study of unexpected infant deaths in England suggested that home visiting by health visitors was directly related to a reduction in mortality of infants scored to be at risk for unexpected infant death (Carpenter, 1983, p. 724). The scoring system for ascertaining who was at risk included factors such as the mother's age, her previous pregnancies, duration of the second stage of labor, mother's blood group, birth weight, single or multiple birth, if the infant was breastfed or bottle-fed, and presence of urinary infection of mother during pregnancy.

Home visits by health visitors were made for SIDS preventive follow-up every 2 weeks for 3 months and every month for up to 6 months to those infants scoring at high risk. "The reduction in mortality attributed directly to the effect of increased visiting of high-risk infants is numerically similar to the number of lives saved by treating cancers in children. This suggests that home visiting by health visitors is highly cost-effective" (Carpenter, 1983, p. 723).

Acute Illnesses

Respiratory diseases and other conditions such as diarrhea result in short-term disability and account for many doctor visits for infants. These diseases caused much death in the past. Today there is less mortality from these conditions, but a tremendous amount of professional time is spent in controlling acute illnesses. The nurse in the pediatric clinic or the nurse who makes home visits will see these kinds of problems and will need the expertise to explain their origin and treatment to parents.

HEALTH RISKS OF CHILDREN AGES 1 TO 5

Children do change in their capacities. As developmental growth occurs, infants and children's needs and problems become different. Figure 15-7 shows the leading causes of death for children between ages 1 and 14 years. As children become mobile, accidental injuries become the major cause of death.

Accidental Injuries

In 1993 about 44% of all deaths among children ages 1 through 4 were caused by injuries (Maternal and Child Health Bureau, 1996, p. 30). Figure 15-8 shows that motor vehicle crashes, fires, and burns caused the greatest number of injury deaths among toddlers and preschoolers, with drownings, suffocation, and firearms also causing a significant number of deaths. Primary prevention of many of these deaths is possible.

Accidental injuries disproportionately strike the young, which is costly to society from many perspectives. Accidental injuries can cause social and emotional stress, significant activity limitation, and financial burdens. "More than half of the impairments caused by injuries result in activity limitations: seventy percent of impairments due to injuries are

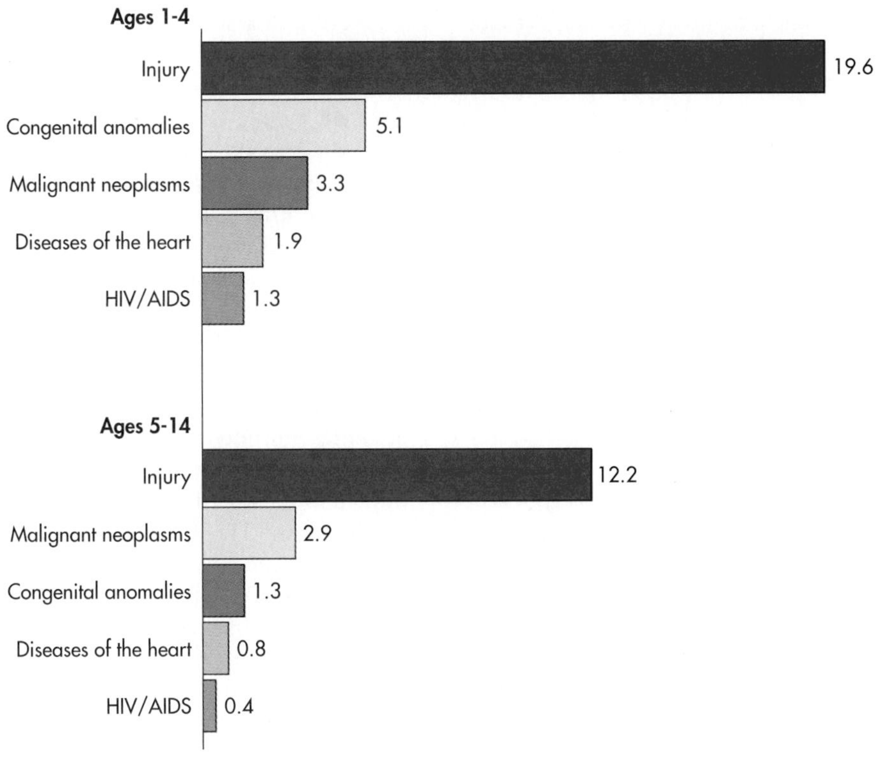

Figure 15-7 Leading causes of death in children ages 1 to 14: 1993. *(From Maternal and Child Health Bureau:* Child health USA '95, *Washington, D.C., 1996, U.S. Government Printing Office, p. 30. Source: National Center for Health Statistics.)*

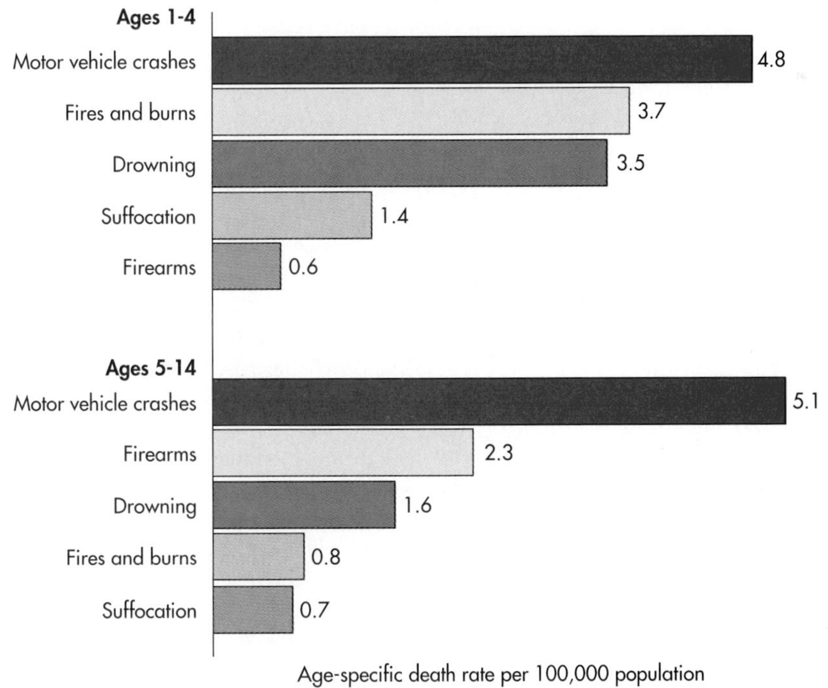

Figure 15-8 Childhood deaths as a result of injury by cause and age: 1993. *(From Maternal and Child Health Bureau:* Child health USA '95, *Washington, D.C., 1996, U.S. Government Printing Office, p. 31. Source: National Center for Health Statistics.)*

deformities or orthopedic impairments" (National Institute on Disability and Rehabilitation Research, 1989, p. 26). It is not difficult to see that accidents are a major health problem and that present education and legislation are not as effective as they should be in combating a problem that is preventable.

Respiratory and Gastrointestinal Problems

Upper respiratory infections become a common cause of illness in the 1- to 5-year-old age group, especially when these children begin to play in groups. Upper respiratory infections can be minor and cause only minimal interference to living. Others can be life-threatening, especially when no treatment is obtained. Lower respiratory tract infections result generally from infections of the upper respiratory tract.

Minor gastrointestinal problems are almost as common as respiratory infections. The use of epidemiology in examining the numbers of cases in a family and a community helps to determine whether the causative agent is communicable. Epidemiological investigation also helps to identify significant environmental conditions that need changing, especially when a child has repeated infections. In one day-care center, for example, repeated episodes of diarrhea among a number of the children led the supervisor to look for a cause. It was discovered that feeding bottles were left in tote bags until the noon feedings and that spoiled milk was the result. After its epidemiological investigation the day-care center began to refrigerate bottles immediately upon the arrival of infants and parents.

Prompt treatment of acute conditions, ongoing medical care, educating parents about good health care practices, and early detection of illness can help to prevent or curtail respiratory and gastrointestinal problems.

Chronic Conditions and Disabilities

Chronic conditions are important because of their long-term effects. They can significantly limit a child's normal activities and increase health care usage. In 1994, almost 5 million children, or 6.7% of all children ages 1 to 18, were limited in their activities as a result of chronic illnesses and impairments (The Institue for Health and Aging, 1996, p. 26). As previously mentioned, children with activity limitations have 3 times as many physician contacts and spend over 10 times as many days in the hospital as do other children (Maternal and Child Health Bureau, 1996, p. 58). "Families of children with chronic conditions share a common set of challenges: high health care costs, greater caretaking responsibilities, obstacles to adequate education, and

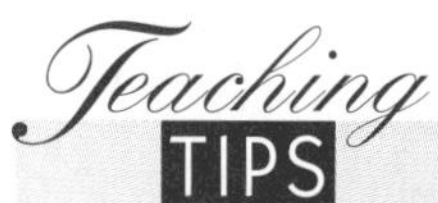

Safety Education Tool

More children die from injuries than any other cause. The good news is that most injuries can be prevented by following simple safety guidelines. Talk with your doctor or other health care provider about ways to protect your child from injuries. Fill out this safety checklist.

Safety Guidelines Checklist

Read the list below and check off (√) each guideline that your family already follows. Work on those you don't.

For All Ages

- Use smoke detectors in your home. Change the batteries every year and check to see that they work once a month.
- Keeping a gun in your home can be dangerous. If you do, make sure that the gun and ammunition are locked up separately and kept out of reach.
- Never drive after drinking alcohol.
- Teach your child traffic safety. Children under 9 years of age need supervision when crossing streets.
- Learn basic life-saving skills (CPR).
- Keep a bottle of ipecac at home to treat poisoning. Talk with a doctor or the local Poison Control Center before using it. Post the Poison Control Center number near your telephone and write it in the space provided on the inside front cover.

Infants and Young Children

- Use a car safety seat at all times until your child weighs at least 40 pounds. When possible, secure it in the center of the back seat.
- Keep medicines, cleaning solutions, and other dangerous substances in childproof containers, locked up and out of reach.
- Use safety gates across stairways (top and bottom) and guards on windows above the first floor.
- Keep hot water heater temperatures below 120° F.
- Keep unused electrical outlets covered with plastic guards.
- Baby walkers can be dangerous. Children using them should be closely supervised. Access should be blocked to stairways and to objects that can fall (such as lamps) or cause burns (such as stoves).
- Keep objects and foods that can cause choking away from your child, such as coins, balloons, small toy parts, hot dogs (unmashed), peanuts, and hard candies.
- Use fences that go all the way around pools and keep gates to pools locked.

A Special Message About SIDS

Sudden Infant Death Syndrome (SIDS) is the leading cause of death for infants. Some authorities believe that placing sleeping infants on the side or back, instead of the stomach, decreases the risk of SIDS.

From USDHHS: *Child health guide: put prevention into practice*, Washington, D.C., 1994, U.S. Government Printing Office, pp. 30-32.

the additional stress these issues create for the entire family" (The Institute for Health and Aging, 1996, p. 26).

Many children who have a chronic condition also have a disability. Causes of disability among children fall under two major categories: diseases and disorders account for approximately 58% of disabling conditions, while impairments account for the remaining 42%. The most common causes of disability among children, in rank order by number of conditions, are asthma (987,000), mental retardation (786,000), mental disorders (440,000), diseases of the nervous system and sense organs (375,000), and speech impairments (335,000) (Wenger, Kaye, LaPlante, 1996). Other causes of disability among children include impairments such as visual and hearing difficulties, learning disabilities, cerebral palsy, spina bifida, and orthopedic impairments. A variety of diseases also cause disability. Examples of these are infectious and parasitic diseases, diseases of the major body systems (e.g., circulatory, genitourinary, and musculoskeletal systems), congenital anomolies, and neoplasms (Wenger, Kaye, LaPlante). Congenital anomalies and neoplasms (Wenger, Kaye, LaPlante). Congenital anomalies and neoplasms are also major killers of children (Figure 15-7).

Chronic conditions and disabilities among children are a major public health concern. It is anticipated that the number of children with activity-limiting chronic conditions will rise as technological advances improve the survival rates for preterm, low birth weight, and drug-affected infants. It is also anticipated that the shift toward caring for children with severe impairments in their homes rather than in an institution will increase the need for home and community-based long-term services (Stucki, 1995, p. 8). A major role for community health nurses who work with families that are dealing with children with disabilities is the case manager role. Community health nurses help these families to deal with chronic grief, obtain needed medical and educational services, and find community resources that can assist them in coping with the demands of the stressors (e.g., financial and emotional) encountered.

Communicable and Preventable Diseases

Preventable communicable diseases are still a major community health problem. The major childhood diseases—poliomyelitis, mumps, tetanus, diphtheria, rubella, pertussis, measles, chickenpox, hepatitis, and *Haemophilus influenzae* (Hib)—can cause permanent disability and death. In spite of the fact that effective immunizations have been available for decades to protect children from several of these diseases, a significant number of preschool children are not adequately immunized.

Figure 15-9 depicts the immunization rates for children aged 19-35 months by selected vaccines. Although vaccination coverage levels among children in this age group are the highest ever recorded in the United States, over 1 million children still lack one or more doses of the recommended vaccines. Immunization coverage levels vary

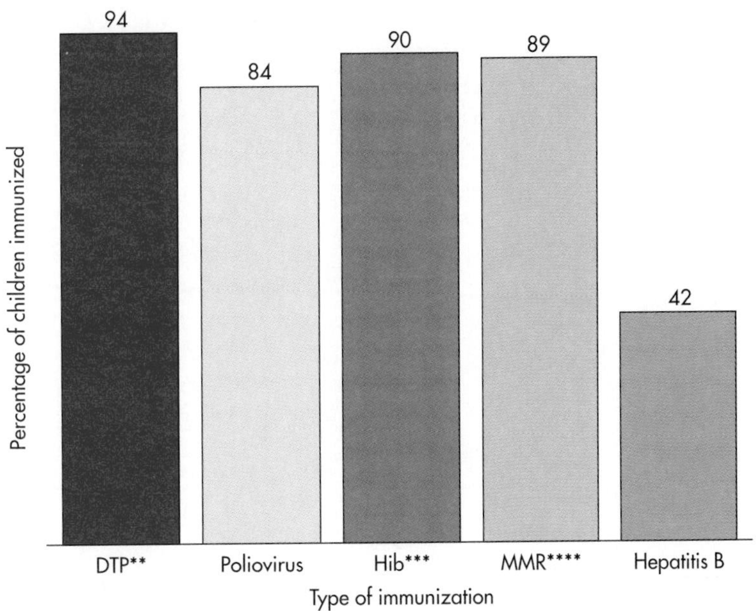

* Data are from April 1994 through March 1995
** DTP: Diphtheria and Tetanus toxoids and pertussis vaccine, ≥3 doses
***Hib: Haemophilus influenzae type b ≥3 doses
****MMR: measles-mumps-rubella ≥1 dose

Figure 15-9 Vaccination coverage levels among children ages 19 to 35 months, by selected vaccines: 1994-1995.*
(From Maternal and Child Health Bureau: Child health USA '95, *Washington, D.C., 1996, U.S. Government Printing Office, p. 52.)*

substantially among the different regions in the country. In some states almost 40% of children are inadequately protected against the vaccine-preventable diseases (Maternal and Child Health Bureau, 1996, p. 52).

Low immunization coverage rates place a community at risk for a major infectious disease outbreak. The recent measles epidemic of 1989-1991 resulted in more than 55,000 reported cases, 11,000 hospitalizations, and more than 130 deaths nationwide. Half of those who died were young children (MDCH, 1997, p. 3). In 1996 pertussis was reported in every state (MDCH, 1997, p. 4). The immunization most likely to be missed by a young child is the fourth DTP on or after the first birthday (MDCH, 1996, p. 4).

Table 15-3, relating complications from childhood diseases, summarizes the problems that can result from the preventable childhood diseases. The contributing factors that allow children, especially preschoolers, to remain unimmunized include the lack of consumer awareness, understanding, and responsibility; the complicated vaccine schedule, which can be easily misunderstood; the increased mobility of families, which can lead to fragmented health care; inadequate funding for immunization research at the federal level; and apathy because the evidences of childhood disease are no longer obvious.

Many reasons for inadequate immunization protection can also be found within the health care system. For example, providers frequently fail to take advantage of opportunities to provide vaccines to at-risk persons, particularly children, during regular visits to health care facilities. Other examples are clinic hours and locations that are not user friendly, fragmented health care services that require parents to make multiple trips to complete well-child care, and caregivers' lack of understanding regarding true contraindications for delaying immunizations.

Pediatric AIDS

Pediatric acquired immunodeficiency syndrome (AIDS) is a major public health problem in the United States. As of December 1996 there were 7629 cases of AIDS among

table 15-3 Some Complications from Selected Childhood Diseases for which Immunizations Are Available

Complications	Mumps	Measles (Rubeola)	Rubella	Rubella (in Utero)	Polio	Tetanus	Pertussis	Diphtheria
Mental retardation		X	X	X			X	
Brain damage		X	X	X			X	
Meningoencephalitis	X	X	X	X				
Paralysis					X			X
Blindness		X	X	X				
Deafness	X	X	X	X				X
Pancreatitis	X							
Juvenile-type diabetes	X							
Orchitis (postpubertal)	X							
Oophoritis (postpubertal)	X							
Sterility (males)	X							
Pneumonia	X	X				X	X	X
Heart damage, pericarditis	X							X
Polyarthritis			X					
Hepatitis	X							
Nephritis	X							X
Cerebral hemorrhage							X	
Muscle spasm						X		
Death	X	X	X	X	X	X	X	X

Modified from Atkinson W, Furphy L, Gantt J, Mayfield M, eds: *Epidemiology and prevention of vaccine-preventable diseases*, ed 2, Atlanta, 1995, CDC; Garner MK: Our values are showing: inadequate childhood immunization, *Health values: achieving high level wellness* 2:130, 1978; Hoekelman RA, Blatman S, Brunell PA et al: *Principles of pediatrics: health care of the young*, New York, 1978, McGraw-Hill; Scipien GM, Barnard MU, Chard MA et al: *Comprehensive pediatric nursing*, ed 3, New York, 1986, McGraw-Hill.

children under 13 years of age, and these numbers continue to grow daily (CDC, 1996, p. 11). In 1996 a total of 678 *new* cases were reported. The majority of pediatric AIDS cases are the result of transmission from infected mothers, with a disproportionate number of cases occurring in black and Hispanic children (see Figure 15-10) (Maternal and Child Health Bureau, 1996, p. 36). In December 1996 90% of the pediatric HIV infection cases to date were acquired from HIV-infected mothers, 5% were associated with transmission of blood and blood products, and 3% were of children who had hemophilia or other coagulation disorders (CDC, 1996).

The epidemiological characteristics of AIDS victims are discussed in Chapter 12. Children with AIDS have characteristics similar to those of heterosexual adults with AIDS, particularly women: the majority of perinatally acquired pediatric AIDS cases are related to intravenous (IV) drug abuse or sexual contact with IV drug abusers. The geographical areas most heavily affected by perinatal transmission of AIDS are New York, Puerto Rico, Florida, and New Jersey. "Children with perinatally acquired AIDS are usually normal at birth and develop symptoms within the first 18 months of life. It is usually manifested as a developmental delay or, after achieving normal development, loss of motor milestones" (Wong, 1995, p. 1601).

Professionals working with families who have children with AIDS must address an array of complex medical, social, and emotional problems. Nursing intervention is primarily focused on providing care for the child, educating the community regarding the *realistic* concerns in terms of communicability of the virus, and preventing disease transmission (Wong, 1995, p. 1603). The goal is to provide a supportive, nurturing environment for the child while

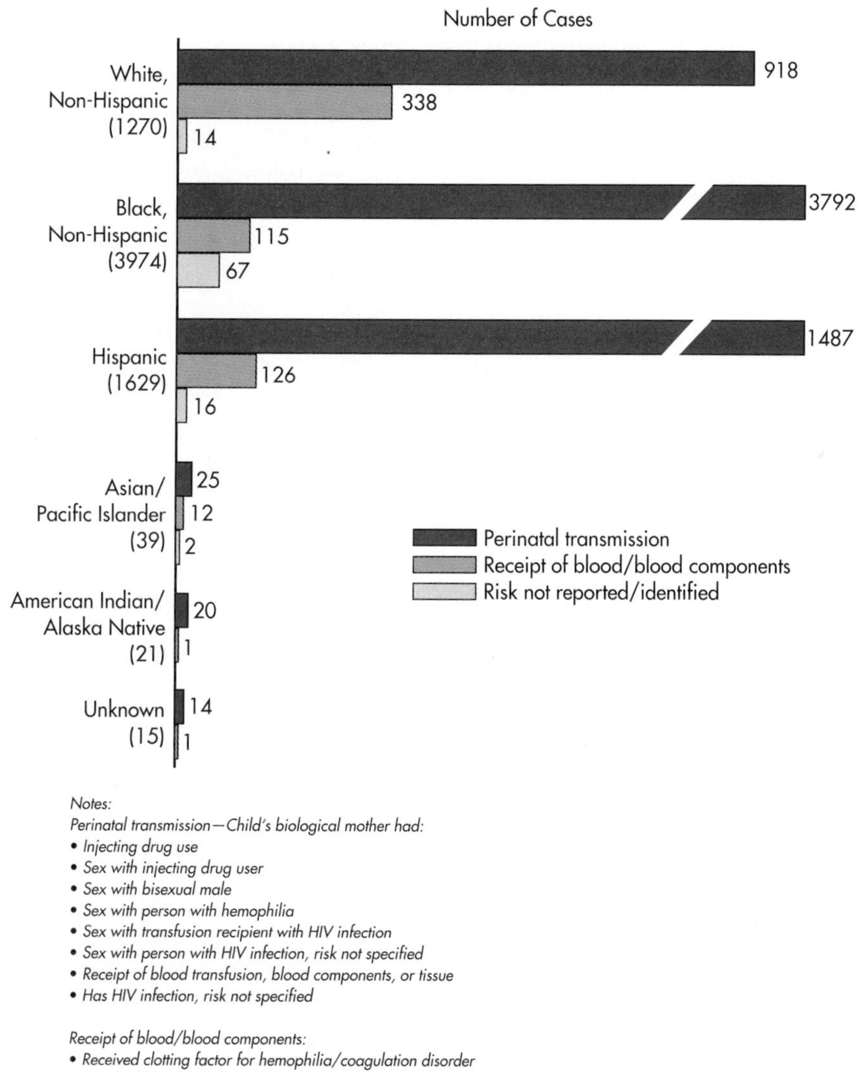

Figure 15-10 Pediatric AIDS cases by race/ethnicity and exposure category: 1981-1995. *(From Maternal and Child Health Bureau:* Child health USA '95, *Washington, D.C., 1996, U.S. Government Printing Office, p. 36.)*

preventing transmission of the virus. Both the community and the child's family are educated about universal precautions (see Chapter 11).

Children with AIDS must be kept comfortable and well nourished and protected from opportunistic infection. In addition, they must receive nurturing parenting that promotes their psychosocial development. Families need supportive assistance to help them handle the physical care needs of their children, obtain adequate financial and health care resources, and cope with the stresses related to the progression of the disease. Family members can experience social isolation, fear, guilt, financial burdens, grief, and physical stress. These families frequently need an advocate in the health care delivery system and the community and help in coordinating health care services. When the AIDS virus was transmitted perinatally, the family faces the additional challenges related to the care of an infected mother. Frequently decisions must be made about who will care for the mother as well as the child, and who will assume guardianship for the child if the mother dies first (Wong).

Community health nurses assume a major role in helping families deal with their emotions and the demands of the stressors encountered. Community health nurses also play a significant role in educating families, professionals, and communities about AIDS prevention. Pediatric AIDS must be prevented! It cannot be cured!

Lead Poisoning

At present, lead poisoning is one of the most common preventable *environmental* diseases of childhood in the United States. Mental retardation, learning disabilities, and other neurological handicaps are the needless results of this condition. Infants and young children are at highest risk for complications of lead toxicity because they absorb lead more readily than do adults and their nervous systems are more susceptible to the effects of lead (CDC, 1997).

Despite the recent and large declines in lead poisoning among children in the United States, 1.7 million American children still have elevated blood lead levels. This represents about 9% of all children under age 6 (Maternal and Child Health Bureau, 1996, p. 35). The risk for lead exposure remains disproportionately high for some groups, including children who are poor, non-Hispanic blacks, Mexican Americans, those living in large metropolitan areas, or those living in older housing (CDC, 1997, p. 144). In one large study examining the extent of lead poisoning among children from birth through 4 years of age, it was found that children living in communities with high rates of poverty, single-parent families, pre1950s housing, and low rates of home ownership were 7 to 10 times more likely to have lead poisoning than other children (Sargent, Brown, Freeman et al, 1995, p. 531).

Lead exposure risk is primarily determined by a child's environmental conditions (CDC, 1997). The most serious remaining sources of lead exposure for children is lead-based paint that has deteriorated into paint chips and lead dust and dust and soil contaminated by residues from emissions of leaded gasoline (Maternal and Child Health Bureau, 1996). These sources of lead exposure continue to plague our children despite the fact that the manufacturing of residential paint with lead was eliminated in 1976 and a phase-out of leaded fuel was initiated in the 1970s (CDC, 1997).

Lead poisoning is not confined to poor children in deteriorated neighborhoods. No economic or racial subgrouping of children is exempt from the risk of adverse health effects from lead toxicity (Sargent, Brown, Freeman et al, 1995). It is estimated that in the United States, approximately 83% of privately owned housing units and 86% of public housing units built before 1980 contain some lead-based paint (CDC, 1997). These homes are found in all types of communities.

Children from some ethnic groups (e.g., Hmong, Chinese, and Hispanic) are exposed to lead through folk remedies used to treat minor ailments. Chinese herbal medicines, Paylooah, an Asian folk medicine used for treating fever in children, and Azarcon, a Mexican folk remedy for "empacho" or chronic indigestion, have been identified as sources of lead poisoning among children (CDC, 1993a). The box below provides a description of these traditional ethnic remedies and how they are used.

Although knowledge about its etiology, pathophysiology, and epidemiology has increased significantly in the past two decades, childhood lead poisoning continues to remain a major public health problem. Each year this condition causes mental retardation and other problems in thousands of children. The long-term effects of lead poisoning can be

Ethnic Sources of Lead Exposure

In some cultures the use of traditional ethnic remedies may contain lead and increase children's risk of lead poisoning. These remedies include:

Azarcon (Mexico)—For digestive problems; a bright orange powder; usual dose is ¼–1 teaspoon, often mixed with oil, milk, or sugar, or sometimes given as a tea; sometimes a pinch is added to a baby bottle or tortilla dough for preventive purposes

Greta (Mexico)—A yellow-orange powder, used in the same way as azarcon

Paylooah (Southeast Asia)—Used for rash or fever; an orange-red powder given as ½ teaspoon straight or in a tea

Surma (India)—Black powder applied to the inner lower eyelid that is used as a cosmetic to improve eyesight

Unknown ayurvedic (Tibet)—Small, gray-brown balls used to improve slow development; two balls are given orally three times a day

Modified from Lead poisoning associated with use of traditional ethnic remedies—California, 1991-1992, *MMWR* 42(27):521-524, 1993a. From Wong DL: *Whaley and Wong's nursing care of infants and children*, ed 5, St. Louis, 1995, Mosby, p. 695.

subtle. The neurological defects may not be discovered until a child enters school and the teacher notes a slight deficiency in the child's performance. The increasing number of children being observed with long-term effects of lead toxicity, with blood levels much lower than previously believed harmful, is an area of major concern.

In 1991 the Centers for Disease Control and Prevention (CDC) revised its childhood lead poisoning prevention policy statement to recommend lowering the blood lead level (BLL) of concern from 25 μg/dl to 10 μg/dl (CDC, 1993c, p. 165). In addition, the CDC introduced a multitiered approach for dealing with the problem that included environmental management, medical follow-up based on elevated BLL, universal screening of all young children, and primary preventive activities such as identification and remediation of sites of lead. Currently CDC is developing new lead poisoning guidelines to assist state and local health departments in designing programs that will address the unique characteristics of the communities served by these departments. It is anticipated that these guidelines will be available by the end of 1997 (CDC, 1997).

A comprehensive, community-wide approach is essential to control lead poisoning among children. To be successful, a lead toxicity prevention program must include environmental management in addition to screening and diagnostic and treatment approaches. These approaches should focus on controlling lead exposure in high-risk areas, epidemiological investigation of environmental hazards, casefinding, early diagnosis and treatment, dissemination of educational materials to professionals and the public, and the passage of effective legal regulations. Community health nurses assume responsibility for many of these activities.

Nutritional Inadequacies

Another condition seen by the community health nurse when working with children age 1 to 5 is nutritional inadequacy and anemia. Inadequate diets can cause growth retardation.

> Although growth retardation is not a problem for the vast majority of young children in the United States, among some age and ethnic subgroups of low-income children up to 16 percent of individuals aged 5 and younger are below the fifth percentile. The prevalence of growth retardation is especially high for Asian and Pacific Islander children aged 12 through 59 months, Hispanic children up to age 24 months, and black infants in the first year of life. The Asian and Pacific Islander children who show the greatest prevalence of low height for age include those of Southeast Asian refugee families. (USDHHS, 1991, pp. 116-117)

The goal for the nation is to reduce growth retardation among low-income children ages 5 and younger to less than 10% by the year 2000.

Two feeding problems commonly seen by the nurse are overfeeding of infants and young children and too-early introduction of foods other than human milk or formula. Feeding solid foods at an early age is viewed by some parents as a developmental milestone and thus they push the infant before he or she is ready. Little evidence appears to support giving solids before the age of 4 to 6 months, because the result of this practice is the replacement by solids of the formula the infant needs for growth. Another result is that the child may be overfed if the amount of formula given is not decreased when solids are given. Solids are not digested well by young children because of their immature gastrointestinal systems. Additionally, infants are not developmentally ready for solid foods. They are unable to avoid feeding by pushing food away, which may result in overeating and lead to excessive weight gain. Early introduction of food also exposes the infant to food antigens that may produce allergies (Wong, 1995).

The most prevalent form of anemia in the United States is dietary iron deficiency (CDC, 1992). Although the prevalence of anemia in U.S. children has declined substantially since 1980, children screened through the Pediatric Nutrition Surveillance System (PedNSS) in 1991 still had a significantly higher prevalence of anemia than other children. The PedNSS uses data from selected public health and nutrition programs such as WIC, Healthy Start, EPSDT, well-child clinics, and other programs funded from maternal and child health block grants. Of the 6,339,720 screened in 1991, the overall prevalence of anemia was 20% to 30% for the PedNSS population, which was much higher than the 5% national prevalence for young children (CDC, p. 21).

Infants and children particularly at risk for anemia are those who are born prematurely, have perinatal blood loss, have congenital heart disease, are irritable and anorexic, have pica or disturbed sleep patterns, and are fed homogenized cow's milk before the age of 9 months. Cow's milk induces enteric blood loss and significantly influences the occurrence of iron-deficiency anemia. Breast-feeding is being promoted to reduce the prevalence of nutritional deficiencies among infants. However, current trends are not encouraging. Although there has been an increase in breast-feeding among women during the early postpartum period, there has been little progress among women breast-feeding 5 to 6 months postpartum (USDHHS, 1995a, p. 95).

Women least likely to breastfeed are those who are employed full-time, low-income (<$10,000/year), black, Hispanic, under 20 years of age, and/or living in the southeastern region (Maternal and Child Health Bureau, 1996, p. 29). The Year 2000 Objective for the Nation is to "increase to at least 75 percent the proportion of mothers who breastfeed their babies in the early post partum period and to at least 50 percent the proportion who continue breastfeeding until their babies are 5 to 6 months old" (USDHHS, 1991, p. 123). In 1994 only 57.4% of mothers were breast-feeding during the early postpartum period, and by 6 months postpartum this percentage declined significantly for white (23.9%), Hispanic (18.9%), and black (10.3%) women (Maternal and Child Health Bureau, 1996, p. 29).

Another major childhood nutritional concern is the problem of obesity, which is the most common nutritional disturbance of children (Wong, 1995). It is a significant public health challenge because it may continue into adulthood, which places adults at risk for cardiovascular disease, morbidity, high blood pressure, and non–insulin-dependent diabetes (Bronner, 1996). Obesity results from an imbalance between dietary intake and caloric requirements and expenditure. Trends reflect that obesity is on the rise: between 1980 and 1994, the percentage of children ages 6 to 11 that were overweight increased from 8% to 14% (Hellmich, 1997). Multiple socioeconomic, cultural, environmental, metabolic, and hereditary factors can influence the development of obesity among children.

Community health nurses play a significant role in preventing nutritional problems among children. They assist families in learning about proper feeding techniques, appropriate dietary requirements, and resources in the community (e.g., WIC and food stamps) that can help them to expand their food budget. They also help families to identify early nutritional problems and to address these problems taking into consideration the family's unique characteristics. Additionally, the community health nurse works with the community to improve nutritional knowledge among populations at risk and nutritional intake in population-focused settings such as schools and Head Start centers.

Dental Problems

Poor dental hygiene is another health problem that begins in the preschool years. Although the prevalence of dental cavities in children has decreased substantially in the past two decades, a significant number of children still have caries in primary and permanent teeth (Figure 15-11). "The ages of greatest vulnerability are 4 to 8 years for the primary dentition and 12 to 18 years for the secondary or permanent dentition" (Wong, 1995, pp. 801-802). The risk for dental caries remains disproportionately high among children who are poor, non-Hispanic black, Mexican American, Native American, and living in rural areas (Edelstein, Douglass, 1995; Maternal and Child Health Bureau, 1996). The prevalence of baby bottle tooth decay (BBTD), a condition caused by sucking on a bottle containing milk or juice at bedtime, is significantly higher among these populations. For example, although it is estimated that 5% of all children in the United States ages 2 through 4 years have BBTD, it has been demonstrated that in some Native American subpopulations BBTD ranges from 17% to 85% (Bolden, Henry, Allukian, 1993). Other causes of dental caries among preschool children include, but are not limited to, eating foods high in carbohydrates, eating frequent between-meal snacks without brushing teeth, and the cariogenicity of some liquid medications such as Pen-Vee-K and phenytoin (Dilantin).

Unfortunately, it is often only after children reach school age that parents become concerned with dental hygiene, and by then significant damage may have already occurred to the teeth. The appearance of their mouths contributes to the way people feel physically and emotionally, and the financial cost of dental repair can be very high.

Behavioral Problems

Disturbance of sleep patterns, toilet training, eating, relationships with strangers, and continual whining and crying are some behavioral problems often seen by the nurse who works with children. Parents will often have questions about problems in these areas that seem minor but can cause daily discomfort to a family and develop into more major problems.

HEALTH PROMOTION NEEDS

Identifying areas where families and larger groups can increase the state of their health, where they are working toward maximizing their potential, is one of the most exciting and challenging aspects of family and community health nursing. Health promotion in the newborn to 5-year-old age group is particularly important because this period provides the foundation for the physical, intellectual, and emotional health for the rest of the child's life.

The nurse needs to remember that behavior changes with age in a patterned, predictable manner. Behavior has form and shape just as physical patterns do. All growth, whether physical or emotional, implies organization. However, norms for various ages can be dangerous if they are used as absolute standards because each child develops with a different rhythm. Making diagnoses from the behavior a child exhibits takes knowledge, skill, and experience. Norms for various ages should be used as guides for planning health promotion programs and for identifying children who may need a comprehensive growth and development assessment.

Health professionals across the nation recognize the value of health promotion services for the newborn to 5-year-old age population group. They also recognize that there is still much to be accomplished to protect our nation's most precious resources—our children.

Health Promotion Before Birth

Good health begins before a child is conceived. Children need to be wanted and planned, and people need to learn how to be parents. Becoming pregnant does not confer readiness for children because an individual does not automatically put aside all personal needs to prepare for a child's world, which is in itself not a rational world.

Parent education needs to start early. It should begin at home and become part of school health curricula and other health education activities in the community. Parenting

Percentage of Children Ages 2-4 with Dental Caries in Primary Teeth, by Race/Ethnicity: 1988-1991

Source (III.14): National Institutes of Health

Percentage of children

13

22

32.3

Non-Hispanic White

Non-Hispanic Black

Mexican-Americans

Race/Ethnicity

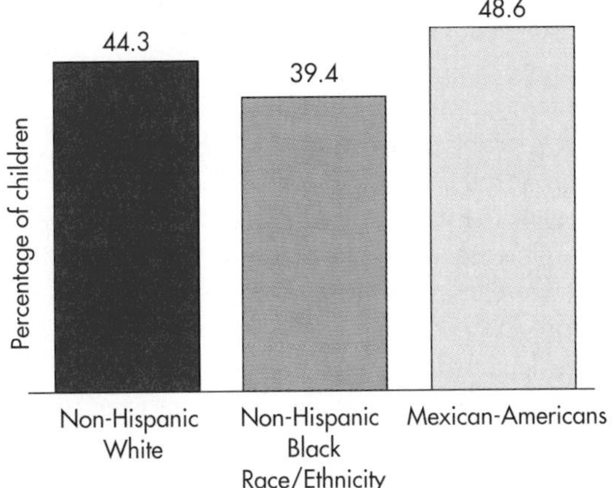

Figure **15-11** Prevalence of dental caries among children ages 2 to 4 and ages 5 to 17. *(From Maternal and Child Health Bureau:* Child health USA '95, *Washington, D.C., 1996, U.S. Government Printing Office, p. 38. Source: National Center for Health Statistics.)*

and family life programs need to include information about planning for pregnancy; lifestyle behaviors that promote or inhibit healthy fetal and child growth; the physical aspects of child care; physical, intellectual, and emotional development of children; and the stresses related to parenting. It is important to include fathers-to-be in family life and parenting programs. Men can play a major role in preventing unintentional pregnancies and sexually transmitted diseases, both of which cause significant problems related to conception and pregnancy. Fathers-to-be also need an opportunity to obtain information necessary to develop nurturing parenting skills.

Health Promotion During Pregnancy

Pregnancy is a developmental task for both parents. Parents need support throughout pregnancy because it is a time of change and of strong emotions, some positive, some negative, and some ambivalent. How people feel about pregnancy varies widely and depends on whether the parents are married, whether they have other children, whether the mother is working, whether memories of their own childhoods are positive or negative, and how they feel about their own parents. Lack of support can cause the parents to feel stress, can delay preparation for the infant, and can retard bond formation. Supportive intervention efforts during and after pregnancy can improve maternal and child health outcomes (Gomby, Larson, Lewit, Behrman, 1993).

Currently many health departments, neighborhood centers, and hospital outpatient clinics have established maternal support services (MSS) to ensure healthy pregnancies for at-risk mothers. These programs provide funding for prenatal care and home visits by a multidisciplinary team, and include social services, health care, and outreach services. With the emphasis on early discharge after birth, the need for community health nursing services for this aggregate is increasing.

Prenatal classes, groups such as LaLèche League, and visits by the community health nurse can help with this kind of support. The nuclear family system of the United States and the mobility of many Americans often means that the parents do not have other family members, close friends, or neighbors who can be helpful in this period.

Concerns that parents have during the time of pregnancy, which should be addressed during prenatal classes, involve preparing for labor and delivery, how to physically prepare the home environment for the new baby, whether to breast-feed, whether the new mother should work outside the home, and how to prepare other siblings for the additional family member. Moreover, the mother needs to know that unhealthy lifestyle behaviors, such as smoking and drinking, can adversely affect the fetus. The mother should begin seeing her obstetrician or family doctor as soon as she suspects she is pregnant.

Parents should know that their genetic backgrounds can play a crucial role in their child's health. Ideally this concern would occur before marriage, but often it does not. Down syndrome, Tay-Sachs disease, sickle-cell anemia, cystic fibrosis, hemophilia, and Huntington's disease are some conditions that have a genetic origin. When parents know that these diseases are in their family constellations, they have several choices. They can have genetic testing before conception, they can adopt, or they can choose not to bear a child. They can also choose to conceive and then have genetic testing to ascertain whether the fetus carries the disease. Another alternative is to conceive and deliver without having genetic tests. If couples know about genetic problems before they marry, they may also make the decision not to marry. The community health nurse needs to be able to help people look at alternatives and provide sources of genetic counseling. There are an increasing number of genetic counseling centers throughout the country.

Expectant parents need more than knowledge to make the transition to parenthood successfully. They need the chance to review the various situations that arise in parenting, compare different ways of dealing with them, and develop their own style of parenting. Nurses have used prenatal class settings to provide clarification about the role of the parent, to do actual role modeling by actively discussing problems and exploring alternatives, and to provide opportunities for role rehearsal. Role rehearsal can be done by using case studies and situations with the opportunity for parents to react and respond. Case studies and sharing of personal experiences to stimulate problem solving can be used with parents throughout any of the developmental and maturational crisis periods they may experience with their children.

Hospitals have created birth centers that involve the family in the birth process and facilitate early discharge to home. This discharge can take place as early as 4 hours postdelivery in some cases. The importance of early discharge for community health nurses is that they need to be skilled in handling nursing care needs of mothers and babies during the immediate postdelivery period. The nurse shown in Figure 15-12 is visiting a family with an infant only 24 hours old. Insurance benefits for this family include coverage for nursing visits, laboratory tests, and homemaking services.

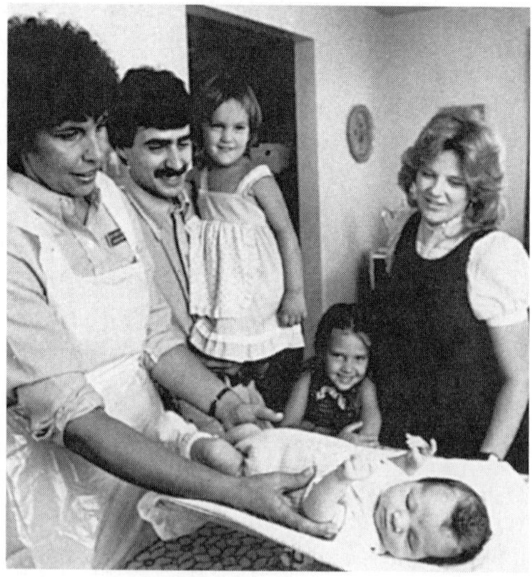

Figure 15-12 A community health nurse whose services are financed under the auspices of the Genessee Region Home Care Association visits an infant only 24 hours old. *(From Genessee Region Home Care Association, Rochester, New York.)*

Health Promotion After Birth

The community health nurse should be aware that sometimes health services are not offered to new parents between the postpartum hospital discharge and the 6-week checkup. The mother is often not in optimum physical condition after experiencing a loss in blood volume, rapid weight loss, and displacement of internal organs during the birth process. Yet she needs to meet the needs of a dependent infant whose respirations are not well established, who is undergoing massive blood changes, and who may be weak, dehydrated, and irritable. In addition, when the mother goes from the protected hospital environment to the home setting, she needs to adjust to role changes and the responsibility of infant care. Nurses in the hospital who work with parents postpartum should make selective referrals of those families needing the services that a community health nurse can offer. The nurse, with observation, is able to "pick up" stresses and provide needed help.

The community health nurse has an important role in the referral process from hospital to home with families who have newborns. The community health nurse can discuss with the hospital nurse the types of families who need referrals. The hospital nurse should assess the entire family situation, assess the parent-child bonding, and make appropriate referrals based on this information. The referral process is based on the hospital nurse's assessment, and it is vital that she or he understand what an appropriate referral is and what the community health nurse can do with families who have newborns.

New parents often have a variety of concerns after taking their infant home. Examples of common concerns the community health nurse addresses with new families are the physical care of the infant, infant feeding schedules, how to know when an infant is ill and should be seen by a doctor, balancing parent and child care schedules, contraceptive methods, weight loss after pregnancy, and dealing with conflicting child care advice from family and friends. Most parents also worry about the infant's growth and development and wonder if it is normal.

Community health nurses help families cope with the emotional and socioeconomic aspects of parenting as well as the physical care of the infant. They also assess the health status of the mother and infant to detect any physical health problems. Additionally, it is not unusual for the community health nurse to educate parents about community resources that can assist them in meeting their basic needs (e.g., food, clothing, or shelter) or that can help them with parenting (e.g., parenting support groups or children's play groups). Nurses who visit new parents in the home often find this to be an extremely rewarding experience.

SUPPORTING FAMILIES

The goal of supporting families is to strengthen them, ensuring the well-being and healthy development of their children. Families are supported by helping parents to cope with the stresses of daily life; giving parents new information about child development and rearing so that parents in turn can better support their own children; reducing the isolation that parents feel, bringing them into contact with other parents; and referring parents to needed services and agencies, ideally before there is a crisis (Allen, Brown, Finlay, 1992, p. 6). In today's complex world no family has all of the knowledge and resources needed to meet their needs. With more births to teens, with declining family incomes, with growing hunger and homelessness, and with increasing lack of access to health care, parenting requires the help of the community. "Parents in different circumstances need different kinds of help and different levels of support, but all parents need some kind of help at one time or another" (Allen, Brown, Finlay, p. 13). Lillian Wald recognized the need to support families when she created the Henry Street Settlement House in New York City in the early part of this century. Her "home" offered health care and helped people with housing and employment and other social service needs.

The most contemporary impetus to the family support movement has been Head Start, the comprehensive preschool program for disadvantaged children. The creators of this program of the 1960s recognized the interrelatedness of health, nutrition, parent involvement, and children's learning. Each parent with a child in Head Start is asked to volunteer time as a classroom aide and to attend parent education meetings with the goal of helping the parents to become better teachers of their own children. Each Head Start program also has a parent council with policy-making responsibilities. "Today more than one-third of the Head Start's paid employees nationwide are former Head Start parents who were inspired to continue their education as a result of their participation in Head Start activities" (Allen, Brown, Finlay, 1992, p. 14).

Supportive family services and interventions are presented in Chapter 8. What is advocated is a holistic approach that emphasizes the importance of the family unit, comprehensively addressing the needs of all family members. Families can have interrelated needs that require coordination of service when numerous resources are used. Community health nurses intervene in this situation and prevent crises by connecting families to support services in the community.

Single Parents

An increasing number of individuals are becoming single parents as a result of divorce, separation, and nonmarital childbearing. Single parenting is occurring among all socioeconomic groups and in all types of communities. It is also occurring among parents in all age groups (USDHHS, 1995b). Although single parents frequently experience special challenges, it is important to realize that single parents can and do provide nurturing environments for their children. A low socioeconomic status can make it more difficult for single parents to address the challenges they face.

Adolescent single parents and their infants are at high risk emotionally, physically, and economically. Help with parenting skills for this age group is a high priority for the community health nurse. Adolescents usually have not completed their own physical, mental, and emotional growth, and becoming responsible for another human being presents both a maturational and a situational crisis for them. Prenatal and postnatal clinics set up for intensive and personal care for this group, as well as alternative education classes within the school system, have been ways in which special support has been provided for adolescent parents. Chapter 16 discusses adolescent parenthood further.

Divorced, single, or separated parents often find themselves fulfilling the roles of individual, father, mother, breadwinner, homemaker, and citizen. This can be an overwhelming situation unless appropriate resources are available and utilized. The community health nurse is able to help single parents look at the reality of their situation and at the options and resources available to them. Community groups, such as Parents Without Partners and parenting support groups, may be helpful. Most single parents are functioning exceptionally well in relation to the responsibilities they encounter. The positive aspects and actions evidenced should be reinforced.

The single father can be at a greater disadvantage for receiving societal supports than the single mother. Many programs have been designed and implemented for maternal-child health, but fathers are frequently neglected when programs are developed to assist single parents. The father, whose involvement with his children has only recently received societal sanction, often finds himself less prepared and with fewer supports in his dual-parent role.

Another dilemma of the single parent is that of the "weekend parent." Many divorced parents are put in the role of seeing their children on a limited basis. They are unsure of their role with their children and have many concerns about how to facilitate their children's developmental growth. The nurse can be helpful in facilitating adjustment to the weekend parent role.

PREVENTIVE INTERVENTION

Newborn Assessment

Assessment of the newborn is viewed as a decisive foundation for early casefinding and preventive care. The kinds of observations that are made help to determine the nursing and medical care that the infant will receive, as well as the kind of parenting that is given.

During the assessment the nurse should get baseline data about the infant's surface features, movement patterns, and general health for comparisons with future examinations. Since health promotion is the concern, systematic periodic assessment over a period of time is important. The developmental approach, rather than the traditional disease-oriented model, should be the focus. Parental involvement in the assessment process helps the nurse to see how the family interacts. It also provides the opportunity to begin anticipatory guidance and problem solving.

The Neonatal Behavioral Assessment Scale developed by T. Berry Brazelton (Brazelton, 1984) is a valid and useful method for observing, making judgments, and scoring selected reflexes, motor responses, and interactive behavioral responses of newborns. The main focus of the scale is on the observation and rating of the infant's interactive behavior. It measures a total of 28 behavioral responses of the infant organized into the following six categories:

1. Habituation—how soon the infant diminishes responding to specific stimuli (e.g., bell) while sleeping
2. Orientation—when and how often the infant attends to auditory and visual stimuli
3. Motor maturity—how well the infant coordinates and controls motor activities
4. Variation—how often the infant coordinates and controls motor activities
5. Self-quieting abilities—how often, how soon, and how effectively the infant uses personal resources to console himself or herself
6. Social behaviors—smiling and cuddling behaviors

Using the Brazelton scale points out vividly that newborns are able to control their responses to external stimuli. Generally, the abilities of newborns have been underestimated by both parents and health professionals.

Anticipatory Guidance

Anticipatory guidance in helping parents to know what to expect of their children at different stages is one of the *most basic and significant* health promotion needs of parents. Through anticipatory guidance parents can gain knowledge about child growth and development and parenting activities that promote a nuturing and safe environment for their children. Parents are able to assess quite accurately their children's strengths and needs when they are given adequate information. This is logical because their proximity makes them frequent observers.

Anticipatory guidance is a process that involves gathering information about the child and his or her environment (see the box, above right), establishing a therapeutic alliance with the parents, and providing education and guidance around normal developmental milestones and parent and child concerns (Foye, 1997, p. 151). Selected topics for anticipatory guidance by developmental age groups are presented in the box on the following page. It is important to focus anticipatory guidance around concerns of the parent and child and identified needs based on an assessment of the child and his or her environment. It is also helpful to anticipate common concerns of most parents (e.g., feeding patterns, toilet training, and discipline), and question parents about their interest in discussing these concerns.

Pertinent Information for Anticipatory Guidance

A. Information about the *child*
   1. *Concerns:* expressed by parent or child
   2. *Health:* current status and follow-up of past problems
   3. *Routine care:* feeding, sleep, and elimination
   4. *Development:* evaluated by school performance or with standardized tests (e.g., Denver Developmental Screening Test, Early Language Milestone Scale)
   5. *Behavior:* temperament and interaction with family, peers, and others

B. Information about the child's *environment*
   1. *Family composition* (at home)
   2. *Caregiving schedule:* who and when
   3. *Family stresses:* (e.g., work, finances, illness, death, moving, marital and other relationships)
   4. *Family supports:* relatives, friends, organizations, material resources
   5. *Stimulation* in the home
   6. *Stimulation/activities* outside the home, (e.g., preschool/school, peers, organizations)
   7. *Safety*

From Foye HR: Anticipatory guidance. In Hoekelman RA, Friedman SB, Nelson NM et al, eds: *Primary pediatric care,* St. Louis, 1997, Mosby, p. 152.

Preventive Health Care Services

Since a child's growth and development is so rapid during the first years of life, it is imperative that a child obtain preventive health care services on a regular basis. These services should include a periodic, comprehensive developmental assessment and immunizations as needed. Periodic assessment helps parents and professionals to evaluate more carefully questionable growth and development and to detect undiagnosed health problems such as hearing loss, anemia, and visual difficulties.

Baseline information compiled through periodic assessment in the home and the physician's office is the key to planning an early intervention program. Baseline data assists parents and professionals in comparing a child's development over time and identifying early deviations from the norm. It is important for a community health nurse to know "normal" expectations for development so that what is unusual, abnormal, or delayed can be quickly recognized.

Numerous schedules are available for preventive child health care services. Appendix 15-1 presents a child preventive care timeline that is recommended by all major pediatric authorities. Immunizations are a crucial component of preventive health care. Figure 15-13 identifies the recommended immunization schedule for infants and children. Providing parents with a written immunization schedule can help to prevent confusion. Effective anticipatory

Topics of Anticipatory Guidance

PRENATAL AND NEWBORN

Prenatal Visit

1. *Health:* pregnancy course; worries; tobacco, alcohol, drug use; hospital and pediatric office procedures
2. *Safety:* infant car seat, crib safety
3. *Nutrition:* planned feeding method
4. *Child care:* help after birth, later arrangements
5. *Family:* changes in relationships (spouse, siblings), supports, stresses, return to work

Newborn Visits

1. *Health:* jaundice, umbilical cord care, circumcision, other common problems, when to call pediatrician's office
2. *Safety:* infant car seat, smoke detector, choking, keeping tap water temperature below 120° F
3. *Nutrition:* feeding, normal weight loss, spitting, vitamin and fluoride supplements
4. *Development/behavior:* individuality, "consolability," visual and auditory responsiveness
5. *Child care:* importance of interaction, parenting books, support for primary caregiver
6. *Family:* postpartum adjustments, fatigue, "blues," special time for siblings

FIRST YEAR

Up to 6 Months

1. *Health:* immunizations, exposure to infections
2. *Safety:* falls, aspiration of small objects or powder, entanglement in mobiles that have long strings
3. *Nutrition:* supplementing breast milk or formula, introducing solids, iron
4. *Development/behavior:* crying/colic, irregular schedules (eating, sleeping, eliminating), response to infant cues, reciprocity, interactive games, beginning eye-hand coordination
5. *Child care:* responsive and affectionate care, caregiving schedule
6. *Family:* return to work, nurturing of all family relationships (spouse and siblings)

6-12 Months

1. *Safety:* locks for household poisons and medications; gates for stairs; ipecac; poison center telephone number; outlet safety covers; avoiding dangling cords or tablecloths; safety devices for windows/screens; toddler car seat when infant reaches 20 pounds; avoiding toys that have small detachable pieces; supervise child in tub or near water
2. *Nutrition:* discouraging use of bottle as a pacifier or while in bed; offering cup and soft finger foods (with supervision); introducing new foods one at a time
3. *Development/behavior:* attachment, basic trust versus mistrust, stranger awareness, night waking, separation anxiety, bedtime routine, transitional object
4. *Child care:* prohibitions few but firm and consistent across caregiving settings: defining discipline as "learning" (not punishment)
5. *Family:* spacing of children

SECOND YEAR

1-2 Years

1. *Health:* immunizations
2. *Safety:* climbing and falls common; supervising outdoor play; ensuring safety caps on medicine bottles; noting dangers of plastic bags, pan handles hanging over stove, and space heaters
3. *Nutrition:* avoiding feeding conflicts (decreased appetite is common); period of self-feeding, weaning from breast or bottle; avoiding sweet or salty snacks
4. *Development/behavior:* autonomy versus shame/doubt, ambivalence (independence/dependence), tantrums, negativism, getting into everything, night fears, readiness for toilet training, self-comforting behaviors (thumb sucking, masturbation), speech, imaginative play, no sharing in play, positive reinforcement for desired behavior
5. *Child care:* freedom to explore in safe place; day care; home a safer place to vent frustrations; needs show of affection, language stimulation through reading and conversation
6. *Family:* sibling relationships, parents modeling of nonaggressive responses to conflict (including their own conflict with their toddler)

PRESCHOOL

2 to 5 Years

1. *Health:* tooth brushing, first dental visit
2. *Safety:* needs close supervision near water or street; home safety factors include padding of sharp furniture corners, fire escape plan for home, and locking up power tools; should have car lap belt at 40 pounds and bike helmet; should know (a) name, address, and telephone number, (b) not to provoke dogs, and (c) to say "no" to strangers
3. *Nutrition:* balanced diet; avoiding sweet or salty snacks; participating in conversation at meals
4. *Development/behavior:* initiative versus guilt; difficulty with impulse control and sharing; developing interest in peers; high activity level; speaking in sentences by age 3; speech mostly intelligible to stranger by age 3; reading books; curiosity about body parts; magical thinking, egocentrism
5. *Child care/preschool:* needs daily special time with parents, bedtime routine; talking about day in day care; limiting TV watching with child; reprimanding privately, answering questions factually and simply; adjusting to preschool, kindergarten readiness
6. *Family:* chores, responsibilities

From Foye HR: Anticipatory guidance. In Hoekelman RA, Friedman SB, Nelson NM et al, eds: *Primary pediatric care*, St. Louis, 1997, Mosby, pp. 153-154.

Continued

Topics of Anticipatory Guidance—cont'd

MIDDLE CHILDHOOD

5 to 10 Years

1. *Health:* appropriate weight; regular exercise; somatic complaints (limb and abdominal pain, headaches); alcohol, tobacco, and drug use; sexual development; physician and child dealings (more direct)
2. *Safety:* bike helmets and street safety; car seat belts; swimming lessons; use of matches, firearms, and power tools; fire escape plan for home; saying "no" to strangers
3. *Nutrition:* balanced diet, daily breakfast, limiting sweet and salty snacks, moderate intake of fatty foods
4. *Development/behavior:* industry versus inferiority, need for successes, peer interactions, adequate sleep
5. *School:* school performance, homework, parent interest
6. *Family:* more time away but continuing need for family support, approval, affection, time together, and communication; family rules about bedtime, chores, and responsibilities; guidance in using money; parents should encourage reading; limiting TV watching and discussing programs seen together; teaching and modeling nonviolent responses to conflict
7. *Other activities:* organized sports, religious groups, other organizations, use of spare time

ADOLESCENCE

Discuss with Adolescent

1. *Health:* alcohol, tobacco, and drug use, health consequences of violence, dental care, physical activity, immunizations
2. *Safety:* bike and skateboard helmet and safety, car seat belts, driving while intoxicated, water safety, hitchhiking, risk taking
3. *Nutrition:* balanced diet, appropriate weight, avoiding junk foods
4. *Sexuality:* physical changes, sex education, peer pressure for sexual activity, sense of responsibility for self and partner. OK to say no, preventing pregnancy and sexually transmitted diseases, breast and testes self-examination
5. *Development/relationships:* identity versus role confusion, family, peers, dating, independence, trying different roles, managing anger other than with verbal and physical attacks
6. *School:* academics, homework
7. *Other activities:* sports, hobbies, organizations, jobs
8. *Future plans:* school, work, relationships with others

Discuss with Parents

1. *Communication:* allowing adolescents to participate in discussion and development of family rules; needs frequent praise and affection, time together, interest in adolescent's activities
2. *Independence:* parent and child ambivalence about independence; expecting periods of estrangement; promoting self-responsibility and independence; still needs supervision
3. *Role model:* actions speak louder than words—parents provide model of responsible, reasonable, nonviolent, and compassionate behavior

guidance assists parents in determining when children should have immunizations and the value of them.

The epidemic of measles in the United States during the period 1989-1991, provided an impetus for the National Vaccine Advisory Committee (NVAC) to establish standards for pediatric immunization practices (see the box on p. 444). These standards have been approved by the U.S. Public Health Service and endorsed by the American Academy of Pediatrics (CDC, 1993b, p. 1). These standards emphasize eliminating barriers that impede the timely receipt of immunizations and the need for health care professionals to learn about true contraindications and precautions to vaccinations (see Appendix 15-2). Timely receipt of immunizations can help to prevent long-term chronic conditions as well as infectious disease outbreaks.

Helping parents to know when a child is ill enough to call a doctor can also help to prevent long-term chronic conditions such as hearing loss from an ear infection. The possibilities for preventive health care are varied and almost endless when helping parents learn to handle childhood illness. Questions such as the following help a community health nurse to determine what information parents need to prevent serious illness: Do the parents have a thermometer and do they know how to use it? Do they understand the meaning of dehydration? Do they know basic first aid? Do they know when to call a physician when the child has a fever?

Accident Prevention

Since accidents are the major cause of death after the age of 1 year, preventing them is critical. Appendix 15-3 summarizes typical actions that cause accidents and lists precautions to take at varying age levels to avoid accidents.

A child's environment significantly influences his or her state of health. A common site of accidental injuries to children under the age of 15 is the home. Human, as well as physical, factors in the home can lead to accidents. For example, parents' lack of knowledge about childhood growth and development can contribute to accidents. Parents who lack this understanding often neglect to "safety-proof" the child's environment. Infants and toddlers need to be protected from hazards in the environment. They lack the cognitive development needed to understand what things or activities could lead to injury. Developmental characteristics that place young children at risk for specific types of accidents are identified in Appendix 15-3. Providing parents with this type of information can help them identify potential hazards in a child's environment.

<table>
<tr><th>Age ► Vaccine ▼</th><th>Birth</th><th>1 mo</th><th>2 mos</th><th>4 mos</th><th>6 mos</th><th>12 mos</th><th>15 mos</th><th>18 mos</th><th>4-6 yrs</th><th>11-12 yrs</th><th>14-16 yrs</th></tr>
<tr><td rowspan="2">Hepatitis B[2,3]</td><td colspan="3">Hep B-1</td><td></td><td></td><td></td><td></td><td></td><td></td><td></td><td></td></tr>
<tr><td></td><td colspan="3">Hep B-2</td><td colspan="4">Hep B-3</td><td></td><td>Hep B[3]</td><td></td></tr>
<tr><td>Diphtheria, tetanus, pertussis[4]</td><td></td><td></td><td>DTaP or DTP</td><td>DTaP or DTP</td><td>DTaP or DTP</td><td></td><td colspan="2">DTaP or DTP[4]</td><td>DTaP or DTP</td><td colspan="2">Td</td></tr>
<tr><td>H. influenzae type b[5]</td><td></td><td></td><td>Hib</td><td>Hib</td><td>Hib[5]</td><td colspan="2">Hib[5]</td><td></td><td></td><td></td><td></td></tr>
<tr><td>Polio[6]</td><td></td><td></td><td>Polio[6]</td><td>Polio</td><td></td><td colspan="3">Polio[6]</td><td>Polio</td><td></td><td></td></tr>
<tr><td>Measles, mumps, rubella[7]</td><td></td><td></td><td></td><td></td><td></td><td colspan="2">MMR</td><td></td><td>MMR[7] or</td><td>MMR[7]</td><td></td></tr>
<tr><td>Varicella[8]</td><td></td><td></td><td></td><td></td><td></td><td colspan="3">Var</td><td></td><td>Var[8]</td><td></td></tr>
</table>

Note: Vaccines[1] are listed under the routinely recommended ages. Bars indicate range of acceptable ages for vaccination. Shaded bars indicate catch-up vaccination: at 11-12 years of age, hepatitis B vaccine should be administered to children not previously vaccinated, and Varicella virus vaccine should be administered to children not previously vaccinated who lack a reliable history of chickenpox.

[1]This schedule indicates the recommended age for routine administration of currently licensed childhood vaccines. Some combination vaccines are available and may be used whenever administration of all components of the vaccine is indicated. Providers should consult the manufacturers' package inserts for detailed recommendations.

[2] **Infants born to HBsAg-negative mothers** should receive 2.5 µg of Merck vaccine (Recombivax HB) or 10 µg of SmithKline Beecham (SB) vaccine (Engerix-B). The 2nd dose should be administered ≥1 mo after the 1st dose.
Infant born to HBsAg-positive mothers should receive 0.5 mL hepatitis B immune globulin (HBIG) within 12 hrs of birth, and either 5 µg of Merck vaccine (Recombivax HB) or 10 µg of SB vaccine (Engerix-B) at a separate site. The 2nd dose is recommended at 1–2 mos of age and the 3rd dose at 6 mos of age.
Infants born to mothers whose HBsAg status is unknown should receive either 5 µg of Merck vaccine (Recombivax HB) or 10 µg of SB vaccine (Engerix-B) within 12 hrs of birth. The 2nd dose of vaccine is recommended at 1 mo of age and the 3rd dose at 6 mos of age. Blood should be drawn at the time of delivery to determine the mother's HBsAg status; if it is positive, the infant should receive HBIG as soon as possible (no later than 1 wk of age). The dosage and timing of subsequent vaccine doses should be based upon the mother's HBsAg status.

[3]Children and adolescents who have not been vaccinated against hepatitis B in infancy may begin the series during any childhood visit. Those who have not previously received 3 doses of hepatitis B vaccine should initiate or complete the series during the 11- to 12-year-old visit. The 2nd dose should be administered at least 1 mo after the 1st dose, and the 3rd dose should be administered at least 4 mos after the 1st dose and at least 2 mos after the 2nd dose.

[4]DTaP (diphtheria and tetanus toxoids and acellular pertussis vaccine) is the preferred vaccine for all doses in the vaccination series, including completion of the series in children who have received ≥1 dose of whole-cell DTP vaccine. Whole-cell DTP is an acceptable alternative to DTaP. The 4th dose of DTaP may be administered as early as 12 months of age, provided 6 months have elapsed since the 3rd dose, and if the child is considered unlikely to return at 15-18 mos of age. Td (tetanus and diphtheria toxoids, absorbed, for adult use) is recommended at 11-12 years of age if at least 5 years have elapsed since the last dose of DTP, DTaP, or DT. Subsequent routine Td boosters are recommended every 10 years.

[5]Three *H. influenzae* type b (Hib) conjugate vaccines are licensed for infant use. If PRP-OMP (PedvaxHIB [Merck]) is administered at 2 and 4 mos of age, a dose at 6 mos is not required. After completing the primary series, any Hib conjugate vaccine may be used as a booster.

[6]Two poliovirus vaccines are currently licensed in the US: inactivated poliovirus vaccine (IPV) and oral poliovirus vaccine (OPV). The following schedules are all acceptable by the ACIP, the AAP, and the AAFP, and parents and providers may choose among them:

1. IPV at 2 and 4 mos; OPV at 12-18 mos and 4-6 yrs
2. IPV at 2, 4, 12-18 mos, and 4-6 yrs
3. OPV at 2, 4, 6-18 mos, and 4-6 yrs

The ACIP routinely recommends schedule 1. IPV is the only poliovirus vaccine recommended for immunocompromised persons and their household contacts.

[7]The 2nd dose of MMR is routinely recommended at 4-6 yrs of age or at 11-12 yrs of age but may be administered during any visit, provided at least 1 month has elapsed since receipt of the 1st dose and that both doses are administered at or after 12 months of age.

[8]Susceptible children may receive Varicella vaccine (Var) at any visit after the first birthday and those who lack a reliable history of chickenpox should be immunized during the 11-12 year-old visit. Children ≥13 years of age should receive 2 doses, at least 1 mo apart.

Figure 15-13 Recommended childhood immunization schedule, United States, January to December 1997. Approved by the Advisory Committee on Immunization Practices (ACIP), the American Academy of Pediatrics (AAP), and the American Academy of Family Physicians (AAFP).

Parents cannot remove all environmental hazards and they *cannot* and *should not* control their children 24 hours a day. However, with a combination of child supervision, education of parents, and legislative and environmental changes to get rid of hazards, accidents can be reduced. Families need an understanding of the philosophy of accident prevention. As specified by the National Safety Council, it is not a barrage of do's and dont's but rather it is doing things the right way in the interest of the welfare of others.

Standards for Pediatric Immunization Practices

1. Immunization services are readily available.
2. There are no barriers or unnecessary prerequisites to the receipt of vaccines.
3. Immunization services are available free or for a minimal fee.
4. Providers utilize all clinical encounters to screen and, when indicated, vaccinate children.
5. Providers educate parents and guardians about immunization in general terms.
6. Providers question parents or guardians about contraindications and, before vaccinating a child, inform them in specific terms about the risks and benefits of the vaccinations their child is to receive.
7. Providers follow only true contraindications.
8. Providers administer simultaneously all vaccine doses for which a child is eligible at the time of each visit.
9. Providers use accurate and complete recording procedures.
10. Providers co-schedule immunization appointments in conjunction with appointments for other child health services.
11. Providers report adverse events following vaccination promptly, accurately, and completely.
12. Providers operate a tracking system.
13. Providers adhere to appropriate procedures for vaccine management.
14. Providers conduct semi-annual audits to assess immunization coverage levels and to review immunization records in the patient populations they serve.
15. Providers maintain up-to-date, easily retrievable medical protocols at all locations where vaccines are administered.
16. Providers practice patient-oriented and community-based approaches.
17. Vaccines are administered by properly trained persons.
18. Providers receive ongoing education and training regarding current immunization recommendations.

From CDC: Standards for pediatric immunization practices, *MMWR* 42 (No RR-5):3, 1993b.

One method the nurse can use to improve the family approach to accident prevention is accident analysis after an accident occurs. What, how, to whom, where, when, and why did the accident happen? Families must understand that the purpose of this is not to fix blame but rather to prevent a recurrence. Often, teaching the parent who is the primary care provider for the child will have an impact on accident prevention. The nurse can help this parent to be alert to hazards in the environment when home visits are made.

The Safe Kids Coalition is a nationwide effort to prevent childhood injury. It is a growing network of 121 state and local coalitions in 41 states, created by the Children's National Medical Center in Washington, D.C. (phone 202-662-0600) with major funding from Johnson and Johnson. The injury intervention strategies used by the coalition are enforcement, engineering, education, and evaluation. An underlying belief of coalition members is that solutions to the injuries sustained by children in accidents will not come from Washington or the media but rather when everyone in a community is involved. For example, in Allentown, Pennsylvania, the local group has sponsored a bike rodeo to teach children and parents about safety in this area. They also sponsored a safety carnival and in-service programs for elementary school teachers. The Safe Kids Coalition is a place for professionals concerned about preventing major problems in the newborn to 5-year-old age group to place their efforts.

The box at right summarizes interventions for preventing child and adolescent injury from preventable accidents as described by the Children's Safety Network. These interventions are part of the efforts of the Safe Kids Coalition as well.

Effective Interventions to Prevent Child and Adolescent Injury

PLANNING AND PRIORITIZING

- A broad-based coalition representing the community of interest;
- surveillance tools and methods to identify and monitor the number of injuries;
- the use of E codes to aid in the ascertainment of injury causes; and
- selection of priority areas for injury control.

COMPREHENSIVE MULTIFACETED APPROACH

- Evaluation of prevention strategies to determine effectiveness;
- dissemination and universal implementation of effective strategies;
- targeting of high-risk groups, such as low income; and
- incorporation of prevention messages and efforts into service systems for children and adolescents.

INSTITUTIONALIZATION AND ACCEPTANCE

- Coordination of local, State and Federal efforts;
- institutionalization of injury prevention programming;
- enforcement of existing legislation protecting children; and
- development of a societal norm of a safe childhood and adolescence.

From Children's Safety Network: *A data book of child and adolescent injury*, Washington, D.C., 1991, National Center for Education in Maternal and Child Health, p. 61.

Prevention of Child Abuse

As previously mentioned in this chapter, abuse and neglect are symptoms of stress in a family. The conditions of poverty, undernutrition, unemployment, overcrowding,

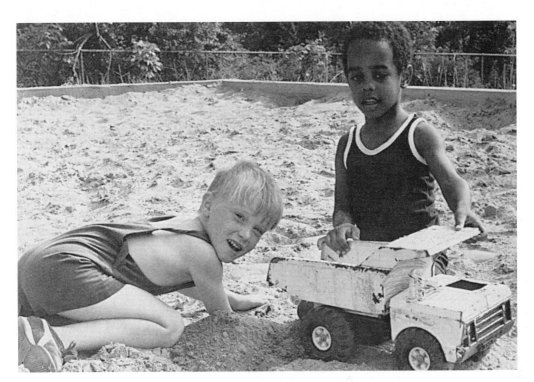

Figure 15-14 Healthy 5-year-old children.

restricted physical surroundings, and inadequate education support this problem. Knowledge currently available tells us that antenatal poverty and nutritional deficits produce a high-risk infant. At the same time, high-quality medical care is least available to the very people who are at highest risk. The high-risk infant and ill-prepared parents have the fewest resources for achieving the best health possible. Communities can deal with these poverty problems at a local level. However, the nation needs to deal with them at a federal level to make the most impact.

To save a child from the serious effects of abuse and neglect, nurses need to be alert when they notice that families are having children very quickly with no relief between pregnancies. The danger signs of marital stress, isolation, and overwhelmed parents need to be seen also. Premature births, where questionable bonding has taken place, indicate a need for priority service, as do families where there are children with developmental disabilities and chronic disease.

Every parent needs to know how children grow and develop. The concept that babies are responsible for their acts and can think and reason like adults is all too commonly believed and must be corrected.

Education of personnel, including judges, attorneys, social workers, and doctors, is necessary so that abused children are found, identified as such, and then given treatment. Parents must not be treated as criminals but rather given help so that their stress is alleviated. Equally important are the rights of children.

Social institutions such as churches and schools need to be used to help support families. In our mobile society where people move frequently, families can feel isolated, alone, and uncared for. Homemaker services, big brothers and sisters, and parent aides, as well as community volunteers, could fill some of the gaps experienced by families who are isolated.

Preschool Assessments

Kindergarten and preschool health assessments are excellent developmental points at which to look at the physical, intellectual, and emotional growth of children. At this time parents are increasingly aware of and concerned about the learning and thought competency of their children. They want to know that their children are ready to begin school. A child's ability to learn, see, perform appropriate gross and fine motor tasks, follow instruction, speak, communicate, and relate socially with others are all indicators of readiness for school (Figure 15-14). The Denver Developmental Screening Test is one method used by community health nurses to look at these areas. Preschool assessments also provide an excellent opportunity to ensure that all children receive immunizations before they are in school.

Day Care for Children

In 1995 more than 60% of all mothers with preschool-age children were in the workforce. This represented a nearly twofold increase since 1970. Figure 15-15 depicts this dramatic increase. Over one fourth of these children spent the time their mothers were working in nonresidential day care centers. Women who work full time tend to use day care centers, whereas women who work part time tend to use in-home care (Maternal and Child Health Bureau, 1996).

Figure 15-15 also depicts the shift in child care arrangements in the past 10 years from in-home care to day care or nursery school settings. The importance of this information for community health nurses is threefold: as parents, nurses may need assistance with finding safe and affordable child care, and further, nurses may be able to assist their clients with this important activity. Additionally, community health nurses can assist day care providers in facilitating a safe and healthy environment for the children they serve. Each year an estimated 7% of all children in day care required medical treatment for injuries (Selecting a safe day care center, 1992, p. 32).

Community health nurses play a significant role in helping day care providers to make the environment safe and prevent the spread of common infectious diseases. They also assist these providers with health education activities, as well as the preparation of nutritionally sound meals. Additionally, they provide suggestions about activities that stimulate growth and development.

The Safe Kids Coalition suggests that parents visit centers, ask questions about services offered, and observe. Look at precautions taken for the prevention of falls from stairs and windows, storage of cleaning supplies, types of toys and their cleanliness—the kinds of concerns that parents have for the safety of children at home. Space for play and the ratio of staff to children are other concerns. The National Association for the Education of Young Children in Washington, D.C., has lists of accredited day care centers across the country.

GENERAL CONCEPTS OF HEALTH PROMOTION

Health promotion needs are based on the developmental tasks and common health problems of the specific population group. For the newborn to 5-year-old and parenting population, the following factors should be considered when developing a health promotion program:

- A monitoring system to identify high-risk infants and parents
- An organized community program to combat problems such as accidents and child abuse

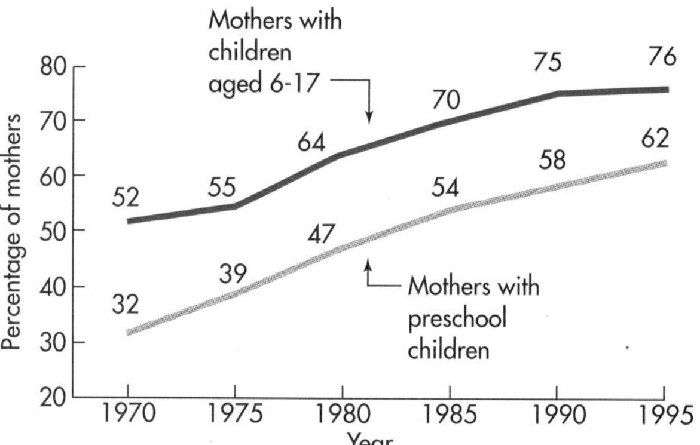

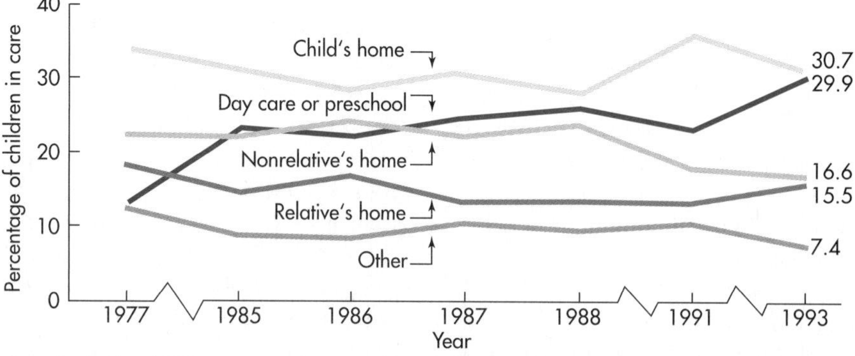

*Data for 1994 and 1995 are not strictly comparable with data for earlier years due to changes in the survey and the estimation process.

Figure **15-15** Mothers in the labor force: 1970 to 1995, and place of care for preschool-aged children: 1977 to 1993. *(From Maternal and Child Health Bureau:* Child health USA '95, *Washington, D.C., 1996, U.S. Government Printing Office, p. 20. Source: U.S. Bureau of the Census and U.S. Bureau of Labor Statistics.)*

- An organized system for provision of preventive health services, such as physical examinations and immunizations
- Health education program to meet anticipatory guidance needs of parents and children
- A well-established procedure for follow-up care of clients with identified health care needs
- Passage and revision of significant legislation, such as immunization and child abuse laws

AGGREGATES AT PARTICULAR RISK AMONG THOSE UNDER 5 YEARS OF AGE

Infants and children cannot speak or act on their own behalf. They are dependent on the adults around them to do for them what must be done to ensure a healthy, happy life. The fact that more than one out of five American children still lives below the poverty line, accompanied by the fact that the number of poor children increased by more than 2.7 million in less than a decade, should strike fear into the thoughts of professionals who care about the health of the children of the United States (Children's Defense Fund, 1996, p. 2). Adults who live around children have not adequately spoken or acted on their behalf. This section discusses three aggregates at particular risk: the homeless, those with fetal alcohol syndrome, and children who are technology-dependent.

The Homeless

Families, mainly mothers with small children, were the fastest-growing group of homeless people in the 1980s. It is difficult to comprehend that thousands of families in this country, headed by women, have no permanent home (Norton, Ridenour, 1995). Having no home hurts children and their families in many ways, but what it obviously does is compromise access to the formal health care system, prenatal care, insurance coverage, sanitary environments, and immunizations. Children in homeless shelters have diarrhea, elevated blood lead levels, and asthma at higher rates than other children. Nutrition and emotional stability are other factors compromised by homelessness. The job of simply being a child must be out of the question in a shelter with dozens of other people and no privacy and certainty about life. It has been found that homeless children are more likely to be developmentally delayed and have depressive and social disorders than those not homeless (Berne, Dato, Mason, Rafferty, 1990; Zima, Wells, Freeman, 1994).

A subgroup at high risk among the homeless is runaway girls. Recent indications are that this population includes increasing numbers of women who are pregnant: one study of homeless girls in 19 cities found that 30% of the girls 16 to 19 years of age were pregnant (Athey, 1989, p. 5). Rarely do these adolescents receive prenatal care, and they are subjected to both physical and sexual abuse. Further, they are vulnerable to drug and alcohol abuse. Athey's report includes descriptions of six programs serving pregnant and homeless adolescents.

The key causes of homelessness are poverty, the shortage of low-income housing, and lack of the support needed by families with special needs or in times of particular stress. Addressing these factors takes initiatives from all levels of government, from corporate and business communities, and from community groups and religious congregations (Mihaly, 1991, p. 220). The American Nurses Association has included homelessness among the issues it advocates for in Washington, D.C., as have many other state associations. Nurses can contact the legislative committee of their state nurses' association for information about what their associations are doing to support this issue.

Fetal Alcohol Syndrome

Fetal alcohol syndrome (FAS) has been called the most common, best known, most preventable cause of mental retardation in the western world. This syndrome is caused by a pregnant woman's heavy use of alcohol, and diagnosis is based on the following symptoms in the infant: retarded growth, a pattern of facial abnormalities, and abnormalities of the central nervous system that can include mental retardation (Masis, May, 1991, p. 484). Fetal alcohol effect and alcohol-related birth defect are manifestations of lower amounts of alcohol ingested during pregnancy. Because there is no cure for this syndrome, primary prevention is of utmost importance. The number of babies born with fetal alcohol syndrome is increasing (USDHHS, 1995a). Accurate statistics are difficult to obtain because women frequently do not report alcohol use during pregnancy because of fear of prosecution (Center for Substance Abuse Treatment, 1993). There is a growing interest in prosecuting mothers who expose their unborn child to drugs. Rhodes (1992) discusses several legal cases where this has occurred.

Female alcoholics are frequently ostracised in our society and thus have been left to produce a number of children with FAS before they themselves die prematurely. Masis and May (1991) describe a hospital-based, comprehensive approach to the prevention of FAS that combines clinical assessment, community outreach, and epidemiological knowledge to attack the resulting birth defects. One of the striking results of this program was its acceptance by the women referred to it: of 48 who were referred, only 3 refused outright. The outstanding success of this program could be a model for others. Poland-Laken and Hutchins (1995) also discuss ways to build and sustain systems of care for substance-using pregnant women and their infants. They describe lessons learned from innovative, community-based demonstration projects.

Children Who Are Technology Dependent

Over the past two decades it has become increasingly possible to save smaller and sicker newborns. Twenty years ago, nine of every 10 babies born weighing less than 1000 grams (2.2 lb) died. Today, with the median birth weight at 7 lb 8 oz, it is not uncommon to find extremely low birth weight babies surviving.

It is the rare low birth weight infant, however, who does not suffer serious complications such as brain or pulmonary hemorrhages, heart failure, or infections—among other problems. Further, the number of babies born each year with multiple defects totals about 30,000. An increasing number of these babies receive sophisticated treatment at birth and grow into young children whose lives are regulated by technology. One such group of children are infants who are ventilator dependent.

Increasing numbers of parents are opting to care at home for their children whose lives are regulated by technology. "Technology-dependent" is a term used to describe a small subset of the disabled child population who rely on life-sustaining medical technology and who typically require complex, hospital-level nursing care. Table 15-4 provides a summary of the most recent large-scale estimate of the size of this population. Both the numbers in this aggregate and the group types are increasing, and the children in groups I, II, and III in Table 15-4 may double in the coming years (U.S. Congress, OTA, 1987, p. 4).

table 15-4 Summary of OTA Estimates of the Size of the Technology Dependent Child Population, 1987

Defined Population	Estimated Number of Children
GROUP I	
Requiring ventilator assistance	680 to 2,000
GROUP II	
Requiring parenteral nutrition	350 to 700
Requiring prolonged intravenous drugs	270 to 8,275
GROUP III	
Requiring other device-based respiratory or nutritional support	1,000 to 6,000
Rounded subtotal (I + II + III)	**2,300 to 17,000**
GROUP IV	
Requiring apnea monitoring	6,800 to 45,000
Requiring renal dialysis	1,000 to 6,000
Requiring other device-associated nursing	Unknown, perhaps 30,000 or more

From U.S. Congress, Office of Technology Assessment: *Technology dependent children: hospital v. home care—a technical memorandum*, OTA-TM-H-38, Washington, D.C., May 1987, U.S. Government Printing Office, p. 4.

Many health care professionals consider the home setting better than the hospital when all the needs of children are considered. This can happen only when parents want their child home, when families can cope with living with the child amid the intrusion of health care providers in the home, and when the effectiveness of home care services including equipment, respite care, social and psychological supports, and professional caregivers are adequate.

The financing of home health care for technology-dependent children is problematic because many of the families frequently lack private insurance. Further, "virtually all very-long-term technology-dependent children requiring a high level of nursing assistance will exceed the limits of their families' private insurance policies, will be uninsurable in the self-purchase insurance market because they are poor risks, and will end up on Medicaid" (U.S. Congress, OTA, 1987, p. 7). As alternatives to hospital care become more widely available, the incentive will be present to discharge these children quicker and sicker into the community, even before adequate preparations have been made. (U.S. Congress, OTA, p. 8). Community health nurses involved in planning for their discharges will need to watch for this scenario. Further, nurses in the community will need high-level technical skills.

In Chapter 10, one mother shares her graphic story of her struggles to keep her ventilator-dependent child at home and the strengths and weaknesses of the health care team who aided the family in its struggle. Families who have children with special needs, such as ventilator-dependent children, need coordinated, comprehensive health care services that ensure continuity of care. They also need to have a clear understanding of the referral process and community resources that can promote family stability and concrete assistance during times of stress. Chapters 8, 10, and 19 are helpful to review when visiting families in the community who have "special" children.

SIGNIFICANT HEALTH LEGISLATION

During the past 70 years there has been significant federal legislation and many demonstration projects concerned with the health of infants and mothers in America. The Children's Bureau was established in 1912. White House Conferences on Children and Youth have been held every 10 years since 1910. The Shepherd-Towner Act of 1921 created federally supported maternal and child health services at the state level. Title V of the Social Security Act of 1935 provided for grants to states for maternal and child health services and services to crippled children. The Emergency Maternity and Infant Care Program existed during the 1930s. The need for community mental health programs was recognized in the 1960s. The Eighty-ninth Congress, during President Johnson's time in office (1963-1968), brought huge changes in child health legislation with the establishment of the Office of Economic Opportunity and its Head Start Program, Medicaid, and the National Institutes of

Child Health and Human Development. Significant current legislation continues to provide funding for maternal and child health services.

Seven major public programs are designed to meet the needs of women and children in this country. These programs are the preventive health and health services block grant; maternal and child health block grant; Early and Periodic Screening, Diagnosis, and Treatment portion of Medicaid; childhood immunization program; childhood lead poisoning prevention; community health centers; and migrant health centers (General Accounting Office, 1992, p. 1). Table 15-5 provides significant data related to each of these programs. A broad range of health, welfare, and environmental services are provided by them. Another significant program that provides needed maternal and child health services is the Women, Infants, and Children Program (WIC). As presented in Chapter 4, WIC is a federal nutrition and health program administered by the U.S. Department of Agriculture that makes food available to at-risk pregnant and lactating women, and infants and children up to the age of 5 years.

Though these programs fill significant needs for many women and children, it is problematic that objectives overlap, that coordination between programs is lacking, and that requirements for the programs are not well defined. Further, resource limitations may result in fewer services than those authorized. When services are listed as optional they may not be made available because grantees may only choose to provide the required services paid for by these

table 15-5 Programs Serving Low-Income Mothers and Children in the United States: Program Objectives and Target Population*

Program and Authority	Program Objectives and Target Population
Community Health Centers Grant (CHC) (Section 330, Public Health Service [PHS] Act)	This program provides preventive and primary health care services and case management of other services to medically underserved populations;† each CHC must demonstrate the capability to serve all age groups, and should be able to identify populations in its service area with special health care needs.
Migrant Health Centers Grant (MHC) (Section 329, PHS Act)	This program provides preventive and management of other services to migrant and seasonal farmworkers and their families; in defining its appropriate role, each center assesses the needs of its target population.
Maternal and Child Health Block Grant (M&CH) (Title V, Social Security Act [SSA])	This block grant program seeks to improve the health of mothers and children who do not have access to adequate health care,‡ particularly those from low-income families: direct services include preventive and primary care for children, prenatal care and delivery services, and postpartum care, but this funding also helps to support the state service delivery infrastructure; other services must also be provided for children with special health care needs (rehabilitative services for certain categories of children under 16 who are disabled).
Childhood Lead Poisoning Prevention Program (CLPPP) (Lead Contamination Control Act, 1988)	This program provides states with resources to establish and expand programs to prevent childhood lead poisoning; program activities may include screening for lead poisoning, referral for medical treatment and environmental intervention, follow-up, and education about lead poisoning. It targets high-risk children under 6 years of age.
Childhood Immunization Program (CIP) (Section 317, PHS Act)	This program provides states with resources to establish and maintain programs to immunize children against vaccine-preventable diseases; CIP funds may be used for the planning and implementation of immunization programs, for vaccine purchase, and for assessment of immunization status.
Preventive Health and Health Services Block Grant (PHHS) (Title XIX, part A of PHS Act)	This block grant program provides states with resources for comprehensive preventive health services. Each state determines the target population to be served.
Medicaid/Early and Periodic Screening, Diagnosis, and Treatment (EPSDT) (Title XIX, SSA)	This program seeks to diagnose physical and mental problems in low-income children under 21 and to provide treatment to correct any conditions found.

From General Accounting Office (GAO): *Federally funded health services: information on seven programs serving low-income women and children*, GAO/HRD-92-73FS, Gaithersburg, Md., May 1992, GAO, pp. 10-11.

*All seven programs are authorized to address the health care needs of women, children, or both, but each targets a slightly different population, and the type of services available under each program varies.

†Medically underserved populations are designated by the Department of Health and Human Services (DHHS) according to the percentage of population with income below the poverty level, percentage of population 65 years of age and over, infant mortality rate, and physicians per 1,000 population.

‡The Maternal and Child Health Block Grant provides both grants to states and funding for set-aside programs. In this fact sheet, we are reporting only on the grants to states.

funds. Thus services provided by one state or grantee may not be provided by another (GAO, 1992, p. 17).

Fragmentation, categorization, and lack of coordinated services were addressed in the late 1980s and early 1990s by private foundations and the federal government. The concept of "One-Stop Shopping" was used to describe a client-centered system that facilitates access to care by enhancing coordination and integration of the many programs available to women (Macro Systems, Inc., 1990, p. iv).

Major issues related to the delivery of maternal and child health services are currently being discussed. These discussions have begun to significantly alter present maternal and child health programs. There is an increasing "number of states turning to managed care as a principal vehicle through which to deliver health care to children, parents, and pregnant women enrolled in Medicaid. As of November 1995, fully half of the states were operating, waiting for approvals of, or developing statewide Medicaid managed care programs, under special, experimental federal waivers that would allow them to make enrollment mandatory" (CDF, 1996, pp. 20-21). Advocates for children are concerned that current discussion about future federal block grants to states could lead to significant reductions in funding for essential maternal and child health services (CDF).

Child Abuse

The Child Abuse Prevention and Treatment Act (Public Law 93-247) was signed into law in 1974 in response to the need for a nationwide effort to solve this complex problem. This act created the National Center on Child Abuse and Neglect as the primary place where the federal government can focus its efforts on identifying, treating, and preventing child abuse and neglect (Combating child abuse, 1988, p. 369). To carry out the mandates of the act, the National Center has begun programs in four areas: demonstration and research, information gathering and dissemination, training and technical assistance, and assistance to states. In 1962 the Children's Bureau developed and promoted a model state child abuse mandatory reporting law that, in effect, states that professionals or child care workers must report suspected child abuse to the appropriate officials. Public Law 93-247 reinforced this mandate.

The Child Abuse Prevention and Treatment Act of 1974 has been amended several times since it was initially passed. In 1988 Congress passed legislation to reauthorize three programs designed to prevent and treat child abuse and domestic violence and to encourage the adoption of hard-to-place children. This legislative act was entitled "The Child Abuse Prevention, Adoption, and Family Services Act of 1988" (Public Law 100-294). It consolidated into one act the Child Abuse Prevention and Treatment Act of 1974, the Child Abuse Prevention and Treatment and Adoption Reform Act of 1978, and the Family Violence Prevention and Services Act of 1984.

Public Law 100-294 mandates funding to support state and local efforts designed to prevent abuse and family violence and to identify and treat the victims. It also ensures funding of the National Center on Child Abuse and Neglect, a national commission on child and youth deaths, a project to study the nationwide incidence of family violence, and initiatives to eliminate barriers to the adoption of older children, minority children, and children with physical and mental handicaps. Additionally, it mandates support of professional training and research activities (USDHHS, 1988).

The states have acted on Public Law 100-294 in various ways. Community health nurses must know the laws that are in effect in the states in which they are working. Health care professionals are directly affected by this law and by state child protection laws that require the reporting of child abuse and neglect.

Developmental Disabilities

Scientific advances in recent decades have made it possible to save infants who previously would have died at birth. However, this phenomenon has created special challenges for health care professionals. The number of infants and children with developmental disabilities is increasing significantly. These children need assistance to help them achieve their maximum potential. Because this assistance was often very costly and not available for many children with developmental disabilities, the Congress has passed, in recent years, two significant pieces of legislation that were designed to promote early intervention with handicapped and at-risk young children.

The Education for All Handicapped Children Act (Public Law 94-142) was enacted in 1975. It was renamed the Individuals with Disabilities Education Act (IDEA) in 1990. IDEA entitles all disabled children between the ages of 6 and 18 to a free and appropriate education regardless of the type of disability or the degree of impairment. It also allows incentive monies for providing services to children beginning at age 3 and for young adults between 18 and 21. This act is discussed more extensively in Chapter 16.

The Education of the Handicapped Act Amendments of 1986 (Public Law 99-457) significantly expanded services to preschool children 3 to 5 years old and at-risk infants and toddlers up to age 3 years. This law created two new federal programs—the preschool grant program and the disabled infants and toddlers program. By 1990-1991 state educational agencies had to provide a free and appropriate education for all disabled children beginning at the age of 3. Significant federal funding was allocated to support the preschool grant program. The disabled infants and toddlers program was established to reduce the potential for developmental delays, help families to meet the special needs of their disabled children and toddlers, minimize institutionalization of disabled individuals, and reduce educational costs to society. Incentive funding for this program has helped states to develop and implement quality early intervention programs and to coordinate early intervention services. Community health nurses are active participants on the multidisciplinary teams that are providing services to infants and toddlers under this program.

On July 26, 1990, President George Bush signed into law the Americans with Disabilities Act, which prohibits discrimination on the basis of disability in employment. For the first time, employers in both the private and public sector cannot discriminate because an individual is disabled (Smith, 1992). Chapter 19 discusses the implications of this act in depth.

BARRIERS TO HEALTH CARE

Major barriers to the delivery of services to the newborn to 5-year-old population and their parents have been discussed earlier in this chapter and in Chapter 14. The following case scenarios illustrate some specific problems parents have in obtaining care for themselves and their children under 5 years of age.

CASE *Scenario*

Sue was 17 years old when she became pregnant. Her husband, Tom, age 18, worked as a gas station attendant. His income provided only the basic necessities of food and rent but was too high to allow them any public assistance. Sue decided to "save" money by waiting for antepartum care until near her EDC. Upon her first antepartum visit to the doctor 1 month before delivery, she was found to be severely hypertensive and diabetic. Her infant weighed 10 lb at birth and required 1 month's hospitalization. Sue and Tom felt that they were severely criticized by the health personnel for not receiving adequate antepartum care.

CASE *Scenario*

Diane and Jim Jones have four children under 5 years of age. Jim has a job-related back injury and is unemployed. The Joneses have a Medicaid card and they use the outpatient department of a large teaching hospital in their city for medical care. They go there only when they absolutely must. The family has no car and uses the city bus line, which involves three transfers for the 4-mile trip. With four children, Mrs. Jones finds this most difficult, especially in cold weather. When she does arrive at the hospital, she must wait several hours and then sees a different physician each time so that she must repeatedly give her family's health histories. Mrs. Jones feels that "the people in that hospital don't care about or understand me and my kids."

As part of the *Healthy Mothers, Healthy Babies* campaign initiated by the U.S. Department of Health and Human Services to help achieve the maternal and infant health objectives for the nation (Bratic, 1982), a study was carried out to document the perceived barriers to seeking health care and information among women of a lower socioeconomic status. Three major barriers were identified ("Healthy Mothers" *Market Research: How to Reach Black and Mexican American Women*, 1982): (1) *low priority of preventive health care*, because it takes considerable energy for many of these mothers to meet basic needs and because government funding sources do not adequately finance preventive health services, (2) *difficulties encountered within the health care system*, including communication barriers, perceived negative attitudes of staff, and the unavailability or inappropriateness of educational materials, and (3) *low motivation to adopt good health practices*, because many clients generally have a day-to-day orientation, multiple life problems, and a support group that does not understand or support certain health habits or practices. These barriers continue to exist and prevent many mothers and children from obtaining basic health care services.

THE ROLES OF THE COMMUNITY HEALTH NURSE

The community health nurse assumes a number of roles in providing service to the newborn to 5-year-old age group. The following section describes some of these roles.

Advocate-Planner

Since the children in the newborn to 5-year-old age group cannot speak for themselves, the nurse becomes an advocate. This can involve pointing out to caregivers the safety hazards in the environment and urging necessary changes. On a broader level, the nurse is an advocate for the development of day care centers in a community and publicizes the inadequacy of health and medical care for economically disadvantaged families. This role of advocate means that the nurse must be involved in the political process to correct issues such as unemployment, lack of adequate income, overcrowding, and the cycle of poverty, which can ultimately be solved only with legislative changes. Attitudes of assertiveness, a knowledge of the political process, and a willingness to take risks are necessary tools for this role.

Teacher

The community health nurse needs to be a teacher. This role includes demonstrating information about child care to families and involving parents in the learning process. Helping parents to understand good nutrition for this age group, or why safety seats and belts are necessary in cars, means involvement of all concerned in the process of teaching and learning and changing values and attitudes. The community health nurse is well versed in the developmental tasks of this age group. Teaching parents about these tasks is a form of anticipatory guidance and assists in task accomplishment.

Group Worker

In order to meet the needs of the newborn to 5-year-old population, the community health nurse needs to be attuned to opportunities for group teaching and counseling.

Working with the LaLèche League or Parents Anonymous, a crisis intervention program set up to help prevent damaging relationships between parents and their children, are options. Other possibilities are numerous. One community health nurse, for example, had in his caseload area a large mobile park. Within the park he found five families who had children in special school classes because of developmental disabilities, each of whom expressed a need for help with their child. This staff nurse helped the parents form a weekly discussion group and the results were that isolated families received mutual supportive help in the form of babysitting, shared meals, and problem solving about how to deal with difficult situations.

Coordinator

Coordinating community resources is another significant role of the community health nurse. Numerous services are available to families, and this is positive. However, families can feel uncared for and torn apart when the department of social services, Medicaid screening clinic, the community health nurse, the school nurse, and the child guidance center all request the same information in detail, or when these same health professionals do not communicate with each other and therefore plan different goals. Professionals need to be careful to ask the permission of a family before they share information regarding that family with another professional or agency. They should seek this permission as soon as they realize that families are working with multiple agencies.

Closely tied to this role is the facilitating role of the nurse. Helping families and the larger community to understand their rights as people and to understand services offered in the community all facilitate the better utilization of these services. The nurse helps families work toward desired change. Every community has persons with ideas and skills; all that needs to be done is to give them direction and reinforcement. Milio's *9226 Kercheval: The Storefront That Did Not Burn* is the classic story of how one community health nurse helped an inner-city area establish its own day care center (Milio, 1970). This nurse found that people saw a great problem with children who were not cared for while mothers worked. She acted as a catalyst to assist in solving the problem and was a facilitator and enabler as well.

Casefinder

Because of the nurse's proximity to infants and children, casefinding has been a strategic role for many years. At-risk children are identified and followed periodically as they develop. Disabilities are lessened when treatment is begun early, and some can be prevented by primary intervention. A system needs to be established in each community to periodically screen all children for problems. The Early Periodic Screening, Diagnosis, and Treatment Program (EPSDT) of Medicaid is one schedule that can be followed.

The North American Nursing Diagnosis Association (NANDA) accepted "altered parenting" and "risk for altered parenting" as appropriate diagnostic terms in nursing and acceptable nursing diagnoses for clinical testing (Gordon, 1997). These diagnoses are presented in the following boxes on the next page. The defining characteristics developed by NANDA provide practitioners with useful parameters for casefinding when working with families with children.

Epidemiologist

Collecting data on health problems and care is an important epidemiological role. Nurses are concerned about why parents do not use available health services and what motivates those who do. They use population-focused practice models to answer these concerns and to develop targeted, aggregate-focused interventions that address the factors that impede service use (Selby, Riportella-Muller, Sorenson, Walters, 1989). Reasons why people do and do not use health care are important elements in planning health services.

When the community health nurse visits parents after accidental poisoning incidents, the nurse can add to the epidemiological understanding of the predisposing and immediate causes of the accident and make recommendations to prevent them from occurring again. If it were the case that 75% of the families who have poisoning accidents have other health problems, there would be evidence that this kind of stress leads to poisoning accidents.

A good record system in the health agency will help nurses to collect data on health problems, to plan interventions, and to evaluate care given. These data can provide information on changing health needs and necessary health services.

A good record system will collect data on the newborn to 5-year-old child that provide the basis for a health history on which later events in the family system can be compared and built.

Clinic Nurse

Community health nurses have long worked in well-baby clinics where, at regular intervals, the health of children up to the age of 5 is assessed, immunizations are given, and parents have the opportunity to discuss concerns of growth and development. This role has been expanded to an assessment and treatment role. Nurses deal with problem behavior such as delayed play, immature social behavior, and temper tantrums. With the nurse's knowledge of child development, behavior modification, and management techniques, the roles of observer, consultant, and counselor to parents, preschool teachers, and day care workers are valuable in dealing with minor problems that can develop into major ones.

Home Visitor

A well-known role of the nurse caring for the needs of the newborn to 5-year-old age group is that of the community

NANDA Nursing Diagnosis: Altered Parenting (Specify Alteration)

DEFINITION

Inability of nurturing figure(s) to create an environment that promotes optimum growth and development of another human being. (NOTE: Adjustment to parenting, in general, is a normal maturation process following birth of a child. This is a broad taxonomic category; specify type of alteration.)

DEFINING CHARACTERISTICS

- Inattentive to infant/child needs
- Inappropriate caretaking behaviors (toilet training, feeding, sleep/rest)
- History of child abuse or abandonment by primary caretaker
- Actual alteration:
  1. Verbalization cannot control child
  2. Abandonment of infant/child
  3. Runaway
- Incidence of physical and psychological trauma
- Lack of parental attachment behaviors
- Inappropriate visual, tactile, auditory stimulation
- Negative identification of infant/child's characteristics
- Negative attachment of meanings to infant/child's characteristics; verbalization of resentment toward infant/child
- Evidence of physical and psychological trauma to infant/child
- Constant verbalization of disappointment in gender or physical characteristics of the infant/child
- Verbalization of role inadequacy
- Verbal disgust at body functions of infant/child
- Noncompliance with health appointments for infant/child or self
- Inappropriate or inconsistent discipline practices
- Frequent accidents (infant/child); frequent illness (infant/child)
- Growth and development lag of infant/child
- Verbalizes desire to have child call parent by first name versus traditional, cultural tendencies
- Child receives care from multiple caretakers without consideration for the needs of the infant/child
- Compulsively seeks role approval from others

ETIOLOGICAL OR RELATED FACTORS

- Knowledge or skill deficit (specify—e.g., parenting skills, developmental guidelines)
- Fear (specify focus)
- Social isolation
- Physical impairment (e.g., blindness)
- Mental or physical illness
- Support system deficit (between/from significant other[s])
- Interrupted parent-infant bonding (e.g., illness of newborn)
- Family or personal stress (financial, legal, recent crisis, cultural change, multiple pregnancies)
- Unmet social, emotional, or developmental needs (of parenting figures)
- Interruption in bonding process (i.e., maternal, paternal, other)
- Unrealistic expectations (self, infant, partner)
- Perceived threat to own survival (physical and emotional)
- Lack of role identity
- Lack of or inappropriate response of child
- Physical or psychosocial abuse (of nurturing figure)
- Limited cognitive functioning

From Gordon M: *Manual of nursing diagnosis, 1997-1998*, St. Louis, 1997, Mosby, pp. 387, 389.

NANDA Nursing Diagnosis: Risk for Altered Parenting (Specify Alteration)

DEFINITION

Presence of risk factors during prenatal or child-rearing period that may interfere with process of adjustment to parenting (specify type of alteration).

RISK FACTORS

- Unavailable or ineffective role model
- History of physical or psychosocial abuse (of nurturing figure)
- Support system deficit (between/from significant others)
- Unmet social, emotional, developmental needs (of parenting figures)
- Interruption in bonding process (maternal, paternal, other)
- Unrealistic expectation (self, infant, partner)
- Perceived threat to own survival (physical, emotional)
- Physical impairment (e.g., blindness)
- Physical or mental illness
- Presence of stress (financial, legal, recent personal crisis, cultural change, multiple pregnancies)
- Knowledge or skill deficit (specify—e.g., parenting skills, developmental progression)
- Limited cognitive functioning
- Lack of role identity
- Lack of, or inappropriate, response of child to relationship
- Social isolation
- Fear (specify focus)

From Gordon M: *Manual of nursing diagnosis, 1997-1998*, St. Louis, 1997, Mosby, p. 391.

health nurse who visits parents and babies in their homes. Each health department sets its own priorities and standards for the care of parents and children. This ranges from the prenatal and postnatal referral of each pregnancy to the referral of only those mothers and infants at high risk. The broad background of community health nurses equips them with skills to help establish the standards as to which newborns and parents will be visited. In particular, families that

A View from the Field LILLY'S ANGER

I am a public health nurse providing home visits to "at risk" pregnant women and infants. The women and infants I see generally live in rural settings.

Perhaps the most challenging aspect of my work is trying to engage the client who, for a combination of reasons, is not initially receptive to help from someone perceived as an "outsider." The following situation provides insight to the challenges and complexities routinely encountered by public health nurses such as myself.

I first encountered Lilly approximately ten months ago. She was eight months pregnant and was found to have some abnormalities in her blood work at the last checkup. She needed to have an ultrasound immediately to determine if the baby was okay. The clinic was unable to reach Lilly by phone and asked me to stop by her home and urge her to get into the clinic as soon as possible for further assessment.

Lilly's need for help on the one hand, and resistance to any kind of intervention on the other hand, quickly surfaced in my initial contact. To begin with, she was very angry. Angry about being awakened from her sleep—I learned she worked nights in a laundry. Angry about having relinquished her first child and the pressure her parents were putting on her to do it again. Angry about her negative experiences with the Department of Social and Health Services. Angry at the prospect of the second ultrasound. "Didn't I just have one a month ago? Can things change all that much in four weeks?"

Speaking in a loud voice and in a forceful manner, Lilly had no difficulty letting me know her thoughts about her pregnancy and her generally less than desirable circumstances. Her anger and frustration were intensified by her imposing figure. Lilly is about six feet tall, large framed, has bright red hair, and is developmentally delayed. I found her presentation rather intimidating, especially in view of the dark and dreary house into which I had been invited to state my business. However, the fact that I allowed Lilly to vent seemed to be having a quieting effect. I tried as much as possible to validate her concerns, and as a result, she gradually became more open to having the second ultrasound. In fact, I actually dialed the number so she could set up the appointment. By the time I left Lilly's home, she was also indicating that she "might" be receptive to another visit. "But don't call until the late afternoon."

Driving away from Lilly's home, I reflected on what had transpired and wondered if I would ever see her again. Given the number of problems in this case, on-going help was certainly needed, but would Lilly be open to it?

Attempts to make contact by phone got nowhere, so I decided to "drop-in" about four weeks after my first visit. My hope was that it was late enough in the day so Lilly would be up from her sleep and receptive to my visit. Apparently, my willingness to listen to her during my first visit rather than retreat during her burst of anger and frustration, earned a certain measure of respect and acceptance. Lilly invited me in and we began to explore in greater detail the concerns and issues touched on during my first contact. This conversation opened the way for me to introduce some thoughts on how she might deal with the problems at hand.

Lilly had followed through with the second ultrasound, which didn't reveal any abnormalities. However, because her blood pressure was up, she was advised to terminate her work and go on bed rest for the balance of her pregnancy—a matter of a week or so. Lilly said she had also decided to keep the baby in spite of the pressure from her parents. With her boyfriend gone, her parents antagonistic, and no apparent circle of friends, it was evident that Lilly had no adequate "support system." Lilly had none of the items she needed for the baby, such as layette and car seat and she was undecided whether to breastfeed or bottle feed. I was relieved and encouraged to hear that Lilly would be receptive to my help in acquiring the necessary items and in obtaining information on how to deal with her bed rest. She also had concerns about how to provide appropriate care for her newborn. Her anxiety was prompted by her complete lack of experience. Having relinquished her first child, the opportunity to learn these skills had been forfeited.

To help expand Lilly's support base, I asked if she might also be willing to see our social worker, who could provide some guidance. She said she was. In fact, at this point in our relationship, she seemed open to exploring whatever ideas and resources I felt might be helpful. The visit ended with the understanding I would return in three days, hopefully with additional information and some of the baby items she needed.

From Dangelmaier A: Lilly's anger. In Zewekh J, Primomo J, Deal L, eds: *Opening doors: stories of public health nursing*, Olympia, Wa., 1992, Washington State Department of Health, Parent-Child Health Services, pp. 41-45.

are poor, uneducated, or headed by teenage parents often face barriers to getting the health care or social support services they need. Many experts believe that providing services in the home reduces these barriers. They also believe that home visiting for prenatal counseling or parenting education for this population group can address problems before they become irreversible or extremely costly (GAO, 1990).

The nurse who visits in the home, especially when both parents are present, is in a privileged position to closely and periodically assess the baby's, the parents', and the family's

A View from the Field LILLY'S ANGER—cont'd

As I left Lilly's, I reflected again on all that had occurred. It was clear we had progressed in our relationship. Lilly was now actively participating in identifying her concerns and exploring resources that could meet her needs. I also thought about one of my primary objectives in this relationship: when possible, to assist Lilly in accomplishing tasks on her own rather than doing them for her. My purpose was to help Lilly gain some much needed confidence and increase her skill level. Hopefully, her trust in me and the strength of our relationship had evolved to the point where she would be comfortable rather than resistant to help. My goals were twofold: assist Lilly to feel competent in meeting the challenges of being a new mother, and help her gain the strengths, confidence and knowledge to seek appropriate help when necessary.

I was able to visit Lilly one more time before the baby was due. I provided her with some information she was interested in and was able to locate both a layette and car seat for the baby. Equally important, the visit provided the opportunity to obtain Lilly's consent for on-going visits in the months following delivery.

Some eight months have passed since Lilly delivered a normal infant girl. The baby is happy and thriving. Monthly visits have allowed me to provide support and the chance to teach Lilly additional skills in caring for her baby. It has been interesting to observe Lilly's increasing ability to cope with problems that have arisen.

In the last few months Lilly has had to deal with being evicted from her rental home, seeing her boyfriend leave again, and continuing criticism from her parents. In spite of this, she interacts positively with the baby and provides good infant care. Lilly has also taken the initiative to find a full-time sitter so that she can work rather than be on welfare. She is comfortable in seeking out resources when needed, as evidenced by her participation in the WIC program, social service counseling, and the low-cost housing authority. She has demonstrated considerable growth in self-confidence and her capacity to function in general. She openly discusses the value of my visits and laughingly reflects back on our shaky beginning. We both agree that our relationship has grown. No longer is getting in touch with Lilly a problem. In fact, she seems quite comfortable in calling me, sharing her concerns, and inviting me to "come and see baby Sarah." I will probably continue regular visits until the baby is a year old. I know that when I no longer provide visits to this family, Lilly and I will both miss the positive working relationship we have come to enjoy. It has been a growing experience for both of us.

I could have given up on Lilly after my first stressful contact. I'm glad I didn't!

development. The nurse can also identify stress, help parents deal with problems of poor bonding, provide role modeling for bonding and parenting, give anticipatory guidance, and help reinforce positive behavior. The nurse aids families in using community resources as necessary. For example, when parents and a new baby with a diagnosis of spina bifida, Down syndrome, or cleft palate come home from the hospital, it is most often the community health nurse who introduces the family to the resources of the Children's Special Health Care Services program, known as crippled children services in some states, for financial aid, to the physical therapy offered by the intermediate school program, or to the interdisciplinary diagnostic services of university-affiliated centers. This same nurse will likely be one of the persons to help parents as they go through the grief process related to having a baby who is less than "perfect." The nurse can also be alert to signs of stress within the family in this situation; living 24 hours a day with a helpless infant who has additional problems can be an overwhelming problem for some families. Homemakers, parent's aides, and parent-support groups are useful when families are in such a situational crisis.

One of the major characteristics of disabled children, and particularly the mentally disabled, is some delay in reaching developmental milestones in self-help skills. It is sometimes assumed that these skills will develop without intervention as a result of physical growth and maturation. Often this is not the case and the child is unable to function independently. This can lead to institutionalization, enormous financial and personal expenditures, and waste of human potential. With the use of behavior modification technology, self-help skills can be attained by disabled persons, including those who are profoundly disabled. The community health nurse is in a unique position to help families with these skills. Beginning immediately after birth with early infant stimulation is essential. The goal is that each person attain his or her own potential. The nurse can aid the family in recognizing this potential and give guidance in the process of reaching it. Time needed to exercise and teach the young child with developmental disabilities can lead to the neglect of other children. Parents and nurse must be cognizant of this situation.

Summary

The years from birth to age 5 provide the foundation for a child's lifelong physical, mental, and social development. The child's health and that of the parents is inextricably interwoven, and both have health care needs that the community health nurse can help to fill.

Utilization of the developmental health promotion model to assess the needs of young children provides a positive way to prevent many of the major health problems of those newborn to 5 years of age, or at least weaken their impact. This is the challenge for community health nurses!

Children are our nation's greatest resource. Decreasing infant and maternal mortality rates reflect this value, as does legislation such as Medicaid, which provides health care for at least a segment of the newborn to 5-year-old population.

CRITICAL *Thinking Exercise*

The View from the Field, "Lilly's Anger" (Dangelmaier, 1992, p. 41), describes a public health nurse whose caseload was at-risk pregnant women and infants. Describe the skills the nurse used as she cared for Lilly and her baby.

REFERENCES

Alexander GR, Korenbrot CC: The role of prenatal care in preventing low birth weight, *The Future of Children* 5(1):103-120, 1995.

Alan Guttmacher Institute: *Teenage pregnancy in the United States: the scope of the problem and state responses*, New York, 1989, The Institute.

Allen M, Brown P, Finlay B: *Helping children by strengthening families: a look at family support programs*, Washington, D.C., 1992, Children's Defense Fund.

Arkin EB: The Healthy Mothers, Healthy Babies, Coalition: four years of progress, *Public Health Rep* 101:147-156, 1986.

Athey J: *Pregnancy and childbearing among homeless adolescents: report of a workshop*, University of Pittsburgh, October 16-17, 1989, Public Health Social Work Training Program, Division of Public and Community Health Service.

Atkinson W, Furphy L, Gantt J, Mayfield M, eds: *Epidemiology and prevention of vaccine-preventable diseases*, ed 2, Atlanta, 1995, CDC.

Berne AS, Dato C, Mason DJ, Rafferty M: A nursing model for addressing the health needs of homeless families, *Image J Nurs Sch* 22:8-13, 1990.

Bolden AJ, Henry JL, Allukian M: Implications of access, utilization and need for oral health care by low income groups and minorities on the dental delivery system, *J Dent Ed* 57:888-899, 1993.

Bratic E: Healthy Mothers, Healthy Babies Coalition—a joint private-public initiative, *Public Health Rep* 97:503-509, 1982.

Brazelton TB: *The neonatal behavioral assessment scale*, ed 2, Philadelphia, 1984, Lippincott.

Bronner YL: Nutritional status outcomes for children: ethnic, cultural, and environmental contexts, *J Am Diet Assoc* 96:891-900, 903, 1996.

Brown S: Drawing women into prenatal care, *Family Planning Perspectives* 21(2):73-80, 88, March/April 1989.

Carpenter RG: Prevention of unexpected infant death, *Lancet* i:723-727, 1983.

Center for Substance Abuse Treatment: *Improving treatment for drug-exposed infant: treatment improvement protocol (TIP) series 5*, Rockville, Md., 1993, Substance Abuse and Mental Health Services Administration.

Centers for Disease Control and Prevention (CDC): Pediatric Nutrition Surveillance System—United States, 1980-1991. In CDC surveillance summaries, *MMWR* 41(No. SS-7):1-24, 1992.

Centers for Disease Control and Prevention (CDC): Lead poisoning associated with use of traditional ethnic remedies—California, 1991-1992, *MMWR* 42(27):521-524, 1993a.

Centers for Disease Control and Prevention (CDC): Standards for pediatric immunization practices, *MMWR* 42:(No RR-5)1-13, 1993b.

Centers for Disease Control and Prevention (CDC): State activities for prevention of lead poisoning among children—U.S., 1992, *MMWR* 42:165-172, 1993c.

Centers for Disease Control and Prevention (CDC): Pediatric AIDS cases by exposure category and race/ethnicity, reported July 1995 through June 1996, United States, *HIV/AIDS Surveillance Report* 8:11, June 1996.

Centers for Disease Control and Prevention (CDC): Update: blood lead levels—United States, 1991-1994, *MMWR* 46(7):142-146, 1997.

Chamberlin RW, ed: *Beyond individual risk assessment: community-wide approaches to promoting the health and development of families and children*, Washington, D.C., 1988, The National Center for Education in Maternal and Child Health.

Chan MM: Sudden infant death syndrome and families at risk, *Pediatr Nurs* 13(3):166-168, 1987.

Chatoor I, Dickson L, Schaefer S, James E: A developmental classification of feeding disorders associated with failure to thrive: diagnosis and treatment. In Drotar D, ed: *New directions in failure to thrive*, New York, 1985, Plenum Press.

Children's Defense Fund (CDF): *The state of America's children yearbook, 1996*, Washington, D.C., 1996, CDF.

Children's Safety Network: *A data book of child and adolescent injury*, Washington, D.C., 1991, National Center for Education in Maternal and Child Health.

Chomitz VR, Cheung LWY, Lieberman E: The role of lifestyle in preventing low birth weight, *The Future of Children* 5(2):121-138, 1995.

Combating child abuse: *Congressional Q Almanac* 44:369, 1988.

Dangelmaier A: Lilly's anger. In Zewekh J, Primomo J, Deal L, eds: *Opening doors: stories of public health nursing*, Olympia, Wa., 1992, Washington State Department of Health, Parent-Child Health Services, pp. 41-45.

Edelstein BL, Douglass CW: Dispelling the myth that 50 percent of U.S. schoolchildren have never had a cavity, *Public Health Rep* 110:522-531, 1995.

Foye HR: Anticipatory guidance. In Hoekelman RA, Friedman SB, Nelson NM et al, eds: *Primary pediatric care*, St. Louis, 1997, Mosby, pp. 151-156.

Garner MK: Our values are showing: inadequate childhood immunization, *Health values: achieving high level wellness* 2:129-133, 1978.

General Accounting Office (GAO): *Home visiting: a promising early intervention strategy for at-risk families*, GAO/HRD-90-83, Gaithersburg, Md., July 1990, GAO.

General Accounting Office (GAO): *Federally funded health services: information on seven programs serving low-income women and children*, GAO/HRD-92-73FS, Gaithersburg, Md., May 1992, GAO.

Gomby DS, Larson CS, Lewit EM, Behrman RE: Home visiting: analysis and recommendations, *The Future of Children* 3:6-22, 1993.

Gordon M: *Manual of nursing diagnosis 1997-1998*, St. Louis, 1997, Mosby.

Hargraves M, Thomas RW: Infant mortality: its history and social construction, *Am J Preventive Medicine* 9(Suppl):17-26, 1993.

"Healthy mothers" market research: how to reach black and Mexican American women, Contract No 232-81-0082, submitted to USDHHS, PHS, September 14, 1982 by Juarez and Associates, Inc., 12139 National Blvd, Los Angeles, Ca.

Hellmich N: Obesity getting worse, especially in kids, *USA Today*, 1997, March 7-9, p. A1.

Hoekelman RA, Blatman S, Brunell PA et al: *Principles of pediatrics: health care of the young*, New York, 1978, McGraw-Hill.

Hughes D, Simpson L: The role of social change in preventing low birth weight, *The Future of Children* 5(2):87-102, 1995.

Institute of Medicine (IOM): *The best intentions: unintended pregnancy and the well-being of children and families*, Washington, D.C., 1995, National Academy of Sciences.

Johnson J, Primas P, Coe M: Factors that prevent women of socioeconomic status from seeking prenatal care, *J Am Acad Nurse Pract* 6(3):105-111, 1994.

Klaus MH, Kennell JH: *Maternal-infant bond*, St. Louis, 1976, Mosby.

Klaus MH, Kennell JH, eds: *Maternal-infant bond*, ed 2, St. Louis, 1982, Mosby.

Kramer MS: The etiology and prevention of low birthweight: current knowledge and priorities for future research. In Berendes H, Kessel S, Yaffe S, eds: *Advances in the prevention of low birthweight: an international symposium*, Washington, D.C., 1991, National Center for Education in Maternal and Child Health.

Lewit EM: Reported child abuse and neglect, *The Future of Children* 4(2):233-242, 1994.

Lewit EM, Baker LS, Corman H, Shiono PH: The direct cost of low birthweight, *The Future of Children* 5:35-56, 1995.

Lowdermilk DL, Perry SE, Bobak IM: *Maternity and women's health care*, ed 6, St. Louis, 1997, Mosby.

Macro Systems, Inc.: *One stop shopping for perinatal services: identification and assessment of implementation methodologies*, Washington, D.C., 1990, National Center for Education in Maternal and Child Health.

Masis KB, May PM: A comprehensive local program for the prevention of fetal alcohol syndrome, *Public Health Rep* 106(5):484-494, 1991.

Mason JO: Today's challenges to the Public Health Service and to the nation, *Public Health Rep* 106(5):473-477, 1991.

Maternal and Child Health Bureau: *Child health USA '95*, Washington, D.C., 1996, U.S. Government Printing Office.

Michigan Department of Community Health (MDCH): *An immunization practice update*, Lansing, Mi., 1997, MDCPH.

Michigan Department of Community Health (MDCH): CDC national immunization survey: individual vaccine levels for children 19-35 months of age, *Michigan Immunization Update* 3:4, 1996.

Mihaly LK: *Homeless families: failed policies and young victims*, Washington, D.C., January 1991, Children's Defense Fund, Child, Youth, and Family Futures Clearinghouse.

Milio N: *9226 Kercheval: the storefront that did not burn*, Ann Arbor, 1970, University of Michigan Press.

Millman M, ed: *Access to health care in America*, Washington, D.C., 1993, National Academy Press.

Murphy E: Celebrating the Bill of Rights in the year of *Rust v. Sullivan*, *Nurs Outlook* 39(5) 238-239, 1991.

National Commission to Prevent Infant Mortality: *Death before life: the tragedy of infant mortality*, Washington, D.C., August 1988, The Commission.

National Commission to Prevent Infant Mortality: *Home visiting: opening doors for America's pregnant women and children*, Washington, D.C., 1989, The Commission.

National Institute on Disability and Rehabilitation Research: *Chartbook on disability in the United States, an Info Use report*, Washington, D.C., 1989, The Institute.

National SIDS Clearinghouse: *Fact sheet: what is SIDS?* McLean, Va., 1989, The Clearinghouse.

Nelson WE, Behrman RE, Kliegman RM, Algin AM, eds: *Nelson textbook of pediatrics*, Philadelphia, 1996, Saunders.

Norton D, Ridenour N: Homeless women and children: the challenge of health promotion, *Nurse Pract Forum* 6:24-33, 1995.

Paneth NS: The problem of low birth weight, *The Future of Children* 5(1):19-34, 1995.

Poland-Laken M, Hutchins E: *Building and sustaining systems of care for substance-using pregnant women and their infants: lessons learned*, Arlington, Va., 1995, National Center for Education in Maternal and Child Health.

Rhodes AM: Criminal penalties for maternal substance abuse, *MCH* 17-11, 1992.

Sargent JD, Brown MJ, Freeman JL et al: Childhood lead poisoning in Massachusetts communities: its association with sociodemographic and housing characteristics, *AJPH* 85:528-534, 1995.

Scipien GM, Barnard MU, Chard MA et al: *Comprehensive pediatric nursing*, ed 3, New York, 1986, McGraw-Hill.

Selby ML, Riportella-Mueller R, Sorenson JR, Walters CR: Improving EPSDT use: development and application of a practice-based model for public health nursing research, *Public Health Nurs* 6:174-181, 1989.

Selecting a safe day care center. Solving the day care puzzle: how to choose the safest center for your child, *Penn Nurse* 47(10):32, Harrisburg, Pa., October 1992, Pennsylvania Nurses Association.

Shiono PH, Behrman RE: Low birth weight: analysis and recommendations, *The Future of Children* 5(1):4-18, 1995.

Singh GH, Yu SM: Infant mortality in the United States: trends, differentials, and projections, 1950 through 2010, *Am J Public Health* 85:957-964, 1995.

Smith LL: Coping with disability. Nurse administrators' obligations under the Americans with Disabilities Act, *J Nurs Adm* 22(3):29-31, 1992.

Stucki BR: *Living in the community with a disability: demographic characteristics of the population with disabilities under age 65*, Washington, D.C., 1995, AARP.

Tedder JL: Using the Brazelton Neonatal Assessment Scale to facilitate the parent-infant relationship in a primary care setting, *Nurse Pract* 16(3):26, 1991.

The Institute for Health and Aging, University of California, San Francisco, *Chronic care in America: a 21st century challenge*, Princeton, N.J., 1996, Robert Wood Johnson Foundation.

U.S. Congress, Office of Technology Assessment: *Technology dependent children: hospital v. home care—a technical memorandum*, OTA-TM-H-38, Washington, D.C., May 1987, U.S. Government Printing Office.

U.S. Congress, Office of Technology Assessment: *Healthy children: investing in the future*, OTA-H-345, Washington, D.C., 1988, U.S. Government Printing Office.

U.S. Congress, Office of Technology Assessment: *Healthy children, investing in the future: summary*, Washington, D.C., 1987, U.S. Government Printing Office.

United States Department of Health and Human Services (USDHHS), Administration for Children, Youth and Families: *Child Abuse Prevention, Adoption and Services Act of 1988*, Washington, D.C., 1988, U.S. Government Printing Office.

United States Department of Health and Human Services (USDHHS), Public Health Service: *Recommendations of the Immunization Practices Advisory Committee: general recommendations on immunization*, Atlanta, 1989, CDC.

United States Department of Health and Human Services (USDHHS), *Healthy people 2000: national health promotion and disease prevention objectives, full report, with commentary*, Washington, D.C., 1991, U.S. Government Printing Office.

United States Department of Health and Human Services (USDHHS), *Healthy People 2000: midcourse review and 1995 revisions*, Washington, D.C., 1995a, U.S. Government Printing Office.

United States Department of Health and Human Services (USDHHS), *Report to congress on out-of-wedlock childbearing*, Washington, D.C., 1995b, U.S. Government Printing Office.

United States Department of Health and Human Services (USDHHS): *Child health guide: put prevention into practice*, Washington, D.C., 1994, U.S. Government Printing Office.

United States Public Health Service (USPHS): *Clinician's handbook of preventive services: put prevention into practice*, Washington, D.C., 1994, U.S. Government Printing Office.

Vaughn VC, McKay RJ, Behrman RE, eds, and Nelson WE, senior ed: *Textbook of pediatrics*, ed 11, Philadelphia, 1979, Saunders.

Wald L: *The house on Henry Street*, New York, 1915, Holt.

Wenger BL, Kaye S, LaPlante MP: Disabilities among children, *Disability Statistics Abstract* 15:1-4, 1996.

Wong DL: *Whaley and Wong's nursing care of infants and children*, ed 5, St. Louis, 1995, Mosby.

World Health Organization (WHO): Progress towards health for all: third monitoring report: health status, *World Health Statistics Q* 48:189-199, 1995.

Zima B, Wells K, Freeman H: Emotional and behavioral problems and severe academic delays among sheltered children in Los Angeles County, *Am J Public Health* 84:260-264, 1994.

SELECTED BIBLIOGRAPHY

Cagle CS, Keen-Payne R: Health promotion teaching in preschools, *MCH* 21:96-99, 1996.

Ferketich S, Mercer R: Predictors of role competence for experienced and inexperienced fathers, *Nurs Res* 44:89, 1995.

Green M, ed: *Bright futures: guidelines for health supervision of infants, children, and adolescents*, Arlington, Va., 1994, Maternal and Child Health Bureau.

Institute of Medicine: *The best intentions: unintended pregnancy and the well-being of children and families*, Washington, D.C., 1995, National Academy of Sciences.

Larroque B, Kaminski M, Dehaene P et al: Moderate prenatal alcohol exposure and psychomotor development at preschool age, *AJPH* 85:1654-1661, 1995.

Killion CM: Special health care needs of homeless pregnant women, *Adv Nurs Sci* 18:44-56, 1995.

Mercer R, Ferketich S: Experienced and inexperienced mothers! Maternal competence during infancy, *Res Nurs Health* 18:333, 1995.

National Institute on Drug Abuse: *Drug use among racial-ethnic minorities*, Rockville, Md., 1995, National Institutes of Health.

Report of the U.S. Preventive Services Task Force: *Guide to clinical preventive services*, ed 2, Baltimore, 1996, Williams and Wilkins.

Rickard KA, Gallahue DL, Gruen GE et al: The play approach to learning in the context of families and schools: an alternative paradigm for nutrition and fitness education in the 21st century, *J Am Diet Assoc* 95:1121-1126, 1995.

The Commonwealth Fund: *Minority Americans do not have equal health opportunities*, New York, 1995, The Fund.

The Commonwealth Fund: *The Commonwealth Fund survey of women's health*, New York, 1993, The Fund.

Tiedje LB, Darling-Fisher C: Fatherhood reconsidered: a critical review, *Res Nurs Health* 19:471-484, 1996.

Rock A: The lethal dangers of the billion-dollar vaccine business, *Money* 25:148-164, 1996.

Wallace HM, Biehl RF, MacQueen JC, Blackman JA: *Mosby's resource guide to children with disabilities and chronic illness*, St. Louis, 1997, Mosby.

16

Care of Children in Schools and Other Settings

Objectives

Upon completion of this chapter, the reader should be able to:

1. Articulate how health care and welfare reform will influence service delivery to children.
2. Describe select demographic characteristics of school-age children.
3. Discuss major health risks among school-age children and nursing interventions to address these risks.
4. Discuss the components of a comprehensive school health program.
5. Describe the role of the community health nurse in the school setting.
6. Summarize how health and educational legislation affect the delivery of health care services to the school-age population.
7. Compare and contrast role responsibilities of select disciplines on the school health team.
8. Formulate guidelines for implementing community health nursing role responsibilities in the school setting.

Our aim is . . . to make an unprecedented commitment to the one priority that I believe ranks above all others—the health and education of our children. Most Ohioans have had enough welfare—enough poverty—enough drugs—enough crimes. Most would love to see that debilitating cycle broken, and the people trapped within it, freed—once and for all. So would I.

The only way to do it is to pick one generation of children—draw a line in the sand—and say to all: This is where it stops.

GOVERNOR GEORGE V. VOINOVICH, 1995
STATE OF OHIO

Although concerted attempts have been made since the turn of the century to improve the health status of all children in the nation, these efforts have fallen far short of their goals. In 1930 the Children's Charter (see the box on the following page) declared that all children, regardless of race, color, or creed (Figure 16-1), should have an environment and life experiences that allow them to develop to their fullest potential. However, as we approach the end of the century, it is becoming increasingly apparent that the nation still has a dramatic number of children who are experiencing many of the maladies implicit in the 1930 Children's Charter. Even today, one in four of the nation's youngest children (children under age 6), and one in five of all children, is living in poverty (National Center for Children in Poverty, 1996). Additionally, significant health and educational disparities exist among American youth (Children's Defense Fund [CDF], 1997; Maternal and Child Health Bureau, 1996). The nation must take measures to stop this trend. The line that is drawn in the sand must be made so unpenetrable that no child crosses over into poverty or is denied essential health and educational services.

Fortunately, there is widespread recognition that a "quiet crisis exists" (Carnegie Task Force on Meeting the Needs of Young Children, 1994) for today's children. Committed citizens and leaders in all walks of life are speaking out and acting on behalf of the United States' most vulnerable citizens. The mid-1990s mark an era of experimentation and national effort to promote healthy family and child growth and development (Knitzer, Page, 1996). National campaign efforts, such as the 1996 Stand For All Children's March described in Chapter 15 and the 1997 Presidents' Summit For America's Future in Philadelphia, which was designed to rekindle the spirit of

The Children's Charter

President Hoover's White House Conference on Child Health and Protection, recognizing the rights of the child as the first rights of citizenship, pledges itself to these aims for the children of America.

I For every child spiritual and moral training to help him to stand firm under the pressure of life

II For every child understanding and the guarding of his personality as his most precious right

III For every child a home and that love and security which a home provides; and for that child who must receive foster care, the nearest substitute for his own home

IV For every child full preparation for his birth, his mother receiving prenatal, natal, and postnatal care; and the establishment of such protective measures as will make childbearing safer

V For every child health protection from birth through adolescence, including: periodical health examinations and, where needed, care of specialists and hospital treatment; regular dental examinations and care of the teeth; protective and preventive measures against communicable diseases; the insuring of pure food, pure milk, and pure water

VI For every child from birth through adolescence, promotion of health, including health instruction and a health program, wholesome physical and mental recreation, with teachers and leaders adequately trained

VII For every child a dwelling-place safe, sanitary, and wholesome, with reasonable provisions for privacy; free from conditions which tend to thwart his development; and a home environment harmonious and enriching

VIII For every child a school which is safe from hazards, sanitary, properly equipped, lighted, and ventilated. For younger children nursery schools and kindergartens to supplement home care

IX For every child a community which recognizes and plans for his needs, protects him against physical dangers, moral hazards, and disease; provides him with safe and wholesome places for play and recreation; and makes provision for his cultural and social needs

X For every child an education which, through the discovery and development of his individual abilities, prepares him for life; and through training and vocational guidance prepares him for living which will yield him the maximum of satisfaction

XI For every child such teaching and training as will prepare him for successful parenthood, homemaking, and the rights of citizenship; and, for parents, supplementary training to fit them to deal wisely with the problems of parenthood

XII For every child education for safety and protection against accidents to which modern conditions subject him—those to which he is directly exposed and those which, through loss or maiming of his parents, affect him indirectly

XIII For every child who is blind, deaf, crippled, or otherwise physically handicapped, and for the child who is mentally handicapped, such measures as will early discover and diagnose his handicap, provide care and treatment, and so train him that he may become an asset to society rather than a liability. Expenses of these services should be borne publicly where they cannot be privately met

XIV For every child who is in conflict with society the right to be dealt with intelligently as society's charge, not society's outcast; with the home, the school, the church, the court and the institution when needed, shaped to return him whenever possible to the normal stream of life

XV For every child the right to grow up in a family with an adequate standard of living and the security of a stable income as the surest safeguard against social handicaps

XVI For every child protection against labor that stunts growth, either physical or mental, that limits education, that deprives children of the right of comradeship, of play, and of joy

XVII For every rural child as satisfactory schooling and health services as for the city child, and an extension to rural families of social, recreational, and cultural facilities

XVIII To supplement the home and the school in the training of youth, and to return to them those interests of which modern life tends to cheat children, every stimulation and encouragement should be given to the extension and development of the voluntary youth organizations

XIX To make everywhere available these minimum protections of the health and welfare of children, there should be a district, county, or community organization for health, education, and welfare, with full-time officials, coordinating with a statewide program which will be responsive to a nationwide service of general information, statistics, and scientific research. This should include:

(a) Trained, full-time public health officials, with public health nurses, sanitary inspection, and laboratory workers

(b) Available hospital beds

(c) Full-time public welfare service for the relief, aid, and guidance of children in special need due to poverty, misfortune, or behavior difficulties, and for the protection of children from abuse, neglect, exploitation, or moral hazard

For every child these rights, regardless of race, or color, or situation, wherever he may live under the protection of the American Flag.

---

volunteerism, have promoted the need for strong *community action* on behalf of all children. Significant federal and state funds are being used to develop special initiatives that address needs of families and children. "Three-quarters of the states (37) are supporting one or more state-funded, comprehensive program strategies explicitly targeted to young children and their families." (Knitzer, Page, p. 10). Emphasis is on increasing efforts to promote the well-being of children at the earliest years, ages birth to 3, to lay a solid foundation for school and other life

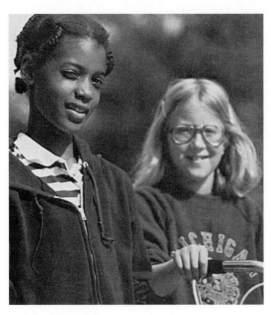

Figure 16-1 All children, regardless of race, color, or creed, need positive life experiences to develop to their fullest potential.

experiences. The importance of all children having a stable relationship with at least one adult, a safe environment, adequate health care, and marketable skills is also being stressed (Abu-Nasr, 1997).

Strategies for promoting the well-being of our youngest children were discussed in Chapter 15. This chapter examines health needs of school-age children and population and community-focused interventions needed to address these needs. An extensive discussion of individual-focused interventions designed to address specific health problems is beyond the scope of this chapter. The reader can obtain a comprehensive understanding of these types of interventions by referring to *Whaley and Wong's Nursing Care of Infants and Children* (Wong, 1995).

CARE OF CHILDREN IN AN ERA OF HEALTH CARE AND WELFARE REFORM

Historically, community health nurses have assumed a major role in developing child health services. At the beginning of the century, Lillian Wald initiated a special project in New York City schools to demonstrate to city officials the value of preventive health counseling in addressing the needs of school-age children (Kalisch, Kalisch, 1995). Since that time, nursing services to meet the needs of our youth have grown steadily. Community health nurses are now working with children in a variety of settings, including their homes, schools, clinics, and residential settings for special aggregates at risk.

Currently, community health nurses face unprecedented challenges and opportunities as they work with children. Although significant shifts in health and welfare policy have provided opportunities for developing innovative child and family health promoting initiatives, it is unclear how the emphasis on cutting health care and welfare costs will affect health outcomes for populations at risk (Andrulis, Acuff, Weiss, Anderson, 1996; CDF, 1997; Collins, Jones, Bloom, 1996; Knitzer, Page, 1996). Community health professionals will play an increasingly significant role in "monitoring the impact of managed care or access to and quality of care for low-income persons" (Rowland, Hanson, 1996, p. 152). They will also play an increasingly important role in assessing the well-being of families as adults receiving Temporary Assistance for Needy Families (TANF) move into the workforce. Evidence to date suggests a need for developing more comprehensive models of care when assisting families leaving welfare for work (CDF, 1997; Collins, Jones, Bloom, 1996).

Community health nurses who work with the school-age population encounter a variety of physical, psychosocial, cultural, environmental, and developmental health problems and concerns. It is obvious to community health professionals that a comprehensive, integrated effort is needed to provide effective and efficient health and welfare services for all segments of this population. Creative partnerships between traditional community health agencies and managed care organizations and community coalitions are emerging at a rapid pace to promote comprehensive service delivery (Brownson, Kreuter, 1997). These partnerships have created a window of opportunity for community health nurses to develop innovative strategies for addressing the needs of children. The community health nurse must have a clear understanding of the demographic characteristics and health risks of the population being served to develop such initiatives.

DEMOGRAPHIC CHARACTERISTICS AND HEALTH RISKS OF SCHOOL-AGE CHILDREN

Since health risks and service needs differ by age, it is important for community health nurses to analyze the demographic characteristics of the population and mortality and morbidity rates specific to the particular age group under consideration. This analysis helps community health nurses to identify health concerns and strengths within their own community. Allocation of resources is based on this knowledge.

Demographic Characteristics

Figure 16-2 displays the resident U.S. population by age group. Trends reflect that while the absolute number of children age 21 or younger is increasing, this age group is declining relative to other age groups in the population. By the year 2000 it is expected that 13% of the population will be 65 or older (Institute for Health and Aging, 1996), whereas the child population is expected to remain at 31.5% (Maternal and Child Health Bureau, 1996). Despite this stabilization, there is a significant number of children residing in our nation. "In 1995, there were almost 83 million children through the age of 21 in the United States, representing

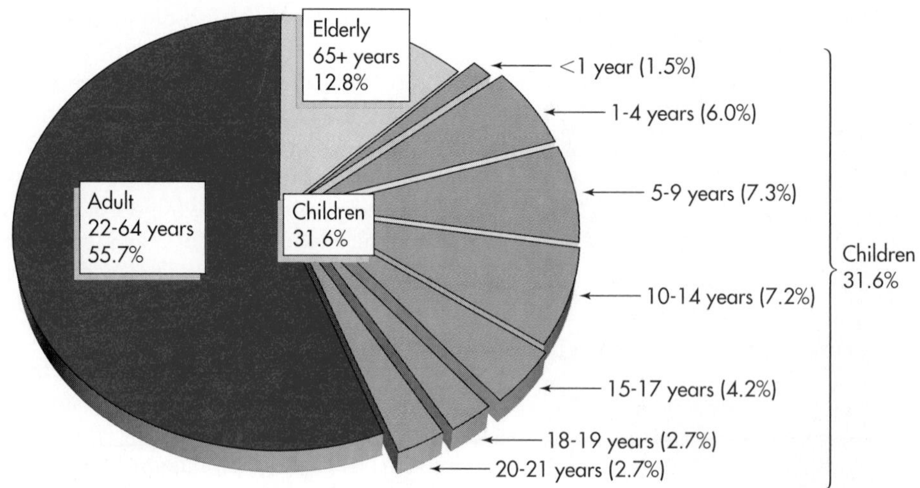

Figure 16-2 U.S. resident population by age group: 1995. *(From Maternal and Child Health Bureau:* Child health USA '95, *Washington, D.C., 1996, U.S. Government Printing Office, p. 17. Source: U.S. Bureau of the Census.)*

table 16-1 Characteristic of U.S. Children through the Age of 17 by Race: 1995, 2000, 2005, 2010, 2025

Of the 78.5 million children through the age of 17 in the United States in 1995, and the projected 82.7 million in 2000, the 85.5 million in 2005, the 87.2 million in 2010, and the 98.8 million in 2025—

	Percentage Distribution				
Race	1995	2000	2005	2010	2025
White	69.5	67.6	65.4	63.4	58.9
Black	13.8	13.9	14.1	14.3	14.7
American Indian, Eskimo, Aleut	1.0	1.0	1.0	1.0	1.1
Asian, Pacific Islander	3.7	4.4	5.0	5.7	7.0
Hispanic	12.1	13.2	14.5	15.5	18.3

From U.S. Bureau of the Census: *Statistical abstract of the United States 1995*, ed 115, Washington, D.C., 1995, U.S. Government Printing Office, pp. 25-26.

31.6% of the total population . . . There were approximately 27 million more children age 21 or younger in 1995 than in 1950" (Maternal and Child Health Bureau, 1996, p. 17). Although the majority of these children through the age of 17 (69.5%) were white in 1995, this ethnic group is declining relative to other ethnic groups (Table 16-1).

The majority of children younger than 6 (62%) and children ages 6 through 17 (76%) have mothers in the workforce (see Figure 15-15). Contrary to stereotypes, the majority of poor families with children work (CDF, 1996). According to the Annie E. Casey Foundation (1996), the fastest growing segment among poor children is children of the working poor.

Disturbingly, when comparing the United States' child poverty rate with those in other major Western industrialized countries, the United States' rate is significantly higher: it is the highest among 18 Western industrialized nations (CDF, 1996). In 1994 14.6 million children under 18 years of age lived in families that had an income below the poverty level. Although the majority of children living in poverty are white, a disproportionately high percentage of black and Hispanic children live in poverty (Figure 16-3). Among Hispanic children the poverty rates vary substantially by place of origin: Puerto Rican and Mexican children are more likely to be living in poverty than Hispanic children from Cuba and Central and South America (National Center for Children in Poverty, 1996). Across ethnic groups, children living with unmarried mothers are particularly at risk for living in poverty. In 1994 23.5% of children under 18 years of age in the United States lived with their mother only. Black and Hispanic children are more likely to live with one parent than white children. Almost two thirds of both black and Hispanic children who reside with a single mother live below the federal poverty level (Maternal and Child Health Bureau, 1996).

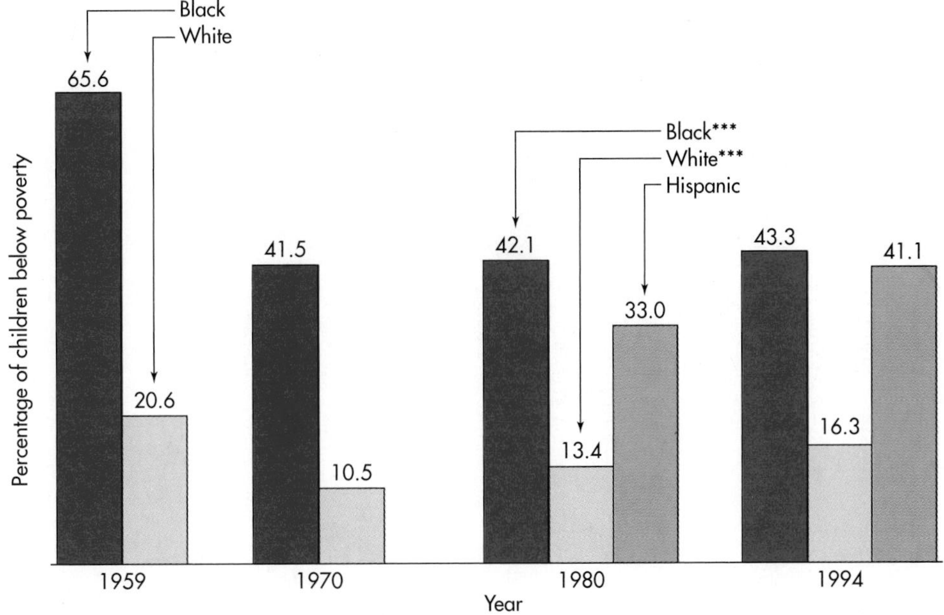

Note: Ethnicity data are not available prior to 1979.

**Related children in a family include householder's own children and all other children in the household who are related to the householder by blood, marriage, or adoption.*

***In 1994, a family of four was considered to be living in poverty if its annual income was below $15,141.*

****Includes Hispanic.*

Figure **16-3** Related children under 18 years of age* living in families below 100% of poverty**: 1994. *(From Maternal and Child Health Bureau:* Child health USA '95, *Washington, D.C., 1996, U.S. Government Printing Office, p. 18. Source: U.S. Department of Commerce.)*

The importance of *comparing* local, state, and national health indicators is vividly illustrated when the poverty rates in the United States are examined. Poverty rates for younger children living in many of America's largest cities, such as Chicago, Dallas, Detroit, Los Angeles, and New York, are significantly higher than the rates for the United States as a whole. There are also significant state-to-state and regional variations in young child (children under 6) poverty rates (YCPRs). For example, "state average YCPRs for the period from 1990 through 1994 ranged from lows of 11 to 12 percent in New Hampshire and Utah to highs of 40 to 41 percent in West Virginia and Louisiana" (National Center for Children in Poverty, 1996, p. 34). The national YCPR for this period was 25%.

Chapters 12 and 15 discussed the influence of poverty on the health status of children. However, the fact that low *"socio-economic status is one of the most powerful risk factors for poor health outcomes"* (Hughes, Simpson, 1995, p. 88) cannot be overstated. Poverty, especially in the earliest childhood years, limits children's future life chances (Korenman, Miller, Sjaastad, 1995).

Childhood Mortality Risks

The 10 leading causes of childhood deaths compared to other age groups are presented in Table 16-2. Although childhood mortality rates have substantially declined over the past several decades, the decline has plateaued in recent years (Maternal and Child Health Bureau, 1996). Additionally, childhood mortality rates for suicide and homicide have significantly increased since the 1960s. AIDS among children emerged during the 1980s. In 1993 HIV infection ranked sixth as the leading cause of death for ages 1 to 4 years, seventh for ages 5 to 14, and sixth for ages 15 to 24 years (U.S. Bureau of the Census, 1996). The epidemiology of AIDS is discussed in Chapter 12. When mortality data are examined, it is important to recognize that death rates vary significantly within segments of the population.

It is striking to note (see Table 16-2) that the majority of childhood deaths could be prevented. It has long been recognized that environmental, social, and behavioral factors greatly influence the occurrence of mortality across the life span. It was noted in our first national health plan that approximately "50 percent of our United States' deaths are due to unhealthy behavior or lifestyle; 20 percent to environmental factors; 20 percent to human biological factors; and only 10 percent to inadequacies in health care" (USDHEW, 1979, p. 9).

INJURIES Although deaths from unintentional injury have declined significantly since 1950, injuries remain the leading cause of death and disability among children and young adults.

table 16-2 Ten Leading Causes of Death by Age Groups—1993

Rank	<1	1-4	5-14	15-24	25-44	45-64	65+	Total
1	Congenital anomalies 7129	Unintentional injuries 2590	Unintentional injuries 3466	Unintentional injuries 13,966	Unintentional injuries 27,277	Malignant neoplasms 133,057	Heart disease 619,755	Heart disease 743,460
2	SIDS 4669	Congenital anomalies 804	Malignant neoplasms 1089	Homicide 8424	HIV 27,228	Heart disease 104,722	Malignant neoplasms 371,549	Malignant neoplasms 529,904
3	Short gestation 4310	Malignant neoplasms 522	Homicide 656	Suicide 4849	Malignant neoplasms 21,834	Cerebrovascular 14,682	Cerebrovascular 131,551	Cerebrovascular 150,108
4	Respiratory distress syndrome 1815	Homicide 464	Congenital anomalies 485	Malignant neoplasms 1738	Heart disease 16,660	Unintentional injuries 14,434	Bronchitis, emphysema, asthma 86,425	Bronchitis, emphysema, asthma 101,077
5	Maternal complications 1343	Heart disease 296	Suicide 321	Heart disease 981	Suicide 12,477	Bronchitis, emphysema, asthma 13,165	Pneumonia & influenza 73,853	Unintentional injuries 90,523
6	Placenta cord membranes 994	HIV 204	Heart disease 303	HIV 609	Homicide 11,815	Diabetes 10,927	Diabetes 40,502	Pneumonia & influenza 82,820
7	Unintentional injuries 898	Pneumonia & influenza 182	HIV 155	Congenital anomalies 472	Liver disease 4477	Liver disease 10,316	Unintentional injuries 27,784	Diabetes 53,894
8	Perinatal infections 772	Perinatal period 100	Bronchitis, emphysema, asthma 138	Pneumonia & influenza 251	Cerebrovascular 3316	HIV 8330	Nephritis 19,743	HIV 37,267
9	Intrauterine hypoxia 549	Septicemia 96	Pneumonia & influenza 135	Cerebrovascular 208	Diabetes 2299	Suicide 7229	Septicemia 16,846	Suicide 31,102
10	Pneumonia & influenza 530	Benign neoplasms 77	Cerebrovascular 79	Bronchitis, emphysema, asthma 206	Pneumonia & influenza 2275	Pneumonia & influenza 5583	Atherosclerosis 16,460	Homicide 26,009

From National Center for Health Statistics: *Health, United States, 1995*, Hyattsville, Md., 1996, Public Health Service, pp. 114, 117-118.

Unintentional injuries claim more than three times as many lives among 5- to 14-year-old children as the next leading cause of death. Motor vehicle accidents are the single largest contributing cause of unintentional-injury deaths for children of any age. Although motor vehicle mortality among teenagers has declined over the last decade, adolescents are particularly at risk for motor vehicle deaths. In 1993 the greatest number of motor vehicle fatalities occurred to persons age 18 (National Safety Council, 1996). White adolescents ages 15 to 19 are more at risk for motor vehicle deaths than their black counterparts (Maternal and Child Health Bureau, 1995).

Following motor vehicle accidents, fires and related burns and drowning are also leading causes of childhood unintentional injury deaths. Children ages 1 to 4 have the highest death rates from these causes, with rates over three times that for children ages 5 to 9 (Maternal and Child Health Bureau, 1995). Drowning fatalities were the second leading cause of unintentional injury death for persons age 9 to 20 in 1993 (National Safety Council, 1996). Among children under 5, drownings occur most frequently in swimming pools and home spas. Household fires are also a particular risk to children, with children under 5 who live in substandard housing at special risk (USDHHS, 1991, p. 13).

Firearms also cause a significant number of injury deaths among children. However, many of these deaths are intentional (Figure 16-4). In 1993 almost 55% of firearm deaths among 5- to 14-year-old children were homicides. In this same year, suicides and homicides accounted for 92% of the firearm deaths among teenagers. "Over the past decade, the proportion of firearm deaths due to homicide has increased by approximately 50%" (Maternal and Child Health Bureau, 1996, p. 41).

A significant challenge for community health professionals in the next decade is to find ways to reduce fatalities from injuries. An important role of the community health nurse is to promote driving safety among adolescents and young adults, including identifying at-risk individuals. Driving without wearing a seat belt or while under the influence of alcohol or other drugs increases an individual's risk for becoming a motor vehicle fatality. Data reflect that a significant number of adolescents engage in these risk-taking behaviors.

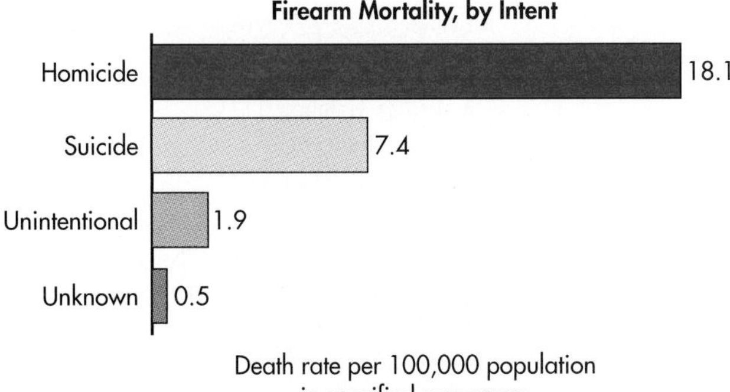

Figure 16-4 Firearms mortality among adolescents, ages 15 to 19: 1993. *(From Maternal and Child Health Bureau:* Child health USA '95, *Washington, D.C. 1996, U.S. Government Printing Office, p. 41.)*

Only one third (34.3%) of all youth (12 to 21 years of age) who participated in the National Health Interview Survey—Youth Risk Behavior Survey (NHIS-YRBS) in 1992 "always" used safety belts when riding in a motor vehicle driven by someone else (Adams, Schoenborn, Moss et al, 1995). Although alcohol-related motor vehicle fatalities have decreased significantly since the mid-1980s, alcohol use among youth is still a major concern. It is estimated that alcohol is involved in 20% to 25% of motor vehicle deaths among teenagers (Maternal and Child Health Bureau, 1996).

The community health nurse can also assume a major role in preventing accidents and injuries in younger school-age children through health education activities designed to prevent poisonings, fires, falls, and other causes of accidents. The Consumer Product Safety Commission (1-800-638-CPSC) provides material on consumer product safety including product hazards, product defects, and injuries sustained in using products. This information can help the nurse to plan sound educational programs. The National Child Safety Council Childwatch (1-800-222-1464) answers questions and distributes literature on safety and sponsors the Missing Kids program (publicized through milk cartons).

HOMICIDE In 1974 homicide became a leading cause of death among children and young adults for the first time in the history of our nation. Since 1960 the rate of homicide has nearly tripled, with firearm use being a major contributor to homicide deaths. If this trend continues, the national mortality rate from firearms will surpass that of motor vehicle crashes by the year 2003 (USDHHS, 1995a). Eight states and the District of Columbia already report more deaths related to firearms than to motor-vehicle crashes (National Center for Injury Prevention and Control [NCIPC], 1995).

In 1993 homicide ranked fourth as the leading cause of deaths for ages 1 to 4 years, third for ages 5 to 14, and second for ages 15 to 24 years (U.S. Bureau of the Census, 1996). The death rate from homicide for black adolescents ages 15 to 19 is over eight times the rate for whites in the same age category (Maternal and Child Health Bureau, 1996). The homicide rate for Hispanic and American Indians/Alaskan Natives is also much higher than the general population (USDHHS, 1991, 1995a). Children at special risk among all ethnic and minority groups are presented in the box on the next page.

Certainly no one factor accounts for the increase in homicide among children. Poverty has been identified as a critical variable because of the high incidence of homicide among impoverished ethnic and minority groups. The use, manufacture, and distribution of drugs is another important factor associated with homicide (USDHHS, 1995a). Family breakup, the accessibility of firearms, characteristics of adolescence that make teenagers prone to violence, and societal attitudes that portray violence as an acceptable conflict resolution strategy are some other factors that should be considered when planning interventions to reduce childhood mortality resulting from violence (NCIPC, 1993b).

Community health nurses must work closely with all agencies in the community to *prevent* homicide in the school-age population. Comprehensive programs to prevent childhood homicide must involve many sectors of the community and multiple approaches to the problem. Activities for preventing youth violence usually employ one of three general prevention strategies: education, legal and regulatory change, and environmental modification (NCIPC, 1993b, p. 11). The box below displays examples of interventions used under each category. Community health nurses assume a significant role in planning and implementing violence control interventions.

Children at Risk for Homicide

YOUTH WITH HIGH-RISK BEHAVIORS

- Juvenile offenders
- Youth with histories of fighting or victimization
- Drug/alcohol abusers
- Drug dealers
- Weapon carriers
- Gang members
- School dropouts
- Unemployed youth
- Homeless youth
- Relocated and immigrant youth
- Youth living in poverty

YOUNG CHILDREN (10 YEARS OR LESS)

- Abused or neglected children
- Children who have witnessed violence
- Children with behavioral problems
- Children living in poverty

From USDHHS: *Healthy people 2000: national health promotion and disease prevention objectives, full report, with commentary:* Washington, D.C., 1991, U.S. Government Printing Office, p. 228-229; NCIPC: *The prevention of youth violence: a framework for community action,* Atlanta, 1993b, CDC, p. 6.

SUICIDE The incidence of suicide among youth has been steadily increasing since 1960. In 1993 suicide ranked fifth as the leading cause of death for ages 5 to 14 years and third for ages 15 to 24 years. The suicide rate has more than tripled among youth in the past 30 years (CDC, 1992c). A major concern of health professionals is the increasing number of suicides among both black and white young males (USDHHS, 1995a). Currently the rate of suicide in 15- to-19-year-olds is about one and one half times as high in white teens as in black teens (Maternal and Child Health Bureau, 1995).

Health professionals view suicide as a problem of extreme importance in the adolescent population because it is an indicator that social, emotional, and physical stress is great. Rapidly changing societal values, population mobility, and economic pressures have presented adolescents with decision-making conflicts that result in uncertainty and stress (Figure 16-5).

The extent of the suicide problem is much greater than the recorded figures indicate. Because suicide is viewed by our culture as a cowardly and disgraceful act, it is often concealed by families and medical personnel. Many suicides are not recorded as such on the death certificate, and it can be difficult to differentiate between suicide and death resulting from an accident. The result is that the recorded incidence reflects only a portion of the deaths caused by suicide. In addition, when one looks at the rate of attempted suicide, the

Activities to Prevent Youth Violence

EDUCATION

Adult mentoring
Conflict resolution
Training in social skills
Firearm safety
Parenting centers
Peer education
Public information and education campaigns

LEGAL/REGULATORY CHANGE

Regulate the use of and access to weapons
- Weaponless schools
- Control of concealed weapons
- Restrictive licensing
- Appropriate sale of guns

Regulate the use of and access to alcohol
- Appropriate sale of alcohol
- Prohibition or control of alcohol sales at events
- Training of servers

Other types of regulations
- Appropriate punishment in schools
- Dress codes

ENVIRONMENTAL MODIFICATION

Modify the social environment
- Home visitation
- Preschool programs such as Head Start
- Therapeutic activities
- Recreational activities
- Work/academic experiences

Modify the physical environment
- Make risk areas visible
- Increase use of an area
- Limit building entrances and exits
- Create sense of ownership

From NCIPC: *The prevention of youth violence: a framework for community action,* Atlanta, 1993b, CDC, p. 11.

problem becomes even more significant because attempts far exceed actual suicides. Of the 12,272 students in grades 9-12 who participated in CDC's Youth Risk Behavior Survey in 1991, 29% had thought seriously about attempting suicide, 19% had made a specific plan to attempt suicide, 7% actually attempted suicide, and 2% made a suicide attempt that resulted in an injury or poisoning that had to be treated by a doctor or nurse (CDC, 1992a, p. 771).

"Suicide clusters" and the possible "contagion" effect of adolescent suicide is a growing public concern. A suicide cluster is the occurrence of suicides or attempted suicides closer together in space and time than is considered usual for a given community. It is estimated that suicide clusters account for approximately 1% to 5% of all suicides among adolescents and young adults. In a cluster, suicides occurring later in the cluster often appear to have been influenced by earlier suicides. Thus a community-wide intervention approach is needed to address this problem. Persons at risk need to be identified and interviewed, personal counseling services should be provided for close friends and relatives of the victims and potentially suicidal adolescents, and the community needs to be supported in a way that minimizes sensationalism (CDC, 1988a).

As with homicide, a comprehensive community-focused approach that emphasizes prevention and is linked as closely as possible with professional mental health resources is needed to combat youth suicide (CDC, 1992c). Currently a broad spectrum of youth suicide prevention programs in the United States use a variety of prevention strategies. The eight strategies outlined in the box below focus on enhancing recognition of suicide, referral, and promoting activities designed to address known or suspected risk factors. Most youth suicide prevention programs target adolescents despite the fact that the suicide rate among young adults 20 to 24 years of age is generally twice as high as the rate among adolescents 15 to 19 years of age. Greater prevention efforts need to be targeted toward young adults (CDC, 1992c, pp. x-xi).

Community health nurses, especially those functioning in the school setting, are in a key position to detect troubled youth and to work with the community in planning a comprehensive suicide prevention program. It is

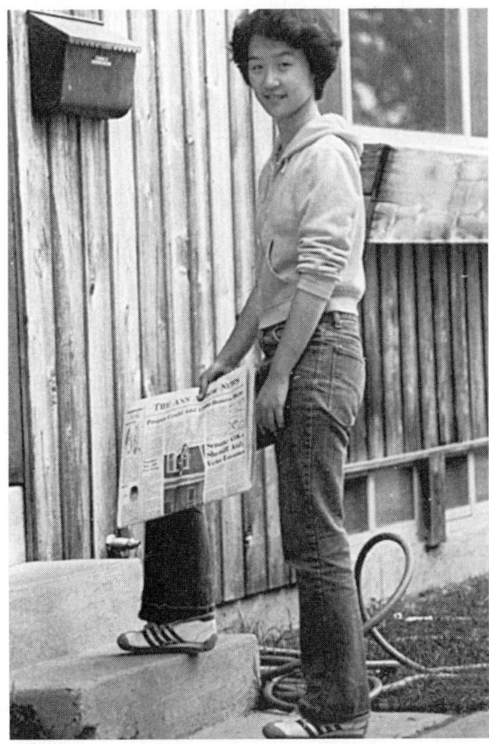

Figure 16-5 Accelerated societal changes have exposed American youth to increased opportunities as well as increased stresses. American youth are exposed much earlier than their previous counterparts to such things as human sexuality concerns, pressures from peers to use alcohol and drugs, and varying lifestyles. Community health nurses are often in a favorable position to detect youth who are having difficulty coping with the demands of life.

Youth Suicide Prevention Strategies

- **School Gatekeeper Training**
  Directed at school staff to help them identify students at risk of suicide, refer such students for help, and respond in cases of a tragic death or other crisis in school.
- **Community Gatekeeper Training**
  Provides training for community members such as clergy, police, and recreation staff to aid them in identifying youths at risk of suicide, and referring these youth for help.
- **General Suicide Education**
  Provides students with facts about suicide, alert them to suicide warning signs, and provide them with information about how to seek help for themselves or for others.
- **Screening Program**
  Involves administration of a standardized instrument to identify high-risk youth in order to provide more thorough assessment and treatment for a smaller, targeted population.
- **Peer Support Programs**
  Designed to foster peer relationships, competency development, and social skills as a method to prevent suicide among high-risk youth.
- **Crisis Centers and Hotlines**
  Provide emergency counseling for suicidal people.
- **Means Restriction**
  Designed to restrict access to firearms, drugs, and other common means of committing suicide.
- **Intervention After a Suicide**
  Designed in part to help prevent or contain suicide clusters and to help youth effectively cope with feelings of loss that come with the sudden death or suicide of a peer.

From CDC: *Youth suicide prevention programs: a resource guide*, Atlanta, 1992c, CDC, pp. ix-x.

important to move beyond an individual-focused approach. A community-oriented approach that targets at risk populations and that uses a variety of intervention strategies is needed to address this alarming problem.

CONGENITAL ANOMALIES Each year approximately 100,000 infants are born in the United States with serious congenital anomalies, and the proportion of these infants who survive into childhood is increasing yearly (USDHHS, 1995a). Many factors increase the risk for congenital anomalies. "One-fourth of all congenital anomalies are caused by genetic factors, suggesting a need for preconception counseling for both men and women" (USDHHS, 1991, p. 10). Poverty, poor housing, malnutrition, pregnancy at a young age, use of alcohol and cigarettes, and inadequate medical care also increase the likelihood that illness, disability, or death will occur. It has been shown that mothers in all age categories who are disadvantaged are at risk for producing an unhealthy child (Chomitz, Cheung, Lieberman, 1995; Paneth, 1995). The risk of having an abnormal birth increases as a mother's consumption of alcohol and tobacco increases (USDHHS, 1991). Young mothers and mothers who have inadequate health care are more likely to have low birth weight babies than other mothers. Low birth weight infants have a high incidence of congenital malformations. These facts suggest that a preventive health program designed to reduce childhood mortality related to congenital malformations must include ways to eliminate poor environmental and social conditions, to expand the use of prenatal services by young and disadvantaged mothers, and to alter unhealthy behaviors (alcohol consumption and smoking) that increase the risk for abnormal births. "Improving women's health before, during, and after pregnancy is the key to reducing the human and economic costs associated with infant mortality and morbidity" (Chomitz, Cheung, Lieberman, 1995, p. 132).

MALIGNANT NEOPLASMS Although cancer is rare among children, it is the chief cause of death *by disease* in youth under age 15. "Common sites include the blood and bone marrow, bone, lymph nodes, brain, nervous system, kidneys, and soft tissues" (American Cancer Society, 1996, p. 15). Over 8000 new cases of cancer are diagnosed yearly among children in the United States. Leukemia accounts for one third of these new cases and one third of the deaths attributed to childhood cancer. Cancer fatality rates for children have declined significantly since 1960. Parents play a significant role in early diagnosis and treatment. Cancer in children can be detected early during regular medical or nursing checkups and by astute parents who observe unusual symptoms in their children that persist (American Cancer Society).

Cancer places a tremendous burden on families and society. The severe nature of this condition and the prolonged treatment needed cause pain and anguish for both the child and the family. Cancer in childhood also causes financial hardship for many families because funding for catastrophic illness is frequently not available. Health planning efforts for cancer should focus on providing early detection, treatment, and supportive services, funding for research, and monies to eliminate individual financial hardships. Community health nurses can significantly assist families in coping with childhood cancer by providing home health care services and by helping them to obtain needed resources from community agencies. For example, the American Cancer Society supplies dressings and equipment free of charge. Other community agencies such as departments of social services provide funds for medical treatment. Helping parents to establish and maintain support networks is an important role for nurses working with families who are coping with childhood cancer (Lynam, 1987).

Childhood Morbidity Risks—Acute Conditions

The incidence of acute conditions in childhood is difficult to ascertain because (1) many acute conditions are not reportable; (2) reportable acute conditions are often not reported; and (3) acute illness is frequently treated at home, and as a result is not brought to the attention of health professionals. Data from the National Health Surveys since 1956 do provide estimated patterns of incidence over time. According to this survey, acute conditions are illnesses and injuries that were first noticed less then 3 months before the reference date of the interview and were serious enough to have had an impact on behavior (Adams, Benson, 1991, p. 3).

The major types of acute conditions for children ages 5 through 17 identified in the National Health Interview Survey fall into five major categories. In order of frequency, these are respiratory conditions, injuries, infective and parasitic diseases, digestive system conditions, and all other conditions. Respiratory conditions, injuries and infective and parasitic diseases will be highlighted below. An extensive discussion of all acute conditions among school-age children is beyond the scope of this book.

The average school-age child misses 5.3 days of school per year because of illness and injury. The number of school-loss days per year per 100 children has not changed significantly over the past two decades (U.S. Bureau of the Census, 1995). Children from families that have an income under $10,000 per year experience more acute conditions than children from families that have an income greater than $10,000 per year (U.S. Bureau of the Census).

RESPIRATORY CONDITIONS Respiratory conditions, including influenza and the common cold, account for over 60% of the reported acute illnesses among school-age children. Influenza causes two thirds of the reported acute respiratory conditions. Diseases of the respiratory system are the major cause of hospitalization of younger children (Figure 16-6). In 1993 these diseases accounted for 36% of hospital discharges of children 1 to 9 years of age. There were 3.4 million hospital discharges of children 1 to 21 years old in 1993. Children under age 18 in families with incomes

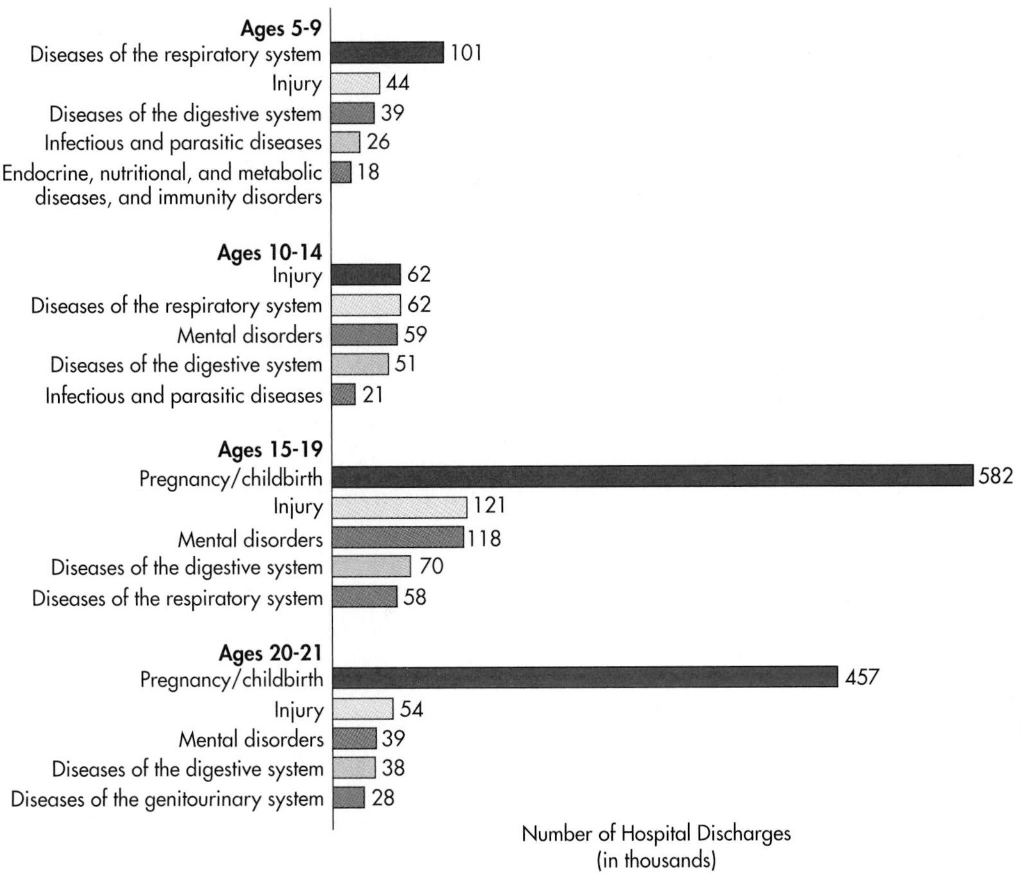

Figure 16-6 Major causes of hospitalization, by age: 1993. *(From Maternal and Child Health Bureau:* Child health USA '95, *Washington, D.C., 1996, U.S. Government Printing Office, p. 32. Source: National Center for Health Statistics.)*

less than $20,000, and black children regardless of income status, are at risk for hospitalization (Maternal and Child Health Bureau, 1996).

Acute respiratory conditions interfere with activities of daily living and may lead to other serious, acute and chronic conditions, such as viral pneumonia, encephalitis, and otitis media. Otitis media can, if untreated, result in permanent hearing loss and chronic ear infection. In 1988 about 25% of the children who responded to the National Health Interview on Child Health reported they had had repeated ear infections during their lifetime (Hendershot, 1989).

INJURIES Injuries disproportionately strike the young and the old (USDHHS, 1991). "Among the leading causes of morbidity in children are medical problems resulting from traumatic injury at home, at school, in an automobile, or associated with recreational activities" (Wong, 1995, p. 1794). Common causes of injury among children are motor-vehicle crashes, violence, falls, poisonings, fires and burns, firearms, sports injuries, and bicycle-related injuries (NCIPC, 1993a).

In 1993 injuries accounted for 11% of the hospital discharges of children 1 to 14 years (Maternal and Child Health Bureau, 1996). "For every injury death, there are about 18 hospitalizations, 233 emergency department visits and 450 office-based physician visits for injuries" (NCIPC, 1995, p. 5). Each year 3.1 million people are treated in emergency departments for sports injuries, 550,000 people are treated for bicycle-related injuries, and 80,000 to 90,000 children are treated for unintentional poisonings (NCIPC, 1993a, 1995).

"In school-age children and adolescents, whose bone growth outstrips muscle growth, difficulty controlling movement can contribute to physical injury" (Wong, 1995, p. 1794). Additionally, many school-age children are vulnerable to engaging in activities beyond their capabilities to keep up with their peers. This places them at risk for injury. Risk-taking among adolescents is common and increases their susceptibility to accidents (Wong). Males have a significantly higher rate of nonfatal injuries than females because of differences in activities and behavior, such as participation in contact sports. Better-planned sports programs might substantially reduce the number of sports-related injuries. Monitoring environmental conditions in homes and schools and promoting highway safety and regulations could also significantly

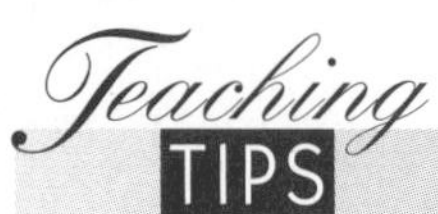

Preventing Intestinal Parasitic Disease

- Always wash hands and fingernails with soap and water before eating and handling food and after toileting.
- Avoid placing fingers in mouth and biting nails.
- Discourage children from scratching bare anal area.
- Use superabsorbent disposable diapers to prevent leakage.
- Change diapers as soon as soiled and dispose of diapers in closed receptable out of children's reach.
- Do not rinse diapers in toilet.
- Disinfect toilet seats and diaper-changing areas; use dilute household bleach (10% solution) or Lysol and wipe clean with paper towels.
- Drink water that is specially treated, especially if camping.
- Wash all raw fruits and vegetables, or food that has fallen on the floor.
- Avoid growing foods in soil fertilized with human excreta.
- Teach children to defecate only in a toilet, not on the ground.
- Keep dogs and cats away from playgrounds or sandboxes.
- Avoid swimming in pools frequented by diapered children.
- Wear shoes outside.

From Wong D: *Whaley and Wong's nursing care of infants and children*, ed 5, St. Louis, 1995, Mosby, p. 684.

decrease childhood injuries. Injury prevention is a major national health priority.

INFECTIVE AND PARASITIC DISEASES Infective and parasitic diseases are of concern to all health professionals because of their contagious nature. Many of them, such as scabies, impetigo, ringworm, head lice, giardiasis, and pinworms, are still considered diseases of the poor and unclean even though this myth has been disproved. Children who have experienced these conditions are often socially isolated and teased by their peers even after treatment ceases. The two most common parasitic infections among children in the United States are giardiasis and pinworms. The prevalence of pinworm infections is highest in school-age children, followed by preschoolers. In some school-age populations the prevalence is near 50%. Giardiasis is the most common protozoan infection in the United States. Its prevalence may range between 1% and 30% depending on the community and age group surveyed. Endemic giardiasis infection in the United States most commonly occurs in July to October among children under the age of 5 and adults 25 to 39 years old. It is associated with drinking contaminated surface water; swimming in bodies of fresh water, such as lakes and rivers; and having a young family member in day care (Benenson, 1995).

The epidemiology of select common infective and parasitic diseases is presented in Appendix 11-3. The reader will find the American Public Health Association handbook *Control of Communicable Diseases Manual* (Benenson, 1995) a valuable resource when identifying and recommending follow-up for any of these conditions. Prevention is the key to effective control of these conditions. Epidemiological investigation to determine the source of infection and to break the chain of transmission is essential. Community health nurses play a significant role in educating families and school personnel about the prevention of infective and parasitic conditions.

Childhood Morbidity Risks—Chronic Conditions

Chronic health problems during childhood are of special concern to health professionals because they can adversely affect a child's growth and development and can cause disability in later life. They can also create considerable emotional and financial stress for children and their families. "Families of children with chronic conditions share a common set of challenges: high health care costs, greater caretaking responsibilities, obstacles to adequate education, and the additional stress these issues create for the entire family" (Institute for Health and Aging, 1996, p. 26).

"Estimates of the prevalence of children with disabilities and chronic illnesses vary from 2% to 32% . . . Larger estimates typically include children with conditions that place few or no limitations on the child's functioning. Smaller estimates include children with conditions that place comparatively severe limitations on the child's functioning" (Ireys, Katz, 1997, p. 3). Figure 16-7 displays the percentage of children ages 1 to 19 years by age, sex, and family income who are limited in their usual activities because of chronic illnesses and impairments. Almost 5 million children had an activity-limiting chronic condition in 1993 (Maternal and Child Health Bureau, 1995).

Disadvantaged children are at risk for chronic conditions. Overall, females report a higher number of activity-limiting conditions than males. However, in youth, males report more limitations than females (Kraus, Stoddard, Gilmartin, 1996). The major activity-limiting conditions among children and adolescents are displayed in Table 16-3. Hyperkinetic syndrome of childhood accounts for two thirds of the mental illness in childhood (Kraus, Stoddard, Gilmartin).

Community health nurses provide supportive assistance in a variety of ways to families whose children have chronic conditions. They assist these families in obtaining adequate health care, in making necessary adjustments in family lifestyle, and in obtaining community resources that will help them to promote their child's growth and development. *Compuplay* is one such resource. Compuplay Resource Centers serve families with children 2 to 14 years of age with physical, mental, sensory, or behavioral disabilities. These centers provide computer play classes, software lending libraries, and local in-service training for

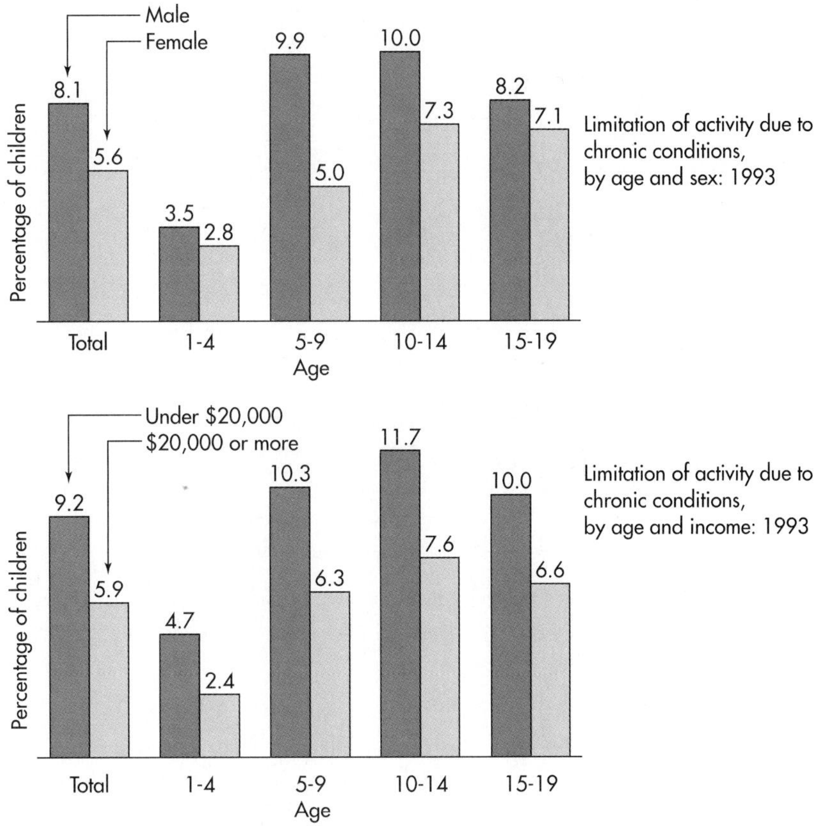

Figure 16-7 Limitation of activity as a result of chronic conditions, by age, sex, and income: 1993. *(From Maternal and Child Health Bureau:* Child health USA '94, *Washington, D.C., 1995, U.S. Government Printing Office, p. 28. Source: National Center for Health Statistics.)*

table 16-3 Five Most Prevalent Causes of Limitations among Persons Under 18 Years

Conditions	Percent of All Limiting Conditions*
1. Asthma	19.8%
2. Learning disability and mental retardation	19.2%
3. Mental illness	8.8%
4. Speech impairments	6.7%
5. Hearing impairments	3.8%

From LaPlante M, Carlson D: *Disability in the United States: prevalence and causes, 1992,* Disability Statistics Report (7), Washington, D.C., 1996, National Institute on Disability and Rehabilitation Research, p. 45.

*Percentage does not total 100% because not all activity-limiting conditions are listed.

professionals. Families interested in this resource can obtain further information by writing to the INNOTEK Director, National Lekotek Center, 2100 Ridge Avenue, Evanston, Il., 60204 or by calling 847-328-0001 (Compuplay Centers, 1988, p. 5). Other resources that may be helpful to families dealing with a chronic illness are identified in Chapter 19.

Community health nurses also assume a significant role in assisting school-age children to accept peers who have a chronic condition. A program to help children adjust to other children with chronic disabling conditions is *Kids on the Block.* This program is a puppet presentation showing puppets in wheelchairs, with assistive devices, and with various physical and mental conditions. This program stimulates discussion of childrens' feelings about peers who are different. Educational and health professionals can obtain more information about *Kids on the Block* by contacting 1-800-368-KIDS.

In addition to chronic diseases, school-age children may experience many chronic social problems that present serious difficulties for both themselves and their families. Homelessness, for example, is becoming increasingly prevalent among families with children. This problem is discussed extensively in Chapter 12. Four other social problems of particular concern to community health nurses who are working with school-age children are child abuse, unintended teenage parenthood, sexually transmitted diseases (STDs), and drug abuse. As reflected in Chapters 12 and 15, none of these concerns is unique to the school-age population.

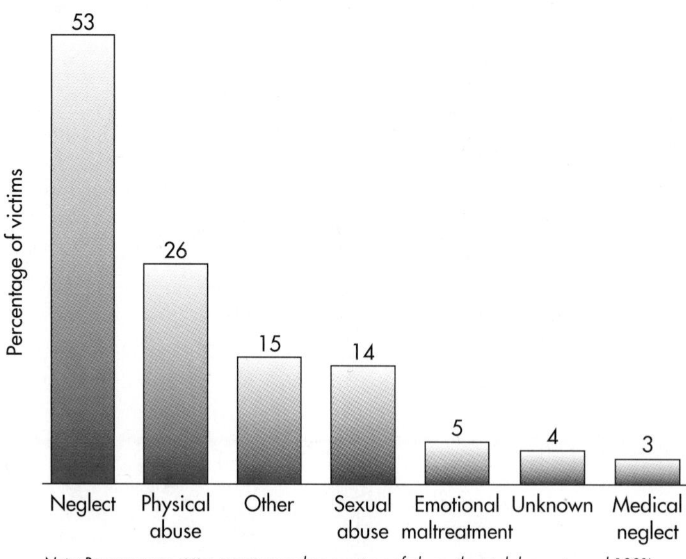

Figure 16-8 Percentage of child abuse and neglect victims, by type of maltreatment: 1994. *(From Maternal and Child Health Bureau:* Child health USA '95, *Washington, D.C., 1996, U.S. Government Printing Office, p. 37. Source: National Center on Child Abuse and Neglect).*

However, they are briefly highlighted here to emphasize the need for health care professionals to evaluate the influence of these problems on child growth and development. The reader is encouraged to review Chapter 12 to gain an understanding of the dynamics associated with child abuse, STDs, and drug abuse.

CHILD ABUSE As a result of increased reporting requirements in recent years, it is now known that child abuse is reaching epidemic proportions among the school-age population. Child abuse can involve physical and/or psychological abuse and neglect and/or sexual abuse.

In 1994 an estimated 2 million reports alleged the maltreatment of 2.9 million children; over 1 million victims of child abuse and neglect were confirmed. A sizable portion of these victims were 3 years old or younger (27%), between the ages of 4 and 6 (20%), and youth ages 13 to 18 (20%) (Maternal and Child Health Bureau, 1996). Generally the highest percentage of victims is in the under-1-year-of-age group. Emotionally maltreated children are on the average 8.1 years old (AAPC, 1986). Except for sexual abuse, maltreatment appears to occur with equal frequency in both sexes (National Center on Child Abuse and Neglect, 1994).

The types of maltreatment children suffered in 1994 are displayed in Figure 16-8. Experts believe that sexual abuse is the most underreported form of child maltreatment because of the conspiracy of silence that characterizes these cases (DePanfilis, Salus, 1992, p. 8). "Most sexual abuse is committed by men (90%) and by persons known to the child (70% to 90%), with family members constituting one-third to one-half of the perpetrators against girls and 10% to 20% of the perpetrators against boys . . . The peak age of vulnerability is between 7 and 13. Girls are victimized more often than boys" (Finkelhor, 1994, p. 31). Children separated from their parents or children whose parents have problems that substantially compromise their ability to supervise and attend to their children are particularly at risk for sexual abuse (Finkelhor).

Although reporting of child maltreatment has improved significantly in the last decade, this problem continues to be underreported and is often not identified (USDHHS, 1996). Preliminary findings from the Third National Incidence Study of Child Abuse and Neglect (a study involving 5700 community professionals who come into contact with children) estimate that almost 44 children per 1000 in the population may be victims of abuse or neglect (USDHHS).

All health care professionals must expand their efforts to identify undetected abuse and neglect in school-age children. The warning signs of abuse are presented in the box on the next page. Clinical manifestations of potential child maltreatment can be found in Appendix 16-1. These indicators assist nurses in identifying victims of abuse and neglect. Strategies aimed at preventing initial maltreatment or its recurrence should be focused on changing risk factors that have been demonstrated to have a major influence on child abuse. For example, strategies designed to reduce marital and financial stresses in families, such as referring families to community agencies for financial aid and counseling, are appropriately aimed at eliminating a significant risk factor of child abuse.

The problems of child abuse and neglect are compounded for professionals who work with the school-age population because often they must deal with the lasting effects of conditions that existed during infancy and the preschool years. Longitudinal studies are beginning to report findings that indicate long-term detrimental consequences of child abuse. Children who are abused during early childhood tend to

WARNING SIGNS OF ABUSE

- Physical evidence of abuse and/or neglect, including previous injuries
- Conflicting stories about the "accident" or injury from the parents or others
- Cause of injury blamed on sibling or other party
- An injury inconsistent with the history, such as a concussion and broken arm from falling off a bed
- History inconsistent with child's developmental level; such as a 6-month-old turning on the hot water
- A complaint other than the one associated with signs of abuse (e.g., a chief complaint of a cold when there is evidence of first- and second-degree burns)
- Inappropriate response of caregiver, such as an exaggerated or absent emotional response; refusal to sign for additional tests or agree to necessary treatment; excessive delay in seeking treatment; absence of the parents for questioning
- Inappropriate response of child, such as little or no response to pain; fear of being touched; excessive or lack of separation anxiety; indiscriminate friendliness to strangers
- Child's report of physical or sexual abuse
- Previous reports of abuse in the family
- Repeated visits to emergency facilities with injuries

From Wong DL: *Whaley and Wong's nursing care of infants and children*, ed 5, St. Louis, 1995, Mosby, p. 705.

have difficulty establishing trust, have more aggessive and behavioral problems than children who have not been abused, and frequently manifest a general air of depression, unhappiness, and sadness. Children who are sexually abused initially exhibit anger, hostility, and sexual problems, but in the long term more serious problems such as diminished self-esteem, fear, and depression emerge (Briere, Elliott, 1994; Dubowitz, 1986). In addition, data suggest that long-term effects of child maltreatment may include other problems such as juvenile delinquency, attempted suicide, substance abuse, truancy, and runaway behavior (Lindberg, Distad, 1985; Powers, Echenrode, Jaklitsch, 1990).

The effects of maltreatment can be devastating and the costs to society extremely high. Professionals and community citizens must join together to deal with this critical problem. To ensure that all children reach their optimal level of functioning, mechanisms must be established for early identification, reporting of actual or suspected abuse situations, and early and adequate intervention. The impact of abuse can be minimized by early recognition and timely response to the child. "Access to good health, education, and social services fosters resilience in children regardless of the specific nature of the stressor" (Humphreys, Ramsey, 1993, pp. 53-54).

Both health professionals and the public need educational opportunities that will increase their knowledge about child abuse and neglect and help them to intervene effectively with abusive families. The *Clearinghouse on Child Abuse and Neglect* (P.O. Box 1182, Washington, D.C., 20013, 1-800-394-3366) was established in 1975 by the federal government to assist communities with their educational needs regarding child abuse. This clearinghouse disseminates information and resource materials on all types of child maltreatment, responds to public inquiries, and has a computerized database that maintains updated statistics. Hotline services are also readily available to help communities and troubled families. The *National Child Abuse Hotline* (1-800-422-4453) provides information, professional counseling, and referrals for treatment. The *Parents Anonymous* National Office (909-621-6184) provides information on self-help groups for parents involved in child maltreatment. Most states have a hotline for Parents Anonymous.

TEENAGE PARENTHOOD National attention is focused on unintended pregnancy (IOM, 1995) and nonmarital childbearing (USDHHS, 1995c) because the consequences associated with both burden children, parents, families, and society. Unintended pregnancies and nonmarital births are widespread in America and have increased significantly over recent decades: It is estimated that almost 60% of all pregnancies are unintended and 30% of all births are to unmarried women. Although unintended pregnancies occur among women of all socioeconomic, marital status, and age groups, the incidence of unintended pregnancy is highest among unmarried and lower-income women and among women at either end of the age span (IOM, 1995; USDHHS, 1995c). Discussion here will highlight pregnancy during the teen years. However, it is important to recognize that teenagers represent only a small part of a larger problem in our nation: "Teenagers account for fewer than a third of all abortions, nonmarital births, and unintended births each year" (Alan Guttmacher Institute, 1994, p. 46).

The *Healthy People 2000* family planning objectives are aimed at reducing pregnancies among teenagers younger than 18 and unintended pregnancies among all women. The emphasis for teenagers is on reducing the incidence of sexual intercourse, increasing effective use of contraceptive methods for the purposes of preventing pregnancy and sexually transmitted diseases, and increasing the opportunities for age-appropriate sexuality education, care, and counseling (USDHHS, 1995a).

Over the past three decades, sexual initiation at a younger age has increased significantly. The increase in the proportion of sexually active young women aged 15 is particularly alarming; this age group shows the largest increase in the proportion of sexually active, from slightly less than 5% in 1979 to nearly 26% in 1988. It is important for health professionals to consider age at initiation of sexual activity, because when first intercourse is early, contraceptive use is lower and pregnancy risk higher (USDHHS, 1995a, p. 47).

Today two thirds of women and three quarters of men have had sexual intercourse before their eighteenth birthday (Figure 16-9). Although contraceptive use among teenagers has increased considerably, most young women are sexually active for a substantial time before going for medical contraceptive services (Alan Guttmacher Institute,

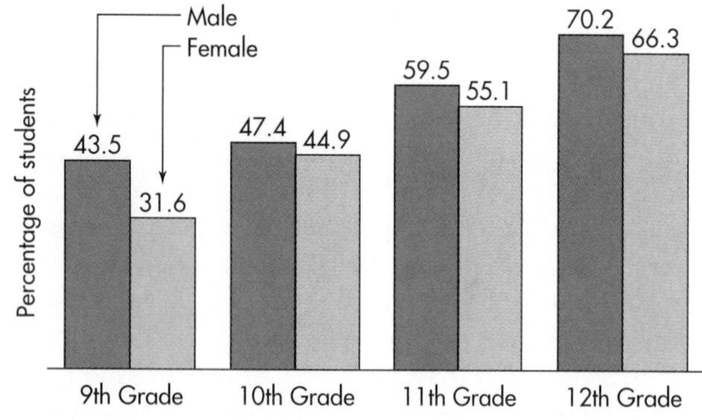

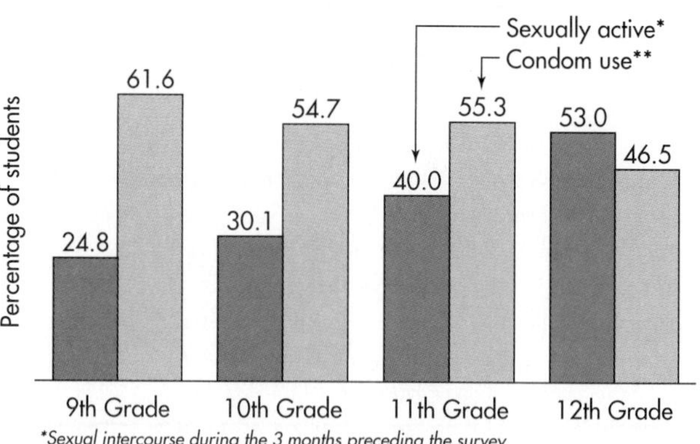

Figure **16-9** Sexual activity of high school students: 1993. *(From Maternal and Child Health Bureau:* Child health USA '95, *Washington, D.C., 1996, U.S. Government Printing Office, p. 43. Source: Centers for Disease Control and Prevention.)*

1994). This places these young women at risk for unintended pregnancy.

Each year one in every 10 American females ages 15 to 19 experience pregnancy. This figure is significantly higher than that of Canada, England, or France, where fewer than one teen in 20 becomes pregnant (Maternal and Child Health Bureau, 1995). The United States also has considerably higher abortion and unintended pregnancy rates among teenagers than those in other Western democracies. Over 85% of the 1 million pregnancies among American adolescent women are unintended (IOM, 1995). One third of adolescent pregnancies in the United States end in an induced abortion: teenagers under 15 years of age report a higher percentage (45%) of abortions. Over half of the pregnancies among American teenage women end in live births (Maternal and Child Health Bureau, 1995, 1996).

The multiplicity and complexity of needs manifested during teenage parenthood mandate close coordination among professionals from all disciplines. Pregnancy can pose serious physical and psychosocial health problems and concerns for the teenage parents, their families, and the community at large. The involved teenagers are dealing with two normative stressors, adolescence and parenthood, which may result in adverse, long-lasting psychosocial consequences if effective intervention is not available.

Medically, both the teenage mother and her baby are at high risk. Children born to teenage parents have a much higher neonatal, postnatal, and infant mortality rate. These babies have a higher incidence of prematurity, low birth weight, and respiratory distress. The mothers tend to have more physical problems throughout their pregnancy. Considering that adolescence is a period when marked physical changes and rapid growth occurs, it is understandable that the additional stress of pregnancy increases a teenage mother's susceptibility to health difficulties. Toxemia, hypertension, nutritional deficiencies, prolonged labor, pelvic disproportion, and cesarean sections are a few complications of pregnancy common to the teenage mother (Alan Guttmacher Institute, 1994; IOM, 1995; USDHHS, 1995c).

Parenthood in adolescence can present a number of special problems. Adolescent mothers face increased risks of single parenthood, incomplete education, poverty, unemployment, and welfare dependency (Hoffman, Foster, Furstenberg, 1993; USDHHS, 1995c). Financially, teenagers are often not able to provide for such basic needs as food, clothing, and shelter. Frequently they need assistance from social service agencies to adequately care for themselves and their children. Because they are not prepared for a career, it is difficult for them to obtain productive employment. Often a pregnant teenager drops out of school, which increases the likelihood that future employment opportunities will be limited and that social isolation from peers will occur.

Individual counseling with teenage parents is necessary but not sufficient to prevent unintended adolescent pregnancies. The Panel on Adolescent Pregnancy and Childbearing (1987) believed that "the responsibility for addressing adolescent pregnancy should be shared among individuals, families, voluntary organizations, communities, and governments, and that public policies should affirm the role and responsibility of families to teach human values" (p. 120). This panel further recommended that prevention of adolescent pregnancy has the highest priority and that needs of young adolescents and disadvantaged youth should be given priority if resources are inadequate to address all the needs. Four indicators have consistently predicted early initiation of sexual activity, adolescent pregnancy, and nonmarital childbearing among teenagers: early school failure, early behavior problems, poverty, and family problems/

family dysfunction (Maternal and Child Health Bureau, 1996, p. 42).

Population- and community-focused programming is needed to address the problems associated with teenage pregnancy. Successful pregnancy prevention programs are comprehensive in nature and provide continuity of care over several years. They also connect adolescents with peer and adult role models, include life skills education, as well as sexuality and contraceptive education and services, and provide mechanisms for buffering youth against the pressures of their environment (USDHHS, 1995c).

Recently, efforts in some communities have been strengthened to prevent the negative outcomes associated with adolescent parenting. A variety of innovative approaches are being used to help teenage mothers complete their education, to prevent repeat pregnancies, and to encourage responsible parenting. "These approaches include alternative schools for pregnant and parenting students within the public school system, residential facilities for homeless teenage mothers on AFDC [now renamed Temporary Assistance to Needy Families], home visiting to assist teenage mothers and their families, and school-based programs that serve mothers as part of a larger effort aimed at all at-risk teenagers" (GAO, 1995b, pp. 2-3). The accompanying box displays the range of services provided by 13 local programs that are recognized by experts as being exemplary in helping disadvantaged teenage mothers complete their high school education. A variety of approaches and services can help mothers to expand life options (GAO, 1995b).

Studies on the consequences of unintended pregnancies and nonmarital childbearing tend to focus on mothers and children. Fathers involved in teenage childbearing tend to be older than the mother. Males and Chew (1996) contend that "what we call schoolage childbearing is predominantly a teen-adult phenomenon" (p. 567). It is estimated that only a minority (26%) of men involved in pregnancies among adolescent women under age 18 are that young: 35% are ages 18 to 19, and 39% are at least 20 (Alan Guttmacher Institute, 1994).

Little is known about the impact of pregnancy on the fathers involved in adolescent childbearing. The limited studies that examine adolescent fathering suggest that educational and emotional problems precede rather than follow the act of fathering (Resnick, Chambliss, Blum, 1993). Some evidence suggests that adolescent fathers may be less affected by the negative impact of early paternity than adolescent mothers, especially in relation to future educational and employment opportunities (Parke, Neville, 1987). However, the adolescent father's involvement with his child is often limited, as a result of others limiting his contact with his child, or by his own choice. This can affect the adolescent father's ability to provide positive parenting (Parke, Neville). Community health professionals must strengthen their efforts in reaching out to fathers involved in adolescent childbearing.

Services to Support High School Completion Among Teenage Mothers

FINANCIAL
- Child care
- Transportation
- Housing
- Small scholarships

SOCIAL
- Parenting education
- Life skills classes
- Counseling
- Anger/stress management
- Support groups
- Teen fathers program
- Recreational activities

EMPLOYMENT/EDUCATION
- Vocational/job skills training
- Job placement
- Job/college fairs
- Tutoring
- Mentor program

HEALTH
- Mental health counseling
- Family planning/pregnancy prevention
- Child development classes
- Home visits by prenatal community nurse
- Substance abuse counseling
- Group therapy
- Health care

SPECIAL FEATURES
- Case management
- Teen parent coordinator/advisor
- Sanctions for repeat pregnancy
- Summer program
- Program for dropouts
- In-home visits
- On-site health clinic

From General Accounting Office (GAO): *Welfare to work: approaches that help teenage mothers complete high school*, Washington, D.C., 1995b, GAO, pp. 11-12.

Chapter 15 discussed extensively the role of the community health nurse in addressing the needs of parents and children. It is important for community health nurses to recognize that when they work with adolescent parents that these parents often need a comprehensive array of interdisciplinary services to avoid the negative consequences associated with early parenthood. Community health nurses play a significant role in helping adolescent parents access these services.

SEXUALLY TRANSMISSIBLE DISEASES (STDs) One alarming consequence of early initiation of sexual activity among adolescents is the dramatic rise in the incidence of sexually transmissible diseases in this age category. As with most social problems, hard data reflect only the tip of the iceberg. Professionals frequently do not accurately report the occurrence of sexually transmissible diseases, and many nonapparent subclinical infections go untreated. "An estimated 85% of women with chlamydial and gonococcal pelvic inflammatory disease (PID) don't seek treatment (Sharts-Hopko, 1997, p. 46). From estimated reports over time, however, it is apparent that sexually transmissible diseases, especially gonorrhea, chlamydial infections, syphilis, herpes, and AIDs have reached epidemic proportions in recent years (USDHHS, 1991, 1995a). Chapter 12 presents information about these and selected other sexually transmitted diseases that affect adolescents and adults.

Although STDs occur among men and women of all socioeconomic and age groups, "STDs disproportionately affect the young, the poor, and minorities" (USDHHS, 1995a, p. 116). Almost 12 million cases of sexually transmitted diseases occur annually, 66% of them in people under the age of 25 years. Of grave concern is the growing segments of young children, adolescents, and young adults affected with AIDS. Young children under the age of 13 are primarily exposed to HIV through perinatal transmission before or during birth (see Chapter 15). Adolescents are primarily exposed to HIV through receipt of blood products and high-risk behaviors, including heterosexual and male-to-male sexual contact and injecting drug use. Young adults are primarily exposed to HIV through high-risk behaviors. Among young adult men, the major exposure category associated with AIDS is male-to-male contact; among young adult women, exposure to HIV is primarily through injecting drug use or through sex with an injecting drug user. The majority of young adults are probably exposed to HIV during adolescence (Maternal and Child Health Bureau, 1996).

It is estimated that for every child with AIDS reported to the CDC, anywhere from 2 to 3 children may be HIV-infected (USDHHS, 1993a). The United States is currently dealing with only the "tip of the AIDS iceberg." However, as discussed in Chapter 11, the portion of the iceberg that is submerged is the most insidious and potentially dangerous portion of the clinical spectrum of disease. Among our nation's youth many STDs are submerged.

STD Action Coalitions and local health departments are valuable resources for the nurse working with adolescents who suspect they may have an STD. Immediate treatment is essential. When diagnosed and treated early, almost all STDs can be treated effectively (USDHHS, 1991). However, many young people suffer serious, permanent complications from these infections. For example, every year an estimated 1 million women have an episode of pelvic inflammatory diseases (PID), the most serious and common complication of STDs among women. About one fifth of these PIDs are experienced by teenagers. PID can lead to infertility, tubal pregnancy, chronic pelvic pain, and other serious consequences. Over 100,000 women become infertile as a result of PID each year (USDHHS).

Community health nurses working with the school-age population must realize that the occurrence of sexually transmitted diseases is a *major* health problem in this age group. Programs that provide preventive, curative, and educative services for all children in the population served by the nurse must be planned. Use of the epidemiological process (Chapter 11) and the principles of health planning (Chapter 14) will facilitate the accomplishment of such a task. For readily accessible STD information, the nurse or client may want to utilize the STD Hotline at 1-800-227-8922, or the AIDS Hotline at 1-800-342-AIDS. These hotlines provide information on STDs and confidential referrals for diagnosis and treatment.

"If adults are going to help teenagers avoid the outcomes of sex that are clearly negative—STDs, unintended pregnancies, abortions, and out-of-wedlock births—they must accept the reality of adolescent sexual activity and deal with it directly and honestly" (Alan Guttmacher Institute, 1994, p. 5). Teenagers encounter a host of stressors that place them at risk for pregnancy and STDs acquisition. They often lack experience in communicating with their partners about contraceptive use. They also frequently fear disclosure and avoid seeking contraceptive services to prevent others from knowing they are sexually active. Additionally, they often lack access to an appropriate source of care and must deal with numerous contradictory messages about responsible sexual behavior. Other Western democracies are much more open with adolescents about sexual relationships (Alan Guttmacher Institute). Our nation needs to learn from these countries.

SUBSTANCE ABUSE Substance abuse among American youth is a major public health problem. Data from national surveys monitoring this problem reflect that it is widespread and on the rise (Johnston, O'Malley, Bachman, 1996b; PRIDE, 1996). In the United States a steady decline—from the late 1970s to the early 1990s—came to a halt in 1991 among 8th-graders and in 1992 among 10th- and 12th-graders. Between 1991 and 1996 the proportion using any illicit drug in the prior 12 months more than doubled for 8th-graders (from 11% to 24%), and between 1992 and 1996 it nearly doubled among 10th-graders (from 20% to 38%) and rose by about half among 12th-graders (from 27% to 40%) (Johnston, O'Malley, Bachman, 1996b, p. 1). The United States ranks highest among all other industrialized countries in its illicit drug use among secondary school students and young adults (Johnston, O'Malley, Bachman, 1996a).

Figure 16-10 displays the prevalence and recency of use of select drugs for 12th-grade students in the United States. The magnitude of the nation's drug problem among secondary school and college students is staggering: sizeable proportions have tried illicit drugs and alcohol and are establishing regular cigarette habits during late adolescence. For example, over a third (38%) of the nation's youth have tried an illicit drug by the end of 8th grade; nearly half (46%) by the end of 10th grade and over half (52%) by the end of 12th grade (Johnston, O'Malley, Bachman, 1996a, p. 28).

The findings from national surveys suggest that our nation cannot afford to be lax in the attention given to the control of drug abuse among youth. Overall, drug use among high school students and young adults remain widespread. Although there are regional and population differences in the use of illicit drugs among young people, no community is free of illegal drug use by secondary and college students (Johnston, O'Malley, Bachman, 1996a). "The drug problem is not an enemy which can be vanquished, as in a war. It is more a recurring and relapsing problem which must be contained to the extent possible on a long-term, ongoing basis; and, therefore, it is a problem which requires an ongoing, dynamic response from our society" (Johnston, O'Malley, Bachman, 1996a, p. 29).

The dynamics associated with substance abuse, as well as the role of community health nurses in addressing this problem, are discussed in Chapter 12. For youth, drug abuse prevention programs have traditionally employed one or both of two strategies: educational or social control through policy, and regulation or legislation (Goodstadt, 1989, p. 247). Goodstadt, based on a review of pertinent research related to preventive drug intervention, promotes the joint development and implementation of educational and policy strategies to combat drug abuse in school settings.

Dusenbury, Falco, and Lake (1997) recently reviewed 47 nationally and currently available drug abuse curricula that focused on primary prevention, were classroom-based, and were designed for any grade level K-12, for which samples could be obtained from program distributors. They found that "prevention curricula which give students training in social resistance skills or how to recognize influences and resist them effectively, and normative education posit-

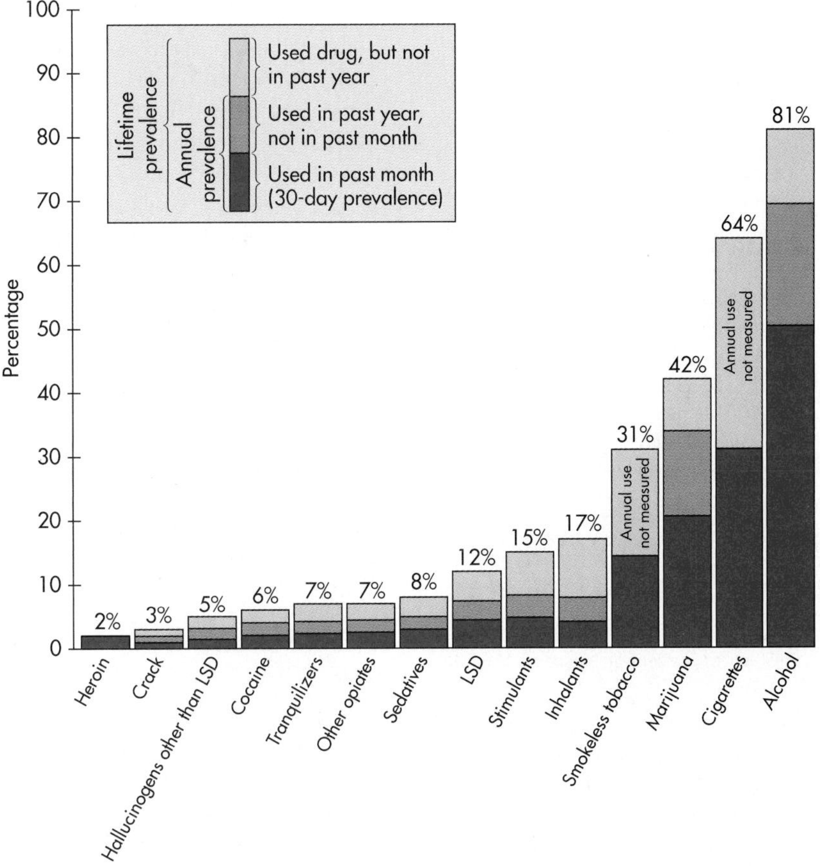

Figure 16-10 Prevalence and recency of use of various types of drugs by twelfth graders, 1995. *(From Johnston LD, O'Malley PM, Bachman JG:* National survey results on drug use from The Monitoring The Future Study, 1975-1995, vol 1, secondary school students, *Washington, D.C., 1996a, U.S. Government Printing Office, p. 49.)*

table 16-4 Drug Abuse Prevention Curricula: Contact Information

Curriculum Name	Contact
Alcohol Misuse Prevention Project	University of Michigan Institute for Social Research Room 2349 Ann Arbor, MI 48106-1248 313/647-0587
DARE	DARE America P.O. Box 2090 Los Angeles, CA 90051-0090 800/223-DARE
Growing Healthy	National Center for Health Education 72 Spring St. Suite 208 New York, NY 10012-4019 800/551-3488
Know Your Body	American Health Foundation 675 Third Ave. 11th floor New York, NY 10017 212/551-2509
Life Skills Training	Institute for Prevention Research Cornell University Medical 411 E. 69th St. New York, NY 10021 212/746-1270
Project Alert	Best Foundation 725 S. Figueroa St. Suite 1615 Los Angeles, CA 90017 800/ALERT-10
Project Northland	University of Minnesota Division of Epidemiology School of Public Health 1300 S. Second St. Suite 300 Minneapolis, MN 55445-1015 612/624-0057
Social Competence Promotion Program	Dept. of Psychology (M/C 285) University of Illinois at Chicago 1007 W. Harrison St. Chicago, IL 60607-7137 312/413-1012
STAR	Institute for Prevention Research 1540 Alcazar St., CHP 207 Los Angeles, CA 90033 213/457-4000
Teenage Health Teaching Modules	Educational Development Center 55 Chapel St. Newton, MA 02158-1060 800/225-4276

From Dusenbury L, Falco M, Lake A: A review of the evaluation of 47 drug abuse prevention curricula available nationally, *J Sch Health* 67:127-132, 1997, p. 131.

ing that drug use is not the norm, have been shown to reduce substance use behavior. In addition, training in broader personal and social skills such as decision-making, anxiety reduction, communication, and assertiveness appears to enhance program effectiveness" (Dusenbury, Falco, Lake, p. 127). Ten of the 47 curricula available to schools have been evaluated in rigorous research studies and have been shown to reduce substance abuse (Table 16-4). However, two curricula (Social Competence Promotion and Teenage Health Teaching Modules) need to be evaluated beyond the posttest to determine the sustained effects on students' drug use. The Project Alert and DARE Curricula had variable success at reducing substance use initially but did not appear to have a long-lasting effect. Dusenbury, Falco, and Lake believe "these [two] programs may still make an important contribution to drug abuse prevention, if done within the context of ongoing and sustained prevention efforts" (p. 130). They stress that reinforcement and follow-up are critical elements of any prevention program. If a program is brief, such as the Project Alert and DARE programs, it appears that the effects diminish over time (Dusenbury, Falco, Lake).

Significant drug prevention and referral service information can be obtained from several national organizations. Alcoholics Anonymous, Cocaine Anonymous, and Narcotics Anonymous answer questions on health risks of substance abuse, provide self-help support services, and assist people in obtaining needed drug treatment services. These organizations are found in local telephone directories. The National Clearinghouse for Alcohol and Drug Information (1-800-729-6686) provides a broad range of educational materials on drug-related issues. The National Parents' Resource Institute for Drug Education (PRIDE: 770-458-9900) also disseminates lay and professional materials on substance abuse and refers families to appropriate service organizations. The National Institute on Drug Abuse hotline (1-800-662-HELP) provides general information on drug abuse and drug prevention programs and offers referrals to drug rehabilitation centers. Most states and local communities have resources that assist youth, adults, and professionals interested in obtaining drug abuse prevention and treatment information. These resources can be accessed by contacting your local health department or community mental health center.

HEALTH PROMOTION DURING THE SCHOOL YEARS

All children must accomplish health promotion tasks that help them to prevent mortality and morbidity, develop healthy lifestyle behaviors, and enhance future development and maturation (see Appendixes 16-2 and 16-3). Sometimes it is a struggle for children to achieve these tasks. The author of *Stuffed Rabbit* (see the box on the next page) dramatically illustrates the stressful process a child goes through to develop independence. Parents, health care professionals, and other interested individuals can help

Stuffed Rabbit

Stuffed rabbit
Seven years my nocturnal security
Now neglected worn and eyeless
Lying in the memory-choked attic
Stabbed by blunt dusty shafts of sunlight
Recalling to me
Evenings of forbidden play beneath giggle-muffling blankets
Recalling to me the day I grew
Too big
Too old
To sleep with innocence while hugging security
I'll leave you here stuffed rabbit,
You're dead
But God, what a long slow funeral we're having!

Gregory Smith, written at age 18

children make the growing process less stressful. They can assist children in achieving a healthy adulthood through preventive and health promoting interventions. Since health risks and needs among children change over time, it is crucial for child caregivers to view health promotion as a longitudinal process that enhances a child's health at critical transition periods (Green, 1994).

Chapter 15 presented a timeline for preventive health care, a recommended schedule for immunizations, and anticipatory guidance health supervision topics for infants, children, and adolescents. Timely anticipatory guidance assists parents and children to understand development needs and health risks. This, in turn, helps parents and children to develop effective strategies for stress management and problem solving. For example, the community health nurse can help parents to discuss sexuality issues openly and honestly with their children by helping them address their fears regarding these issues.

Both individual-focused and population-focused interventions are used by health care professionals to guide a child through the growth process. Individual-focused interventions are aimed at monitoring growth and development on a continuous basis, helping children to develop healthy lifestyle patterns, and creating a supportive environment to enhance growth and development. The topics of anticipatory guidance presented in Chapter 15 assist health care providers to identify family and child strengths and health service needs. A family-centered approach to care is essential for health providers to successfully promote a child's health. "Because families are the ones who see their child on a continuous basis, and in a variety of settings, through different developmental stages, they really are the *experts*" (Shelton, Stepanek, 1994, p. 8).

From a population-focused perspective, health care providers work in partnership with communities to design health promotion programs based on community needs and national and local health objectives. Illustrative of this are the innovative cardiovascular health promotion projects developed to promote children's heart health. These programs are grounded in the belief that primary prevention is the key to successfully reduce major problems in adulthood.

The National Heart, Lung, and Blood Institute has funded several culturally relevant programs to address children's heart health. For example, the HIP HOP TO HEALTH program, designed to honor the African-American heritage, reflects children's interest in the inner city–bred phenomenon of hip-hop music. This project uses ethnic traditions and tastes in music, dancing, food, clothing, and sports to promote healthy heart eating and activity among inner-city African-American children. The PATHWAYS program is another example of a culturally relevant health promotion heart project. It uses traditional Native American games, such as "the coyote has smelly feet," an Apache version of tag, to promote an understanding of different tribal cultures and to increase physical activity among Native American children. It also helps families to prepare healthy traditional tribal foods and children to develop healthy nutritional habits. The 1996 special edition of the *Heart Memo* published by the National Heart, Lung, and Blood Institute (301-251-1222), discusses both the HIP HOP TO HEALTH program and the PATHWAYS program, as well as several other heart healthy projects for children. This Heart Memo provides valuable tips for developing effective population-focused interventions for children.

When working with children it is critical for all health care professionals to observe for lags in normal growth and development. Early casefinding and intervention can prevent permanent disability. A comprehensive biopsychosocial and cultural assessment should be done with every child and family when the child is not performing at the appropriate developmental age level. Intervention should be started immediately if a developmental disability is confirmed.

Developmental Disabilities

Developmental disabilities are increasingly common among school-age children and present significant stresses to those affected. Although estimates of the number of children with developmental disabilities vary significantly, it is known that several million children and their families are dealing with this problem. A diagnosis of a disabling condition constitutes a crisis for families and may require multiple adjustments in their lifestyle. Community health nurses frequently assume a significant role in promoting physical and psychosocial well-being among families by addressing the issues related to developmental disabilities.

As with average children, the degree to which children with developmental disabilities adjust successfully as healthy individuals varies. The nature and quality of their previous and current life experiences and their physical, emotional, and cognitive status greatly influence how well children with developmental disabilities progress. Typically these children have different life experiences from average children, and these differences are weighted in a negative direction. Numerous variables affect the socioadaptive capacity of children with developmental disabilities. An overwhelming number of the factors are influenced by environmental conditions. Few of them are inherent in the child or immutable to change (Clemen, Pattullo, 1980, p. 226).

Since the passage of Public Law 94-142, Education for All Handicapped Children Act in 1975 (renamed the Individuals With Disabilities Education Act, or the IDEA, in 1990), the number of children receiving special education services in elementary and secondary public schools has increased from 3.7 million to 4.6 million (Snyder, 1993). One in every 10 students in public schools today receives special education under the Individuals With Disabilities Education Act (Office of Special Education Programs, 1994). Over half of all children receiving special education services in public schools are identified as having a learning disability. Almost one fourth are identified as having speech or language impairments; over one tenth are identified as having mental retardation; and almost one tenth are identified as having serious emotional disturbances (Office of Special Education Programs). Lyon (1996) contends that "the influence of advocacy has contributed to a substantial proliferation in the number of children who have been identified with learning disabilities relative to other handicapping conditions" (p. 57).

Public Law 94-142 mandated that every school system receiving special federal educational funds must provide a "free, appropriate education for all handicapped children between the ages of six and eighteen, regardless of the type of handicap or the degree of impairment." It also provided incentive monies to extend services to children beginning at age 3 and for young adults between 18 through 21. Public Law 99-457 (the Education for All Handicapped Children Act Amendments of 1986) amended Public Law 94-142 and created a new Preschool Grant Program (currently reauthorized under P.L. 102-119). This program mandates that children, beginning at the age of 3, have the "right to education." It also created a new Handicapped Infants and Toddlers Program that provides incentive monies to enhance educational services for disabled and at-risk infants and toddlers. Provisions of this law require that each child have an Individual Educational Plan (IEP) and families have an Individualized Family Service Plan (IFSP). These plans specify educational goals and strategies for achieving these goals (Winstead-Fry, Bishop, 1997).

School systems that receive IDEA funds are required to purchase whatever is needed to meet a child's educational needs. Other major mandates covered by IDEA are:

- A "child-find plan" to identify all children within the state who have special needs;
- Appropriate educational opportunities in the least restrictive environment;
- Due process safeguards that help parents provide input concerning their child's educational needs and challenge decisions regarding their child;
- An individualized education program (IEP); and
- Assurance that tests and other evaluation materials do not reflect cultural or racial bias.

Like other young persons, children with developmental disabilities need coordinated, comprehensive community health services designed to foster optimal growth. No one community system can provide the entire spectrum of services needed by the school-age population. Current emphasis is on developing integrated service delivery models that link preventive health care and educational programming to prevent duplicated and fragmented service delivery. Since most children attend school, the school is a logical environment in which to provide a comprehensive array of health services (USDHHS, 1993b). However, it is important to remember that school health cannot be separated from the ecological and social conditions of the home and the community.

A COMPREHENSIVE SCHOOL HEALTH PROGRAM

As early as 1850, educators and health professionals recognized that the school was an important focal point for health promotion activities. At that time Lemuel Shattuck (1850, pp. 178-179) wrote the following:

> Every child should be taught, early in life, that, to preserve his own life and his own health and the lives and health of others, is one of his most important and constantly abiding duties. Some measure is needed which shall compel children to make a sanitary examination of themselves and their associates, and thus elicit a practical application of the lessons of sanitary science in the everyday duties of life. The recommendation now under consideration is designed to furnish this measure. It is to be carried into operation in the use of a blank schedule, which is to be printed on a letter sheet, in the form prescribed in the appendix, and furnished to the teacher of each school. He is to appoint a sanitary committee of the scholars, at the commencement of school, and, on the first day of each month, to fill it out under his superintendence. . . . Such a measure is simple, would take a few minutes each day, and cannot operate otherwise than usefully upon the children, in forming habits of exact observation, and in making a personal application of the laws of health and life to themselves. This is education of an eminently practical character, and of the highest importance.

Shattuck was advanced in his thinking about school health programming. He promoted self-care through education and "sanitary examination," or physical inspection. His writings also reflected current epidemiological emphasis on the responsibility that all citizens have for preserving life and promoting health. Additionally, he recognized that health education was an appropriate function of the school and that this function can best be coordinated by a "sanitary committee," or health council.

Today comprehensive school health programming incorporates Shattack's ideas and other concepts aimed at promoting healthy living. Schools are envisioned as an important "hub" for the integration of social health, mental health, and support services for children and families" (Elders, 1993, p. 312). This vision is reflected in current definitions and models for comprehensive school health.

Recently, the Institute of Medicine's Committee on Comprehensive School Health Programs adopted an interim statement that provides a definition of a comprehensive school health program. This definition is given below (Allensworth, Wyche, Lawson, Nicholson, 1995):

> A comprehensive school health program is an integrated set of planned, sequential, school-affiliated strategies, activities, and services designed to promote the optimal physical, emotional, social, and educational development of students. The program involves and is supportive of families and is determined by the local community, based on community needs, resources, standards, and requirements. It is coordinated by a multidisciplinary team and accountable to the community for program quality and effectiveness. (p. 2)

Currently no one single model is used to guide health programming in the school setting. Recently Resnicow and Allensworth (1996) proposed a coordinated eight-component model (Figure 16-11) that is a refinement of the comprehensive school health program (CSHP) model developed by Allensworth and Kolbe (1987) in the late 1980s. The CSHP model "extended the classic triad of health services, health education, and healthful environment to include physical education, counseling, psychology, and social services, food service, staff wellness, and family/community involvement" (Resnicow, Allensworth, 1996, p. 59). Resnicow and Allensworth refined the CSHP model by including the school health coordinator as an essential element in the model. They believe that the school health coordinator plays a central role in the integration, coordination, and management of school health programming. They also propose that this coordinator intervene with staff, parents, students, and the community to promote school- and community-based health programming that supports and enhances school health activities. Resnicow and Allensworth believe that in the classic school health model, healthy environment, staff wellness, and community activities were often neglected because no one had the designated responsibility for addressing them. Links to the community are extremely important because they help school service providers identify community needs and plan, implement, and evaluate school health activities. The school often assumes a central role in promoting community action for health.

The Centers for Disease Control and Prevention, Division of Adolescent and School Health (USDHHS, 1993b) also identifies eight components in a comprehensive school health program. These components are identified and briefly described in the box on the next page. When communities develop school health programs, they focus on the most pressing health issues of the students in their communities,

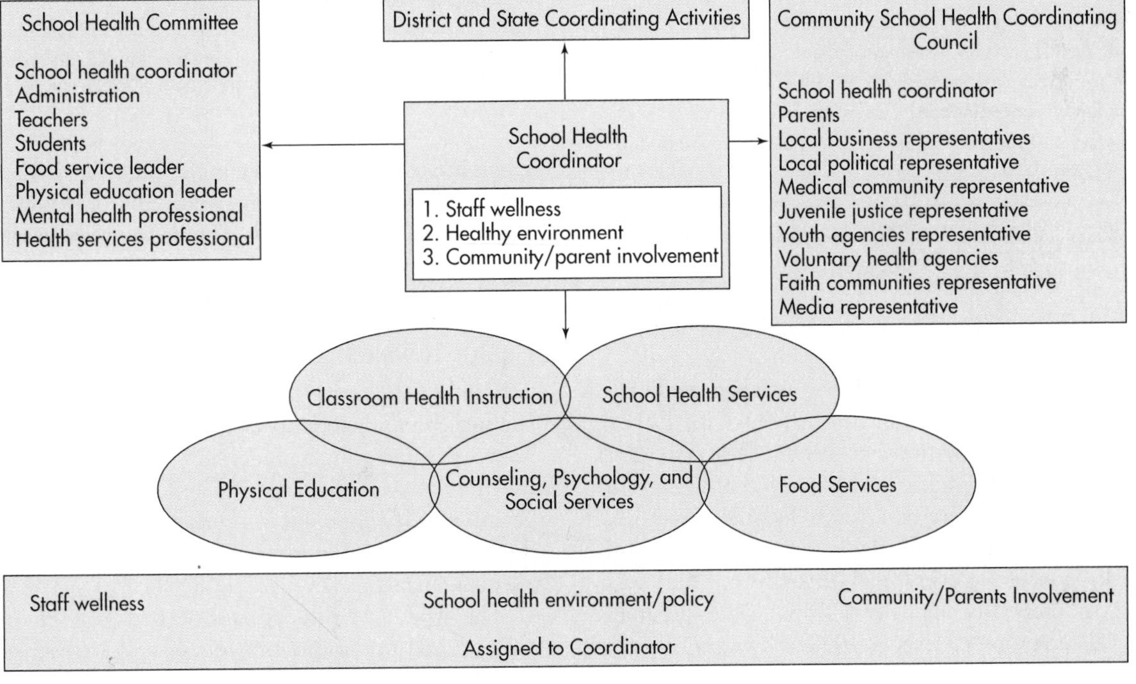

Figure **16-11** The comprehensive school health program revisited. *(From Resnicow K, Allensworth D: Conducting a comprehensive school health program,* J Sch Health 66:59-63, 1996, *p. 61.)*

Key Components of a Comprehensive School Health Program

Addressing the full range of health needs of school-aged children calls for a broad and comprehensive approach. A comprehensive school health program includes eight key components:

- **Health education,** providing planned, sequential instructional programs for prekindergarten through twelfth-grade students. Health education programs are designed to impact positively the knowledge, attitudes, beliefs, and behaviors of the intervention group.
- **Clinical services,** offering first aid and other clinical services to students and sometimes their families, through school-based or school-linked programs. Screening, diagnosis, and treatment are frequently performed as well as case management for children with special health care needs.
- **Counseling and mental health services,** providing vocational guidance and psychological assessments. Consultations and interventions are also conducted. Issues involving self-esteem, self-control, and peer pressure are addressed with students.
- **School environment,** ensuring a safe and secure setting for learning. Aspects of a healthy environment include prevention of lead poisoning; removal of asbestos; the regulation of noise, heating, and lighting; as well as fostering secure, nonthreatening relationships among students and faculty.
- **School food programs,** providing school food services offering healthy choices, as well as education on healthy eating habits and food preparation.
- **Physical education and physical fitness,** providing age-appropriate activities for students to improve their health status, reduce stress, and increase social development.
- **Faculty and staff health promotion,** placing schools in the role of the worksite and offering a range of health promotion and disease prevention services to school faculty and staff. Adult participation in health promotion activities may also serve to model healthful behavior to students.
- **Community coordination,** increasing the school's constituency of supporters and building coalitions within the community.

From Office of Disease Prevention and Health Promotion: *School health: findings from evaluated programs*, Washington, D.C., 1993b, U.S. Government Printing Office, pp. 1-1 - 1-2.

table 16-5 Single Most Significant Health Problem Reported by Districts by Grade Level (%)

Problem	Elementary School	Middle School	High School
Accident/injury prevention	6.4	3.1	0.8
Chronic health problem	11.2	5.2	2.9
Communicable disease	5.6	1.9	1.0
Dental problems	1.2	0.6	0.0
Drug/substance abuse	0.6	2.7	6.8
Environmental concerns	0.6	0.0	0.0
High-risk social behaviors	18.9	33.8	45.6
Inadequate immunizations	1.9	0.6	0.2
Infectious disease	3.3	0.8	1.0
Lack of access to health care	9.5	4.1	2.9
Mental illness/ emotional problems	4.8	6.4	5.0
Poor school attendance	2.3	2.3	2.9
Poverty	5.8	2.1	2.1
Self-esteem problems	8.7	19.9	7.7
Special health needs	9.1	2.9	1.9
Suicide	0.6	1.0	0.2
Teen pregnancy	0.0	1.7	6.6
Unhealthy lifestyle habits	6.4	8.1	8.5
Violence	0.0	1.2	2.3
Vision problems	0.6	0.2	0.4

From Fryer G, Igoe J: Functions of school nurses and health assistants in U.S. school health programs, *J Sch Health* 66:55-58, 1996.

such as sexual activity, substance abuse, violence, cardiovascular health risks, and poor nutrition (USDHHS, 1993b). Results from a recent nationwide survey of a systematic random sample of school districts reflect that although student health problems vary remarkably by grade level (Table 16-5), high-risk social behavior is the single most significant health concern at every level (Fryer, Igoe, 1996).

Other comprehensive models for school health programming have been proposed (Nader, 1992). However, "there is no special definition of school health to which all the various professions and organizations involved in this field subscribe . . . There is general consensus that school health programs are composed of three major functional areas: health services, health education, and environmental health" (Igoe, Parcel, 1992, p. 307). There is also a general consensus that a successful school health program uses an interagency, interdisciplinary approach to service delivery.

Health Services

School health services are designed to protect and promote the health of all students and all school personnel. Health service programming includes such things as periodic screenings for hearing and vision disorders and scoliosis, emergency care, development of a care management plan for children with disabilities, and the preparation of nutritionally adequate meals.

The type of health services needed in a school setting varies based on community needs and strengths and the characteristics of the population being served. Before developing a school health program, health professionals, school personnel, and community citizens jointly assess their community to identify specific health service needs. School health services should not duplicate services already available in the community. Rather, they should augment community resources to enhance health care service delivery in the community. For example, if a community lacks accessible health services for children and youth, the school may provide primary health care services through a school-based clinic. Currently over 500 school-based clinics operate in elementary, middle, and high schools in the United States (GAO, 1995a), and this number is growing. There are also school-linked clinics and other health service models for children in many states (Center for the Future of Children, 1992; Ferretti, Verhey, Isham, 1996; Passarelli, 1994). These types of clinics are located in many major cities and rural areas to improve children's access to health care. However, in some school settings primary health care services are not needed because the community has an adequate number of health personnel, accessible clinic services for disadvantaged populations, and families in the school district who are financially stable.

Regardless of the resources available in the community, certain basic health services should be provided in all school systems. Strategies should be established to achieve the following objectives:

- To appraise the health status of students and school personnel on a continual basis
- To counsel students, parents, teachers, and others regarding appraisal findings
- To encourage health care to correct remedial defects
- To provide emergency care for injury or sudden illness
- To prevent and control infectious diseases
- To identify children with disabling conditions and to arrange for educational programming that will enhance the maximum potential of these children
- To maintain a record-keeping system that complies with state laws (e.g., documentation of immunization status) and that documents the health needs of special children

To accomplish these objectives health education, health promotion, and environmental inspection activities must be integrated. Having one person in the school system responsible for coordinating this integration is essential.

Health Education

Health education is a process that helps people make sound decisions about personal health practices and about individual, family, and community well-being. Knowledge alone does not necessarily foster appropriate health habits. To facilitate effective decision making in health matters, the school system should provide every child with the opportunity to acquire *knowledge* essential for understanding healthy functioning, develop *attitudes* and *habits* that promote healthy lifestyle behaviors, and practice health *skills* conducive to effective living (Stone, Perry, Luepker, 1989). To achieve these goals, the child, the family, and the community must be involved in the educational process. This is essential because a variety of forces influence the development of healthy lifestyle behaviors.

A *planned* series of *integrated* health educational activities based on input received from students, parents, community citizens, health care professionals, and educators is needed to ensure that health education will become an integral component of a school's curriculum. Informal health counseling with individual students and special health projects such as "know your heart" and "maturational processes" are valuable but not sufficient to adequately prepare children to make sound decisions about all the personal, family, and community health needs they will encounter. "Rigorous studies show that comprehensive health education in schools is effective in reducing the prevalence of health risk behaviors among youth" (CDC, 1995, p. 3).

National health objectives provide a framework for developing a sound health education program in the school setting. They help schools to develop curriculum offerings that target critical health issues among school-age children such as substance abuse, violence, and sexuality concerns (see the *Healthy People 2000* box). They also provide support for developing a planned, sequential preschool-to-12 comprehensive curriculum. Health educational activities in the school should be aimed at promoting both physiological and psychosocial functioning. Students must be helped to analyze how normal growth and development progresses and to discuss their needs in relation to the maturational process. The emphasis in a sound health education curriculum is on developing healthy lifestyle patterns.

Curriculum planning for health instruction is the responsibility of all professionals in the school system. The school nurse is often asked to assume a major role in organizing health education activities. A school nurse's educational preparation and clinical experience and contact with the community puts her or him in a favorable position for understanding the essential concepts of health and illness and for coordinating activities between the school and the community. However, it is crucial to remember that a school nurse alone cannot implement a sound health education program. Without administrative support and active involvement of all teachers, it would be impossible to achieve appropriate selection and sequencing of health content throughout the grade levels or to obtain sufficient time for health educational activities.

Healthy School Environment

Environmental factors that affect the health and well-being of children in the school setting are numerous. Psychosocial and physical aspects of the environment need to be monitored to ensure an optimal setting for student learning. A healthy school environment is one that promotes optimum

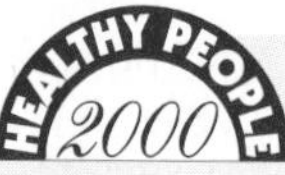

Objectives Related to School Health Education

2.19:* Increase to at least 75 percent the proportion of the Nation's schools that provide nutrition education from preschool through 12th grade, preferably as part of quality school health education.

3.10: Establish tobacco-free environments and include tobacco use prevention in the curricula at all elementary, middle, and secondary schools, preferably as part of quality school health education.

4.9: Increase the proportion of high school seniors who perceive social disapproval associated with the heavy use of alcohol, occasional use of marijuana, and experimentation with cocaine.

4.10: Increase the proportion of high school seniors who associate risk of physical or psychological harm with the heavy use of alcohol, regular use of marijuana, and experimentation with cocaine.

4.13: Provide to children in all school districts and private schools, primary and secondary school educational programs on alcohol and other drugs, preferably as part of quality school health education.

5.8: Increase to at least 85 percent the proportion of people aged 10 through 18 who have discussed human sexuality, including values surrounding sexuality, with their parents and/or have received information through another parentally endorsed source, such as youth, school, or religious programs.

7.16: Increase to at least 50 percent the proportion of elementary and secondary schools that teach nonviolent conflict resolution skills, preferably as a part of quality school health education.

8.4: Increase to at least 75 percent the proportion of the Nation's elementary and secondary schools that provide planned and sequential kindergarten through 12th grade quality school health education.

9.18: Provide academic instruction on injury prevention and control, preferably as part of quality school health education, in at least 50 percent of public school systems (grades K through 12).

18.10: Increase to at least 95 percent the proportion of schools that have age-appropriate HIV education curricula for students in 4th through 12th grade, preferably as part of quality school health education.

19.12: Include instruction in sexually transmitted disease transmission prevention in the curricula of all middle and secondary schools, preferably as part of quality school health education.

From USDHHS: *Healthy People 2000: national health promotion and disease prevention objectives, full report, with commentary*, Washington, D.C., 1991, U.S. Government Printing Office.
*The objective number in the *Healthy People 2000* document. Baseline data are available in this document.

psychosocial and physical growth and development among school-age children and school personnel. It provides an atmosphere that fosters sound mental health and favorable social conditions. It is organized in a way that reduces unhealthy stress and eliminates safety hazards for all students and school personnel.

A healthful school environment has the following features (Comer, 1992; Igoe, 1992; Nader, 1992):

- An architectural design that takes into consideration the developmental characteristics of the population being served, the needs of disabled students and staff, and the needs of the instructional program
- A comfortable environment that has adequate seating, lighting, heating, ventilation, toilet facilities, and drinking fountains
- An organized safety program, including procedures for emergency care
- An established procedure to ensure safe, sanitary conditions free from environmental hazards
- A recreational program that allows all students to participate
- A planned schedule of school activities that takes into account the physical and psychosocial needs of children at varying grade levels
- An organized school lunch program that provides nutritious foods, adequate time for good personal hygiene, and sufficient facilities for comfortable eating
- An established program that provides psychosocial counseling and consultation services for staff and students

No one professional discipline can plan and implement all the services described in these three components—health services, health education, healthy school environment—of a total school health program. The role of nursing in the school setting is described in the following section. The reader should keep in mind, however, that effective teamwork is essential for successful school health programming.

THE ROLE OF THE COMMUNITY HEALTH NURSE IN THE SCHOOL HEALTH PROGRAM

The role of nursing in the school health program has been evolving since the beginning of the century when Lillian Wald placed Lina Rogers, the first school nurse, in the New York City schools. Control of communicable disease is no longer the primary emphasis of nursing service in the school setting. It is now recognized that the school nurse has a significant contribution to make in all aspects of the comprehensive school health program. School nurses are currently providing a complex array of school health services, such as case management for chronic health problems, primary health care services, and family counseling. The challenging nature of the role of the nurse in the school setting was illustrated by Burton (1992) as she provided an accounting of the "A Day in the Life of a School Nurse" (see A View from the Field). It is becoming increasingly apparent to the nursing professional that the scope of school nursing practice will expand in the future as a growing number of communities use school-based health centers to provide primary care services to children.

The Essence and Standards of School Nursing

"School nursing, as a specialty branch of professional nursing: (1) seeks to prevent or identify client health or health-related problems [primary and secondary prevention]; and (2) intervenes to modify or remediate these problems [secondary and tertiary prevention]" (NASN, 1988). "These purposes are accomplished through the provision or facilitation of health services and health education in, or as part of, the school. In so doing, school nursing contributes directly to the student's education, as well as to the health of the family and the community" (Proctor, Lordi, Zaiger, 1993, p. 11).

The National Association of School Nurses (NASN) has provided standards for practice to guide nurses' efforts in the school setting (see the box on p. 488). Criteria to measure the achievement of these standards can be found in the document *School Nursing Practice: Roles and Standards* (Proctor, Lordi, Zaiger, 1993). "Standards define a set of rules, actions, or outcomes" (Katz, Green, 1997, p. 9). For example, in the NASN standards one identified outcome is "to contribute to the education of the client with special health needs by assessing the client" (NASN Standard 3). A specific criterion to measure the degree to which this standard is met might be "the school nurse completes a health history and physical assessment including vision, hearing, nutritional, and developmental appraisals on each student with health needs" (Proctor, Lordi, Zaiger, 1993, p. 29). Standards and criteria are used to guide quality measurement. Quality measurement is discussed extensively in Chapter 24.

School nursing is an exciting, rewarding field of nursing practice that provides numerous opportunities for creative, independent functioning. Needs of the population being served, community resources, patterns for delivery of service, and federal, state, and local funding and regulations influence how each of these nurses functions.

Legislative and Legal Issues

Federal and state legislation significantly influence nursing practice in the school setting. To function effectively in the schools, the nurse must be familiar with the legal issues involved in delivering care to children and knowledgeable about legislative programs that finance health care services for our youth. Chapters 4 and 15 discussed the major federal assistance programs that support the delivery of services to children, including Medicaid, Temporary Assistance to Needy Families, the Children With Special Health Care Needs Title V Program, SSI, WIC, and the Food Stamp Program. Legislation related to school nutrition programs (e.g., National School Lunch Program and School Breakfast Program) is also designed to safeguard the health and well-being of American children. These programs provide nutritionally adequate food and encourage the development of healthy lifestyle behaviors through education. For many children in the United States, the school nutrition programs provide their major source of food.

From a state perspective, laws that govern school health vary significantly. It is important for all school nurses to understand their state laws, because these laws provide the legal basis for the scope of nursing practice, malpractice, the reporting of abuse and neglect, and health service delivery. All school personnel are required to report suspected abuse and neglect.

"The legal basis for the (school) health program is either mandated or recommended, or no policy exists. Data suggest a relationship between economic investment in children (e.g., health insurance and mandated school health programs) and children's well-being" (Baker, 1994, p. 182). State mandated school health requirements cover programs like health screening for scoliosis, hearing and vision, immunizations, disaster management, and food handling and preparation. As discussed previously, both state and federal laws mandate special education programming for children with disabilities. School nurses actively participate in the educational planning for children with special needs.

School nurses also actively participate in implementing the provisions of the Occupational Safety and Health Act (OSHA). In many school districts the nurse assumes major responsibility for in-servicing staff on OSHA's bloodborne pathogens standards. Chapters 11 and 18 discuss the mandates of OSHA.

One of the nation's strongest privacy protection laws, the Family Educational Rights and Privacy Act (FERPA) mandates safeguarding of student records (Policy Studies Associates, 1997). FERPA "defines education records as *all* records that schools or education agencies maintain about students. It guarantees parents' review and appeal of the records about their child, and restricts release of students' records" (Policy Studies Associates, p. 139). Schools that do not comply with FERPA regulations will lose their federal education funds.

All nurses working with children must also address informed consent issues. Informed parental consent is generally required for children to receive health care services, including immunizations, medical treatment by a physician, and special psychological testing for learning difficulties. An exception to this requirement occurs when children need emergency care and a parent is not readily available to

A View *from the* Field — A Day in the Life of a School Nurse

If you had told me 10 years ago that I would be working for a public school system, I would have said you were crazy! But here I am, in 1992, working in a field that I believe is truly on the "cutting edge" of health care—school nursing.

When I took this job, I really had no idea what I was getting into. In fact, my husband encouraged me to take this position because he thought that it would be a "fluff" position supervising nurses as they handed out band-aids, and that the vacation time looked good.

For the past five years, I have held the position of nursing supervisor for the Lawrence Public Schools in Lawrence, Mass.

Lawrence is a poor city of 63,000 people, known for its negative health status indicators and largely minority population. The public school population of 11,000 students is 77 percent minority, mostly Hispanic newcomers. Lawrence has the highest teen pregnancy rate and one of the worst drug abuse problems in Massachusetts. Those problems, combined with a 44 percent high school dropout rate and the lowest basic skills scores in the state, make our youth some of the neediest in the country.

A solid grasp of the nursing process has been the cornerstone of my practice. In the first months of employment as the nursing supervisor for the school district, I undertook a complete needs assessment that included interviews with principals, nursing staff and the community as a whole. I then invited these people to work with me on the Lawrence School Health Advisory Council. When the assessment was completed, I developed a plan for comprehensive health education and school health services, including school-based health centers at the high school, and at the elementary/middle level, developed and implemented a comprehensive health education program in grades K-12, integrated AIDS education into the health education program, and developed a comprehensive substance abuse program. I am proud to say that even with severe budget cuts, five years later, we are right on target.

What I have discovered is that school nursing is truly an opportunity to practice primary prevention at its best. It is exciting, challenging and fun! Every day is different, so it is difficult to choose one day to describe my life.

This day begins at 7:30 AM. I need to deliver syringes and sharps containers to a middle school and make sure everything is in order for the school nurse to immunize 6th grade students with the second dose of MMR vaccine. I have arranged for two other school nurses to help. There are about 100 students who need to be immunized today.

The next stop is an 8 AM. meeting with my boss, the assistant superintendent of schools. I am meeting with him to bring him up to date on the Drug Free Schools Project. We have been fortunate this year to have received over $1 million in grants to develop and implement a comprehensive substance abuse prevention program in the schools. The project includes curriculum development, setting up student assistance teams, peer leadership, children of alcoholics support groups, parent education groups, teacher and administrator training and policy development. Since I am the "health person" in the school district, anything to do with health, AIDS, drugs, sex, teen pregnancy or violence gets directed to me. This is primary prevention!

It is now 9 AM. On the way to my office I stop at the community health center to meet with staff who serve the teen health center at the high school. I need to bring them up to date on Medicaid billing issues and new forms that were presented at a meeting with the state health department last week.

I arrive at my office that is located in a K-8 elementary school around 10 AM. There is a stack of messages waiting for me that need to be returned. I answer these calls. One of the calls is to a parent who needs bus transportation for her child who just had surgery. I need to approve all medical transportation. Another call is from the superintendent's office. "Send over copies of our AIDS curriculum . . . another school district is interested in what we are doing." They need the information yesterday! Another call is from a principal—she needs a nurse in the building every day for a child with a G-tube. Still another call is from one of the school nurses—there are 15 cases of chicken pox in her school today!

It is now 10:30 AM, and I need to prepare for a School Health Advisory Council meeting scheduled for this afternoon.

At noon, I attend a meeting of the Lawrence Violence Prevention Coalition. This community coalition was formed to develop a community response to increasing violence in the city. The question here, as in most community groups, is "What are the schools doing, and why are they not doing more?"

At 2 PM, the School Health Advisory Council meets. This council is made up of students, parents, teachers, school administrators, school nurses, as well as health and human services professionals from the community. This group of people provide me with the guidance and support I need to do my job. Because several parents on the council are more comfortable speaking Spanish, I meet with them 30 minutes before the meeting to provide them with an orientation to the agenda so that they will feel more comfortable and be able to provide input during the meeting.

From Burton PT: A day in the life of a nurse: school nursing on cutting edge of prevention, *Am Nurse* 24:23, 1992, September.

A View from the Field — A Day in the Life of a School Nurse—cont'd

At this council meeting, I present our health services budget as well as a review of the health services staffing pattern and health status of our kids. Today, I do not have good news to report. I have been instructed to present a level-funded budget to the school committee, but this actually means a budget cut. A nurse who left the system five months ago will probably not be replaced.

We have 1,218 children with some type of health problem, an increase of more than 200 since last year. This includes 428 children with asthma, an increase of 125 students since last year. We also have a significant increase in the number of students with active seizure disorders, kidney disease, heart disease and leukemia. The need for direct nursing services has increased with twice the number of children requiring medication in school this year. Also with the mandates of Special Education, more children with complex needs are being brought into the system. The needs of these children range from intermittent catheterization and G-tube feedings to case management and clinical services. The council discusses my report in detail. They are concerned about decreases in staff with the increased need for services. Council members, including parents, offer to speak at upcoming school committee meetings in support of the health program.

It has been a busy day, but a good one. I believe that, at least for this day, I have shown how effective school nurses can be, and what a vital role nurses play in bridging the gap between the health care and education communities. With the severe fiscal constraints faced by school districts, difficult decisions are made everyday. The purpose of the school system is to educate children. However, the basic health and safety needs of children must be met in order for them to learn. Because attitudes and health behaviors that school-age children develop will be carried into adulthood, the schools need to accept responsibility for educating the whole child.

School nurses play a vital role in helping the school meet this responsibility. They are truly on the cutting edge of health promotion and health services. They practice primary prevention at its best!

As a final note, I add that my husband now says I am the only person he knows who can take a perfectly simple job and make it complicated.

Peg Trainor Burton is the nursing supervisor for the Lawrence Public Schools in Lawrence, Mass. A diploma graduate of St. Mary's School of Nursing in Clarksburg, W. Va., Burton earned a BSN at Duquesne University, Pittsburgh, Pa., and a master's degree at Boston University School of Nursing, where she specialized in community health nursing. She holds current certification as a family nurse practitioner. Burton is a member of ANA, the National Association of School Nurses, the American School Health Association and the American Public Health Association.

give consent or refuses to give consent (Wong, 1995). However, since it is very difficult to establish what constitutes an emergency, every school needs well-developed policies that address emergency situations.

Laws that allow minors to seek treatment without parental consent usually deal with human sexuality problems, drug abuse, and mental health services. In almost all states, minors can receive medical treatment for STDs on their own. In some states physicians can diagnose pregnancy and provide prenatal care, contraceptive services, and drug abuse and other mental health assistance without parent consent. Although emancipated minors can give informed consent for certain types of health care, it is important for school nurses to recognize there are significant variations in state laws regarding this issue (OTA, 1991).

State and federal legislation is written to promote and protect the health of children. A knowledge of federal and state laws helps school nurses to speak out on behalf of children when required services are not provided or when a child's rights are being violated. Advocating for strong health policy is a significant nursing intervention.

Patterns for Providing School Nursing Services

Two administrative patterns are commonly used to provide nursing services in the school setting: specialized and generalized. Specialized services are provided by school nurses who are usually employed by the board of education. These nurses are accountable to school administrators and work only with the school-age population. Some health departments are developing special school-health units within the health department. These specialized school nurses are accountable to the community health nursing director as well as to school administration. Generalized services are often provided by community health nurses hired by health departments or visiting nurse associations. These nurses function part time in the school setting as part of a generalized community health nursing program. They work with all at-risk populations in their assigned area. Some schools of nursing are developing nursing practice or research centers in the school environment. These centers provide practice and/or research opportunities for nursing students and faculty and nursing services for the school community.

There is controversy about which pattern for delivering school nursing services is most appropriate. Clinical

Standards of School Nursing Practice

NASN STANDARD 1: CLINICAL KNOWLEDGE

The school nurse utilizes a distinct knowledge base for decision-making in nursing practice.

NASN STANDARD 2: NURSING PROCESS

The school nurse uses a systematic approach to problem-solving in nursing practice.

NASN STANDARD 3: CLIENTS WITH SPECIAL HEALTH NEEDS

The school nurse contributes to the education of the client with special health needs by assessing the client, planning and providing appropriate nursing care, and evaluating the identified outcomes of care.

NASN STANDARD 4: COMMUNICATION

The school nurse uses effective written, verbal and nonverbal communication skills.

NASN STANDARD 5: PROGRAM MANAGEMENT

The school nurse establishes and maintains a comprehensive school health program.

NASN STANDARD 6: COLLABORATION WITHIN THE SCHOOL SYSTEM

The school nurse collaborates with other school professionals, parents, and caregivers to meet the health, developmental, and educational needs of clients.

NASN STANDARD 7: COLLABORATION WITH COMMUNITY HEALTH SYSTEMS

The school nurse collaborates with members of the community in the delivery of health and social services, and utilizes knowledge of community health systems and resources to function as a school-community liaison.

NASN STANDARD 8: HEALTH EDUCATION

The school nurse assists students, families, and the school community to achieve optimal levels of wellness through appropriately designed and delivered health education.

NASN STANDARD 9: RESEARCH

The school nurse contributes to nursing and school health through innovations in practice and participation in research or research-related activities.

NASN STANDARD 10: PROFESSIONAL DEVELOPMENT

The school nurse identifies, delineates, and clarifies the nursing role, promotes quality of care, pursues continued professional enhancement, and demonstrates professional conduct.

From Proctor ST, Lordi SL, Zaiger DS: *School nursing practice: roles and standards*, Scarborough, Me., 1993, National Association of School Nurses, Inc., p. 18.

experience has shown that a variety of service delivery patterns can be used effectively to promote the health of the school community. Regardless of the administrative pattern used for delivering nursing services in the school setting, the nurse should establish strategies for ensuring that he or she is a sanctioned member of the school health team. The school nurse should also develop strategies for obtaining professional mentoring.

The activities of generalized and specialized school nurses vary among school systems. Some educational systems use the nurse in limited ways. Others use the nurse in a comprehensive manner, such as Burton (1992) described earlier in this chapter.

Roles of the Nurse on the School Health Team

School nurses assume a variety of roles and carry out a complex array of activities to promote health and prevent disease within a school community. Rustia's school health promotion model (Figure 16-12) clearly illustrates the range of interventions used by nurses to promote healthy living and to improve quality of life. It also reflects the comprehensive nature of school nursing and can be used by the school nurse as a framework for articulating roles and functions. A school nurse who is able to clearly articulate her or his role and functions and who demonstrates clinical expertise to all members of the school health team is more likely to be used appropriately than one who has trouble defining what it is a school nurse has to offer.

ADVOCATE Many disadvantaged families have inadequate resources to obtain essential health care services for their children. The school nurse becomes an advocate for these children to help them to obtain the health care they deserve. This can involve reaching out to families to assist them in understanding their child's health care needs. It may also involve working with other service providers to improve a child's access to service. On a broader level, the school nurse becomes actively involved in influencing funders to allocate funds for needed health care services. For example, school nurses frequently advocate for community-based adolescent health care services. Despite the fact that developmentally the adolescent has different needs than younger school-age children, services that specifically address the needs of the adolescent are lacking or inadequate (National Commission on the Role of the School and the

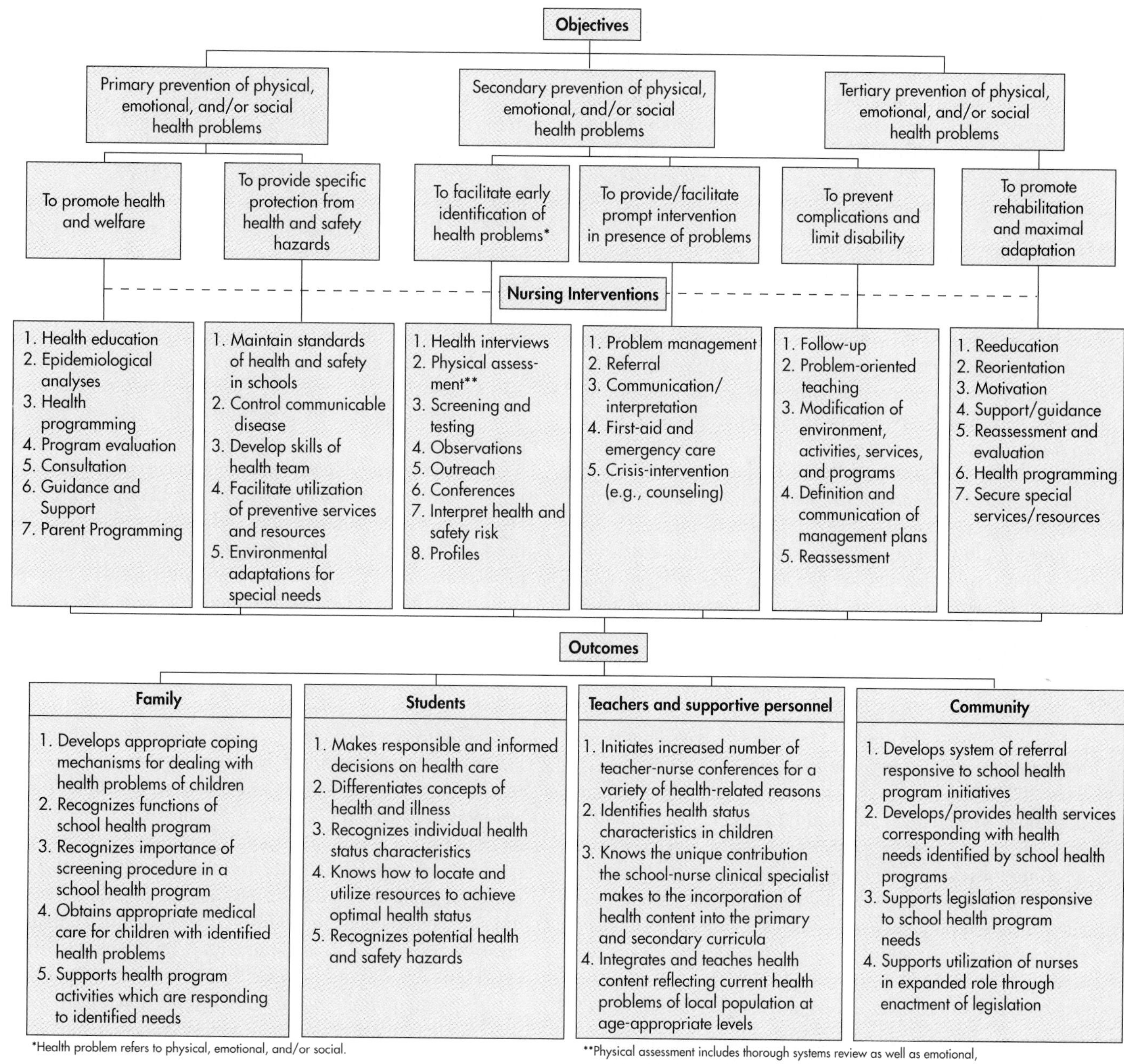

Figure **16-12** Rustia's school health promotion model: delineation of nursing interventions and client outcomes. *(From Rustia J: Rustia school health promotion model,* J Sch Health *52(2):109, 1982.)*

Community in Improving Adolescent Health, 1990). On a broader level, the nurse also advocates for health in the school setting. It is not uncommon for the school nurse to identify environmental conditions that are unsafe, or gaps in health education programming, or deficiencies in the delivery of personal health services. A concerned school nurse does not ignore these situations.

CASEFINDER "Every child has a right to have an education which will meet his individualized needs and to have care and treatment for handicapping [disabling] conditions so that he can learn more effectively" (1930 Children's Charter). Casefinding is essential if these goals are to be accomplished. All personnel in the school system have a responsibility to identify as early as possible children at risk for physical, behavioral, social, or academic disabilities.

School nurses use a variety of methods to identify at-risk children. They observe children during their normal school activities, work with parents and school personnel to identify students in need of assessment and evaluation services, and review medical records to identify indicators of poor health. The school nurse also plans screening programs for the purpose of casefinding. Additionally, it is not unusual for the school nurse to casefind through incidental observation. For example, many orthopedic problems have been picked up by an alert school nurse who has watched children walking down the hall during recess. Eating lunch in the school cafeteria has helped other school nurses to identify children with poor dietary habits. Walking out on the playground during recess frequently assists school nurses in determining which children are having difficulty relating to their peers.

Incidental observations do not replace the need for periodic, systematic health observations. School nurses meet regularly with every teacher in the school system to encourage them to observe regularly the health status of all students in the classroom. Teachers play an important role in a health appraisal program. Their position in the classroom setting provides them with frequent opportunities to make significant observations of each child's health status. One teacher, for example, assisted the school nurse in identifying a child with an undiagnosed congenital health defect. This teacher became concerned because this child always "looked pale and tired and took longer than most children to get up after a fall on the playground." The teacher shared her concerns with the school nurse, who referred the child to her family physician. Medical follow-up revealed that the child had a heart problem.

School nurses also establish procedures that allow them to systematically observe the children on a regular basis. They plan comprehensive screening programs to evaluate developmental changes and health needs over time. Height and weight measurements, hearing and vision tests, dental examinations, and immunization checks have traditionally been conducted in the school setting. In many school settings a more comprehensive screening is done to identify children at risk. In addition to the traditional procedures, screening for scoliosis, urinary tract infections, anemia, and psychosocial difficulties is completed by some school nurses.

School nurses find that by reviewing medical records and absenteeism reports, they can frequently identify children who need follow-up. For example, one school nurse noted on a kindergarten child's medical record that the child's blood pressure was extremely high. She followed up on this situation by talking with the child's parents and teacher. This assessment revealed that the child's father had hypertension and that the teacher had noticed that the child's ears turned bright red with physical exertion. The child's blood pressure was also high when the nurse took it in the clinic setting. The physician had not followed up on the child's blood pressure after his school physical, because he believed that it was high as a result of the child being anxious about seeing a physician. This child was indeed hypertensive and was placed under the care of a cardiac specialist.

Review of absenteeism records can help school nurses to identify children at risk for future illnesses and absenteeism and, often, families that need nursing interventions. It is not unusual for families that are ineffectively dealing with stress to neglect family functions, including helping children to attend school regularly. Assisting these families to problem solve in relation to their current stresses is probably the best way to help their children.

COMMUNITY COORDINATOR School nurses must engage in community liaison activities to meet the needs of all school-age children. No school system has adequate resources to handle all the health problems experienced by the children it serves. Cooperative planning and collaboration between the educational system and other community agencies who are assisting children can serve only to enhance the effectiveness of the school's health program.

Community involvement should be sought by the school nurse during all stages of the health-planning process. Health programs conducted at school that fulfill health needs as identified by the community are far more successful than programs that ignore community priorities. Perceptions of health problems and community needs vary among communities. Thus it is important for community health nurses working in the school setting to ascertain from their clients what constitutes the communities' most pressing health needs.

Community coordinating activities can be challenging and rewarding. For example, working with others in parent-teacher organizations or community agencies can help the school nurse make the school health program more culturally relevant. Community coordinating activities also expose school nurses to different viewpoints, which help nurses expand their range of alternative solutions for addressing health needs. In addition, these activities enhance creative thinking through stimulation by others, facilitate continuity of care, and increase community participation in health programming. Community interest groups are more motivated to implement a health program if they have participated in designing that health program. School nurses, through their involvement with groups, can gain a greater appreciation of community issues, demands, and needs.

CONSULTANT Nurses bring to the school setting a unique set of skills that allow them to become valuable, contributing members of the school health team. Specifically, nursing differs from other disciplines in the school setting in three major areas. First, nurses have been prepared to assess comprehensively all the variables that have an influence on a child's health status. Nurses' understanding of normal growth and development, as well as disease processes, provides them with the knowledge needed for identifying both physical and psychosocial health problems and for determining how to handle health concerns. Teachers frequently ask school nurses questions about disease conditions such as diabetes, epilepsy, hepatitis, or scabies.

They may question whether a child is ill, when to send a child home when he or she is not feeling well, or whether a child with a chronic condition should be allowed to participate in recreational activities. Children with chronic conditions are frequently overprotected by school personnel until medical recommendations are interpreted by the nurse. It is also not uncommon for the school nurse to encounter fear when infectious diseases are present in the school system and school personnel do not understand the etiology of communicable diseases or how to prevent the spread of these diseases. One teacher, for example, became so upset after she heard that one of her students had hepatitis that she moved the child's desk into the hall and immediately called the school nurse. She wanted the nurse to talk with her class about "what to do when they got hepatitis." The teacher was sure that everyone in the classroom would become ill, because all she knew about this condition was that it was contagious. Her anxiety was reduced once the nurse explained the etiology and the mode of transmission of this disease process and the treatment needs of the ill child. Appendix 11-3 summarizes some of the common communicable diseases encountered by community health nurses in the school settings.

The nurse's preparation for dealing with the family as the unit of service is a second major area of uniqueness. Family problems can affect a child's functioning in school and often these problems must be addressed before a child's ineffective functioning is changed. Problem behavior such as poor school attendance, aggressive behavior, use of drugs, or withdrawal from school activities often signals that a child's family is having difficulty. The adolescent depicted in the following case scenario illustrates this point. The child had a consistently high absenteeism record until the school nurse provided family-centered nursing intervention.

CASE *Scenario*

Pattie Lynne Babcock was a 14-year-old junior high school student who was missing an average of 2 days of school per week when the school social worker referred her to the generalized school nurse. Even though Pattie only had a functional heart murmur, her mother would relate any illness she had to her "bad heart." The school social worker felt that Pattie Lynne's mother needed help with understanding how her fears were affecting Pattie Lynne's perceptions of her health. Mrs. Babcock was very receptive to the nurse's visit. She had been widowed recently and "wasn't sure how to care for Pattie Lynne properly." During the nurse's first home visit, Mrs. Babcock related that she hadn't been feeling well lately. Her heart pounded so fast at times that she feared she might have a heart attack. She had trouble with her vision but felt it was because she was getting old. Mrs. Babcock had a history of hypertension but had stopped taking her blood pressure medication "because it made her feel worse." The nurse found her blood pressure to be 210/116 and stressed the need for immediate medical follow-up. Mrs. Babcock reluctantly made an appointment with her family physician while the nurse was in the home. She felt she had too many other things to take care of to worry about herself. Using crisis intervention principles, the school nurse in this situation helped Mrs. Babcock identify what it was she had to handle and then encouraged her to work on one thing at a time. The nurse's promise to return motivated Mrs. Babcock to seek medical care. During the nurse's second visit the following week, Mrs. Babcock reported that she was feeling better physically and was also able to verbalize that she thought she was going to die. She could identify that when she was afraid, "it was nice to have Pattie Lynne home with me." She also saw how her fear of having a heart attack altered her perceptions of Pattie Lynne's heart murmur. The school nurse continued to make home visits until Mrs. Babcock developed mechanisms to cope with the changes in her life. Like all school-age children, Pattie Lynne continued to miss a day of school periodically. Her attendance record improved dramatically, however, once the nurse assisted Mrs. Babcock in dealing with her problems.

Extensive knowledge of community resources and the referral process is the third unique skill the school nurse has to contribute in the school setting. Many families within school systems do not have a regular source of medical supervision. Other families have their own physician and dentist but cannot afford to use these services. One student community health nurse came back to the health department disturbed following her second visit to an inner-city junior high school. She was appalled at the number of children who had obvious dental caries and questioned why their parents did not care enough about them to obtain dental care. A staff nurse suggested to her that limited financial resources might be preventing many of these families from obtaining the dental care that was needed. When the student contacted the parents of these children, she found that financial difficulties were indeed the problem. After she discussed the services available at the health department dental clinic, two families requested that all of their children be referred to this resource. School personnel were appreciative of these referrals and identified several other children who needed dental aid. Parents and school personnel do *care*. If school nurses demonstrate that they are willing to use the unique skills they have, both families and other members of the school health team will confer with them regularly.

EPIDEMIOLOGIST Health services in a school setting should be designed to meet the needs of the total school population. Health counseling and instruction with individual students reach only the tip of the iceberg in a given population. Nurses must become epidemiologists. They need to identify *aggregates at risk* to plan effective school health programs.

Effective school nurses organize the data they have to identify factors that influence the health status of school-age populations. The characteristics of populations are studied to determine the most appropriate intervention strategies to meet their needs. One school nurse used health record information, data obtained during home visits, contact with students in the health clinic, and census tract information to substantiate the need for a breakfast program in the school system. The combined information from all of these data sources revealed that the children in this school had significant nutritional deficiences (e.g., there was a high prevalence of nutritional anemia among the children) and had difficulty functioning in the classroom setting as a result of not eating breakfast. Additionally, this information showed that a large percentage of the children came from poor families that had difficulty meeting the families' basic needs. When the school nurse shared these facts with the school administrator, she agreed with the nurse that federal funds should be sought to support a breakfast program.

An epidemiological approach to school health is a prevention-oriented approach. In the situation just mentioned, the nurse worked to prevent nutritional problems such as anemia and to prevent learning difficulties in the future. Children who are ill often do not learn well. Prevention is far less costly than curative care.

Accurate and complete record-keeping is essential for epidemiological studies to be effective. A record system must be designed to allow for complete and efficient recording of data. A cumulative record of each child's health status should be maintained, and records of children with special health problems tagged. A tagging system allows for quick analysis of the needs of the population as a whole. For example, if 50 children in a school system have problems with obesity, group counseling sessions and changes in curriculum planning may be warranted.

It is imperative for community health nurses in the school setting to evaluate the results of their interventions. When nurses work with aggregates, the epidemiological process is the tool that most appropriately helps them to examine the results of their group intervention strategies (see Chapter 11). *Until nurses begin to document what they have accomplished, they will not be used to their fullest potential.*

HEALTH COUNSELOR Children and youth are currently facing difficult and complex health problems and concerns. They are exposed much earlier than their previous counterparts to issues such as sexuality concerns, varying lifestyles, pressures from peers to use alcohol and drugs, decisions regarding future career planning in a highly unstable employment environment, and family disruption and disorganization. Often they have knowledge about these issues but lack experience in dealing with them. They have a need to discuss their feelings and emotions with a nonthreatening adult. Because the school nurse does not evaluate a student's academic performance, which helps students to view her or him as nonthreatening, and because students may have physical health complaints when experiencing emotional stress, the school nurse is frequently the first member of the school health team to identify a student's need for counseling. In these situations the nurse makes the appropriate referral in consultation with the student and his or her family.

As in other settings, the nurse in the school uses the family-centered nursing process to determine appropriate management goals and intervention strategies. When the child visits the health center, the nurse assesses the situation to identify actual as well as presenting needs. Problems can easily be missed by the nurse if insufficient data form the basis for her or his nursing diagnoses. The case scenario that follows illustrates the need to collect adequate data to diagnose a child's actual health problems and to plan a variety of intervention strategies to resolve these problems.

CASE *Scenario*

Lindsey Elizabeth, a first-grader, was lying on the cot in the health clinic when the community health nurse arrived for her weekly visit. The school secretary reported to the nurse that Lindsey had just come into her office crying because she had a stomach ache. When asked by the school nurse how she was feeling, Lindsey sobbed and stated, "My stomach hurts." The school nurse completed a physical examination to rule out a serious health problem. However, when she provided Lindsey with a little attention, the child stopped crying. When she was asked if her parents knew she did not feel well this morning, her answer was, "My mother doesn't love me anymore. She went away." The nurse helped Lindsey to verbalize her feelings of rejection and let her know that she understood how much it hurts to lose someone you love. A hug by the nurse provided the support Lindsey needed to return to class. The nurse realized that Lindsey needed other types of assistance to deal with the demands of the encountered stressor. She discussed with Lindsey's teachers interventions to reduce stress. In addition, the nurse contacted Lindsey's father. He was very angry that his wife had left and found it extremely difficult to talk to his children about what was happening. Fortunately he was concerned about how his separation was affecting his children and agreed to seek family counseling at a local mental health clinic. Lindsey's mother never returned home. Her father, however, learned how to deal with his anger and gradually was able to allow his children to talk about their mother. This, coupled with support from an empathic teacher, helped Lindsey to function more effectively in the school setting.

Younger school children often verbalize their feelings more readily than older children. Since one of the developmental tasks of adolescence is to achieve emotional independence from parents and other adults, students at the junior or senior high level may test the school nurse before they share their real concerns. One such case is described here:

CASE *Scenario*

Noel, a 14-year-old junior high student, wandered into the health clinic during class breaks 3 weeks in a row with minor physical complaints. Finally he asked the nurse if he could talk with her alone. He wanted to know "how a person could tell if he had VD." Further discussion revealed that Noel was having nocturnal emissions and thought he had gonorrhea because he had learned in a health class that a purulent discharge occurred with this disease. Noel had never heard about nocturnal emissions and was fearful that his wet discharges at night were caused by gonorrhea. He was greatly relieved when he found out that he was normal. The nurse encouraged him to return to the clinic if he had other questions and suggested that his father might be able to talk with him about other developmental changes that occur during adolescence. The need to discuss normal developmental changes, as well as to review how STDs are transmitted, was also shared with the teacher responsible for the eighth-grade health class.

Health counseling opportunities such as the ones described above are numerous and present in all school settings. Nurses who are attuned to the developmental needs and the social characteristics of the population they are serving will not be "Band-Aid pushers." Rather, they will take time to find out from other school personnel which students have health problems and will be alert for students who need health counseling.

HEALTH EDUCATOR The ultimate goal of nursing intervention is to help the client to help himself or herself. Through health education activities in the school setting, school nurses are preparing children and their families, school personnel, and the community to make sound health decisions. They recognize that the population they serve needs adequate knowledge and the opportunity to explore values and attitudes about health matters before they can assume responsibility for maintaining their personal health status.

The National Association of School Nurses views health education as an important function for nurses in the school setting. It believes that the school nurse should be involved in a broad range of health education activities. The Teaching Tips box reflects this belief and provides examples of health education activities carried out by nurses in the school setting.

Health education is a significant nursing intervention that can promote the well-being of students, families, and the school community. "To make the most of the opportunities schools offer, schools should be viewed in their larger context. They are not only places for instruction, but also places where over 3 million of our nation's working adults and essentially all of its young people spend a major portion of their lives" (CDC, 1995, p. 3). Viewed from this perspective, school nurses take advantage of both informal as well as formal opportunities to educate people about health.

HOME VISITOR Parents are vital members of the school health team. They are ultimately responsible for the health care of their children and they greatly influence their children's health practices. Contact with parents in the home environment is a most effective way of increasing their understanding and involvement with their child's health problems. Home visits also demonstrate that the school nurse cares about parents as individuals and respects their parental rights.

At times home visiting is the only way to obtain a comprehensive picture of a child's health status. This is particularly true if the nurse perceives that family dynamics are adversely affecting a child's level of functioning. Assessment of parent-child relationships is best obtained in the client's natural setting. Observations of how the child is physically handled, of environmental conditions, and of interactions between a child, the parents, and siblings are more easily assessed in the home environment. These observations provide a different type of data than a conference with a parent in the health clinic.

The school nurse cannot possibly visit at home every child served in the school system. Children who manifest needs or difficulties such as the following should receive priority for home visits:

- History of many absences as a result of illness
- Behavioral problems that interfere with academic functioning or that adversely affect social relationships with peers
- Adjustment difficulties related to a chronic condition such as diabetes, epilepsy, heart defects, or obesity
- Suspected child abuse or neglect
- Special programming needs in relation to a developmental disability
- Lack of medical follow-up on an identified health problem
- Pregnancy
- Frequent exposure to infectious diseases

Home visiting can be rewarding and extremely beneficial. It frequently is the key that opens the door to a happier life for many children. The following case scenario describes how a home visit helped one 8-year-old child to positively increase her interactions with her peers:

CASE *Scenario*

Tammie Baxter was referred to the school nurse because she had a pronounced body odor. Her peers shunned her, and she appeared to be a lonely child. Tammie's teacher had many questions about her home environment and the health status of her parents. She had heard that Tammie's father was ill as a result of complications of diabetes. A very receptive mother answered the door when the school nurse made her first home visit. The nurse discovered that a family of seven was living in a five-room

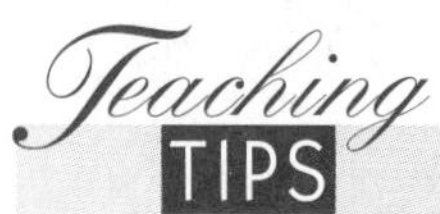

Nursing Opportunities for Health Education in the School Setting

Advocate

School nurses act as advocates for sound health education practices within the school and the larger community. They work with school personnel to ensure that certified health education teachers are employed by the school district. They also lobby for a planned, comprehensive, sequential pre-K to 12 curriculum, based on students' needs and current and emerging societal and health trends. Additionally, they lobby in the community to promote community action for health. This action might include health education activities that promote healthy lifestyles or contact with governmental officials to encourage increased funding for school health education.

Classroom Instruction

School nurses provide formal health instruction within the classroom on a variety of subjects such as health careers, substance abuse, violence prevention, consumer self-help, and sexuality. They may also provide formal health instruction for parents and other community residents within classes open to the community. Some school districts, for example, offer health career and consumer self-help classes after school hours to community residents. Additionally, the school nurse is involved in providing formal instruction to employees, especially in relation to universal precautions for bloodborne pathogens. Generally, the school nurse does not assume total responsibility for teaching a health class unless she or he was specifically hired for that purpose. Usually the nurse guest lectures or assume responsibility for a health unit within a class.

Client Teaching

Nurses in the school setting work with several client groups, including students, teachers, parents, and communities. In relation to these client groups, they have numerous health instruction opportunities. The school nurse, for example, would help a 14-year-old junior high student to understand body changes during adolescence after frequent visits to the health clinic with menstrual cramps. Or she or he would talk with individual teachers about the need for medical follow-up after a health screening for hypertension. Additionally, the school nurse would talk with parents about the neurological signs and symptoms of brain concussion if their child was hit on the head by a swing in the playground. On a broader level, the school nurse might provide health instruction for a group of community residents who expressed an interest in learning about resources to assist with the care of elderly parents.

Curriculum Planning

School nurses actively participate in planning and evaluating a school health curriculum that addresses major community needs. They also assist school personnel to select age-appropriate, culturally relevant instructional materials that are scientifically sound. Frequently they develop an instructional resource file to help teachers address common health issues in the classroom.

Resource Person

School nurses frequently consult with teachers, parents, and school administrators about concerns they may have about their own health status or the health status of one of the children in the school. They also consult with teachers who request assistance with developing a health education class. Additionally, they provide inservice programming for all staff regarding student health concerns, or for parents who are interested in gaining knowledge about what their children are learning in school.

Role Modeling

School nurses can educate students, staff, and parents by role modeling positive health behaviors. They might reinforce nutritional instruction by the foods they select for lunch. Or they might promote healthy relationship building by the way they interact with others. They may also role model effective infectious disease control measures. It is important for the school nurse to recognize that their health actions can significantly influence the health actions of others.

Modified from Bradley BJ: The school nurse as health educator, *J Sch Health* 67:3-8, 1997; Proctor ST, Lordi SL, Zaiger DS: *School nursing practice: roles and standards*, Scarborough, Me., 1993, National Association of School Nurses, Inc.

home that was composed of a living room, a kitchen, two bedrooms, and a bath. All five Baxter children, ages 8, 6, 4, 2, and 1, were sleeping on mattresses on the floor in one bedroom. Tammie smelled like urine, not because she was ill, but because three of her siblings had enuresis. She had limited clothes because the family was having severe financial problems. Tammie's difficulties with personal hygiene were resolved quickly once her mother discovered how the other children were treating her. A referral was made to a community clothes closet so that Tammie could be dressed like her peers. Tammie's teacher was amazed at how quickly her personal hygiene changed after this referral. A little extra attention from the teacher also helped to alter Tammie's relationships with her classmates.

A long-term helping relationship between the Baxter family and the school nurse evolved from this one simple teacher referral. Tammie was not, however, the focus of the conversation on subsequent visits. Her father was indeed in need of medical care. Mr. Baxter was laid

table 16-6 Role Descriptions for Selected Members of the School Health Team

Discipline	Role Description
Principals	School administrators who are responsible for planning and providing direction for all activities carried out to meet the goals of the school, including nursing services.
Teachers	Staff members who are responsible for the educational aspects of the school program. Teachers enhance the total school health program by conducting health education activities in the classroom and by identifying children who have physical and emotional health problems that impede learning.
Teacher consultants	Pupil personnel specialists* who have advanced training for handling educational programming for children with special learning needs such as reading problems, mental disabilities, and emotional disturbances.
Teachers, homebound	Pupil personnel teachers, specially trained to deal with physical disabilities and the educational implications of these conditions. These persons work in the home with children who have been certified by a physician as being unable to attend school. These individuals provide both educational instruction and counseling services for homebound students.
School social workers	Pupil personnel specialists who provide direct counseling services for a child and family, if the child is demonstrating adjustment difficulties in the school setting. School social workers apply the principles and methods of social casework to help students to enhance their social and emotional adjustment and to adapt to change. The primary purpose of their intervention is to reduce impediments to learning. These individuals are often used as resource persons by all other members of the school health team.
Screening technicians	Pupil personnel staff trained to identify particular health problems, usually vision and hearing difficulties, through the use of screening tests.
Volunteers	Lay staff who receive in-service education to carry out defined tasks for other staff members. Responsibilities should relate to the in-service training they have received. Careful selection, training, and supervision by professional staff is a must if these individuals are to be utilized successfully in the school setting.
Therapists, physical	Pupil personnel specialists who treat muscular disabilities of children on a prescriptive order from the child's physician. Their services are designed to enable students to improve their physical health status so that their physical health problems do not impede learning.
Therapists, speech	Pupil personnel specialists who work with children who have difficulty producing and combining certain sounds in words, who are unable to speak with reasonable fluency, who speak with an abnormally pitched voice, or who have physical anomalies such as cerebral palsy. Speech therapists help children to develop normal speech patterns that help them to more effectively develop social relationships and to advance academically.
School psychologists	Pupil personnel specialists whose major responsibility is to determine the reasons for a child's inability to learn. These specialists are often known as the school diagnosticians because the primary purpose of their service is to identify or diagnose causes of learning problems. These individuals use psychological tests, such as IQ and personality tests, during the psychological assessment. Parental permission must be obtained before a child can be tested by these specialists. The amount of direct counseling a psychologist does with a child varies from one school to another. Usually, however, this person functions as a consultant to other school personnel. Psychologists in other settings are often more involved in direct counseling services.

Modified from Jackson County Intermediate School District: *Special education services available to Jackson County*, Jackson, Mi., undated, The School District.

*Pupil personnel division—a special service division of a local board of education. Pupil personnel specialists in this division are accountable to the superintendent of schools.

off from work at an industrial plant because he was showing sugar in his urine. A telephone call between the community health nurse working in the school and the industrial nurse clarified that Mr. Baxter could return to work as soon as his diabetes was under control. Several community referrals helped this family to obtain medical care.

TEAM MEMBER No one discipline can meet the needs of all the school-age children. Team cooperation and collaboration are essential for children to receive the health services they deserve. The school nurse who has a "me" philosophy rather than a "we" philosophy will quickly become frustrated and will find that it is impossible to achieve school health goals.

Successful school nurses function within the framework of the total school health program, working cooperatively with other school personnel. Understanding the roles of each member of the school team can facilitate planning and implementation of nursing services. The role definitions presented in Table 16-6 are guidelines. When entering a new school system, every nurse should spend time to identify specified role responsibilities for each discipline in her or his school district. For an interdisciplinary team to function effectively, all team members must define how they can integrate their specific skills into an effective group effort that emphasizes a common endeavor. No team effort will be successful unless the central figures on the team are the child and involved family.

PRACTICAL TIPS FOR ROLE IMPLEMENTATION

Implementing multiple and varied roles is a formidable task. It is important for school nurses to avoid panic or withdrawal when they do not initially accomplish their goals. It takes time to develop a meaningful role in any setting. Provided below are some suggestions for facilitating the role implementation process in the school setting.

Define Your Philosophy of Nursing Practice

If school nurses cannot articulate the role of the nurse in the school health program, they cannot expect other members of the health care team to use them as they would like to be used. Reviewing the literature devoted to school nursing and the school health policies developed by your agency will provide you with information needed to formulate a philosophy of practice with which you can feel comfortable.

Study Your Community

Understanding the needs of the population you are serving is essential. Children, families, and school personnel will respond more quickly to your suggestions if you demonstrate a sensitivity to their concerns and if you support your comments with data. Review the students' health records to identify their pressing health problems. Analyze census tract data to determine the characteristics of the families in the school district. Talk with students and teachers as you walk around the school building. Avoid sitting in the health clinic. Leave the school setting and drive through the area in which your school is located. Do a community analysis (see Chapters 3 and 13).

Contact Key People

A school nurse who takes the initiative to contact school personnel and community groups responsible for the implementation of the school health program is more likely to become quickly involved than one who functions in isolation. Meet with the school principal before school starts. Explain your role and determine a time when you can orient teachers to the nursing services you have to offer. Find out the name of the president of the PTA and the student health council. A telephone call to these individuals may open the doors to the community and the student body.

Demonstrate Your Skills

The best way to help others to understand what it is you do is to show them what you can do. Follow up quickly on the referrals sent to you by other school personnel. Share with them the results of your interventions. A nurse who too quickly states that an activity is not the nurse's responsibility is apt to make other members of the team hesitant to use her or him. Often the nurse is requested to provide first aid or to inspect for communicable disease because individuals making these requests are afraid to handle these situations. Respond to their concerns by first caring for the children and then providing school personnel with information so that they can handle these situations in the future.

Communicate with All Members of the School Health Team

Do not wait for others to come to you. Relate with teachers in their lounge and in their classroom. Ask questions about the students that will help you to determine where your services are most needed. Share in writing or in person when you have followed up on a referral. Use the bulletin board to provide health information to students. *Talk with the school secretary.* She or he probably knows the students and their families as well as any other person in the building.

Organize Your Activities

A school nurse who just lets things happen frequently does not accomplish goals. Establish a calendar of activities for the year. Be specific about the goals you want to accomplish. Know when you will orient the teachers to your services, when you will provide inservice education, when you will review student records, and when you will follow up on student health problems. A tickler system (see Chapter 23) can help you to monitor student follow-up needs. *A calendar is a must.* If you do not plan your time, others will plan it for you.

Set Priorities

A nurse cannot be all things to all people. Identify what needs to be done and then determine what you can handle, considering the time you have available. Request consultation from the school health team to establish priorities significant to the needs of the population being served.

Document Your Activities

People respond favorably to concrete data. Keep a daily record of your activities. Use these records with others to substantiate what you have done, to support the need to set priorities, and to document the need for a new health program or changes in the existing health program. *Remember, changes generally do not occur when concrete data are lacking.*

SUMMARY

Traditionally, community health nurses have assumed a major role in planning health services for school-age children. Currently they work with this population group in a variety of settings such as the home, the school, clinics, and residential settings for children with special needs. A family-centered, prevention-oriented, interdisciplinary approach is the most effective way to meet the needs of school-age children, regardless of the setting in which the nurse is functioning.

Community health nurses who work with school-age children encounter an array of physical, psychosocial, cultural, environmental, and developmental health problems and concerns. A well-organized, comprehensive health care system that takes into consideration the developmental characteristics of children and adolescents is essential if youth are to reach their maximum potential.

Since most children attend school, the school is a logical environment in which to promote the health of all children. The role of the community health nurse in the school health program has been evolving since the turn of the century. Initially a school nurse was seen as the professional who provided first aid, gave injections, inspected for communicable diseases, or counseled "dirty" children. Now she or he is an advocate, a health counselor, a health educator, an epidemiologist, a consultant, a community health planner, and a coordinator. Teamwork is essential for successful implementation of these roles. The central figures on the team *must* be the school-age child and his or her family.

Working with school-age children and their families can be challenging and rewarding. Nurses who have a philosophy of nursing that stresses the need to help others help themselves and focuses on the client's strengths find school nursing particularly rewarding.

CRITICAL *Thinking Exercise*

Considering the characteristics of the students in the high school you attended and the school environment, discuss the health needs of this group of adolescents and strategies you would use to address these needs. Additionally, identify factors in that environment that would facilitate or hinder the implementation of health education efforts, health services programming, and environmental engineering strategies.

REFERENCES

Abu-Nasr D: Volunteer vision turns into reality, *The Ann Arbor News*, April 27, 1997, pp. A-1, A-11.

Adams PF, Benson V: Current estimates from the National Health Interview Survey: National Center for Health Statistics, *Vital Health Stat* 10(181), 1991.

Adams PP, Schoenborn CA, Moss AJ et al: Health risk behaviors among our Nation's youth: United States, 1992, *Vital and Health Statistics Report* Series 10, No. 192, Hyattsville, Md., 1995, Public Health Service.

Alan Guttmacher Institute (AGI): *Sex and America's teenagers*, New York, 1994, AGI.

Allensworth D, Kolbe J: The comprehensive school health program: exploring an expanded concept, *J Sch Health* 57:409-412, 1987.

Allensworth D, Wyche J, Lawson E, Nicholson L, eds: *Defining a comprehensive school health program: an interim statement*, Washington, D.C., 1995, National Academy Press.

American Association for Protecting Children (AAPC): *Highlights of official child neglect and abuse reporting—1984*, Denver, 1986, American Humane Association.

American Cancer Society (ACS): *Cancer facts and figures—1996*, Atlanta, 1996, ACS.

Andrulis DP, Acuff KL, Weiss KB, Anderson RJ: Public hospitals and health care reform: choices and challenges, *AJPH* 86:162-165, 1996.

Annie E. Casey Foundation: *Kids count data book, 1996: state profiles of child well-being*, Baltimore, Md., 1996, The Foundation.

Baker C: School health policy issues, *Nurs Health Care* 15:178-184, 1994.

Benenson AS, ed: *Control of communicable diseases manual*, ed 16, Washington, D.C., 1995, American Public Health Association.

Bradley BJ: The school nurse as health educator, *J Sch Health* 67:3-8, 1997.

Briere JN, Elliott DM: Immediate and long-term impacts of child sexual abuse, *The Future of Children* 4(2):54-69, 1994.

Brownson RC, Kreuter MW: Future trends affecting public health: challenges and opportunities, *J Public Health Management Practice* 3(2):49-60, 1997.

Burton PT: A day in the life of a nurse: school nursing on cutting edge of prevention, *Am Nurse* 24:23, 1992, September.

Carnegie Task Force on Meeting the Needs of Young Children: *Starting points: meeting the needs of our youngest children*, New York, 1994, Carnegie Corporation of New York.

Center for the Future of Children: School linked services, *The Future of Children* 2(1)6-144, 1992.

Centers for Disease Control (CDC): The effectiveness of school health education, *MMWR* 35(38):593-595, 1986.

Centers for Disease Control (CDC): CDC recommendations for a community plan for the prevention and containment of suicide clusters, *MMWR* 37(S-6):1-12, 1988a.

Centers for Disease Control and Prevention (CDC): Behaviors related to unintentional and intentional injuries among high school students—United States, 1991, *MMWR* 41:771-772, 1992a.

Centers for Disease Control and Prevention (CDC): *Youth suicide prevention programs: a resource guide*, Atlanta, 1992c, CDC.

Centers for Disease Control and Prevention (CDC): *School health programs: an investment in our future: at-a-glance, 1995*, Atlanta, 1995, CDC.

Children's Defense Fund (CDF): *The state of America's children yearbook 1996*, Washington, D.C., 1996, CDF.

Children's Defense Fund (CDF): *The state of America's children yearbook 1997*, Washington, D.C., 1997, CDF.

Chomitz VR, Cheung LWY, Lieberman E: The role of lifestyle in preventing low birth weight, *The Future of Children* 5(1):121-138, 1995.

Clearinghouse on Child Abuse and Neglect Information: *Child abuse and neglect: a shared community concern*, Washington, D.C., 1992, U.S. Government Printing Office.

Clemen S, Pattullo A: The adolescent with mental retardation. In Howe J, ed: *Nursing care of the adolescent*, New York, 1980, McGraw-Hill.

Collins A, Jones S, Bloom H: *Children and welfare reform: highlights from recent research*, New York, 1996, National Center for Children in Poverty.

Comer JP: Environmental health: the psychosocial climate. In Wallace HM, Patrick K, Parcel GS, Igoe SB, eds, *Principles and practices of student health*, vol II, Oakland, Ca., 1992, Third Party Publishing, pp. 377-392.

Compuplay Centers provide computer resources, *NARICQ* 1(3):5, 1988.

DePanfilis D, Salus MK: *A coordinated response to child abuse and neglect: a basic manual,* Washington, D.C., 1992, U.S. Government Printing Office.

Dubowitz H: *Child maltreatment in the United States: etiology, impact and prevention,* Washington, D.C., 1986, U.S. Congress, Office of Technology Assessment.

Dusenbury L, Falco M, Lake A: A review of the evaluation of 47 drug abuse prevention curricula available nationally, *J Sch Health* 67: 127-132, 1997.

Elders MJ: Schools and health: a natural partnership, *J Sch Health* 63:312-315, 1993.

Ferretti CK, Verhey MP, Isham MM: Development of a nurse-managed, school-based health center, *Nurs Educ* 21(5):35-42, 1996.

Finkelhor D: Current information on the scope and nature of child sexual abuse, *The Future of Children* 4(2):31-53, 1994.

Finkelhor D, Araji S: *A source book on child sexual abuse,* Beverly Hills, Ca., 1986, Sage.

Fryer G, Igoe J: Functions of school nurses and health assistants in U.S. school health programs, *J Sch Health* 66:55-58, 1996.

General Accounting Office (GAO): *Health care: school-based health centers can expand access for children,* Gaithersburg, Md., 1995a, GAO.

General Accounting Office (GAO): *Welfare to work: approaches that help teenage mothers complete high school,* Washington, D.C., 1995b, GAO.

Goodstadt MS: Substance abuse curricula vs. school drug policies, *J Sch Health* 59:246-250, 1989.

Green M, ed: *Bright futures: guidelines for health supervision of infants, children, and adolescents,* Arlington, Va., 1994, National Center for Education in Maternal and Child Health.

Hendershot GE: *The 1988 National Health Interview Survey on Child Health: new opportunities for research,* Atlanta, 1989, National Center for Health Statistics.

Hoffman SD, Foster EM, Furstenberg FF: Reevaluating the costs of teenage childbearing, *Demography* 30:1-13, 1993.

Hughes D, Simpson L: The role of social change in preventing low birth weight, *The Future of Children* 5(2):87-102, 1995.

Humphreys J, Ramsey AM: Child abuse. In Campbell J and Humphreys J: *Nursing care of survivors of family violence,* St. Louis, 1993, Mosby, pp. 36-67.

Igoe JB: Environmental health: the physical environment. In Wallace HM, Patrick K, Parcel GS, Igoe JB, eds: *Principles and practices of student health,* Vol II, Oakland, Ca., 1992, Third Party Publishing, pp. 369-377.

Igoe J, Parcel G: Contemporary issues of school health: mechanisms for change. In Wallace HM, Patrick K, Parcel GS, Igoe JB, eds: *Principles and practices of student health, vol II,* Oakland, Ca., 1992, Third Party Publishing, pp. 306-328.

Institute for Health and Aging, University of California, San Francisco: *Chronic care in America: a 21st century challenge,* Princeton, N.J., 1996, The Robert Wood Johnson Foundation.

Institute of Medicine (IOM): *The best intentions: unintended pregnancy and the well-being of children and families,* Washington, D.C., 1995, National Academy of Science.

Ireys HT, Katz S: The demography of disability and chronic illness among children. In Wallace HM, Biehl RF, MacQueen JC, Blackman JA, eds: *Mosby's resource guide to children with disabilities and chronic illness,* St. Louis, 1997, Mosby.

Jackson County Intermediate School District: *Special education services available to Jackson County,* Jackson, Mi., undated, The District.

Johnston LD, O'Malley PM, Bachman JG: *National survey results on drug use from The Monitoring The Future Study, 1975-1995, Vol 1, secondary school students,* Washington, D.C., 1996a, U.S. Government Printing Office.

Johnston L, O'Malley P, Bachman J: *News release, the rise in drug use among American teens continues in 1996,* Ann Arbor, Mi., 1996b, December 19, University of Michigan's Institute for Social Research.

Kalisch P, Kalisch BJ: *The advance of American nursing,* ed 3, Boston, 1995, Little, Brown.

Katz J, Green E: *Managing quality: a guide to system-wide performance management in health care,* St. Louis, 1997, Mosby.

Knitzer J, Page S: *Map and track: state initiatives for young children and families,* New York, 1996, National Center for Children in Poverty.

Korenman S, Miller JE, Sjaastad JE: Long-term poverty and child development in the United States, *Children and Youth Services Review* 17(1-2):127-151, 1995.

Kraus LE, Stoddard S, Gilmartin D: *Chartbook on disability in the United States, 1996,* National Institute on Disability and Rehabilitation Research.

LaPlante M, Carlson D: *Disability in the United States: prevalence and causes, 1992,* Disability Statistics Report (7), Washington, D.C., 1996, National Institute on Disability and Rehabilitation Research.

Lindberg FH, Distad LJ: Survival response to incest: adolescents in crisis, *Child Abuse and Neglect* 9:521-526, 1985.

Lynam MJ: The parent network in pediatric oncology, supportive or not? *Cancer Nurs* 10:207-216, 1987.

Lyon GR: Learning disabilities, *The Future of Children* 6(1):54-76, 1996.

Males M, Chew KSY: The ages of fathers in California adolescent births, 1993, *Am J Public Health* 86:565-568, 1996.

Maternal and Child Health Bureau: *Child health USA '94,* Washington, D.C., 1995, U.S. Government Printing Office.

Maternal and Child Health Bureau: *Child health USA '95,* Washington, D.C., 1996, U.S. Government Printing Office.

Nader PR: Comprehensive school health. In Wallace HM, Patrick K, Parcel GS, Igoe JB, eds: *Principles and practices of student health, vol II,* Oakland, Ca., 1992, Third Party Publishing, pp. 273-279.

National Association of School Nurses (NASN): *Philosophy of school health services and school nursing,* Scarborough, Me., 1988, NASN.

National Center for Children in Poverty: *One in four: America's youngest poor,* New York, 1996, The Center.

National Center for Health Statistics (NCHS): *Health, United States, 1995,* Hyattsville, Md., 1996, Public Health Service.

National Center for Injury Prevention and Control (NCIPC): *Injury control in the 1990s: a national plan for action,* Atlanta, 1993a, NCIPC.

National Center for Injury Prevention and Control (NCIPC): *The prevention of youth violence: a framework for community action,* Atlanta, 1993b, CDC.

National Center for Injury Prevention and Control (NCIPC): *Injury in the United States fact sheet,* Atlanta, 1995, NCIPC.

National Center on Child Abuse and Neglect: *A report to the Congress: joining together to fight child abuse,* Washington, D.C., 1986, U.S. Government Printing Office.

National Center on Child Abuse and Neglect: *Child maltreatment 1992: report from the states to the National Center on Child Abuse and Neglect,* Washington, D.C., 1994, U.S. Government Printing Office.

National Commission to Prevent Infant Mortality: *Home visiting: opening doors for America's pregnant women and children,* Washington, D.C., 1989, The Commission.

National Commission on the Role of the School and the Community in Improving Adolescent Health: *code blue: uniting for healthier youth,* Alexandria, Va., 1990, National Association of State Board of Education, pp. 1-52.

National Safety Council: *Accident facts 1996*, Itasca, Il., 1996, The Council.

Office of Disease Prevention and Health Promotion: *School health: findings from evaluated programs*, Washington, D.C., 1993, U.S. Government Printing Office.

Office of Special Education Programs: *Implementation of the Individuals with Disabilities Education Act; sixteenth annual report to Congress*, Washington, D.C., 1994, U.S. Department of Education.

Office of Technology Assessment (OTA): *Adolescent health, vol. III: crosscutting issues in the delivery of health and related services*, Washington, D.C., 1991, U.S. Government Printing Office.

Panel on Adolescent Pregnancy and Childbearing, National Research Council: *Risking the future: adolescent sexuality, pregnancy, and childbearing*, Washington, D.C., 1987, National Academy Press.

Paneth NS: The problem of low-birth weight, *The Future of Children* 5(1):19-34, 1995.

Parents' Resource Institute for Drug Education (PRIDE): *Press release: student use of most drugs reaches highest level in nine years*, Atlanta, 1996, September 25, PRIDE.

Parke RD, Neville B: Teenage fatherhood. In Itofferth SL, Hays CD, eds: *Risking the future: adolescent sexuality, pregnancy, and childbearing, Vol. II, working papers and statistical appendices*, Washington, D.C., 1987, National Academy Press.

Passarelli C: School nursing trends for the future, *J Sch Health* 64:141-146, 1994.

Policy Studies Associates: Protecting the privacy of student education records, *J Sch Health* 67:139-140, 1997.

Powers JL, Echenrode J, Jaklitsch B: Maltreatment among runaway and homeless youth, *Child Abuse and Neglect* 14:87-98, 1990.

Proctor ST, Lordi SL, Zaiger DS: *School nursing practice: roles and standards*, Scarborough, Me., 1993, National Association of School Nurses, Inc.

Resnick MD, Chambliss SA, Blum RN: Health and risk behaviors of urban adolescent males involved with pregnancy, *Fam Soc* 366-374, 1993.

Resnicow K, Allensworth D: Conducting a comprehensive school health program, *J Sch Health* 66:59-63, 1996.

Rowland D, Hanson K: Medicaid: moving to managed care, *Health Affairs* 15:150-152, 1996.

Rustia J: Rustia school health promotion model, *J Sch Health* 52(2) 108-115, 1982.

Sharts-Hopko NC: STDs in women: what you need to know, *AJN* 97(4):46-55, 1997.

Shattuck L: *Report of the Sanitary Commission of Massachusetts*, Boston, 1850, Dutton & Wentworth.

Shelton TL, Stepanek JJ: *Family-centered care for children needing specialized health and developmental services*, Bethesda, Md., 1994, Association for the Care of Children's Health.

Snyder TD, ed: *120 years of American education: a statistical portrait*, Washington, D.C., 1993, National Center for Education Statistics.

Stone EJ, Perry CL, Luepker RV: Synthesis of cardiovascular behavioral research for youth health promotion, *Health Educ Q* 16:155-169, 1989.

U.S. Bureau of the Census: *Statistical abstract of the United States 1995*, ed 115, Washington, D.C., 1995, U.S. Government Printing Office.

U.S. Bureau of the Census: *Statistical abstract of the United States 1996*, ed 116, Washington, D.C., 1996, U.S. Government Printing Office.

U.S. Department of Health, Education and Welfare (USDHEW): *Healthy people: the Surgeon General's report on health promotion and disease prevention*, DHEW Pub No. PHS 79-55071, Washington, D.C., 1979, U.S. Government Printing Office.

U.S. Department of Health and Human Services (USDHHS): *Healthy people 2000: national health promotion and disease prevention objectives, full report, with commentary*, Washington, D.C., 1991, U.S. Government Printing Office.

U.S. Department of Health and Human Services (USDHHS): National Institute of Child Health and Human Development: *The new face of AIDS: a maternal and pediatric epidemic*, Washington, D.C., 1993a, The Institute.

U.S. Department of Health and Human Services (USDHHS): *School-based health centers and managed care*, Washington, D.C., 1993b, Office of Inspector General.

U.S. Department of Health and Human Services (USDHHS): *Healthy People 2000: midcourse review and 1995 revisions*, Washington, D.C., 1995a, U.S. Government Printing Office.

U.S. Department of Health and Human Services (USDHHS): *Report to Congress on out-of-wedlock childbearing*, Hyattsville, Md., 1995c, U.S. Government Printing Office.

U.S. Department of Health and Human Services (USDHHS): *Child maltreatment 1994: reports from the states to the National Center on Child Abuse and Neglect*, Washington, D.C., 1996, U.S. Government Printing Office.

Winstead-Fry P, Bishop KK: Nurses and Public Law 102-119: a family-centered continuing education program, *J Contin Educ Nurs* 28(1):26-31, 1997.

Wong DL: *Whaley and Wong's nursing care of infants and children*, ed 5, St. Louis, 1995, Mosby.

SELECTED BIBLIOGRAPHY

American Medical Association: AMA *guidelines for adolescent preventive services (GAPS): recommendations and rationale*, Baltimore, Md., 1994, Williams & Wilkins.

Atwood JD, Donnelly JW: Adolescent pregnancy: combating the problem from a multi-systemic health perspective, *Health Educ* 40(4):219-227, 1993.

Botvin GJ, Schinke S, Orlandi MA: *Drug abuse prevention with multiethnic youth*, Thousand Oaks, Ca., 1995, Sage.

Braddock D, Hemp R, Bachelder L, Fujiura G: *The state of the states in developmental disabilities*, ed 4, Washington, D.C., 1995, American Association on Mental Retardation.

Breckon DJ: *Managing health promotion programs*, Gaithersburg, Md., 1997, Aspen Publishers.

Center for the Future of Children: School linked services, *The Future of Children* 2(1), 6-144, 1992.

Center for the Future of Children: U.S. health care for children, *The Future of Children* 2(2):4-212, 1992.

Children's Defense Fund: *The state of America's children 1992*, Washington, D.C., 1997, The Fund.

Collins J, Jones S, Bloom H: *Children and welfare reform: highlights from recent research*, New York, 1996, Nation Center for Children in Poverty.

Errecart MT, Walberg HJ, Ross JG et al: Effectiveness of teenage health teaching models, *J Sch Health* 61:26-30, 1991.

General Accounting Office (GAO): *School safety, promising initiatives for addressing school violence*, HEHS-95-106, Washington, D.C., 1995, General Accounting Office.

General Accounting Office (GAO): *Early childhood programs: local perspectives on barriers to providing head start services*, Washington, D.C., 1994, GAO.

Irwin CE, Brindis C, Holt KA, Langlykke K, eds: *Health care reform: opportunities for improving adolescent health*, Arlington, Va., 1994, National Center for Education in Maternal and Child Health.

Josten L, Wedeking L, Block D et al: Linking high-risk, low-income, pregnant women to public health services, *J Public Health Management Practice* 3(2):27-36, 1997.

National Maternal and Child Health Clearinghouse: *Boosting immunization rates within comprehensive child health systems: a report on state title V program activities (FY '91)*, Washington, D.C., 1994, Association of Maternal and Child Health Programs.

Spencer N: *Poverty and child health*, New York, 1996, Radcliffe Medical Press.

Strasburger VC: *Adolescents and the media: medical and psychological impact*, Thousand Oaks, Ca., 1995, Sage.

U.S. Department of Health and Human Services (USDHHS): *School-based health centers and managed care: examples of coordination*, Washington, D.C., 1993, Office of Inspector General.

U.S. Department of Health and Human Services (USDHHS): *Clinician's handbook of preventive services: put prevention into practice*, Washington, D.C., 1994, U.S. Government Printing Office.

World Health Organization (WHO): *The health of young people: a challenge and a promise*, Geneva, 1993, WHO.

Yawn BP, Yawn RA: Adolescent pregnancy: a preventable consequence, *The Prevention Researcher* 4(1):1-4, 1997.

Health Promotion Concerns of Adult Men and Women

Ella Mae Brooks, RN, PhD

Objectives

Upon completion of this chapter, the reader should be able to:

1. Discuss how achievement of developmental milestones can enhance growth in adulthood.
2. Describe common stressors experienced during adulthood and nursing interventions that assist adults in coping with these stressors.
3. Discuss nursing interventions for wellness in relation to adult roles and developmental tasks.
4. Use *Healthy People 2000* objectives to identify health risks among adults.
5. Analyze the major causes of mortality and morbidity for adult men and women.
6. Understand gender influences on health needs and behaviors.
7. Evaluate factors that increase adults' risk for mortality and morbidity.
8. Discuss the community health nurse's role in maintaining the health of adult men and women.
9. Describe aggregates at risk among adult males and females.
10. Develop primary, secondary, and tertiary interventions to promote and maintain the health of adult men and women.

Along with the multiple roles and responsibilities of adulthood, adults are developing as individuals and need to be concerned with their health. This chapter discusses adult aggregates at risk for high mortality and morbidity, examines health behaviors that increase mortality and morbidity risks, and discusses nursing interventions to promote health and reduce mortality and morbidity risks. Other chapters present the health needs of parents of the newborn, infant, and young child (Chapter 15); occupational health issues (Chapter 18); the adult with a disabling condition (Chapter 19); and older adulthood (Chapter 20). Other contemporary issues such as minority health status and trends, sexually transmitted diseases, substance abuse, and accidents/injuries are discussed in Chapter 12.

HEALTHY PEOPLE 2000 AND ADULT HEALTH

Adulthood is usually a time of relatively good physical and mental health when people have the opportunity to assume personal responsibility for their health behaviors. Taking personal responsibility in physical fitness and healthy eating are known to have an effect in preventing many health problems such as coronary heart disease, hypertension, stroke, diabetes, colon cancer, and obesity. Many of the leading causes of morbidity and mortality for adults are preventable through changes in lifestyle and health habits. *Healthy People 2000* examined health habits and risk factors for the adult and established national health objectives for improving adult health.

Health Habits/Health Risks

Healthy People 2000 stated that risk factors such as poor nutrition, overweight, lack of exercise, smoking, alcohol consumption, and failure to use seatbelts and preventive health and screening services all contribute significantly to the five major causes of death in the United States: cancer, heart disease, stroke, injury, and chronic lung disease. *Healthy People 2000* issued a major challenge for adults to modify their lifestyles to maintain health and prevent disease (USDHHS, 1991a, p. 23). Nurses intervene with adults to reduce health risks and promote health. For example, a community health nurse might develop a smoking cessation program for adults in the community; a community health nurse may also identify high-risk aggregates for developing coronary heart disease and may develop a worksite fitness program to help these adults address coronary heart disease risk factors such as lack of physical activity and poor dietary habits.

Many risk factors are long-established habits that are hard to break. Such habits provide challenges for nurses to

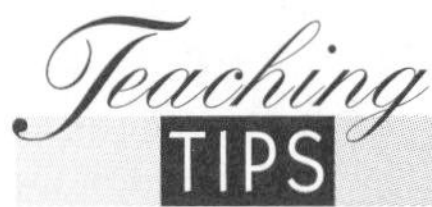

Educational Topics for Promoting Adult Health

1. Cessation of smoking
2. Not drinking to excess
3. Adequate nutritional intake
4. Control of environmental hazards
5. Promotion of worksite health and safety
6. Prevention and control of hypertension
7. Pap smear at least every 2 years
8. Regular self-examination of the breasts and testicles
9. Knowledge of and action on cancer warning signs
10. Counseling to promote mental health
11. Regular exercise
12. Regular use of car seatbelts
13. Preventive dental care
14. Preventive health care (including immunizations and screening procedures)

Modified from USDHHS: *Healthy People 2000: national health promotion and disease prevention objectives, full report, with commentary*, Washington, D.C., 1991a, U.S. Government Printing Office, pp. 152-154.

develop creative interventions and teaching strategies that are effective in helping adults reduce health risks and develop healthy behaviors. The Teaching Tips box lists some selected educational topics from *Healthy People 2000* for reducing risk factors and promoting healthy living among adults. These educational topics can be used by community health nurses as a guide for developing nursing interventions that promote the health of adults.

The Nation's Objectives for Adult Health

Healthy People 2000 has an overall goal to reduce the death rate for adults by 20% to no more than 340 per 100,000 people age 25 to 64 (baseline: 423 per 100,000). Numerous adult health objectives are scattered throughout the document's 22 priority areas. A summary of major focus areas for *Healthy People 2000* adult health objectives is given in the box on the next page. These objectives address health status measures, risk reduction activities, and services utilization and protection.

Progress toward achieving the year 2000 adult health objectives is illustrated by accomplishments such as a reduction in the incidence of coronary heart disease and cancer deaths, a decline in overall adult smoking rates, an increased incidence in women having Pap smears and mammograms, a small decline in fat consumption, reductions in alcohol consumption and alcohol-related cirrhosis, a decrease in motor vehicle deaths, a decrease in work-related injury and deaths, and an increase in worksite stress management programs (USDHHS, 1995a). Despite the nation's accomplishments, lifestyle behaviors continue to adversely influence the health of adults in the United States.

The prevalence of obesity has increased, and fewer people who are overweight appear to be taking steps to control their weight through measures such as eating less and exercising more. For both men and women, adopting sound dietary practices combined with regular physical activity has declined (USDHHS, 1995a, p. 25). A survey showed that only about one quarter of Americans were aware of the dietary requirements for fruits and vegetables, and those who were aware of these ate more fruits and vegetables than those who were unaware (USDHHS, 1995a, p. 30). However, the survey showed that nurse practitioners routinely inquired about exercise habits in only 30% of their patients and formulated an exercise plan for only 14% of their patients (USDHHS, 1995a, p. 25). Such information should be gathered on a routine basis.

Community health nurses can play a significant role in helping the nation accomplish the year 2000 health objectives. Having an understanding of these objectives can assist nurses in developing individual and aggregate health interventions that address these objectives. When developing interventions, nurses take into consideration the developmental tasks of adulthood as well as health risk factors.

DEVELOPMENTAL TASKS OF ADULTHOOD

It has long been established that significant personality growth and development occurs during adulthood (Erikson, 1963, 1982; Havighurst, 1972; Stevenson, 1977). Human beings change, learn, and pass through developmental stages that require achievement of predictable tasks. Accomplishment of these tasks provides a foundation for growth; if they are not accomplished, future development can be jeopardized or altered.

Adult development is influenced by numerous variables including individual needs, interpersonal relationships (including family roles), established patterns of coping, support systems, community roles, and societal expectations. Table 17-1 illustrates the complexity of the developmental stages and tasks of adulthood. These stages are not absolute with age and they may overlap as adults progress through the life span.

Erikson's Intimacy, Generativity, and Ego Integrity

Erik Erikson's (1963) classic work on developmental theory stressed the importance of psychosocial aspects of development. Erikson wrote that development was a continuous process and that delays or crisis at one developmental stage could diminish successful achievement of other stages of development. His psychosocial theories address stages of development, developmental goals and tasks, psychosocial crises, and coping processes. Erikson described eight

HEALTHY PEOPLE 2000 Objectives Targeting Adults: Focus Areas

HEALTH STATUS OBJECTIVES

- Reduce coronary heart disease deaths
- Reduce lung cancer deaths
- Reduce the number of unintended pregnancies
- Reduce the prevalence of mental disorders
- Reduce the incidence of homicides
- Reduce deaths from work-related injuries
- Reduce destructive periodontal disease
- Reverse the rise in cancer deaths
- Reduce diabetes incidence
- Reduce diabetes-related deaths
- Reduce the most severe complications of diabetes (e.g., end-stage renal disease, blindness, lower extremity amputation, perinatal mortality, congenital malformations)
- Reduce the incidence of viral hepatitis
- Reduce the incidence of tuberculosis

RISK REDUCTION OBJECTIVES

- Reduce dietary fat intake
- Reduce dietary sodium intake
- Increase dietary calcium intake
- Increase the use of dietary complex carbohydrate and fiber-containing foods
- Reduce alcohol consumption
- Increase the effective use of family planning methods
- Increase the proportion of people who seek help in coping with personal and emotional problems
- Increase the proportion of people with high blood pressure who report blood pressure is under control
- Reduce the mean serum cholesterol level

SERVICES AND PROTECTION OBJECTIVES

- Increase the proportion of postsecondary institutions with institution-wide health promotion programs for students, faculty, and staff
- Increase the proportion of women age 40 and older who (a) have ever received a clinical breast examination and a mammogram and (b) have received these examinations within the last 2 years
- Increase the proportion of women age 18 who (a) have ever received a Pap test and (b) received a Pap test within the preceding 1 to 3 years
- Increase the proportion of people age 50 and older who (a) have received fecal occult blood testing within the preceding 1 to 2 years and (b) have ever received sigmoidoscopy
- Increase the proportion of adults who have received all of the screening and immunization services and at least one of the counseling services recommended by the U.S. Preventive Services Task Force

In addition to the focus areas listed, other objectives address aspects of adult health such as stress reduction and weight management programs, community and worksite fitness facilities, infertility, using food labels to assist in nutritional planning, use of community mental health support programs, decreasing family violence, home testing for radon and environmental lead, reducing sun exposure, hearing and vision protection programs, increasing access to services, and removing financial barriers to health care.

From USDHHS: *Healthy People 2000: national health promotion and disease prevention objectives, full report with commentary,* Washington, D.C., 1991a, U.S. Government Printing Office, pp. 19-23.

developmental stages from birth to death, three of which apply to the 18- to 65-year-old population. According to Erikson (1963, 1982) these stages are intimacy (young adult), generativity (middle adult), and ego integrity (older adult).

INTIMACY Young adults are involved in an intense search of self. At the same time they are at the developmental stage of *intimacy* and need to begin to relate to others, become partners in friendships, and develop sexual, work, and community relationships. Young adulthood is a time for development of close personal relationships and commitment to others. Young adults may experience conflicting values, attitudes, and ideas as they sort out what life means to them and develop the ethical strength to abide by their commitments. The young adult who is successful in achieving intimacy will develop the ability to love and commit to others; unsuccessful resolution can result in isolation and self-absorption.

GENERATIVITY As life continues into middlescence, it is expected that the middle adult will guide and care for the younger generation and assist the older one. This involves an ability to care and do for others, and when these attributes exist the adult becomes *generative* in nature. Generativity is viewed in terms of caring and sharing, as well as procreativity, productivity, and creativity. The generative person extends herself or himself to others outside the family. One does not have to be a biological parent to be generative! Generative adults help guide others on a path to their own generativity. If this task is not reached, stagnation can occur. Stagnated adults do not demonstrate the need or inclination to care for others. Instead they are likely to be egocentric and self-absorbed.

table 17-1 Developmental Tasks of the Adult (Ages 18-65): Major Goals—to Develop Intimacy, Generativity, and Ego Integrity

Young Adult	Middlescent: Middlescence I	Middlescent: Middlescence II
AGE: 18-29 YEARS	AGE: 30-50 YEARS	AGE: 51-70 YEARS*
1. Establishing autonomy from parents or parent surrogates	1. Developing socioeconomic consolidation	1. Maintaining flexible views in occupational, civic, political, religious, and social positions
2. Choosing and preparing for an occupation	2. Evaluating one's occupation or career in light of a personal value system	2. Keeping current on relevant scientific, political, and cultural changes
3. Developing a marital relationship or other form of companionship	3. Helping younger persons to become integrated human beings	3. Developing mutually supportive (interdependent) relationships with grown offspring and other members of the younger generation
4. Developing and initiating parenting behaviors for use with own, and other's, offspring	4. Enhancing or redeveloping intimacy with spouse or most significant other	4. Reevaluating and enhancing the relationship with spouse or most significant other or adjusting to his or her loss
5. Developing a personal lifestyle and philosophy of life	5. Developing a few deep friendships	5. Helping aged parents or other relatives progress through the last stage of life
6. Accepting one's role as a citizen and developing participatory citizen behaviors	6. Helping aging persons progress through the later years of life	6. Deriving satisfaction from increased availability of leisure time
	7. Assuming responsible positions in occupational, social, and civic activities, organizations, and communities	7. Preparing for retirement and planning another career when feasible
	8. Maintaining and improving the home and other forms of property	8. Adapting self and behavior to signals of the accelerated aging process
	9. Using leisure time in satisfying and creative ways	
	10. Adjusting to biological or personal system changes that occur	

Material on middlescence from Stevenson JS: *Issues and crises during middlescence*, New York, 1977, Appleton-Century-Crofts, pp. 18, 25.
*In her text, Stevenson assigns the age range for Middlescence II to be 50-70 years.

EGO INTEGRITY In older adulthood *ego integrity* is established. This is a contemplative process that involves self-assessment, evaluating where one has been, where one is going, and examining personal values, decisions, and lifestyles. One also strives to accomplish personal and civic aspirations during this stage of life and to become self-fulfilled. If life aspirations are not fulfilled, adulthood can be a time of disillusionment, disenchantment, and despair. The person who has achieved ego integrity knows and likes himself or herself and is able to accept individual strengths and weaknesses, distinguish the things over which he or she has control, and accept those things that cannot be changed. Despair is likely to occur if ego integrity is not reached.

To promote wellness and to enhance an adult's self-care capabilities, the community health nurse needs to have an understanding of the processes involved in developing intimacy, generativity, and ego integrity. Adults should be facilitated in moving toward accomplishment of these developmental tasks. Helping adults understand developmental tasks can facilitate their achievement, promote self-esteem and personal growth, and ultimately lead to self-fulfillment.

Life for an adult is complex and changing, and adults play many interdependent "roles." Some roles assumed by the adult include parent, grandparent, individual, spouse or companion, son or daughter, citizen, friend, and worker. The box on the next page delineates some of these adult roles. Usually these roles are developmentally sequential or complementary. However, a person may not be ready to assume a role when it arises. Examples of role changes that people may not be prepared to make are unplanned parenthood and mandatory retirement, especially if retirement is not desired. Role changes that occur abruptly may create frustration and personal crises in the adult. Nurses must assess for stressors that may precipitate adult crises and be prepared to intervene appropriately.

Facilitating Role Performance Among Adults

INDIVIDUAL

Adults need to define what is personally important to them and set personal life goals. At times this can create conflict for the nurse, especially when client goals differ from the nurse's. The nurse who is sensitive and accepts the client's right of self-determination generates trust and facilitates a more collaborative working relationship. Nurses need to "individualize" care to meet client needs.

PARENT

The generative aspect of middlescence is explicit when the roles of parent and grandparent are discussed. In the role of parent the adult is expected to maintain the family physically, emotionally, and financially and assist in the socialization process. Parenting issues in the middle years often involve adolescent children and launching of adult children. It is helpful for the nurse to discuss children's developmental tasks with parents. Such discussions can assist parents in understanding what is normal (e.g., being rebellious is a part of normal adolescent behavior). The community health nurse can assist parents in achieving generational balance and understanding.

GRANDPARENT

Grandparenting is often part of life's middle years. Some middlescents are delighted, eagerly await grandchildren, and look forward to being involved with grandchildren—others do not. Grandparents may find that they have more time to spend with their grandchildren than they did with their own children. A grandparent can enhance the growth of younger generations. In classic writings on the family, Duvall said, "When those who are at the beginning of the journey hold hands with those who have travelled a long way and know all the turns in the road, each gains the strength needed by both" (Duvall, 1962, p. 409).

SPOUSE OR COMPANION

In adulthood time is spent in developing and redeveloping relationships with a spouse or significant other and spending time in companionship relationship. A significant other can be anyone with whom the adult has a close, meaningful relationship. With today's many lifestyles it is completely possible that there will be a significant other who is not a spouse. This significant other may be part of a heterosexual or homosexual relationship. Being nonjudgmental about various lifestyles is essential if the community health nurse is to help the adult achieve self-fulfillment.

SON OR DAUGHTER

Adults are trying to maintain meaningful relationships with parents and may be experiencing role reversal with them. In these "reversed" roles some adult children become caretakers of their elderly parents. Adult children need to assist aged parents in maintaining their dignity and must refrain from dominating them, taking over their decision making, and robbing them of their independence.

It is important for the adult to deal with the eventual death of aging parents. Plans for burial arrangements and the handling of personal affairs should be considered. Health care professionals need to be comfortable in teaching and talking about death and dying. It is also crucial for adults to realize that it is normal for aging parents to talk about death. Assisting aging parents to resolve their feelings about death and articulating advanced directives can help adults in accepting their own eventual death and other grief, dying, death, and loss situations.

CITIZEN/LEADER

Adults are expected to take an active role in civic activities and hold local, state, and national offices. They are sought as community leaders and often serve as community volunteers. Adults are valuable resources as volunteer staff and supporters for health projects in the community. Community health nurses can assist adults in understanding the need for balancing citizen commitments with family and individual responsibilities.

FRIEND

Adulthood is a time of life when developing and maintaining a few deep friendships is beneficial and rewarding. Having friends that one can count on, enjoy being with, and share activities with helps provide support and pleasure when family contacts are limited.

WORKER

The health of the worker and the role of the occupational health nurse are discussed in Chapter 18. Working is generally essential to one's economic stability and has psychological implications for the individual as well.

The young adult is in a stage of training for, and deciding on, a career. The middlescent may be at a career peak and derives much satisfaction from her or his job. This is usually the time of maximum power and influence. Americans in executive positions are often 40 to 65 years old and earn a large part of the nation's income.

SELECTED STRESSORS OF ADULTHOOD AND NURSING INTERVENTION

Adult life is usually healthy, productive, and fulfilling, but it may also include frustration, confusion, and lack of direction. Nurses can provide adults with anticipatory, supportive guidance and interact with them to promote health. Providing adults with information about community resources, preventive health practices, and developmental expectations are several ways to promote health in adults.

The life span comprises a series of life change events. Chapter 8 elaborates on experiences that signify life change events. The number, duration, and type of these events will vary with individuals. Because of the uniqueness of individuals, a life event that is major for one person may not be considered major for another.

Unlike young children, who have parents or others to support and guide them through the experience of life change events, the adult often does not have adequate support available during times of heightened stress or may not use the help that is available because dependency is feared. Our society emphasizes self-sufficiency during adulthood, but even a mature adult may experience feelings of insecurity at various times and need assistance from others. Many adults must learn that *interdependency* is a mature state.

Examples of some life change events that affect adults include the following: leaving the parental home, obtaining job education and training, pursuing a career, marriage, childbearing, child rearing, child launching, providing for an aging parent, pursuing leisure-time activities, and experiencing the death of a parent. Life change events that are more or less expected usually evoke what could be termed *normative stress*. However, other life change events induce stress that goes beyond what could be considered normative and may necessitate developing new interpersonal relationships, coping mechanisms, and resources. Examples of some of these life change events are divorce or separation, loss of a child, loss of a job, development of a chronic health condition, and career changes. If these events occur in rapid succession, the adult may have difficulty adapting and may experience crisis.

An example of what can happen when major life events occur in rapid succession is seen in the Stephen Johns case scenario.

CASE *Scenario*

In a period of less than 14 years, Mr. Johns, 32 years old, left home to enter college, completed a college education, entered a career, married, bought a house, had a child, changed jobs, moved to a new residence, became divorced, moved to another residence, changed jobs again, and experienced the death of a parent. These were all significant life events for Mr. Johns, and the rapid succession of their development left him in a confused and disorganized state. He was overwhelmed with his life and began to question whether it had meaning. Thus he sought counseling at a local mental health clinic. Through work with a psychiatric nurse therapist, Mr. Johns was able to establish life goals and take action to achieve these goals. This made him comfortable about himself as a person and gave direction and meaning to his life. He began to recognize his own strengths and to work within and accept his limitations. He began to reach out to others and saw that interdependency can be therapeutic.

Although major life events may not always be experienced this rapidly, or in this magnitude, significant stresses do occur during adulthood. While experiencing these stresses adults are also trying to achieve a balance between their responsibilities to family and society, to develop as individuals, and to maintain health. These tasks by themselves produce stress. Thus when sudden or unexpected situational difficulties arise, such as divorce, death, or changes in job and residence, the individual is at risk for crisis.

Helping Clients in Crisis

Crisis may be experienced at any time throughout adult life. When mobilizing coping mechanisms during times of stress, the adult has many life experiences from which to draw. However, these experiences do not necessarily prepare one to handle all situations. At each developmental stage new or different events require adaptation.

When adults are in crisis, they should be helped to look at the circumstances that precipitated the crisis and modify them to reduce future occurrences. The nurse is supportive of the client without leveling judgment and helps the client and family to assess the resources and support systems they have available and to make plans for the immediate future. As discussed in Chapter 8, the mastery of a crisis provides opportunities for personal growth and development.

The resources people use during crisis and time of need will vary. Emotional support, encouragement, assistance with problem solving, companionship, and tangible aid have been shown to be helpful to people who are dealing with a crisis. Individuals experiencing a crisis may look for caregivers who can provide these interventions. Sometimes individuals under stress need help in identifying the need for supportive assistance.

A major goal of community health nursing practice in relation to crisis is prevention. To achieve this goal, the community health nurse recognizes early signs and symptoms of heightened stress (see Chapter 8) and helps individuals who are experiencing these symptoms to mobilize appropriate coping mechanisms and prevent major developmental crises.

Selected Examples of Normative Crises

As adults in contemporary society move through the life span they may experience overwhelming stress that leads to normative crises. As previously mentioned, these crises may occur at any time throughout the adult life. Selected examples of the most common normative crises are addressed in this section. These examples include adults dissatisfied with work, those with leisure time needs, parents who are launching their children, and adults who are caretakers of aging parents.

ADULTS DISSATISFIED WITH WORK Job dissatisfaction is often related to other personal difficulties. Stresses at work can be compounded when an adult has home pressures to handle. This was the case with Ed Sorka.

CASE *Scenario*

Ed Sorka was a 29-year-old husband and father of two daughters, ages 3 and 5. He became disillusioned with his job because "his boss demanded too much and gave too few rewards." Ed's wife had multiple sclerosis that was getting progressively worse. She required help with activities of daily living and found it hard to participate in social events. Ed was a devoted husband and father. All his spare time was spent with his family. He found it difficult to talk about his wife's condition or his need for leisure activities; verbalizing stress encountered at work was much easier for him to handle. When the community health nurse helped him to examine both work and home stresses, Ed discovered that he really did not want to change jobs but that he did need time for himself. Arrangements were made for homemaker services to reduce the demands on Ed's time.

The stress caused by job dissatisfaction can appear in all aspects of health and family life. When a person's job starts making him or her physically or emotionally ill and takes a toll on family life, it is time to take a serious look at the situation. The nurse can guide the family in assessing the situation and refer them to appropriate community resources.

ADULTS WITH LEISURE TIME NEEDS *Leisure* is not an easy word to define. It means many things to many people. Leisure is antithetical to work as an economic pursuit. It is a planned activity that promotes growth and is pleasurable. *Internal motivation* is a key factor in planning and implementing leisure activities.

Many adults are too busy to engage in regular leisure-time activity. Leisure activities can be relaxing, rejuvenating, and refreshing. They can help to provide a link between responsibilities that cannot be ignored and a need to pursue something of personal value or interest. People need time in which to enjoy themselves and relax.

Adults need leisure time. Using leisure time in satisfying and creative ways is a developmental task for adulthood. The community health nurse should encourage the adult to make a conscious effort to devote time to leisure activities. The great amount of free time that often accompanies retirement and later life will be better spent if individuals have developed leisure-time activities that are satisfying in adulthood.

Frequently the adult needs help in examining why he or she does not engage in leisure activities. Often it will be found that many adults do not know how to use the free time they have and thus they devote all their time to work or other responsibilities. The nurse can assist people by helping them identify interests they would like to develop or redevelop, as demonstrated in the following scenario.

CASE *Scenario*

Sara Washington was a 40-year-old divorced woman with no children. She was referred to the community health nurse for health supervision visits by her family physician following hospitalization for severe hypertension. After her divorce Sara devoted herself to work. She was an interior designer who was well respected in her field; promotion came very rapidly. Most of her social involvements were work-related.

Sara's recent hospitalization scared her. When the community health nurse took a social history on her first home visit, she replied, "I know I can't keep working like I have been, but I get bored when I don't have something to do. There is very little social life for a woman my age in this town. My peers are all married or divorced themselves. Those who are divorced are like me, they work all the time."

Community health nursing intervention helped Sara to discover how much she missed contact with people on a personal level, the types of social activities she might explore, her fears about getting involved, and the middlescent's need for leisure-time activities to achieve normal growth and development. Sara had enjoyed cooking, entertaining friends, art, and drama before her divorce. Supportive encouragement by the community health nurse facilitated her involvement once again in these activities. She especially enjoyed dance lessons and found that they provided several opportunities for socializing. "You know, when one takes the time, it really isn't that difficult to find something fun to do," stated Sara during one of the nurse's home visits.

Adults who have experienced a stressful life event such as divorce may use work to reduce their tension and anxiety, overlooking leisure activities. An astute community health nurse might prevent this from happening by providing anticipatory guidance and supportive encouragement when encountering adults during times of heightened stress.

PARENTS WHO ARE LAUNCHING CHILDREN A primary task of the parent in the middle years is launching children from the parental home. Launching is a normal part of growth and development and a time when the young adult becomes independent and autonomous. It can be a brief or prolonged period.

Parents who have accomplished the developmental tasks of middlescence are more likely to foster independence in their children and relinquish control than those who have not. Middlescent parents who have not faced the developmental issues of their life period find it difficult to launch their adult children and "let go."

The nurse can help parents through this process by discussing it with them and assisting parents in identifying ways to achieve satisfaction. Adolescents and young adults have a greater chance of achieving healthy independence when their parents support their efforts.

The community health nurse can help parents become aware of how involvement with their children changes during launching. In successful launching parents become less directive and recognize that young adults need time to sort out what they want from life.

Launching is often a time when parents reflect on how they have raised their children. They frequently evaluate their parenting on the basis of how their children have progressed toward financial independence and whether or not they have established a stable, happy home. Many parents do not consider a child fully launched until these two tasks have been achieved.

Duvall and Miller (1985, p. 276) have discussed the family developmental tasks involved in launching as follows:

- Adapting physical facilities and resources for releasing young adults

- Meeting launching-center families' costs
- Reallocating responsibilities among grown and growing offspring and their parents
- Developing increasingly mature roles within the family
- Interacting, communicating, and appropriately expressing affection, aggression, disappointment, success, and sexuality
- Releasing and incorporating family members satisfactorily
- Establishing patterns for relating to in-laws, relatives, guests, friends, community pressures, and impinging world pressures
- Setting attainable goals, rewarding achievement, and encouraging family loyalties within a context of personal freedom

It is important that children recognize the stresses their parents may be experiencing during the launching period. Too often the focus of nursing intervention is only on the parent. Parents are frequently made to think that what they are doing is "all wrong." Adolescents and young adults need to understand that they are not the only ones experiencing stress and that they need to take responsibility for their own actions. The rights of the parents, as well as those of the children, should be protected. This is illustrated in the following case scenario.

CASE *Scenario*

John Michael, age 22, decided to live with his parents because he wanted to save money to buy a condominium. He expected to live free of charge, to have no household responsibilities in his parents' home, and to come and go as he pleased. Conflicts arose when John's parents did not agree with his plans. His parents were experiencing financial stress. They had two other children in college and had just finished spending a considerable amount of money for John's education. John was making an adequate salary and they expected him to contribute financially toward family expenses. They also felt that he should assume responsibility for some of the household chores. John became angry. He wanted the freedom of adulthood without having to assume the responsibilities that went along with this freedom.

The community health nurse was involved with John's family because Mrs. Michael was a newly diagnosed diabetic. It was during her third home visit that the nurse identified the stress between John and his parents. During the visit, John's mother was tense, to the point of being in tears. Observing her distressed state, the nurse encouraged her to verbalize her feelings and afterward made arrangements to meet jointly with John and his parents. During this conference, the nurse requested that each family member share his or her perceptions of what was happening. Emphasis was also placed on identifying alternative ways to resolve the family conflict and on assisting each family member to see his or her needs and responsibilities.

One issue that became apparent during this conference was that John realized his parents also had needs and were experiencing stress. Just as parents must examine the developmental needs of their children, adult children must also be capable of looking at the developmental needs of their parents. Children often fail to do this, especially when they are working toward establishing self-identity. The child at launching age is able to relate, at least partially, to the needs of his or her parents, but may need some help in recognizing this fact.

ADULTS WHO ARE CARETAKERS FOR AGING PARENTS

This role is becoming more prevalent, and although it can be rewarding and gratifying, it can also precipitate stress and crisis situations (see Chapter 21). Many middlescent and even older adults are caring for older parents and at the same time working and caring for children at home. Caretaking can mean less leisure time and even feelings of guilt about not doing enough or having to place a parent in a nursing home when home care is no longer feasible. The nurse can encourage families to verbalize their feelings about caretaking, assess the caretaker situation, realistically look at what they can do, and utilize appropriate community resources. Sometimes utilizing community resources means that the caretaker needs to obtain adult day care services or have someone assist in the home during the day. Caregiver support can assist families in making these difficult decisions.

In addition to the developmental tasks, stresses, and crises that are occurring in adulthood, the physical nature of the human body is changing. Some of these physical changes provide a challenge for adults in achieving and maintaining health.

THE HUMAN BODY IN ADULTHOOD

Achieving health for the adult involves maintaining physical, social and mental well-being (including successful achievement of developmental tasks). Since most adults are considered healthy, the health care needs of adults may be overlooked. Often adults are frequently "too busy" or "too involved" to look after personal health. It can be a challenge for the nurse to persuade the well adult to obtain health care and to practice preventive health practices. The human body during adulthood is briefly discussed to help illustrate some of the physical and mental changes that the adult experiences.

The human body is constantly undergoing physical and mental changes. During adulthood the person begins to develop an acute awareness of growing older and is faced with adjusting to a changing body image as physical alterations occur. This adjustment is often difficult in American society because the beauty and stamina of youth are prized. The incidence of chronic and physically disabling conditions increases with age, and these conditions can also affect how one views oneself.

Several physical changes occur in the human body during adulthood. The senses of taste and smell begin to diminish. Vision is usually well maintained in early adulthood, but presbyopia (farsightedness) is extremely common by middlescence. Presbyopia is caused by a decreased lens elasticity that reduces the power of accommodation. It hinders the ability of the individual to view objects at close range, and glasses may be necessary for reading or close work. After age 30 the cornea begins to lose transparency and the pupil decreases in size. These changes allow less light to be admitted to the eye and result in poor illumination.

Permanent sensorineural hearing loss as a result of aging (presbycusis) accelerates during middlescence. The person experiencing presbycusis has decreased auditory acuity for higher tones and may have difficulty engaging in normal conversation, including talking over the telephone. The duration and type of noise exposure that a person encounters during earlier life influences how soon presbycusis begins. For example, the person exposed to industrial noise or the avid hunter may experience presbycusis earlier than others because of more extensive sensorineural hearing damage during youth.

Metabolic function—combining food with oxygen to create energy—decreases during adulthood. This, coupled with the fact that the person is often becoming more sedentary, can mean increased weight. The basal metabolism rate gradually decreases by middle age with a resultant need for reduction in caloric intake.

Decreasing elasticity of the blood vessels, especially the coronary arteries, predisposes the middlescent to cardiovascular disease. Many middlescents evidence the symptomatology of cardiac conditions, such as shortness of breath, chest pains, and dyspnea on exertion. Incidence of death from cardiovascular disease is on the rise in adulthood.

In middlescence the female's ovarian estrogen production and menstruation cease. This event is called *menopause;* it usually occurs between the ages of 45 and 55 years but can be earlier or later. Menopause is a normal transition for midlife women but is often viewed negatively. Nurses can assist women in addressing the negative aspects of menopause by helping them realize that their sexuality does not end with menopause and, after menopause, they may experience a new zest and vitality in life (Greenwood, 1996). The symptoms that woman experience during menopause are an interplay of psychological and physiological changes that are largely a result of decreased ovarian activity and the resultant estrogen deficiency. These symptoms generally subside after menopause. The accompanying box lists some of the symptoms experienced by women during menopause.

It is important to note that a woman does not necessarily experience all of these symptoms. Some women may experience many of them and others may experience very few or pass through menopause without any symptoms. However, for some women the symptoms create havoc. It is not unusual for women to fear dementia because experiencing short-term memory loss and lack of concentration during this time is common (Peters, 1996). Community health nurses have an important role in alleviating fears such as these by educating people about the normal changes with menopause. Women do not have to suffer menopausal symptoms silently. Some therapies such as hormone replacement, estrogen vaginal creams, and vaginal lubricants may be indicated (Greenwood, 1996; Hofland, Powers, 1996).

Common Menopausal Symptoms

- Hot flashes
- Sweating
- Chills
- Palpitations
- Headaches
- Vaginal dryness
- Vaginitis
- Atrophic vaginitis
- Decreased libido
- Skin changes
- Fatigue
- Insomnia
- Dizziness
- Mood swings
- Depression
- Irritability
- Poor concentration
- Short-term memory loss
- Weight gain

Altering behaviors, physical activity, and dietary intake may also lessen the menopausal symptoms. This includes activities such as smoking cessation and minimal alcohol intake, since both may contribute to irregular bleeding and increased tension; decreasing caffeine intake because it stimulates the central nervous system, which increases tension and irritability; engaging in frequent and regular exercise, which may help reduce frequency and severity of hot flashes as well as aid in weight control; avoiding stressful situations that may increase symptoms; and being cognizant of nutritional intake such as calcium, fats, sugars, salt, and carbohydrates for weight control, as well as prevention of health problems such as osteoporosis and hypertension (Greenwood, 1996).

Once a woman passes through menopause her childbearing capabilities cease. This often has greater psychological meaning than physical significance. To be safe, it is often recommended that a woman continue to use a reliable method of birth control for at least 1 year after she has gone 12 consecutive months without a menstrual period.

In middlescence the male passes through a period called the *climacteric* in which the testes decrease but do not cease testosterone production. During this time the testes may atrophy slightly, frequency of sexual activity may tend to decline, and prostate problems are common (Thompson, Wilson, 1996). The male usually goes through this period between ages 50 and 60. He may or may not experience any physical symptoms. Some symptoms such as irritability, easy frustration, depression, and change in sexual drive are sometimes evidenced. Often it is more difficult for men than women to admit to these changes or talk about them. This was profoundly described when Gail Sheehy (1996) stated, "if menopause is the silent passage [for women], male menopause is unspeakable" (p. 292). Many people are not aware that this period exists for men and are often bewildered by male behavior during the climacteric.

The human responses to menopause and the climacteric can cause stress and affect relationships. Educating adult men and women about normal life change events that occur during the menopause and climacteric can help alleviate interpersonal stresses that may negatively influence their relationships. Community health nurses have an important educative role in this area.

With menopause a woman's estrogen level drops drastically, which increases the risk for calcium loss and osteoporosis. Decalcification of the bones, a condition called *osteoporosis*, begins in middlescence. Not all older adults will develop osteoporosis, although there is a decrease in bone mass that occurs with aging (Arnaud, 1996). With osteoporosis the bones become fragile and are easily broken. Bone fractures and vertebral compression that cause back pain and other problems can occur (Greenwood, 1996). Before menopause estrogen helps to protect the bones from losing calcium (Greenwood). Estrogen replacement therapy may be advised to decrease bone loss and fracture rate associated with menopause (Arnaud, 1996). Lack of exercise, low dietary calcium intake, excess alcohol intake, and smoking are also factors that contribute to osteoporosis (Greenwood, 1996). Adequate dietary intake of calcium should begin early in young women to help increase maximum bone strength. The National Institutes of Health has recommended that adult women ages 25 to 50 should have 1000 mg, and those over age 50 should have 1500 mg, of calcium per day (Greenwood, p. 72).

As a person ages, the amount of skeletal muscle decreases and muscle cells are replaced by adipose and connective tissue. As a result of these changes, adults have decreased muscle tone, a flabbier appearance, and decreased muscle strength. Exercise will help maintain muscle tone and strength and increase calcium absorption. The adult can engage in a variety of activities and sports, but it is advised that individuals check with a physician before beginning any vigorous exercise routine. The adult should exercise consistently, gradually increasing the amount to avoid overexertion.

An example of how an adult undergoing the physical changes of middlescence can be affected by these changes is seen in the following case scenario.

CASE *Scenario*

Marge, a 50-year-old widow and mother of three daughters, ages 24, 27, and 30, is a typical example of how many people react to body changes during middlescence. When Marge's oldest daughter celebrated her thirtieth birthday she became concerned about her own "aging" process. She sought help at a local adult screening clinic because she perceived that the physical changes she was undergoing were making her look older than her chronological age. She wanted to maintain a youthful look and stated, "I am having a hard time getting old. I fear the physical changes and the dependency associated with aging."

Marge had an established career and had just recently developed an intimate relationship with a man that could lead to marriage. She was loved and respected by her children. Friends enjoyed being with her and described her as intellectually stimulating and fun. However, Marge could focus only on her physical changes and was experiencing anxiety in relation to them.

The community health nurse who saw Marge at the adult screening clinic made arrangements to visit her at home. Marge was helped to identify her strengths and to look more realistically at the changes in her appearance. The nurse discussed normal physical and emotional change associated with middlescence. Marge gradually began to realize that if she focused on her physical appearance alone, she could jeopardize some of the other joys in her life that provided self-fulfillment.

The physical changes of the aging process can be difficult to handle, and the community health nurse works with many adults who share Marge's concerns. Some adults may seek mental health counseling to assist them in adapting to the changes and demands of adulthood, and nurses can refer clients to appropriate community resources for help. The development of generativity, intimacy, and ego integrity helps an individual to adapt to physical changes associated with the aging process.

Even though physical functioning changes or decreases, mental functioning can be maintained or increased during adulthood. Cerebral capacity begins to weaken relatively slowly, unless other factors such as cerebrovascular occlusion or depression occur. General intelligence of the middlescent is often greater than at any other time of life.

SELECTED HEALTH RISKS AND CAUSES OF MORBIDITY AND MORTALITY AMONG ADULT MEN AND WOMEN

Many diseases and conditions of adults can be prevented with changes in lifestyle and are amenable to community health nursing intervention. Figure 17-1 portrays graphically the leading causes of death for adults. Heart disease and cancer were the two leading causes in 1993. Accidents, including motor-vehicle accidents, all other accidents, and adverse effects, were the third highest cause (CDC, 1996a, p. 161). This section discusses health risks, as well as major morbidity and mortality for men and women in adulthood.

Smoking and Health

One major risk factor for morbidity and mortality among adults is smoking. It was 1964 when Americans were first seriously presented with information that linked smoking and lung cancer. In that year the classic report of *Smoking and Health: Report of the Advisory Committee to the Surgeon*

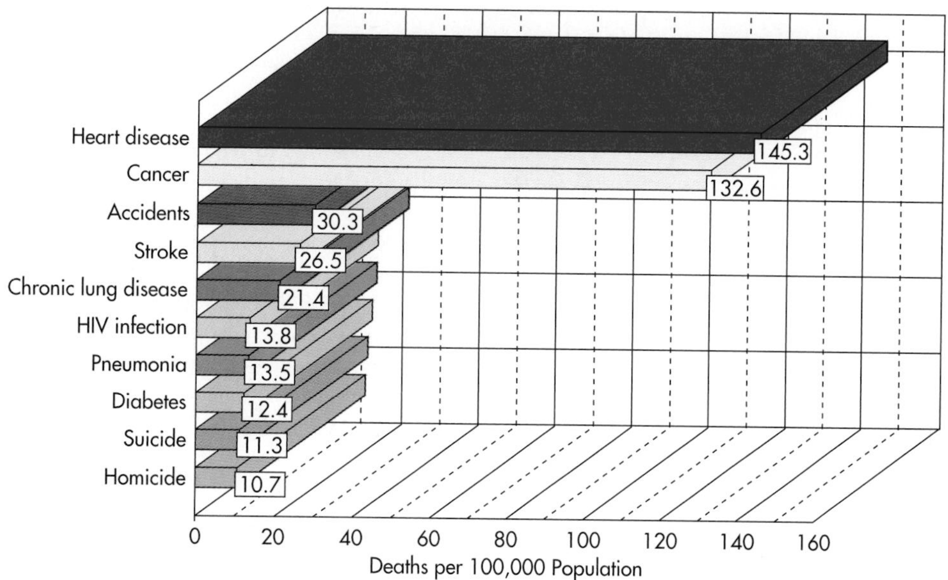

Figure 17-1 Leading causes of death, 1993, age-adjusted. *(Modified from CDC: Mortality patterns—United States, 1993, MMWR 45(8):162, March 1, 1996a.)*

General of the Public Health Service (USDHEW, 1964), often referred to as the *Surgeon General's Report on Smoking and Health*, was published. The report, prepared by an independent body of scientists approved by the Tobacco Institute and eight health organizations, reviewed more than 7000 studies and noted a causal relationship between cigarette smoking, lung cancer, and other serious diseases (USDHHS, 1989, p. viii). As a result, it was determined that remedial action was necessary to curtail cigarette smoking. Since that report every Surgeon General of the United States has promoted smoking cessation and has reinforced the knowledge that smoking is one of the most significant causes of disease and death.

Use of tobacco products is the single leading preventable cause of illness and premature death in the United States today (USDHHS, 1995a, p. 36). An estimated 46 million Americans smoke, and 14% of high school students are already frequent smokers (American Cancer Society, 1996a, p. 24). Smoking cessation becomes more difficult when the habit is developed early in life because of the nicotine tolerance that is built up through years of smoking (Henningfield, Schuh, 1996). Hence prevention efforts must target young adults before they ever begin smoking.

Congress has passed legislation that requires health warnings be printed on cigarette packages, cigarette advertising be banned in the broadcast media, and public awareness on the hazards of smoking be proliferated. The U.S. Public Health Service conducts research and regularly publishes reports on smoking and health. Radio and television advertisements for cigarettes are no longer allowed; programs and literature aimed at helping the smoker to stop smoking have been circulated; the rights of nonsmokers are being stressed; nonsmoking areas have been designated in many public places and on public transportation; smoking is banned on domestic airline flights and higher cigarette taxes have been levied. Many communities have adopted laws or regulations banning smoking in public places, such as worksites, or have restricted smoking to designated specific areas.

According to the World Health Organization 3 million people die worldwide each year as a result of smoking (ACS, 1996a, p. 24). Smoking is related to more than 400,000 U.S. deaths each year (ACS, 1996a, p. 24). In the U.S. smoking accounts for 30% of all cancer deaths, 90% of lung cancers among men, and 79% of lung cancers among women (ACS, 1996a, p. 21). Those who smoke two or more packs of cigarettes a day have a lung cancer mortality rate 12 to 25 times greater than that of nonsmokers (ACS, 1996a, p. 24).

Today the relationship between smoking and cardiovascular disease and lung cancer is well established. Smoking is a major risk factor linked to other diseases and cancers, including oral, laryngeal, esophageal, pancreatic, and urinary bladder cancer, respiratory problems, and some forms of cerebrovascular disease (Harris, 1996, p. 59). Smoking is a serious health risk in pregnancy and has been linked to retarded growth and fetal and neonatal death. Furthermore, and alarmingly, environmental tobacco smoke (including second-hand smoke) is linked to approximately 3000 lung cancer deaths each year among *nonsmokers* (USDHHS, 1995a, p. 36). Clearly, this demonstrates the need to create a smoke-free society. The former U.S. Surgeon General, C. Everett Koop, was the first prominent public official to advocate a smoke-free society by year 2000 (Glantz, 1996, p. 156). Creating a smoke-free society continues to be a primary concern with community health nurses and other public health professionals. Smoking prevention and smoking cessation is a major goal in the *Healthy People 2000* document.

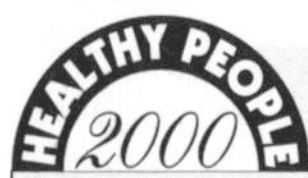

Tobacco: Focus Areas of Objectives

- Decrease tobacco-related coronary heart disease deaths.
- Decrease tobacco-related lung cancer deaths.
- Slow the rise in chronic obstructive pulmonary disease (COPD).
- Reduce the prevalence of cigarette smoking among all ages.
- Promote smoking cessation during pregnancy.
- Reduce the number of children regularly exposed to tobacco smoke.
- Reduce smokeless tobacco use.
- Establish tobacco-free environments.
- Include tobacco prevention in the school curricula.
- Promote worksite smoking policies.
- Enact state laws to prohibit smoking in workplaces and public places or limit it to designated areas.
- Enact and enforce state laws that prohibit distribution of tobacco products to youth younger than 18 years of age.
- Severely restrict all forms of tobacco product advertising targeting youth or to which youth younger than 18 are likely to be exposed.
- Encourage primary care providers to routinely explain smoking risks and promote smoking cessation.

Modified from USDHHS: *Healthy people 2000: national health promotion and disease prevention objectives, full report, with commentary*, Washington, D.C., 1991a, U.S. Government Printing Office, pp. 137-154.

HEALTHY PEOPLE 2000 AND SMOKING *Healthy People 2000* highlights the significance of smoking as a major health problem. Tobacco use is one of 22 priority areas in the *Healthy People 2000* document (USDHHS, 1991a). Numerous objectives address tobacco use. The accompanying box lists the focus areas of these objectives. Six core components of tobacco control are targeted: preventing tobacco use, treating nicotine addiction, protecting nonsmokers from exposure to environmental tobacco smoke, limiting the effect of tobacco advertising and promotion on young people, increasing the price of tobacco products, and regulating tobacco products (USDHHS, 1995a, p. 36). Each of these areas can guide community health nurses when they develop primary, secondary, and tertiary preventions to decrease tobacco use. Table 17-2 provides some examples of primary, secondary, and tertiary nursing interventions designed to address smoking cessation.

Overall, at midcourse review, smoking cessation has increased among the general public. Significant progress has been made in achieving all objectives except smoking cessation among pregnant women, high school seniors, and young people aged 20 to 24 (USDHHS, 1995a, p. 36). Smoking cessation among pregnant women and young adults has moved away from the *Healthy People 2000* target. Hence smoking cessation among high school youth and pregnant women are major areas targeted in *Healthy People 2000* revisions (USDHHS, 1995a, p. 36).

SMOKING AND PREGNANCY Smoking during pregnancy increases the risk of stillbirth, miscarriage, premature birth, and low birth weight infants (USDHHS, 1989, p. 19). There is evidence that heavy smoking (two or more packs per day) by pregnant women can cause serious birth defects such as mental retardation, facial anomalies, and heart defects. Infants born to women who smoked during pregnancy are more likely to die of sudden infant death syndrome (ACS, 1996a, p. 25). The effects of smoking endanger not only the health of the pregnant woman but also that of her fetus. Pregnant women must be taught about these risks and helped to understand the enormous responsibility they have toward the health of their unborn child. With the knowledge of these risks it is imperative that nurses make a concerted effort to work with pregnant women to prevent and cease smoking. Nurses must work diligently to achieve the *Healthy People 2000* objective to increase smoking cessation among pregnant women. Community health nurses can intervene at all levels of prevention by educating women about the risks of smoking during pregnancy and working with them to complete smoking cessation programs.

ENVIRONMENTAL TOBACCO SMOKE The Environmental Protection Agency (EPA) has stated that passive inhalation of smoke is a serious public health concern. This health problem is elaborated on in Chapter 6. About 3000 adult deaths each year have been attributed to nonsmokers breathing the smoke from other smokers (ACS, 1996a, p. 25). The box on the next page provides some additional facts about environmental tobacco smoke. Community health nurses must consider these facts when developing nursing interventions that promote a smoke-free society.

SMOKELESS TOBACCO Use of smokeless tobacco, such as snuff and chewing tobacco, is a health concern. About 5 million U.S. adults use smokeless tobacco (ACS, 1996a, p. 26). The use of smokeless tobacco is increasing among adolescent and young adult males—20% of male high school students use it (ACS, 1996a, p. 26). Although overall progress has been made toward the *Healthy People 2000* objective of reducing smokeless tobacco use among youth, it is still an area of focus to prevent movement away from the *Healthy People 2000* objective.

Smokeless tobacco has been linked to oral cancer. Annually there are 29,000 new cases of oral cancer and more than 8000 deaths (ACS, 1996a, p. 19). Teenagers as well as

table 17-2 Primary, Secondary, and Tertiary Preventive Nursing Interventions to Combat Tobacco Use

Prevention Level	Primary Prevention	Secondary Prevention	Tertiary Prevention
-Goal -Objective	-Smoke-Free Society -Don't Smoke/Use Tobacco	-Smoke-Free Society -Stop Smoking/Tobacco Use	-Smoke-Free Society -Avoid Relapse
Examples of Nursing Interventions	• Develop community public awareness programs to alert public to health problems associated with dangers of tobacco use and nicotine addiction. • Support state and community efforts that limit tobacco sales and restrict smoking to areas that would decrease effects of environmental tobacco smoke. • Provide tobacco use prevention education that is population and developmentally specific. • Advocate against products that are packaged to resemble tobacco products (e.g., bubble gum and candy), which may entice youth to experiment with tobacco use. • Provide health promotion education at schools and worksites that address the value of not smoking.	• Casefind to identify smokers in a selected population and refer smokers to a smoking cessation group in community. • Assess smoking-related health statistics in a select community, public areas in community, and worksites where nonsmokers are at risk for environmental tobacco smoke. • Collaborate with primary health care providers in local community to routinely screen, advocate smoking cessation, and assist with cessation measures. • Casefind by routinely questioning pregnant women about tobacco use and work with them to stop smoking. • Assess population to identify and eliminate risk behaviors related to smoking (such as peer pressure).	• Coordinate follow-up programs to prevent former smokers from relapse. • Collaborate with community providers to establish community support groups to help former tobacco users to successfully resist smoking/tobacco use. • Provide follow-up and self-help materials to encourage continued smoking cessation. • Assess smoking habits during routine health encounters to prevent former smokers from relapse.

adults are dying of oral cancers related to smokeless tobacco. All 50 states and the District of Columbia have enacted laws prohibiting the sale of tobacco products to youth under age 18. However, enforcement varies from state to state (USDHHS, 1995a, p. 37). Although the *Healthy People 2000* objective of enacting laws to prohibit sale of tobacco products to children is considered 100% achieved, it continues to be monitored.

The Comprehensive Smokeless Tobacco Education Act of 1986 (Public Law 99-252) established a program of public education to inform people of the health dangers of smokeless tobacco products. It supports educational programs, public service announcements, and research on the effects of smokeless tobacco on human health. It also regulates the advertising and labeling of smokeless tobacco products.

TOBACCO USE AND THE COMMUNITY HEALTH NURSE The ultimate goal in relation to tobacco use is to create a smoke-free society. Community health nurses can provide great influence toward developing a smoke-free society because they have easy access to populations at risk in communities and health care agencies. Nurses can intervene at all levels of prevention (see Table 17-2). The most effective

Facts About Environmental Tobacco Smoke (ETS)

- The risk of dying from lung cancer is 30% higher for a nonsmoker living with a smoker compared with a nonsmoker living in a smoke-free environment.
- Approximately 35,000 to 40,000 excess heart disease deaths among people who are not current smokers are caused by ETS.
- ETS contains essentially all of the same carcinogens and toxic agents that are inhaled by the smoker.
- ETS can result in aggravated asthmatic conditions, impaired blood circulation, bronchitis, and pneumonia.
- ETS poses additional health hazards for unborn and young children.
- Children born in secondhand smoke environments have increased risks of respiratory illness and infections, impaired development of lung function, and middle ear infections.
- Infants born to women who smoked during pregnancy are more likely to die of sudden infant death syndrome (SIDS).

Modified from American Cancer Society (ACS): *Cancer facts and figures—1996*, Atlanta, 1996a, ACS, p. 25. Reprinted by permission of the American Cancer Society.

intervention is primary prevention. Primary prevention is accomplished through awareness and education that instills in populations the health hazards of tobacco use and motivates them to avoid using tobacco products.

Secondary prevention is accomplished through identifying those at risk, those who are using tobacco products, and those who are addicted to nicotine (ACS, 1996a, p. 25). Secondary interventions focus on cessation of tobacco use and breaking the addiction. Guiding individuals through smoking cessation groups and educating regarding alternative activities to smoking (e.g., exercise, hobbies) is helpful.

Tertiary prevention focuses on helping persons to remain smokefree by preventing relapse. Chapter 12 discusses the principles used in breaking the cycle of addiction, which can include nicotine addiction. Similar to other drugs, cigarette smoking tends to be a progressive addiction. People do not start out with the intention of becoming addicted to tobacco but instead addiction develops gradually (Henningfield, Schuh, 1996, p. 114). Most people are capable of quitting smoking, but the key is to prevent relapse (Miller, 1996, p. 34). Tertiary prevention is perhaps the greatest challenge because smoking cessation relapse rates tend to be high (Henningfield, Schuh, 1996; Shiffman, 1993). In some cases nicotine replacement (such as gum or patch) is used to aid in immediate nicotine withdrawal, although results are mixed about the effectiveness of nicotine replacements (Miller, 1996). Tertiary prevention must focus on methods that prevent smoker relapse and help rehabilitated smokers to abstain from smoking. Often smokers who have undergone smoking cessation have a single episode of relapse, which engenders feelings of weakness and failure. It affects their self-confidence and ultimately may escalate into full-blown relapse (O'Connell, Gerkovich, Cook, 1995). This should be considered when nurses develop tertiary interventions. It is important to help former smokers realize that smoking cessation is a difficult process and that relapses should not be viewed as failures. Often involvement in support groups can help former smokers recognize the struggle with smoking cessation. Community health nurses must be aware of resources in the community. The American Lung Association is one example of an excellent community resource for smoking cessation.

AMERICAN LUNG ASSOCIATION The American Lung Association is one of the oldest private, voluntary health agencies in the United States. Its mission is to prevent and control lung disease. The association provides numerous classes and publications on smoking, smoking cessation, and lung cancer. The nurse can obtain many useful teaching tools and resources from the association. The association has state affiliates all over the country and thousands of local offices.

Gender Influences on Health

As discussed in Chapter 11, personal factors, including gender, age, race, socioeconomic status, stress, lifestyle, and health behavior, influence the epidemiology of disease occurrence and resolution. Of these factors, gender has frequently been neglected in health care practice and research. There is, however, a growing recognition that the differences in women and men produce unique health risks and needs that often require special health planning and programming. Much of the research done in the past has used male subjects. Recently the Women's Health Initiative Project, started in 1991 by the National Institutes of Health, brought about a focus on women's issues and is providing valuable data that can facilitate health planning for women. Additionally, *women's health* has emerged as a specialty focus for practitioners.

Health status statistics demonstrate that mortality and morbidity risks of females and males differ. In America women live longer than men. The life expectancy for women in the United States has been continuously higher than that of men since before 1900. In 1993 life expectancy at birth was 78.8 years for women, 6.6 years longer than that for men (National Center for Health Statistics, 1996, p. 17).

Socioeconomic status (SES) and lifestyle patterns have a great influence on the overall life expectancy of both men and women (Dennerstein, 1995, p.56). Genetic and biological forces also have a significant impact on certain disease-specific mortality rates according to gender and race (e.g. cancer of prostate, uterine cancer, and sickle-cell anemia).

In general, women have a higher prevalence of chronic conditions than men. For example, arthritis is more prevalent among women than men, and women experience more limitations from arthritis than men (National Center for Health Statistics, 1996, p. 29). Conversely, men have a higher incidence of Parkinson's disease (LeMone, Burke, 1996, p. 1825). Gender differences related to selected other chronic conditions are discussed throughout this chapter.

Women also have issues that arise from their gender and roles in society such as childbirth, menstruation, and menopause. Previously seen as "diseases," these conditions are now viewed as part of the normal female physiological processes. Historically, women were treated differently and more apt to be mislabeled with a mental disorder than men (Cowan, 1996). The pain of labor, nausea in pregnancy, and menopausal changes are no longer dismissed as psychogenic. As data emerge from research on women's health issues new light is continuously being shed on many previously mislabeled "problems" or "diseases" of women.

The Jacob Institute of Women's Health (4409 12th Street SW, Washington, D.C. 20024-2188) is an organization committed to excellence in women's health care. The Institute publishes *The Women's Health Data Book: A Profile of Women's Health in the United States*, which compiles in a single publication much of the available national data on the issues central to understanding women's health (Horton, 1995). It is highly readable and informative.

Men also have health issues that arise from their gender and their roles in society. Death rates among men from accidents, homicides, and suicides are much higher than those of women (National Center for Health Statistics, 1996, p. 18). However, women are more often the victims of domestic violence than men. Violence, including domestic violence, is discussed in Chapter 12. AIDS is a disease that at first was more prevalent among men, but its prevalence is increasing among women. AIDS is also discussed in Chapter 12.

Women and men in our culture are frequently taught that certain roles and traits are not "gender" acceptable. Nurses need to understand how gender affects the incidence and prevalence of diseases and conditions, as well as their treatments. Gender bias may exist within the caregiver or client role and may interfere with therapeutic relationships and treatments (Hawthorne, 1994, p. 79). Nurses must be aware of their own gender biases, remain sensitive to gender issues, and confront those issues as they arise.

Cardiovascular Disease

Cardiovascular diseases are the number one killer in America (American Heart Association, 1995c). They are among the leading causes of disability and have modifiable risk factors, which include diabetes, hypertension, elevated blood cholesterol, cigarette smoking, obesity, and physical inactivity (USDHHS, 1995a). Prevention and control of heart disease and stroke is a priority area in the *Healthy People 2000* document. Several health objectives address this goal.

Cardiovascular diseases kill almost one million Americans each year—close to one person every 33 seconds (AHA, 1994, p. 1). If statistics hold true, close to one in two Americans will die of cardiovascular disease. Since 1900, in the United States cardiovascular disease has been the number one killer disease every year except 1918 (AHA, p. 1).

The accompanying box lists the risk factors associated with heart disease and stroke. Americans are becoming increasingly aware of these risk factors. Major risk factors that cannot be changed include heredity, age, and sex (presently American men are at greater risk of experiencing a heart attack than women). Other risk factors can be alleviated through changes in behaviors, habits, and lifestyle.

With all cardiovascular diseases community health nurses should fervently focus on primary prevention activities by attending to modifiable risk factors. Community health nurses promote increased awareness of cardiovascular risk factors and interventions to decrease them, encourage clients to have regular medical supervision, and inform them of available community resources. The health education activities of the nurse in this area cannot be overestimated. Americans have remarkable knowledge gaps about how to protect themselves against the disease that is most likely to kill them (USDHHS, 1995a). The accompanying box provides some examples of nursing interventions that focus on preventing cardiovascular diseases.

Risk Factors Associated with Heart Disease and Stroke

- Smoking
- Elevated blood cholesterol
- High blood pressure
- Physical inactivity
- Diabetes
- Obesity
- Stress
- Heredity
- Sex (male)
- Age

Modified from USDHS: *Facts about blood cholesterol*, NIH Pub No. 94-2694, Bestheda, Md., 1994, U.S. Government Printing Office, pp. 1-2.

Examples of Community Health Nursing Interventions to Prevent Cardiovascular Disease in Adults

EDUCATE CLIENTS ABOUT:

- Cardiovascular risk factors
- Stroke risk factors
- Signs of heart attack and stroke
- Benefits of regular exercise
- Role of nutrition in cardiovascular disease
- Role of stress and cardiovascular disease

CASEFIND BY:

- Hypertension screening
- Cholesterol screening
- Stress assessment
- Nutrition and weight assessment
- Assessing familial histories for cardiovascular diseases
- Assessing worksite populations to identify workers at risk

COLLABORATE WITH COMMUNITY HEALTH PROVIDERS AND CLIENTS TO DEVELOP:

- Smoking cessation groups
- Worksite exercise, smoking cessation, blood pressure, and stress management programs
- Referral resources for adults at risk
- Aggregate exercise and weight reduction programs

HEART DISEASE Heart disease is the number one cause of death in America. The leading cause of death from heart disease is heart attacks. Although the death rate from heart attacks has dropped significantly in the last decade, more than 1.5 million Americans suffer heart attacks each year, about one third will die from them, and about 250,000 will die within 1 hour of the onset of symptoms (AHA, 1994, p. 9).

The American Heart Association's (AHA) warning signals of heart attack are in the box on the next page. The AHA notes that not all these warning signs occur in every heart attack, and if any of these begin, the person should not wait, but seek help immediately. About half of all heart

American Heart Association: Warning Signs of Heart Attack

- Uncomfortable pressure, fullness, squeezing, or pain in the center of the chest lasting more than a few minutes
- Pain that spreads to the shoulders, neck, or arms
- Chest discomfort with lightheadedness, fainting, sweating, nausea, or shortness of breath

From American Heart Association (AHA): *Heart attack and stroke: signals and action*, Dallas, 1996, AHA, p. 4. Reproduced with permission. *Heart attack and stroke: signals and action*, 1989, 1992, 1994. Copyright American Heart Association.

attack victims wait 2 hours or longer before deciding to get help. This greatly reduces their likelihood of survival because most heart attack victims who die do so within 2 hours of the first awareness of symptoms (AHA, 1994, p. 9).

The risk of smokers having a heart attack is more than twice that of nonsmokers, and smokers' risk for sudden cardiac death is two to four times the risk of nonsmokers (AHA, 1995b, p. 19). Smoking is the greatest risk factor for peripheral vascular disease and environmental tobacco smoke increases death risk of nonsmokers. (AHA, 1995b, p. 19). It is important to promote nonsmoking and a smoke-free society. Regardless of how long persons have smoked, their risk of heart disease declines rapidly when they stop smoking (AHA, p. 20).

Coronary heart disease and heart attacks are much more frequent in those who are inactive than in people who are active. Elevated serum cholesterol levels put one at risk for developing cardiovascular disease. Regular exercise can have a significant impact on reducing the risk of heart attacks and disease.

Community health nurses can be instrumental in reducing the morbidity and mortality from heart attacks through interventions that focus on primary and secondary prevention. Community health nurses can educate people about the risk factors and warning signals of heart attacks, develop risk modification programs, teach families cardiopulmonary resuscitation, and familiarize them with emergency community resources. Educating adults and families regarding the importance of immediate action when a heart attack is suspected is critical to reduce the risk of mortality. For successful risk modification (e.g., activity, nutrition counseling, and hypertension control), interventions must include awareness of personal barriers to risk modification and strategies for motivating people to change lifestyle behaviors (Biggs, Fleury, 1996). Interventions that focus on prevention and early intervention are crucial to reducing the morbidity and mortality from heart attacks.

STROKES As previously noted in Figure 17-1, strokes rank fourth among all causes of death in the United States. Annually more than 500,000 Americans suffer a stroke (AHA, 1994, p. 11). Strokes are a major cause of serious disability, and more than half of all stroke survivors need some type of assistance to manage daily activities (AHA, p. 11).

Many stroke victims are disabled by paralysis and suffer resultant speech/language and memory deficits. Frequently early signs and warnings are ignored, and as a result the stroke takes a higher toll. Often a stroke can be prevented by heeding early warning signs and seeking early treatment. The box on the next page lists the early warning signs of a stroke. Community health nurses have an important role in health promotion by educating people about the signs of a stroke and encouraging early intervention.

Through all levels of prevention community health nurses can do much to decrease morbidity and mortality through health education activities about risk factor reduction, behavior modification, and rehabilitation services. The long-term rehabilitation needs of persons with stroke can cause great emotional and psychological distress for both client and family. When strokes occur, the community health nurse can be instrumental in helping the family work through the adaptation and rehabilitation process and assist in community resource referral, coordination, and utilization.

HYPERTENSION Hypertension is a risk factor for heart attack and stroke. More than 50 million Americans have hypertension. In 1993 high blood pressure killed 37,520 Americans and contributed to the deaths of thousands more (AHA, 1995a, p. 4). These statistics are not surprising, since more than a third of people who have high blood pressure do not know they have it; more than half of all clients who are hypertensive are not on treatment; about 27% are on inadequate therapy; and only about 21% are on adequate therapy (AHA, 1995a, p. 4). Table 17-3 shows the normal and abnormal blood pressure categories for adults age 18 and older.

High blood pressure is easy to detect, and through appropriate management easy to control. Controlling high blood pressure has been shown to be one of the most effective means available for reducing mortality in the adult population. Community health nurses have a major role in prevention and control through teaching, early detection and screening activities, risk modification programs, referral for medical treatment, and facilitating clients in complying with treatment regimens. Table 17-4 provides some general guidelines for hypertension screening and referral.

AMERICAN HEART ASSOCIATION The AHA is the leading voluntary, national agency actively involved in cardiovascular education, treatment, and research. The association was founded in 1924, and its mission is to reduce disability and death from cardiovascular diseases and stroke. It is actively engaged in research and has more than 2250 local affiliates in all 50 states. Since 1949 the association has invested more than $1.4 billion in cardiovascular research (AHA, 1995c, p. 1). The AHA offers classes, publications, and numerous services to the general public. Nurses can use the

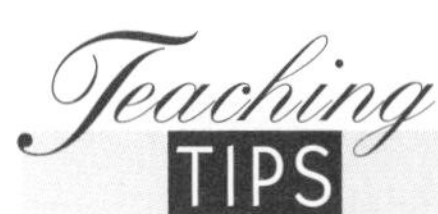

Heart-Healthy Cooking

The way you cook is just as important as what you cook. Discuss your current cooking habits with your nurse or dietitian. Set goals for the future.

WHEN I COOK I WILL:

1. **Trim** the fat from meat before cooking it.
2. **Remove** the skin and fat before cooking chicken or turkey.
3. **Bake,** roast, grill, broil, or boil foods instead of frying.
4. **Place** meat on a rack to roast so the fat drips off.
5. **Brown** ground meat and drain off the fat before adding it to a recipe.
6. **Use** a nonstick pan and a small amount of cooking spray, oil, or margarine if frying.
7. **Use** fat-free ingredients such as wine, tomato juice, lemon juice, or bouillon to baste meats and poultry.
8. **Use** defatted beef or chicken broth to make gravy.
9. **Cool** sauces or soups in the refrigerator and skim off the fat.
10. **Substitute** low-fat ingredients for high-fat ingredients in recipes using the table below.
11. **Add** pasta, rice, dry peas, or beans to main dishes and decrease the meat.
12. **Use** small amounts of lean meats, herbs, or flavored seasoning (such as Butter Buds) to flavor vegetables, rather than fatback, saltpork, or butter.
13. **Make** large batches of foods and freeze meal-sized portions if you live alone. Supplement with fruit, vegetables, and breads.

RECIPE INGREDIENT	SUBSTITUTION
Whole milk, light cream	Skim or 1% milk
Evaporated milk	Evaporated skim milk
1 whole egg	¼ cup egg substitute or 2 egg whites
1 cup butter	1 cup margarine or ⅔ cup vegetable oil
Shortening	Margarine
Mayonnaise or salad dressing	Nonfat or light varieties
Cheese	Low-fat or fat-free cheese
Sour cream	Nonfat or low-fat sour cream or yogurt
1 square unsweetened baking chocolate	3 tbsp. cocoa powder and 1 tbsp. oil or margarine
Fat for "greasing" the pan	Nonstick cooking spray

From Martin KS, Larson BJ, Gorski LA, Hayko DM, eds: *Mosby's home health client teaching guides: R_x for teaching*, St. Louis, 1997, Mosby, p. V-A-1-9.

SIGNS OF STROKE

- Sudden weakness or numbness of the face, arm, or leg on one side of the body.
- Sudden dimness or loss of vision, particularly in one eye.
- Loss of speech, or trouble talking or understanding speech.
- Sudden, severe headaches with no apparent cause.
- Unexplained dizziness, unsteadiness, or sudden falls, especially along with any of the previous symptoms.

From American Heart Association (AHA): *Heart attack and stroke: signals and action*, Dallas, 1996, AHA, p. 8. Reproduced with permission. *Heart attack and stroke: signals and action*, 1989, 1992, 1994. Copyright American Heart Association.

association as a resource for developing health promotion activities.

Cancer

Cancer is the leading cause of death in men and women ages 25 through 64 and is associated with a variety of risk factors. The financial costs of cancer are enormous. The National Cancer Institute estimates the yearly costs for cancer at $104 billion (ACS, 1996a, p. 5). However, dollars cannot begin to measure the toll cancer takes on human suffering and mortality. Although cancer mortality rates have not changed significantly over time, there have been changes in mortality for some age groups and for some types of cancers. Mortality could be significantly reduced by reducing risk factors. Smoking is a primary risk factor that accounts for 30% of all cancer deaths (USDHHS, 1995a, p. 36). By eliminating one single risk factor, such as smoking, the cancer incidence and mortality rates could be significantly reduced! Other risk factors can also make a difference in the incidence of cancer. Table 17-5 presents the risk factors associated with cancer at the primary and secondary levels of prevention. Community health nurses have a key role in developing interventions to reduce these risk factors.

The box on page 520 presents selected epidemiological data about the five leading cancers of concern to adult men

table 17-3 Classification of Blood Pressure for Adults Age 18 Years and Older*

Category	Systolic (mm Hg)	Diastolic (mm Hg)
Normal†	<130	<85
High normal	130-139	85-89
Hypertension‡		
Stage 1 (mild)	140-159	90-99
Stage 2 (Moderate)	160-179	100-109
Stage 3 (Severe)	180-209	110-119
Stage 4 (Very Severe)	≥210	≥120

From U.S. Department of Health and Human Services (USDHHS): *The fifth report of the joint national committee on detection, evaluation, and treatment of high blood pressure*, NIH Pub No. 95-1088, Bethesda, Md., 1995b, Public Health Service, p. 4.

**Not taking antihypertensive drugs and not acutely ill. When systolic and diastolic fall into different categories, the higher category should be selected to classify the individual's blood pressure status. For instance, 160/92 mm Hg should be classified as stage 2, and 180/120 mm Hg should be classified as stage 4. Isolated systolic hypertension (ISH) is defined as SBP ≥140 mm Hg and DBP <90 mm Hg and staged appropriately (e.g., 170/85 mm Hg is defined as stage 2 ISH).*

†Optimal blood pressure with respect to cardiovascular risk is SBP <120 mm Hg and DBP <80 mm Hg. However, unusually low readings should be evaluated for clinical significance.

‡Based on the average of two or more readings taken at each of two or more visits following an initial screening.

Note: In addition to classifying stages of hypertension based on average blood pressure levels, the clinician should specify presence or absence of target-organ disease and additional risk factors. For example, a patient with diabetes and a blood pressure of 142/94 mm Hg plus left ventricular hypertrophy should be classified as "stage 1 hypertension with target-organ disease (left ventricular hypertrophy) and with another major risk factor (diabetes)." This specificity is important for risk classification and management.

table 17-4 Recommendations for Follow-up Based on Initial Set of Blood Pressure Measurements for Adults Age 18 and Older

Initial Screening Blood Pressure (mm Hg)*		
Systolic	**Diastolic**	**Follow-up Recommended†**
<130	<85	Recheck in 2 years
130-139	85-89	Recheck in 1 year‡
140-159	90-99	Confirm within 2 months
160-179	100-109	Evaluate or refer to source of care within 1 month
180-209	110-119	Evaluate or refer to source of care within 1 week
≥210	≥120	Evaluate or refer to source of care immediately

From U.S. Department of Health and Human Services (USDHHS): *The fifth report of the joint national committee on detection, evaluation, and treatment of high blood pressure*, NIH Pub No. 95-1088, Bethesda, Md., 1995b, Public Health Service, p. 6.

**If the systolic and diastolic are different, follow recommendation for the shorter time follow-up (e.g., 160/85 mm Hg should be evaluated or referred to source of care within 1 month).*

†The scheduling of follow-up should be modified by reliable information about past blood pressure measurements, other cardiovascular risk factors, or target-organ disease.

‡Consider providing advice about lifestyle modifications.

and women. Overall, cancer incidence and mortality rates are generally higher for blacks than for whites (ACS, 1996a, p. 20). Incidence and mortality for cancers of the lung, female breast, colon, and rectum are lower among Native Americans, Asian and Pacific Islanders, and Hispanics than for whites (ACS, 1996a, p. 20).

Cancer disproportionately strikes minority groups. A report, by the U.S. Public Health Service, *Health Status of Minorities and Low-Income Groups*, found wide gaps in cancer death rates between minorities and whites (USDHHS, 1991b). Comparisons in relation to cancer incidence and ethnicity revealed the following data related to minority health when compared to whites: Japanese living in the United States have a higher incidence of stomach cancer; Chinese living in the United States have a higher incidence of cervical and stomach cancers; Hawaiians have a higher incidence of lung and stomach cancers and the highest rate of breast cancer; Native Americans have higher rates of gallbladder, stomach, and cervical cancers; and blacks have a higher rate of lung cancer.

Differences in survival rates and mortality among ethnic groups are illustrated in Tables 17-6 and 17-7. Table 17-6 shows cancer deaths, by race, for the 10 leading causes of cancer. Table 17-7 portrays the trends in cancer survival by race and cancer sites. Varying lifestyles, including nutritional patterns among ethnic groups, screening behaviors, values and belief systems, socioeconomic status, lack of insurance, and lack of access to health services are all associated with cancer risks and may provide some explanation for the differences in health care utilization and cancer mortality among various ethnic populations (ACS, 1996a, p. 20).

Gender differences also become evident when examining mortality and survival rates for many cancers. Figure 17-2 shows the 1996 estimates of new cancer cases and deaths by site and sex. It is encouraging to note that the survival rates for many cancers, with the exception of lung cancer, are increasing. Although skin cancer has the

table 17-5 Cancer Prevention: Risk Factors Associated with Cancer

Risk Factor	Risk and Prevention Information
Alcohol	Oral cancer and cancers of the larynx, throat, esophagus, and liver occur more frequently among heavy drinkers of alcohol, especially when accompanied by smoking cigarettes or chewing tobacco.
Smokeless tobacco	Use of chewing tobacco or snuff increases risk of cancer of the mouth, larynx, throat, and esophagus and is a highly addictive habit.
Estrogen	Estrogen treatment to control menopausal symptoms can increase risk of endometrial cancer. However, including progesterone in estrogen replacement therapy helps to minimize this risk. Consultation with a physician will help each woman to assess personal risks and benefits. Continued research is needed in the area of estrogen use and breast cancer.
Occupational hazards	Exposure to several different industrial agents (nickel, chromate, asbestos, vinyl chloride, etc.) increases risk of various cancers. Risk of lung cancer from asbestos is greatly increased when combined with cigarette smoking.
Smoking	Cigarette smoking is responsible for 90% of lung cancer cases among men and 79% among women—about 87% overall. Smoking accounts for about 30% of all cancer deaths. Those who smoke two or more packs of cigarettes a day have lung cancer mortality rates 12 to 25 times greater than nonsmokers.
Sunlight	Almost all of the more than 800,000 cases of basal and squamous cell skin cancer diagnosed each year in the U.S. are sun-related (ultraviolet radiation). Epidemiological evidence shows that sun exposure is a major factor in the development of melanoma and that incidence increases for those living near the equator.
Ionizing radiation	Excessive exposure to ionizing radiation can increase cancer risk. Most medical and dental x-rays are adjusted to deliver the lowest dose possible without sacrificing image quality. Excessive radon exposure in homes may increase risk of lung cancer, especially in cigarette smokers. If levels are found to be too high, remedial actions should be taken.
Nutrition and diet	Research is showing the important role nutrition plays in preventing cancer. Evidence indicates that people may reduce their cancer risk by observing these nutrition guidelines: 1. **Maintain desirable weight.** Individuals 40% or more overweight increase their risk of colon, breast, prostate, gallbladder, ovary, and uterus cancers. Weight maintenance can be accomplished by reducing total caloric intake and adopting a physically active lifestyle. 2. **Eat a varied diet.** A varied diet eaten in moderation offers the best hope for lowering the risk of cancer. 3. **Include a variety of vegetables and fruits in the daily diet.** Studies have shown that daily consumption of vegetables and fresh fruits is associated with a decreased risk of lung, prostate, bladder, esophagus, colorectal, and stomach cancers. 4. **Eat more high-fiber foods such as whole grain cereals, breads, and pasta, vegetables, and fruits.** High-fiber diets are a healthy substitute for fatty foods and may reduce the risk of colon cancer. 5. **Cut down on total fat intake.** A diet high in fat may be a factor in the development of certain cancers, particularly breast, colon, and prostate. The American Cancer Society recommends reducing total fat intake to 30% or less of total caloric intake. 6. **Limit consumption of alcohol, if you drink at all.** The heavy use of alcohol, especially when accompanied by cigarette smoking or smokeless tobacco use, increases the risk of cancers of the mouth, larynx, throat, esophagus, and liver. 7. **Limit consumption of salt-cured, smoked, and nitrite-cured foods.** In areas of the world where salt-cured and smoked foods are eaten frequently, there is higher incidence of cancer of the esophagus and stomach. Modern methods of food processing and preserving appear to avoid the cancer-causing by-products associated with older methods of food treatment.

Modified from American Cancer Society (ACS): *Cancer facts and figures—1996*, Atlanta, 1996a, ACS, pp. 21-22.
Reprinted by permission of American Cancer Society.

highest incidence it is amenable to prevention and treatment and does not carry a high mortality rate. Lung cancer and colon/rectum cancer carry relatively high mortality rates. Lung cancer now rivals breast cancer as the leading cause of cancer death in American women (ACS, 1996a, p. 10). Unfortunately, diagnostic procedures such as chest x-ray films and sputum examinations usually do not reveal lung cancer until it has already spread. In adult men, 90% of all lung cancer deaths have a direct relationship to smoking (ACS, 1996a, p. 21). Fortunately several effective screening procedures are now available to detect breast cancer and cancers of the colon or rectum. For example, women can do regular self-examination of the breasts (Figure 17-3) and can have a physical examination and mammography.

Five Leading Cancers of Concern for Adult Men and Women

1. ***Lung cancer*** is the most common and most preventable cancer. There were an estimated 158,700 deaths in 1996 from lung cancer. Cigarette smoking is by far the most important risk factor in the development of lung cancer. The incidence of lung cancer has declined slightly among men but is continuing to increase among women. Early detection is crucial and often difficult because symptoms do not appear until the disease has advanced. Symptoms include persistent cough, sputum streaked with blood, chest pain, and recurring pneumonia or bronchitis. Survival rate is increased greatly with early detection and treatment.
2. ***Colorectal cancer*** is the second leading cause of cancer deaths among men and women. There were approximately 133,500 new cases in 1996. Overall there has been a decrease in colorectal cancer in recent years. The incidence is higher among men than women. The primary risk factors include personal or family history of colorectal cancer or polyps, inflammatory bowel disease, physical inactivity, and high fat and/or low-fiber diet. Some recent studies have shown that estrogen replacement therapy and non-steroidal antiinflammatory drugs may reduce colorectal cancer risk. Symptoms include rectal bleeding, blood in stool, diarrhea, or a change in bowel habits. With early detection it is possible to have a survival rate as high as 91%.
3. ***Breast cancer*** is the second leading cause of cancer death among women with an estimated 44,560 deaths in 1996 (44,300 women, 260 men). Since 1987 the incidence of breast cancer has leveled off, and this is thought to be due to the increase in early detection methods (i.e., mammography) before cancer has spread. Risk factors include age, family history of breast cancer, some forms of benign breast disease, early menarche, extended use of estrogen, never having children or having first child late in life, and socioeconomic status. Symptoms may include mammography changes, breast changes such as lump, thickening, swelling, dimpling, skin irritation, distortion, retraction, scaliness, pain, tenderness of the nipple, or nipple discharge. Survival rate may be as high as 96% with early detection. Survival rate decreases with cancer metastases. ACS recommends mammography for asymptomatic women ages 40 to 49 every 1 to 2 years and yearly beginning age 50; clinical breast exam every 3 years for women 20 to 40 years of age, and yearly beginning age 40; and monthly self-exams by all women 20 years or older.
4. ***Prostate cancer*** is the second leading cause of cancer death in men, with an estimated 41,400 deaths in 1996. The incidence is almost two times higher among black men than white men. Between 1980 and 1990 there was a dramatic increase in the incidence of prostate cancer, which is thought to be due to improved methods of detection. Primary risk factors include age (over 80% are diagnosed in men over age 65), family history of prostate cancer, and racially black. Early detection and treatment of cancer in localized stage may result in survival rate as high as 98%! ACS recommends every man over age 40 should have digital rectal exam annually as part of a regular physical exam; beginning age 50 every man should have prostate-specific antigen blood test annually; and a transurethral ultrasound if either test is suspicious.
5. ***Cervical cancer*** has decreased steadily over the past two decades largely due to use of the Pap test and improved methods of detection. There were an estimated 4900 deaths from cervical cancer in 1996. The mortality rate is more than two times higher in blacks than whites. Risk factors include sexual practices, history of sexually transmitted diseases, women who have intercourse at early age, multiple sexual partners, cigarette smoking, and socioeconomic status. Early detection and treatment of localized cancer can have a 91% survival rate. ACS recommends a Pap test with pelvic exam annually for all women who are, or have been, sexually active or are age 18 or older.

Modified from American Cancer Society: *Cancer facts and figures—1996*, Atlanta, 1996a, ACS, pp. 10-14. Reprinted by permission of American Cancer Society.

Community health nurses have an important educative role in teaching people about risk factors, providing nursing care, and assisting families in utilizing community resources. Using the principles of crisis intervention and grieving, as discussed in Chapter 8, the nurse can facilitate family coping and adjustment. If the need for hospice care arises, the nurse can make appropriate referrals to available resources (hospice care is discussed in Chapter 21). Many nurses are providing hospice care and are developing new hospice programs around the country. Hospice services are also provided by many home health care agencies, which provide a range of home care services.

NATIONAL CANCER INSTITUTE The National Cancer Institute is the federal government's chief source of cancer information, education, and research. This Institute has numerous publications, including pamphlets on different types of cancer and supportive care for cancer victims such as *Taking Time: Support for People with Cancer and the People Who Care about Them*. *Taking Time* is an excellent resource for nurses to share with families. It covers topics including sharing the diagnosis, sharing feelings, coping within the family, assistance in obtaining equipment and/or supplies, self-image, the world outside, living each day, and resources.

By dialing 1-800-4-CANCER (1-800-638-6070 in Alaska) one can access the Cancer Information Service of the National Cancer Institute. This service provides information on community agencies and services, answers questions, and provides publications and a publication list for different types of cancer. It also provides information about active treatment centers for specific types of cancer.

The National Cancer Institute has developed the PDQ (Physician Data Query), a computerized data base designed

table 17-6 Reported Cancer Deaths, 10 Leading Causes of Cancer Death, and Percent of Total Cancer Deaths, by Race, U.S., 1992

	White	African American	Native American*,†	Asian & Pacific Islander†	Hispanic‡
	All Sites 454,516 (100%)	All Sites 58,401 (100%)	All Sites 1,473 (100%)	All Sites 6,173 (100%)	All Sites 15,218 (100%)
1	Lung 128,704 (28.3%)	Lung 15,472 (26.5%)	Lung 381 (25.9%)	Lung 1,371 (22.2%)	Lung 2,674 (17.6%)
2	Colon & Rectum 50,516 (11.1%)	Colon & Rectum 6,073 (10.4%)	Colon & Rectum 119 (8.1%)	Colon & Rectum 668 (10.8%)	Colon & Rectum 1,466 (9.6%)
3	Female Breast 37,797 (8.3%)	Prostate 5,485 (9.4%)	Female Breast 105 (7.1%)	Liver & Other Biliary 653 (10.6%)	Female Breast 1,297 (8.5%)
4	Prostate 28,430 (6.3%)	Female Breast 4,779 (8.2%)	Liver & Other Biliary 87 (5.9%)	Stomach 523 (8.5%)	Liver & Other Biliary 913 (6.0%)
5	Pancreas 22,519 (5.0%)	Pancreas 3,180 (5.4%)	Prostate 87 (5.9%)	Female Breast 387 (6.3%)	Stomach 885 (5.8%)
6	Lymphoma 20,074 (4.4%)	Stomach 2,213 (3.8%)	Stomach 67 (4.5%)	Pancreas 309 (5.0%)	Prostate 873 (5.7%)
7	Leukemia 17,405 (3.8%)	Esophagus 1,897 (3.2%)	Pancreas 63 (4.3%)	Lymphoma 263 (4.3%)	Lymphoma 851 (5.6%)
8	Ovary 12,142 (2.7%)	Leukemia 1,587 (2.7%)	Leukemia 55 (3.7%)	Prostate 238 (3.9%)	Pancreas 850 (5.6%)
9	Liver & Other Biliary 11,283 (2.5%)	Multiple Myeloma 1,543 (2.6%)	Kidney 53 (3.6%)	Leukemia 225 (3.6%)	Leukemia 739 (4.9%)
10	Brain & CNS 11,132 (2.4%)	Liver & Other Biliary 1,476 (2.5%)	Ovary 41 (2.8%)	Oral Cavity 156 (2.5%)	Ovary 454 (3.0%)

From American Cancer Society (ACS): *Cancer facts and figures—1996*, Atlanta, 1996a, ACS, p. 20. Reprinted by permission of American Cancer Society.

Note: Since each column includes only the top 10 cancer sites, site-specific numbers and percentages do not add up to the All Sites totals.

*Includes American Indians and Native Alaskans.

†Numbers are likely to be underestimates due to underreporting of Asian, Pacific Islander, and Native American race on death certificates.

‡Persons classified as of Hispanic origin on death certificates may be of any race. Hispanic origin is reported for all states except New Hampshire and Oklahoma. In 1990, the 48 states from which data were collected accounted for about 99.6% of the Hispanic population in the United States.

to give quick and easy access to the latest treatment information for most types of cancer, descriptions of clinical trials that are open for patient entry, and the names of organizations and physicians involved in cancer care (National Cancer Institute, 1989, p. 11). Patients can call 1-800-4-CANCER to get PDQ information.

AMERICAN CANCER SOCIETY The American Cancer Society is at the forefront of private sector cancer education and research in the United States. It is the largest private source of cancer research funds in the United States and is one of the largest voluntary health agencies in the country today, with more than 3400 local chapters. It traces its origins to 1913, when the American Society for the Control of Cancer was founded to disseminate knowledge concerning the symptoms, treatment, and prevention of cancer; to investigate conditions under which cancer occurs; and to compile statistics on cancer (ACS, 1996a, p. 26). The increased survival rates for many types of cancer may be a result of the support and funding of cancer research by the ACS. In 1946, when the ACS provided its first research grant, only one in four cancer patients was alive 5 years after diagnosis. Today about 50% of newly diagnosed cancer patients are alive 5 years later (ACS, 1996b, p. 3).

The American Cancer Society's public education programs and publications reach millions of Americans each year. The society is involved in professional education, publishes *Cancer Nursing News* (sent to about 90,000 nurses around the country), supports professorships in clinical oncology, and offers clinical oncology awards. The ACS's service and rehabilitation activities include the following resource and information services: *CanSurmount*—a short-term home visitor program for patients and their families; *Reach to Recovery*—a patient visitor program that addresses the needs of women who have had breast cancer; *Man to Man*—a group program that provides information about prostate cancer and related issues; *Look Good . . . Feel Better*—a program designed to teach women cancer patients beauty techniques to help restore their appearance

table 17-7 Trends in Cancer Survival by Race

Cases Diagnosed in 1960-63, 1970-73, 1974-76, 1980-82, 1986-91

	White Relative 5-Year Survival Rate (Percent)					Black Relative 5-Year Survival Rate (Percent)				
Site	1960-63[1]	1970-73[1]	1974-76[2]	1980-82[2]	1986-91[2]	1960-63[1]	1970-73[1]	1974-76[2]	1980-82[2]	1986-91[2]
All sites	39	43	50	52	58*	27	31	39	40	42*
Oral cavity & pharynx	45	43	55	55	55	—	—	36	31	33
Esophagus	4	4	5	7	11*	1	4	4	5	7*
Stomach	11	13	15	16	19*	8	13	16	19	20
Colon	43	49	50	56	62*	34	37	45	49	53*
Rectum	38	45	49	53	60*	27	30	42	38	52*
Liver	—	—	4	4	6*	—	—	1	2	5*
Pancreas	1	2	3	3	3*	1	2	3	5	5*
Larynx	53	62	66	69	68	—	—	58	59	52
Lung & bronchus	8	10	12	14	14*	5	7	11	12	11
Melanoma of skin	60	68	80	83	87*	—	—	66†	60‡	70†
Breast (female)	63	68	75	77	84*	46	51	63	66	69*
Cervix uteri	58	64	69	68	71	47	61	64	61	56*
Corpus uteri & unspecified	73	81	89	83	85*	31	44	61	54	56
Ovary	32	36	36	39	44*	32	32	40	38	38
Prostate	50	63	68	74	87*	35	55	58	65	71*
Testis	63	72	79	92	95*	—	—	76†	90†	86†
Urinary bladder	53	61	74	79	82*	24	36	47	58	59*
Kidney & renal pelvis	37	46	52	51	59*	38	44	49	55	54
Brain and nervous system	18	20	22	25	28*	19	19	27	31	31
Thyroid gland	83	86	92	94	95*	—	—	88	95	91
Hodgkin's disease	40	67	71	75	81*	—	—	69	71	70
Non-Hodgkin's lymphoma	31	41	47	52	52*	—	—	48	51	45
Multiple myeloma	12	19	24	28	28*	—	—	27	29	29
Leukemia	14	22	35	39	41*	—	—	31	33	32

From American Cancer Society: *Cancer facts and figures—1996*, Atlanta, 1996a, ACS, p. 18. Reprinted by permission of American Cancer Society.
Source: Cancer Statistics Branch, National Cancer Institute.
[1]Rates are based on End Results Group data from a series of hospital registries and one population-based registry.
[2]Rates are from the SEER program. They are based on data from population-based registries in Connecticut, New Mexico, Utah, Iowa, Hawaii, Atlanta, Detroit, Seattle–Puget Sound and San Francisco–Oakland. Rates are based on follow-up of patients through 1993.
*The difference in rates between 1974-76 and 1986-91 is statistically significant ($p < 0.05$).
†The standard error of the survival rate is between 5 and 10 percentage points.
‡The standard error of the survival rate is greater than 10 percentage points.
—Valid survival rate could not be calculated.

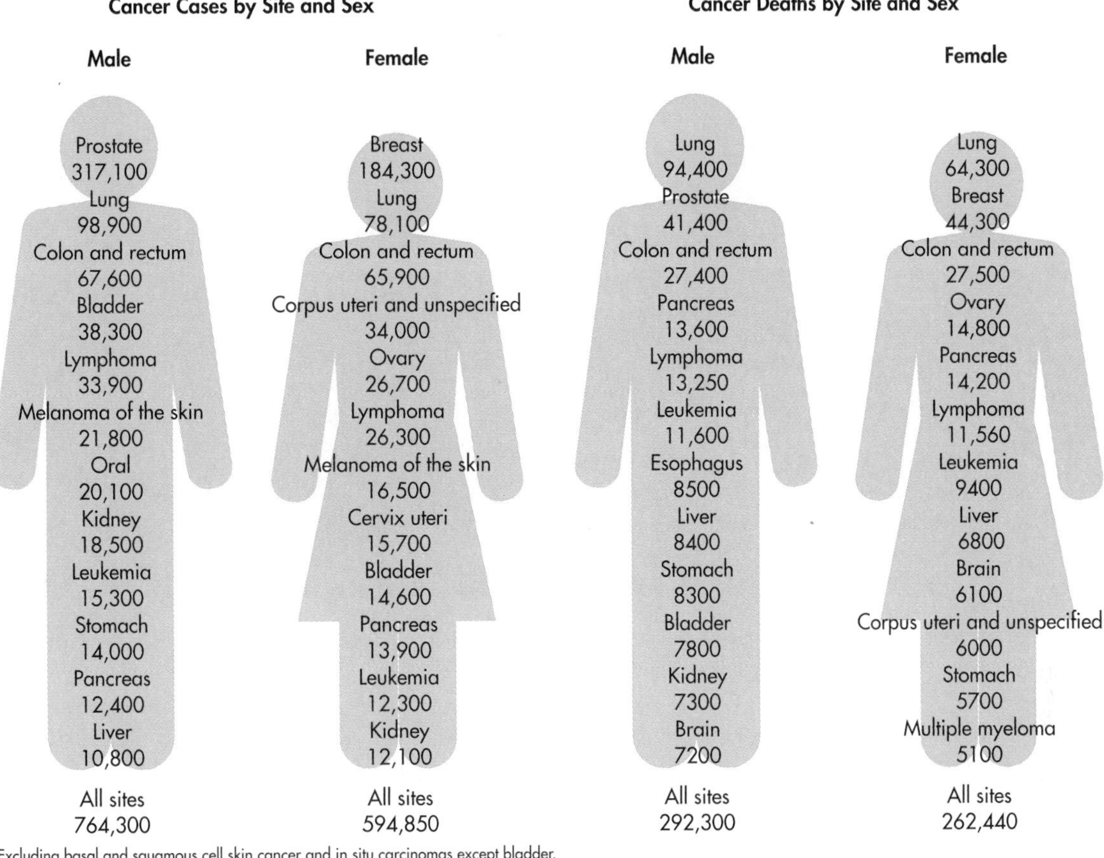

Figure 17-2 Leading sites of new cancer cases and deaths—1996 estimates. *(From American Cancer Society: Cancer facts and figures—1996, Atlanta, 1996a, ACS, p. 11.) Reprinted by permission of American Cancer Society.*

and self-image during chemotherapy and radiation treatments; laryngectomy rehabilitation volunteers in coordination with the International Association of Laryngectomies (IAL); ostomy rehabilitation volunteers in coordination with the United Ostomy Association; and children's camps.

Accidents

Accidents are the leading cause of death among all persons ages 1 to 37 and are the fifth leading cause of death among people of all ages (National Safety Council, 1995, p. 10). Accidents and the term *unintentional injury* are often used interchangeably. When death occurs under "accidental" circumstances, the preferred term within the public health community is *unintentional injury* (CDC, 1996a, p. 162). Unintentional injury does not include suicides and homicides, which are separate categories and are discussed in Chapter 12. The economic costs of fatal and nonfatal unintentional injuries are immense. In 1994 the estimated costs for unintentional injuries, including wages lost, medical, vehicle damage, fire losses, administrative, and employer costs were almost $4.5 billion (National Safety Council, 1995, p. 4)! However, what cannot be measured in dollars is the physical pain and suffering that results from unintentional injuries.

Table 17-8 graphically details the leading causes of mortality among adults, including the kinds of unintentional injuries that kill people ages 15 to 75. Note that unintentional injuries are the leading causes of death until age 35, when cancer, HIV, and heart disease begin to rank above accidents as leading causes of death. As persons age, diseases become more prevalent and rank higher than accidental deaths as leading causes of death. Age is a significant risk factor for developing many cardiovascular diseases, cancer, and other chronic conditions. Gender differences are also noted when reviewing the leading causes of death for adults. For example, accidental deaths are much higher for men than for women of all age groups (see Table 17-8). This may be attributed to numerous factors such as lifestyle patterns and occupations. Men increase their risk for unintentional injury because they are more likely than women to engage in risky behaviors and work in dangerous occupations.

Community health nurses have a major educative role in primary prevention of unintentional injuries. Health promotion interventions that are developmentally specific and

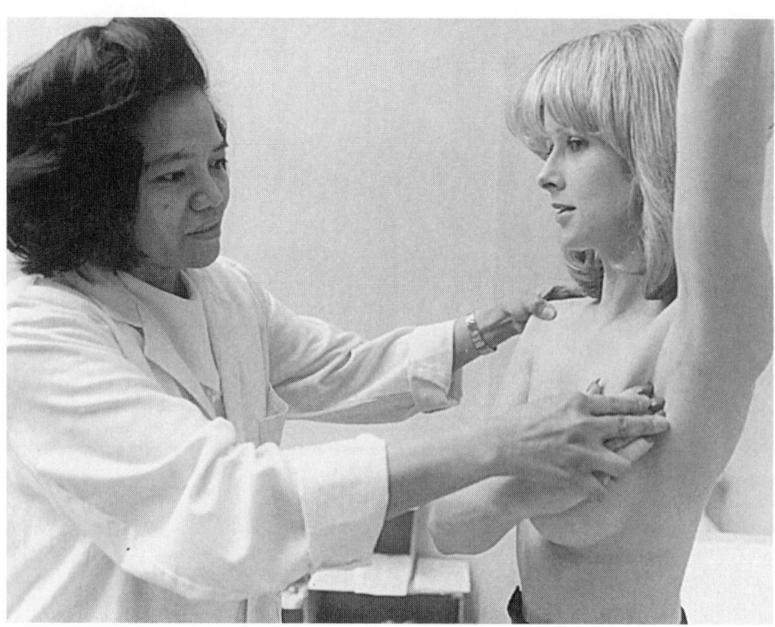

Figure 17-3 Breast self-examination being taught by a health care worker. *(Courtesy American Cancer Society.)*

tailored to each community will be the most effective. Like many other health problems, the most effective intervention for accidents is *prevention*. Health education interventions that are geared toward fire safety, home safety, firearm safety, water safety, seat belt use, driver safety, CPR training, health risk information awareness, stress reduction, health education, and poison control and treatment are just some examples of nursing activities that can help decrease unintentional injury rates in this country.

AGGREGATES AT RISK IN THE ADULT MALE AND FEMALE POPULATION

As with any age group, there are persons at special risk in the adult population who require concentrated community health nursing intervention. Throughout this text the special health needs of minorities are addressed, and minority health has been extensively discussed in Chapter 12. Several groups of adults who are at risk for increased mortality and morbidity, including the homeless and those living in poverty, those who abuse drugs, those at risk for STDs and those exposed to domestic violence, were discussed in Chapter 12. Other selected aggregates that will be discussed here include those who suffer from depression, adults changing jobs or careers, those experiencing unemployment, adults with chronic illness, adults in marital crisis, adult gays and lesbians, and adult men and women who are incarcerated.

Adult Men and Women Who Suffer from Depression

Depression is the most common, most treatable, and possibly the most painful of mental illnesses in the United States (Thompson, McFarland, Hirsch, Tucker, 1993, p. 1321). "Depression is often unrecognized and untreated in older adults" (Reynolds, 1996, p. 28). Major depression is the most common severe mental disorder in women. Approximately 7 million women in the United States suffer from major depression (Horton, 1995, p. 82). The onset of depression in women is most common between ages 25 and 44 and there is some evidence, such as the increased incidence of suicide attempts in young adults, that depression may be occurring at an earlier age (Horton, p. 83).

Freud viewed depression as aggression turned inward. Depression has been described as chronic frustration stemming from environmental stresses in family, social, or work environments beyond the coping ability and resources of the client. Depression can result when stress is intensified. All persons experience times when they feel low or discouraged, but these depressed feelings are usually acute and self-limiting. Depression becomes a serious problem when it is chronic and affects the ability to cope with the events, roles, and responsibilities of daily living. Depression is often precipitated by a loss of some kind: death, separation, or loss of job, status, or health.

Some symptoms of depression include general sadness and despair, difficulty in making decisions, difficulty in carrying on a conversation, trouble concentrating, trouble sleeping, tiredness, listlessness, loss of appetite, eating binges, social regression, loss of or decreased libido, and decreased self-esteem. People who are depressed may be overly sensitive to what other people say or do, may be angry with others and not trust them, and may withdraw from others because of a fear of being among people.

Persons who are depressed are often not aware that they are suffering from this condition. They know that they do

table 17-8 Adult Deaths and Death Rates by Age and Sex, 1992

	Number of Deaths			Death Rates*		
Cause by Age	Total	Male	Female	Total	Male	Female
AGES 15 TO 24						
All causes	35,548	26,207	8,341	95.6	141.8	47.2
Unintentional injuries	13,662	10,253	3,409	37.8	55.5	19.3
Motor vehicle	10,305	7,438	2,867	28.5	40.3	16.2
Drowning	771	706	65	2.1	3.8	0.4
Firearms	519	476	43	1.4	2.6	0.2
Poison (solid, liquid)	454	339	115	1.3	1.8	0.7
Falls	242	203	39	0.7	1.1	0.2
All other	1,371	1,091	280	3.8	5.9	1.6
Homicide	8,019	6,891	1,128	22.2	37.3	6.4
Suicide	4,693	4,044	649	13.0	21.9	3.7
Cancer	1,809	1,084	725	5.0	5.9	4.1
AGES 25 TO 34						
All causes	58,481	42,895	15,586	137.8	202.0	73.5
Unintentional injuries	13,798	10,746	3,052	32.5	50.6	14.4
Motor vehicle	8,229	6,163	2,066	19.4	29.0	9.7
Poison (solid, liquid)	1,848	1,454	394	4.4	6.8	1.9
Drowning	706	632	74	1.7	3.0	0.3
Fires, burns	399	287	112	0.9	1.4	0.5
Falls	398	330	68	0.9	1.6	0.3
All other	2,218	1,880	338	5.2	8.9	1.6
HIV	10,426	8,965	1,461	24.6	42.2	6.9
Homicide	7,343	5,832	1,511	17.3	27.5	7.1
Suicide	6,172	5,102	1,070	14.5	24.0	5.0
Cancer	5,303	2,571	2,732	12.5	12.1	12.9
Heart disease	3,423	2,274	1,149	8.1	10.7	5.4
AGES 35 TO 44						
All causes	91,290	62,995	28,295	228.8	318.7	140.5
Cancer	16,882	7,524	9,358	42.3	38.1	46.5
HIV	14,203	12,544	1,659	35.6	63.5	8.2
Heart disease	12,698	9,455	3,243	31.8	47.8	16.1
Unintentional injuries	12,010	9,235	2,775	30.1	46.7	13.8
Motor vehicle	5,842	4,164	1,678	14.6	21.1	8.3
Poison (solid, liquid)	2,453	1,990	463	6.1	10.1	2.3
Drowning	578	500	78	1.4	2.5	0.4
Falls	522	422	100	1.3	2.1	0.5
Fires, burns	397	299	98	1.0	1.5	0.5
All other	2,218	1,860	358	5.6	9.4	1.8
Suicide	6,009	4,680	1,329	15.1	23.7	6.6
Homicide	4,460	3,479	981	11.2	17.6	4.9

Modified from National Safety Council: *Accident facts, 1995 ed*, Itasca, Il., 1995, The Council, pp. 11-12.
*Deaths per 100,000 population in each age group

Continued

not feel well and often only seek medical help for minor physical problems. That is why it is so important for the community health nurse to systematically collect a complete health history (see Chapter 9) when working with adult clients. If data are collected only on the client's physical health complaints, depression can be overlooked.

Maintaining two-way communication between the client and nurse is essential. People who are depressed generally appreciate feedback on what is going on, to know that someone has listened to them, and that someone is available for support and assistance. Unfortunately, all too often the depressed client is excluded from social contacts; family,

table 17-8 ADULT DEATHS AND DEATH RATES BY AGE AND SEX, 1992—CONT'D

	NUMBER OF DEATHS			DEATH RATES*		
CAUSE BY AGE	TOTAL	MALE	FEMALE	TOTAL	MALE	FEMALE
AGES 45 TO 54						
All causes	125,030	79,271	45,759	456.1	591.7	326.4
Cancer	41,206	20,603	20,603	150.3	153.8	147.0
Heart disease	31,413	23,273	8,140	114.6	173.7	58.1
Unintentional injuries	7,485	5,488	1,997	27.3	41.0	14.2
Motor vehicle	3,721	2,550	1,171	13.6	19.0	8.4
Poison (solid, liquid)	789	578	211	2.9	4.3	1.5
Falls	613	472	141	2.2	3.5	1.0
Fires, burns	345	254	91	1.3	1.9	0.6
Drowning	338	298	40	1.2	2.2	0.3
All other	1,679	1,336	343	6.1	10.0	2.4
HIV	5,575	5,104	471	20.3	38.1	3.4
Stroke	4,791	2,589	2,202	17.5	19.3	15.7
Chronic liver disease	4,569	3,322	1,247	16.7	24.8	8.9
Suicide	4,018	2,999	1,019	14.7	22.4	7.3
AGES 55 TO 64						
All causes	240,991	146,880	94,111	1,151.7	1,481.5	854.7
Cancer	91,609	50,898	40,711	437.8	513.4	369.7
Heart disease	72,516	49,956	22,560	346.5	503.9	204.9
COPD	10,098	5,582	4,516	48.3	56.3	41.0
Stroke	9,709	5,270	4,439	46.4	53.2	40.3
Diabetes	7,109	3,557	3,552	34.0	35.9	32.3
Unintentional injuries	6,397	4,438	1,959	30.6	44.8	17.8
Motor vehicle	2,876	1,859	1,017	13.7	18.8	9.2
Falls	808	579	229	3.9	5.8	2.1
Fires, burns	393	272	121	1.9	2.7	1.1
Medical complications	304	171	133	1.5	1.7	1.2
Poison (solid, liquid)	259	167	92	1.2	1.7	0.8
All other	1,757	1,390	367	8.4	14.0	3.3
Chronic liver disease	5,780	3,981	1,799	27.6	40.2	16.3

friends, and even professionals may isolate depressed clients in an attempt to protect the client from further hurt or stress. This social isolation serves to reinforce the client's feelings that no one cares.

Depressed individuals who are identified as potentially suicidal should be referred for psychotherapy. Some nurses are afraid to assess for suicide potential because they fear their questioning may precipitate a suicide attempt. However, suicide is not prevented by avoiding conversation about it. It is prevented by helping clients get the assistance they need to deal with stresses in their daily lives.

Encountering clients who are depressed is common in community health nursing practice. At times the client is able to resolve the depressed state by using the supportive assistance of the community health nurse and significant others, such as family, friends, relatives, and lovers. At other times additional mental health counseling is necessary. However, depression will continue to exist until the individual is able to successfully mobilize coping mechanisms that enhance growth. Most chronic depressions are related to unresolved psychosocial difficulties. Crisis and normative stress are self-limiting; chronic depression is not.

The nurse can refer the client to community resources such as community mental health centers and self-help groups. Other sources of information and referral for the client and family are groups such as the Foundation for Depressive Illness (1-800-248-4344) and the National Mental Health Association (703-684-7722). On the federal level, the National Institute of Mental Health (NIMH) is charged with improving the understanding, treatment, and rehabilitation of the mentally ill; preventing mental illness; and fostering the mental health of the people. NIMH is involved in prevention activities. It sponsors Project D/ART (Depression/Awareness, Recognition, and Treatment). Project D/ART is concerned with ameliorating the public health problem of depression and aims to improve the identification, assessment, treatment, and clinical management of depressive disorders through an educational program focused on the general public, primary care providers, and mental health specialists. Project D/ART is involved with many voluntary and professional organizations and provides information and materials for the general public as well as professional audiences. A national goal is to "increase to at least 45 percent the proportion of people with major depressive disorders who obtain treatment" (USDHHS, 1991a, p. 215). Several other mental health national goals focus on stress management and the establishment of community resources to assist people who have mental disorders.

Men and Women Changing Jobs or Careers

When changing jobs or careers a major reorganization is required in one's life, and the stresses encountered should not be underestimated. The process can involve significant stress, particularly if changing a job or a career was not a voluntary decision (e.g., being fired or laid off), and unemployment may result. Even if the decision was a voluntary one, the individual may have doubts about the decision and may not have consensus within the family.

When some people change jobs or careers it may mean going back to school. An example of the health stresses that this could cause is seen in the McSweeney family. The family had an increased incidence of health problems when Mr. McSweeney returned to college to prepare for another career.

CASE *Scenario*

George McSweeney was a 38-year-old engineer, husband, and father of three school-age children. As a result of industrial noise he lost 50% of his hearing. Unable to continue functioning at his job, he returned to college to prepare for another career. Financially his family had few difficulties. Although Mr. McSweeney was not eligible for workers' compensation he received federal scholarship monies and his wife had a part-time job. The community health nurse encountered the McSweeney family after they had repeatedly taken Lisa, their 10-year-old daughter, into the emergency room for treatment of an asthmatic condition. The nurse was well received by the family because both parents were unsure of when to seek medical care for their daughter. The nurse discovered that Lisa's condition had been under good control until the family moved and she had to change schools. In addition, she found that Mr. McSweeney was having tension headaches regularly; a medical evaluation ruled out organic problems. Lisa had fewer asthma attacks and Mr. McSweeney had fewer headaches as the family began to verbalize the frustrations associated with the multiple changes they had recently experienced.

To assist the adult in dealing with change and stress the nurse needs to assess individual and/or family perceptions of the situation. Is it viewed as a new and challenging adventure? Is it a threat to personal and economic security? Is it causing problems within the family structure?

Community health nurses should be especially sensitive to the stresses that can occur when an individual is changing jobs or careers. The nurse assesses the situation, listens to the client's concerns, and refers the client to appropriate resources (e.g., stress management, counseling services, vocational rehabilitation).

From an aggregate perspective, the number of adults experiencing the need for a job or career change is increasing drastically. As organizations downsize and new technology emerges the need for job or career changes is becoming a normal occurrence. The current trend in our nation reflects a need for workers to prepare for multiple careers throughout their lives. Community health nurses can assist with this process by developing support groups for those who need to make immediate changes and through preventive intervention with children and adults just starting their careers.

Adults Experiencing Unemployment

No one is exempt from loss of employment, and this can create devastation for a family; however, some groups are more at risk for unemployment than others. The unemployment rate varies significantly by race and ethnicity. Unemployment is higher among blacks than whites (U.S. Bureau of the Census, 1995, pp. 48-49).

When unemployment occurs, regardless of reason, it can be very disruptive and stressful for families involved. Family stress can mount as work responsibilities are redistributed, roles are altered, and family goals are modified. Role reversal between husband and wife may occur, and there can be increased frequency of marital disruption and role conflict. In addition to economic deprivation, unemployment can cause increased family violence, instability, and economic deprivation. Social stigma is often attached to unemployment. The unemployed family may become socially isolated and suffer altered self-esteem.

People who are unemployed are often unable to afford health care services because they lose insurance and health care benefits. Unemployment generates stress that can cause health problems. The unemployed worker may not feel well physically and have symptoms such as chest pains, shortness of breath, dizziness, dry mouth, eczema, weakness, and inability to sleep. Psychological stress among the unemployed may be evidenced by lowered self-esteem, anxiety, apathy, decreased appetite, inertia, and feelings of helplessness. The unemployed suffer from a variety of psychosomatic conditions. Family members of the unemployed can also evidence health problems and stress related to the unemployment. Although unemployment necessitates family adjustment, change, and adaptation, the stress experienced can be minimized and positive growth can occur.

Unemployment is a major crisis physically, socially, emotionally, and financially. Community health nurses can help families understand what is happening and encourage them to use appropriate community resources. They can also work with community groups to mobilize resources for the unemployed and make referrals for job training or new employment. Community partnerships may be needed to address issues related to unemployment particularly if a community has a significantly high unemployment rate. Chapter 14 discusses mobilizing community partnerships for social and health action.

Adults with Chronic Illness

Chronic illness is a major health problem in the American population (see Chapters 11 and 19). Illness for the individual or family is a normal part of the life cycle. Everyone expects at some point in time to have a case of the flu, a cold, or even minor surgery. Acute, nondisabling illness can often be handled by normal resources and coping mechanisms. It does not involve major lifestyle adaptation. If the illness becomes chronic, disabling, or terminal, however, the family situation can become stressful.

When the adult is afflicted with a chronic health condition, major life changes occur. These changes can involve increased health care tasks, the possibility of strained family relationships, modifications in family goals, financial stress, need for housing adaptation, and social isolation. The grieving process in relation to such conditions is discussed in Chapter 19. The individual and family may also demonstrate changes in work, school, and community experiences as a result of the illness.

The extent to which lifestyle changes occur during chronic illness varies, depending on the degree of disability encountered and the adult's perception of the event. Role reversal, changes in sexual behavior, and alterations in self-image are a few examples of the problems experienced by clients who have developed debilitating chronic illness during adulthood. The adult who is not progressing well along the developmental continuum may regress, become depressed, or become dependent when chronically ill. He or she may resist treatment or become self-absorbed, and may use the illness as an escape from responsibility.

Research has shown that families who adjusted well to chronic illness viewed the illness in a positive light—that is, a greater appreciation of life for the present was developed (Hough, Lewis, Woods, 1991). Further, these families viewed themselves as competent and effective and stated that they were more sensitive and empathic about the needs of others.

Use of both the educative and problem-solving approaches to nursing intervention is essential when nurses work with families and aggregates who are dealing with a chronic condition. They need increased knowledge to realistically evaluate the changes that are occurring and that may occur. These clients also need to problem-solve to determine the most appropriate ways for them to adapt to changes, especially permanent ones. Different coping mechanisms and resources must be mobilized to reduce tension.

The possibility of death may also be a matter for the nurse to work through with chronically ill adults and their families. Families should be encouraged to articulate advance directives, express their fears and, if the client's situation warrants it, to prepare for death. Reading materials such as the classics on death and dying written by Kubler-Ross (1974, 1975) can enhance a community health nurse's skill in working with clients who are dying.

Situations involving death and dying are inevitable. Yet for many Americans death education comes late in life, and they are often not equipped to deal with it in relation to themselves or others. Knowledge of the grief process may assist the adult in resolving grief associated with death. A great number of middlescents experience death for the first time with the loss of a parent. Death education and helping a family work through the grieving process are important community health nursing interventions.

When working with any chronically ill adult, the community health nurse will more than likely use the referral process. A variety of community resources, including ostomy clubs, Multiple Sclerosis Association, American Cancer Society, American Lung Association, American Heart Association, Goodwill Industries, the division of vocational rehabilitation, and the department of social services, will help clients and their families to adapt to chronic illness. Chapter 21 discusses support and education for the caregiver and the client when chronic illness is present.

The nurse can assist the client and family by making them aware of the medical course of the client's condition, giving anticipatory guidance, and encouraging them to take an active role in health care decision making. Nurses can help the chronically ill adult accept the interdependency needed to deal successfully with his or her condition and should not make unrealistic promises of recovery or an optimistic prognosis if this is not the case. There may be no guarantee that treatment will improve the level of disability, and false hopes prevent the client from confronting and working through the crisis.

People Who Are Experiencing Marital Crises

It is not uncommon for the community health nurse to encounter families who are experiencing some form of marital crisis such as divorce and domestic violence (discussed in Chapter 12). The divorce rate has increased dramatically in the past three decades (U.S. Bureau of the Census, 1995, pp. 54-55) and when experienced, marital crisis is a major life stress for the adult. As a result of divorce, as well as an increase in the number of never married parents, there has been a rise in single-parent households, which creates additional stress for many adults (U.S. Bureau of the Census, p. 58).

Marital disenchantment, separation, and divorce occur throughout adulthood. For instance, during middlescence spouses find that they have more time together, and if they are unable to reestablish intimacy or reinforce it they may become disenchanted with their marital relationship. In addition, the sexual changes (menopause and climacteric) that occur during middlescence can also adversely affect the way in which spouses relate in the marital relationship.

Disenchantment, separation, and divorce have an impact on all family members. Adults, as well as children, need to make major changes. Experiencing feelings of uncertainty, betrayal, insecurity, failure, and loss is common during this time. As with all crises, the primary focus of the community health nurse with clients who are experiencing marital stress is on helping them to achieve crisis resolution and growth. Resolution could require divorce or separation, but it also may occur through renegotiation and alteration of family patterns that are ineffective. A therapeutic approach that encourages problem solving rather than blaming can best facilitate successful resolution during this time of crisis.

From both an aggregate and family perspective, anticipatory guidance activities by community health nurses may be instrumental in preventing marital crises. Preparing young adults to handle the stresses of parenthood, or middlescent couples to deal with the conflicts during launching, may decrease the amount of stress experienced at these times. Parenting and life stress management groups are commonly found in communities throughout the country. Community health nurses frequently have an active role in establishing and conducting these groups.

Gays and Lesbians

Gays and lesbians experience the same health needs and stresses as heterosexual adults throughout their lives (Carlson, 1996, p. 66). However, gays and lesbians have health care issues that create added stress related to disclosing their sexual identity, seeking health care, and confronting attitudes from health care providers. Bias and discrimination are a reality for gays and lesbians and many "have experienced lifelong rejection from family, peers, and co-workers" (Denenberg, 1995, p. 83). Despite the fact that homosexuality was declassified as a mental illness over 20 years ago, most gays and lesbians continue to be victims of prejudice and discrimination (Carlson, 1996, p. 71; Eliason, 1996, p. 5; Hellman, 1996, p. 1094).

Deciding when or *if* they should disclose their identity to health care providers can be a highly stressful ordeal, because many gays and lesbians fear that they will be negatively viewed by health care providers (Eliason, 1996, p. 91). In traditional health care settings gay and lesbian partners are often not afforded the same recognition and partner support status as is granted their heterosexual counterparts. This adds personal stress for the client because many fear their partners may not be allowed to provide the desired emotional support. Gays and lesbians are often unable to freely express themselves in the health care setting (Hellman, 1996, p. 1095). Research has shown that many gays and lesbians, upon disclosure of their sexual identity to health care providers, have experienced reactions such as ostracism, condescension, shock, pity, disapproval, fear, avoidance, and even rough physical handling (Eliason, 1996, p. 121; Stevens, Hall, 1990, p. 24). As a result of these types of reactions, gays and lesbians may be reluctant to seek health care, which can put them at risk for the development of health problems and disease progression by delaying early treatment (Denenberg, 1995; Eliason, 1996).

Eliason and Randall (1991) reported that lesbians were reluctant to seek care when they had health concerns because of negative past experiences and even harm. Lesbians are less likely than their heterosexual counterparts to seek regular gynecological examinations, Pap smears, breast examinations, mammograms, and other preventive services (Denenberg, 1995; Eliason, 1996). This increases their risk for development and progression of adult health problems such as cardiovascular diseases, hypertension, and cancer, which are often detected through preventive activities such as screening and Pap smears. Lesbians also have fewer pregnancies than heterosexual women, which places them at a higher risk for breast cancer. Additionally, lesbians may receive unscreened insemination or have sexual intercourse with a stranger in order to have children, which puts them at high risk for HIV (Denenberg, 1995, p. 82). Safe-sex education is as pertinent to lesbian clients as heterosexual clients because they are not immune to sexually transmitted diseases and bacterial infections.

Gay men have health needs similar to the heterosexual men. Like lesbians, gay men are often reluctant to seek preventive health and treatment services for fear of discrimination. Gay men are more likely to experience violent discrimination, such as "gay bashing," than lesbian women, which makes them more reluctant to disclose their sexual identity and to seek health care for fear of additional violence (Eliason, 1996, pp. 189-192). Gay men have higher rates of HIV/AIDS and are more apt to engage in casual sex than their lesbian counterparts, which places them at a high risk for STDs and other infections (Eliason, p. 200). Hence safe-sex education is extremely important to this population. It is also recommended that gay men of all ages have yearly rectal examinations that screen for cancer or other infections (Eliason, p. 201).

Both gays and lesbians have higher rates of substance abuse, depression, and suicide than that of the general population (Eliason, 1996; Hall, 1993; Hellman, 1996). There is a real need for preventive and mental health treatment services for gay and lesbian adults. However, many are reluctant to seek such services because of the stigmatizing effects of receiving treatment. Many feel that they cannot be open and expressive in their treatment setting and fear further stigmatization related to their mental health (Hellman). Clearly an open environment and increased sensitivity on the part of health care providers is essential.

Perhaps the greatest health need for this population is for health care providers to accept gays and lesbians without prejudice and in a positive manner. Community health nurses have an opportunity to foster positive attitudes in meeting the needs of gay and lesbian adults. Clinicians need to examine their own biases and fears regarding gays and lesbians so that they do not negatively jeopardize their health care (Carlson, 1996, p. 73). No person should ever be afraid of seeking out health care providers to meet their health needs. "Health care providers need to find ways to alleviate pain and suffering, not to compound them" (Eliason, 1996, p. 187). If quality nursing care is to be given nonjudgmentally, nurses must recognize their own homophobias and identify their inaccurate knowledge base in order for all persons to receive the health care they need. Community health nurses can intervene at various levels of health promotion and prevention. Some examples of interventions include education regarding safe sexual practices that are tailored to gays and lesbians, preventive screening practices such as regular Pap smears for lesbians and anal examinations for men, suicide prevention education, screening for depression and suicide risks, and referral for treatment.

Individuals Who Are Incarcerated

The number of individuals who are incarcerated is increasing each year. The prison population spans all ages, including both men and women, and minorities are disproportionately represented. The majority of inmates are between 18 and 34 years of age, with elderly inmates being in the minority (LaMere, Smyer, Gragert, 1996). The number of women incarcerated has increased substantially. Since 1980 the number of persons in federal and state prisons more than tripled, from 329,821 persons in 1980 to a record 1,104,074 at mid-year 1995 (CDC, 1996b). As the rate of crime has escalated and as more criminals are being incarcerated, the number of prison beds needed has also increased. As a result, prisons have become overcrowded. In 1995 state prisons were filled 17% to 29% above capacity, and federal prisons were 25% above capacity (Meddis, 1995, p. A3).

Incarceration and overcrowding places inmates at risk for many health problems. Demographic data reflect that incarcerated persons are primarily from low socioeconomic backgrounds, have had problems with substance abuse, have had little health care before incarceration, and experience high rates of mental illness. Incarcerated persons also engage in unhealthy lifestyles that increase the risk of developing illness and disease (National Institute of Justice, 1995, p. xi).

Numerous health risks and health problems exist among incarcerated populations. As a result of the previous lifestyles of the inmates and the prison environment, many sexually transmitted diseases and other communicable diseases, as well as chronic illnesses, are prevalent. HIV/AIDS is rapidly increasing in the prison population, and HIV transmission is a serious concern (CDC, 1996c, p. 268). Many inmates who have also been IV drug users are HIV-infected before incarceration and, in some instances, incarceration may be the first time prisoners have received any health care or preventive education (Gaiter, Doll, 1996, p. 1201). Because of the diversity of the prison population, interventions must be specific to gender, cognitive, and developmental levels, and culturally sensitive (Gaiter, Doll, p. 1202). This can only be accomplished by a comprehensive understanding of risk factors (e.g., drug use, consensual as well as nonconsensual unprotected sex, alcohol use, ignorance) surrounding the HIV/AIDS-infected prison population.

The incidence and prevalence of tuberculosis (TB) in prisons has also increased significantly. The prison environment is a high risk environment due to overcrowding, inadequate ventilation, and coinfection with HIV, which allows TB to easily spread among inmates. Many prisoners have latent TB, and coinfection with HIV increases the risk of developing active TB. The strongest known risk for converting latent TB to active TB is coinfection with HIV (CDC, 1996b). Since TB is spread through the air it takes only one prisoner with active TB to infect numerous others sharing the same crowded air space (CDC, 1996b, p. 5). CDC has recommended stronger regulations to control the spread of TB in federal, state, and local prisons (CDC, 1996b).

State and local health departments have an active role in carrying out standards and practices to control TB. As a result, community health nurses are active participants in screening, intervention, and the referral process. Concern about the spread of communicable disease also extends beyond the prison walls. When prisoners are released it is imperative that there are community support services for a follow-up process to control the spread of communicable disease to others in the community. Community health nurses have a role in managed care that will ensure ongoing care of prisoners when they are released to the community.

Nursing in prisons encompasses a wide variety of interventions that range from acute emergency care, casefinding, health education, treatment for STDs, psychiatric care, and substance abuse intervention to treatment for chronic illnesses such as arthritis, hypertension, and diabetes. A number of chronic illnesses and mobility problems require ongoing treatment and evaluation during incarceration. Table 17-9 presents some self-reported and physician-diagnosed illnesses of a number of inmates. Nurses must be able to work independently and be able to meet chronic, as well as acute, health needs of the incarcerated.

As mentioned above, more women have also become incarcerated. Incarcerated women have health needs that are similar to their male counterparts such as substance abuse, STDs, HIV/AIDS, TB, and mental and chronic illnesses. However, pregnancy can have societal implications, as well as personal implications. Pregnant women in federal prisons

table 17-9 Percentage of Male Inmates with Lifetime History of Specific Self-Reported Physician-Diagnosed Illness

	Age, y		
	50-59 (N = 82)	>59 (N = 37)	Overall (N = 119)
Arthritis	40.2	56.8	45.4
Hypertension	36.7	45.9	39.7
Any venereal disease	21.5	21.6	21.6
Stomach or intestinal ulcers	18.3	27.0	21.0
Prostate problems	17.1	27.0	20.2
Myocardial infarction	17.7	21.6	19.0
Emphysema	14.6	27.0	18.5
Diabetes	10.1	13.5	11.2
Asthma	8.5	10.8	9.2
Stroke	3.8	16.2	7.8
Cancer	6.3	8.1	6.9
Cirrhosis or liver disease	4.9	2.7	4.2
Injury requiring medical care	78.5	73.0	76.7

From Colsher PL, Wallace RB, Loeffelholz PL, Sales M: Health status of older male prisoners: a comprehensive survey, *Am J Public Health* 82(6):882, 1992.

may not participate in the direct care of their infants, and the birth mother has to make a choice of either placing her infant up for adoption or seeking someone who will assume guardianship responsibilities (Huft, 1992). Frequently grandparents and other relatives care for the children of incarcerated adults. Community health nurses frequently help these guardians access appropriate community services. Incarceration not only affects incarcerated individuals but, most powerfully, their children. Care of pregnant women involves gynecological and obstetrical care, as well as other services such as WIC and well-child care.

Care of pregnant women in prisons is complicated by stress, restrictive environments, alterations in social supports, and the displacement of the maternal role functions after birth (Huft, 1992). The environment, coupled with distorted maternal role functioning, can contribute to depression. Fogel and Martin (1992) have studied incarcerated women who are mothers and who are not mothers: both groups had high levels of depression that did not mitigate over time, but the mothers had higher levels of anxiety that remained high. Women in prisons are in need of services that would enhance their emotional and psychological health as well as their physical health.

Just as the number of individuals who are incarcerated has increased, so has the cost of prison health care. The high rate of HIV/AIDS, TB, and an increasingly aging prison population has also added to the increase in prison health costs (McDonald, 1995). To contain costs, prisons are contracting with community agencies to provide health care to the prisoners (McDonald).

Community health nurses and nurses in acute-care settings may be providing direct care in addition to preventive services as part of a collaborative effort to provide quality care to the incarcerated. Community placement concerns upon prison release may also be addressed by the community health nurse. Community health nurses must know the resources in the community to make appropriate referral and follow-up. They must also be knowledgeable about family dynamics and how to address changes in these dynamics as a released prisoner reenters the home environment. Like other problems that have been discussed in this chapter, providing competent care for the incarcerated will require sensitivity to issues involved with caring for the incarcerated. This will also require nurses to solve personal issues and be aware of biases that may interfere with providing quality care.

THE ROLE OF THE NURSE WITH PEOPLE WHO ARE INCARCERATED The ANA has articulated several position statements for nurses working in prisons. The ANA's Council of Community Health Nurses developed the *Scope and Standards of Nursing Practice in Correctional Facilities* in 1985 and revised them in 1995. The purpose of these standards is to guide professional nurse practice in correctional facilities, for the general incarcerated prison population, and in specialty facilities such as those for women, juveniles, and the mentally ill. Specific ANA guidelines exist for nurses' management and care of inmates with HIV (ANA, 1996, pp. 17-20) and TB throughout the United States (ANA, pp. 59-62). The American Public Health Association has also published *Standards for Health Services in Correctional Institutions* (1986).

Perhaps more than any other environment where nurses practice, the prison environment may present the greatest challenge to providing quality care. Prison nurses' personal attitudes and beliefs must be explored so they do not interfere with their role in providing the highest standard of professional care. The role of the nurse in the prison is to provide health care services that are within the scope of practice for each particular state, and the standards specifically point out that the role excludes involvement in disciplinary procedures (including execution), except for regulations that apply to nursing personnel (ANA, 1995). Primary health services in this field include using the nursing process in screening, providing direct health care services, teaching, counseling, and assisting prisoners to manage their own health care.

It has long been recognized that nurses can have role conflict when working in prisons. Alexander-Rodriguez (1983) wrote that there is a basic conflict between the goals of correctional health care and correctional institutions. A prison nurse must meet the demands of perhaps two philosophically opposite corporate cultures (Stevens, 1995, p. 8). In the public health care culture there is a prevailing belief of basic goodness, whereas in the prison system the presence of evil prevails, and as a result nurses can be polarized between the two directions (Stevens, pp. 7-8). To provide competent care in the prison environment the prison nurse must understand the differences in values, beliefs, and norms between a corporate health care environment and a prison correctional environment. Self-awareness of issues related to caring for incarcerated populations can help allay conflict in achieving health goals and providing quality nursing care for the incarcerated.

Prisoners struggle to survive, and times of illness make them vulnerable to suffering and in need of humanistic health care (Berkman, 1995). "The biggest challenge for a nurse working in a prison, is to remain true to the humanistic philosophy of nursing and not be slowly and imperceptibly converted to the role of prison keeper. When that happens it is time to get out of prison health care" (Alexander-Rodriguez, 1983, p. 116).

Some nursing schools are providing clinical and preventive services to prisoners (Fontes, 1991; Hall, Ortiz-Peters, 1986; Roell, 1985). Increasingly, community health nurses are expanding their services to prisoners in city and county jails. In these settings the nurse may conduct health education programs, screen for and follow-up on sexually transmitted diseases, act as a health care resource to staff, assist prisoners in finding health care resources upon discharge, and provide supportive and problem-solving counseling. Prison systems are in need of strong primary health prevention programs, especially related to communicable disease prevention and mental health services.

THE COMMUNITY HEALTH NURSE'S ROLE IN MAINTAINING THE HEALTH OF ADULT MEN AND WOMEN

Although community health nurses' interventions have been discussed throughout this chapter, further emphasis is needed here to highlight the significant role nurses perform in promoting the health of adults. Health is a blend of developmental, physiological, psychological, spiritual, and social factors. When one of these factors becomes out of balance, all are affected. Community health nurses take into consideration all of these factors when developing interventions to comprehensively address the needs of adult clients. Implementing comprehensive interventions requires an awareness of available resources and frequently involves collaborative and interdisciplinary team work.

Various approaches are often needed to plan nursing interventions that address the health needs of well adults. It is not an easy task to motivate adults to participate in health activities, especially if they consider themselves to be well. Well adults do not always recognize or act on health needs, and may ignore primary prevention activities. The community health nurse implements interventions at all levels of prevention. Use of the referral process (discussed in Chapter 10) is an integral part of promoting the health of the adult. Nurses can help adults become aware of the available resources that meet their health care needs and refer them to these resources when appropriate. However, many health care resources are organized to deal with acute health care episodes rather than with preventive health care measures.

Health Promotion Through Preventive Intervention

As discussed in earlier chapters, health promotion begins with people who are basically healthy and encourages the development of lifestyles that maintain and support health and well-being. Although little is known about how individuals and families achieve health and well-being, or about what factors influence them in the process, a great deal is known about many health promotion activities such as smoking cessation, regular exercise, and dietary modifications that enhance a healthy lifestyle. Although we are well aware of the risk factors that enhance disease occurrences in adulthood, more effective strategies are needed to assist adults in addressing these risk factors. Community-based research intervention projects, such as work-site cancer prevention that includes smoking cessation and nutrition habits (Sorensen, Thompson, Glanz et al, 1996), are emerging to address this need.

Some examples of selected health promotion activities that help healthy adult clients to improve or maintain their well-being were previously displayed in the Teaching Tips box on page 502. Other areas of health promotion, such as environmental health and occupational health and safety, are matters of legislation and enforcement as well as individual decision making. Obtaining documented data about health promotion and nursing interventions that produce successful health outcomes is critical when working toward influencing legislation and health policy. Legislative and health policy action, such as laws related to smoking in public places, are needed to comprehensively address the health needs of adult populations in the community.

Community health nurses carry out many primary prevention activities to comprehensively address the personal health needs of adults. They are particularly interested in helping the adult learn about preventable health problems and about health behaviors that can promote wellness and decrease personal health risks. A major primary prevention activity with adults is health teaching and counseling about family and personal health risk factors, accident prevention and safety, nutrition, personal hygiene, health examinations, family planning, STDs, disease transmission, and immunizations. Such health teaching, with use of resources as appropriate, may help to prevent an illness or injury, dental caries, an unwanted pregnancy, marital disenchantment, a suicide attempt, a case of tetanus, a case of flu, an incident of child abuse, or an STD. Health teaching activities help the adult to look at health in relation to present and future functioning.

Primary prevention and health risk appraisal are major goals of health promotion but are not always easily attainable. In recent years increased emphasis has been placed on primary prevention. However, many preventive health care measures, such as yearly physical examinations, are not covered under many forms of health insurance and become out-of-pocket expenses for the client. Therefore cost is a factor that often impedes adults taking advantage of preventive services. Health screening programs can provide valuable health services to persons who otherwise would not obtain them.

The community health nurse can assess individual and family health risk factors and encourage health actions which decrease these risks. Health risk appraisal can also be handled through an automated process in which an individual's health-related behaviors and personal characteristics are compared to mortality statistics and other epidemiological data. Relating individual and group data helps individuals to identify their risk of dying from a specific condition by a specified time and the amount of risk that could be eliminated by making appropriate behavioral changes in health practices. This automated approach is increasingly accessible to the general public and can have beneficial health consequences. However, the real challenge for health professionals is to help people act on personal health risks.

When counseling about health promotion activities, nurses should be sensitive and keep in mind that people bring their own beliefs, attitudes, and values to health care situations. Beliefs about individual and family susceptibility to illness, the severity of illness in terms of health and lifestyle disruption, the perceived effectiveness of diagnostic and health prevention activities, and perceived barriers to care will affect the health promotion and prevention activities in which a person engages (Pender, 1996).

Health teaching with the young adult should focus on violence in addition to accident prevention (see Chapter 12). Accidents, suicide, and homicide are the leading causes of death for persons 20 to 29 years of age. It is important to try to determine the nature and timing of critical precedents that place individuals at high risk for committing violent acts against themselves or others and to identify significant persons or groups in contact with high-risk individuals who could save the individual's life.

To prevent certain conditions, nurses can help adults look at their own personal health habits and risk factors. Smoking, excessive intake of alcoholic beverages, lack of sufficient rest, an inadequate diet, and other risk factors all have an impact on an adult's present and future health status.

When nurses practice from a prevention perspective they stress the importance of medical, dental, and ophthalmological examinations for prevention, early diagnosis, and treatment of disease. Secondary preventive health measures for the adult include practicing self-examination of the breasts and testicles, yearly Pap smears, and adherence to prescribed medical and dental regimens. The adult should be assisted to see the value of monitoring and screening for conditions for which he or she has a familial or individual predisposition, such as cardiovascular accidents, diabetes, cancer, or hypertension. Appendix 17-1 summarizes adult screening procedures used with adult clients and the age at which they should be done. Information in this appendix provides parameters for discussion when the community health nurse is carrying out health counseling.

Tertiary prevention health activities that the nurse may use with the adult are related to rehabilitation activities that minimize the degree of disability of the condition. These activities are discussed in Chapter 19, where the nurse's role in rehabilitation of the disabled adult is covered. They involve interdisciplinary functioning and focus on encouraging client compliance with prescribed medical and dental regimens, as well as exploring ways to promote healthy coping behaviors.

Pender, Barkauskas, Hayman et al (1992, p. 108) have described three points at which a person or a group may be highly receptive to input about health promotion and disease prevention. These points are derived from a developmental and a person-environment interaction perspective that address developmental and situational stress. The three points include the following: age-specific times that are the same for most people, including menarche, parenthood, and retirement; historically specific times in the life of a society, including changes in the roles of men and women and insecurity in the labor market; and, finally, events that vary among individuals and families, including death of a partner or geographical relocation. These points can help the community health nurse develop aggregate-specific interventions aimed at reducing selected health risks.

The health risks and morbidity and mortality data for adults mandate that community health nurses continue lifelong education. Family violence, homelessness, tuberculosis, HIV/AIDS, unemployment, chronic illness—these are topics that are overwhelming in scope and that can affect practitioners themselves. Dealing with them means that nurses be well-informed; that they build in supports, both informal and formal, for the stressful times in their lives; and that political involvement at some level is crucial to ensure a basic level of health care for all.

LEGISLATION AFFECTING ADULT HEALTH

The legislation that influences the adult also makes an impact on other age groups. The Social Security Act of 1935 and its amendments provide maternal-child health programs, which are discussed in Chapters 4, 15, and 16. The Social Security Act also provides for Medicaid and Medicare, for which the medically indigent or terminally ill adult may qualify. The Public Health Service Act of 1944 and its amendments have helped to provide adult health care services. Health planning and environmental health legislation have also benefitted adult health (see Chapters 6 and 14).

Among legislation that specifically addresses the adult population is the Occupational Safety and Health Act of 1970, which is discussed in Chapter 18. It deals with maintaining the health of the adult in the workplace and focuses on maintaining wellness. Two pieces of legislation passed in the early part of this decade, The Americans with Disabilities Act and The Family and Medical Leave Act, have the potential to positively influence the health of adults in the coming years. These acts are discussed in Chapter 4. However, recent welfare reform efforts in the later half of the current decade will likely significantly stress many families. Increasing community and aggregate focus strategies will be needed to assist people in obtaining meaningful employment and health care resources.

Summary

The breadth of the health issues affecting adult men and women is vast. Of all of the population groups presented in this text, adults have the greatest opportunity to improve their health status because they have monetary and physical independence. The fact that younger and older people depend on them can present burdens and challenges.

Adults who financially and emotionally support other age groups are vulnerable to unique pressures and stresses. It is often hard for them to admit that they have health problems or are experiencing stress.

The role of the nurse in helping adults achieve their developmental tasks is an important one. Understanding human development and its impact on health is essential. It is easier for adults to promote and maintain health when they know about health behaviors that enhance wellness and prevent stress. Major goals of the community health nurse when working with adults are to increase health promotion, prevent illness, and promote self-care capabilities. To accomplish these goals nurses need a supportive work environment, engagement in the politics of health care, and a belief in lifelong learning.

The author acknowledges the work from previous editions of this text in the development of this chapter.

CRITICAL *Thinking Exercise*

Consider the community where you live. Identify the groups of adults at risk and their health promotion needs. Prioritize the health promotion needs and describe your reasoning. Using the three levels of prevention, outline a plan for your health promotion priority. Identify the community agencies and the resources they could provide to help address the health needs among the adult population. Describe barriers that may impede implementation of your health promotion plan. Describe factors that would facilitate implementation of your planned interventions.

REFERENCES

Alexander-Rodriguez T: Prison health—a role for professional nursing, *Nurs Outlook* 31(2):115-118, 1983.

American Cancer Society (ACS): *Cancer facts and figures—1996*, Atlanta, 1996a, ACS.

American Cancer Society (ACS): *Research Program Report 1995*, Atlanta, 1996b, ACS.

American Heart Association (AHA): *Heart and stroke facts: 1995 statistical supplement*, Dallas, 1994, AHA.

American Heart Association (AHA): *Fact sheet on heart attack, stroke, and risk factors*, Dallas, 1995a, AHA.

American Heart Association (AHA): *Heart and stroke facts*, Dallas, 1995b, AHA.

American Heart Association (AHA): *1996 research facts*, Dallas, 1995c, AHA.

American Heart Association (AHA): *Heart attack and stroke: signals and action*, Dallas, 1996, AHA.

American Nurses Association (ANA): American Nurses Association position statement on tuberculosis and HIV. In *Compendium of American Nurses Association position statements*, Washington, D.C., 1996, ANA.

American Nurses Association (ANA): *Scope and standards of nursing practice in correctional facilities*, Washington, D.C., 1995, ANA.

American Nurses Association (ANA): *Scope and standards of nursing practice in correctional facilities*, Kansas City, 1985, ANA.

American Public Health Association (APHA): *Standards for health services in correctional institutions*, Washington, D.C., 1986, APHA.

Arnaud C: Osteoporosis: using bone markers for diagnosis and monitoring, *Geriatrics* 51(4):24-30, 1996.

Berkman A: Prison health: the breaking point, *Am J Public Health* 85:1616-1618, 1995.

Biggs J, Fleury J: An exploration of perceived barriers to cardiovascular risk reduction, *Cardiovasc Nurs* 30(6):41-46, November/December 1996.

Carlson K: Gay and lesbian families. In Harway M, ed: *Treating the changing family*, New York, 1996, Wiley, pp. 62-76.

Centers for Disease Control and Prevention (CDC): HIV/AIDS education and prevention programs for adults in prisons and jails and juveniles in confinement facilities—United States, 1994, *MMWR* 45(13):268-270, 1996c.

Centers for Disease Control and Prevention (CDC): Mortality patterns—United States, 1993, *MMWR* 45(8):161-164, March 1, 1996a.

Centers for Disease Control and Prevention (CDC): Prevention and control of tuberculosis in correctional facilities, *MMWR* 45(RR-8):1-6, June 7, 1996b.

Colsher PL, Wallace RB, Loeffelholz PL, Sales M: Health status of older male prisoners: a comprehensive survey, *Am J Public Health* 82(6):881-883, 1992.

Cowan P: Women's mental health issues: reflections on past attitudes and present practices, *J Psychosoc Nurs Ment Health Serv* 34(4):20-24, 1996.

Denenberg R: Report on lesbian health, *WHI* 5(2):81-91, 1995.

Dennerstein L: Gender, health, and ill-health, *WHI* 5(2):53-59, 1995.

Duvall EM: *Family development*, ed 2, New York, 1962, Lippincott.

Duvall EM, Miller BC: *Marriage and family development*, ed 6, New York, 1985, Harper & Row.

Eliason MJ: *Who cares? institutional barriers to health care for lesbian, gay, and bisexual persons*, Pub No. 14-6742, New York, 1996, NLN.

Eliason MJ, Randall CE: Lesbian phobia in nursing students, *West J Nurs Res* 13(3):363-374, 1991.

Erikson EH: *Childhood and society*, ed 2, New York, 1963, Norton.

Erikson EH: *The life cycle completed: a review*, New York, 1982, Norton.

Fogel CI, Martin SL: The mental health of incarcerated women, *West J Nurs Res* 14(1):30-47, 1992.

Fontes HC: Prisons: logical innovative clinical nursing laboratories, *Nurs Health Care* 12(6):300-303, 1991.

Gaiter J, Doll LS: Editorial: Improving HIV/AIDS prevention in prisons is good public health policy, *Am J Public Health* 86(9):1201-1203, 1996.

Glantz SA: Editorial: Preventing tobacco use—the youth access trap, *Am J Public Health* 8(2):156-157, 1996.

Greenwood S: *Menopause, naturally, preparing for the second half of life*, Volcano, Ca., 1996, Volcano Press.

Hall C, Ortiz-Peters R: Faculty practice in a prison setting: implications for teaching, *J Nurs Educ* 25(7):306-309, 1986.

Hall M: Lesbians and alcohol: patterns and paradoxes in medical notions and lesbians' beliefs, *J Psychoactive Drugs* 25(2):109-119, 1993.

Harris JE: Cigarette smoke components and disease: cigarette smoke is more than a triad of tar, nicotine and carbon monoxide. In National Cancer Institute: *The FTC cigarette test method for determining tar, nicotine, and carbon monoxide yields of U.S. cigarettes*, NIH Pub No. 96-4028, Washington, D.C., 1996, The Institute, pp. 59-79.

Havighurst RJ: *Developmental tasks and education*, New York, 1972, David McKay.

Hawthorne MH: Gender differences in recovery after coronary artery surgery, *Image J Nurs Sch* 26(1):75-80, 1994.

Hellman RE: Issues in the treatment of lesbian women and gay men with chronic mental illness, *Psychiatric Services* 47(10):1093-1098, 1996.

Henningfield JE, Schuh LM: Pharmacology and markers: nicotine pharmacology and addictive effects. In National Cancer Institute: *The FTC cigarette test method for determining tar, nicotine, and carbon monoxide yields of U.S. cigarettes*, NIH Pub No. 96-4028, Washington, D.C., 1996, The Institute, pp. 113-125.

Hofland SL, Powers J: Sexual dysfunction in menopausal woman: hormonal causes and management issues, *Geriatr Nurs* 17(4):161-165, 1996.

Horton JA, ed: *The women's health data book: a profile of women's health in the United States*, Washington, D.C., 1995, The Jacob Institute of Women's Health.

Hough EE, Lewis FM, Woods NF: Family response to a mother's chronic illness: case studies of well-and poorly adjusted families, *West J Nurs Res* 13(5):568-596, 1991.

Huft AG: Psychosocial adaptation to pregnancy in prison, *J Psychosoc Nurs Ment Health Serv* 30(4):19-23, 1992.

Kubler-Ross E: *Questions and answers on death and dying*, New York, 1974, Collier Books.

Kubler-Ross E: *Death: the final stage of growth*, Englewood Cliffs, N.J., 1975, Prentice-Hall.

LaMere S, Smyer T, Gragert M: The aging inmate, *J Psychosoc Nurs Ment Health Serv* 34(4):25-29, 1996.

LeMone P, Burke KM: *Medical-surgical nursing: critical thinking in client care*, Menlo Park, Ca., 1996, Addison-Wesley.

Martin KS, Larson BJ, Gorski LA, Hayko DM, eds: *Mosby's home health client teaching guides: R_x for teaching*, St. Louis, 1997, Mosby, p. V-A, 1-9.

McDonald DC: *Managing prison health care costs*, Washington, D.C., 1995, U.S. Department of Justice.

Meddis SV: An unprecedented level of imprisonment in USA, *USA Today*, August 10, 1995, p. A3.

Miller NH: Tips for smoking cessation, *Cardiovasc Nurs* 32(5):33-35, 1996.

National Cancer Institute: *Questions and answers about PDQ, the National Cancer Institute's computerized database for physicians*, Washington, D.C., 1989, The Institute.

National Center for Health Statistics: *Health, United States, 1995 Chartbook*, DHHS Pub No. (PHS) 96-1232-1, Hyattsville, Md., 1996, Public Health Service.

National Institute of Justice: *Issues and practices: 1994 update, tuberculosis in correctional facilities*, Washington, D.C., 1995, National Institute for Justice.

National Safety Council: *Accident facts, 1995 ed*, Itasca, Il., 1995, The Council.

O'Connell KA, Gerkovich MM, Cook MR: Reversal theory's mastery and sympathy states in smoking cessation, *Image J Nurse Sch* 27(4):311-316, 1995.

Pender N: *Health promotion in nursing practice*, ed 3, 1996, Appleton & Lange.

Pender NJ, Barkauskas VH, Hayman L et al: Health promotion and disease prevention: toward excellence in nursing practice and education, *Nurs Outlook* 40(3):106-113, 1992.

Peters SL: Some women on fast track feel derailed, *USA Today*, February 1, 1996, pp. 1A, 2A.

Reynolds CF: Depression: making the diagnosis and using SSRIs in older adults, *Geriatrics* 51(10):28-34, 1996.

Roell S: Prison practicum scores points with students and inmates, *Nurs Health Care* 6(2):103-105, 1985.

Sheehy G: *New passages: mapping your life across time*, New York, 1996, Ballantine Books.

Shiffman S: Smoking cessation treatment: any progress? Special section: clinical research in smoking cessation, *J Consulting Clin Psychol* 61:718-722, 1993.

Sorensen G, Thompson B, Glanz K et al: Work site-based cancer prevention: primary results from the working well trial, *Am J Public Health* 86(7):939-947, 1996.

Stevens PE, Hall JM: Abusive health care interactions experienced by lesbians: cases of institutional violence, *Response* 13(3):23-27, 1990.

Stevens R: When your clients are in jail, *Nurs Forum* 28(4):5-8, 1995.

Stevenson JS: *Issues and crises during middlescence*, New York, 1977, Appleton-Century-Crofts.

Thompson JM, Wilson SF: *Health assessment for nursing practice*, St. Louis, 1996, Mosby.

Thompson JM, McFarland GK, Hirsch JE, Tucker SM: *Mosby's clinical nursing*, ed 3, St. Louis, 1993, Mosby.

U.S. Bureau of the Census: *Statistical abstract of the United States, 1995*, ed 115, Washington, D.C., 1995, U.S. Government Printing Office.

U.S. Department of Health, Education and Welfare (USDHEW): *Smoking and health: report of the advisory committee to the Surgeon General of the Public Health Service*, Washington, D.C., 1964, U.S. Government Printing Office.

U.S. Department of Health and Human Services (USDHHS): *Facts about blood cholesterol*, NIH Pub No. 94-2694, Bethesda, Md., 1994, U.S. Government Printing Office.

U.S. Department of Health and Human Services (USDHHS): *Healthy people 2000: national health promotion and disease prevention objectives, full report, with commentary*, Washington, D.C., 1991a, U.S. Government Printing Office.

U.S. Department of Health and Human Services (USDHHS): *Healthy people 2000: midcourse review and 1995 revisions*, Washington, D.C., 1995a, U.S. Government Printing Office.

U.S. Department of Health and Human Services (USDHHS): *Health status of minorities and low-income groups*, ed 3, Washington, D.C., 1991b, U.S. Government Printing Office.

U.S. Department of Health and Human Services (USDHHS): *The fifth report of the joint national committee on detection, evaluation, and treatment of high blood pressure*, NIH Pub No. 95-1088, Bethesda, Md., 1995b, Public Health Service.

U.S. Department of Health and Human Services (USDHHS): *The Surgeon General's 1989 report on reducing the health consequences of smoking: 25 years of progress*, Washington, D.C., 1989, U.S. Government Printing Office.

U.S. Public Health Service: *Put prevention into practice*, Waldorf, Md., 1994, American Nurses Publishing.

SELECTED BIBLIOGRAPHY

Allen DG, Whatley M: Nursing and men's health: some critical considerations, *Nurs Clin North Am* 21(1):3-13, 1986.

Breslau N, Peterson EL: Smoking cessation in young adults: age at initiation of cigarette smoking, *Am J Public Health* 86(2):214-220, 1996.

Desmond AM: The relationship between loneliness and social interactions in women prisoners, *J Psychosocial Nurs* 29(2):5-9, 1991.

DiFranza JR, Savageau JA, Aisquith BF: Youth access to tobacco: the effects of age, gender, vending machine locks and "it's the law" programs, *Am J Public Health* 86(2):221-224, 1996.

Duffy ME: Determinants of health promotion in midlife women, *Nurs Res* 37(6):358-362, 1988.

Escobedo LG, Peddicord JP: Smoking prevalence in U.S. birth cohorts: the influence of gender and education, *Am J Public Health* 86(2):231-236, 1996.

Goldstein AO, Bearman NS: State lobbyists and organizations in the United States: crossed lines, *Am J Public Health* 86(8):1137-1142, 1996.

Hitchcock JM, Wilson HS: Personal risking: lesbian self-disclosure of sexual orientation to professional health care providers, *Nurs Res* 41(3):178-183, 1992.

LeVay S: A difference in hypothalamic structure between heterosexual and homosexual men, *Science* 253:1034-1037, August 1991.

Lipp EJ, Deane D, Trimble N: Cardiovascular risks in adolescent males, *Appl Nurs Res* 9(3):102-107, 1996.

National Cancer Institute: *The FTC cigarette test method for determining tar, nicotine, and carbon monoxide yields of U.S. cigarettes*, NIH Pub No. 96-4028, Washington, D.C., 1996, The Institute.

National Mental Health Association: *Depression: what you should know about it*, Alexandria, Va., 1988, The Association.

Notelovitz M, Tonnessen D: *Menopause and midlife health*, New York, 1993, St. Martin's Press.

Peterson E, Schultz L, Andreski P, Chilcoat H: Are smokers with alcohol disorders less likely to quit? *Am J Public Health* 86(7):985-990, 1996.

Shea S, Basch CE, Wechsler H, Lantigua R: The Washington Heights-Inwood Healthy Heart program: a 6-year report from a disadvantaged urban setting, *Am J Public Health* 86(2):166-171, 1996.

Sheehy G: *Menopause: the silent passage*, New York, 1993, Simon & Schuster.

Tobacco and health, *Am J Public Health*, special issue, 79:2, 1989.

U.S. Department of Health and Human Services (USDHHS): *Physical activity and health: a report of the Surgeon General*, Atlanta, 1996, Centers for Disease Control and Prevention, National Center for Chronic Disease Prevention and Health Promotion.

U.S. Department of Health and Human Services (USDHHS): *Women's health: report of the Public Health Service Task Force on Women's Health Issues*, DHHS Pub No. (PHS) 85-5026, Washington, D.C., 1985, U.S. Government Printing Office.

Warner KE: Smoking and health: a 25-year perspective, *Am J Public Health* 79(12):141-142, 1989.

Women's health—report of the Public Health Service Task Force on women's health issues, *Public Health Rep* 100:73-106, 1985.

Zapka JG, Bigelow C, Hurley T et al: Mammography use among sociodemographically diverse women: the accuracy of self-report, *Am J Public Health* 86(7):1016-1021, 1996.

18

Occupational Health Nursing

Objectives

Upon completion of this chapter, the reader should be able to:

1. Discuss the *Healthy People 2000* national health objectives for occupational health.
2. Summarize the purpose, intents, and mandates of the Occupational Safety and Health Act of 1970.
3. Discuss the evolution of occupational health nursing in the United States.
4. Describe recommended educational preparation and professional opportunities for the occupational health nurse.
5. Understand the objectives and functions of the occupational health nurse.
6. Discuss the 10 leading work-related diseases/injuries in the United States.
7. Discuss communicable diseases that are contemporary workplace concerns.
8. Discuss smoking and violence as occupational health concerns.
9. Understand some major health concerns of agricultural workers.

Occupational health is the application of public health principles and medical, nursing and engineering practice for the purpose of conserving, promoting and restoring the health and effectiveness of workers through their place of employment.

MARY LOUISE BROWN, *OCCUPATIONAL HEALTH NURSING*, New York, 1956, Springer, p. 1.

The first census in 1790 revealed the United States to be an agricultural nation; however, the Industrial Revolution rapidly changed this. Between 1870 and 1910 the U.S. population rose 132%, whereas the number of persons working in industry rose almost 400% (Morris, 1976, p. 109). Today there are approximately 110 million workers in the United States (USDHHS, 1991a, p. 65). Work is an important part of American life, and Americans are working more hours than ever before (NIOSH, 1995, p. 2). Americans spend one fourth to one third of their time at work (Rogers, 1994a, p. 1).

The American workforce is diverse, representing all socioeconomic levels, ethnic and racial groups, and cultural and religious backgrounds. Women now make up 46% of the labor force, and 23% of the workforce are minorities (USDHHS, 1995, p. 74). The median age of the American worker is 37.9 years (USDHHS, p. 74); and the working population is basically a well adult population. Occupational health professionals strive to make the workplace safe and healthy, and emphasize primary prevention activities such as health education, health promotion, and worker protection. The workplace environment profoundly affects health (NIOSH, 1995, p. 2). This chapter addresses occupational health in the United States and the role of the occupational health nurse in promoting the health of workers and their families.

OCCUPATIONAL HEALTH IN THE UNITED STATES

Historically, the workplace was not always a healthy place. By the mid-1800s many Americans worked under unsafe or unhealthy conditions, and workers rallied for shorter work days, health and safety measures, and child labor laws. During these years almost half of all employees in New England factories were children from 7 to 16 years of age. Massachusetts was a leader in implementing occupational safety and health provisions. In 1836 Massachusetts became the first state to enact a child labor law; in 1850, the first to study occupational health; in 1879, the first to pass legislation requiring factory safety inspections; and in 1886, the first to require reporting of industrial accidents.

Around the turn of the century, *occupational medicine* and *occupational health nursing* began to emerge in the United States: the Homestake Mining Company sponsored the first industrial medical department in the United States in 1887 (U.S. Department of Labor [USDL], 1977, p. 15). In 1888

Betty Moulder, a nurse, was hired by a group of Pennsylvania coal mining companies to care for the miners and their families, but little is known of her duties or accomplishments (Haag, Glazner, 1992, p. 56; Parker-Conrad, 1988, p. 156). At this time, public awareness of occupational health hazards also increased, and physicians began to write about occupational disease.

The federal government issued its first major report on occupational safety and health in 1903 (USDL, 1977, pp. 15-16). About this time a pioneer in occupational medicine, Dr. Alice Hamilton, began her work. In 1910 she became the chair of the Occupational Disease Commission in Illinois; it was the first such commission in the country. In 1911 she was chosen to head the newly formed *Federal Occupational Disease Commission*.

Dr. Hamilton achieved international recognition for her research and writings on occupational diseases and conditions. She is considered by many to be the founder of occupational medicine in this country. Among her numerous publications are the classic *Industrial Poisons in the United States* (1925) and *Exploring the Dangerous Trades: the Autobiography of Alice Hamilton, M.D.* (1943). Dr. Hamilton lived a long and remarkable life. She died the year that the Occupational Safety and Health Act of 1970 was passed, at the age of 101.

During Dr. Hamilton's time the emergence of labor unions and the formation of the U.S. Department of Labor placed new emphasis on occupational health and safety. Although for different reasons, workers and employers agreed on the value of maintaining worker health. Workers were concerned about their health, and if they were not healthy their economic security was threatened. Employers wanted healthy workers because unhealthy ones threatened the economic stability of the workplace. Who was financially responsible for lost wages and health care when an employee died or became ill, injured, or disabled because of work-related conditions was a major point of difference between workers and employers.

In the early 1900s workers began to take a firm stand on the right to be compensated for job-related illness, injury, or disability, and state workers' compensation legislation came into being. The first workers' compensation acts met with much resistance from employers, and many were ruled to be unconstitutional. In 1911 New Jersey passed the first workers' compensation act to be upheld by the courts. Other states quickly followed, with nine more acts in 1911; 11 in 1912; 11 in 1913; and all states by 1948 (USDL, 1977, p. 77). This legislation sparked new interest in employers to keep workers healthy and signaled the development of industrial health services in the workplace (Haag, Glazner, 1992, p. 56).

At this time much was happening in occupational health. Cornell University Medical College established an occupational disease clinic in 1910, and soon others opened around the country (Felton, 1976, p. 814). The U.S. Department of Labor was elevated to a cabinet-level position in 1913, the Office of Industrial Hygiene and Sanitation in the U.S. Public Health Service and the Industrial Hygiene Section of the American Public Health Association were both established in 1914, and in 1916 the American Association of Industrial Physicians and Surgeons was organized in Detroit, Michigan (Felton, pp. 812-813).

Almost 25 years after workers' compensation began to be legislated, the Social Security Act of 1935 enacted unemployment insurance and made funds available to expand industrial hygiene programs—leading to the establishment of divisions of industrial hygiene in many state and local health departments (McGrath, 1945, p. 123). Selected legislation and events in occupational health in the United States since 1935 are given in the box on the next page. Work is a part of life, and unfortunately many work-related injuries, diseases, and conditions exist. More than $115 billion is spent in the United States on workplace injuries and illnesses each year (Sattler, 1996, p. 233), and national health objectives have been developed to promote health at the workplace.

WORK AS A DEVELOPMENTAL TASK

A developmental framework is used throughout this text, and developmental tasks are discussed. Work has been described as a developmental task for the adult (Duvall, Miller, 1985; Stevenson, 1977), and it is also a basic part of life and social roles (Rogers, 1994a, p. 1). Our nation promotes the work ethic and expects that adults will work and be self-sufficient. Work becomes a source of productivity, social contact, personal development, and self-expression. Work is a major means of establishing individual, family, and national economic security. People often identify closely with work, and their personal identity may be intertwined with their work life.

The developmental tasks of work are carried out simultaneously with family and individual developmental tasks. If work-related developmental tasks are interrupted or left undone, sequential development can be affected and stress can occur. For example, being out of work (unemployment) can be stressful and carry with it negative experiences and societal connotations. Unemployment as a crisis for the adult is discussed in Chapter 17.

Duvall and Miller (1985) described the young adult as facing the work-related task of selecting and training for an occupation; the adult and middlescent as carrying out a socially adequate worker role and creating a balance between family, community, work, and leisure; and the aged adult as adjusting to retirement. The developmental tasks of the young adult involve integrating personal values with career development and socioeconomic constraints; the early-middle-years adult as developing socioeconomic consolidation and assuming responsible positions in occupational activities; the late-middle-years adult as maintaining flexible views in occupational positions, preparing for another

Selected Legislation and Events in Occupational Health in the United States—1936 to Present

1936 *Walsh-Healy Act* sets occupational safety and health standards and minimum age limitations for workers employed in government contract work.

1938 *Fair Labor Standards Act* sets a minimum age for child labor: 16 years old for general work and 18 years old for hazardous work, applicable to most industrial settings. Also establishes maximum hours and minimum wages for interstate commerce workers.

1939 American Industrial Hygiene Association established.

1941 *Federal Mine Inspection Act* passes, helping to ensure greater safety in the mining industry.

1946 American Academy of Occupational Medicine established. It merges with the American Occupational Medicine Association to form the American Academy of Occupational and Environmental Medicine in 1988.

1948 All states have enacted *Workers' Compensation* acts.

1952 *Coal Mine Safety Act* is passed, ensuring greater coal mine safety.

1966 *Mine-Safety Act* is passed, requiring mandatory inspections and health and safety standards.

1969 *Coal Mine Health and Safety Act* is passed, setting mandatory health and safety standards for underground mines.

1970 *Occupational Safety and Health Act of 1970* is passed. It is the most significant piece of occupational safety and health legislation in the U.S., establishing the Occupational Safety and Health Administration (OSHA) and the National Institute of Occupational Safety and Health (NIOSH).

1972 *Black Lung Benefits Act* provides benefits to black lung victims.

1977 *Federal Mine Safety and Health Act* is passed, consolidating all existing mine legislation into one act.

1979 *Healthy People* is published by the U.S. Public Health Service, establishing occupational health as a national health priority area and setting national occupational health objectives.

1990 The *Americans with Disabilities Act* is passed, safeguarding the rights of the disabled worker.

1991 *Healthy People 2000* is published by the U.S. Public Health Service, continuing occupational health as a national health priority area.

1993 *Family Leave Act* provides protection from loss of employment when time is needed by an employee to care for ill children, spouse, parent or the employee's own illness—employees are entitled to up to 12 weeks unpaid leave during the year.

career when feasible, and preparing for retirement; and the adult in late adulthood as pursuing a second or third career and/or adjusting to retirement. Maintaining the health of the worker is an important role of occupational health and occupational health nursing.

OCCUPATIONAL HEALTH AND THE *HEALTHY PEOPLE 2000* OBJECTIVES FOR THE NATION

As reflected in the box on the next page, occupational health is a priority area in *Healthy People 2000*. These national objectives address the areas of improving health status, reducing risk factors and improving services/protection, and targeting reduction of work-related death, injuries, cumulative trauma disorders, back injury, skin disorders, lead poisoning, lung disease, hearing loss, and communicable diseases. One objective, "to implement state occupational safety and health plans for the identification, management, and prevention of leading work-related diseases and injuries in all 50 states," was an especially aggressive undertaking since only 10 states had such programs when the objectives were determined (A Public Health Service, 1992). Today more than 30 states have such plans in place (USDHHS, 1995, p. 76).

Progress on achieving national occupational health objectives is mixed. The objective related to reducing the incidence of hepatitis B infections among occupationally exposed workers has been reached. Progress has been made in the following areas: reducing work-related deaths, having occupationally exposed workers receive hepatitis B immunizations, the implementation of occupational health and safety plans by states, state development of occupational lung disease exposure standards, and increasing the number of worksite back injury and promotion programs. However, the incidence of cumulative trauma disorders has more than tripled, the incidence of occupational skin disorders has greatly increased, and increases have occurred in the incidence of nonfatal work-related injuries (notably among nurses, personal care workers, and transportation workers) (USDHHS, 1995, p. 74). Motor vehicle crashes are the leading cause of fatal injury in the workplace (USDHHS, p. 75).

National health objectives focus on protecting worker health, keeping workers healthy, and providing a safe and healthful work environment. Accomplishment of these objectives will require implementation of occupational safety and health education—not just in the workplace, but also in schools and homes. "The time has come to protect one of our most valuable resources: the American worker" (NIOSH, 1995, p. 2).

OCCUPATIONAL HEALTH LEGISLATION IN THE UNITED STATES

In comparison with other industrial nations, the United States was slow to enact occupational safety and health legislation. By 1884 Germany had already enacted a law that provided for a comprehensive system of occupational

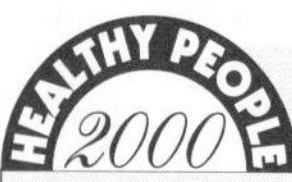

Objectives Targeting Occupational Safety and Health

HEALTH STATUS OBJECTIVES

1. Reduce deaths from work-related injuries to no more than 4 per 100,000 full-time workers.
2. Reduce work-related injuries resulting in medical treatment, lost time from work, or restricted work activity to no more than 6 cases per 100 full-time workers.
3. Reduce cumulative trauma disorders to an incidence of no more than 60 cases per 100,000 full-time workers.
4. Reduce occupational skin disorders or diseases to an incidence of no more than 55 per 100,000 full-time workers.
5. Reduce hepatitis B infections among occupational exposed workers to an incidence of no more than 1,250 cases.

RISK REDUCTION OBJECTIVES

6. Increase to at least 75 percent the proportion of worksites with 50 or more employees that mandate employee use of occupant protection systems, such as seatbelts, during all work-related motor vehicle travel.
7. Reduce to no more than 15 percent the proportion of workers exposed to average daily noise levels that exceed 85 dBA.
8. Eliminate exposures which result in workers having blood lead concentrations greater than 25 μg/dL of whole blood.
9. Increase hepatitis B immunization levels to 90 percent among occupationally exposed workers.

SERVICES AND PROTECTION OBJECTIVES

10. Implement occupational safety and health plans in 50 states for the identification, management, and prevention of leading work-related diseases and injuries within the State.
11. Establish in 50 States exposure standards adequate to prevent the major occupational lung diseases to which their worker populations are exposed (byssinosis, asbestosis, coal workers' pneumoconiosis, and silicosis).
12. Increase to at least 70 percent the proportion of worksites with 50 or more employees that have implemented programs on worker health and safety.
13. Increase to at least 50 percent the proportion of worksites with 50 or more employees that offer back injury prevention and rehabilitation programs.
14. Establish in 50 States either public health or labor department programs that provide consultation and assistance to small businesses to implement safety and health programs for their employees.
15. Increase to at least 75 percent the proportion of primary care providers who routinely elicit occupational health exposures as a part of patient history and provide relevant counseling.
16. Reduce deaths from work-related homicides to no more than 0.5 per 100,000 full-time workers.
17. Reduce the overall age-adjusted mortality rate for four major preventable occupational lung diseases (byssinosis, asbestosis, coal workers' pneumoconiosis, and silicosis).
18. Increase to 100 percent the proportion of worksites with a formal smoking policy that prohibits or severely restricts smoking at the workplace.
19. Enact in 50 States and the District of Columbia comprehensive laws on clean indoor air that prohibit smoking or limit it to separately ventilated areas in the workplace and enclosed public places.

From USDHHS: *Healthy people 2000: midcourse review and 1995 revisions,* Washington, D.C., 1995, U.S. Government Printing Office.

health, including compensation for occupational illness, injury, or disability irrespective of who was responsible for the occurrence of the condition (McCall, 1977, p. 21).

For years occupational health nurses, occupational physicians, and countless workers stressed the hazards in the American workplace. In 1968 the Surgeon General, Dr. William Steward, told Congress that U.S. Public Health Service studies showed that 65% of industrial workers were exposed to toxic or harmful substances or conditions in their place of employment (Stellman, Daum, 1973, pp. xiii-xiv). The same year an occupational health law was defeated by Congress.

Many Americans thought that legislation in the workplace would endanger the free enterprise system. However, with the support of workers and labor unions, the *Occupational Safety and Health Act of 1970* was passed. The act was passed to ensure Americans the right to "safe and healthful working conditions" (NIOSH, 1995, p. 2). It is the most significant piece of occupational safety and health legislation in the United States.

Occupational Safety and Health Act of 1970

The Occupational Safety and Health Act of 1970 (Public Law 91-596) made the health of workers a public concern and made a national commitment to maintaining worker health and preventing work-related disease, disability, and death. Since the passage of the act progress has been made, yet workplace hazards continue to inflict a tremendous toll in both human and economic costs (NIOSH, 1995, p. 2).

INTENTS AND MANDATES OF THE ACT The intents of this act were (1) to prevent placing toxic substances in the workplace, (2) to regulate exposure to toxic and dangerous substances already in the workplace, and (3) to compensate workers for occupational illness and injury. To carry out these intents, the act had specific mandates that delineated the formation of agencies to carry them out:

- *Occupational Safety and Health Administration (OSHA).* This administration sets and enforces standards for occupational safety and health. It is under the jurisdiction of the Department of Labor.

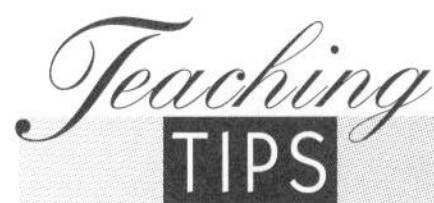

Worksite Educational Topics That Address Healthy People 2000 Objectives

- Violence prevention in the worksite, including a plan for handling disruptive employees and visitors.
- Techniques to decrease psychological stress in the work environment.
- Prevention of infectious diseases, including a discussion of universal precautions and importance of hepatitis B immunization for at-risk employees.
- Health promotion programs that address the major health problems among adults (e.g., healthy heart cooking, weight control, exercise activities, and smoking cessation).
- Worksite policies for stringent use of occupational protective equipment (e.g., safety belts, hearing protection devices, and protective clothing that is resistant to chemical and physical hazards).
- Worksite hazards for the pregnant woman.
- Prevention of back injuries.
- Prevention of cumulative trauma disorders.
- Characteristics of adolescents that increase their risk for occupational injuries.
- Motor vehicle safety in the work setting.

- *National Institute for Occupational Safety and Health (NIOSH)*. This institute conducts research and training and makes recommendations for the prevention of work-related illnesses and injuries and occupational health standards to OSHA. It is under the jurisdiction of the Department of Health and Human Services and has a toll-free number for information (1-800-35-NIOSH). Its philosophy is reflected in its vision statement: "Delivering on the nation's promise: safety and health at work for all people . . . through research and prevention" (NIOSH, 1995, p. 3).
- *Occupational Safety and Health Review Commission*. A quasijudicial agency charged with ruling on cases forwarded to it by the Department of Labor when disagreements arise over the results of safety and health inspections performed by OSHA.
- *National Advisory Council on Occupational Safety and Health*. A consumer and professional council that makes occupational safety and health recommendations to OSHA and NIOSH.
- *National Commission on State Workers' Compensation Laws*. A temporary evaluative commission to study and make recommendations on the adequacy of state workers' compensation laws to the President. *Official termination date: October 30, 1972.*

The act also established federal occupational safety and health standards and imposed fines and sentences for violation of federal occupational safety and health regulations.

OSHA requires employers to keep records of work-related deaths, injuries, and illnesses for review. Under the act, states can develop their own occupational safety and health administrations as long as the state standards meet or exceed the federal standards. The occupational health nurse works frequently with OSHA and NIOSH.

SOME PROBLEMS WITH THE ACT There have been a number of problems with the act, including the following:

FUNDING. Funding for the act has been grossly inadequate, and has affected the ability of OSHA to carry out its intents and mandates. According to the *Budget of the United States, Fiscal Year 1994*, estimated funding is set at approximately $294 million for OSHA with an additional $68 million available in grants to states for the cost of their OSHA programs, and $112 million to NIOSH. This amounts to less than $2 per citizen per year in federal occupational safety and health spending.

COORDINATION OF SERVICES. OSHA and NIOSH are under the jurisdiction of two different federal departments; their resources and services have not always been well coordinated, and interagency problems have existed (OSHA is under the Department of Labor and NIOSH is under the Department of Health and Human Services). NIOSH researches occupational safety and health standards, and OSHA has the authority to set and enforce them.

FINES AND SENTENCES. Extremely low fines and sentences were set by the original provisions of the act. Even though recent increases have been made, fines and sentences still may not be severe enough to act as incentives to employers to improve working conditions.

ECONOMIC IMPACT STATEMENTS. Economic impact statements became policy in 1975. They are an occupational cost analysis study of a proposed OSHA standard or regulation. If a company can show that it would not be economically feasible to comply with a standard or regulation, it can appeal the proposed regulation.

SCOPE OF THE PROBLEM. Hundreds of thousands of workplaces are covered under the act. Added to this is the fact that there are more than 80,000 chemicals in the workplace (Greaves, 1992, p. 1333), and thousands of these chemicals are considered to be toxic or carcinogens. The enormity of problems such as work-related injuries, illness, disability, and death add to the scope. A look at the 10 leading causes of work-related illness later in this chapter helps to illustrate the enormity of the problem.

LEGAL CHALLENGES. In the first year of the act approximately 100 bills were introduced in Congress to amend or repeal it (McNeely, 1992, p. 19). Almost every occupational health standard established by OSHA has been challenged in the courts, leading to costly and time-consuming delays in establishing standards (McNeely, p. 19). Legal arguments challenging the right of OSHA to set and enforce occupational safety and health standards continue.

LACK OF TRAINED PERSONNEL. There is no minimum qualification for the personnel responsible for interpreting the complex OSHA regulations and implementing compliance activities (Sattler, 1996, p. 233). There are severe shortages of industrial hygienists, occupational health nurses, and physicians. Currently only 1500 physicians and 4000 nurses are certified in occupational health—that equates to one occupational physician and fewer than three occupational health nurses to care for every 80,000 active workers and 20,000 retired or disabled workers (NIOSH, 1995, p. 8). With its present workforce, OSHA can inspect only about 2% of the nation's workplaces in any given year (McNeely, 1992, p. 20). It has been noted that there are more park rangers than OSHA inspectors, and that typical workplaces will see an inspector once every 77 years—about as often as we see Halley's Comet! (McNeely, p. 20). NIOSH Educational Resource Centers are making strides to train and educate professionals in the field. The American Public Health Association (APHA) and the American Association of Occupational Health Nurses (AAOHN) advocate educational programs that prepare health professionals in occupational health and safety.

RULE-MAKING PROCESS. NIOSH first researches standards, then OSHA establishes the proposed standard, or "rule." The OSHA rule-making process is cumbersome, time-consuming, and often slow. It includes public hearings on proposed standards (with a pre-hearing public comment period provided), and a post-hearing public comment period before the final rule is posted. OSHA is working on developing a streamlined process that will reduce the time required to produce a regulation (Smith, 1995a).

DISSEMINATION OF INFORMATION. Once a regulation is promulgated the only requirement of the federal government is to place the final standard in the Federal Register; the vast majority of employers do not have ready access to this document, and the federal government does not have any systematic mechanism to identify affected parties or to send information to targeted audiences (Sattler, 1996, p. 233). Also, there is no mandate that training materials be developed to help employers implement standards (Sattler, p. 233).

The Occupational Safety and Health Act and the Occupational Health Nurse

The provisions of the Occupational Safety and Health Act of 1970 affect occupational health nursing practice. The nurse needs to have a knowledge of the standards established under the act and make certain that the workplace is in compliance with the act's rules and regulations. The nurse will often participate in OSHA on-site workplace visits, assist workers in understanding their rights under the act, and implement health education programs. A survey of occupational health nurses indicated that an important challenge facing them in the workplace is keeping up with OSHA regulations (Rogers, Cox, 1994, p. 161). The nurse may take part in NIOSH education and training programs.

OCCUPATIONAL HEALTH NURSING IN THE UNITED STATES

In her classic text *Occupational Health Nursing*, Mary Louise Brown defined occupational health nursing as "The application of nursing and public health procedures for the purpose of conserving, promoting and restoring the health of individuals and groups through their places of employment" (Brown, 1956, p. 15). Today's occupational health nurses continue to practice these concepts and principles, as well as others that have evolved over time.

The contemporary role of the occupational health nurse emphasizes independent functioning, health promotion, prevention, investigative skills, and management of health care services (Rogers, 1994a, p. 34). Occupational health nursing practice is a synthesis of knowledge from nursing, medicine, public health, occupational health, social/behavioral sciences, as well as knowledge from management/administration theories and legal principles (Rogers, 1994a, p. 34). According to the American Association of Occupational Health Nurses (1994a), occupational health nursing practice is defined as:

> The specialty practice that provides for and delivers health care services to workers and worker populations. The practice focuses on promotion, protection and restoration of workers' health within the context of a safe and healthy work environment. Occupational health nursing practice is autonomous, and occupational health nurses make independent nursing judgements in providing occupational health services. The foundation for occupational health nursing practice is research-based with an emphasis on optimizing health, preventing illness and injury, and reducing health hazards.

A model for contemporary occupational health nursing practice is given in Figure 18-1. The occupational health nurse is considered a key figure in the management and delivery of occupational health services at the worksite (Rogers, 1994a, p. 39). As illustrated in Figure 18-1, the occupational health nurse's practice is affected by a variety of internal and external factors. These factors influence nursing interventions. For example, in some occupational health settings comprehensive health promotion programs are implemented, but in others the emphasis is on the care of ill and injured workers, with little attention placed on health promotion. These differences are influenced by such

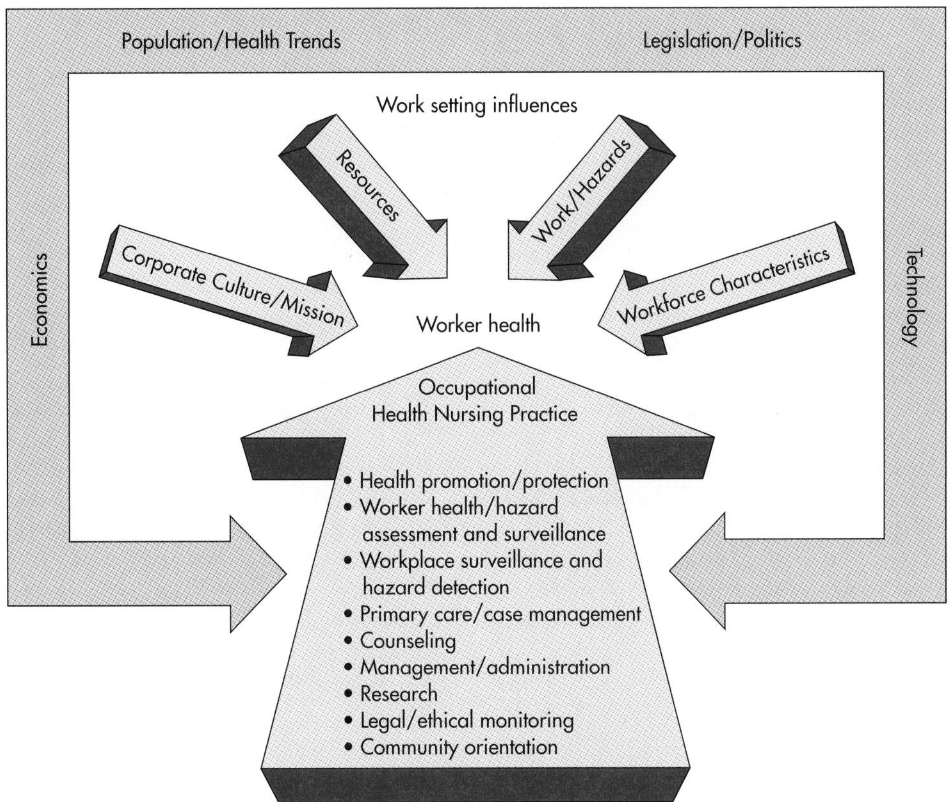

Figure 18-1 Conceptual model for occupational health nursing practice. *(From Rogers B: Occupational health nursing: concepts and practice, Philadelphia, 1994a, Saunders, p. 39. Copyright © by Bonnie Rogers.)*

things as resources allocated for occupational health services and the values of the organization.

The History of Occupational Health Nursing in the United States

Occupational health nurses originally were called *industrial nurses*. As the scope of practice broadened the title was changed. The box on the following page gives a chronological overview of occupational health nursing in the United States. The evolution of occupational health nursing closely follows advances in public health and occupational health.

In 1895 the woman considered by many to be the first occupational health nurse in the United States, *Ada Mayo Stewart,* was hired by the Vermont Marble Company. Much has been written about Miss Stewart. Her sister Harriet, also a nurse, worked with her during the first year of her practice (Rogers, 1994a, p. 23). The Vermont Marble Company was ahead of its time. It hired an occupational health nurse years before other companies and provided worker benefits such as housing, a library, profit-sharing, general accident insurance, and a company store (Felton, 1988; Pinkham, 1988, p. 20). When the company decided to offer nursing services Miss Stewart was an outstanding candidate for the job. She had studied the classics, history, mathematics, English, and Latin, and had graduated from Waltham Training School for Nurses where she had received training in "district nursing" (see Chapter 1) (Pinkham, p. 20).

Miss Stewart was employed as a visiting nurse who gave care in the home to sick company employees and family members, and went into the schools to teach health practices to the children of employees. She often traveled through town on a bicycle and "conversed" in a form of sign language with many non–English-speaking residents (Markolf, 1945, p. 127). In addition to her other nursing responsibilities she learned about the health care customs of the native countries of the people she cared for and taught health education in the schools (Markolf, pp. 127-128), making her an early practitioner of both transcultural and school nursing. The March 1945 issue of *Public Health Nursing* celebrated the 50th anniversary of Miss Stewart's work. For that issue Miss Stewart, now Ada Markolf, wrote a manuscript titled "Industrial Nursing Begins in Vermont." This interesting article was written in third person, as she told the story of the "first" occupational health nursing experience in the United States (Brown, 1988, p. 434).

An Overview of Occupational Health Nursing in the United States

1895 Ada Mayo Stewart (Markolf) is hired by the Vermont Marble Company.
1897 Anna B. Duncan is hired by the Benefit Association of John Wanamaker Company (New York).
1913 First registry for industrial nurses originates in Boston.
1915 Boston Industrial Nurses' Club organized.
1916 Factory Nurses' Conference organized (forerunner of the American Association of Industrial Nurses).
1917 First training course to educate occupational health nurses: *Industrial Service for Nurses,* offered at Boston College.
1919 Florence S. Wright writes *Industrial Nursing.*
1920 The National Organization for Public Health Nursing (NOPHN) establishes an Industrial Nursing section.
1942 American Association of Industrial Nurses is founded (becomes the American Association of Occupational Health Nurses in 1977).
1945 *Industrial Nursing* journal begins publication (1945-1949).
1946 Bertha McGrath writes a manual on industrial nursing, *Nursing in Industry,* in collaboration with the National Organization for Public Health Nursing.
1953 *American Association of Industrial Nurses Journal* established (Becomes *Occupational Health Nursing* in 1969 and *AAOHN Journal* in 1986).
1956 Mary Louise Brown writes the classic book *Occupational Health Nursing.*
1970 *Occupational Safety and Health Act of 1970* passes, having numerous implications for occupational health nursing practice.
1971 American Board of Occupational Health Nurses (ABOHN) formed to establish certification standards and examinations; first examination given in 1974.
1979 *Healthy People* establishes occupational health as a national health priority area, and national health objectives are developed for occupational safety.
1981 American Association of Occupational Health Nurses (AAOHN) establishes a research committee.
1982 First research session held at the annual AAOHN Conference, and the following year the first research award is given.
1989 AAOHN established priority research areas in occupational health nursing (see box on p. 550).
1991 *Healthy People 2000* continues occupational health as a national health priority area.
1994 Dr. Bonnie Rogers writes *Occupational Health Nursing: Concepts and Practice.*

In the early part of the twentieth century many significant events occurred in occupational health nursing. At this time retail stores, cotton mills, and the mining industry began to have programs staffed by nurses (Felton, 1976, p. 814; Gardner, 1916, p. 301; McGrath, 1946; Waters, 1919, p. 728). Florence S. Wright wrote the first book on industrial nursing in 1919. In 1920 the National Organization for Public Health Nursing established an Industrial Nursing Section that defined industrial health nursing (Brown, 1988, p. 435; Pravikoff, 1992, p. 532).

In 1941 Olive Whitlock Kulp became the first industrial nurse to work for the federal government (Parker-Conrad, 1988; Parrish, Allred, 1995). In 1942 the *American Association of Industrial Nurses* (AAIN) was founded with Catherine Dempsey as the first president. The new association published the journal *Industrial Nursing.* At its foundation the AAIN had annual membership dues of 50 cents (Parker-Conrad, 1988, p. 158), and its membership numbered approximately 300 nurses from 16 states (Martin, 1977, p. 10).

In 1945 the National Organization for Public Health Nursing and the AAIN took a position that specific courses in industrial nursing should *not* be a part of the undergraduate nursing program, and recommended that *specialty education* be at the graduate level (AAIN, 1976; Olson, Kochevar, 1989, p. 33). However, these organizations recommended that schools of nursing place more emphasis on examining industrial influences on the health of workers and their families, and advised *integration* of such content throughout the student's educational program (Markolf, 1945, p. 129).

Historically, short courses were a primary form of instruction in occupational health nursing (Rogers, 1991, p. 101). One of the first such courses was offered by Boston University College of Business Administration in 1917 (Barlow, 1992, p. 464; Parker-Conrad, 1988, p. 159). It consisted of 10 lectures per week for 16 weeks, a 2-week practicum, and assistance with job placement (Parker-Conrad, p. 159). Early course content frequently focused on industrial injuries and medical problems common to the worksite (Barlow, 1992, p. 464; Rogers, 1991, p. 101). Early occupational health nurses recieved most of their education on the job, and few specialized educational opportunities existed. Although discussions on integrating occupational health nursing content into baccalaureate curricula have been under way for almost 50 years, today integration of occupational health nursing theory and concepts into undergraduate nursing education remains limited.

Several significant changes in the 1970s and 1980s have advanced OHN practice. In the 1970s the Occupational Safety and Health Act provided an impetus to occupational health nursing education and practice when NIOSH Educational Resources Centers were established. On January 1, 1977, the AAIN changed its name to the *American Association of Occupational Health Nurses* (AAOHN) to help reflect the increasing range of opportunities in the field. In 1983 the AAOHN established the first research award in occupational health nursing and in 1990 established research priorities. In 1988 the first occupational health nurse consultant was hired by OSHA, and in 1993 the Office of Occupational Health Nursing was established at OSHA. The 1990s and beyond look promising for occupational health nursing, and more nurses are receiving specialty education in occupational health.

Occupational Health Nursing Education and Certification

Occupational health nursing is grounded in public health and nursing theory, with an emphasis on community health nursing (Rogers, 1994a, p. 31). The AAOHN supports the baccalaureate degree in nursing as basic preparation for entry into occupational health nursing practice (AAOHN, 1996b). In a recent survey 42% of the occupational health nurses responding reported a diploma in nursing as their level of nursing education, and 22% reported a bachelor of science degree in nursing as their highest level of education—28% were certified as an occupational health nurse (Rogers, Cox, 1994, p. 159).

The USDHHS has recommended that the professional education of all primary health care providers should include instruction in occupational safety and health and give them an understanding of the relationship between work and health (USDHHS, 1991a, p. 297). In a study done by Rogers (1991) of baccalaureate schools of nursing in the United States, 58% of the responding schools indicated they had integrated curricular content on worker health and 47% had integrated content on basic occupational health nursing services. Graduate education in occupational health nursing is available in several universities across the country.

GRADUATE EDUCATION The National Institute for Occupational Safety and Health Educational Resource Centers (NIOSH ERCs) offer graduate and continuing education in occupational health and safety for health professionals. They operate under federal grants, with student stipends often available.

Currently 14 ERCs are at major universities across the nation (a listing can be obtained by contacting NIOSH at 1-800-35-NIOSH). All ERCs have a nursing component, and some offer doctoral education in nursing. Graduate education in occupational health nursing, especially on the doctoral level, is in its infancy.

Many occupational health nurses cannot take advantage of graduate education because they are not prepared at the baccalaureate level. A study by Lusk, Disch, and Barkauskas (1988) showed that approximately 65% of the respondents were prepared at the associate degree or diploma level and only 2% had a master's degree in nursing. A significant role of an occupational health nurse (OHN) leader at the worksite is to help nursing staff to advance their practice through education.

CERTIFICATION Certification for OHNs has been available since 1974. It involves a combination of work experience, coursework, and written examination. Areas involved in certification testing include knowledge of toxicology, treatment of chemical exposures, ergonomics, the Occupational Safety and Health Act and workers' compensation legislation, and competence in physical assessment (Maciag, 1993, p. 39). Since 1996 a baccalaureate degree is required for OHN certification (Maciag, p. 39). Further information can be obtained by contacting AAOHN.

American Association of Occupational Health Nurses (AAOHN)

The AAOHN is the specialty organization for occupational health nurses. It has chapters in every state and a membership of more than 12,500 nurses. AAOHN works in close cooperation with the American Nurses Association (ANA), its membership, and the more than 23,000 practicing occupational health nurses in the United States.

The mission of AAOHN is to promote occupational health nursing, maintain professional integrity, and enhance its professional status (AAOHN, 1989b). AAOHN has divisions of professional affairs, governmental affairs, public affairs, and membership. The association establishes standards of occupational health nursing practice, assists nurses in providing quality care, and serves as an advocate for occupational health and occupational health nursing (AAOHN, 1989b).

AAOHN assisted in developing the *Healthy People 2000* occupational health objectives. The association was instrumental in having occupational health nurses placed on the staff of OSHA (Barlow, 1992, p. 465; Haag, Glazner, 1992, p. 59). The *AAOHN Journal* is published by the association. For further information on the association contact the American Association of Occupational Health Nurses at 50 Lenox Pointe, Atlanta, Georgia 30324 (404-262-1162).

AAOHN recommends a minimum of 2 years of professional nursing experience in a primary care setting, such as community health, ambulatory care, emergency, or critical care units before entering occupational health nursing practice (AAOHN, 1986). Additional experience in areas such as community health, mental health, rehabilitation, and medical-surgical nursing is desirable.

STANDARDS OF PRACTICE Standards of practice are a baseline against which nursing actions can be measured. AAOHN (1994a) has developed standards for occupational health nursing practice that address policy, personnel, resources, nursing practice, and evaluation. They are periodically revised to reflect the changing scope and essence of practice and can be obtained through AAOHN.

Objectives of Occupational Health Nursing

Primary objectives for the occupational health nurse are to:

1. Protect the worker from occupational safety and health hazards
2. Promote a safe and healthful workplace
3. Facilitate efforts of workers and workers' families to meet their health and welfare needs
4. Promote education and research in the field

The nurse must work cooperatively with the worker, his or her family, the workplace, and the community to accomplish occupational safety and health objectives. The nurse realizes that successful fulfillment of these objectives will promote high-level wellness, enhance quality of life, increase job productivity, and produce a safer work environment. Although many occupational health nurses work alone, often without direct medical supervision, they recognize the need for interdisciplinary collaboration and support. A philosophy of occupational health nursing is given in the accompanying box.

The number of nurses needed at a work setting is determined by the size of the company, the type of workplace, the number of employees, employee health status, and actual, as well as potential, health and safety problems (AAOHN, 1991b). Staffing recommendations for an effective occupational nursing program are given in the box on the next page. If these staffing recommendations are not met it can be difficult to achieve nursing objectives and effectively implement nursing roles and functions.

Functions of the Occupational Health Nurse

The functions of the occupational health nurse are oriented heavily toward prevention, protection, and health promotion (Barlow, 1992, p. 464). These functions focus on keeping the worker healthy. Occupational health nursing functions can be classified into the categories of administration and management, environmental surveillance, direct nursing care, health education, counseling, and research.

Confidentiality and ethics play an important role in all occupational health nursing functions. The AAOHN (AAOHN, 1991a) has published a *code of ethics* for occupational health nurses to help guide their practice. Ethical issues confronting the occupational health nurse include informed consent, confidentiality of health care records, worker rights, resource allocation, drug testing in the workplace, right-to-know issues, and concerns related to AIDS. The AAOHN code of ethics stresses the need to protect and promote the health and safety of the worker and safeguard workers' rights.

The confidential treatment of health information and records and the worker's right to privacy are professional obligations of the occupational health nurse (AAOHN, 1996c, 1996d). Unjustified disclosure can damage the client, damage the nurse-client relationship, inhibit the client from freely disclosing pertinent health matters, and put the nurse at legal risk (AAOHN, 1994b, p. 1). Confidentiality can be a difficult issue for the occupational health nurse. The nurse is frequently caught between management's demands to know medical information about an employee and the nurse's responsibility to protect employee privacy.

To protect employees from unauthorized or indiscriminate access to their health information, it is recommended

Philosophy of Occupational Health Nursing Service

The occupational health service contributes to a safe and healthful work environment through programs aimed at reducing and eliminating work-related hazards and enhancing health promotion. Occupational health services are provided to individual workers and the collective workforce within an environment that considers and meets the needs of a diverse workforce.

The occupational health nursing service is central and integral to an effective occupational health program. The occupational health nurse professional is an advocate for the worker and often manages the occupational health service. As such the occupational health nurse is concerned not only with how the worker's health is affected or influenced by the worksite and organization but also by how the worker, her or his family, the community, and the environment interact to affect worker health and productivity.

To protect worker rights, workers are given information regarding work-related hazards so that informed decisions can be made. In addition, confidentiality of health records and information is safeguarded.

The occupational health nurse professional is part of a collaborative team that has the responsibility to inform the employer of unsafe and unhealthful working conditions and practices and of the need for workplace controls. The employer has the responsibility to provide a safe and healthful work environment and to recognize and support the occupational health nurse as a professional with specialized knowledge and skills.

The occupational health nurse professional has an obligation to maintain and improve knowledge and skills relative to her or his position and to keep current with research and legislation affecting occupational health and nursing practice; the occupational health nurse professional is accountable for interventions, judgments, and decisions made according to practice standards.

The occupational health nursing service encourages a mutually supportive relationship with the community through referrals and utilization of resources and by being a productive part of the larger ecosystem that enhances the environment.

High-quality occupational health care is provided in a cost-effective manner that promotes productivity through good health.

From Rogers B: *Occupational health nursing: concepts and practice*, Philadelphia, 1994a, Saunders, p. 34. Copyright © 1994 by Bonnie Rogers.

Staffing Recommendations for an Effective Occupational Health Nursing Program

- One occupational health nurse for up to 300 employees in an industrial setting and up to 750 in a nonindustrial setting
- Two or more occupational health nurses for up to 600 industrial employees
- Three or more occupational health nurses for up to 1,000 employees in an industrial setting
- One occupational health nurse for each additional 1,000 employees in either setting

NOTE: Larger and more hazardous occupational settings require more nursing personnel. Smaller organizations can implement an effective program with part-time nursing services.

From American Association of Occupational Health Nurses: *Occupational health nursing: the answer to health care cost containment*, Atlanta, 1991b, AAOHN.

that written policies and procedures be developed on record access; that educational activities be carried out to let employees, employers, and other health care providers know about policies regarding record access; and that legal counsel be sought by the nurse in instances of unclear or questionable practices (AAOHN, 1996c).

The following section describes the specific roles and functions of the occupational health nurse. In performing these functions occupational health nurses are involved in activities ranging from health promotion to rehabilitation, and they emphasize primary prevention.

ADMINISTRATION AND MANAGEMENT Research by Lusk (1990) examined corporate expectations for the occupational health nurse currently and in the future. Lusk found that management viewed occupational health nursing activities as focusing on care of illness and emergencies, counseling, follow-up on workers' compensation claims, and performing health assessments. Lusk noted that expansion of the occupational health nurse's role was expected and that many "future" activities selected by management were related to cost-containment, as well as developing health programs, analyzing health trends, conducting research, and meeting with other disciplines to solve health problems.

The operation of the occupational health service at the workplace is a major part of the nurse's administrative and management function. Administration and management activities include managing the occupational health service, keeping an up-to-date occupational health nursing policy and procedure manual, training and supervision of auxiliary health personnel, cooperation with federal and state occupational health regulatory bodies, maintenance of occupational health records, student supervision, community resource collaboration, quality assurance activities, and familiarity with legal/ethical issues related to practice.

RECORD KEEPING. Keeping records is an important administrative function. Just as in the hospital setting, the nurse has both legal and professional responsibilities to keep accurate, comprehensive, up-to-date written records. OSHA regulations and company policy require specific record keeping activities (AAOHN, 1996d; Maddux, 1995); inadequate recordkeeping often results in OSHA citations (Smith, 1995b). Records should note all employee contacts with the health service, beginning with the preemployment physical and interview, including the reason for the visit, nursing plans of care, results of screening procedures, periodic health appraisals, health risk assessments, rehabilitation activities, community referrals, and participation in worksite educational programs. *These records are confidential!*

STUDENT SUPERVISION/EDUCATION. The nurse is involved in the educational programs of nursing students (Thomas, 1995) and may be involved in the educational programs of other disciplines, such as occupational safety and health, social work, vocational rehabilitation, toxicology, public health, and audiology. The occupational health nurse also helps to supervise physicians involved in occupational medicine residency programs (Bertsche, Sanborn, Jones, 1989).

One still relatively "uncharted" educational area that occupational health nurses can develop is that of educating school children about occupational safety and health. Comprehensive school health education curricula that incorporate concepts of occupational health were recommended more than 15 years ago in the document *Promoting Health, Preventing Disease: Objectives for the Nation* (USDHHS, 1980, p. 42); they continue to be encouraged in *Healthy People 2000*. To date, little progress has been made in this endeavor.

COMMUNITY RESOURCE COLLABORATION/UTILIZATION. Collaborating with and using community resources is crucial to providing comprehensive care to workers and their families. The nurse needs to be knowledgeable about community resources, establish effective networks with community agencies, and refer clients to agencies as appropriate (see Chapter 10). Resources of particular interest to the occupational health nurse include state and local health departments; vocational rehabilitation agencies; counseling services for problems such as alcoholism, drug abuse, and domestic violence; voluntary organizations such as the American Heart Association, American Lung Association, American Diabetic Association, and American Cancer Society; and home health care agencies.

QUALITY MANAGEMENT AND ACCOUNTABILITY. Chapter 24 presents concepts of quality management that can be applied in all aspects of community health nursing practice. Figure 18-2 depicts interacting elements working together to define the scope of nursing practice and promote accountability and quality care. Standards of practice assist

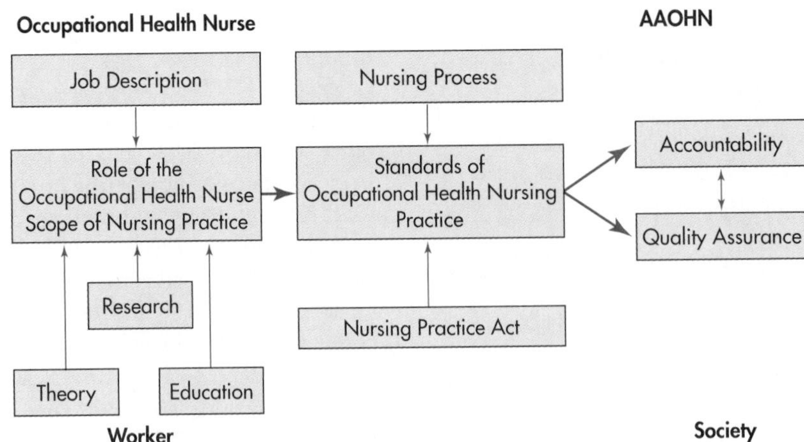

Figure 18-2 Quality care in occupational health nursing. *(From Randolph SA: Occupational health nursing: a commitment to excellence,* AAOHN J *36:166, 1988.)*

the OHN in providing quality nursing care and in assuring accountability for nursing functions.

Quality management activities include such activities as peer review, self-evaluation and audit, and overall program evaluation (see Chapter 24). Part of the quality improvement process is anticipating problems before the delivery of care (Widtfeldt, 1992, p. 329). One measure of quality of care is employee satisfaction with the services. Research has indicated that employees are generally satisfied with the occupational health nursing services (Rogers, Winslow, Higgins, 1993, p. 61). As nurses implement quality management activities, they frequently find themselves advocating for additional occupational health programs.

CASE MANAGEMENT. Case management is discussed in Chapter 10. It is a process of coordinating a client's health care services to achieve optimal, quality care delivered in a cost-effective manner. Occupational health nurses are in a unique position to implement such coordination, recommend treatment plans that assure quality and efficacy while controlling costs, monitor care outcomes, and maintain collaborative communication (AAOHN, 1996e). Occupational health nurses are becoming increasingly involved in case management interventions (AAOHN, 1996e; Dyck, 1996; O'Brien, 1995).

ENVIRONMENTAL SURVEILLANCE The nurse continuously surveys the work environment for existing and potential health hazards and works to establish cause-and-effect relationships between such hazards and occupational health conditions. These surveillance activities are usually implemented in conjunction with other members of the occupational health team: members of management, occupational safety personnel, industrial hygienists, physicians, and OSHA inspectors. An example of a nurse carrying out environmental surveillance is given in the following scenario.

CASE *Scenario*

An occupational health nurse suspected that one area of the plant in which she worked had a higher-than-average noise area. After obtaining permission from the plant management to do periodic audiometric testing on the workers in this area in combination with testing on a control group, she began to collect data to confirm her hypothesis. Employees in both areas were tested every 6 months. Over time the nurse was able to show that the workers in this one area had increasingly abnormal audiograms and that the control group had consistently normal ones. The workers themselves had not noticed any change in hearing, but the audiograms told a different story. As a result of the study corrective measures were taken. In this example, the nurse's actions assisted in facilitating the health of the workers.

Appendix 18-1 represents an assessment guide that assists occupational health nurses to systematically complete an environmental survey. Occupational health nurses apply the principles of epidemiology, primary prevention, and community assessment when they implement surveillance activities at the worksite (see Chapters 11 and 13).

DIRECT NURSING CARE The direct nursing care functions of the occupational health nurse are diverse and demand a high level of nursing skill, professional flexibility, and independence. This care encompasses primary, secondary, and tertiary prevention, with nursing interventions ranging from assessment to rehabilitation. The direct nursing care activities of the OHN include, but are not limited to, physical assessment and screening, communicable disease control, emergency care, treatment of nonoccupational injuries and illnesses, treatment of acute and chronic conditions, and rehabilitation.

Occupational injuries and illnesses can be life threatening. It is estimated that more than 100,000 deaths, and an incalculable number of diseases and illnesses, occur each year as a direct result of occupational disease and illness (USDHHS, 1995). Each year more than 10 million traumatic injuries occur on the job; over 3 million of these are severe, and more than 1.8 million result in permanent disabilities (USDHHS, 1991a, pp. 296, 299). Although fatal occupational injuries have gradually declined, injuries resulting in permanent disabilities are increasing (USDHHS, 1995).

The nurse is in an excellent position to promote health in the workplace. Workers often comply with nursing plans of care and view the nurse as someone who is concerned about them. To carry out these functions, the nurse must be able to assess both the worker and the workplace and implement a range of nursing interventions.

PHYSICAL ASSESSMENT, SCREENING, AND RISK IDENTIFICATION. The occupational health nurse needs to be skilled in physical assessment and frequently does preemployment and return-to-work physicals. The nurse is involved in screening procedures such as audiometrics, electrocardiograms, vision screening, and pulmonary function analysis. These procedures provide baseline and follow-up data that assists in diagnosis and treatment. The nurse frequently conducts health risk appraisals (see Chapter 9) to identify individual health risks, guide health counseling, and provide direction for health educational programs (Adams, Mackey, Lindenberg, Baden, 1995). For example, in analyzing a compilation of health risk data it is found that 70% of the workers smoke. As a result, the nurse works with plant management and the workers to explore the possibility of providing a smoking cessation program at the workplace.

REHABILITATION. The nurse is often involved in developing and implementing employee rehabilitation plans and activities (see Chapter 19). Rehabilitation activities should begin as soon as possible, and many of these activities may be carried out in the workplace. Rehabilitation planning incorporates the worker and his or her family and appropriate community resources. Following rehabilitation, the nurse may be involved in assessing and facilitating the employee's ability to return to work.

COMMUNICABLE DISEASE CONTROL. Numerous communicable diseases are of concern in the workplace, including colds and influenza, tuberculosis, hepatitis B, and AIDS (TB, hepatitis B, and AIDS are discussed later in this chapter). It is estimated that as many as 80% of American adults are not fully immunized. The workplace can serve as a setting to maintain adult immunization schedules (AAOHN, 1996a; Lukes, 1995, pp. 625-626). The occupational health nurse uses the epidemiological process described in Chapter 11 to prevent and control communicable disease at the worksite.

EMERGENCY CARE. Emergency care is probably the most dramatic of the occupational health nurse's direct care functions. The nurse must be skilled in cardiopulmonary resuscitation, first aid, and emergency care techniques. The nurse is often the first health professional in the workplace to have contact with the ill or injured worker, and has to make a decision about what immediate action to take.

TREATMENT OF NONOCCUPATIONAL ILLNESS AND INJURIES. These conditions are a part of the nurse's direct care function and can take a large part of the nurse's time. Although they occur outside the workplace, they have an effect on work and the work setting. The occupational health nurse will initially treat these conditions and refer the client to appropriate community agencies.

Among the nonoccupational conditions the nurse encounters are alcoholism and drug abuse. If an employee comes to work under the influence of drugs and/or alcohol and the employer allows the individual to remain in the worksite, workers' compensation laws in many states rule in favor of the worker in the event of occupational injury. For the safety of the worker, and to protect the employer from liability, employees who are unfit to work should not be permitted at the worksite. In some cases the worker's supervisor will make the decision regarding fitness for work, and in other cases the nurse will. The challenge for the occupational health nurse is to influence management to initiate effective interventions and treatment programs. Employee assistance counseling is an integral component of the occupational health service (Rogers, 1994a, p. 256).

ACUTE AND CHRONIC CONDITIONS. These conditions are daily occurrences for the occupational health nurse and range from the common cold to the crippling effects of arthritis or work-related injuries. Chronic conditions are discussed throughout the text and are specifically addressed in Chapter 19. Many community agencies (e.g., American Heart Association, American Lung Association) provide excellent services and information about chronic conditions that help the nurse to link people with community resources.

HEALTH EDUCATION AND HEALTH PROMOTION Health education interventions are often utilized by the occupational health nurse (O'Brien, 1995, p. 152). These interventions focus on primary prevention, wellness, and improving quality of life. Employers sponsor such worksite programs, realizing that it often costs less to educate workers about health care risks than to pay for illness, injury, and disability. Such programs help to reduce workers' compensation costs, result in fewer medical benefits being used and less time lost from work, and enhance worker productivity. For example, each employee who smokes costs his or her employer $960 per year in excess illness costs (Sorensen, Lando, Pechacek, 1993, p. 121). If successful smoking cessation programs can be implemented in the workplace, this cost can be greatly reduced.

Healthy People 2000 has an objective to increase to at least 70% the number of worksites that provide programs on worker health and safety; presently only about 64% of worksites have such programs (USDHHS, 1995, p. 209). These programs focus on smoking cessation (35.6%), health risk assessment (29.5%), back care (28.6%), stress management (26.6%), and exercise/fitness (22.1%). Other worksite health promotion programs include blood pressure control, weight control, nutrition education, and lifestyle and behavioral change. Employers are quick to use nurses in such health education programs (Davidson, Widtfeldt, Bey, 1992, p. 181).

The Occupational Safety and Health Act of 1970 requires that workers have the right to know the health hazards they are exposed to in the workplace. Making the worker aware of these hazards is frequently a role of the occupational health nurse. Another important aspect of health education and health promotion is the interpretation of health and welfare benefits to the employee. This means interpreting benefits offered through the employer, as well as providing information about available community resources and services.

Educating the worker to the hazards of the workplace and actions that can be taken to minimize them is a critical step in illness and injury reduction. One problem related to this can be the difficulty of overcoming the attitudes and actions of the workers themselves. Many people who are exposed to occupational hazards deny the risks of working around such hazards and do not take steps to lessen their chances of developing health problems. It may also be difficult to get the worker to realize that a stressor exists, especially if the stressor is invisible to the human eye (e.g., gases, asbestos). People are less suspicious of, and tend to minimize the effects of, hazards they cannot see.

Finding time at the workplace to implement health education activities can be a challenge because employers may not be willing to grant work time, and employees have little free time on the job except for lunch and coffee breaks. Distributing educational materials in the lunchroom or in pay envelopes and using posters, fliers, and short videos are examples of efficient and effective methods of health education in the worksite. The nurse can also coordinate health education activities in the workplace with those going on in the community. For example, if the community is celebrating health and fitness week, or having a smoking cessation activity such as a "Smokebusters Program," the nurse can build on these activities in the workplace.

COUNSELING Health counseling is an important occupational health nursing function that focuses on normal growth and development, family health, workplace stressors, at-risk health behaviors, and results of tests and screenings. If the counseling required is beyond the scope of the nurse and the client is in agreement, a referral can be made to a counseling resource in the community.

RESEARCH "Not all nurses need to conduct research but all nurses need to use research findings in their practice" (Lusk, 1993, p. 153). Research links theory, education, and practice (LoBiondo-Wood, Haber, 1994, p. 6). Further, research tests theory, builds a knowledge base in the field, and serves as the basis for practice in the profession. Occupational health nurses can play a vital role in the conduct of research to improve worker health and productivity and prevent illness and injury (Rogers, 1994b, p. 190). Nurse researchers, management, and practicing nurses need to work collaboratively to use research findings in nursing practice (Rogers, 1992b, p. 41).

The National Center for Nursing Research was established in 1986 and in 1993 became the National Institute for Nursing Research (NINR) (see Chapter 1). This institute has assisted nursing researchers in making significant strides in the development of knowledge for guiding nursing practice. In 1981 the AAOHN established a research committee for the purpose of promoting occupational health nursing research, and in 1983 its first research award was given. Vigorous strides have been made in occupational health nursing research over the last decade. The AAOHN encourages nursing research, and the *AAOHN Journal* regularly publishes research articles and information. In 1989 research priorities were established by AAOHN; they are given in the accompanying box. National occupational health research priorities are given in Table 18-1. These

American Association of Occupational Health Nurses: Research Priorities in Occupational Health Nursing

- Effectiveness of primary health care delivery at the worksite
- Effectiveness of health promotion nursing intervention strategies
- Methods for handling complex ethical issues related to occupational health (e.g., confidentiality of employee health records, truth telling)
- Strategies that minimize work related health outcomes (e.g., back injuries)
- Health effects resulting from chemical exposures in the workplace
- Occupational hazards of health care workers
- Factors that influence worker rehabilitation and return to work
- Mechanisms to assure quality and cost effectiveness of occupational health programs (e.g., effects of employee assistance programs or health surveillance programs on improving employee health)
- Effectiveness of occupational health nursing programs on employee productivity and morale
- Factors that contribute to behavioral changes among health care workers for self-protection from occupational hazards (e.g., HIV/AIDS)
- Factors that contribute to sustained risk reduction behavior related to lifestyle choices (e.g., smoking, substance abuse, nutrition)
- Effectiveness of ergonomic strategies to reduce worker injury and illness

From American Association of Occupational Health Nurses (AAOHN): *AAOHN research priorities in occupational health nursing*, Atlanta, February, 1990, AAOHN. Used with permission of the author.

research priorities focus on occupational health stressors and promoting worker health.

OCCUPATIONAL HEALTH STRESSORS AND WORKER HEALTH

Though most occupational illnesses, injuries, and deaths are preventable, there are more than 3 million disabling work injuries and 370,000 cases of occupational illness each year in the United States (NIOSH, 1995, p. 2). An average of 17 Americans die each day from injuries on the job, and an additional 137 workers die each day from workplace diseases (NIOSH, p. 2). The stressors in the workplace that cause occupational illness and injury are extensive and diverse and can be categorized as:

Chemical: liquids, gases, dusts, particles, fumes, mists, and vapors

Physical: electromagnetic and ionizing radiation, noise, pressure, vibration, heat, and cold

Biological: insects, mold, fungi, and bacteria

Ergonomic: monotony, fatigue, boredom, stress; the effects of the environment on humankind

It can be difficult to formulate cause-and-effect relationships between occupational stressors and specific illnesses and conditions. Factors such as long latency periods, multiple stressors, and lack of comprehensive, up-to-date statistics complicate the process of linking occupational stressors to diseases and conditions.

table 18-1 NATIONAL OCCUPATIONAL RESEARCH AGENDA

CATEGORY	PRIORITY RESEARCH AREAS
Disease and injury	Allergic and irritant dermatitis
	Asthma and chronic obstructive pulmonary disease
	Fertility and pregnancy abnormalities
	Hearing loss
	Infectious diseases
	Low back disorders
	Musculoskeletal disorders of the upper extremities
	Traumatic injuries
Work environment and workforce	Emerging technologies
	Indoor environment
	Mixed exposures
	Organization of work
	Special populations at risk
Research tools and approaches	Cancer research methods
	Control technology and personal protective equipment
	Exposure assessment methods
	Health services research
	Intervention effectiveness research
	Risk assessment methods
	Social and economic consequences of workplace illness and injury
	Surveillance research methods

From National Institute of Occupational Safety and Health (NIOSH): *National occupational research agenda,* Cincinnati, Oh., 1996, NIOSH.

Long Latency Periods

A primary problem in formulating cause-and-effect relationships is that no immediate, observable effect of the stressor may be apparent. Long latency periods may exist between contact with the stressor and stressor effects. For example, occupational cancers usually do not become evident until 5 to 40 years after the initial exposure to the carcinogen (CDC, 1984, p. 127). Asbestosis often has a 30-year or longer latency period. In diseases and conditions with long latency periods, the worker may already have left the job where contact occurred by the time the condition is apparent, making it increasingly difficult to identify and trace the stressor.

Multiple Stressors

The influence of multiple stressors affects establishing cause-and-effect relationships. A person may have been occupationally and environmentally exposed to many stressors; the interactions between them may greatly increase the risk of contracting the condition, and their effects may not be easily separated (CDC, 1984, p. 126). It can be difficult to determine which stressor caused the problem. How can the miner with emphysema prove that mine work, rather than a heavy smoking habit, was the primary factor in the causation of the disease?

Lack of Comprehensive, Up-to-Date Statistics

Current, comprehensive occupational health statistics are often not readily available (USDHHS, 1991a, p. 309; USDHHS, 1995, p. 209). Birth and death certificates are commonly used in this country to obtain health statistics, but occupational information such as job and place of employment is generally missing or incomplete. In an attempt to develop preventive strategies for conditions such as low birth weight infants, to determine teratogens, and to decrease the incidence of infant mortality, parental employment has become a part of the standard *U.S. fetal death certificate*.

The national health objectives in *Healthy People 2000* address the need for primary care health professionals to routinely elicit occupational health data as part of a client's health history. Health professionals need to collect and analyze work-related injury and illness data from primary care visits, workers' compensation claims, and hospital discharge and admission data. These data should include known or potential workplace stressors to which the worker has been exposed. Until occupational health data are routinely collected and analyzed it will be difficult to formulate cause-and-effect relationships for work-related diseases and injuries, develop prevention plans, and have comprehensive occupational health statistics.

LEADING CAUSES OF WORK-RELATED DISEASES AND INJURIES

In 1983 NIOSH developed a "classic" list of the 10 leading work-related diseases and injuries in the United States, which continues to guide occupational health practice (Table 18-2). Problems were placed on the list because of the frequency of their occurrence, severity of effect, and likelihood that preventive strategies could be developed and implemented (NIOSH, 1988f). National strategies to prevent these diseases and injuries have been developed, and prevention of these diseases has been integrated into *Healthy People 2000*.

Occupational disease and injury are significant national concerns, and occupational health has become a health priority for the nation (USDDHS, 1995). Occupational health affects the quality of life for individuals, families, and communities. From a financial standpoint it is estimated that billions of dollars are lost annually as a result of work-related diseases and injuries through wages, medical expenses, insurance claims, and production delays. Millions of workdays are lost each year to work-related illness and absenteeism. In addition to their potential for causing serious physical illness and injury, they have an impact on the worker's psychosocial well-being. For personal, societal, and economic reasons there is a great need to reduce the incidence of work-related disease, injury, and death.

Occupational Lung Diseases

Occupational lung diseases encompass a number of pulmonary diseases, including byssinosis (brown lung), asbestosis, coal workers' pneumoconiosis (black lung), and silicosis. Today, as a result of *Healthy People 2000* activities, almost all states have exposure standards adequate to prevent these major occupational lung diseases. However, fewer than half of the states have implemented occupational safety and health plans for the management and prevention of such diseases (USDHHS, 1995, p. 73). Other occupational lung diseases include farmer's lung, lung cancer, emphysema, asthma, and chronic industrial bronchitis.

The illness, disability, and death caused by these diseases is enormous, and early recognition of them is often difficult because of long latency periods before they are detectable. Two occupational lung diseases with exceptionally long latency periods are silicosis (latency period of approximately 15 years) and asbestosis (latency period of approximately 30 years). Once long periods of time have elapsed it becomes increasingly difficult to link the occupational stressor to the occupational disease. Other factors, such as smoking, can contribute to the disease process and obscure the link between disease and toxic exposure at work.

Prevention strategies for occupational lung disease include stricter standards and regulations, increased surveillance of regulation compliance by employers, hazard removal, health education and training, and technology such as engineering designs for better ventilation and substance isolation (NIOSH, 1986a, pp. 4-7; USDHHS, 1991a, p. 306).

Musculoskeletal Injuries

Factors that contribute to musculoskeletal injuries in the workplace are *environmental hazards; human biological factors*, such as size, strength, or range of motion; *behavioral or lifestyle factors*, such as insufficient sleep, mental lapses, and lack of adequate fitness; and *inadequacies in health care diagnosis and treatment* (NIOSH, 1986b, pp. 1-2). Musculoskeletal workplace injuries are often a result of traumatogens (NIOSH, 1986b, p. 1). A "traumatogen" is a

table 18-2 The 10 Leading Work-Related Diseases and Injuries—United States

Diseases/Conditions	Examples
1. Occupational lung diseases	Asbestosis, byssinosis, silicosis, coal workers' pneumoconiosis, lung cancer, occupational asthma
2. Musculoskeletal injuries	Disorders of the back, trunk, upper extremity, neck, lower extremity; traumatically induced Raynaud's phenomenon
3. Occupational cancers (other than lung)	Leukemia, mesothelioma; cancers of the bladder, nose, and liver
4. Traumatic injury and death	Amputations, fractures, eye loss, lacerations
5. Cardiovascular diseases	Hypertension, coronary artery disease, acute myocardial infarction
6. Disorders of reproduction	Infertility, spontaneous abortion, teratogenesis
7. Neurotoxic disorders	Peripheral neuropathy, toxic encephalitis, psychoses, extreme personality changes (exposure-related)
8. Loss of hearing	Noise-induced hearing loss
9. Dermatological conditions	Dermatoses, burns (scaldings), chemical burns, contusions (abrasions)
10. Psychological disorders	Neuroses, personality disorders, alcoholism, drug dependency, stress reactions

From Centers for Disease Control (CDC): Leading work-related diseases and injuries—U.S. (occupational lung diseases), MMWR 32:25, January 21, 1983a; USDHHS: *Healthy people 2000: health promotion and disease prevention objectives for the nation, full report, with commentary*, Washington, D.C., 1991a, U.S. Government Printing Office.

source of biomechanical stress stemming from job demands that exceed the worker's strength and/or endurance, such as heavy lifting or repetitive, forceful manual twisting (NIOSH, 1986b, p. 1). Although these injuries result in few work-related deaths, they account for a great deal of human suffering and loss of productivity.

Back injuries are a major component of musculoskeletal injuries. A national health objective is to increase to at least 50% the number of worksites offering back injury prevention programs. Back injuries account for one third of all workers' compensation claims (Karas, Conrad, 1996, p. 189). Almost 50% of back injuries occur in the health care field (DiBenedetto, 1995, p. 134). At least 1 in 15 nurses will experience back injury serious enough to interfere with their professional career, and each year more than 40,000 nurses will report illness caused by back pain, resulting in a loss of more 764,000 work days (DiBenedetto, p. 134).

Back injuries are associated with ineffective job and equipment design, improper body mechanics, repetitive motion, and vibration injuries. Preventive interventions include health education, employer compliance with regulations, improved equipment design, limiting biomechanical stresses on the worker, and rotation of workers to jobs with different physical demands. Occupational health nurses play an active role in implementing prevention and control measures in relation to musculoskeletal injuries.

Occupational Cancers

More than 200 years have passed since Sir Percivall Pott, a physician, linked cancer of the scrotum in chimney sweeps to their occupational exposure to soot. Estimates of the percentage of cancers related to the workplace are as high as 20%. Table 18-3 lists some occupational cancers and carcinogens by industry and occupation.

The incidence rate of some cancers among occupational groups is obvious and significant (e.g., cancer of the bone in radium dial workers, mesothelioma in asbestosis workers); however, some occupationally induced cancers such as mesothelioma have long latency periods and can appear decades after exposure. Also, many cancers have multiple etiologies, and it may be difficult to determine if the workplace was the cause (e.g., lung cancer). Another problem in documenting occupationally induced cancers is that significant differences in the rates of cancer among small subgroups of a population may be overlooked because these rates affect the overall rate in the larger population only slightly, if at all—creating a "dilution factor" that obscures the occupational cancer.

Thousands of suspected carcinogens in the workplace are not regulated. Exposure to carcinogens does not always cause cancer, and not everything is a carcinogen. The *dose*, *frequency of exposure*, and *duration of contact* are often the key to the toxicity of a substance. For example, many chemicals such as zinc, nickel, tin, and potassium are essential for health in small quantities but are toxic in larger quantities.

table 18-3 Selected Occupational Cancers

Cancer	Industry/Occupation	Agent
Hemangiosarcoma of the liver	Vinyl chloride polymerization	Vinyl chloride monomer
	Industry vintners	Arsenical pesticides
Malignant neoplasm of nasal cavities	Woodworkers, cabinet/furniture makers	Hardwood dusts
	Boot and shoe producers	Unknown
	Radium chemists, processors, dial painters	Radium
	Nickel smelting and refining	Nickel
Malignant neoplasm of larynx	Asbestos industries and utilizers	Asbestos
Mesothelioma	Asbestos industries and utilizers	Asbestos
Malignant neoplasm of bone	Radium chemists, processors, dial painters	Radium
Malignant neoplasm of scrotum	Automatic lathe operators, metalworkers	Mineral/cutting oils
	Coke oven workers, petroleum refiners, tar distillers	Soots and tars, tar distillates
Malignant neoplasm of bladder	Rubber and dye workers	Benzidine, alpha and beta naphthylamine, auramine, magenta, 4-aminobiphenyl, 4-nitrophenyl
Malignant neoplasm of kidney	Coke oven workers	Coke oven emissions
Lymphoid leukemia, acute	Rubber industry	Unknown
	Radiologists	Ionizing radiation
Myeloid leukemia, acute	Occupations with exposure to benzene	Benzene
	Radiologists	Ionizing radiation

From Centers for Disease Control and Prevention (CDC): Leading work-related diseases and injuries—U.S. (occupational cancers other than lung), *MMWR* 33:126, March 9, 1984. Modified from Rutstein DD, Mullan RJ, Frazier TM et al: Sentinel health events (occupational): a basis for physician recognition and public health surveillance, *Am J Public Health* 73:1054-1062, 1984.

Nursing screening and risk identification interventions include a comprehensive occupational history that addresses potential exposure to occupational carcinogens by type, dose, frequency of exposure, and length of exposure can assist in documenting occupationally induced cancers.

Traumatic Injury and Death

NIOSH estimates that at least 10 million traumatic injuries occur on the job each year (USDHHS, 1991a, p. 299), that every 5 seconds a worker is injured badly enough to require a hospital visit, and that 17 workers lose their lives in the workplace every day (Sattler, 1996, p. 233). Occupational trauma is second only to motor vehicle accidents as a reported cause of unintentional death in the United States (NIOSH, 1986d, p. 1). Occupational traumatic injuries include amputations, fractures, lacerations, eye loss, acute poisonings, burns, and death.

The *Healthy People 2000* occupational health objectives address the need for reduction of deaths from work-related injuries; reducing work-related injuries that require medical treatment, lost time from work, or restricted work activity; reducing cumulative trauma disorders; and increasing the number of worksites that offer back injury prevention and rehabilitation programs. Progress has been made on national health objectives in relation to decreasing work-related injury death, but nonfatal work-related injuries have increased (USDHHS, 1995, p. 73).

Construction workers, nursing and personal care workers, and farm workers have the highest rates of work-related injury in the United States (USDHHS, 1995, p. 208), and injuries among nurses and personal caregivers have actually increased in recent years. Back injuries account for 40% of the injuries occurring in health care workers (USDHHS, 1991a, p. 299), and fewer than 20 states offer worksite back injury and rehabilitation programs (USDHHS, 1995, p. 73).

Cumulative trauma disorders are on the rise in the workplace, almost doubling between 1987 (100 cases per 100,000 workers) and 1989 (192 cases per 100,000 workers) (A Public Health Service progress, 1992). These disorders often occur as a result of repetitive motion and repeated pressure in the workplace. Repetitive motions may lead to disorders such as carpal tunnel syndrome, tendinitis, ganglionitis, and bursitis, as well as damage to muscles, tendons, ligaments, and joints. The prevention of traumatic injury is related to implementing engineering controls, practicing safe work habits, using personal protective equipment, and monitoring the workplace for emerging hazards. The occupational health nurse assumes an important role in assessing and reinforcing the need for such measures and helping to implement them in the workplace.

Cardiovascular Disease

Cardiovascular diseases are the leading cause of death in the United States. Although personal risk factors play an important role in developing these diseases, factors in the workplace such as stress and exposure to cardiotoxins also contribute their effects (USDHHS, 1987, p. 74).

The acute cardiac effect of carbon monoxide is well known. Research has linked workers exposed to carbon disulfide with cardiovascular symptoms and arteriosclerotic heart disease, and associated acute episodes of anginal pain, myocardial infarction, and even cardiovascular death with occupational exposures to nitroglycerine and other aliphatic nitrates (Fine, 1992, pp. 593-594). Other occupational exposures that may increase the risk of cardiovascular disease include cobalt, lead, antimony, and cadmium (NIOSH, 1986e, p. 2). Environmental smoke in the workplace needs to be considered in relation to cardiovascular disease, and many workplaces are placing restrictions on smoking or prohibiting it all together.

Control of cardiovascular disease is addressed in the *Healthy People 2000* occupational health objectives under implementation of programs on worker health and safety. The worksite is an excellent location for teaching individuals about positive health practices and implementing preventive programs on personal risk factors such as smoking cessation, proper diet, blood pressure control, exercise, and stress reduction. An increasing number of workplaces have established health promotion and wellness programs designed to prevent premature deaths related to cardiovascular disease. These programs often work in partnership with community resources such as the American Heart Association.

Reproductive Disorders

As early as the late 1800s reproductive disorders related to industrial exposures were noted. At that time unusually high rates of infertility, spontaneous abortion, stillbirth, neonatal death, and macrocephaly were noted in European communities where lead-working was a primary occupation; more recently links have been made between industrial chemicals and reproductive disorders (LeMasters, 1992, p. 151). According to some estimates, 20 million American workers are exposed to reproductive hazards each year in the workplace (Barrett, Phillips, 1995, p. 40). Such hazards can be physical hazards (e.g., ionizing radiation), chemical hazards (e.g., ethers), biological hazards (e.g., bacteria and viruses) and ergonomic hazards (e.g., stress). Chapter 6 examines some known teratogens in the environment.

Ionizing radiation profoundly affects reproductive function in both men and women. It is estimated that 1.3 million persons are exposed to ionizing radiation at work and that 44% of these workers are in health care, including a disproportionate number of nurses (Barrett, Phillips, 1995, p. 43). Research has shown sterility in male dibromochloropropane workers, impotence in workers exposed to specific neurotoxins, increased birth defects among children born to female pharmaceutical workers, and excessive spontaneous abortions and chromosomal alterations among health care personnel exposed to anesthetic gases (USDHHS, 1987, p. 74; NIOSH, 1988a, p. 1). Nurses and other health care workers are at special risk of reproductive disorders caused by exposure to anesthetic gases, antineoplastic drugs, antiviral drugs, viruses, bacteria, and ionizing radiation (Shortridge-McCauley, 1995).

More women than ever before are in the workplace, and maternal exposure to some toxicants can cause infertility, menstrual disorders, illness during pregnancy, chromosome or breast milk alteration, early onset of menopause, and libido suppression (LeMasters, 1992, p. 153). Fetal exposure to some toxicants can result in preterm delivery, fetal death, low birth weight, congenital malformation, and developmental disabilities (LeMasters, p. 153). The occupational health nurse needs to advise workers of such hazards and of the risks of continuing work in an environment that may be considered unsafe in regard to reproductive health (Barrett, Phillips, 1995, p. 46). The nurse also needs to give special attention to pregnant workers and provide counseling about good nutrition, proper rest, prenatal care, and hazards outside of the work environment such as fetal alcohol syndrome and drug abuse. The key to promoting the reproductive health of American workers is primary preventive education and counseling workers about reproductive hazards so that they can make informed decisions about their reproductive health (Barrett, Phillips, p. 48).

Neurotoxic Disorders

Disorders of the nervous system that result from toxic exposures in the workplace have been recorded throughout history. As early as the first century palsy in workers exposed to lead dust was noted (NIOSH, 1988b, p. 1). More than 850 chemicals in the American workplace have been identified as toxic to the central nervous system, and the number of workers exposed to neurotoxic chemicals has been estimated at 8 million (USDHHS, 1987, p. 74). *Healthy People 2000* addresses worker exposure to neurotoxins.

Peripheral neuropathy, characterized by numbness and tingling in the feet or hands followed by clumsiness and/or incoordination, is one of the most common and serious problems in workers exposed to neurotoxins. These workers may find their ability to work impaired on either a temporary or permanent basis. Behavioral neurotoxicity and changes in behavior resulting from chemical exposure can also occur. Chemicals well known for causing neurotoxic symptoms include arsenic, carbon disulfide, carbon monoxide, kepone, lead, manganese, and mercury. The Mad Hatter of Lewis Carroll's *Alice in Wonderland* was not purely a figment of Carroll's imagination. In Carroll's time hatters used mercury in hatmaking, and many of them went mad as a result of mercury poisoning. Nursing interventions should include screening workers exposed to neurotoxic agents to detect the early symptoms of central nervous system damage (Baker, 1992, p. 570).

Psychological Disorders

Psychological stressors are present on all jobs. Psychological disorders in the workplace include affective disturbances such as anxiety, depression, and job dissatisfaction; maladaptive behavioral or lifestyle patterns; and chemical dependencies and alcohol abuse (NIOSH, 1988e, p. 2). Psychological disorders can be brought on by anxiety, boredom, stress, monotony, and fatigue. They are heavily concentrated among workers with lower income, lower education, fewer skills, and less prestigious jobs (NIOSH, 1988e, p. 4). Workers who are balancing the responsibilities of employment and family caregiving are also at risk for experiencing psychological stress (McGovern, Matter, 1992, p. 35).

One interesting work-related psychological phenomenon is *mass psychogenic illness*. Mass psychogenic illness occurs when a number of workers simultaneously experience similar symptoms seemingly contagious in nature but whose etiology can only be linked to a psychological stressor. Symptoms of mass psychogenic illness include headaches, nausea, chills, blurred vision, muscular weakness, and difficulty breathing (Colligan, Stockton, 1978; Moss, 1992, p. 671); the illness is frequently linked with workers being overcome by strange odors (Colligan, Murphy, 1979; Moss, 1992, p. 671). Epidemics of mass psychogenic illness typically occur in controlled social settings, such as workers on a factory assembly line (Moss, p. 671), and it has been routinely linked with stressful job situations.

When outbreaks of mass psychogenic illness occur it is recommended that symptomatic persons be removed to an out-of-the-way area and that the situation be handled as quietly as possible to prevent mass spread of the symptoms (CDC, 1983b). The nurse must be sensitive to the needs of the worker while maintaining a focus on the reality of the situation. It is important to remember that the symptoms are real to those who are experiencing them. *The nurse must evaluate each situation carefully, since there may actually be a hazardous occupational stressor present.*

Nursing interventions in relation to work-related psychological disorders can address improving working conditions to minimize stress, surveillance of psychological disorders and work factors, education and training activities, and advocating for increased psychological services for workers. The occupational health nurse should be sensitive to the fact that family members are often the victims of the effects of work stress and psychological disturbance. Nursing interventions such as group sessions on stress awareness and management may be especially helpful for workers and their families. The nurse should refer workers to appropriate community mental health resources, as well as resources in the community that can assist the worker in balancing the responsibilities of caregiving and work.

Hearing Loss

Approximately 10 million American workers are exposed to potentially harmful noise levels (McCunney, 1992, p. 1121)

(Figure 18-3). Noise is a physical stressor that can result in hearing loss. Noise-induced hearing loss in the workplace was recognized in the early 1700s by Bernardo Ramazzini in his writings on the diseases of occupations. By the early twentieth century boilermakers' deafness, caused by riveting inside metal boilers, was an occupational hazard of considerable magnitude (NIOSH, 1988c, p. 1). Federal efforts to regulate occupational noise began in 1955. Noise-induced hearing loss is one of the most common and preventable occupational health problems. Many research studies indicate that worker hearing loss is directly related to worker noise exposure levels and increases with the noise level and duration (McGuire, 1994).

Hearing loss caused by industrial noise is often represented on audiograms by a descending slope with a "notch" at 3000 Hz to 4000 Hz, which is often referred to as the industrial noise trauma notch (Figure 18-4). The person suffering from industrial hearing loss may initially notice *tinnitus*, which is a ringing or hissing sound in the ear. The onset of hearing loss is usually gradual and painless, and the individual may not be aware of the hearing loss until the damage is permanent or communication is affected (McGuire, 1996).

The occupational health nurse plays a key role in an industrial hearing conservation program and frequently has primary responsibility for the implementation, administration, coordination, and evaluation of the hearing conservation program (McGuire, 1991, pp. 233, 239). A successful industrial hearing conservation program complies with the OSHA hearing conservation program regulations and plant site regulations. Some activities implemented by the nurse in these programs are given in the box on the following page.

Nursing interventions include obtaining the workers' medical and occupational histories, audiometric testing, referring employees with hearing complaints or questionable audiograms to a physician, educating and counseling employees about industrial noise, supplying employees with hearing protection muffs or plugs, and encouraging employees to wear the protection in and outside the work environment as appropriate. Other activities to prevent work-related hearing loss include the development of noise abatement methods and plant design to make work processes quieter, attenuating workplace noise sources, implementing effective hearing conservation programs (including the use of hearing protection by workers), and research on noise-induced hearing loss.

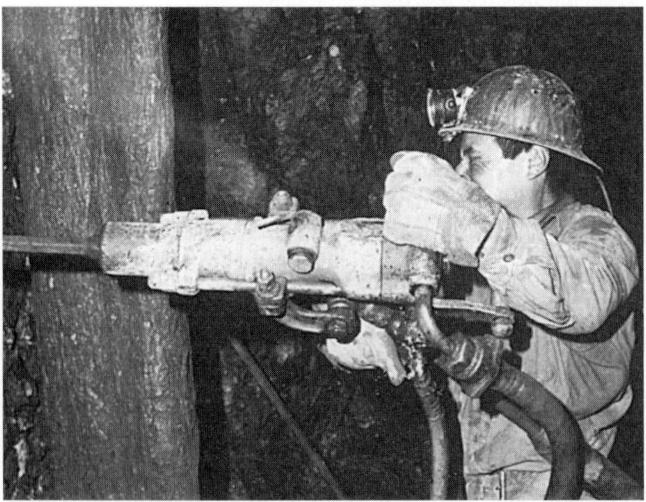

Figure 18-3 Many American workers are exposed to dangerous levels of noise. *(Courtesy World Health Organization.)*

Dermatological Disorders

Reduction of workplace dermatological disorders is a national health objective. Unfortunately, occupational skin disorders are on the increase and are the most prevalent causes of occupational illness and lost time from work

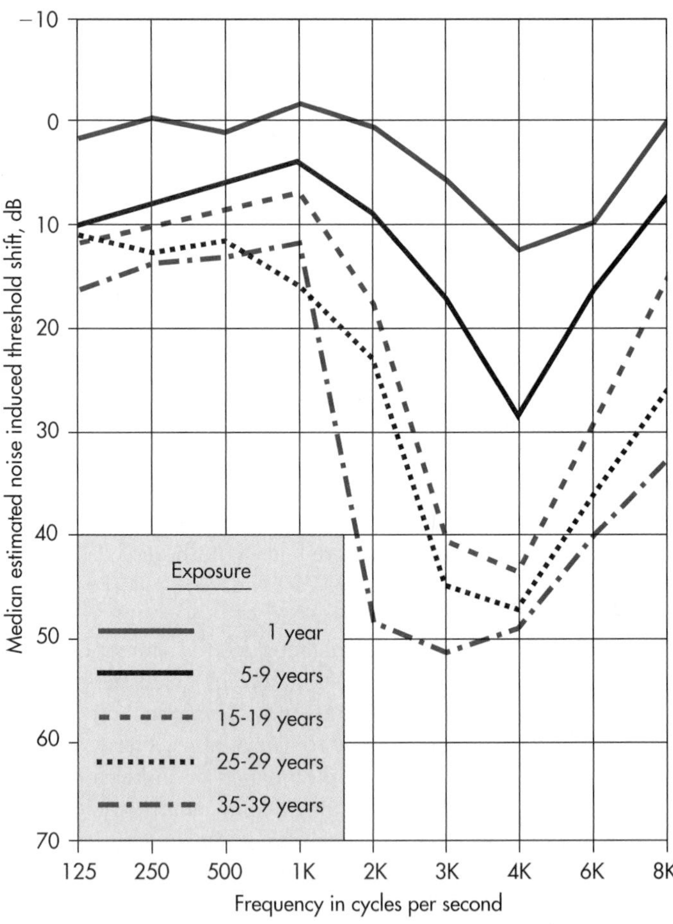

Figure 18-4 Median permanent threshold shifts in hearing levels as a function of exposure years to jute weaving noise. *(Data from Taylor WA, Mair A, Burns W: Study of noise and hearing in jute weaving,* Acoustical Society of America *48:524-530, 1965, as cited in USDHHS:* NIOSH publication on noise and hearing: criteria for a recommended standard—occupational exposure to noise, *Cincinnati, Oh., 1991b, NIOSH, p. 511.)*

(USDHHS, 1995, p. 75). The skin is often directly exposed, making this organ especially vulnerable to occupational diseases; dermal absorption of some chemicals may be more serious than absorption by inhalation (NIOSH, 1988d, p. 1). Occupational dermatoses can be divided into four major categories: (1) mechanical—friction and pressure, (2) chemical, (3) physical—heat, cold, radiation, and (4) biological—viruses, bacteria, fungi, and parasites (Tucker, Key, 1992, p. 557). Fortunately, dermatological conditions are usually amenable to early diagnosis and treatment.

Preventive measures include engineering controls that eliminate or reduce skin exposure, containment or redesign of industrial processes, use of personal protective clothing, and the use of less toxic chemicals in the workplace (USDHHS, 1991a, p. 301). Nursing interventions to prevent such conditions include health education activities, encouraging workers to use protective clothing, and early assessment and treatment.

OTHER CONCERNS IN THE WORKPLACE

The 10 leading work related diseases and conditions are relatively well-known. *Healthy People 2000* notes a number of additional conditions that also need attention, including hepatitis B, smoking in the workplace, and violence in the workplace.

Hepatitis B in the Workplace

In 1990, *Healthy People 2000* noted that each year approximately 12,000 health care workers become infected with hepatitis B (HBV), resulting in 6200 clinical HBV infections, 600 hospitalizations, and 1200 people becoming carriers (USDHHS, 1991a, p. 301). National health objectives addressed reducing the incidence of HBV in the workplace, and increasing the rate of immunization among occupationally exposed workers. The national objective to reduce the incidence of hepatitis B in the workplace has been reached, and progress has been made toward the objective of hepatitis B immunizations being obtained by occupationally exposed workers—the immunization level for these workers has increased to more than 70% (USDHHS, 1995, pp. 74-75). Employers must provide HBV vaccine free of charge to employees who are occupationally at risk for the disease.

Nursing interventions to prevent HBV in the workplace include encouraging safe work practices, such as the use of gloves, masks, and protective clothing; vaccinating workers against the disease; and health education activities, such as teaching workers about proper handling of blood products and disposal of contaminated waste. As health care workers, nurses are at a much higher risk for exposure to HBV than the general public.

NURSING ACTIVITIES IN HEARING CONSERVATION PROGRAMS

- Assesses the workers' environment for noise exposure and coordinates with management work areas where hearing protection should be worn.
- Determines employees who may be predisposed to hearing loss.
- Performs audiometric testing on prospective employees, continues to measure employees' hearing periodically, and examines audiometric data for accuracy and reliability.
- Provides effective hearing protection for employees, including individually fitting employees for such hearing protection.
- Provides ongoing educational programs on hearing conservation and noise abatement in the workplace.
- Assists in implementing administrative and engineering controls to reduce noise levels and prevent noise in the workplace.

AIDS in the Workplace

A separate priority area in *Healthy People 2000* was devoted to HIV infection. Since there is no known cure for AIDS, the first priority of the public health system is to prevent it (USDHHS, 1991a, p. 480). Although acquired immunodeficiency syndrome (AIDS) has been discussed in Chapter 12, the role of the occupational health nurse in AIDS treatment and prevention is discussed here.

The AAOHN has the following recommendations for AIDS: workers with AIDS should be employed for as long as possible, confidentiality of HIV testing results and records should be maintained, management should take aggressive action to establish AIDS policy and education at the workplace, and discrimination against the HIV-positive employee should be discouraged (AAOHN, 1989a). There is no indication that people who test HIV-positive and are asymptomatic are any less capable of performing on the job than noninfected workers (Jaffe, Schmitt, 1992, p. 693).

Research by Hansen, Booth, Fawal, and Langer (1988) showed that most workers held some negative attitudes and myths about HIV-positive coworkers. There is a great need for health education programs to educate workers and employers about AIDS and to dispel myths. Research by Nyamathi and Flaskerud (1989) revealed statistically significant improvements in AIDS knowledge following an AIDS education program with employees.

The occupational health nurse is a key figure in AIDS policy development and educational programming (Harris, 1990, p. 11). This requires that the nurse keep up to date with rapidly changing AIDS research, information, and statistics. Nursing intervention frequently involves implementing AIDS education in the workplace and referring workers to community resources for confidential testing and follow-up. In the workplace the risk of HIV infection is directly related to potential exposures to blood or body fluids from coworkers or clients (Jaffe, Schmitt, 1992, p. 693). Nurses play a significant role in reducing exposure by educating employers and employees about OSHA's regulation of bloodborne pathogens (see Chapter 11).

Tuberculosis in the Workplace

Millions of people in the United States are infected with M. *tuberculosis*, but infection with the bacilli does not mean that a person has active disease (see Chapter 11). However, active cases of tuberculosis (TB) are diagnosed in the United States. The epidemiology of TB was discussed in Chapter 11. Although there has been a recent decline in the annual incidence of TB after a 7-year upward trend, TB continues to remain a significant health problem in the United States.

Workers—health care workers in particular—are a significant at-risk group. Tuberculosis is transmitted by airborne, droplet nuclei that disperse throughout the air and can be carried on air currents throughout a building; transmission of disease is facilitated by prolonged exposure in relatively small, enclosed spaces with inadequate ventilation (Doyle, 1995, p. 476). Several hundred workplace-originated cases of TB have occurred in the United States (USDHHS, 1993).

Nursing intervention in preventing workplace exposure to TB combines health education and disease prevention activities, early detection (TB skin tests and x-rays), and follow-up on treatment. OSHA is developing a standard and protocols for controlling TB exposure in the workplace (Smith, 1995a). The occupational health nurse must be involved in prevention and surveillance interventions that can help prevent the spread of this disease.

Smoking in the Workplace

Smoking and health is discussed in Chapter 17. Smoking in the workplace is a serious health problem for smokers and nonsmokers alike. Recent research has shown that passive inhalation of smoke is also damaging to health. *Healthy People 2000* now has objectives in relation to smoking cessation. One national health objective is to increase to 100% the proportion of worksites with a formal smoking policy that severely restricts smoking at the workplace. Another objective is to have all states enact laws on clean indoor air that prohibit or limit smoking to separately ventilated areas in the workplace (USDHHS, 1995, p. 211). The benefits of a smoke-free work force include better health, reduced absenteeism, and increased worker productivity (Caplan, 1995, p. 634).

To effectively intervene with workers who smoke, the nurse must understand the physiological, behavioral, social, and addictive aspects of smoking (Caplan, 1995, p. 634). Nursing intervention involves providing smoking cessation programs at the worksite, individual counseling on smoking and health, and referring workers to community smoking cessation resources.

Violence in the Workplace

In the 1995 revisions to the *Healthy People 2000* national health objectives, an objective was added under occupational health to reduce deaths from work-related homicides. Homicide is the second leading cause of fatal injury for all workers and the leading cause of fatal injury in the workplace for women (Gates, 1996, p. 171). Homicide accounts for 39% of all fatal injuries for women at work (Levin, Hewitt, Misner, 1996, p. 326).

Workers at greatest risk of work-related homicide are employees in the taxi industry, law enforcement officers, security guards, and employees of liquor stores, gasoline stations, restaurants, and bars (USDHHS, 1995, p. 210). The highest risk occurs in occupations where money is exchanged (Levin, Hewitt, Misner, 1996, p. 327). Violence includes harassment, assaults, and threats, as well as injury and death. Research is beginning to examine the epidemiology of violence (Gates, 1996, p. 171). Health care workers are at risk for verbal and physical aggression, and violence toward health care workers is an important emerging issue (DiBenedetto, 1995, p. 134; Felton, 1993).

Workplace violence is a public health problem that occupational health nurses need to address (Levin, Hewitt, Misner, 1996, p. 326). A recent study by Gates (1996) found that many occupational health nurses believe their companies are at risk for violence and that their job responsibilities place them at an increased risk for violence. In the study 58% of the nurses surveyed said they had been harassed at their current workplaces, 15% had been threatened, and almost 5% had been physically assaulted; 70% of the nurses surveyed stated that they considered their companies to be at risk for violence; and when asked if their job responsibilities placed them at risk for violence, 55% answered "yes" (Gates). Although almost 40% of the nurses in the study stated that their companies had conducted some type of violence prevention program in the last year, only 14% of these programs had actually been conducted by nurses, and most employers did not view workplace violence prevention education as part of the nurses' job responsibilities (Gates, p. 173).

Employers need to take steps to ensure a safe workplace and to educate workers about safety. Nurses need to work to maintain and create nonviolent workplaces. Violence prevention research is in its infancy; further research with occupational health nurses and workplace violence is needed. Such research will facilitate an increased awareness of violence prevention and the development of appropriate nursing interventions, as well as the development of policies, procedures, and security measures in relation to violence at the workplace (Gates, 1996, p. 175).

MINORITY WORKERS AND OCCUPATIONAL HEALTH

Employment in hazardous occupations is much more common among minority workers (African Americans,

Hispanics, Asians, and Native Americans) than their white counterparts. This results in a disproportionate number of occupational diseases, injuries, and deaths within these population groups. These workers are less likely to receive adequate health care and often are not even properly diagnosed. Nurses need to consider this in their plans of care and implementation of health education and safety programs.

African-American and Hispanic workers tend to be underrepresented in low-risk occupations and highly overrepresented in dangerous high-risk ones (Morris, 1989, p. 53). Fifteen percent of the 7 million African-American workers are permanently disabled from work-related causes, compared to 10% of white workers. African Americans have a 37% greater likelihood of suffering work-related illness or injury and a 20% greater likelihood of dying from a job-related condition than whites (Morris, p. 53).

Eighty-five percent of the migrant and seasonal farmworker populations are composed of minorities (Fact sheet, 1993). Minorities are at particular risk for agricultural work-related fatal injury: the risk for work-related death among Hispanic and African-American agricultural workers is almost 30% greater than among whites, and for all other minorities the risk is twice as great as for whites (CDC, 1992b, p. 11). Farm work has one of the highest occupational fatality rates in the United States, and many of these deaths and injuries occur among seasonal migrant farm workers. For this reason agricultural workers have been selected for further discussion.

AGRICULTURAL WORKERS

The term *agricultural worker* is not universally defined and encompasses several groups, including farm owners and their families; migrant and seasonal workers; and agricultural service workers (CDC, 1992b, p. 11). Approximately 13.1 million persons in the United States derive some income from farming; in addition, 6 million persons are considered to be members of farm families (Olson, Bark, 1996, p. 198). Major differences in the agricultural work force, compared to workforces in general industry, are that the workplace is often the farmer's home (Connon, Freund, Ehlers, 1993, p. 427), and occupational exposures change as the production process, equipment, weather, and conditions change (Olson, Bark, p. 198).

Historically, farm workers have not been protected well by federal laws including the National Labor Relations Act (which guarantees the right to join a union and bargain collectively), the Fair Labor Standards Act (which governs minimum wage and child labor), and the Occupational Safety and Health Act (which governs standards of health and safety in the workplace), due to enforcement issues such as inadequate funding for surveillance activities (Kelsey, 1994; Pollack, Rubenstein, Landrigan, 1994). It is difficult to monitor the safety, environmental health, and labor practices of farmers.

Occupational Health Nurse in Agricultural Communities Program (OHNAC)

To prevent illness, injury, and death with agricultural workers, NIOSH started the "agricultural initiative" that includes the OHNAC Program, the Farm Family Health and Hazard Survey, Agricultural Health Promotion System, Cancer Screening in Farmers, and Agricultural Research Centers (Connon, Freund, Ehlers, 1993, p. 422). The OHNAC Program created a new role for occupational health nurses. This program is carried out in 10 states by nurses with the cooperation of local health departments, rural hospitals, migrant health centers, county cooperative extension offices, and clinics (Randolph, Migliozzi, 1993, p. 431). Using an epidemiological framework, the nurse draws on knowledge from both community health and occupational health nursing (Randolph, Migliozzi, p. 430).

The OHNAC Program goals are to conduct active surveillance of injuries and illness affecting agricultural workers and their families; identify preventable health events; and develop interventions directed at reducing or eliminating these events (Dobler, 1995). Nursing interventions include collecting data; writing prevention-oriented articles; making presentations to farm groups, schools, and individuals; addressing the sociocultural aspects of health; and conducting farm safety programs that include educating workers about farm hazards, agricultural respiratory conditions, and hearing conservation (Dobler). OHNAC nurses must know the communities in which they work and develop community partnerships (see Chapters 3 and 14). The nurse is in a unique position to teach about risk awareness, safety principles, and community resources (Olson, Bark, 1996, p. 203).

Some Health Concerns of Agricultural Workers

Agriculture is one of the most hazardous occupations in the United States, and it is also one of the most underserved (Connon, Freund, Ehlers, 1993, p. 427). Although the agricultural industry employs only 2% of U.S. workers, it ranks fourth in the number of work-related fatalities (CDC, 1992b, p. 11). Farming injuries and fatalities have become so frequent that they are sometimes accepted by the farming community as unavoidable (Lexau, Kingsbury, Lenz et al, 1993, p. 441). Nurses must work to prevent injuries and change attitudes.

Agricultural workers have an injury rate four times the number of all other occupations (Dobler, 1995). Injury and disease associated with physical, chemical, and biological hazards occur disproportionately among agricultural workers and their families. Agricultural machinery, especially farm tractors, is a major cause of work-related deaths among farm workers.

Among the major industrial classifications, workers in agriculture have the highest rate of occupational illnesses (CDC, 1992b, p. 12). They rank first in occupational skin disorders (largely as a result of their exposure to pesticides and chemicals), and are at increased risk for a variety of malignant and nonmalignant chronic diseases (CDC, p. 12).

Protecting farm children, who are often agricultural workers, from injury is problematic. Children are frequently involved in aspects of operating the farm from a very young age. Nurses need to promote childhood farm safety and protection (Lexau, Kingsbury, Lenz et al, 1993, p. 447). An estimated 23,000 injuries and 300 fatalities on U.S. farms involve children (Ehlers, Connon, Themann et al, 1993, p. 414).

Agricultural workers have a high incidence of respiratory illnesses (CDC, 1992b, p. 12). These illnesses include (1) airway inflammatory responses to organic dust exposure (e.g., rhinitis, pharyngitis, laryngitis, bronchitis, asthma, toxic organic dust syndrome), (2) airway immunological responses to organic dust exposures (e.g., allergic rhinitis, extrinsic asthma), (3) interstitial immunological responses to certain fungi and bactreria (e.g., hypersensitivity pneumonitis ("farmer's lung"), pneumonia, and (4) respiratory injury responses to chemical exposures (e.g., laryngeal edema, pharyngitis, pulmonary edema, interstitial fibrosis, bronchitis, and respiratory depression or arrest (American Lung Association of Iowa, 1986, p. 2).

Frequently, respiratory illnesses are diagnosed incorrectly, and farmers return to a work setting that further induces or aggravates the condition (American Lung Association of Iowa, 1986, p. 1). Permanent lung damage can be prevented by eliminating the exposures. Farm management and engineering changes that reduce exposure to dusts are advisable for all farmers (American Lung Association of Iowa, p. 1). "Farmer's lung" is a respiratory condition that is gaining increased attention.

FARMER'S LUNG Farmer's lung is one of many respiratory conditions to which agricultural workers are susceptible. Farmers tend to inhale a significant amount of bacterial and fungal spores that can lead to a condition called "farmer's lung," or hypersensitivity pneumonitis. Farmer's lung was first described in the literature almost 40 years ago (Dickie, Rankin, 1958; Totten, Reid, Davies, Moran, 1958) and is a form of allergic alveolitis. Like coal miner's black lung and textile worker's brown lung, it is an occupationally related disease; unlike these diseases there is often an immediate recovery when the person is removed from the causative environment (Reyes, Wenzel, Lawton, Emanuel, 1982, p. 146). Residual lung damage in the form of pulmonary fibrosis can occur (American Lung Association, 1989, p. 4).

Symptoms of an acute attack are similar to those of the flu and appear some 4 to 6 hours after the person breathes the offending dust; they may persist for as little as 12 hours or as long as 10 days (American Lung Association, 1989, p. 1). After repeated exposure to the dust, chronic cough may develop with excessive sputum production, cough, dyspnea, myalgia, and malaise (American Lung Association, p. 1). The changes are those of hypersensitivity pneumonitis, and the disease is characterized by unresolved pneumonia, interstitial pneumonitis, pleural fibrosis, and granuloma and edema (Reyes, Wenzel, Lawton, Emanuel, 1982). Most drugs are of limited value in treatment (American Lung Association, 1989, p. 4). Avoidance of the offending dust is the most important treatment and control measure.

Migrant Farm Workers

Migrant farm workers are a special group of agricultural workers. There are approximately 4.2 million migrant farm workers and their dependents in the United States (CDC, 1992a, p. 2). They face numerous health hazards (Figure 18-5) and are not protected well by many of the laws that govern the health and welfare of other workers. Migrant farm workers encounter problems that include financial instability, child labor, poor housing, lack of education, and impaired access to health and social services.

Migrant farm work is one of the most hazardous occupations in the United States. A major problem with estimating occupational injury among migrant farm workers is that few reliable statistics are kept. Two well-documented occupational health hazards for the migrant farm worker are injuries from farm machinery and exposure to agricultural chemicals such as pesticides.

The stresses the migrant worker must face, such as poor working conditions, problems with access to health services, decreased educational opportunities for themselves and their children, and low wages, all contribute to poverty and poor health beyond what most Americans will ever experience. Because the migrant worker is often concerned with immediate, day-to-day survival, planning for the future is difficult. The nurse working with migrant families can facilitate their efforts in obtaining health care and improve

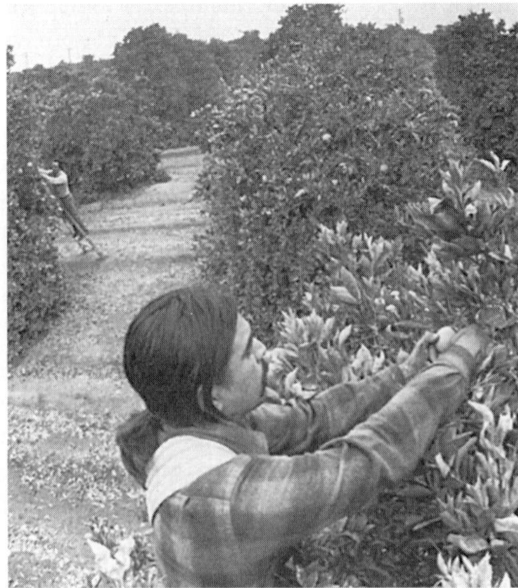

Figure 18-5 Migrant farm workers are exposed to many health risks. *(Courtesy U.S. Department of Agriculture.)*

their quality of life. The nurse often needs to assume the role of client advocate. Helping to ensure the health of migrant workers is a challenging endeavor, as well as a social and professional responsibility that cannot be ignored.

FINANCIAL STABILITY Migrant farm workers represent a large, mobile supply of cheap labor. Their work is characterized by low wages, long hours, few benefits, and poor working conditions. They are the working poor, without many of the health and welfare benefits that other workers have. Many migrant farm families have incomes below the poverty level and live in chronic poverty. Many migrant families have incomes of less than $7500 a year (Migrant health, 1993).

CHILD LABOR Child labor has all but disappeared from U.S. industry except in the agricultural sector. Many migrant children work to supplement the family income. Employers use child labor because it is inexpensive and available. Children who work are subjected to the same agricultural hazards and health risks as adults, including long hours, hazardous or faulty equipment, exposure to the elements, and toxic chemicals. Working children have a high rate of accidental injury on the job. Working keeps children from normal childhood activities and often from school.

HOUSING Migrant farm workers often live in substandard housing that is crowded, inadequate, and unsanitary (Fact sheet, 1993; Watkins, Larson, Harlan, Young, 1990, p. 567). Migrant housing is continually described as horrible and dehumanizing, without adequate heat, light, or ventilation, and often without plumbing or refrigeration (Fact sheet, 1993; Goldfarb, 1981, p. 42). In eight major agricultural states, more than 35% of this housing lacked inside running water, and few employers provided even minimal toilet facilities in the field for farm workers (Fact sheet, 1993). These unsanitary and unsafe housing conditions are breeding grounds for diseases, disability, hopelessness, and death.

EDUCATION Many migrant children never enter high school and, of those who do, few graduate. It is not that migrant families do not want an education for their children; they just have great difficulty obtaining it. Their mobility and the seasonal nature of farm work necessitate frequent school change and absences. School officials are often lax in enforcing school attendance and other regulations for migrant children. Migrant children may be labeled slow, retarded, uncooperative, or uninterested when actually the situation is more a social problem than a question of educational ability. The aspirations of migrant families for their children to receive a good education often go unfulfilled. As long as migrant children are poorly educated, it will be difficult for them to escape their present living conditions.

ACCESS TO SERVICES Migrant families face language, cultural, financial, immigration, educational, and other barriers to obtaining health and welfare services (CDC, 1992a, p. 2). Communities may be indifferent to issues of migrant health and welfare. Migrant workers generally have no voice in community planning and decision making and often do not feel a sense of belonging to the communities in which they work. Although migrant families may qualify for federal aid programs and services, they may not be aware of them. In 1969 a Supreme Court decision (*Shapiro v. Thompson*, 394 U.S. 618) ruled that a state could not exclude persons from welfare benefits because they were not residents of that state. As a result of this ruling many migrant families are eligible for services such as Temporary Assistance to Needy Families, food stamps, and Medicaid. However, the 1996 welfare reform law allows states the option to bar or limit current residents and new immigrants from several welfare benefits (National Immigrant Law Center, 1996).

HEALTH The transient nature of their work makes it difficult to provide continuous, comprehensive health services; many migrant families are uninsured and are not aware of the health care services available to them. They often do not have a regular source of primary health care, have numerous and complex health problems, and evidence higher rates of diseases and conditions than other Americans. Migrant farm workers suffer as much as twenty times the rate of diarrhea found among the urban poor; and up to 78% suffer from parasitic infection, as compared to 2% to 3% of the general population (Fact sheet, 1993). They suffer and die from heat stress and dehydration, and more than 40% have positive TB skin test results (Fact sheet). In addition, in relation to the general population, migrant farm workers have higher incidence of diabetes, digestive diseases, hypertension, malnutrition, high-risk pregnancies, infant mortality, and dental disease (CDC, 1992a, p. 2). They are six times more likely to develop tuberculosis than other employed adults (CDC, 1992a, p. 1).

Although they have a higher incidence of high-risk pregnancies, migrant women are less likely to have adequate prenatal care than their white counterparts. The majority of preschool farm children are not appropriately vaccinated for their age level (Fact sheet, 1993). Migrant children have a high incidence of hospitalization and chronic illness (Watkins, Larson, Harlan, Young, 1990, p. 568). Research has shown that migrant workers are at high risk for developing malignant lymphoma, leukemia, multiple myeloma, testicular cancer, and cancer of the gastrointestinal tract (Moses, 1989, pp. 121-122). Goldfarb (1981) found that the average life expectancy for the migrant worker was 49 years, while the average life expectancy for the nation as a whole was 74 years. This figure is statistically and *morally* significant. Migrant health is an important area that needs to be addressed in the United States.

Thousands of farm workers are affected each year from exposure to pesticides. Acute health effects from exposure to pesticides range from contact dermatitis to systemic poisoning and death. The primary route of exposure to pesticides, except for fumigants, is through the skin, and they may persist on the skin for several months (Moses, 1989,

p. 116). Few studies have been done on the chronic health problems related to pesticide exposure, and surveillance and record keeping on these exposures is lacking.

MIGRANT HEALTH CENTERS Since the Migrant Health Act was passed in 1962, these centers have striven to provide comprehensive health services to migrant and seasonal farm workers and are an important source of health care for workers and their families. Services provided by these centers include mental health, substance abuse, transportation, pharmacy, dental, emergency, environmental health, prenatal, pediatric, and social services (National Association of Community Health Centers, 1991, p. 19). Preventive services provided by these centers include health education and counseling, immunizations, blood lead screening, antepartal care, developmental and physical assessments, hearing exams, and the supplemental food program for Women, Infants, and Children (WIC) (National Association of Community Health Centers, p. 19). Approximately 500,000 migrant workers are served by 100 such centers each year (CDC, 1992a, p. 2). The nurse plays a major role in service provision in these centers, and many services are provided by primary care nurses.

OCCUPATIONAL HEALTH: A LOOK TO THE FUTURE

As a priority area in *Healthy People 2000*, occupational health will remain at the forefront of the nation's health agenda. AAOHN was instrumental in the development of the national occupational health objectives and continues to play an active role in promoting occupational health. More than any other health profession, the nurse has been at the forefront of occupational health in the United States.

Our national health agenda is now emphasizing community-based care and preventive health services. The occupational health nurse has historically been involved in these activities. Nurses will be called on to develop, implement, and evaluate worksite health promotion programs. The occupational health programs of the future must incorporate employees into the planning and implementation of occupational health programs, recognize the importance of prevention versus treatment, use state-of-the-art information and surveillance systems, and improve quality while controlling costs (Newkirk, 1996; Rest, 1996).

AAOHN has made a firm commitment to research, and occupational health nurses will expand their research agendas. Educational opportunities will increase in occupational health nursing, and more occupational health nurses will obtain graduate education. In addition, they will be involved in educating school children and the general public about occupational health.

Ethical issues will increase in scope and individual nurses, as well as their professional organizations, will need to monitor them closely. Issues such as AIDS, hepatitis B, tuberculosis, and violence in the workplace; confidentiality; legal/ethical dilemmas; and right-to-know will continue to need to be addressed. Case management techniques will be increasingly utilized, and cost containment and efficiency of service will remain important issues. Standards of care will be updated and revised and continue to guide the profession.

International occupational health concerns will increasingly emerge. Rapid industrialization, lack of occupational safety and health legislation, inadequate control measures for communicable disease, and inadequate health care systems place many countries at risk for worker health problems (Levy, 1996). Levy noted that in some countries where workers are unprotected and plentiful, managers know that for every worker who cannot work because of illness or injury incurred at work, several people are waiting to be hired for the same job. Nurses need to be proactive in national and international occupational health issues and advocate for better occupational health policies. Nurses need to remain politically and socially active, advocate for effective occupational health legislation and services, and help shape national and international health objectives reflective of current occupational health issues.

SUMMARY

Occupational health influences not only the status of the individual worker but also the health of society as a whole. Maintaining the health of the working population is an important task for all health professionals. Historically, nursing has been at the forefront of occupational health activities and has served as a role model to other professions in the field.

This chapter has addressed many occupational health concerns of workers, their families, and the community, illustrating that occupational health is a rapidly emerging and changing field. It is notable that there have been more advances in the protection of workers from occupational health hazards in the United States in the last 25 years than in the entire history of the nation. Our country now has federal and state legislation to protect the health and safety of the worker, occupational health is a national health priority, and national occupational health objectives are being implemented. Occupational health nursing will provide many opportunities for future practitioners. Increasingly, community-based initiatives for health promotion will be directed toward workers in the occupational health setting. Occupational health nursing will be an important part of the nursing of the future; it is an exciting, challenging field with unlimited potential.

CRITICAL *Thinking Exercise*

Taking into consideration that nurses are workers, analyze some of the occupational stressors that nurses are exposed to in the workplace and identify primary prevention activities to protect nurses from their effects. What are some of the occupational stressors you are concerned about in your nursing career? Formulate guidelines addressing these concerns.

REFERENCES

Adams J, Mackey T, Lindenberg J, Baden T: Primary care at the worksite: the use of health risk appraisal in a nursing center, *AAOHN J* 43(1):17-22, 1995.

American Association of Industrial Nurses (AAIN): *The nurse in industry*, New York, 1976, AAIN.

American Association of Occupational Health Nurses (AAOHN): *Educational preparation for entry into professional practice* (position statement), Atlanta, 1986, AAOHN.

American Association of Occupational Health Nurses (AAOHN): A year of progress... American Association of Occupational Health Nurses 1988 Annual Report, *AAOHN J* 37(4), 1989a.

American Association of Occupational Health Nurses (AAOHN): *A commitment for excellence*, Atlanta, 1989b, AAOHN.

American Association of Occupational Health Nurses (AAOHN): *AAOHN research priorities in occupational health nursing*, Atlanta, February, 1990, AAOHN.

American Association of Occupational Health Nurses (AAOHN): *AAOHN code of ethics and interpretive statements*, Atlanta, 1991a, AAOHN.

American Association of Occupational Health Nurses (AAOHN): *Occupational health nursing: the answer to health care cost containment*, Atlanta, 1991b, AAOHN.

American Association of Occupational Health Nurses (AAOHN): *Standards of occupational health nursing practice*, Atlanta, 1994a, AAOHN.

American Association of Occupational Health Nurses (AAOHN): *Confidentiality*, Atlanta, 1994b, AAOHN.

American Association of Occupational Health Nurses (AAOHN): *Adult immunizations*, Atlanta, 1996a, AAOHN.

American Association of Occupational Health Nurses (AAOHN): *Educational preparation for entry into professional practice*, Atlanta, 1996b, AAOHN.

American Association of Occupational Health Nurses (AAOHN): *Confidentiality of health information*, Atlanta, 1996c, AAOHN.

American Association of Occupational Health Nurses (AAOHN): *Employee health records: requirements, retention, and access*, Atlanta, 1996d, AAOHN.

American Association of Occupational Health Nurses (AAOHN): *The occupational health nurse as a case manager*, Atlanta, 1996e, AAOHN.

American Lung Association: *Facts about... hypersensitivity pneumonitis: lung hazards on the job*, Washington, D.C., 1989, The Association.

American Lung Association of Iowa: *Agricultural respiratory hazards: education series for the health professional*, Des Moines, Ia., 1986, The Association.

A *Public Health Service progress report on* Healthy People 2000: *occupational safety and health*, Washington, D.C., 1992, CDC.

Baker EL: Neurologic disorders. In Rom WR: *Environmental and occupational medicine*, ed 2, Boston, 1992, Little, Brown, pp. 561-572.

Barlow R: Role of the occupational health nurse in the year 2000, *AAOHN J* 40:463-467, 1992.

Barrett V, Phillips JA: Reproductive health in the American workplace, *AAOHN J* 43:40-51, 1995.

Bertsche PK, Sanborn JS, Jones ER: Occupational medicine residency training programs: the role occupational health nurses play, *AAOHN J* 37:316-320, 1989.

Brown ML: *Occupational health nursing*, New York, 1956, Springer.

Brown ML: An historical perspective: one hundred years of industrial or occupational health nursing in the United States, *AAOHN J* 36:433-435, 1988.

Caplan D: Smoking: issues and interventions for occupational health nurses, *AAOHN J* 43:633-645, 1995.

Centers for Disease Control (CDC): Leading work-related diseases and injuries—U.S. (occupational lung diseases), *MMWR* 32:24-27, January 21, 1983a.

Centers for Disease Control (CDC): Leading work-related diseases and injuries—U.S. (occupational cancers other than lung), *MMWR* 33:125-128, March 9, 1984.

Centers for Disease Control (CDC): Epidemic psychogenic illness in an industrial setting—Pennsylvania, *MMWR* 32:189-190, 1983b.

Centers for Disease Control and Prevention (CDC): Prevention and control of tuberculosis in migrant farm workers, *MMWR* 41:1-15, June 5, 1992a.

Centers for Disease Control and Prevention (CDC): Surgeon General's Conference on Agricultural Safety and Health, 1991, *MMWR* 41:5, 11-12, 1992b.

Colligan MJ, Murphy LA: Mass psychogenic illness in organizations: an overview, *J Occup Psychol* 52:77-90, 1979.

Colligan MJ, Stockton W: The mystery of assembly-line hysteria, *Psychology Today*, June 1978, pp. 93-99, 114-116.

Connon CL, Freund E, Ehlers JK: The occupational health nurses in agricultural communities program: identifying and preventing agriculturally related illnesses and injuries, *AAOHN J* 41:422-428, 1993.

Davidson G, Widtfeldt A, Bey J: On-site occupational health nursing services: estimating the net savings: part I, *AAOHN J* 40:172-181, 1992.

DiBenedetto DV: Occupational hazards of the health care industry, *AAOHN J* 43:131-137, 1995.

Dickie HA, Rankin J: Farmer's lung: an acute granulomatous interstital pneumonitis occuring in agricultural workers, *JAMA* 167:1069-1078, 1958.

Dobler LK: Occupational health nurses in agricultural communities, *Prairie Rose* June, July, August:11-12, 1995.

Doyle AJ: Tuberculosis. Preventing occupational transmission to health care workers, *AAOHN J* 43:475-481, 1995.

Duvall EM, Miller BC: *Marriage and family development*, ed 6, New York, 1985, Harper & Row.

Dyck D: Managed rehabilitative care: overview for occupational health nurses, *AAOHN J* 44:18-27, 1996.

Ehlers JK, Connon C, Themann CL et al: Health and safety hazards associated with farming, *AAOHN J* 41:414-420, 1993.

Fact Sheet: basic health, Austin, Tx., 1993, National Migrant Resource Program.

Felton JS: 200 years of occupational medicine in the U.S., *J Occup Med* 28:809-814, 1976.

Felton JS: The genesis of American occupational health nursing: part II, *AAOHN J* 34:31-35, 1988.

Felton JS: Occupational violence—an intensified work concomitant, *OEM Report* 7(12):101-103, 1993.

Fine LJ: Occupational heart disease. In Rom WR: *Environmental and occupational medicine*, ed 2, Boston, 1992, Little, Brown, pp. 593-600.

Gardner MS: *Public health nursing*, New York, 1916, MacMillan.

Gates DM: Workplace violence: occupational health nurses: beliefs and experiences, *AAOHN J* 44:171-176, 1996.

Goldfarb RL: *Caste of despair*, Ames, Ia., 1981, Iowa University Press.

Greaves WW: The toxic substances control act. In Rom WR: *Environmental and occupational medicine*, ed 2, Boston, 1992, Little, Brown, pp. 1333-1338.

Haag AB, Glazner LK: A remembrance of the past, an investment for the future, *AAOHN J* 40:56-60, 1992.

Hamilton A: *Exploring the dangerous trades: the autobiography of Alice Hamilton, M.D.*, Boston, 1943, Little, Brown.

Hamilton A: *Industrial poisons in the United States*, New York, 1925, MacMillan.

Hansen B, Booth W, Fawal HJ, Langer RW: Workers with AIDS: attitudes of fellow employees, *AAOHN J* 36:279-283, 1988.

Harris J: AIDS policy and education in the workplace, *AAOHN J* 38:6-11, 1990.

Jaffe HA, Schmitt J: AIDS in the workplace. In Rom WR: *Environmental and occupational medicine*, ed 2, Boston, 1992, Little, Brown, pp. 685-713.

Karas BE, Conrad R: Back injury prevention interventions in the workplace, *AAOHN J* 44:189-196, 1996.

Kelsey TW: The agrarian myth and policy responses to farm safety, *Am J Public Health* 84:1, 171, 177, 1994.

LeMasters G: Occupational exposures and effects on male and female reproduction. In Rom WR: *Environmental and occupational medicine*, ed 2, Boston, 1992, Little, Brown, pp. 147-170.

Levin PF, Hewitt JB, Misner ST: Workplace violence: female occupational homicides in metropolitan Chicago, *AAOHN J* 44:326-331, 1996.

Levy BS: Global occupational health issues, *AAOHN J* 44:244-248, 1996.

Lexau C, Kingsbury L, Lenz B et al: Building coalitions: a community wide approach for promoting farming health and safety, *AAOHN J* 41:440-449, 1993.

LoBiondo-Wood G, Haber J: *Nursing research: methods, critical appraisal, and utilization*, ed 3, St. Louis, 1994, Mosby.

Lukes E: Childhood immunizations. an update for occupational health nurses, *AAOHN J* 43:622-626, 1995.

Lusk SL: Corporate expectations for occupational health nurses' activities, *AAOHN J* 38:368-374, 1990.

Lusk SL: Linking practice and research, *AAOHN J* 41:153-157, 1993.

Lusk SL, Disch JM, Barkauskas VH: Barriers to advanced education for occupational health nurses, *AAOHN J* 36:457-463, 1988.

Maciag ME: Occupational health nursing in the 1990s: a different model of practice, *AAOHN J* 41:39-45, 1993.

Maddux J: OSHA gears up for more streamlined, user-friendly record keeping standard, *Occup Safety Health* 64(1):34-36, 1995.

Markolf AS: Industrial nursing begins in Vermont, *Public Health Nurs* 37:125-129, 1945.

Martin G: New roles for the occupational health nurse, *Job Safety and Health* 5(4):9-15, 1977.

McCall B: How West Germany protects its workers, *Job Safety and Health* 5(7):21-25, 1977.

McCunney RJ: Occupational exposure to noise. In Rom WR: *Environmental and occupational medicine*, ed 2, Boston, 1992, Little, Brown, pp. 1121-1132.

McGovern P, Matter D: Work and family: competing demands affecting worker well being, *AAOHN J* 40:24-35, 1992.

McGrath BJ: *Nursing in commerce and industry*, New York, 1946, The Commonwealth Fund.

McGrath BJ: Fifty years of industrial nursing in the United States, *Public Health Nurs* 37:119-124, 1945.

McGuire JL: Hearing conservation and employee conservation. In Hansen DJ, ed: *The work environment: occupational health fundamentals*, vol I, Chelsea, Mi., 1991, Lewis, pp. 209-240.

McGuire JL: Nuisance noise in the office. In Hansen DJ, ed: *The work environment: occupational health fundamentals*, vol III, Ann Arbor, Mi., 1994, Lewis.

McGuire JL: Conversation with author: worker hearing conversation, July 26, 1996.

McNeely E: Tracking the future of OSHA, *AAOHN J* 40:17-23, 1992.

Migrant health status: profile of a population with complex health problems, Austin, Tx., 1993, National Migrant Resource Program.

Morris LD: Minorities, jobs, and health, *AAOHN J* 37:53-55, 1989.

Morris R: *The American worker*, Washington, D.C., 1976, U.S. Government Printing Office.

Moses M: Pesticide related health problems and farm workers, *AAOHN J* 37:115-130, 1989.

Moss L: Mental health and the changing workplace environment. In Rom WR: *Environmental and occupational medicine*, ed 2, Boston, 1992, Little, Brown, pp. 667-684.

National Association of Community Health Centers, Inc.: *Community and migrant health centers: a key component of the U.S. health care system—overview and status report 1991*, Washington, D.C., 1991, The Association.

National Immigration Law Center: *Overview of benefit restrictions to immigrants in 1996 welfare and immigration laws*, Washington, D.C., 1996, The Center.

National Institute of Occupational Safety and Health (NIOSH): *Proposed national strategies for the prevention of leading work-related diseases and injuries: occupational lung diseases* (NIOSH Pub No. 89-128), Cincinnati, Oh., 1986a, NIOSH.

National Institute of Occupational Safety and Health (NIOSH): *Proposed national strategies for the prevention of leading work-related diseases and injuries: musculoskeletal injuries* (NIOSH Pub No. 89-129), Cincinnati, Oh., 1986b, NIOSH.

National Institute of Occupational Safety and Health (NIOSH): *Proposed national strategies for the prevention of leading work-related diseases and injuries: severe occupational traumatic injuries and diseases* (NIOSH Pub No. 89-131), Cincinnati, Oh., 1986d, NIOSH.

National Institute of Occupational Safety and Health (NIOSH): *Proposed national strategies for the prevention of leading work-related diseases and injuries: occupational cardiovascular diseases* (NIOSH Pub No. 89-132), Cincinnati, Oh., 1986e, NIOSH.

National Institute of Occupational Safety and Health (NIOSH): *Proposed national strategies for the prevention of leading work-related diseases and injuries: disorders of reproduction* (NIOSH Pub No. 89-133), Cincinnati, Oh., 1988a, NIOSH.

National Institute of Occupational Safety and Health (NIOSH): *Proposed national strategies for the prevention of leading work-related diseases and injuries: neurotoxic disorders* (NIOSH Pub No. 89-134), Cincinnati, Oh., 1988b, NIOSH.

National Institute of Occupational Safety and Health (NIOSH): *Proposed national strategies for the prevention of leading work-related diseases and injuries: noise-induced hearing loss* (NIOSH Pub No. 89-135), Cincinnati, Oh., 1988c, NIOSH.

National Institute of Occupational Safety and Health (NIOSH): *Proposed national strategies for the prevention of leading work-related diseases and injuries: dermatological conditions* (NIOSH Pub No. 89-136), Cincinnati, Oh., 1988d, NIOSH.

National Institute of Occupational Safety and Health (NIOSH): *Proposed national strategies for the prevention of leading work-related diseases and injuries: psychological disorders* (NIOSH Pub No. 89-137), Cincinnati, Oh., 1988e, NIOSH.

National Institute of Occupational Safety and Health (NIOSH): *List of ten leading work-related diseases and injuries*, Cincinnati, Oh., 1988f, NIOSH.

National Institute of Occupational Safety and Health (NIOSH): *New directions at NIOSH*, Cincinnati, Oh., 1995, NIOSH.

National Institute of Occupational Safety and Health (NIOSH): *National occupational research agenda*, Cincinnati, Oh., 1996, NIOSH.

Newkirk WL: Occupational health programs: envisioning the next generation, *AAOHN J* 44(5):228-232, 1996.

Nyamathi A, Flaskerud JH: Effectiveness of an AIDS education program on knowledge, attitudes and practices of state employees, *AAOHN J* 37:397-403, 1989.

O'Brien S: Occupational health nursing roles: future challenges and opportunities, *AAOHN J* 43:148-154, 1995.

Office of Management and Budget: *Budget of the United States government FY 1997*, Washington, D.C., 1996, U.S. Government Printing Office.

Olson DK, Bark SM: Health hazards affecting the animal confinement farm worker, *AAOHN J* 44:198-206, 1996.

Olson DK, Kochevar L: Occupational health and safety content in baccalaureate nursing programs, *AAOHN J* 37:33-38, 1989.

Parker-Conrad J: A century of practice: occupational health nursing, *AAOHN J* 36:156-161, 1988.

Parrish RS, Allred RH: Theories and trends in occupational health nursing, *AAOHN J* 43:514-521, 1995.

Pinkham J: 100 years of industrial nursing has vastly improved workplace safety, *Occup Safety Health* 57(4):20-23, 1988.

Pollack S, Rubenstein H, Landrigan P: Child labor. In Last J, Wallace R, eds: *Public health and preventive medicine,* Norwalk, Ct., 1994, Appleton-Lange.

Pravikoff DS: General nursing and occupational health nursing, *AAOHN J* 40:531-537, 1992.

Randolph SA: Occupational health nursing: a commitment to excellence, *AAOHN J* 36:166-169, 1988.

Randolph SA, Migliozzi AA: The role of the agricultural health nurse: bringing together community and occupational health, *AAOHN J* 41(9):429-433, 1993.

Reyes CN, Wenzel FJ, Lawton BR, Emanuel DA: The pulmonary pathology of farmer's lung disease, *Chest* 81(2):142-146, 1982.

Rest KM: Worker participation in occupational health programs: establishing a central role, *AAOHN J* 44:221-227, 1996.

Rogers B: Occupational health nursing education: curricular content in baccalaureate programs, *AAOHN J* 39:101-108, 1991.

Rogers B: Research corner: research utilization, *AAOHN J* 40:41, 1992b.

Rogers B: *Occupational health nursing: concepts and practice,* Philadelphia, 1994a, Saunders.

Rogers B: Research, prevention and practice, *AAOHN J* 42:190-191, 1994b.

Rogers B, Cox AR: Advancing the profession of occupational health nursing, *AAOHN J* 42:158-163, 1994.

Rogers B, Winslow B, Higgins S: Employee satisfaction with occupational health services, *AAOHN J* 41:58-65, 1993.

Rutstein DD, Mullan RJ, Frazier TM et al: Sentinel health events (occupational): a basis for physician recognition and public health surveillance, *Am J Public Health* 73:1054-1062, 1984.

Sattler B: Occupational and environmental health: from the back roads to the highways, *AAOHN J* 44:233-237, 1996.

Serafini P: Nursing assessment in industry, *Am J Public Health* 66(8): 755-760, 1976.

Shortridge-McCauley LA: Reproductive hazards: an overview of exposures to health care workers, *AAOHN J* 43:614-621, 1995.

Smith RB: OSHA's TB rulemaking, *Occup Safety Health* 64(4):48-49, 51, 1995a.

Smith RB: Where is OSHA going? *Occup Safety Health* 64(10):41-46, 1995b.

Sorensen G, Lando H, Pechacek TF: Promoting smoking cessation at the workplace: results of a randomized controlled intervention study, *J Occup Med* 35(2):121-126, 1993.

Stellman JM, Daum DM: *Work is dangerous to your health,* New York, 1973, Vintage Books.

Stevenson JS: *Issues and crisis during middlescence,* New York, 1977, Appleton-Century-Crofts.

Taylor WA, Mair A, Burns W: Study of noise and hearing in jute weaving, *Acoustical Society of America* 48:524-530, 1965.

Thomas PA: Preparing nursing students for practice: successful implementation of a clinical practicuum in occupational health nursing, *AAOHN J* 43:412-415, 1995.

Totten RS, Reid DS, Davies HO, Moran TJ: Farmers' lung, *Am J Med* 25:803-810, 1958.

Tucker SB, Key MM: Occupational skin disease. In Rom WR: *Environmental and occupational medicine,* ed 2, Boston, 1992, Little, Brown, pp. 551-560.

Ubell E: How dangerous is your job? *Parade* January 8, 1989, pp. 4-7.

U.S. Department of Health and Human Services (USDHHS): *Promoting health, preventing disease: objectives for the nation,* Washington, D.C., 1980, U.S. Government Printing Office.

U.S. Department of Health and Human Services (USDHHS): *The national health survey of workplace health promotion activities,* Washington, D.C., 1987, U.S. Government Printing Office.

U.S. Department of Health and Human Services (USDHHS): *Healthy people 2000: health promotion and disease prevention objectives for the nation, full report, with commentary,* Washington, D.C., 1991a, U.S. Government Printing Office.

U.S. Department of Health and Human Services (USDHHS): *NIOSH publications on noise and hearing: criteria for a recommended standard—occupational exposure to noise,* Cincinnati, Oh., 1991b, NIOSH.

U.S. Department of Health and Human Services (USDHHS): Initial therapy for tuberculosis in the era of multidrug resistance: recommendations for the Advisory Council for the elimination of tuberculosis, *MMWR* 42(RR7): 1-8, 1993.

U.S. Department of Health and Human Services (USDHHS): *Healthy people 2000: midcourse review and 1995 revisions,* Washington, D.C., 1995, U.S. Government Printing Office.

U.S. Department of Labor (USDL): *Labor firsts in America,* Washington, D.C., 1977, U.S. Government Printing Office.

Waters Y: Industrial nursing, *Public Health Nurs* 11:728-731, 1919.

Watkins EL, Larson K, Harlan C, Young S: A model program for providing health services for migrant farmworker mothers and children, *Public Health Rep* 105(6):567-576, 1990.

Widtfeldt AK: Quality and quality improvement in occupational health nursing, *AAOHN J* 40(7):326-332, 1992.

Wright FS: *Industrial nursing,* New York, 1919, MacMillan.

SELECTED BIBLIOGRAPHY

American Association of Occupational Health Nurses (AAOHN): *Comment on OSHA's voluntary guidelines for workplace violence prevention for health care workers,* Atlanta, 1995, AAOHN.

Ashford NA: *Crisis in the workplace,* Cambridge, Ma., 1976, MIT Press.

Babbitz MA: Approaching the 21st century: congressional agenda for health care and occupational health, *AAOHN J* 40:12-15, 1992.

Brodeur P: *Expendable Americans,* New York, 1974, Viking.

Brown ML: *Occupational health nursing: principles and practice,* New York, 1981, Springer.

Brown ML, Meigs JW: Occupational health nursing services, *Industrial Medicine and Surgery* 24:84-88, 1955.

Burgel BJ: Primary care at the worksite: policy issues, *AAOHN J* 44:238-243, 1996.

Charley IH: *The birth of industrial nursing,* Baltimore, 1954, Williams & Wilkins.

Cochran LB: Occupational health nursing—past, present, and future, *Ga Nurs* 53(5):6, 1993.

Felton JS: Teaching occupational health at the secondary level, *J Occup Med* 23:27-29, 1981.

Finn PL: Occupational safety and health education in the public schools: rationale, goals, and implementation, *Preventive Med* 7(3):245-249, 1978.

Goldstein DH: The occupational safety and health act of 1970, *Am J Nurs* 71:1535-1538, 1971.

Goldwater LJ: From Hippocrates to Ramazzini, *Annals of Medical History* 8:27, 1936.

Hart BG: The aging workforce: challenges for the occupational health nurse, *AAOHN J* 40:36-40, 1992.

Kidd P, Townley K, Cole H et al: The process of chore teaching: implications for farm youth injury, *Fam Community Health* 19:78-89, 1997.

Kuhar MB, Kuhar B: Over the counter medications and nursing mothers: a guide for occupational health nurses, *AAOHN J* 44:345-348, 1996.

Lee JA: *The new nurse in industry* (NIOSH Pub), Washington, D.C., 1978, U.S. Government Printing Office.

Lessure LJ, Griffith HM: Putting prevention into clinical practice, *AAOHN J* 43:72-76, 1995.

Lukes E, Wachs S: Keys to disability management, *AAOHN J* 44:141-148, 1996.

Nelson ML, Olson DK: Health care worker incidents reported in a rural health care facility: a descriptive study, *AAOHN J* 44:115-122, 1996.

Page JA, O'Brien MW: *Bitter wages*, New York, 1973, Grossman.

Rees PG, Hays BJ: Fostering expertise in occupational health nursing, *AAOHN J* 44(2):67-72, 1996.

Saphire LS, Doran B: International travel preparedness: a guideline for occupational health professionals, *AAOHN J* 44:123-128, 1996.

Saxe JM: Adult immunization update, *AAOHN J* 44:349-359, 1996.

Scott R: *Muscle and blood*, New York, 1974, Duncan.

Smith RB: Recordkeeping rule aims for accuracy, wiser use of injury and illness data, *Occ Safety Health* 64(1):37, 40, 41, 68, 1995.

Thompson MC, Holihan E, MacNeal B: Health on the road: developing a program for international travelers, *AAOHN J* 44:300-311, 1996.

U.S. Department of Labor: *Important events in American labor history, 1778-1975*, Washington, D.C., 1976, U.S. Government Printing Office.

19

The Adult Who Is Disabled

OBJECTIVES

Upon completion of this chapter, the reader should be able to:

1. Summarize five national health objectives for chronic disabling conditions.
2. Distinguish between the terms *chronic condition, disability,* and *handicap.*
3. Discuss the concepts of normalization and mainstreaming.
4. Explain individual, family, and societal variables that influence adaptation to a disability.
5. Discuss the grieving process in relation to chronic conditions.
6. Identify the critical elements of chronic sorrow.
7. Describe areas of major concern for persons who are disabled.
8. Discuss the role of community health nurses when working with adults who are disabled.
9. Identify federal, state, and local agencies that provide services to persons who are disabled.
10. Identify legislation that provides health care resources and services for adults who are disabled.

When working with persons who are disabled, remember that first they are persons and, secondarily, they have a disabling condition.

Since early in recorded history people have noted the disabling conditions that existed among them. Disabling conditions were recorded as early as the fourth century BC (Buscaglia, 1983, p. 152). Hippocrates, Aristotle, Galen, and others studied such conditions and sought explanations for their existence. Many people who were disabled died in childhood, and few lived to adulthood.

Throughout history societies have dealt in various ways with their members who were disabled. Attitudes toward the disabled have ranged from acceptance to rejection and from understanding to fear. In early times disabling conditions were sometimes viewed as a punishment for sin, and the Elizabethan Poor Law of 1601 (see Chapter 4) equated such conditions with crime. Under this law people who were disabled were often publicly punished and imprisoned (Sussman, 1966, p. 3). The classic story of the *Hunchback of Notre Dame* illustrates society's reaction to disfigurement during the eighteenth century.

Today being disabled is no longer considered a sin or a crime. However, people who are disabled may be socially stigmatized, socially isolated, and face discrimination.

Disabilities are disproportionately represented among minorities, the elderly, and people of lower socioeconomic status (Pope, Tarlov, 1991, p. 1). The World Health Organization (WHO) estimates that 10% of the world's population, 400 million people, are disabled (Frye, 1993, p. 43). It is estimated that as many as 50 million Americans are disabled (U.S. Department of Commerce, 1995, p. 139; Wenger, Kaye, LaPlante, 1996, p. 1). Approximately 10% of Americans are limited in activity because of a chronic disabling condition (USDHHS, 1995, p. 108). Such conditions are a serious health problem for Americans.

HEALTHY PEOPLE 2000 AND CHRONIC DISABLING CONDITIONS

Chronic disabling conditions lead to physical, emotional, social, and economic costs to individuals, families, and the nation (USDHHS, 1995, p. 108). They are one of the priority areas addressed in *Healthy People 2000.* National health objectives for them are given in the box on the following page. Of the 10 leading causes of death in the United States, all are either chronic disabling conditions or related to such conditions.

National health objectives focus on the need to prevent disabilities; early diagnosis and treatment of chronic conditions; and provision of information, skills training, and support services to increase the ability of people to manage their conditions, to live independently, and to participate fully in their communities (USDHHS, 1995, p. 108). Limited progress has been made in reaching the year 2000 national health objectives in relation to chronic disabling conditions. Activity limitation from these conditions is on the rise, end-stage renal disease has increased, and the prevalence of diabetes and obesity is increasing (USDHHS,

HEALTHY PEOPLE 2000 Objectives Targeting Chronic Disabling Conditions

1. Increase years of healthy life to at least 65 years.
2. Reduce to no more than 8 percent the proportion of people who experience a limitation in major activity due to chronic conditions.
3. Reduce to no more than 90 per 1,000 people the proportion of all people aged 65 and older who have difficulty in performing two or more personal care activities, thereby preserving independence.
4. Reduce to no more than 10 percent the proportion of people with asthma who experience activity limitation.
5. Reduce activity limitation due to chronic back conditions to a prevalence of no more than 19 per 1,000 people.
6. Reduce significant hearing impairment to a prevalence of no more than 82 per 1,000 people.
7. Reduce significant visual impairment to a prevalence of no more than 30 per 1,000 people.
8. Reduce the prevalence of serious mental retardation in school-aged children to no more than 2 per 1,000 children.
9. Reduce diabetes-related deaths to no more than 34 per 100,000 people.
10. Reduce the most severe complications of diabetes as follows:

End-stage renal disease	1.4/1,000
Blindness	1.4/1,000
Lower extremity amputation	4.9/1,000
Perinatal mortality	2%
Major congenital malformations	4%

11. Reduce diabetes to an incidence of no more than 2.5 per 1,000 people and a prevalence of no more than 25 per 1,000 people.
12. Reduce overweight to a prevalence of no more than 20 percent among people aged 20 and older and no more than 15 percent among adolescents aged 12 through 19.
13. Increase to at least 30 percent the proportion of people aged 6 and older who engage regularly, preferably daily, in light to moderate physical activity for at least 30 minutes per day.
14. Increase to at least 40 percent the proportion of people with chronic and disabling conditions who receive formal patient education including information about community and self-help resources as an integral part of the management of their condition.
15. Increase to at least 80 percent the proportion of providers of primary care for children who routinely refer or screen infants and children for impairments of vision, hearing, speech and language and assess other developmental milestones as part of well-child care.
16. Reduce the age at which children with significant hearing impairment are identified to no more than 12 months.
17. Increase to at least 60 percent the proportion of providers of primary care for older adults who routinely evaluate people aged 65 and older for urinary incontinence and impairments of vision, hearing, cognition, and functional status.
18. Increase to at least 90 percent the proportion of peri-menopausal women who have been counseled about the benefits and risks of estrogen replacement therapy for prevention of osteoporosis.
19. Increase to at least 75 percent the proportion of worksites with 50 or more employees that have a voluntary established policy or program for the hiring of people with disabilities.
20. Increase to 50 the number of States that have service systems for children with or at risk of chronic and disabling conditions.
21. Reduce the prevalence of peptic ulcer disease to no more than 18 per 1,000 people aged 18 and older by preventing its recurrence.

From USDHHS: *Healthy people 2000, midcourse review and 1995 revisions*, Washington, D.C., 1995, U.S. Government Printing Office, pp. 241-246.

p. 108). Communities across the nation have much work to do if the year 2000 objectives are to be met.

The National Center for Chronic Disease Prevention and Health Promotion (NCCDPHP), part of the Centers for Disease Control and Prevention, is a lead federal agency in chronic disease prevention. It advocates for healthier lifestyles, facilitates nationwide efforts to prevent chronic diseases, and works with communities to translate research findings into effective community health programs. It actively supports initiatives that promote good nutrition, tobacco-free lifestyles, physical activity, adolescent and school health, reproductive health, health promotion, and early disease detection. NCCDPHP programs target populations, such as older Americans and minorities, that have a disproportionate share of chronic diseases, and assists states in developing surveillance systems to monitor and track chronic diseases and related risk factors.

CHRONIC, DISABLING, AND HANDICAPPING CONDITIONS: RELATED BUT DISTINCT PHENOMENA

Words such as *disabled* and *handicapped* often carry with them negative societal stereotypes and can be personally devaluing. Over the years numerous "labels" such as *disabled*, *impaired*, *crippled*, *people with special needs*, *exceptional people*, and *handicappers* have been used with varying levels of success to describe people with chronic disabling conditions. U.S. legislation frequently uses the word *disability* in title and text, and local communities still frequently use the word *handicap* when providing services such as parking and access. Whatever descriptors are used, the important value is the "people first" philosophy: put the person first—before the condition; treat people with respect; and facilitate personal growth and independence. Putting the person first is not just a matter of semantics, it is a matter of value and belief. If clients prefer the use of one term over another, such as *handicapable* rather than *handicapped*, then that is the term that should be used. The use of the terms *chronic, disabling,* and *handicapped* in this chapter reflect what has been legislated and how services are often provided and described.

Patrick (1994) has discussed the concept of disablement. The epidemiology of disablement covers the triad of impairment, disability, and handicap (Patrick, 1994, p. 1723; WHO, 1980). *Impairment* refers to dysfunction at the organic level; *disability* refers to physical or psychological dysfunction resulting in functional limitations at the person level; and *handicap* refers not so much to an individual but to a social state—a status assigned to the person with impairment or disability by societal expectations that shape interactions (Patrick, 1994, p. 1724). A disability becomes a handicap based on the level of disability it imposes on an individual and by societal definition.

According to the World Health Organization (1981, p. 8) chronic disease conditions become disabling and handicapping conditions, according to the following schema:

Disease/condition→impairment→disability→handicap

Although this schema can frequently be applied, progression from one stage to another is not always linear or unidirectional and an individual might skip stages. An example of this is the public's attitude toward disfiguring impairments—these impairments often cause no functional limitation but impose a disability by affecting social acceptance and interaction (Pope, Tarlov, 1991, pp. 9-10, 91).

The Institute of Medicine (IOM) (Pope, Tarlov, 1991, pp. 102-103, 273, 275) has recommended that a conceptual framework, standard measures of disability, and a national disability surveillance system be developed. The IOM also recommends that longitudinal studies that assist in determining the causes and rates of transition between pathology, impairment, functional limitation, and disability be conducted; and that priorities be established for disability prevention. A model of disability that shows the interaction of the disabling process, quality of life, and risk factors is given in Figure 19-1. In this model the heading of *disability* incorporates all levels of disabilities, including handicaps. Various personal, societal, and environmental variables that influence the progression of a condition from pathology to disability affect the degree of limitation or disability a person experiences and the occurrence of secondary conditions, as well as adaptation to the disability (Pope, Tarlov, p. 10).

Chronic Conditions that Cause Significant Morbidity and Mortality among Americans

Ten chronic diseases take the greatest toll in U.S. lives and quality of life and are highly preventable:

1. Coronary heart disease
2. Cerebrovascular disease
3. Lung cancer
4. Chronic obstructive lung disease
5. Colorectal cancer
6. Breast cancer
7. Diabetes
8. Cirrhosis/alcoholism
9. Cervical cancer
10. Chronic musculoskeletal disease (including arthritis, osteoporosis, and lower back pain)

From NCCDPHP: *CDC/NCCDPHP: turning research findings into effective community programs*, Atlanta, 1996, CDC.

Chronic Conditions

Chronic conditions were defined in Chapter 11 as impairments or deviations from normal that have at least one of the following characteristics: permanency, residual disability, irreversible pathological causation and alteration, need for special rehabilitation and training, and need for a period of long-term supervision and care (Commission on Chronic Illness, 1957, p. 4). When you think about it, many people have at least one chronic condition.

Ten major chronic diseases in the United States and common risk factors for them are given in the accompanying boxes. Other risk factors include genetic disorders, violence, educational deficiencies, perinatal complications, injury, environmental factors, unsanitary living conditions, and stress (Pope, Tarlov, 1991, p. 84). In Figure 19-1 risk factors are classified as biological, environmental, and lifestyle.

Three chronic diseases—cardiovascular disease, cancer, and diabetes—greatly diminish the quality of life for millions of Americans and account for about 75% of U.S. deaths annually (National Center for Chronic Disease Prevention and Health Promotion, 1996). Other chronic conditions include asthma, skin conditions, arthritis, cerebral palsy, mental retardation, deafness, speech defects, visual impairment, drug addiction, alcoholism, epilepsy, spinal cord injury, mental or emotional illness, multiple sclerosis, muscular dystrophy, orthopedic impairments, and perceptual handicaps such as dyslexia, brain dysfunction, and developmental aphasia. The health of the nation will be profoundly affected by the outcome of the fight against chronic disease.

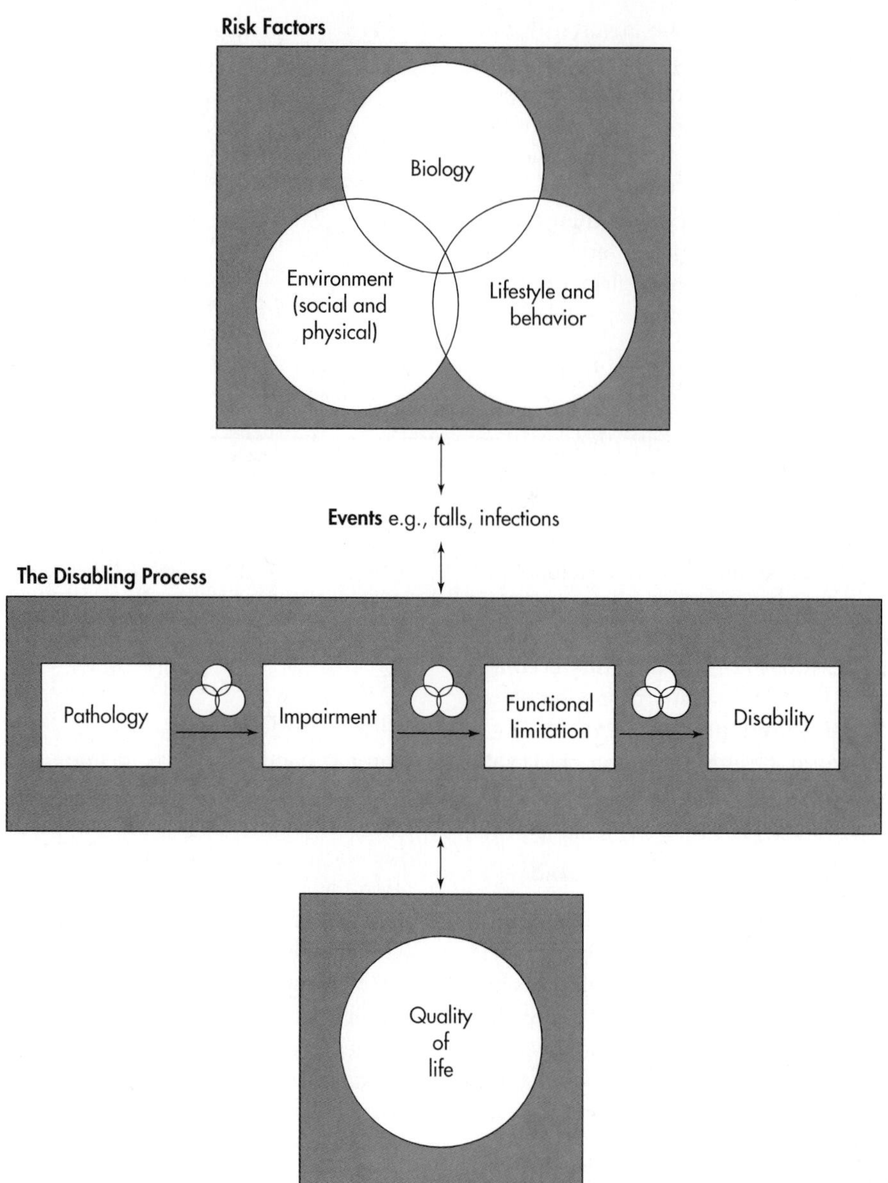

Figure 19-1 Model of disability showing the interaction of the disabling process, quality of life, and risk factors. The potential for additional risk factors is shown between the stages of the model (e.g., falls, infections). *(Reprinted with permission from Pope AM, Tarlov AR, (eds):* Disability in America: toward a national agenda for prevention, *Washington, D.C., 1991, National Academy Press, p. 9, 85. Copyright © 1991 by the National Academy of Sciences. Courtesy of the National Academy Press, Washington, D.C.).*

Not all chronic conditions are disabling or handicapping. People can have a condition for a lifetime and not consider themselves disabled. Chronic conditions become disabling when they cause functional limitations, or "impairments," and adversely affect an individual's ability to carry out one or more *major life activities*.

Although the prevalence of chronic conditions increases with age, they occur across the life span (Figure 19-2). People under the age of 18 are likely to have chronic conditions associated with mental impairment, mental illness, asthma, orthopedic conditions, or speech and hearing disorders; young adults are more likely to have orthopedic and back impairments; and at older ages degenerative diseases such as arthritis and heart disease are prevalent (USDHHS, 1992, p. 23). Interestingly, 70% of visual impairments and 58% of hearing impairments are found among individuals under age 65, and although developmental disability is commonly associated with children, the majority of people with devel-

Common Risk Factors for Chronic Disease

Many chronic diseases and conditions share common risk factors, all of which can be controlled to some extent through intervention:

- Smoking
- Poor nutrition
- Sedentary lifestyle
- Alcohol misuse
- Inadequate preventive health services (e.g., inadequate prenatal care and immunizations)
- Unprotected sexual intercourse

From NCCDPHP: *CDC/NCCDPHP: turning research findings into effective community programs*, Atlanta, 1996, CDC.

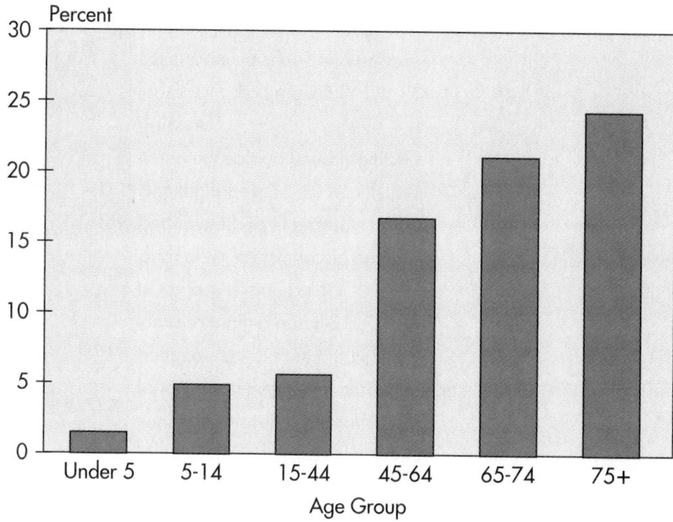

Figure 19-2 Percentage of people experiencing limitations of major activity as a result of disability. *(From USDHHS:* Healthy People 2000: national health promotion and disease prevention objectives, full report, with commentary, *Washington, D.C., 1991, U.S. Government Printing Office, p. 41.)*

opmental disability are 22 to 49 years old (Stucki, 1995, pp. 12, 18). Traumatic injuries to the spinal cord occur most often to young men between the ages of 16 and 30 (Stucki, p. 10).

What Is Disability?

Consensus is lacking on a definition of disability. WHO (1981, p. 8) has defined a disability as any restriction or lack of ability to perform an activity in the manner, or within the range, considered to be normal for a human being. The National Institute on Disability and Rehabilitation Research (NIDRR) (Max, Rice, Trupin, 1996, p. 1) defines disability as a limitation in activity caused by a chronic condition or impairment. Using this definition a child under age 5 with a disability is one who is unable to participate in play activities; a child or adolescent age 5 to 17 with a disability is one who needs to attend a special school or is limited or unable to attend school; and an adult with a disability is one who cannot work or do housework, is limited in the amount of kind of work or housework, or is limited in other activities (Max, Rice, Trupin, p. 1). Nursing interventions focus on preventing disability, diminishing the severity of disabling conditions, and improving the quality of life for people who are disabled.

In 1990 the Americans with Disabilities Act defined a disability as a physical or mental impairment that substantially limits one or more of an individual's major life activities. Included under this definition are individuals who have a record of an impairment or are regarded as having such an impairment. It includes the triad of disablement previously mentioned and gives legal sanction to a definition of disability that includes both the individual's disability and the societal response (Patrick, 1994, p. 1724).

The *level* of a person's disability is determined by combining the results of the health history, clinical evaluation, assessment of client and family perception of the situation, and measurement of ability to carry out activities of daily living (ADL) and instrumental activities of daily living (IADL). ADLs include self-care activities necessary to survive such as eating, dressing, bathing, transferring, and toileting. IADLs include activities such as performing housework, managing finances, cooking/meal preparation, doing laundry, shopping, running errands, taking medicine without help, and using the telephone. Below are four general levels of functional disability, taking into consideration ADL, IADL, and employment abilities:

Level I: Partial disability characterized by slight limitation in one or more of the major life activities; able to take part in school, competitive employment, and self-care

Level II: Partial disability characterized by moderate limitation in one or more of the major life activities; generally able to attend school, work regularly or part-time (but the employment may need to be modified); may need assistance with self-care

Level III: Partial disability characterized by severe limitation in one or more of the major life activities; usually unable to attend school or work regularly (considered occupationally disabled); often requires assistance with self-care

Level IV: Total disability characterized by complete, or almost complete, dependency on others for activities of daily living, self-care, and economic support; usually unable to work or attend regular school

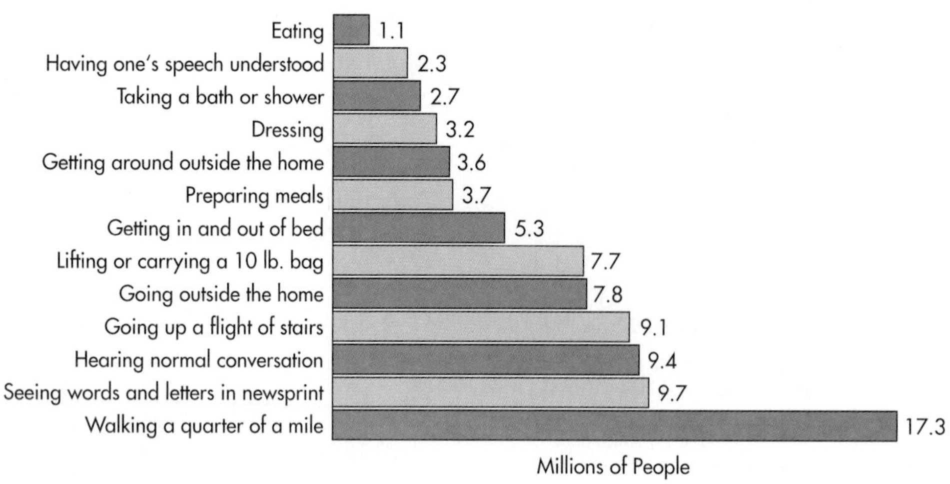

Figure 19-3 Some functional limitations of adults with disabilities. *(From U.S. Department of Commerce:* Statistical abstract of the United States 1995, *Washington, D.C., 1995, U.S. Government Printing Office, p. 138.)*

A condition can encompass the entire range of disability. People with similar underlying pathologies can present varying degrees of limitation and disability (Lafata, Koch, Weissert, 1994, p. 1813). For example, a person with cerebral palsy may evidence functional abilities ranging from independence to total dependence. Figure 19-3 illustrates some functional limitations of adults with disabilities. The chronic conditions of mental retardation, emphysema, heart disease, orthopedic conditions, and arthritis have some of the highest rates of disability.

Disabling conditions frequently result from injuries, chronic conditions, the aging process, and developmental disabilities such as cerebral palsy, mental retardation, and birth defects. More than one third of people with disabilities have two or more disabling conditions (Trupin, Rice, 1995, p. 1). Multiple disabling conditions increase with age (Pope, Tarlov, 1991, p. 191). Overall only 40% of people with disabling conditions rate their health as fair or poor (Trupin, Rice, 1995, p. 2). However, people with multiple disabling conditions have poorer health and use more medical services than those with only one condition (Trupin, Rice, p. 1).

Frequently a secondary disabling condition will develop in relation to an existing disabling condition (e.g., decubitus ulcers in a person with quadriplegia). These *secondary conditions* can result in further deterioration such as decubitus ulcers, contractures, physical deconditioning, cardiopulmonary conditions, and mental depression (Pope, Tarlov, 1991, p. 13). Nursing interventions play an important role in keeping secondary conditions from occurring; some common secondary conditions are given in Table 19-1.

Handicapping Conditions

A handicap is a condition that *substantially* limits one or more of an individual's major life activities (President's Committee on Employment of the Handicapped, 1978; WHO, 1981), resulting in "functional limitations" that affect an individual's ability to fulfill normal societal roles. Functional limitations adversely affect an individual's ability to carry out one or more major life activity defined as communication, ambulation, self-care, socialization, education, vocational training, transportation, housing, and employment. A handicap involves some form of societal devaluation and results in physical and emotional pain and expenditure of time, effort, and money. The level of disability caused by a handicapping condition determines client needs, intervention strategies, and appropriate community resources. Individuals with handicapping conditions have complex social, emotional, physical, educational, and financial needs that involve redefining family and community roles, relationships, and responsibilities.

Mainstreaming and Normalization

The concepts of mainstreaming and normalization are important to discuss in relation to the person who is disabled. Legislation, such as the Americans with Disabilities Act of 1990, the Individuals with Disabilities Education Act of the same year, and the Rehabilitation Act Amendments of 1992 have helped to ensure the rights of Americans with disabilities, assisting them in living as normal a life as possible. Increasingly, Americans with chronic disabling conditions are encouraged to be independent and are being integrated into the mainstream of community life (Chappell, 1994, p. 23). Normalization and mainstreaming reinforce the philosophy that people who are disabled are people first and that, secondarily, they have a disabling condition.

Mainstreaming refers to integrating the person who is disabled into the everyday life of the community. The person functions in the "mainstream" of the community and is not

table 19-1 Causes of Some Common Secondary Conditions

Secondary Condition	Causes
Decubitus ulcers	Inaccessibility to adequate health care, improper seating for those with the disuse syndrome, lack of continuous personal hygiene.
Genitourinary tract disorders	Inaccessibility to adequate health care, genetic disorders, alcohol and drug abuse, nutritional disorders, lack of personal hygiene, acute and chronic illness.
Cardiovascular disorders	Alcohol and drug abuse, tobacco use, nutritional disorders, stress, inaccessibility to adequate health care, acute and chronic illness, lack of physical fitness.
Stroke	Lack of physical fitness, nutritional disorders, tobacco use, stress, alcohol and drug abuse, inaccessibility to adequate health care (hypertension control).
Musculoskeletal problems	Lack of physical fitness, injuries, stress, genetic disorders, perinatal complications, acute and chronic illness, inaccessibility to adequate health care.
Arthritis	Speculated lack of physical fitness, nutritional disorders, stress and possibly genetic disorder.
Respiratory problems	Lack of physical fitness, acute and chronic illness, environmental quality problems, alcohol and drug problems, tobacco use, unsanitary living conditions, genetic disorders.
Hearing loss	Genetic disorders, acute and chronic illness, injuries, violence, environmental quality problems (noise pollution).
Speech and language problems	Genetic disorders, acute and chronic illness, injuries, environmental quality problems, neurological deficits (such as strokes), cancer and respiratory problems.
Vision problems	Genetic disorders, acute and chronic illness, injuries, violence, nutritional disorders, environmental quality problems, inaccessibility to adequate health care.
Emotional problems	Genetic disorders, stress, alcohol and drug abuse, deleterious child-rearing practices and familial-cultural beliefs, inaccessibility to adequate mental health care.
Skin disorders	Genetic disorders, acute and chronic illness, injuries (fires and burns), nutritional disorders, unsanitary living conditions, stress.

Reprinted with permission from Pope AM, Tarlov AR, (eds): *Disability in America: toward a national agenda for prevention*, Washington, D.C., 1991, National Academy Press, p. 216. Copyright © 1991 by the National Academy of Sciences. Courtesy of the National Academy Press, Washington, D.C.

separated from it. Many people who are disabled are already in the mainstream of the community and are difficult to distinguish from other community members. For others, special efforts need to be taken for this integration to occur (e.g., persons who are mentally retarded, persons with spinal cord injury, and persons who are severely physically handicapped).

Normalization refers to helping people live as normal a life as possible. It involves assisting people in participating in the same activities of daily living as other members of the community such as employment, home maintenance, school, and social and recreational activities.

Mainstreaming and normalization focus on maximizing the strengths of people who are disabled, enhancing their quality of life, and reducing their social isolation. Social isolation can be personally devaluing and developmentally devastating. Nurses' interventions focus on assisting individuals who are disabled in becoming integrated into the mainstream of community life and living as normal a life as possible. Successful accomplishment of such outcomes requires care management, utilization of community resources, and recognition that people who are disabled are entitled to the same rights and respect as everyone else.

ADAPTATION TO DISABLEMENT

Adaptation to chronic, disabling, and handicapping conditions is a complex process and is influenced by individual, family, community, and societal variables. How these variables interact with each other will determine how well the individual and family adapts. The attitudes and expectations of family, friends, and health care professionals significantly influence the self-perceptions of people with disablement (Oermann, Lindgren, 1995, p. 6). Limiting the disablement and improving the quality of life are part of the adaptation process.

Societal Attitudes

Society creates disabilities (Buscaglia, 1983; Patrick, 1994), and societal attitudes play a major role in individual and family adaptation to disabling and handicapping conditions. In fact, the debilitating aspects of a disability result not so much from the condition itself but from the manner in which others define and respond to it. Societal barriers can be more handicapping to individuals than the disability itself (ARN, 1994a, p. 5) and can increase the social isolation of people who are disabled. The nurse promotes quality of life for people who are disabled through nursing interventions that alter society's adverse values and attitudes (ARN, 1994a, p. 5).

Disabling conditions are defined and viewed differently by various cultures, as is shown in the example of Donald Sims (Figure 19-4), who has impaired functioning of his lower extremities following a motorcycle accident. He found that when he visited the Choco Indians in Panama his strengths were respected and his differences accepted. The attitudes of the Choco Indians helped him to realize his potential, and Sims stated:

> An unbelievable experience! They treated me as though I was no different—I was accepted as a person—a people, a culture with no concept of handicapped. I did what I could, they did their thing, and we all worked and played together. No one shied away from the chair. The Choco Indians made my Panama trip the most wonderful experience since my accident. They helped reinstate my faith in people, life itself, and a positive attitude toward all things.

Societal attitudes have been described as "invisible barriers" (Kendrick, 1983, p. 17). The impact of these barriers is seen in the quote from Deborah Kendrick, a mother who is blind:

> The difficulty is neither in being blind nor in being a mother. It is in the attitudes of others, the invisible barriers which can separate me from other mothers and my children from their children. (p. 18)

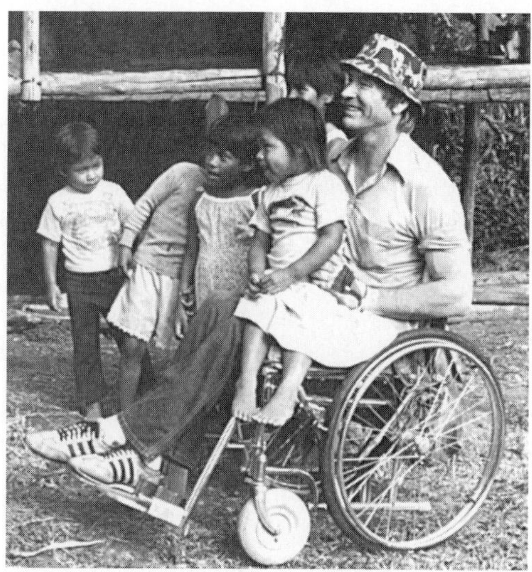

Figure 19-4 Societal attitudes influence how individuals, families, and groups perceive differences among individuals in a society and can facilitate or inhibit individual growth and development. *(Courtesy Donald Sims and photographer H. Morgan Smith, Explorations, Brigade Quartermasters. Morgan Smith is an honorary member of the Choco Indian tribe, and is an anthropologist and naturalist who has conducted numerous archeological excavations.)*

Lack of knowledge and misconceptions about the cause, treatment, and prognosis of disabling conditions contributes to nonfacilitative attitudes. Persons who are disabled are often characterized as being helpless, suffering, dependent, and emotionally unstable. They may be held at least partially responsible for their disability (Seifert, 1981). Buscaglia (1983) described an interesting study about such attitudes. In the study, nonhandicapped people were viewed in two different situations: (1) in a wheelchair or with leg braces, giving the impression of being handicapped, and (2) without the wheelchair or leg braces in a normal situation. In the first instance the individual was described as helpless, hopeless, and of decreased value; however, the same person in the second situation was described positively. Studies have shown that even people with handicapping conditions have negative attitudes toward people who are handicapped.

Safilios-Rothschild (1982), in her classic work on disability, identified a number of societal variables that affect attitudes toward people who are disabled. These variables are presented in the box on the next page. Societal attitudes have a significant impact on the residential, educational, social, occupational, and health services available to the person who is disabled.

Attitudes of Health Care Professionals

The attitudes of health professionals greatly influence a person's response to treatment and adaptation to the disability (Oermann, Lindgren, 1995, p. 8). Too often health care professionals look on people who are disabled in terms of their limitations, not their strengths. When health professionals interact with a family based on their perceptions about disabled individuals and their cultural context rather than interactions with the family, the family's needs may not be met (Weeks, 1995, p. 256). Nurses need to assess and overcome their own attitudinal barriers toward disabling conditions and develop facilitative attitudes toward clients regardless of the level of disability and potential for rehabilitation (Oermann, Lindgren, 1995, p. 8).

Individual and Family Variables Influencing Adaptation

Individual and family variables also affect adaptation to a disability. These variables interact with each other and the attitudinal variables previously discussed, and it can be difficult to separate the effects of one from another.

THE FAMILY WITH A MEMBER WHO IS DISABLED Family-centered nursing interventions play a key role in promoting client progress and rehabilitation outcomes (Reeber, 1992, p. 332; Watson, 1992, p. 51; Weeks, 1995, p. 256; Youngblood, Hines, 1992, p. 325). Families are often the primary caregivers for people who are disabled. It is important to identify strategies that promote family stability and growth after a disabling condition has been diagnosed. Reactions to a disabled family member usually develop within

Variables Affecting Societal Attitudes Toward People Who Are Disabled

BELIEFS REGARDING THE VALUE OF PHYSICAL AND MENTAL INTEGRITY

The value a society places on physical and mental integrity will greatly affect societal acceptance of people who are disabled and the scope of services offered to them. If a society highly values physical and mental integrity and "devalues" people who are disabled, they may experience prejudice, discrimination, and be isolated from the mainstream of society in placements such as institutions for the mentally ill and mentally retarded and other long-term care facilities.

BELIEFS IN RELATION TO ILLNESS

In most societies, people who are acutely ill are usually allowed to be "sick" for the duration of their illness. However, once the condition becomes chronic the person may be expected to "adjust," and may even be expected to perform "normally" in relation to societal roles and expectations, even when achieving such behavior may be difficult.

BELIEFS REGARDING CONDITION OCCURRENCE

If it is believed that the individual had a high degree of responsibility in the occurrence of the condition, less aid and assistance may be given. Obesity, alcoholism, mental illness, AIDS, domestic violence, and drug abuse are examples of this.

THE ROLE OF THE GOVERNMENT IN ALLEVIATING SOCIAL PROBLEMS

If a society does not believe that the government should assume an active role in alleviating social problems, there may be little public assistance or social support for people who are disabled. Also the government may assume a treatment or assistance role rather than a preventive one.

BELIEFS REGARDING THE ORIGINS OF POVERTY

Many people who have disabling conditions live in poverty. If a society believes that poverty is generally a matter of self-will, there may be less willingness to assist people who are disabled.

THE RATE OF UNEMPLOYMENT AND ECONOMIC DEVELOPMENT

When unemployment is high and/or the economy is unstable, people who are disabled may be at a disadvantage in hiring and employment practices; and there may also be less inclination to financially subsidize those who are disabled.

Modified from Safilios-Rothschild C: *The sociology and social psychology of disability rehabilitation*. New York, 1982. University Press of America, p. 4.

1 to 4 weeks of diagnosis and are difficult to change later (Weeks, 1995, p. 256).

Nursing interventions should include assessing the entire family unit (see Chapters 7 and 9). The family assessment process includes examining family dynamics and characteristics and perceptions of roles, disability, health care, coping skills, and support systems (Youngblood, Hines, 1992, p. 325). The box on the following page presents some questions that help the nurse to assess the family's perception of the disability.

Knowing how caregivers and prospective caregivers view their situation and what they want to know and learn is essential to provide effective nursing care for the family with a disabled member (Davidhizer, 1992, p. 66; Weeks, 1995, p. 256). Research by Weeks has shown perceived educational needs of prospective family caregivers (see the Teaching Tips box on p. 577). Nurses need to be aware of these needs, provide client and family education, and refer clients to appropriate resources. Some information resources are given in the box on page 578.

Disabling conditions require that a family reallocate goals and priorities, division of labor, use of time, family roles, financial resources, and caregiving—sometimes on a long-term basis. This frequently happens in families with a member who is severely physically or mentally disabled. Take, for example, parents of a child who is severely mentally disabled.

CASE Scenario

With the help of community supports such as school programs and community health nursing services Mr. and Mrs. Zelinski had been able to care at home for Joshua, their 19-year-old son who is severely mentally retarded, since his birth. Mrs. Zelinski gave up her job when Joshua was born so that she would be available to take care of him. Joshua's medical care frequently strained family finances. Respite care was not readily available in their community, and the Zelinskis rarely traveled or did things together without Joshua. Joshua has reached the age of adulthood and is unable to live independently. Except for a state institution there are no other local residential placements for him, and the Zelinskis had mutually decided that institutional placement was not an acceptable option for them. When other parents were launching their adult children Mr. and Mrs. Zelinski were reassessing family goals, roles, finances, and resources and prepared to continue to care for their adult child at home.

Situations like this are not uncommon, and lack of appropriate community resources and supports takes a toll on many families caring for members who are disabled. Respite

Assessment of Family's Perception of Disability

I. Family Characteristics
- What are the biological characteristics of each family member?
- What is the family's cultural/ethnic background?
- What are the socioeconomic resources available to family members?
- What are the personality characteristics of each family member?

II. The Family's Perception of Rules and Roles
- What are the rules that govern family interactions?
- How do family members interact with each other?
- What is the structure of the family unit?
- How are rules and roles assigned?
- What events cause rules and/or roles to change?

III. The Family's Perception of the Disability
- What meaning does the disability have for each family member?
- What responsibility does each member have for the management of the disability?
- How are decisions made about the management of the disability?
- How are family interactions affected by the disability?

IV. The Family's Perception of Health Care
- What experiences have family members had with health care systems?
- What experiences with health care systems have resulted from the disability?
- What expectations do family members have in regard to the management of the disability?
- How do family members expect to interact with health care professionals?

V. The Family's Perception of Coping Skills and Support Systems
- How have family members reacted to crisis in the past?
- What information does the family need about the disability?
- What resources are available to family members?
- What support systems are available to family members?

From Youngblood NM, Hines J: The influence of the family's perception of disability on rehabilitation outcomes, *Rehabil Nurs* 17(6):325, 1992. Reprinted from Rehabilitation Nursing, Vol 17, Issue 6, with permission of the Association of Rehabilitation Nurses, 4700 Lake Avenue, Glenview, Il., 60025-1485. Copyright © 1992, Association of Rehabilitation Nurses.

services are a particularly pressing need (Montgomery, 1995).

FAMILY STRESS When persons become disabled they and their families experience stress (Winterhalter, 1992, p. 23). As discussed in Chapter 8, such conditions are often stressful to families because they may be required to compromise or accept a less-than-perfect solution to adapt to the situation (McCubbin, McCubbin, 1993).

Each family will adapt and cope differently. As indicated in Chapter 8, some families are more vulnerable to stress than others, and disabling conditions can produce stress for the entire family. The availability of appropriate community resources can assist the family in adapting to the disability and prevent family burnout. Family adaptation is a significant factor in client progress and outcomes (Thomas, Ellison, Howell, Winters, 1992, p. 186; Weeks, 1995, p. 256).

Research has found that families of persons who are disabled may be treated as if they were different from other families or somehow to blame for the disability (Buzinski, 1980). This creates even more stress and can make it more difficult for families to adjust. Also, families may be forced to organize priorities around the needs of the disabled member and, frequently, the financial demands of the condition place economic hardships and additional stress on the family. While caring for a disabled family member families are expected to carry out other day-to-day activities and responsibilities, such as school, work, and household maintenance. The stress of these multiple roles and activities can be overwhelming and result in caregiver burnout.

If the stress of caregiving becomes too great a decision may be made to place the disabled family member outside the home. Studies have shown that families are more likely to place handicapped members outside the home when the following variables exist: the person is severely disabled; the family structure is incapable of providing adequate time, care, and resources; there is a high level of family conflict and discord, such as marital dissatisfaction; and community support systems are insufficient (Giele, 1984; Sherman, Cocozza, 1984). Supportive interventions can help to alleviate some of the stress the family is experiencing as a result of such variables.

VARIABLES AFFECTING ADAPTATION TO A DISABILITY The impact of a disabling condition on the individual and family is influenced by a number of variables. Some of these variables are listed in the box on page 578 and discussed here.

The *stage of grief and mourning* the individual and family have reached in relation to the condition is important. The person and family have suffered a loss. This loss may take many forms, such as loss of independence, control over life, privacy, body image, body functioning, social status, financial stability, employment, material possessions, and predetermined self-fulfillment. Losses in terms of changes in personal relationships and roles may also occur. The process may be compounded by the fact that there may be no

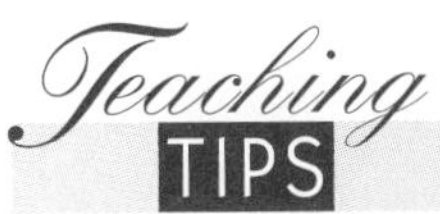

Educational Wants of Prospective Family Caregivers of Newly Disabled Adults*

RANK	ITEM (LEARNING TO . . .)	MEAN SCORE
1	Normalize the daily routine of a disabled adult within the bounds of his or her disabilities.	4.86
2	Ensure that assistance is available when a disabled adult needs help.	4.83
3	Evaluate the strengths and capabilities of a disabled adult.	4.81
4	Supervise or carry out prescribed treatments and other recommendations for maintaining a disabled adult's well-being.	4.80
5	Anticipate the needs of a disabled adult for future assistance and services.	4.77
6	Evaluate options for treatment and services for a disabled adult.	4.71
7	Monitor the course of the disease (or condition) and evaluate the significance of changes in a disabled adult.	4.67
7	Communicate adequately with a disabled adult.	4.67
7	Maintain or gain up-to-date knowledge of the health and human services systems and the options within these systems.	4.67
7	Maintain or gain up-to-date knowledge of payment mechanisms for services provided to disabled adults.	4.67
8	Perform basic personal care procedures for a disabled adult.	4.65
9	Provide structure for a disabled adult's activities.	4.64
10	Manage the current and future costs related to being a caregiver.	4.63
10	Give appropriate consideration to a disabled adult family member's opinions and preferences.	4.63
11	Accept emotionally the likelihood of a progressive decline in the health of a person who is significant to you.	4.59
12	Work through changes in the lifelong relationship between you and another person.	4.54
13	Avoid severe drain on your own physical strength and health.	4.53
13	Interact with medical and other human service providers.	4.53
14	Be creative in decreasing the tediousness of the daily routines of providing care to a disabled adult.	4.52
14	Compensate for emotional drain due to your constant responsibilities.	4.52

Reprinted from Weeks SK: What are the educational needs of prospective family caregivers of newly disabled adults, *Rehabil Nurs*, 20(5):256-260, 1995, with permission of the Association of Rehabilitation Nurses, 4700 W. Lake Avenue, Glenview, Il., 60025-1485. Copyright © 1995. Association of Rehabilitation Nurses.
*Scores ranged from 1 (no importance) to 5 (high importance).

immediate end in sight, and the individual is grieving personally while experiencing the effects of significant others grieving as well. Until grieving has been successfully accomplished, treatment, rehabilitation, and adaptation cannot be fully successful. Unresolved grief can seriously alter and affect interpersonal relationships and family functioning.

Community health nurses play a major role in helping families to experience a healthy grieving process. Being able to accept the fact that *grief is normal* helps the nurse to assist families in working through the process in a constructive manner.

The stages in the grief and mourning process in relation to a handicap closely resemble the stages discussed by Kubler-Ross (1969), who studied death and dying. The following list describes the grief and mourning process that a person and family experience while adapting to a disabling condition:

- *Denial*. The individual/family is not prepared to accept the reality and ramifications of the disability and deny that it is occurring.
- *Awareness*. The individual/family realizes that the disability is real, the loss becomes real, and feelings of hostility, bitterness, and anger can arise in response to it.
- *Mourning*. The individual/family actively grieves for the loss that has occurred.
- *Depression*. The individual/family realizes the permanency, long-term nature, or other ramifications of the condition and experiences feelings of rejection, helplessness, altered self-esteem, and despair. This is often a very encompassing and time-consuming stage.

Some Information Resources for People Who Are Disabled

Accent on Living (AOL)
P.O. Box 700
Bloomington, Illinois 61702
(309) 378-2961
This organization has a computerized retrieval system containing information on products and devices and how-to information in areas such as eating, bathing, grooming, clothing, furniture, home management, toilet care, sexuality, mobility, and written and oral communication. For a nominal charge, a search is made on the requestor's topic. The *Buyer's Guide* is available from AOL and lists equipment and devices that assist people who are disabled in activities of daily living. The organization's *Accent on Living* quarterly magazine contains practical and inspiration articles as well as information on products, techniques, and money saving ideas for people who are disabled.

Access/Abilities
P.O. Box 458
Mill Valley, California 94942
(415) 388-3250
This organization is dedicated to linking people who are disabled to appropriate resources to enhance their quality of life and assist them in being independent. It has a database of information about accessible travel opportunities, aid and appliances, sports and recreation programs, clothing that really fits, shopping and other customized services, and social services. It offers consulting services concerning architectural barriers and accessibility, provides needs assessments and ideas for access solutions, and offers sensitivity and awareness training regarding disability issues.

Clearinghouse on Disability Information
U.S. Department of Education
Washington, D.C.
1-800-328-0272
This clearinghouse responds to inquiries on a wide range of topics including federal programs and legislation affecting the disabled community. The clearinghouse refers people to appropriate sources.

DIRECT LINK for the Disabled, Inc.
P.O. Box 1036
Solvang, California 93464
(805) 688-1603
The organization provides information and resources on disability related questions. Its mission is to improve the quality of health and human services information to meet the unique needs of people who are disabled and their families. The LINKUP database contains listings of over 11,000 organizations such as independent living centers, employment programs, support groups, device assessment centers, financial assistance programs, government offices, national organizations, community information centers, agencies offering direct services to disabled people and their families, information on technology, and resource notebooks on conditions such as head injury/coma, stroke, spinal cord injury, and neuromuscular disease.

Beach Center on Families and Disabilities
University of Kansas
Institute for Lifespan Studies
3111 Haworth Hall
Lawrence, Kansas 66045
(913) 864-7600
The center is sponsored by the National Institute on Disabilities and Rehabilitation Research (NIDRR). Its research focuses on individualizing services to families, enhancing family capabilities, providing advocacy services, and reducing family stress. For further information contact Beach Center on Families and Disabilities.

Variables Affecting Adaptation to a Disability

The stage of grief and mourning
Age at which the disabling condition occurred
Age-appropriateness of the disability
Rapidity of onset of the disability
Level of disability caused by the disabling condition
Visibility of the disability
Value of the disabled area
Attitudes regarding self
Attitudes of significant others
Community resources available and used
Coping mechanisms used
Prognosis and/or expected duration of the disability

- *Adaptation*. The individual/family becomes capable of coping with the disability. Although periods of depression may occur periodically, the goal of this stage is equilibrium and rehabilitation.

Related to the grieving process is the concept of chronic sorrow. *Chronic sorrow* is a term used to describe the long-term periodic sadness and depression the client and family experience in relation to chronic illness (Lindgren, Burke, Hainsworth, Eakes, 1992, p. 27). The critical attributes of chronic sorrow are given in the box on the following page. Chronic sorrow is a form of unresolved grieving. Although it is natural for some chronic sorrow to occur, the nurse should work with the client and family to help achieve grief resolution and promote successful coping and adaptation.

Critical Attributes of Chronic Sorrow

There is a perception of sorrow or sadness over time in a situation that has no predictable end.

The sadness or sorrow is cyclic or recurrent.

The sorrow or sadness is triggered either internally or externally and brings to mind the person's losses, disappointment or fears.

The sadness or sorrow is progressive and can intensify even years after the initial sense of disappointment, loss or fear.

From Lindgren CL, Burke ML, Hainsworth MA, Eakes GG: Chronic sorrow: a lifespan concept, *Scholar Inq Nurs Pract* 6(1):31, 1992. Used by permission of Springer Publishing Co., Inc., N.Y., 10013.

The *age* at which a disabling condition occurs and the age-appropriateness of the condition are also critical to adaptation. Disabling conditions that occur after the development of personal self-image frequently cause more difficulty with coping and adaptation. A child born without an arm will have a different adjustment process than the child who loses an arm at age 5 or the adult who loses an arm at age 50. The internalized body image of the adult makes it difficult to accept, much less incorporate, drastic alterations of body structure. An "age-appropriate" disability is often more easily accepted. For example, an elderly person with a hearing impairment or arthritis is often more readily accepted by others than a preschooler with the same condition.

The *rapidity of a condition's onset* is also critical to adjustment. A sudden alteration that affects personal functioning and self-image, as well as the image held by others, is difficult to absorb. If a condition develops gradually, as does rheumatoid arthritis, the adjustment time is lengthened and there is an opportunity to develop skills, resources, support systems, and coping mechanisms. If the occurrence is sudden, as with traumatic injury (e.g., spinal cord injury), there is little or no adjustment time. Sudden change is difficult to incorporate into one's body image. People need time to adapt, and treatment and rehabilitation techniques may need to be delayed until adaptation begins to take place.

The *level of disability* associated with a condition makes an impact on the adjustment the individual/family is able to make. Generally, the higher the level of disability, the more difficult it is to adjust. An individual with a paralyzed hand will likely have less difficulty in adjustment than a paraplegic or a person who is severely mentally retarded. The level of disability will be a major determinant of the functional capacity of the individual and the response of society to the disability.

The *visibility* of the condition affects the adjustment made to it. People generally have stronger reactions to visible conditions than to invisible signs and symptoms. Visible conditions will generally elicit more discriminating individual and societal responses than a nonvisible or slightly visible condition.

The *value of the disabled part* is of major importance. The personal and social value placed on body parts or functions significantly affect the type and degree of stigma attached to the disability. The value placed on body parts will vary from individual to individual and between societies; however, some parts seem to have a higher value than others. The example of facial disfigurement helps illustrate the value placed on specific body parts. Although facial disfigurement usually causes few functional limitations, it is one of the most difficult disabling conditions to adjust to because of the high value placed on facial characteristics. Conditions that create sexual disabilities are also difficult for most people to accept.

Attitudes regarding self and the *attitudes about oneself held by significant others* have an important effect on an individual's social and psychological adjustment to a disabling condition. The nurse can assist the person in building positive attitudes by looking at their strengths and enhancing their self-esteem. The box on the next page provides nursing activities that assist clients in increasing their judgment of self-worth.

Community resources play a key role in disability outcome, and adjustment is impeded if necessary services are not available and accessible. Nurses need to be familiar with community resources and know how to utilize the referral process (see Chapter 10).

Coping abilities of the individual and family are crucial, and how well the family is able to cope with the disabling condition will influence the client's recovery and adaptation (Reeber, 1992, p. 333). Using effective coping strategies can moderate the psychological impact of the condition (Miller, 1992, p. 19). Effective coping helps to reduce tension and maintain equilibrium, promote family growth, enhance sound decision making, maintain autonomy, avoid the use of negative self-evaluation, and control potential stressors before they become a problem (Miller, p. 21). Having a responsive health care delivery system and appropriate community resources aids the family in successful coping.

The *prognosis* of the condition is an important variable in adaptation. If the long-term prognosis does not show much hope of cure or recovery it can be discouraging, and even devastating, to the client and family. Conditions where the prognosis is more encouraging make it easier for the family to cope and adapt.

It is crucial for the community health nurse to identify variables that may hamper successful adaptation. Once such variables are identified the nurse can develop interventions to counteract their effect and facilitate adaptation.

NIC Nursing Intervention: Self-Esteem Enhancement

DEFINITION

Assisting a patient to increase his/her personal judgment of self-worth

ACTIVITIES

Monitor patient's statements of self-worth
Determine patient's locus of control
Determine patient's confidence in own judgment
Encourage patient to identify strengths
Encourage eye contact in communicating with others
Reinforce the personal strengths that patient identifies
Provide experiences that increase patient's autonomy, as appropriate
Assist patient to identify positive responses from others
Refrain from negatively criticizing
Refrain from teasing
Convey confidence in patient's ability to handle situation
Assist in setting realistic goals to achieve higher self-esteem
Assist patient to accept dependence on others, as appropriate
Assist patient to reexamine negative perceptions of self
Encourage increased responsibility for self, as appropriate
Assist patient to identify the impact of peer group on feelings of self-worth
Explore previous achievements of success
Explore reasons for self-criticism or guilt
Encourage the patient to evaluate own behavior
Encourage patient to accept new challenges
Reward or praise patient's progress toward reaching goals
Facilitate an environment and activities that will increase self-esteem
Assist patient to identify significance of culture, religion, race, gender, and age on self-esteem
Instruct parents on the importance of their interest and support in their children's development of a positive self-concept
Instruct parents to set clear expectations and to define limits with their children
Teach parents to recognize children's accomplishments
Monitor frequency of self-negating verbalizations
Monitor lack of follow-through in goal attainment
Monitor levels of self-esteem over time, as appropriate

From McCloskey JC, Bulechek GM, eds: *Nursing interventions classification (NIC)*, ed 2, St. Louis, 1996, Mosby, p. 492.

SOME AREAS OF CONCERN FOR PEOPLE WHO ARE DISABLED

Some areas of concern for people who are disabled are listed in the accompanying box, above right, and discussed here. Many of these concerns focus on improving the quality of life and allowing the person who is disabled to lead as normal a life as possible. The degree to which these concerns are evidenced is highly individual.

Some Areas of Concern for People Who Are Disabled

Education
Financial stability
Employment
Access to resources and services
Health care
Social, recreational, and athletic opportunities
Sexuality
Guardianship
Community residential opportunities
Attendant services
Respite care
Civil rights

Education

Historically, people who are disabled have been at an educational disadvantage in the United States. It was not until 1975 that the federal government enacted a law mandating a free, appropriate education for all children, regardless of their disabilities (see Chapter 16). Before 1975, if a person did not fit into existing local school district programs, the school district was not responsible for the person's education, and many persons who were disabled were denied an education unless their families could afford to send them to private schools. Today, local public school districts *must* provide a free education for all children with disabilities from ages 6 through 21, and other provisions of the law can enable services from birth through 21. However, once the age of 21 is reached, educational opportunities are limited. This can pose a special hardship for families, especially families with disabled members who may not be eligible for other training, higher education, or employment (e.g., people who are mentally disabled).

By law, when a person who is disabled applies for college entrance, job training, or adult basic education he or she must be considered on academic records and cannot be discriminated against because of the disability. Also, educational programs cannot limit the number of disabled students admitted and are required to accommodate the student who is disabled (e.g., provision of access, translators for the deaf).

Other resources to facilitate the educational endeavors of people who are disabled include homebound and computerized instruction, libraries, Braille and audiobooks for the visually impaired, closed caption educational programming for people who are hard of hearing, and modified classrooms for the physically impaired. The U.S. Department of Education recognizes the Distance Education and Training Council (1601 Eighteenth Street, N.W., Washington, D.C. 20009-2529) and its *Directory of Accredited Institutions* as a resource for locating quality schools of home study. Also, the National Library Service for the Blind and Physically Handicapped has a network of libraries throughout the United States that produce, distribute, and loan educational materials.

The federal government operates the National Library Service for the Blind and Physically Handicapped, and Gallaudet University (Washington, D.C.) is funded by the federal government to provide a college education for people who are deaf. The HEATH Resource Center, located in Washington, D.C., is the national clearinghouse for postsecondary education information for individuals with disabilities (Clearinghouse, 1993, p. 10).

Numerous resources exist in the private sector to facilitate educational endeavors of people who are disabled. Both Apple Computer and International Business Machines (IBM) offer special services for people who are disabled. Apple Computer established the *Disability Solutions Group* (Disability Solutions Group, 20525 Mariani Avenue, Cupertino, Ca. 95014) to help make computers more accessible to people with disabilities and to provide a database that describes adaptive devices, software programs, disability-related organizations, publications, and networks. IBM offers educational assistance to people with disability through the *Independence Special Needs Systems* (1000 N.W. 51st Street, Boca Raton, Fl. 33432, 1-800-426-4832). This center helps individuals learn how health technology and computers can enhance life at school, home, and work.

Education in the arts is often overlooked when planning care for people who are disabled. Organizations exist today to enable artistic expression for people who are disabled (see the accompanying box). Also, professional and public education about disabling conditions and disability prevention is needed. More education must be carried out by public health agencies, schools, and at home to instill in people the importance of healthful, disability preventing behaviors (Pope, Tarlov, 1991, p. 211).

Financial Stability

Financial stability is a major concern for people who are disabled. An adult who is disabled is financially responsible for himself or herself. Although many adults who are disabled are financially independent, some are unable to achieve this independence and must rely on assistance programs for financial support. Many families with a disabled member have financial problems as a result of the disabling condition.

Financial assistance programs for the adult who is disabled are offered through the state Department of Social Services (DSS) or the federal Social Security Administration (SSA) (see Chapter 4). Under the Social Security Administration the person who is disabled may be eligible for Social Security Disability Insurance benefits or Supplemental Security Income (SSI). Under DSS the person may be eligible for all forms of aid such as General Assistance, Temporary Assistance to Needy Families (TANF), and Medicaid. The individual may also receive private disability insurance benefits.

Disability and the Arts

Very Special Arts (VSA)
1331 F Street, NW
Suite 800
Washington, D.C. 20004
(202) 628-2800
VSA is an affiliate of the John F. Kennedy Center for the Performing Arts in Washington, D.C. It creates and supports learning opportunities through the arts for people with disabilities. It sponsors arts programs, awards, and festivals for people with physical and mental disabilities. VSA programs are implemented through an extensive network of state, local, and international organizations. A program of special interest to health care professionals is its *Arts for Children in Hospitals Program*. The Very Special Arts Gallery in Washington, D.C. showcases the work of artists with disabilities.

National Institute of Art and Disabilities (NIAD)
551 Twenty-Third Street
Richmond, California 94804
(510) 620-0290
The institute operates programs, provides professional training and consultation, and helps establish art centers and programs for children and adults with disabilities. It offers creative opportunities in painting, sculpture, and printing and promotes exhibitions of creative art of people with disabilities. Publications include *Freedom to Create, The Creative Spirit* and *Art and Disabilities, Disabled Artist at Work,* as well as a quarterly newsletter. It has served as a prototype for similar programs nationwide.

Kardon Institute of the Arts for People with Disabilities (KIA)
10700 Knights Road
Philadelphia, Pennsylvania 19154
(215) 637-2077
The mission of KIA is to make the joys and benefits of participation and education in the arts accessible to persons with disabilities. Its programs include instrumental and vocal instruction and music therapy. It provides information on establishing music programs for people who are disabled and has an extensive library collection on the topic of music for the disabled, including a collection of large print and braille music, textbooks, and supportive materials on all areas of teaching music to people who are disabled. It publishes *Guide to the Selection of Musical Instruments with Respect to Physical Ability and Disability,* the first reference book of its kind on the subject.

Employment

Whatever the employment setting, the skills and talents of persons with disabilities can be utilized, and the majority of industries across the country employ people with disabilities (President's Committee on Employment of People with Disabilities, 1996). However, many adults who are disabled remain unemployed or underemployed, despite their ability to

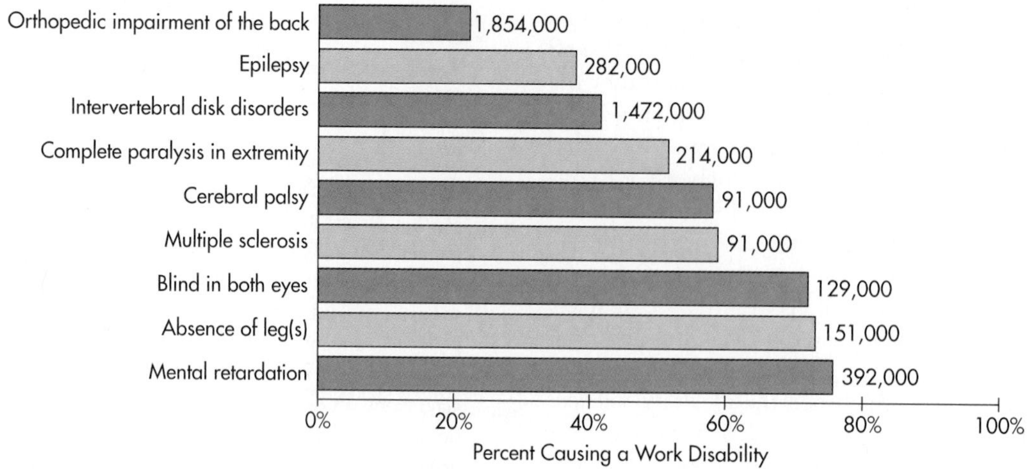

Figure **19-5** Chronic conditions with a high risk of causing a work disability among people age 18-69. *(From Kraus LE, Stoddard SL:* Chartbook on work disability in the United States, an InfoUse report, *Washington, D.C., 1991, National Institute on Disability and Rehabilitation Research, p. 55.)*

take part in meaningful work in the community (Employment, 1996, p. 4).

The President's Committee on Employment of the Handicapped was established by President Harry Truman in 1947 to facilitate employment of disabled war veterans and other handicapped Americans. That committee is now the President's Committee on Employment of People with Disabilities. The committee sponsors the Job Accommodation Network (JAN), which assists employers in accommodating the workplace to the disabled worker; has publications dealing with employment opportunities and issues; sponsors an annual conference where disability issues are addressed; and takes part in public education and affirmative action.

Many states have a Governor's Committee on Employment of People with Disabilities. Across the nation there are more than 2000 local branches of state Employment Service (ES) offices that are mandated by law to employ a specialist trained in working with people who are disabled to assist them in finding employment.

As a result of the Americans with Disabilities Act (ADA), employers are prohibited from discriminating against any qualified individual with a disability in terms of job hiring, training, compensation, and advancement and are required to make reasonable accommodations to hire workers who are disabled. Under ADA provisions employers cannot ask job applicants about the existence, nature, or severity of a disability; medical history; health insurance claims; or work absenteeism (Reno, 1993, p. A9). Employers who discriminate against the disabled face legal action, fines, and penalties.

Disabling conditions can limit a person's ability to work (Figures 19-5 and 19-6). Adults who are disabled are found in competitive, modified, and sheltered employment. *Competitive employment* is work with nondisabled members of the workforce on an equal basis, such as a job on the assembly line at an automotive factory. *Modified employment* is work done with nondisabled members of the workforce to meet the needs of the workers who are disabled. *Sheltered employment* (Figure 19-7) is work that is available specifically for people who are disabled and is done under direct supervision and guidance. Private organizations such as Associations for Retarded Citizens and Goodwill Industries sponsor such employment, and legislation provides for special preference being given in bidding on government contracts to workplaces offering sheltered employment.

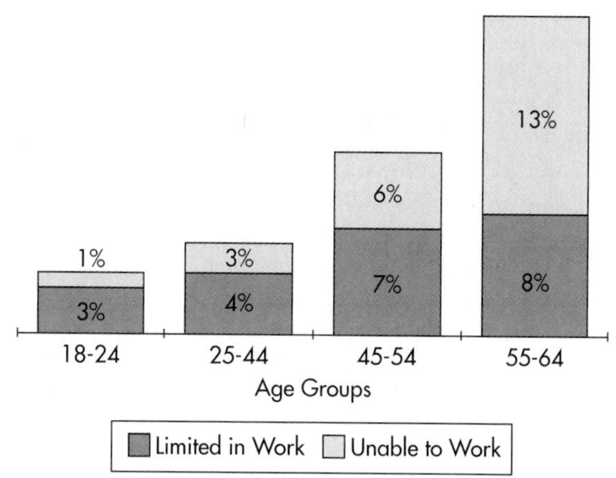

Figure **19-6** Percentage of adult population unable to or limited in work, by age. *(From Stucki BR:* Living in the community with a disability: demographic characteristics of the population with disabilities under age 65, *Washington, D.C., 1995, American Association of Retired Persons, p. 55.)*

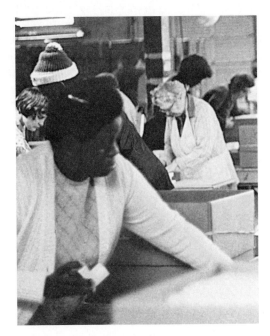

Figure **19-7** The majority of adults who are disabled can achieve skills that permit them to be gainfully employed. Sheltered workshops provide job training and placement services that enhance an individual's ability to function in competitive as well as noncompetitive work environments. *(Courtesy Sunshine Industries, a nonprofit voluntary agency, sponsored by the Association of Retarded Citizens, Knox County, Tennessee, and Mary Louise Peacock, photographer.)*

Persons who are disabled have proven to be loyal, trustworthy, capable, dependable employees who are willing to work, have good job performance, and reliable attendance records. Our country's work ethic makes employment a central part of life. It is a societal expectation that people will work and be self-sufficient. Work has a great deal to do with how people identify themselves, as well as how they are identified by others. Employment offers the possibility of improving an individual's and family's quality of life and increasing self-esteem.

Access to Resources and Services

A major barrier to employment and other life activities for the person who is disabled is limited access to community services, resources, and employment. Access has both transportation and physical accessibility components.

Accessible transportation is critical to maintaining independence and self-sufficiency. Many persons who are disabled are unable to drive, and the United States does not generally have good public transportation. Provisions of the Americans with Disabilities Act provided for increased accessibility to public transportation.

In the United States a shortage of available and reliable public transportation prevents persons who are disabled from taking part in employment and many other activities and necessitates heavy reliance on friends, relatives, Dial-A-Rides, and other voluntary transportation services. Medicaid may provide transportation to medical appointments. To assist the person who is disabled in independent driving, the American Automobile Association (AAA) publishes *The Handicapped Driver's Mobility Guide*. Other countries have made much greater strides in meeting transportation needs of disabled persons than has the United States. By the 1980s Sweden had all public vehicles made accessible to people who are disabled, France had a rail system that has specially equipped cars for people who are disabled, Japan had a totally accessible rail system, and Great Britain required that all taxis be accessible (Dietl, 1983). The United States has still not reached the level of accessibility experienced by other countries almost two decades ago.

Accommodations such as ramps, elevators, wide aisles, and doorways assist persons who are disabled in gaining access to buildings. The Americans with Disabilities Act has helped to ensure physical access to buildings. Under the law workplaces are required to make reasonable accommodations to accommodate workers who are disabled. Such accommodations are rarely expensive. Data collected by the President's Committee on Employment of People with Disabilities showed that 18% of employers reported that making such accommodations cost them nothing, 50% said the cost was $500 or less, and only 5% reported costs greater than $5000 (Reasonable accommodation, 1995, p. 6). Overall, companies have an average return of $28.69 in benefits for every dollar invested in making an accommodation (President's Committee on Employment of People with Disabilities, 1996) and the accommodations usually qualify for employer tax credits.

Health Care

Americans with disabilities, one sixth of the U.S. population, account for almost half of medical spending (Max, Rice, Trupin, 1996, p. 1). Almost 45% of this medical spending is for hospital care (Max, Rice, Trupin, p. 1). Adults who are unable to perform their major activity (paid work or keeping house) contact their physicians five times more each year than people who are able to perform their major activity (20 physician contacts versus 4) (LaPlante, Rice, Wenger, 1995, p. 1).

ACCESS TO CARE Americans with disabilities often have difficulty gaining access to health care. They may not be able to afford regular medical care; doctors may refuse to take Medicaid or Medicare; transportation to health care is often difficult to arrange; facilities may not be accessible; and assistive devices are often too expensive or not available. Shopping for health care supplies can be difficult for the person who is disabled. Sears has a shop-at-home *Home Health Care Catalog* (1-800-326-1750), J.C. Penney has a shop-at-home *For Your Special Needs: Home Health Care and Easy Dressing Fashions* catalog (1-800-222-6161) and *Maxi* is a catalog of aids and appliances for independent living (1-800-522-6294).

ATTITUDES OF HEALTH CARE PROFESSIONALS Persons who are disabled report that they often do not use health care services because of professionals who are insensitive and unaware of the special needs imposed by a disability (deBalcazar, Bradford, Fawcett, 1988, p. 32). They also report that health care professionals sometimes do not seem knowledgeable about their conditions and are disinterested in them. During health care procedures personal dignity and privacy need to be taken into consideration, and special positioning and comfort measures may be necessary.

HEALTH INSURANCE Other industrialized nations have national health programs where people have health insurance regardless of whether they have a disabling condition. Americans with disabilities often have a difficult time obtaining private health insurance because their condition preceded their insurance application, a "preexisting" condition; because they are considered high risk; or because they cannot afford insurance. Some persons with disabilities are eligible for Medicaid and Medicare. Whatever the form of health insurance, it is often inadequate to meet their special health needs (e.g., assistive devices, physical and occupational therapy, and prescriptions).

Social, Recreational, and Athletic Opportunities

Few social, recreational, and athletic programs are designed for persons who are disabled, and they may have difficulty accessing such programs in the community. A problem with many people who are disabled is that of social isolation.

Some adults who are disabled, especially those who are mentally retarded, find great enjoyment in participating in social and recreational activities planned especially for them (e.g., parties, camp, athletic activities). Others, such as the unstable diabetic, may readily integrate into existing community activities. Whatever the level of disability, people should have social and recreational opportunities available to them.

Activities such as the Special Olympics and the Paralympics provide opportunities for athletes who are disabled to participate in sporting events. The Paralympic games draw elite athletes from all over the world and immediately follow the Olympic games. Disabled Sports USA is an organization that works to ensure that persons of all ages with physical disabilities have access to sports, recreation, and physical education programs. With almost 100 local chapters nationwide, the organization offers year-round sports programs and can be reached at 451 Hungerford Drive, Suite 100, Rockville, Md. 20850 (301-217-0960).

The Itinerary, a magazine for travelers with disabilities, specializes in helping people who are disabled know about "accessible" vacations. To make national parks more accessible, the National Park Service has travel guides for people who are disabled. Mobility International USA and the Society for the Advancement of Travel for the Handicapped (SATH) represent the interests of disabled travelers, provide information on travel for the disabled throughout the world, offer travel tips, and have listings of travel agents who are experienced in dealing with people who are disabled. Mobility International USA can be reached at P.O. Box 10767 Eugene, Or. 97403 (541-343-1284), and SATH can be reached at 347 Fifth Avenue, Suite 610, New York, N.Y. 10016 (212-447-SATH).

Sexuality

Persons who are disabled are just as interested in romance, and sex, as nondisabled people (Duffy, 1996, p. R1). Unfortunately, health care professionals sometimes ignore or have difficulty dealing with the sexual aspects of disability (Greco, 1996, p. 594). Adding to this, many misconceptions surround the sexuality of people who are disabled, and they are often treated as if they were asexual. Yvonne Duffy, an author who is disabled, writes:

> Of all the nuances of acceptance that people with disabilities seek, the opportunity to be considered worthy of love—as spouses and lovers—has remained the most elusive. We have discovered that though we may be considered fine neighbors, co-workers or even friends, the line is often drawn when it comes to intimate relationships. (Duffy, 1996, p. R1)

Duffy goes on to state that as a teenager:

> I felt uncomfortable at the few social functions to which I was invited . . . Occasionally, a young man approached me to inquire about the state of my health—as though having a disability meant that I was sick. Conversation seldom progressed beyond that point . . . Times are changing though. As an adult, I have known men who looked beyond my disability to find the real me.

Health care professionals need to look closely at their own attitudes about sexuality and not let their attitudes deny, limit, or inhibit the person from sexual expression and fulfillment.

The Council on Sexuality and Disability provides extensive information and counseling on sexuality and disability (122 E. 23rd Street, New York, N.Y. 10010). The Sexuality Information and Education Council of the United States (SIECUS) advocates that persons with disabilities receive sexuality education, sexual health care, and opportunities for socializing and sexual expression, and that health care professionals work with people who are disabled and their families to help them understand and support the sexual development and expression of people who are disabled (SIECUS, 1996, p. 22).

SIECUS recommends that social and health care agencies develop policies and procedures to ensure the protection of the sexual rights of people who are disabled. SIECUS (1995) regularly publishes an annotated bibliography on sexuality and disability. The SIECUS journal *Sexuality and Disability* offers the health care professional insightful readings.

Alterations in sexual function can accompany disabling conditions. Physiologic alterations in sexual function can occur in relation to impaired physical mobility, increased or decreased sensation, pain, bowel and/or bladder incontinence, fatigue, genital sexual dysfunction, endocrine dysfunction, and the effects of medications (Greco, 1996, pp. 605-606).

Psychosocial alterations in sexual function can occur as a result of social isolation, impaired self-concept, partner issues, and cognitive and behavioral alterations (Greco, 1996, pp. 607-608).

A sexual history should be part of the nurse's assessment. When the client is asked questions concerning sexuality the nurse "leaves the door open for any questions or discussion by the client" (Greco, 1996, p. 596). The sexual implications of the client's disability should routinely be addressed. The box below gives a sexual history format that can be helpful to the nurse in obtaining assessment information from clients who are disabled. Nursing interventions include education and counseling for the client and partner, compensation strategies, and making the client aware of available resources (Greco, p. 611).

Being disabled does not change a person's need for intimacy. Achievement of intimacy with a partner can lead to increased self-esteem and fulfillment. If sexual dysfunction

Sexual History Form

Name ______________________ Age ____
Marital/partnership status (includes quality, duration)
____
Occupation ____________ Highest education ______
Religion ____________ Interests/hobbies ______
____

MEDICAL HISTORY

Psychological/psychiatric problems ____________
Behavioral/emotional problems ____________
Renal insufficiency ____________
Diabetes ____________
Neurologic conditions ____________
Hereditary disorders ____________
Hypertension ____________
Endocrine disorders ____________
Sexually transmitted diseases ____________

CURRENT MEDICATIONS

Antihypertensives ____________
Antipsychotics ____________
Antihistamines ____________
Alcohol ____________
Analgesics ____________
Narcotics ____________
Recreational drugs ____________

PREMORBID SEXUAL FUNCTION

Description of sexual activities preferred ____________
Frequency of sexual activity ____________
Partner who generally initiates sexual activity ____________
Sexual preferences of the client ____________

SPECIFIC CONCERNS OF THE COUPLE

Fertility ____________
Birth control ____________
Importance of sex in the relationship ____________

Physical issues that impact sexual function ____________
Transfers ____________
Ability to dress/undress ____________
Hemiplegia/hemiparesis ____________
Paraplegia/quadriplegia ____________
Range-of-motion limitations ____________
Hypertonicity ____________
Hypotonicity ____________
Endurance ____________
Balance ____________
Presence of sensation versus being hypersensitive ____________
Presence of pain and location ____________
Presence of bowel and/or bladder incontinence ____________
Presence of genitourinary or gastrointestinal collection devices and their position
____
Difficulty with vision, hearing, oral motor control
____
General and genital hygiene and cleanliness ____________

SEXUAL RESPONSE ISSUES

Female
- Menstrual history ____________
- Sexual interest ____________
- Frequency of sexual interaction ____________
- Vaginal lubrication ____________
- Sensation present ____________
- Orgasmic capacity ____________
- Fertility ____________

Male
- Sexual interest ____________
- Presence of morning erections ____________
- Presence of erections with manual stimulation ____________
- Process for ejaculation ____________
- Sensation present ____________
- Type of ejaculation and volume ____________
- Fertility ____________

From Greco SB: Sexuality and education counseling. In Hoeman SP: *Rehabilitation nursing: process and application*, ed 2, St. Louis, 1996, Mosby, p. 609.

exists, the person can be helped to find avenues of sexual expression and fulfillment. Unfortunately, the lack of counseling resources and the reluctance of professionals to deal with the topic of sexuality can leave the client with unanswered questions and little assistance in working out problems and concerns.

Guardianship

Most persons who are disabled do not need guardians and are able to go through their entire lives making their own decisions. This is especially true of people who are physically disabled. However, guardianship is often considered for individuals who are severely disabled, especially those who are mentally ill or mentally retarded.

Guardianship can be either plenary (complete) or partial. Partial guardianship implies that the person is able to carry out some functions independently but needs assistance in carrying out other functions. If no guardian is appointed the person is responsible for making his or her own decisions—including decisions regarding health care.

Parents are "natural" guardians of their own minor children and can make legal decisions for them. Parents are *not* natural guardians of their adult offspring, even if they are disabled, and cannot make legal decisions for them without having guardianship. Once the age of majority is reached, a person is legally responsible for himself or herself unless a legal guardian has been appointed by the court. Many parents are unaware of this fact, and anticipatory guidance about guardianship needs is helpful.

Handling guardianship issues can be difficult for families. Families frequently experience a crisis when they realize that their adult offspring are not able to take care of their own decision making at the age of maturity. At this point parents may have to accept the reality that their offspring may never develop the skills to function independently, and feelings of sadness and hopelessness are not uncommon. Helping families identify the strengths their adult offspring have, the potential they have for benefitting from experiences that are developmentally within their reach, and linking them with appropriate resources can reduce parents' anxiety and increase their ability to plan for the future.

In some families siblings, relatives, or friends may be asked to assume guardianship responsibility for an adult who is disabled. In some situations this is a feasible solution and in others it is not. At times community health nurses have found that families assume that adults who are disabled are unable to care for themselves just because they are disabled. It is important to remember that not all adults who are disabled need guardians. In fact, most of them do not. The nurse can assist the family in looking at guardianship options and determining what is best for everyone involved.

Community Residential Opportunities

It is the right of people who are disabled to live their lives as normally and independently as possible in the mainstream of the community. Many people who are disabled do not require any specialized form of housing and live independently in the community.

Historically, people who were disabled, especially people who were mentally impaired, were placed in state residential facilities. For example, in the 1950s hundreds of thousands of people resided in psychiatric mental hospitals in the United States (Shadish, Lurigio, Lewis, 1989, p. 2). During the last 35 years more than 100 such residential institutions have closed (Hayden, Abery, 1994). Conversely, the number of people with disabilities living in community settings has increased by almost 200,000 in the last 15 years (Giordano, D'Alonzo, 1995, p. 15), and the numbers continue to increase. States and local communities are developing innovative ways to assist people who are disabled to live in the mainstream of community life.

In 1972 the nation's first independent living center was established in Berkeley, California (Smith, Smith, Richards et al, 1994, p. 14). The nation's independent living centers help people to live independently by providing services such as wheelchair repair, training of attendants, and referrals for employment and housing (Robert Wood Johnson Foundation, 1992, p. 76). A publication, *Independent Living*, assists people who are handicapped with independent living needs and is available through Equal Opportunity Publications, 150 Motor Parkway, Suite 400, Greenlawn, N.Y. 11740.

Table 19-2 presents some of the community residential alternatives for people who are disabled. Today voluntary agencies and state and local governments have increased funding for such alternative, community-based facilities (Giordano, D'Alonzo, 1994, p. 3). Unfortunately, at the same time federally subsidized housing for people who are disabled has decreased (Aronson, 1996). Community living arrangements should meet the needs of the individual. When selecting a residential placement, objectives for the individual should be established and the placement carefully evaluated.

ADAPTING THE LIVING ENVIRONMENT For some persons who are disabled, especially those with mobility limitations or those who are wheelchair bound, independent living means that housing needs be accessible. Persons with disabilities who need to adapt their homes may be eligible for home improvement loans insured by the Department of Housing and Urban Development (HUD). The HUD-insured loan can be used to remove architectural barriers or hazards in the home and make home adaptations. They may also be eligible for rental assistance through HUD. The box on page 588 lists some resources for accessible housing.

table 19-2 Residential Alternatives for Persons with Disabilities

Residential Model	Characteristics
Public residential facilities	Institutionalized facilities with trained staff and full-time supervision for residents. Residents are segregated from the community.
Sheltered villages	Institutionalized facilities with trained staff and full-time supervision for residents. Privately supported, the facilities are often located in rural areas where the residents are segregated from the community.
Public community facilities	Institutionalized facilities with trained staff and full-time supervision for residents. (These residences are also referred to as *Intermediate Care Facilities.*) Residents are segregated from the community for some activities but integrated for other activities.
Public group homes	Government operated homes that are shared by groups of persons and supervised by a staff which may be part time. Residents may be segregated from the community for some activities but integrated for other activities.
Private group homes	Privately operated homes that otherwise have the same characteristics as *public group homes.*
Cooperatively owned group homes	Homes that are owned jointly by residents and for which full-time or part-time staff may be employed. Residents may be segregated from the community for some activities but integrated for other activities.
Foster care	Persons with disabilities live in the home and under the supervision of a caregiver. The caregiver may be paid a stipend for these services. The degree to which residents are integrated can vary according to the attitudes of caregivers.
Publicly managed supervised apartments	Government operated apartments that are leased to individuals. Persons are supervised or assisted by an apartment manager who may be part time. Residents may be segregated from the community for some activities but integrated for other activities.
Privately managed, supervised apartments	Privately managed apartments that have the same characteristics as *publicly managed, supervised apartments.*
Cooperatively owned, supervised apartments	Cooperatively owned apartments or condominiums that are leased to individuals. Otherwise, this type of residence has the same characteristics as *publicly or privately owned supervised apartments.*
Independent living	A wide range of residential options that could include renting or purchasing a residence in ways similar to those by which residences are selected and maintained by persons without disabilities. Persons with disabilities would have unrestricted access to community activities and could request assistance from agency personnel as appropriate.

From Giordano G, D'Alonzo BJ: The link between transition and independent living, *Am Rehabil* 20(1):2-7, 1994, p. 4.

FUNDING AND MONITORING The funding and monitoring of residential placements will vary from state to state. People looking for specific placements can check with local departments of human or social services, departments of mental health, HUD, or specialty agencies dealing with the conditions involved. Some examples of such agencies are the local Association for Retarded Citizens, the National Association for Multiple Sclerosis, and associations for the blind. These agencies are often aware of community placement opportunities and can refer people to appropriate resources.

ZONING AND BUILDING REGULATIONS In many areas restrictive zoning regulations do not allow group homes for persons who are disabled. Restrictive zoning policies have led to the clustering of community residential facilities for persons who are disabled (often persons who are mentally ill or mentally retarded) in areas where zoning regulations were not restrictive; these are often less desirable residential areas. Some communities have gone to court to prevent, remove, or restrict residences for the disabled.

The effective community health nurse educates the community and its leaders regarding the residential needs of a person who is disabled. Actively participating on community advisory boards that facilitate community residential programs provides opportunities to work with community leaders, educate the public, and establish new and innovative community residential opportunities.

Attendant Services

The person who is disabled may not be able to carry out all the activities of daily living. When this happens the person can benefit from attendant services. The attendant assists the person in such activities as maintaining personal appearance and hygiene (e.g., feeding, dressing, grooming), mobility, household maintenance, safety, companionship, and resource utilization.

Unfortunately, no comprehensive, uniform system for providing such services exists, and services vary greatly from state to state. Many persons who need attendant services are unable to obtain them, often because of the cost involved. These services are sometimes funded through

Some Resources for Accessible Housing

Accessible housing is essential if persons with disabilities are to be able to live independently in the community. Builders and contractors are often unaware of modifications or regulations involving handicap accessibility, and individuals are often not aware of how to adapt housing to meet their needs. Some resources for accessible housing are:

Center for Universal Design
North Carolina State University
Box 8613
Raleigh, North Carolina, 27695-8613
1-800-647-6777, (919) 515-3082
The nation's first research and training center focused on making housing accessible and available to people with handicaps is funded by the National Institute on Disability and Rehabilitation Research (NIDRR) of the U.S. Department of Education. The center offers design solutions (including floor plan designs), training, information, referral, and technical assistance to improve the quality and availability of residential environments for people with disabilities.

Adaptive Environments Center
374 Congress Street Suite 301
Boston, Massachusetts 02110
(617) 695-1225
Offers consultation, workshops, courses, conferences, and resource materials on accessible and adaptive design. Its goal is to eliminate barriers that limit education, employment, recreational, and cultural life to people who have disabilities and to create environments that are universally accessible to all. It has developed numerous programs and publications, including *A Consumer's Guide to Home Adaptation* and *Teaching Strategies for Universal Design*. It offers a technical assistance hotline in relation to compliance with the Americans with Disabilities Act (ADA) and ADA technical assistance programs (1-800-893-1225).

National Handicap Housing Institute
1050 Thorndale Avenue
New Brighton, Minnesota 55112
(612) 639-9799
Provides services related to the development of barrier-free housing, specializes in housing, and assists architects, builders, and owners with many of the problems in creating accessible new buildings and adapting and retrofitting older structures. Provides information on various housing assistance programs for which persons with disabilities may be eligible, as well as design and product information.

Medicaid, Department of Social Services (Social Services Block Grant Title XX), Older Americans Act provisions, Veterans Administration, and various state and locally funded programs. If attendant services are not available some people who are disabled may not be able to live independently, and without these services persons who are disabled may be needlessly placed in nursing homes and other institutional settings (Kafka, 1993, p. 14). The community health nurse can be instrumental in helping to link clients with such services.

Respite Care

It is unfair to expect the caretakers of persons who are disabled to provide 24-hour-a-day care and to assume all the burden for this care. However, this frequently happens, and caretakers experience burnout.

Respite care is one solution to the problem of caretaker overload. It is short-term, 24-hour-a-day care, including, but not limited to, the following settings: nursing homes, clients' homes, private homes, foster care, group homes, hospitals, and institutions. Respite care provides temporary relief for the caretaker and may prevent institutionalization. It is also successful in decreasing stress, increasing coping ability, and improving the quality of life for both caretakers and persons who are disabled. A caretaker may request respite care for personal reasons such as illness, vacation, or mental health. Whatever the reason, it is legitimate for the caretaker to request time away.

Most people are unfamiliar with the concept of respite care, and in the United States it is difficult to obtain. As with attendant services, when it exists privately, the costs are often prohibitive. Some families and organizations have developed respite co-op groups where they exchange periods of time in caring for their respective disabled family members. The Omnibus Budget Reconciliation Act of 1981 allowed Medicaid waivers for reimbursement of respite care if the cost is the same or less than institutional care, realizing that it can be more economical to finance respite care services than it is to provide institutional care or long-term care.

When nurses assist a client in looking for respite care, agencies that deal with the specific condition(s) involved should be contacted, along with the local department of social services. The community health nurse can be instrumental in advocating for respite care services for clients and in making this very important need known to the community. If only from a cost-effectiveness standpoint, the community should be interested.

Civil Rights

The Americans with Disabilities Act has sometimes been referred to as the Civil Rights Act for People with Disabilities. This law and others legally guarantee the civil rights of people who are disabled. Before this law the civil rights of people who were disabled were often in peril.

It is the responsibility of the Office for Civil Rights in the U.S. Department of Education and the Office for Civil Rights in the U.S. Department of Health and Human Services to enforce federal laws prohibiting discrimination against persons who are disabled in federally assisted programs or activities and to investigate discrimination complaints brought by individuals under these statutes. Many states have protection and advocacy agencies to help ensure that the civil rights of people who are disabled are upheld.

SOME RESOURCES FOR PEOPLE WHO ARE DISABLED

The federal, state, and local governments offer many services to persons who are disabled. Federal resources remain rather constant across the nation, but state and local resources can vary greatly. Federal programs are enabled largely through legislation that will be discussed later in this chapter. The IOM (Pope, Tarlov, 1991, p. 195) has recommended that collaborative projects involving primary care providers, public health agencies, voluntary associations, and the community should be developed to coordinate disability prevention programs that implement interventions centered on individual needs with a goal of improving an individual's physical, mental, and social well-being over the life course. On an international level the World Health Organization, World Institute on Disability, and Rehabilitation International (a federation of national, regional, and international organizations and agencies working together to prevent disability) address issues related to health and disability.

Federal Government Resources

On the federal level many different departments offer services to persons who are disabled. The U.S. Department of Education and the Department of Health and Human Services offer numerous services.

U.S. DEPARTMENT OF EDUCATION The department is involved in information, education, and advocacy programs for people with disabilities. It oversees compliance with federal legislation for the education of children with disabilities and houses the Office of Special Education Programs and the National Institute on Disability and Rehabilitation Research (NIDRR). The Office of Special Education Programs under the Rehabilitation Services Administration publishes the quarterly periodical *American Rehabilitation*. NIDRR contributes to the independence of people with disabilities and sponsors Rehabilitation Research and Training Centers (RRTCs), Rehabilitation Engineering Centers (RECs), and research and demonstration projects, research training, and career development grants (Seelman, Levesque, 1995, pp. 32-33). NIDRR also gathers disability data and publishes a series, *Disability Statistics Abstract*, that highlights information on disabling conditions.

The National Rehabilitation Information Center (NARIC) (1-800-34-NARIC) describes itself as serving the nation's disabled community and providing "information for independence" (NARIC, 1996). It was established in 1977 and is funded by NIDRR to collect and disseminate disability information, including the results of federally funded research projects. NARIC publishes a directory of national disability information resources, a guide to disability and rehabilitation periodicals, resource guides, and fact sheets on rehabilitation topics. NARIC's computerized databases include REHABDATA, ABLEDATA, and ABLE INFORM (ABLE INFORM, 1995, p. 1). REHABDATA (1-800-346-2742) contains bibliographical information on the NARIC library; ABLEDATA (1-800-227-0216) provides information about commercial rehabilitation products; and ABLE INFORM (301-589-3563) is an electronic bulletin board of assistive technology, disability, and rehabilitation information. ABLEDATA has become one of the most important national sources of information on assistive technology and the manufacturers of products for persons with disabilities (Seelman, Levesque, 1995, p. 35).

U.S. DEPARTMENT OF HEALTH AND HUMAN SERVICES The department provides services to persons who are disabled, including grants to states for maternal and child health. The Medicaid and Medicare programs administered by the department provide funding for numerous health care services used by people with disabilities. The department's Centers for Disease Control and Prevention (CDC) works to prevent chronic disabling conditions among Americans and collects national statistics on disabling conditions. As previously mentioned, *Healthy People 2000*, a publication of the department, has national objectives for limiting the prevalence of chronic disabling conditions.

NATIONAL COUNCIL ON DISABILITY The council is presidentially appointed and has made prevention of disability one of its highest priorities. It works closely with the Office of Disease Prevention and Health Promotion in the CDC and its efforts include promoting the development of a national disabilities prevention plan.

NATIONAL INFORMATION CENTER FOR CHILDREN AND YOUTH WITH DISABILITIES The center provides information services and lists of resources to aid parents in accessing services. Resource sheets with names and addresses of state agencies are available by writing the center at P.O. Box 1492, Washington, D.C. 20013-1492 or calling 1-800-695-0285.

State Government Resources

Numerous offices and departments on the state level offer services to people who are disabled. Programs are administered by each state and will vary from one state to another. The nurse is encouraged to explore the organization and provision of services in the state in which she or he is practicing.

STATE DEPARTMENTS OF EDUCATION These departments are responsible for special education and related services in their state for preschool-, elementary-, and secondary-age children; they provide consultation, information services, and funding for such programs. They also answer individual questions about special education and related services and may have manuals explaining the services.

STATE VOCATIONAL REHABILITATION AGENCY These agencies provide medical, therapeutic, counseling, education, training, and other services needed to prepare people with disabilities for work. They can provide individuals with the address of the nearest rehabilitation office and refer them to the states' various community living programs—including independent living.

STATE HEALTH AUTHORITY (SHA) SHAs often fund and administer children's special health care services (CSHCS) programs. Previously these state programs were often referred to as "Crippled Children's Services." The services are primarily funded through federal grants to states to provide health care services to children who are disabled or who have chronic health problems. Services usually provided include payment for direct care, counseling, genetic disease testing, training and education for health care professionals and caregivers, and research funding. SHAs and local health departments work collaboratively to provide these services to families. The National Center for Maternal and Child Health compiles information on state programs receiving these federal funds.

OFFICE OF STATE COORDINATOR OF VOCATIONAL EDUCATION FOR STUDENTS WITH DISABILITIES States that are receiving federal funds for vocational education must ensure that funding is used in programs that include students with disabilities (Parent guide, 1996). These offices help to link students with current programs.

STATE MENTAL RETARDATION/DEVELOPMENTAL DISABILITIES AGENCIES Such agencies plan, administer, and develop standards for mental retardation/developmental disabilities programs provided in state-operated facilities and state-funded community-based programs (Parent guide, 1996). They provide information on programs and program eligibility.

STATE MENTAL HEALTH AGENCIES These agencies often finance and administer community mental health centers and state residential facilities for people who are mentally ill and mentally retarded. They develop standards for state and local mental health programs and provide information on community and residential treatment programs and placement options (Parent guide, 1996). They may compile community resource lists.

STATE PROTECTION AND ADVOCACY AGENCIES Protection and advocacy agencies are responsible for pursuing legal, administrative, and other remedies to protect the rights of persons who are developmentally disabled or mentally ill (Parent guide, 1996). As advocates they protect and guard the individual's human and civil rights. They usually compile resource lists about housing, health, social, and recreation programs; support groups; and social services available in local communities. They are an excellent source of information and referral on all aspects of disabling conditions.

UNIVERSITY-AFFILIATED PROGRAMS State universities may have institutes that study disabling conditions (e.g., Institute for the Study of Mental Retardation and Related Disabilities) and frequently provide education and training for health, education, and social service professionals in working with people who are disabled. They may also provide direct services to people with disabilities through specially designated programs and institutes. Information and listings of university-affiliated programs can be obtained by contacting the American Association of University Affiliated Programs for Persons with Developmental Disabilities at 8630 Felton Street, Suite 410, Silver Spring, Md. 20910 (301-588-8252).

Legislation and the Person Who Is Disabled

- Developmental Disabilities Act (1971)
- Rehabilitation Act of 1973
- Developmental Disabilities and Bill of Rights Act (1975, 1984)
- Education for All Handicapped Children Act (1975)
- Mental Health Systems Act (1980)
- Civil Rights of Institutionalized Persons Act (1980)
- Protection and Advocacy for Mentally Ill Individuals Act (1986, 1988)
- Americans with Disabilities Act (1990)
- Individuals with Disabilities Education Act (1990)

Local Resources

Local school districts, health departments, and practitioners in private practice offer numerous services to persons who are disabled. Many of the state services previously described are provided on a local level. Private, voluntary agencies such as the American Cancer Society, American Lung Association, American Heart Association, Associations for Retarded Citizens, American Cerebral Palsy Association, and Handicapped Veterans program provide services directly to American communities. The organization of these resources has been discussed in Chapter 5, and locating and utilizing resources has been presented in Chapter 10.

LEGISLATION

An overview of federal legislation and voluntary efforts that facilitate service provisions for persons with disabilities is presented in Appendix 19-1. Several major pieces of legislation have provided the mechanisms for meeting many needs of persons who are disabled and are given in the box above.

Today many people consider the most significant piece of legislation for Americans who are disabled to be the Americans with Disabilities Act of 1990 (Public Law 101-336). This act helps to ensure the civil rights of persons who are disabled; empower them; and offer them opportunities, promise, and dignity. The act is designed to provide a clear mandate to end discrimination against individuals with disabilities and deals with issues such as housing, employment, public transportation, and communication services. As a result of this legislation, all across America access to transportation, buildings, and recreational areas has been enhanced; interpreters are being provided; workplaces are accommodating people who are disabled; and people are becoming more sensitive to the needs of the disabled community and are helping to make a difference in the lives of persons who are disabled. The act calls on everyone to remove barriers to access (Reno, 1993). According to Attorney General Janet Reno, this law is helping to break down not only physical barriers but also social barriers, and has helped people with and without disabilities work together to eliminate the barriers that have kept people who are disabled from being treated equally.

The nurse needs to be knowledgeable about legislation that affects persons who are handicapped and to advocate for necessary legislation. The nurse needs to be able to assist clients in knowing their rights under the law and how to proceed when these rights are violated.

REHABILITATION

Rehabilitation activities are an important part of the treatment plan for many persons who are disabled. Rehabilitation is the process of restoring an individual to the fullest physical, mental, social, vocational, and economic usefulness possible. Major goals of rehabilitation are to integrate the individual into society and provide as normal a life as possible. Rehabilitation is often a long-term process demanding a high level of commitment. Some predicted developments in rehabilitation during the next 25 years are given in the box, above right.

Predicted Developments in Rehabilitation During the Next 25 Years

1. Community-based rehabilitation services will increase.
2. Supported employment programs will increase.
3. Individuals with disabilities will assume greater control of the programs that affect them.
4. Models of culturally sensitive rehabilitation counseling will emerge.
5. Private-sector businesses will become increasingly involved in rehabilitation.
6. Tolerance and acceptance of disabilities will expand among persons without disabilities.
7. Rehabilitation technology will have an increased impact on persons with disabilities.
8. Services for older persons with disabilities will expand.
9. Programs built on partnerships between agencies, communities, and businesses will expand.
10. Life span approaches will permeate rehabilitation.
11. Rehabilitation services will become less agency focused and more client centered.
12. Models for developing rehabilitation personnel through nontraditional programs will emerge.
13. Services for persons with severe disabilities will expand.
14. Independent living opportunities will broaden for persons with disabilities.
15. Federal and state regulations, and the implementation of those regulations, will be directed increasingly to local levels.

From Giordano G, D'Alonzo BJ: Challenge and progress in rehabilitation: a review of the past 25 years and a preview of the future, *Am Rehab* 21(3):14-21, 1995, p. 18.

Individuals, their families, and significant others are essential members of the interdisciplinary rehabilitation team (Association of Rehabilitation Nurses [ARN], 1994a, p. 2). Comprehensive rehabilitation programs combine medical treatment with such things as home health nursing services, social services, psychological services, and physical, occupational, and speech therapy. A key component of many rehabilitation programs is vocational rehabilitation.

VOCATIONAL REHABILITATION A major goal of vocational rehabilitation is to have a client in an appropriate, satisfying job with a stable employer. Vocational rehabilitation efforts involve assessment of the client's work potential, vocational education, and training; obtaining the assistive devices necessary for employment; vocational counseling and employment placement; evaluation; and follow-up. Lengthy unemployment can be devastating, and it is important to return people to work as soon as possible (Breese, Mikrut, 1995, p. 39).

Many vocational rehabilitation services are provided under the Rehabilitation Act of 1973 as amended (see the box on the next page) through its vocational rehabilitation programs. To qualify for these programs a person must be at least 16 years old, have a physical or mental disability that constitutes an employment handicap, and be able to become employable as a result of the education, training, and rehabilitation. To apply for rehabilitation services the person should contact the local office of the state Department of Education, Division of Vocational Services. Other rehabilitation programs are offered through hospitals, long-term care facilities, and outpatient settings.

COMMUNITY REHABILITATION FACILITIES Rehabilitation facilities in the United States arose out of a concern by local leaders, parents, and advocates who perceived a real need for resources and services to assist people with disabilities in their home communities (Geigel, 1995, p. 24). Starting in the nineteenth century, the private sector began to develop rehabilitation facilities, workshops, work centers, and extended employment facilities—the evolution was a uniquely American phenomenon (Geigel, p. 24). Today such facilities make up a national network of private association and service providers such as local school districts, universities, Goodwill Industries, National Easter Seal Society, Jewish

Rehabilitation Act of 1973 (P.L. 93-112) as Amended

The purposes of this Act are: 1) to empower individuals with disabilities to maximize employment, economic self-sufficiency, independence, and inclusion and integration into society through comprehensive and coordinated state-of-the-art programs, independent living centers and services; research; training, demonstrations projects; and the guarantee of equal opportunity; and 2) to ensure that the federal government plays a leadership role in promoting the employment of individuals with disabilities, especially individuals with severe disabilities, and in assisting states and providers of services in fulfilling the aspirations of such individuals with disabilities for meaningful and gainful employment and independent living.

This act replaced the Vocational Rehabilitation Act of 1920 and was a landmark piece of legislation for individuals with disabilities. It was the genesis of many fundamental concepts such as individuals being included in the development and implementation of their rehabilitation plans, guaranteed civil rights of individuals with disabilities and advocacy programs for individuals with disabilities.

From Stafford BJ: A legislative perspective on the Rehabilitation Act, *Am Rehabil* 21(3):37-41, 1995.

Rehabilitation Nursing Practice

Rehabilitation nurses rely on sound theoretic foundations and scientific knowledge as they work with clients and their families to:

- Set goals for maximum levels of interdependent functioning and activities of daily living
- Promote self-care, prevent complications or further disability
- Reinforce positive coping behaviors
- Ensure access with continuity of services and care
- Advocate for optimal quality of life
- Improve outcome for clients
- Contribute to reforms in the character, structure, and delivery of health care in the United States

From Hoeman SP: Conceptual bases for rehabilitation nursing. In Hoeman SP: *Rehabilitation nursing: process and application*, ed 2, St. Louis, 1996, Mosby, p. 3.

Vocational Services, Associations for Retarded Citizens, United Cerebral Palsy Association, and the American Rehabilitation Association and provide homebound programs, sheltered workshops, and training. These facilities provide many valuable services to the person who is disabled. Innovations in rehabilitation service provision have recently provided services such as "rehabilitation on wheels," mobile rehabilitation units that take rehabilitation services into rural and underserved areas (Lavallee, Crupi, 1992).

The Nurse and the Rehabilitation Process

Nurses who practice in rehabilitation must possess the special knowledge and clinical skills that help them to deal with the profound impact of disability on individuals and their families, and must realize that individuals with disabilities have intrinsic worth that transcends their disability (ARN, 1994a, p. 3). To facilitate care of clients who are disabled the rehabilitation nurse must have knowledge of growth and development, functional status, family and crisis theory, group process, role theory, adaptation and coping, learning theory, and the change process (ARN, 1994a, p. 4).

Rehabilitation nurses intervene to prevent disability, reduce the stigma of disability, restore optimal functioning, enhance quality of life, promote independence, help the individual and family adapt to an altered lifestyle, and assist people in looking beyond the disability (ARN, 1994a, p. 3). The box above right presents some additional nursing interventions.

Early intervention results in successful care outcomes and the smooth transition between phases of rehabilitation and community reintegration (Breese, Mikrut, 1995, p. 39). There is a direct correlation between the time the injury or illness occurred, when the rehabilitation referral was made, and the success of the rehabilitation program. The longer the time lapse between condition occurrence and rehabilitation services, the less chance that rehabilitation efforts will be optimally effective. Early involvement with a skilled support person, such as a community health nurse, will help bridge gaps in service and help to reduce frustration and lessen the likelihood of secondary disabilities occurring.

Both hospital and community health nurses are in key positions to help the client and family accept and implement the rehabilitation program. The rehabilitation process follows the same steps as the nursing process (see Chapter 9). It involves data gathering, formation of diagnoses and rehabilitation prognoses, goals, plans, follow-up, and evaluation. Records are kept and discharge planning is done (see Chapter 10). It is an interdisciplinary process that involves counseling and case management (see Chapter 10). It often involves vocational rehabilitation, restorative services, retraining, and ongoing utilization of community resources. Diagnoses frequently used by rehabilitation nurses are given in the box on the next page.

When a disability strikes one family member, all members are affected in some way, and family variables such as coping patterns, expectations, ability to utilize community resources, and economic status will affect the family's ability to adapt. As a result of the effects of protracted stress in providing for the needs of family members with disabling conditions, often with limited access to community resources, families may dissolve or develop secondary psychosocial issues such as emotional difficulties or substance abuse, frustration, and isolation (Breese, Mikrut, 1995, p. 39). Nursing interventions focus on minimizing family stress and promoting adaptation. The nurse serves as a case manager, coordinating activities, maintaining communication with the client and family, and linking clients to community resources.

Nursing Diagnoses Used Most Frequently in Rehabilitation Nursing Practice

*Impaired physical mobility
*Self-care deficit
*Alteration in urinary elimination pattern
*Impaired skin integrity
*Alteration in bowel elimination pattern
*Potential for physical injury
*Knowledge deficit
*Impaired verbal communication
*Decreased activity tolerance
Alterations in comfort
Impaired thought process
Ineffective family coping
Noncompliance
Body image disturbance
Self-esteem disturbances
Alteration in nutrition: Less than required
Health management deficit
Impaired home maintenance management
Sensory perception alterations
Uncompensated swallowing impairment

From Sawin KJ, Heard L: Nursing diagnoses used most frequently in rehabilitation nursing practice, *Rehabil Nurs* 17(5):257, 1992. Reprinted from *Rehabilitation Nursing,* Vol 17, Issue 5, with permission of the Association of Rehabilitation Nurses, 4700 W. Lake Avenue, Glenview, Il., 60025-1485. Copyright © 1992, Association of Rehabilitation Nurses.
*Top 9 diagnoses.

Client and family involvement in the rehabilitation process is essential. If families are supported and included during the initial phase of rehabilitation they are often more effective in supporting the client and have better long-term adaptation to the disability (Winterhalter, 1992, p. 23). Provision of early interventions, stabilization of psychosocial function, case management, and utilization of community resources (see Chapter 10) assist a family in adapting to the disability and having successful rehabilitation outcomes. Some factors related to adaptation have been previously discussed in this chapter.

The rehabilitation plan of care is mutually established with the client and family. If the rehabilitation plan does not promote active client participation and is under the control of professionals the process can be ineffective and inhibit client independence. Lack of client participation can also affect the client's self-esteem and can disrupt the therapeutic process. Motivation to follow through on a rehabilitation plan is often increased if the client is involved in the plan and believes it will result in increased independence and quality of life. In providing care, nurses must be careful to be empathetic, not sympathetic, and encourage independence and self-care.

Caretakers should be helped to use anticipatory guidance (The Teaching Tips box on p. 577 listed some perceived needs of prospective caretakers). They also need assistance in planning for the long-term implications associated with the condition, setting realistic expectations, and using self-management techniques. Nurses can provide support, guidance, knowledge, and assistance, but only the client and his or her family can evoke change.

Allowing for meaningful expression of feelings that can range from despair and hopelessness to unrealistic optimism is a significant contribution of the community health nurse. Also, nurses need to assess their personal feelings, which can inhibit or enhance their ability to function effectively with persons who are disabled. Numerous studies have shown that health care providers have many inaccurate perceptions and negative attitudes about persons who are disabled (Lindgren, Oermann, 1993, p. 121). Lindgren and Oermann conducted a study to examine the attitudes of nursing students toward the disabled to determine the effect of an educational program on these attitudes. Study results showed that students had significantly higher scores and more positive attitudes following the education program.

CHRONIC PAIN Chronic pain is pain that recurs or persists over an extended period of time and interferes with functioning (Simon, McTier, 1996, p. 20). Chronic pain is described by some health experts as the major cause of disability in the nation—affecting more than 50 million Americans (Simon, McTier, p. 20). It is a common element of many disabling conditions, and chronic pain syndrome is in itself a disabling condition. Chronic pain has a significant effect on individuals and their families and impedes a person's ability to work and to perform role function. Rehabilitation programs have been designed specifically to address chronic pain (Vines, Cox, Nicoll, Garrett, 1996, p. 25). The goal of a nurse in pain management is to improve the level of functioning for those affected by pain (ARN, 1994b).

People suffering from chronic pain evidence inactivity, depression, disruption of marital and family relationships, use of drugs to control the pain, disruptions in sleep patterns, and disruptions in eating (weight gain or loss) (Simon, 1996, p. 14). Research by Simon (Simon, McTier, 1996) has resulted in the development of a Chronic Pain Assessment tool for nurses. The pain history section of the tool is given in Figure 19-8.

Research by Simon (1996) found three common nursing diagnoses for clients with chronic pain: (1) ineffective coping related to chronic pain, (2) activity intolerance related to decreased muscle tone and strength from inactivity secondary to chronic pain, and (3) sleep pattern disturbance related to pain and distress. Nursing roles in pain management include those of educator, clinician, and case manager. Interventions should be directed at assessing and monitoring the pain, pain control and reduction, and

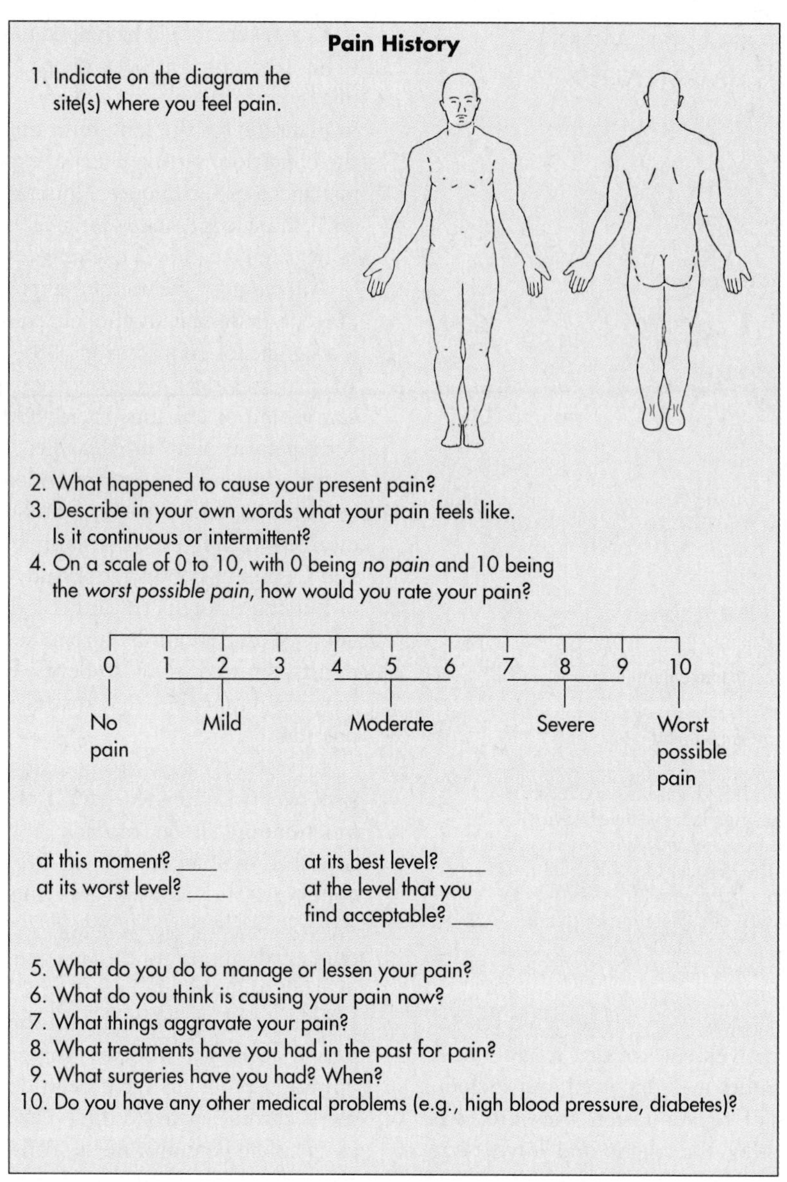
Pain History

1. Indicate on the diagram the site(s) where you feel pain.

2. What happened to cause your present pain?
3. Describe in your own words what your pain feels like. Is it continuous or intermittent?
4. On a scale of 0 to 10, with 0 being *no pain* and 10 being the *worst possible pain*, how would you rate your pain?

0 1 2 3 4 5 6 7 8 9 10

No pain | Mild | Moderate | Severe | Worst possible pain

at this moment? ____
at its worst level? ____
at its best level? ____
at the level that you find acceptable? ____

5. What do you do to manage or lessen your pain?
6. What do you think is causing your pain now?
7. What things aggravate your pain?
8. What treatments have you had in the past for pain?
9. What surgeries have you had? When?
10. Do you have any other medical problems (e.g., high blood pressure, diabetes)?

Figure 19-8 Pain history section of a chronic pain assessment tool. *(Reprinted from Simon JM, McTier CL: Development of a chronic pain assessment tool,* Rehabil Nurs *21(1):20-24, 1996c, with permission of the Association of Rehabilitation Nurses, 4700 W. Lake Avenue, Glenview, Il., 60025-1485. Copyright © 1996 Association of Rehabilitation Nurses.)*

educating the client and the family about chronic pain. This education includes information on the physiology of the affected body systems, pain cycle, exercise and body mechanics in relation to pain, the purpose and side effects of the pain medication, problem-solving skills and communication techniques, good nutrition, and sleep enhancement (Simon, p. 16). Research has shown that rehabilitation programs for pain, managed and evaluated primarily by professional rehabilitation nurses, have been successful in helping clients control their pain and achieve a higher level of physical functioning and role performance (Vines, Cox, Nicoll, Garrett, 1996, p. 30).

GROUP LEARNING INTERVENTIONS Nursing interventions that involve group learning for adults with chronic disabilities have proved to be successful (Payne, 1995, p. 268). It appears that the commonality of emotional and physical problems shared by clients in groups is conducive to learning (Payne, p. 268). Nursing research on the use of groups with adults who are disabled has shown that group members received the following benefits from others in the group: learning from each other, reduced feelings of isolation, and enjoyment of hearing other's experiences, goals, and problems (Payne, 1993). Other studies have shown that group sessions have been helpful in treating the social isolation and loneliness often experienced by people with disabilities (Acorn, Bramptom, 1992, p. 22).

SELF-CARE, SELF-MANAGEMENT, AND SELF-ADVOCACY Nursing interventions should focus on self-care, self-management, and self-advocacy. Self-care interventions help to keep the person independent. Self-management techniques are directed toward helping clients to make appropriate decisions about their life and health care. Self-advocacy interventions help the person to be in control of the situation and be able to act effectively on his or her own behalf. Some self-advocacy behaviors are given in the box at right. Nurses who promote self-advocacy work in partnership with clients, assisting them in obtaining the knowledge needed to make informed decisions and in learning negotiation skills.

SELF-ADVOCACY

Self-advocacy enables persons who are disabled and their families to:

- Control the type and source of treatment received
- Be free to refuse treatment or services
- Have access to all relevant information about their own treatment
- Comprehend the process of appealing any decision which affects them
- Make informed choices
- Rely on service providers to be catalysts and resources rather than decision makers
- Take reasonable risks and have the right to fail but to take responsibility for change
- Acquire skills that will maximize independence
- Engage in productive activity commensurate with their needs, abilities, and interests

Modified from Breese P, Mikrut S: Survivor training and empowerment program (S.T.E.P.), *Am Rehab* 21(3):38-42, 1995, pp. 41-42.

THE COMMUNITY HEALTH NURSE'S ROLE WITH THE ADULT WHO IS DISABLED

In working with clients with disabilities nurses carry out many roles, including case manager, counselor, teacher, advocate, and caregiver. On a daily basis the community health nurse will work with people who have disabling conditions and assist them in living successfully in the community.

The community health nurse is involved in primary, secondary, and tertiary preventive activities in relation to chronic conditions. Nurses carry out primary prevention activities such as teaching clients about risk factors and healthy lifestyles. Nurses must also focus on prevention strategies for people who already have potentially disabling conditions (e.g., a disease, impairment, or functional limitation) and try to prevent a disability from occurring. According to the IOM (Pope, Tarlov, 1991, p. 3), health professionals should look at the risks for developing a disability or secondary condition related to the disability, assess how quality of life is affected by disabling conditions, and work toward improving it.

Community health nurses build on client strengths, establish mutually acceptable goals, and link the client with community resources. Assisting clients with utilizing community resources is an important role. The nurse assists the client and family in adjusting to changes imposed by the condition and assists families in enhancing their abilities to cope, grow, and adapt. Because of the complexities of providing therapeutic services to people who are disabled, community health nurses often use an interdisciplinary approach to providing care and may be part of a multidisciplinary team. Many community health nursing interventions involve health education activities.

Health Education Activities

Health education has historically been a community health nursing role. It enables persons who are disabled and their families to become as independent as possible (Wilson, 1995).

Nursing interventions include teaching clients about their conditions, community resources, self-management, self-care, and self-advocacy. Community health nurses also "educate" communities about people who are disabled and disabling conditions. Nurses may promote community awareness by focusing on primary prevention of disabling conditions. Health education activities in schools and workplaces can assist people in understanding disabling conditions and accepting people who are disabled. For example, in the school setting programs that discuss disabilities, such as "New Kids on the Block," can be an effective way to help children learn about disabling conditions. School nurses can help children understand disabling conditions and why these conditions exist, and assist children in accepting each others' differences. Local health departments and community agencies have numerous health education materials available to assist the nurse in working with families and the community.

The Nurse and Community Resource Utilization

Resources on the federal, state, and local level have been previously discussed in this chapter. Crucial to the successful adaptation to chronic and handicapping conditions is the utilization of community resources. (ARN, 1994a, p. 20). The knowledgeable community health nurse refers clients to appropriate community resources (see Chapter 10), because clients often are not aware of the resources available to them or how to work with these resources.

The box below tells a story of survivors of traumatic brain injury (TBI) and resource utilization. Almost 2 million Americans experience TBI each year; at least half of the cases result in at least short-term disability, and more than 50,000 people die as a result of their injuries (Forkosch, Kaye, LaPlante, 1996, p. 1). Almost one third of TBIs involve motor vehicles, and household accidents account for one fourth (Forkosch, Kaye, LaPlante, p. 1). Both are areas for nursing health education interventions in relation to use of seatbelts, household safety, and accident prevention.

Although many excellent resources are available, it is often difficult for the client to locate them. The nurse can help link the client and family to resources, assist them in being persistent when exploring resources, and encourage them in their search. Searching out available resources can be a trying experience. Clients often hear of resources from other people experiencing the same condition, such as meetings with self-help groups.

If the search for resources becomes too harrowing the nurse may want to make contacts on behalf of the client. This should be done in such a way as to help the client avoid discouragement but not encourage dependence. Resources others take for granted, such as appropriate clothing and household furnishings, tools, and appliances, can be difficult to obtain for the person who is disabled (information listings have previously been given throughout the chapter).

Some helpful publications are *Health Information Resources in the Federal Government,* published by the Office of Disease Prevention and Health Promotion, as well as directories of national disability organizations published by the National Institute on Disability Research and Rehabilitation. These publications provide listings of many resources that can be of assistance to the person who is disabled.

The local telephone directory and mail-order catalogs are other sources of information. Some telephone directories include specific sections on community resources. Many agencies are located under the government phone listings, or under specific headings in the yellow pages such as hospitals, hospital equipment, rehabilitation, and mental health. Local health departments and departments of human or social services, federal Social Security Administration offices, state developmental disability councils, United Way, and public libraries are all sources of information. Shop-at-home catalogs (previously mentioned under Health Care in this chapter) have many items that can be useful to the person who is disabled.

A Story of Survival and Resource Management

Survivors of traumatic brain injury (TBI) and their families face an extremely complex and potentially confusing array of services, medical professionals, and human service delivery systems. The course of rehabilitation is extensive, sometimes encompassing many years, numerous medical disciplines, service delivery systems, and bureaucratic entities. The process of rehabilitation and community reintegration following brain injury often requires years of effort and major medical and rehabilitative expenses. Survivors of TBI emerge from the medical milieu concerned about the future but unaware and uninformed of the bureaucratic and medicolegal challenges that lie ahead.

Most of the survivors of TBI receive time-limited case management services through the insurance carrier responsible for covering the accident or through a facility-based case manager who acts as an internal coordinator of the rehabilitation team. However, once the injured person leaves the facility and insurance monies are depleted, case management (service coordination) either stops or is abruptly transferred to the family. Therefore, upon transfer to the home or community families, by default, begin to face the reality of providing long-term support and service coordination with limited financial and emotional resources.

Survivors, through extensive hospitalizations and indoctrination into the role of the client, frequently learn to passively accept medical treatment and rehabilitation options available to them. After discharge from the medical setting they are thrust into the role of fending for themselves with few supports and are often unable to obtain information on existing service or programs that address their unique needs.

Unfortunately, little preparation is given to people with brain injury and their families to adequately function in their new role as "service coordinator." Forced to fill the role of self-advocate or service coordinator, survivors and their families learn about available services and procurement of those services in a lengthy piecemeal process that may never reveal the full spectrum of assistance available. The process is a time-consuming, frustrating, and potentially overwhelming endeavor for a family already taxed by the advent of a traumatic event.

Human service delivery systems and state social service systems, which typically assume responsibility for the provision of long-term support and case management, are unable to keep pace with the ever-increasing demand for service to a population of Americans who live longer and have more severely disabling conditions. Case management—or service coordination—specifically for people with brain injury has not been developed in most states and is not readily available to these individuals who have difficulty accessing other social service systems. As a result, many survivors of brain injury "fall through the bureaucratic cracks," are unable to access services available to people with other disabilities, and become exhausted by running the gauntlet of social services before they realize any success for their efforts.

Modified from Breese P, Mikrut S: Survivor training and empowerment program (S.T.E.P.), *Am Rehab* 21(3):38-39, 1995.

Evaluating the Client's Rehabilitation Regimen

Evaluating the client's rehabilitation regimen is an important role for the community health nurse. The nurse needs to consider components of the rehabilitation plans such as appropriateness of resources and client satisfaction with the plan of care. Questions that address client outcomes and satisfaction should be raised. Use of a client satisfaction survey can be helpful. It can provide data about client perceptions of their care, serve as a basis for decision making about patient care, and help to show clients and families that their opinions are valued (Courts, 1988, p. 79). Sample items for such a survey are given in Figure 19-9.

The nurse's role in working with the client who is disabled is varied and comprehensive. She or he will need to be flexible and adaptable in implementing rehabilitation care and sensitive to the needs of the client and family.

THE NURSE AND CLIENT ADVOCACY

The person who is disabled is vulnerable and at risk for having unmet health care needs. The nurse uses advocacy skills to facilitate the development of relevant public policies and community services, decrease societal barriers for people who are disabled, and facilitate more positive societal attitudes. Nurses are frequently involved in advocacy for clients who are disabled; however, many health professionals hesitate to put themselves in client advocacy positions for reasons including:

- *Unfamiliar role*. Professionals have generally not been trained to be advocates and often do not have the skills to undertake such a role. The advocate may find advocacy difficult, awkward, and uncomfortable.
- *Fear of reprisal*. Often, the greater the impact of the advocacy action, the greater the risk of reprisal. The advocate must be aware of the possibility of reprisal and must evaluate the possible outcomes of his or her behavior.
- *Role conflict*. It is difficult to take stands contrary to the stand of other professionals in the field or contrary to the organization for which one works, and the advocate may be pressured to "conform." The advocacy role may be in conflict with the professional role or personal beliefs.
- *Apathy*. It is easier not to be involved, especially when one is not personally or directly affected.
- *Lack of support*. If one lacks the support of others, the advocacy stand becomes more difficult and sometimes risky (e.g., job security).
- *Change implications*. Advocacy often means change, and change can mean stress.

Concerns such as not enough time or money, no one to help, not wanting to get involved on an emotional level, and the system not being ready for change all are common reasons for not assuming an advocacy role. It is easy to feel empathy with these concerns, and most people have probably voiced them at one time or another. Taking an advocacy stand requires time, a commitment to client rights, and the belief that clients have a right to essential health care services. The impact that a nurse can have on the system as an advocate should not be underestimated. An example of this is the case of a nurse working with a local association of parents of disabled children.

CASE *Scenario*

The parents in a local association for disabled citizens were increasingly aware of instances of suspected abuse of their children in the institutional setting in which they resided. The parents had talked with the institution administration and felt that they were not receiving adequate information; some of the parents felt intimidated. The parents were concerned about the implications of their actions on their children. If they continued to press for information, they were worried about reprisals. If they did not press for information, they were worried that the situation would get worse. A nurse who was a member of the association was able to act as an advocate and take action.

The nurse met with the parents and the institution administration. After assessing and concluding that there was a problem and that the administration was resistant to change, the nurse examined the laws of the state regarding child abuse. One section of the law clearly stated that an institution must be independently investigated when there were suspected cases of child abuse or neglect. The nurse knew that state institutions were not adhering to that section of the law and were doing their own investigations of abuse and neglect. By obtaining legal counsel, working with the parent group, and using the established grievance procedure for state mental health clients, the community health nurse was able to help effect change in the system. The state now has impartial investigations of all cases of child abuse in state institutions and residential facilities, and parents or guardians have access to the results.

The advocacy efforts of this community health nurse had many positive effects. Reporting procedures for institutional cases of suspected abuse and neglect were clearly written and implemented in that state. The state legislature appropriated a large sum of money to be used in further protection and advocacy services for people who are developmentally disabled. In addition, the general public became increasingly aware of the needs of people who are mentally disabled and some of the conditions under which they live.

Nurses are in a position to correct public misconceptions about people who are disabled. They can work to gain greater acceptance of individuals who are disabled in whatever setting they reside. The nurse can be instrumental in

Preadmission information

How did you find out about the rehabilitation unit? (Check one)

- ❑ Doctor
- ❑ Nurse
- ❑ Other health person
- ❑ Friend
- ❑ Other (please name) ______________________________

Did the nurse or doctor talk to you before you came? ❑ Yes ❑ No

If yes, did you get your questions answered? ❑ Yes ❑ No

If yes, did you understand what the unit was like? ❑ Yes ❑ No

What should patients know about the rehabilitation unit before coming to the unit?

About your care	**Always**	**Often**	**Sometimes**	**Rarely**	**Never**	**NA**
I was included in planning my care.	❑	❑	❑	❑	❑	❑
The staff listened to my problems.	❑	❑	❑	❑	❑	❑
Questions about sex were answered.	❑	❑	❑	❑	❑	❑
My call light was answered quickly.	❑	❑	❑	❑	❑	❑
I learned about my medications.	❑	❑	❑	❑	❑	❑
Nurses explained things to be done to me.	❑	❑	❑	❑	❑	❑
Therapists explained things to be done to me.	❑	❑	❑	❑	❑	❑
Family						
My family was included in planning my care.	❑	❑	❑	❑	❑	❑
My family was taught how to care for me.	❑	❑	❑	❑	❑	❑
My family had their questions answered.	❑	❑	❑	❑	❑	❑
My family went to family support group.	❑	❑	❑	❑	❑	❑
My family rated this group as helpful.	❑	❑	❑	❑	❑	❑
If you had speech problems, please answer the following:						
Therapist helped me learn to talk.	❑	❑	❑	❑	❑	❑
My speech improved.	❑	❑	❑	❑	❑	❑
Staff understood my speech problem.	❑	❑	❑	❑	❑	❑
I learned to talk with the staff.	❑	❑	❑	❑	❑	❑
Family was taught to understand my speech.	❑	❑	❑	❑	❑	❑

Results and evaluation

Did you have special things to learn before you came? ❑ Yes ❑ No

Did you learn what you wanted to learn? ❑ Yes, definitely. ❑ Yes, I think so. ❑ No, I don't think so. ❑ No, definitely not.

If needed, would you return to the unit? ❑ Yes ❑ Probably ❑ No

Would you tell others to come to the unit? ❑ Yes ❑ Probably ❑ No

What I liked most about the rehabilitation center:

____

____

____

What I liked least about the rehabilitation center:

____

____

____

Figure **19-9** Sample items on a patient satisfaction survey. *(Reprinted from Courts NF: A patient satisfaction survey for a rehab unit,* Rehabil Nurs *13(2):80, 1988, with permission of the Association of Rehabilitation Nurses, 4700 W. Lake Avenue, Glenview, Il., 60025-1485. Copyright © 1988 Association of Rehabilitation Nurses.)*

promoting a positive attitude toward people who are considered disabled by the general public.

NURSING ORGANIZATIONS AND DISABILITY

A number of specialty nursing organizations focus on disabling conditions. The Association of Rehabilitation Nurses (ARN) is a professional organization for rehabilitation nurses and an excellent resource on rehabilitation nursing practice. ARN sponsors research and educational opportunities in rehabilitation nursing. It offers numerous publications, including *Standards and Scope of Rehabilitation Nursing Practice* (1994a) (see the box on the next page) and the journals *Rehabilitation Nursing* and *Rehabilitation Nursing Research*. ARN promotes research-based rehabilitation nursing practice (Hoeman, Dayhoff, Thompson, 1993, p. 40) and has offered certification in rehabilitation nursing

Standards of Rehabilitation Nursing Practice

The goal of rehabilitation nursing is to assist the individual who has a disability and/or chronic illness in restoring, maintaining, and promoting his or her maximal health. This includes preventing chronic illness and disability. The rehabilitation nurse is skilled at treating alterations in functional ability and lifestyle that result from physical disability and chronic illness.

STANDARDS OF CARE

Standard I. Assessment
The rehabilitation nurse collects client health data.

Standard II. Nursing Diagnosis
The rehabilitation nurse analyzes the assessment when determining diagnoses.

Standard III. Outcome Identification
The rehabilitation nurse identifies expected outcomes individualized to the client.

Standard IV. Planning
The rehabilitation nurse develops a plan of care that prescribes interventions to attain expected outcomes.

Standard V. Intervention
The rehabilitation nurse implements the interventions identified in the plan of care.

Standard VI. Evaluation
The rehabilitation nurse evaluates the client's progress toward attainment of outcome.

STANDARDS OF PROFESSIONAL PERFORMANCE

Standard I. Quality of Care
The rehabilitation nurse systematically evaluates the quality and effectiveness of rehabilitation nursing practice.

Standard II. Performance Appraisal
The rehabilitation nurse evaluates his or her own nursing practice in relation to professional practice standards and relevant statutes and regulations.

Standard III. Education
The rehabilitation nurse acquires and maintains current knowledge in nursing practice.

Standard IV. Collegiality
The rehabilitation nurse contributes to the professional development of peers, colleagues, and others.

Standard V. Ethics
The rehabilitation nurse's decisions and actions on behalf of clients are determined in an ethical manner.

Standard VI. Collaboration
The rehabilitation nurse collaborates with the client, significant others, and health care providers in providing client care.

Standard VII. Research
The rehabilitation nurse uses research findings in practice.

Standard VIII. Resource Utilization
The rehabilitation nurse considers factors related to safety, effectiveness, and cost in planning and delivering client care.

Reprinted with permission from Association of Rehabilitation Nurses: *Standards and scope of rehabilitation nursing practice*, ed 3, Glenview, Il, 1994a, The Association. Copyright © 1994 Association of Rehabilitation Nurses, 4700 W. Lake Avenue, Glenview, Il., 60025-1485.

since 1984. Other nursing organizations in specialty areas of practice that work with people with disabling conditions are given in the box on the next page.

Summary

The number of individuals in society who are characterized as disabled can be expected to increase, and demand for services to these individuals will increase concomitantly. Adults who are disabled are confronted with adapting to their disability amidst societal, family, and individual variables—influencing adaptation and personal growth and development. Many disabling conditions are long term and require ongoing use of community resources. The need for case management interventions is great, as is the need for greater accessibility to services and greater availability of services for people who are disabled.

Community health nurses are in a unique position to assist clients who are disabled in obtaining services that will enhance adaptation and promote growth. They assist clients with rehabilitation and work cooperatively with the clients and their families to establish plans of care. A sensitivity to the needs of this population group and an awareness that there are individual differences among clients who are disabled are both essential for the community health nurse to function effectively with clients who have special needs.

Increasingly, health care professionals are becoming actively involved in advocacy for this population group. Advocacy has been critical in the procurement of many essential services for these clients. While legislation in the last decade has reflected a more positive attitude toward people who are disabled, numerous needs remain unmet. Professionals must continue to facilitate public awareness about disabling conditions and the needs of people who are experiencing them. Americans who are disabled have the same human and civil rights as everyone else and deserve their share of the country's health resources.

Critical *Thinking Exercise*

In this chapter the effect of societal values on adaptation to a disability was discussed. What are some of the values the American society holds that affect adaptation to a disability and the quality of life for people who are disabled? As a nurse, what are some things that you could do to facilitate positive attitudes toward persons who are disabled? What are your own attitudes about persons who are disabled, and how do you think these attitudes will affect your nursing practice?

Nursing Organizations and Disability

Association of Rehabilitation Nurses
4700 West Lake Avenue
Glenview, Illinois 60025-1485
1-800-229-7530 or (817) 375-4710

American Association of Spinal Cord Injury Nurses
75-20 Astoria Boulevard
Jackson Heights, New York 11370-1177
(718) 803-3782

American Nephrology Nurses' Association
East Holly Avenue
Box 56
Pitman, New Jersey 08071-0056
(609) 256-2320

American Society for Long Term Care Nurses
660 Lonely Cottage Drive
Upper Black Eddy, Pennsylvania 18972-9313
(610) 847-5396

American Society of Pain Management Nurses
11512 Allecingie Parkway
Richmond, Virginia 23235
(804) 378-0072

Developmental Disabilities Nurses Association
1720 Willow Creek Circle, Suite 515
Eugene, Oregon 97402
1-800-888-6733

Drug and Alcohol Nursing Association
660 Lonely Cottage Drive
Upper Black Eddy, Pennsylvania 18972-9313
(610) 847-5396

National Association of Orthopaedic Nurses
East Holly Avenue
Box 56
Pitman, New Jersey 08071-0056
(609) 256-2310

Oncology Nursing Society
501 Holiday Drive
Pittsburgh, Pennsylvania 15220
(412) 921-7373

REFERENCES

ABLE INFORM: New, improved information center for assistive technology, disability news and resources, *NARIC Q* 4(4):1, 10, 1995.

Acorn S, Bramptom E: Patients, loneliness: a challenge for rehabilitation nurses, *Rehabil Nurs* 17(1):22-25, 1992.

Association of Rehabilitation Nurses (ARN): *Standards and scope of rehabilitation nursing practice*, Skokie, Il., 1994a, ARN.

Association of Rehabilitation Nurses (ARN): *The pain management rehabilitation nurse: role description*, Skokie, Il., 1994b, ARN.

Aronson L: The housing crisis faced by people with disabilities—analysis and options (Part I), *Access* 8(1):2, 1996.

Breese P, Mikrut S: Survivor training and empowerment program (S.T.E.P.), *Am Rehab* 21(3):38-42, 1995.

Buscaglia LF, ed: *The disabled and their parents: a counseling challenge*, ed 2, Thorofare, N.J., 1983, Slack.

Buzinski P: Groups for brothers and sisters of developmentally disabled children: one component of a family-centered approach, *Issues Compr Pediatr Nurs* 4(1):45-50, 1980.

Chappell JA: The whole is greater than the sum of its parts, *Am Rehab* 20(1):23-29, 1994.

Clearinghouse on Disability Information: *Pocket guide to federal help for individuals with disabilities*, Washington, D.C., 1993, U.S. Government Printing Office.

Commission on Chronic Illness: *Chronic illness in the United States, vol I: prevention of chronic illness*, Cambridge, Ma., 1957, Harvard University Press.

Courts NF: A patient satisfaction survey for a rehab unit, *Rehabil Nurs* 13(2):79-81, 1988.

Davidhizer R: Understanding powerlessness in family members of the chronically ill, *Geriatr Nurs* 13(2):66-69, 1992.

deBalcazar YS, Bradford B, Fawcett SB: Common concerns of disabled Americans: issues and options, *Soc Policy* 19(2):29-35, 1988.

Dietl D: The phoenix: from the ashes and looking to the ultimate barrier: our own attitude, *J Rehabil* 49(3):12-17, 1983.

Duffy Y: Disability shouldn't be a bar to romance, *The Atlanta Journal Constitution*, August 11, 1996, p. R1.

Employment: spotlighting . . . the ARC of Tennessee's position statements, *The Arc Connection*, Spring:4, 1996.

Forkosch JA, Kaye S, LaPlante MP: The incidence of traumatic brain injury in the United States, *Disabil Stat Abstract*, Number 14, Washington, D.C., 1996, National Institute on Disability and Rehabilitation Research.

Frye BA: Review of the World Health Organization's report on disability prevention and rehabilitation, *Rehabil Nurs* 18(1):43-44, 1993.

Geigel W: Rehabilitation facilities: a perspective, *Am Rehab* 21(3):28-30, 1995.

Giele JZ: A delicate balance: the family's role in the care of the handicapped, *Fam Relations* 33(1):85-94, 1984.

Giordano G, D'Alonzo BJ: The link between transition and independent living, *Am Rehab* 20(1):2-7, 1994.

Giordano G, D'Alonzo BJ: Challenge and progress in rehabilitation: a review of the past 25 years and a preview of the future, *Am Rehab* 21(3):14-21, 1995.

Greco SB: Sexuality and education counseling. In Hoeman SP: *Rehabilitation nursing: process and application*, ed 2, St. Louis, 1996, Mosby, pp. 594-627.

Hayden MF, Abery BH, eds: *Challenges for a service system in transition: ensuring quality community experiences for persons with developmental disabilities*, Baltimore, Md., 1994, Brookes.

Hoeman SP: Conceptual bases for rehabilitation nursing. In Hoeman SP: *Rehabilitation nursing: process and application*, ed 2, St. Louis, 1996, Mosby, pp. 3-20.

Hoeman SP, Dayhoff NE, Thompson TC: The initial ANF research survey: rehabilitation nursing research interests of ARN members, *Rehabil Nurs* 18(1):40-41, 1993.

Kafka B: A civil rights or interdependence perspective on attendant services, *Rehab Gazette* 33(1):13-14, 1993.

Kendrick D: Invisible barriers: how you can make parenting easier, *Disabled USA* 1:17-19, 1983.

Kraus LE, Stoddard S: *Chartbook on work disability in the United States, an InfoUse Report*, Washington, D.C., 1991, National Institute on Disability and Rehabilitation Research.

Kubler-Ross E: *On death and dying*, New York, 1969, MacMillan.

Lafata JE, Koch GG, Weissert WG: Estimating activity limitation in the noninstitutionalized population: a method for small areas, *Am J Public Health* 84(11):1813-1817, 1994.

LaPlante MP, Rice DP, Wenger BL: Medical care use, health insurance and disability in the United States, *Disabil Stat Abstract*, Number 8, Washington, D.C., 1995, National Institute on Disability and Rehabilitation Research.

Lavallee DJ, Crupi CD: Rehabilitation takes to the road, *Holistic Nurs Pract* 6(2):60-66, 1992.

Lindgren CL, Burke ML, Hainsworth MA, Eakes GG: Chronic sorrow: a lifespan concept, *Scholar Inq Nurs Pract* 6(1):27-40, 1992.

Lindgren CL, Oermann MH: Effects of an educational intervention on students' attitudes toward the disabled, *J Nurs Educ* 32(3):121-126, 1993.

Max W, Rice DP, Trupin L: Medical expenditures for people with disabilities, *Disabil Stat Abstract*, Number 12, Washington, D.C., 1996, National Institute for Disability and Rehabilitation Research.

McCloskey JC, Bulechek GM, eds: *Nursing interventions classification (NIC)*, ed 2, St. Louis, 1996, Mosby.

McCubbin MA, McCubbin HI: Families coping with illness: the resiliency model of family stress, adjustment, and adaptation. In Danielson CB, Hamel-Bissell B, Winstead-Fry P, eds: *Families health and illness: perspectives on coping and intervention*, St. Louis, 1993, Mosby.

Miller JF: *Coping with chronic illness: overcoming powerlessness*, ed 2, Philadelphia, Pa., 1992, F.A. Davis.

Montgomery RJV: Examining respite care: promises and limitations. In Kane RA, Penrod JD, eds: *Family caregiving in an aging society: policy perspectives*, Thousand Oaks, Ca., 1995, Sage.

National Center for Chronic Disease Prevention and Health Promotion (NCCDPHP): *CDC/NCCDPHP: turning research findings into effective community programs*, Atlanta, 1996, Centers for Disease Control and Prevention.

National Institute on Disability and Rehabilitation Research: *Directory of national information sources on disabilities*, Washington, D.C., 1995, Department of Education.

National Rehabilitation Information Center (NARIC): *Factsheet on the National Rehabilitation Information Center, Information for Independence*, Silver Spring, Md., 1996, NARIC.

Oermann MH, Lindgren CL: An educational program's effects on students' attitudes toward people with disabilities: a 1-year follow-up, *Rehabil Nurs* 20(1):6-10, 1995.

Parent guide form NICHCY, *The Helping Hand*, July:2-3, 1996.

Patrick DL: Toward an epidemiology of disablement, *Am J Public Health* 84(11):1723-1724, 1994.

Payne JA: The contribution of group learning to the rehabilitation of spinal cord injured adults, *Rehabil Nurs* 18(7):375-379, 1993.

Payne JA: Group learning for adults with disabilities or chronic disease, *Rehabil Nurs* 20(5):268-272, 1995.

Pope AM, Tarlov AR, eds: *Disability in America: toward a national agenda for prevention*, Washington, D.C., 1991, National Academy Press.

President's Committee on Employment of the Handicapped: *Affirmative action to employ handicapped people*, Washington, D.C., 1978, U.S. Government Printing Office.

President's Committee on Employment of People with Disabilities: *Ability for hire: educational kit 1996*, Washington, D.C., 1996, The Committee.

Reasonable accommodation: what consumers and employers want to know, *NARIC Q* 4(4):2, 6, 1995.

Reeber BJ: Evaluating the effects of a family education intervention, *Rehabil Nurs* 17(6):332-336, 1992.

Reno J: Disability law will be enforced, *USA Today*, Monday, July 26, 1993, p. A9.

Robert Wood Johnson Foundation: *Challenges in health care*, New York, 1992, The Foundation.

Safilios-Rothschild C: *The sociology and social psychology of disability rehabilitation*, New York, 1982, University Press of America.

Sawin KJ, Heard L: Nursing diagnoses used most frequently in rehabilitation nursing practice, *Rehabil Nurs* 17(5):256-262, 1992.

Seelman K, Levesque CA: Rehabilitation research: its beginnings and ongoing contributions, *Am Rehab* 21(3):31-36, 1995.

Seifert KH: The attitudes of working people toward disabled persons, especially in regard to vocational rehabilitation. In Spiegel AD, Podair S, eds: *Rehabilitating people with disabilities into the mainstream of society*, Park Ridge, N.J., 1981, Noyes Medical.

Sexuality Information and Education Council of the United States (SIECUS): Sexuality and disability: a SIECUS annotated bibliography of available print and audiovisual materials, *SIECUS Report* 23(4):26-36, 1995.

Sexuality Information and Education Council of the United States (SIECUS): SIECUS position statements on human sexuality, sexual health and sexuality education and information 1995-96, *SIECUS Report* 24(3):21-23, 1996.

Shadish WR, Lurigio AJ, Lewis DA: After deinstitutionalization: the present and future of mental health long-term care policy, *J Soc Issues* 45(3):1-15, 1989.

Sherman BR, Cocozza JJ: Stress in families of the developmentally disabled: a literature review of factors affecting the decision to seek out-of-home placements, *Fam Relations* 33(1):95-103, 1984.

Simon JM: Chronic pain syndrome: nursing assessment and intervention, *Rehabil Nurs* 21(1):13-19, 1996.

Simon JM, McTier CL: Development of a chronic pain assessment tool, *Rehabil Nurs* 21(1):20-24, 1996.

Smith LW, Smith QW, Richards L et al: Independent living centers: moving into the 21st century, *Am Rehab* 20(1):14-22, 1994.

Stafford BJ: A legislative perspective on the Rehabilitation Act, *Am Rehab* 21(3):37-41, 1995.

Stucki BR: *Living in the community with a disability: demographic characteristics of the population with disabilities under age 65*, Washington, D.C., 1995, American Association of Retired Persons.

Sussman MB, ed: *Sociology and rehabilitation*, Washington, D.C., 1966, American Sociological Association.

Thomas VM, Ellison K, Howell EV, Winters K: Caring for the person receiving ventilatory support at home: caregiver's needs and involvements, *Heart & Lung* 21:180-186, 1992.

Trupin L, Rice DP: Health status, medical care use, and number of disabling conditions in the United States, *Disabil Stat Abstract*, Number 9, Washington, D.C., 1995, National Institute on Disability and Rehabilitation Research.

U.S. Department of Commerce: *Statistical abstract of the United States 1995*, Washington, D.C., 1995, U.S. Government Printing Office.

U.S. Department of Health and Human Services (USDHHS): *Healthy people 2000: national health promotion and disease prevention objectives, full report, with commentary*, Washington, D.C., 1991, U.S. Government Printing Office.

U.S. Department of Health and Human Services (USDHHS): *Health United States 1991*, Washington, D.C., 1992, U.S. Government Printing Office.

U.S. Department of Health and Human Services (USDHHS): *Healthy people 2000, midcourse review and 1995 revisions*, Washington, D.C., 1995, U.S. Government Printing Office.

Vines SW, Cox A, Nicoll L, Garrett S: Effects of a multimodal pain rehabilitation program: pilot study, *Rehabil Nurs* 21(1):25-30, 1996.

Watson PG: Family issues in rehabilitation, *Holistic Nurs Pract* 6(2):51-59, 1992.

Weeks SK: What are the educational needs of prospective family caregivers of newly disabled adults? *Rehabil Nurs* 20(5):256-260, 272, 1995.

Wenger BL, Kaye S, LaPlante MP: Disabilities among children, *Disabil Stat Abstract*, Number 15, National Institute on Disability and Rehabilitation Research, March 1996.

Wilson JA: Rehabilitation nurses: be proud of who you are and the job you perform, *Rehabil Nurs* 20(3):168, 1995.

Winterhalter JG: Group support for families during the acute phase of rehabilitation, *Holistic Nurs Pract* 6(2):23-31, 1992.

World Health Organization (WHO): *International classification of impairments, disabilities, and handicaps*, Geneva, 1980, WHO.

World Health Organization (WHO), Expert Committee on Disability Prevention and Rehabilitation: *Disability prevention and rehabilitation*, Technical Report Series 668, Geneva, 1981, WHO.

Youngblood NM, Hines J: The influence of the family's perception of disability on rehabilitation outcomes, *Rehabil Nurs* 17(6):323-326, 1992.

SELECTED BIBLIOGRAPHY

Biordi B, Oermann MH: The effect of prior experience in a rehabilitation setting on students' attitudes toward the disabled, *Rehabil Nurs* 18(2):95-98, 1993.

Blake K: The social isolation of young men with quadriplegia, *Rehabil Nurs* 20(1):17-22, 1995.

Boxtel AM, Napholz L, Gnewikow D: Using a wheelchair activity as a learning experience for student nurses, *Rehabil Nurs* 20(5):265-267, 1995.

Derstine JB: The rehabilitation clinical nurse specialist of the 1990s: roles assumed by recent graduates, *Rehabil Nurs* 17(3):139-140, 1992.

Garee B, Cheever R, eds: *Marriage and disability*, Bloomington, Il., 1992, Cheever Publishing.

Gibbons KB: A model for professional rehabilitation nursing practice, *Rehabil Nurs* 20(1):23-28, 1995.

Hoeman SP: Community-based rehabilitation, *Holistic Nurs Pract* 6(2):32-41, 1992.

Holmes GE, Karst RH, Kuehn MD: Community resource utilization in rehabilitation: the shape of the future, *Am Rehab* 18(3):23-25, 1992.

Hwu Y-J: The impact of chronic illness on patients, *Rehabil Nurs* 20(4):221-225, 1995.

Kirk K: Chronically ill patients' perceptions of nursing care, *Rehabil Nurs* 18(2):99-104, 1993.

Leahy MJ, Habeck RV, VanTol B: Doctoral dissertation research in rehabilitation: 1980-1989, *Rehab Counseling Bull* 35(4):253-288, 1992.

Lishner DM, Richardson M, Levine P, Patrick D: Access to primary health care among persons with disabilities in rural areas: a summary of the literature, *Rural Health Policy* 12(1):45-53, 1996.

Makas E: Positive attitudes toward disabled people: disabled and nondisabled persons' perspectives, *J Soc Issues* 44(1):49-61, 1988.

McDonald SE, Lloyd WM, Murphy D, Russert MG: *Sexuality and spinal cord injury*, Milwaukee, Wi., 1993, The Spinal Cord Injury Center.

Neal LJ: The rehabilitation nursing team in the home health care setting, *Rehabil Nurs* 20(1):32-36, 1995.

Penrose J: Double handicap: does he take sugar? *Nurs Times* 79:52-54, 1983.

Provan KG: Services integration for vulnerable populations: lessons from community mental health, *Fam Community Health* 19:19-30, 1997.

Reed KL: History of federal legislation for persons with disabilities, *Am J Occup Ther* 46(5):397-408, 1992.

Rothenberg RB, Koplan JP: Chronic disease in the 1990s, *Annu Rev Public Health* 11:267-296, 1990.

Russell NK, Roter DL: Health promotion counseling of chronic-disease patients during primary care visits, *Am J Public Health* 83(7):979-982, 1993.

Sheppard B: Patient's views of rehabilitation, *Clin Elderly Care* 9(10):27-30, 1994.

The Americans with Disabilities Act questions and answers, Washington, D.C., 1991, U.S. Equal Employment Opportunity Commission and U.S. Department of Justice Civil Rights Division.

Topolnicki DM: The gulag of guardianship, *Money* 18(3):149-152, 1989.

Weiss DV: Accessible vacations, *J Rehabil* 54(3):8-9, 1988.

The Well Elderly: Needs and Services

OBJECTIVES

Upon completion of this chapter, the reader should be able to:

1. Construct a personal philosophy of aging.
2. Articulate societal values and attitudes in relation to aging.
3. Discuss the *Healthy People 2000* initiative in relation to aging.
4. State major causes of mortality and morbidity for the elderly.
5. Describe health promotion and wellness activities for the elderly.
6. Identify significant legislation in relation to older Americans.
7. Describe barriers to health care for the elderly.
8. Conceptualize the community health nurse's role in promoting healthy aging.

There's no shame in growing old—we're all doing it. Age is, after all, the one thing we all share.

MAGGIE KUHN

Meet Art Johnson, a retired school principal from Waterford, Michigan. At 80 years of age he taught adult education at a local high school, golfed competitively, continued postgraduate education, and helped with coaching Little League baseball. He was known and loved in his community.

Meet Hattie Harris of Rochester, New York, where the city declared a "Hattie Harris Day." At 91 years of age she was described as the "elder statesman of the Republican Party" and the "Mayor of Strathallan Park." In those positions she advised political candidates, sought financial backing from business leaders, and set up neighborhood political rallies.

Meet Herbert Kirk of Bozeman, Montana. At 97 years of age he received his bachelor's degree from Montana State University. At the graduation ceremony Mr. Kirk received a standing ovation from the thousands of people gathered at the university fieldhouse. Part of the ceremony included the reading of a congratulatory letter sent by President Bill Clinton. The year before he had won two gold medals in the International Track Athletic Congress in Finland.

Individuals like Art Johnson, Hattie Harris, and Herbert Kirk can be found in any American community. They are examples of older Americans who have lived life to its fullest and best. They exemplify successful aging!

AGING DEFINED

Aging and "old age" are relatively contemporary phenomena. The average Stone Age human lived 15 years. By the late 1700s people lived into their 30s, and the life expectancy for turn-of-the-century Americans was less than 50 years (Painter, 1993, p. D1).

Aging is a natural and lifelong process of growing and developing. Everyone is aging! Aging is a universal phenomenon that begins at birth and continues throughout life, as well as an individual process that incorporates personal life experiences. In the United States a chronological marker, the age of 65, is often used to denote the advent of "old age."

The designation of old age in the United States was legislatively determined by the Social Security Act of 1935, which set eligibility for federal old age retirement benefits at age 65. In 1935 many Americans did not live to reach their 65th birthday. Today over 2 million Americans celebrate their 65th birthday each year—more than 5500 each day (American Association of Retired Persons [AARP], 1996, p. 1). With this "graying of America" old age is being redefined both socially and politically.

Nurses are providing care to more older people than ever before. Nurses can facilitate healthy aging. The box on the following page highlights a number of active older people.

SOME PERSPECTIVES ON AGING

Older people are the gatekeepers of a nation's history, values, culture, and traditions. They are "those who have gone before" and made today's technology and lifestyles possible.

Go for It—Healthy, Active Aging

Mary Baker Eddy directed the Christian Science Church at 89.
Harold and Bertha Soderquist joined the Peace Corps and learned a foreign language when he was 80 and she was 76.
Thomas Edison, the inventor of the electric light bulb, filed for his 1033rd patent at the age of 81.
Albert Schweitzer was in charge of an African hospital at 89 and helped build a half-mile road near the hospital at 87.
George Bernard Shaw was writing at 91.
Claude Pepper served as a U.S. Congressman at 88.
Ronald Reagan served as President of the United States in his 70s.
Maggie Kuhn headed the Gray Panthers at 88.
Anna Mary Moses, better known as Grandma Moses, illustrated an edition of *'Twas the Night Before Christmas* when she was 100.
Frank Lloyd Wright began his most creative and prolific work at the age of 69 and was active until his death at 91.
Herbert Kirk graduated from Montana State University in 1993 at age 97. The university was 100 years old that year.

Excerpts from Harris DK: *Sociology of aging*, ed 2, New York, 1990, Harper & Row; and Comfort A: *Say yes to old age: developing a positive attitude toward aging*, New York, 1990, Crown.

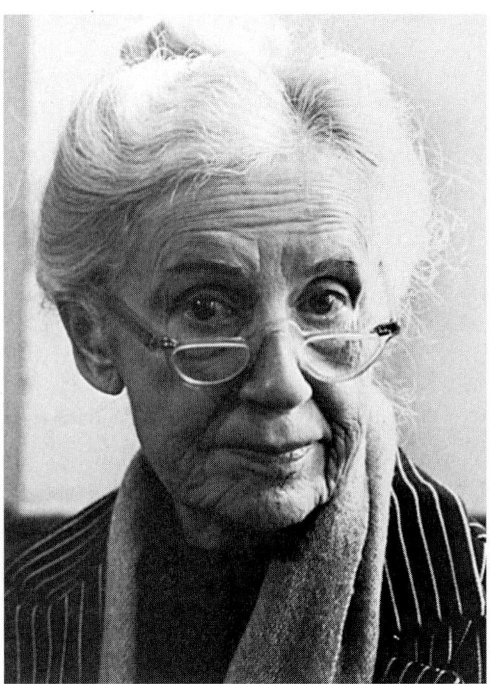

Figure 20-1 Maggie Kuhn, founder of the Gray Panthers. *(Courtesy Julie Jensen, Photographer.)*

Throughout history aging persons have been portrayed in literature and art as wise individuals, strong in character, and leaders of their people. However, cultures vary in how older people are cared for and respected.

American Attitudes toward Age and Aging

America is often described as an ageist society. Robert Butler, a renowned gerontologist, coined the term *ageism* in 1968 and defined it as a process of systematic stereotyping of, and discrimination against, people because they are old (Sheppard, 1990, p. 4). The Gray Panthers (Figure 20-1), an organization that staunchly advocates the rights of older people, view ageism as the use of age to define capability and role. The costs of ageism are great: as with other forms of prejudice it is dehumanizing and inhibits people from maximizing their potential.

Biases against aging are so deeply ingrained in our society that they unintentionally surface in everyday life—in writing, films, and even conversation—denying older persons their individuality and the opportunity to maximize their potential (AARP, 1984, pp. 3, 6). Descriptors such as *vigorous*, *active*, *attractive*, and *independent* are often used to describe a person of 20, 30, or 40, but rarely one of 70, 80, or 90.

In general, Americans are not educationally, socially, or emotionally prepared for old age (McGuire, Gerber, 1996) and many myths and misconceptions about aging exist. The box on the next page looks at some common myths about aging. People need to become knowledgeable about the aging process; develop realistic, positive attitudes toward aging; and realize that older people are valuable and contributing members of society. Nurses need to evaluate their attitudes about age and aging and how these attitudes affect nursing care and facilitate healthy aging.

Community health nurses have unique opportunities to facilitate healthy aging. For example, they can implement aging education programs in schools, teach elderly clients about available resources in the community, work with area agencies on aging to enhance service provision to the elderly (e.g., senior centers, local offices on aging, senior apartments), provide direct nursing care, and develop creative learning opportunities and programs. Innovative nurses have developed nurse-run clinics for senior citizens that provide essential health services; developed community aging education programs; and participated in community planning activities for the elderly. Nurse-managed centers for older adults can provide quality, comprehensive care and can be a vital part of the plan to help meet the health needs of the rapidly expanding elderly population (Yoder, 1996, p. 18).

Cross-Cultural Aging

Six percent of the world's population, 357 million people, are older than 65 (U.S. Bureau of the Census, 1996, p. v). By the year 2000 there will be more than 426 million elderly in the world (U.S. Bureau of the Census, 1992, p. v).

Various countries and cultures differ in how they view and define elderly. In some cultures elderly people are given elevated status and treated with great respect. In other cultures elders deal with significant social hardships. The

Myths About Aging

ALL OLDER PEOPLE ARE ALIKE

Fact: Older people are uniquely individual.

MOST OLDER PEOPLE LIVE IN INSTITUTIONAL SETTINGS

Fact: Only 5% of older people are in institutional settings.

THE MAJORITY OF OLDER PEOPLE ARE LONELY AND ISOLATED FROM THEIR FAMILIES

Fact: The majority of older people live in a family setting. Many older people live near their children and have regular contact with friends and family.

OLDER PEOPLE CANNOT LEARN

Fact: Older people are capable of learning and enjoy learning. The senior "Elderhostel" program is a good example of this.

THE MAJORITY OF OLDER PEOPLE VIEW THEMSELVES AS BEING IN POOR HEALTH

Fact: The majority (71%) of older people report their health as being good or excellent.

OLDER PEOPLE CANNOT WORK

Fact: Approximately 3.6 million older Americans are in the labor force.

THE MAJORITY OF OLDER PEOPLE HAVE INCOMES BELOW THE POVERTY LEVEL

Fact: Only 20% of older Americans are classified as poor or near-poor.

MOST OLDER PEOPLE HAVE NO INTEREST IN SEXUAL ACTIVITY

Fact: The need for sexual activity does not stop with old age.

OLD AGE BEGINS AT 65

Fact: In this country 65 was legislated as the age for Social Security Retirement benefits; but when "old age" begins is very individual.

Excerpts from Harris DK: *Sociology of aging*, ed 2, New York, 1990, Harper & Row, p. 5; and American Association of Retired Persons: *A profile of older Americans 1995*, Washington, D.C., 1996, AARP.

box above right illustrates some of the cultural and ethnic diversity and disparity in the elderly population in the United States.

Cultural sensitivity helps the nurse to elicit values, attitudes, and health practices that affect how clients respond during times of stress and illness and aids in developing and implementing effective health promotion strategies. The cultural assessment guide found in Appendix 7-1 assists "the community health nurse in obtaining cultural data. Understanding different cultural values and attitudes in relation to aging and health is essential for community health nurses to develop strategies that enhance the quality of life for the aged.

A Look at Cultural/Ethnic Diversity in the Elderly—U.S.

Racial diversity within the elderly population is increasing in the U.S. Presently, 1 in 10 elderly are of races other than white, and by 2050 this is expected to increase to 2 in 10.

Black (2.7 million) and Hispanic (1.5 million) elderly Americans are the most heavily represented ethnic minority groups among the aged.

Between 1990 and 2050 the number of black elderly is expected to quadruple and the Hispanic elderly population is expected to be seven times larger.

There is a *disparity in longevity* between ethnic groups. Life expectancy at birth is 80 years for white females, 74 years for black females, 73 years for white males, and 65 years for black males. However, longevity is increasing in U.S. ethnic groups. (About one fifth of elderly blacks and elderly Hispanics were 80 + in 1990 and this is expected to increase to about one third for blacks and over one third for Hispanics by 2050).

There is *economic disparity* between ethnic groups. Approximately 33 percent of elderly blacks, 22 percent of elderly Hispanics, and 11 percent of elderly whites live in poverty. The lifetime employment earnings for elderly whites are significantly higher than the earnings for elderly blacks and Hispanics. This implies fewer retirement resources for blacks and Hispanics.

From U.S. Bureau of the Census: *Sixty-five plus in the United States*, Special Studies, P 23-190, Washington, D.C., 1996, U.S. Government Printing Office, pp. v, vi, 2-4.

Developmental Tasks of Aging

Aging is a stage of human development and has specific *developmental tasks*. Accomplishing these tasks assists the individual in self-fulfillment and personal growth (Figure 20-2). Developmental tasks for the elderly person include maintaining appropriate and satisfying living arrangements, adjusting to retirement, safeguarding physical and mental health, continuing a social network of friends and family, and maintaining an active role in the community. Accomplishing developmental tasks often involves role reorientation as children are launched from the home, retirement occurs, reverse caregiver roles are assumed with elderly parents, and changes in health status alters one's functional abilities.

According to Erikson (1982), older persons are faced with resolving the psychological conflict of *integrity versus despair*. The successful accomplishment of integrity occurs when individuals review their lives, accept what they have done, and feel satisfied with what they have accomplished. If this does not occur the older person may experience despair and depression and may become dissatisfied with life.

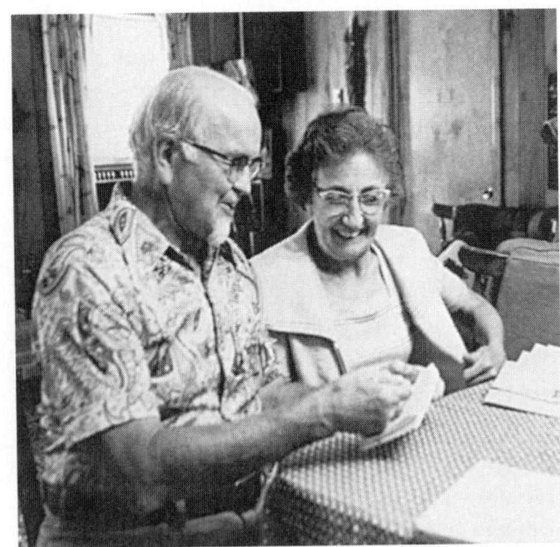

Figure 20-2 An aging couple.

The end result of the aging process is death, and nurses, the aged, and their families must come to terms with helping the client and family work through this final stage of life and human development. Nurses should evaluate their own feelings and thoughts about death and dying to enhance client care.

HEALTHY PEOPLE 2000 AND AGING

Healthy People 2000 (USDHHS, 1991) addressed the health of older Americans and formulated a national health goal to increase the span of healthy life for all Americans (USDHHS, p. 6). Almost 30 specific national health objectives for the elderly are integrated throughout the document. These objectives are displayed in the box on the next page. The nurse should be familiar with these objectives, understand their impact on nursing care, and be at the forefront of their accomplishment.

According to *Healthy People 2000*, the most important aspect of health promotion for older people is to maintain health and functional independence (USDHHS, 1991, pp. 24, 587). The document notes that a significant number of the health problems evidenced with aging are either preventable or can be controlled by preventive activities, and that strong social support is important in promoting the health of older adults (USDHHS, p. 587).

Unfortunately, many older people are not adequately participating in preventive health activities in relation to exercise, nutrition, immunizations, and health care visits, and many communities across the nation do not have programs that adequately meet the needs of older adults. Less than a third of the noninstitutionalized elderly report participation in moderate physical activity, such as walking and gardening on a regular basis; less than 10% routinely engage in vigorous physical activity; only 10% receive pneumococcal vaccine and 20% receive influenza vaccines; and many do not have adequate nutritional intake or regular physical examinations and screenings (USDHHS, 1991, p. 587). Changing unhealthy lifestyle patterns can improve health and reduce the likelihood of disability. Nurses need to encourage elderly clients to take part in preventive health activities.

Across the the nation agencies are working to meet national health objectives and promote healthy aging. In the public sector numerous federal, state, and local agencies are working to promote healthy aging. The National Institute on Aging has provided significant leadership in this endeavor. In the private sector, the American Association of Retired Persons (AARP) has been a lead organization in promoting health promotion activities that assist older Americans in reaching *Healthy People 2000* objectives (USDHHS, 1995, p. 156). Both AARP and the National Council on the Aging (NCOA) have developed health promotion programs and publications targeting older Americans. These programs frequently address leading causes of morbidity and mortality among the elderly and provide strategies for reducing health risks.

ELDER MORBIDITY AND MORTALITY

Major causes of death among people aged 65 and older are heart disease, cancer, stroke, chronic obstructive pulmonary disease, pneumonia, and influenza (USDHHS, 1991, p. 587; U.S. Preventive Services Task Force, 1996). In relation to morbidity, the most frequently occurring chronic problems among noninstitutionalized elderly persons include arthritis (50%), hypertension (36%), heart disease (32%), hearing impairments (29%), orthopedic impairments (16%), sinusitis (15%), and diabetes (10%) (AARP, 1996, p. 13). Other chronic conditions include depression, osteoporosis, incontinence, digestive disorders, constipation, chronic pain, sleep disturbance, Alzheimer's disease, and dementia. Principal reasons for office visits to primary care providers and common diagnoses in older clients are given in Table 20-1.

Chronic conditions can have a great impact on quality of life and a person's ability to carry out activities of daily living. As discussed in Chapter 19, the incidence of chronic conditions increases with age, and these conditions can significantly affect physical functioning and activities of daily living (Figure 20-3). Elderly persons most affected by health limitations are women, the poor, and minorities. However, income has a greater effect than race and gender on activity limitation. Improving functional independence in late life and limiting the effects of chronic conditions is an important part of health promotion for older adults. The number of days in which usual activities are restricted because of illness or injury increases with age. Older people average 35 days a year of restricted activity (AARP, 1996, p. 12). Many elderly Americans are on medication regimens.

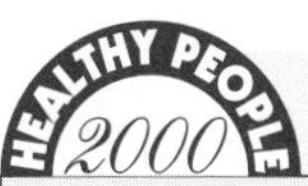

Objectives Targeting Older Adults

HEALTH STATUS OBJECTIVES

Reduce suicides among white men aged 65 and older to no more than 39.2 per 100,000.

Reduce deaths among people age 70 and older caused by motor vehicle crashes to no more than 20 per 100,000.

Reduce deaths among people aged 65 through 84 from falls and fall-related injuries to no more than 14.4 per 100,000.

Reduce deaths among people aged 85 and older from falls and fall-related injuries to no more than 105 per 100,000.

Reduce residential fire deaths among people aged 65 and older to no more than 3.3 per 100,000.

Reduce hip fractures among people aged 65 and older so that hospitalizations for this condition are no more than 607 per 100,000.

Reduce to no more than 20 percent the proportion of people aged 65 and older who have lost all of their natural teeth.

Increase years of healthy life to at least 65 years.

Reduce to no more than 90 per 1,000 people the proportion of all people aged 65 and older who have difficulty in performing two or more personal care activities, thereby preserving independence.

Reduce significant hearing impairment among people aged 45 and older to a prevalence of no more than 180 per 1,000.

Reduce significant visual impairment among people aged 65 and older to a prevalence of no more than 70 per 1,000.

Reduce epidemic-related pneumonia and influenza deaths among people aged 65 and older to no more than 7.3 per 100,000.

Reduce pneumonia-related days of restricted activity for people aged 65 and older.

RISK REDUCTION OBJECTIVES

Increase to at least 30 percent the proportion of people aged 65 and older who engage regularly, preferably daily, in light to moderate physical activity for at least 30 minutes per day.

Reduce to no more than 22 percent the proportion of people aged 65 and older who engage in no leisure-time physical activity.

Increase immunization levels for pneumococcal pneumonia and influenza immunization among institutionalized chronically ill or older people to at least 80 percent.

Increase to at least 40 percent the proportion of adults aged 65 and older who have received, as a minimum within the appropriate interval, all of the screening and immunization services and at least one of the counseling services appropriate for their age and gender as recommended by the U.S. Preventive Services Task Force.

SERVICES AND PROTECTION OBJECTIVES

Increase to at least 80 percent the receipt of home food services by people aged 65 and older who have difficulty in preparing their own meals or are otherwise in need of home-delivered meals.

Increase to at least 90 percent the proportion of people aged 65 and older who had the opportunity to participate during the preceding year in at least one organized health promotion program through a senior center, lifecare facility, or other community-based setting that serves older adults.

Increase to at least 30 the number of States that have design standards for signs, signals, markings, lighting, and other characteristics of the roadway environment to improve the visual stimuli and protect the safety of older drivers and pedestrians.

Increase to at least 75 percent the proportion of primary care providers who routinely review with their patients aged 65 and older all prescribed and over-the-counter medicines taken by their patients each time a new medication is prescribed.

Extend to all long-term institutional facilities the requirement that oral examinations and services be provided no later than 90 days after entry into these facilities.

Increase to at least 60 percent the proportion of people aged 65 and older using the oral health care system during each year.

Increase to at least 80 percent the proportion of women aged 40 and older who have ever received a clinical breast examination and a mammogram, and to at least 60 percent those aged 50 and older who have received them within the preceding 1 to 2 years.

Increase to at least 95 percent the proportion of women aged 70 and older with uterine cervix who have ever received a Pap test, and to at least 70 percent who received a Pap test within the preceding 1 to 3 years.

Increase to at least 50 percent the proportion of people aged 50 and older who have received fecal occult blood testing within the preceding 1 to 2 years, and to at least 40 percent those who have ever received proctosigmoidoscopy.

Increase to at least 40 percent the proportion of people aged 50 and older visiting a primary care provider in the preceding year who have received oral, skin, and digital rectal examinations during one such visit.

Increase to at least 60 percent the proportion of providers of primary care for older adults who routinely evaluate people aged 65 and older for urinary incontinence and impairments of vision, hearing, cognition, and functional status.

Increase to at least 90 percent the proportion of perimenopausal women who have been counseled about the benefits and risks of estrogen replacement therapy.

From USDHHS: *Healthy People 2000, full report, with commentary*, Washington, D.C., 1991, U.S. Government Printing Office, pp. 588-590.

table 20-1 Primary Care Office Visits Among Older Patients

	Age (Years) 65-74	75 and Older
10 PRINCIPAL REASONS FOR VISIT		
	1. Postoperative visit	1. General medical examination
	2. General medical examination	2. Vision dysfunction
	3. Vision dysfunction	3. Postoperative visit
	4. Glaucoma	4. Glaucoma
	5. Cough	5. Blood pressure check
	6. Diabetes mellitus	6. Cough
	7. Back symptoms	7. Cataract
	8. Hypertension	8. Vertigo or dizziness
	9. Blood pressure check	9. Hypertension
	10. Skin lesion	10. Back symptoms
10 MOST COMMON DIAGNOSES		
	1. Essential hypertension	1. Essential hypertension
	2. Diabetes mellitus	2. Glaucoma
	3. Glaucoma	3. Cataract
	4. Cataract	4. Diabetes mellitus
	5. Chronic ischemic heart disease	5. Chronic ischemic heart disease
	6. Osteoarthritis	6. Osteoarthritis
	7. Dermatoses	7. Cardiac dysrhythmias
	8. Cardiac dysrhythmias	8. Organ or tissue replacement
	9. Lipid disorders	9. Dermatoses
	10. Bronchitis	10. Heart failure

From U.S. Department of Health and Human Services, Public Health Service: National Ambulatory Medical Care Survey: 1991 Summary, *Vital Health Statistics*, Series 13, No. 116, May 1994. In Ham RJ, Sloane PD: *Primary care geriatrics: a case-based approach*, ed 3, St. Louis, 1997, Mosby, p. 5.

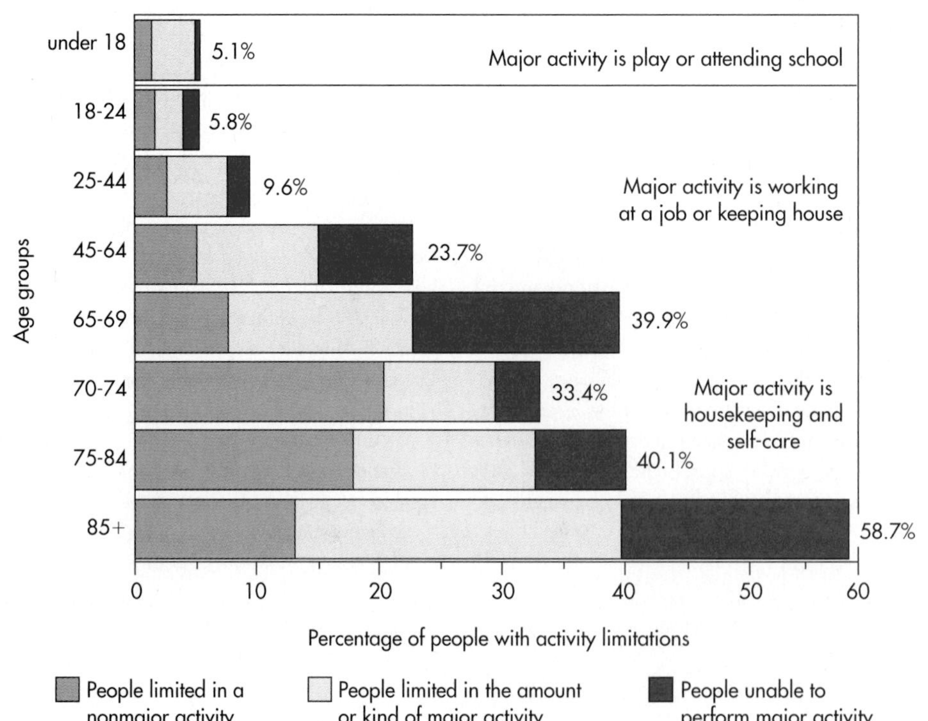

Figure 20-3 Activity limitations of all degrees by age groups. *(From Kraus LE, Stoddard S:* Chartbook on disability in the United States, an InfoUse Report, *Washington, D.C., March 1989, U.S. National Institute on Disability and Rehabilitation Research, p. 10.)*

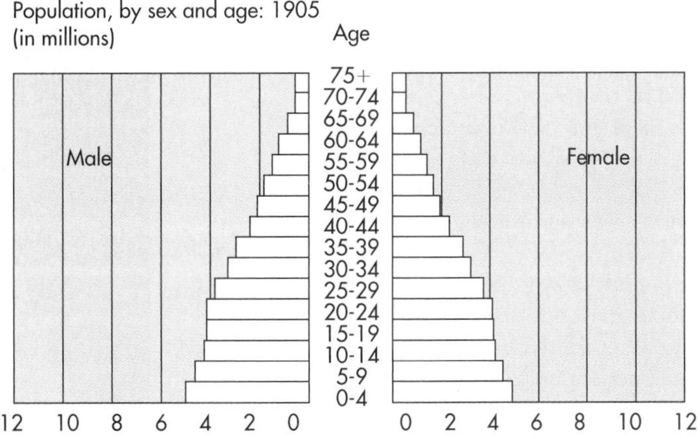

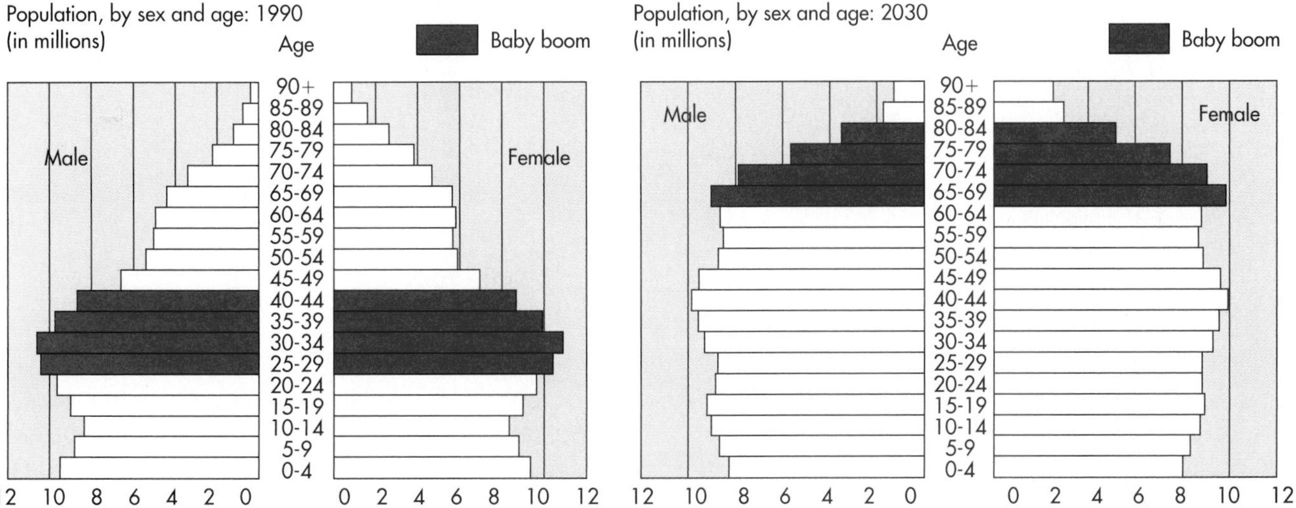

Figure 20-4 Population characteristics by age and sex, United States 1905, 1990, and 2030. *(From U.S. Bureau of the Census:* Sixty-five plus in America, *Washington, D.C., 1992, U.S. Government Printing Office, pp. 1-2, 2-4, 2-9.)*

HEALTH CARE EXPENDITURES

Although the 65 and older age group represents 12% of the U.S. population, it accounts for 36% of total personal health care expenditures. This amounts to $5360 per older person per year and includes $72 billion in Medicare expenditures and $20 billion in Medicaid expenditures (AARP, 1996, p. 14). About $1500 of these expenditure came from direct payment "out-of-pocket" expenditures by the elderly individual (AARP, p. 14). These expenditures are more than four times the amount spent by younger persons on personal health care (AARP, p. 14). Older people account for 37% of all hospital stays and 47% of all hospital days (AARP, p. 14). Hospital expenses (42%) are the largest part of health expenditures for the elderly, followed by physicians (21%) and nursing home care (20%) (AARP, p. 14).

DEMOGRAPHICS AND AGING: UNITED STATES

In colonial times half the U.S. population was under age 16, and only a few people lived to the age of 65 (U.S. Bureau of the Census, 1992, p. 2-1). Since 1900 there has been over a tenfold increase in older people (from 3 million to 32 million), and the percentage of the population age 65 and older has tripled (from 4% to 12%). Figure 20-4 illustrates the aging of America and how it is expected to continue. Analysis of this figure shows that by the year 2030 there will be as many people 65 and older in the United States as there are people under the age of 20. The box on the next page gives some descriptive information on aging and the elderly in the United States.

Of particular interest is the most rapidly growing age group in the United States, Americans age 85 and older, the "oldest old." Figure 20-5 displays the growth of this age group in the United States from 1900 to 2050. Today there are more than 50,000 centenarians in the United States, and it is predicted that there will be more than 1 million within the next 50 years (U.S. Bureau of the Census, 1992, p. 1). A rapidly growing population of older Americans has significant implications for nursing and health care.

Aging in the United States

A child born today can expect to live to be 75+ years of age, compared to age 47 for a child born in 1900.

The elderly population increased more than 20% over the last decade. (Among American elderly, 19 million are age 65 to 74, 11 million are age 75 to 84, and 4 million are 85+.)

Elders age 85+ are the most rapidly growing segment of our population.

From 2010 to 2030 the elderly population is expected to **increase** 73% while the population under age 65 will **decrease** almost 3%. By 2040 we could have more people aged 65 or older than we have persons under 20 years of age.

More than half of the elderly live in the nine states of California, New York, Florida, Pennsylvania, Texas, Illinois, Ohio, New Jersey, and Michigan. Each of these states has more than 1 million elderly residents, and California has the largest number (over 3 million) while Florida has the largest proportion (18.6%).

Elderly women outnumber elderly men three to two.

Only 5% of American elderly reside in institutional settings such as nursing homes.

The majority of noninstitutionalized elderly (68%) live in a family setting, and about 30% live alone.

Data from American Association of Retired Persons: *A profile of older Americans 1995,* Washington, D.C., 1996, AARP; and U.S. Bureau of the Census: *Sixty-five plus in America,* Washington, D.C., 1992, U.S. Government Printing Office, pp. v, 1-1 to 1-2.

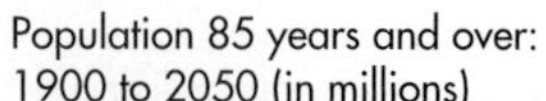

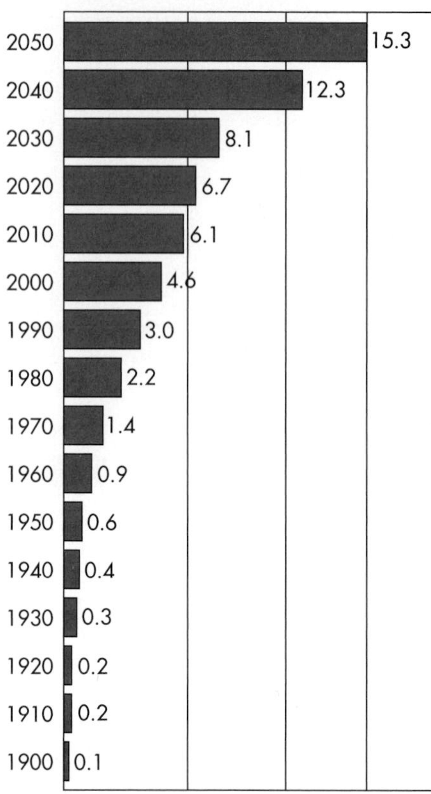

Figure 20-5 U.S. population 85 years and over: 1900 to 2050. *(From U.S. Bureau of the Census:* Sixty-five plus in America, *Washington, D.C., 1992, U.S. Government Printing Office, p. 2-10.)*

Employment and Retirement

The number of older workers increased by almost 1 million in the last decade, and almost 4 million older Americans are working (Upward Trend, 1996). The National Council on the Aging (NCOA) offers the Senior Community Service Employment Program and works with employers in helping them to see the advantages of hiring older workers and keeping them in the workplace.

Retirement is a rather contemporary phenomenon. Before the passage of the retirement provisions of the Social Security Act of 1935 (see Chapter 4), few Americans could afford to retire. With the advent of retirement benefits people were able to retire from work and enjoy life's later years. Today people are spending more years than ever before in retirement.

Many older people work and provide community service in voluntary positions. Programs such as the Retired Senior Volunteer Programs (RSVP) and the Service Corps of Retired Executives (SCORE) are active in many communities. Information on such programs can usually be obtained through local Area Agencies on Aging. It has been estimated that one in four older Americans performs volunteer community services.

A strong correlation exists between successful retirement and retirement planning. The nurse can be instrumental in helping people recognize the need for retirement planning and can assist persons in seeing the options open to them, make them aware of community resources, and offer support and guidance during this stage of transition.

NCOA and AARP have information available that assists in planning for retirement, and many workplaces have retirement planning programs. Planning for retirement is more than just financial planning; it is planning for the entire retirement experience. Retirement is a time for role restructuring and major decisions such as choosing where one will live; deciding on a new or part-time career; determining educational, recreational, and leisure pursuits; addressing relationships with friends and family; and reassessing finances. For many, retirement is the first time they have significant amounts of time for leisure and recreational pursuits.

Income

In old age, especially after retirement, many Americans live on relatively fixed incomes. The median income of older persons is approximately $16,500 a year for men and

$9400 for women (AARP, 1996, p. 9). Almost 4 million older Americans live in poverty, and another 2 million are classified as "near-poor" (having incomes between the poverty level and 125% of this level) (AARP, p. 10). Older women, minorities, and the "oldest old" are more likely to live in poverty.

The major source of income for older Americans is Social Security (AARP, 1996, p. 10). Private pension plans provide approximately 19% of the income of those 65 and older (AARP, p. 10). However, less than half of the elderly are receiving such pensions (USDHHS, 1992, p. 8). Only 8% of the elderly receive public assistance, 6% receive food stamps, and 12% receive Medicaid (AARP, 1996, p. 10).

Housing

Safe, appropriate housing is a major concern for the elderly. Many elders continue to live independently in their own homes. Of the almost 21 million households headed by older Americans, 78% were owners and 22% were renters (AARP, 1996, p. 11). About one third of older renter households live in publicly subsidized housing (AARP, p. 10). Many communities offer "senior housing" units to the elderly that are rented on a sliding scale basis. However, recent budget cuts in federal spending for housing and community development have placed close to 1 million older adults on waiting lists for subsidized housing (NCOA, 1993, p. 18).

NCOA has a national goal of decent, affordable, safe, and appropriate housing for senior citizens (NCOA, 1993, p. 18). Innovative housing ideas for the elderly are being developed, including home sharing, home equity conversion, group homes, "granny flats," and home renovations that suit the individual's changing needs. The Center for Independent Living discussed in Chapter 19 helps develop innovative floor plans and interior designs that aid the elderly person in independent living.

Whether to live in their own homes or apartments, live with relatives, or live in a long-term care facility are just some of the many issues that confront the elderly. Appropriate housing helps promote self-esteem, provides comfort, encourages socialization, and prevents or delays the costly alternative of institutionalization (NCOA, 1993, p. 18).

Education

The educational level of the older population is increasing. In the last 25 years the percentage of elders who had completed high school in the United States rose from 28% to 62%, and about 13% of these had a bachelor's degree or higher (AARP, 1996, p. 12). It is not uncommon for older people to return to school or have advanced degrees. Programs such as Elderhostel have emerged around the country and enable elders to continue their education throughout life. Better-educated consumers are scrutinizing their health care more and demanding care appropriate to their needs.

NORMAL BODY CHANGES IN AGING

Aging is a natural and lifelong process. As we age, physical, psychosocial, and emotional changes occur. The physical, mental, and psychological changes associated with aging occur very gradually and are highly individual (e.g., less than 1% of the physical function an individual has at age 30 is lost each succeeding year). Listed in Table 20-2 are some physical changes that occur with aging and their implications for care. These changes must be taken into account if the client's potential for health and wellness is to be maximized. For instance, smooth muscle weakness and muscle atrophy often lead to constipation with older people. However, diet and exercise can help to overcome this problem.

Other changes that come with aging include thinning of the vaginal walls, increasing vaginal dryness, and atrophy of the testes. As a result of physical changes, sexual experiences may differ from those of earlier years but can still be fulfilling and pleasurable. In a research study by Johnson (1996) elders were found to be interested, active, and satisfied with a variety of sexual activities even in the presence of a number of health concerns. Sexuality is an important component of the lives of elders; however, it is often overlooked by health care professionals. Some questions that the nurse can ask in obtaining a sexual health history from the older adult are given in the box on page 613. The community health nurse can help answer clients' questions and assist them in fulfilling their sexuality.

Numerous books have been written for elders who wish to remain healthy and enjoy old age. The noted psychologist B.F. Skinner has written (with M.E. Vaughn) *Enjoy Old Age: A Program of Self-Management* (1983) out of his own life experience; Maggie Kuhn has written *Maggie Kuhn on Aging* (1977); Alex Comfort has written *Say Yes to Old Age: Developing a Positive Attitude Toward Aging* (1990); and Lydia Bronte has written *The Longevity Factor* (1993). A common theme in all of these books is that aging is individual and old age can be a time of continued growth, development, and fulfillment. Americans are fortunate to live in a country where they are able to grow old. They need to take advantage of, and look forward to, this opportunity for a long and active life.

SOME CONSIDERATIONS IN HEALTH PROMOTION OF THE AGED

Most older people generally view their health positively. More than 70% of older people living in the community describe their health as excellent, very good, or good (AARP, 1996, p. 12). There was little difference between the sexes on their rating of health; however, older blacks were much more likely to relate their health as fair or poor (43%) than older whites (27%) (AARP, p. 12).

Although most elders consider themselves healthy, a medical model that focuses on secondary and tertiary prevention and disease pathology has historically dominated the provision of health care. In line with *Healthy People*

table 20-2 Physical Changes with Age

Change	Implications
SKELETAL SYSTEM	
1. Drying out of vertebral disks	1. Postural changes and decreased stature (average loss of 2 inches)
2. Muscle atrophy	2. Diminished strength and balance
3. Decalcification of bones	3. Osteoporosis, increased risk of fractures
4. Ossification of joint cartilage	4. Joint pain and stiffness
GASTROINTESTINAL SYSTEM	
1. Diminished production of hydrochloric acid	1. Impaired digestion and absorption
2. Decreased salivary gland secretion	2. Impaired digestion
3. Delayed emptying of the stomach and esophagus	3. Feeling of "fullness," gastric reflux
4. Decreased peristalsis	4. Slowed digestion and absorption
RESPIRATORY SYSTEM	
1. Increase in residual lung volume and decrease in vital capacity	1. Impaired ventilation and reduced ability to cough or breathe deeply
2. Loss of elasticity of lung tissue and decrease in muscle structure	2. Difficulty breathing; increased episodes of shortness of breath and dyspnea on exertion
3. Decrease in oxygen exchange between the alveoli and capillaries	3. Less oxygen available; dyspnea on exertion
NEUROLOGICAL SYSTEM	
1. Decrease in size and weight of brain and in number of neurons	1. Slower nerve transmission; thought and memory changes
2. Spinal cord synapse degeneration	2. Diminished coordination
3. Optic and auditory nerve degeneration	3. Diminished vision and hearing
GENITOURINARY SYSTEM	
1. Bladder: loss of muscle tone	1. Incomplete bladder emptying that can result in urinary retention and cystitis
2. Pelvic muscle and sphincter relaxation	2. Urinary incontinence
3. Kidney: reduced blood flow and filtration; interstitial fibrosis	3. Fluid and electrolyte imbalance
4. Atrophy of ovarian, uterine, vaginal tissues; thinning of vaginal walls	4. Decreased vaginal lubrication; decreased vaginal elasticity; loss of fertility; stress incontinence
5. Diminished spermatogenesis; atrophy of testes, enlargement of prostrate	5. Increased time for erection; reduced volume of seminal fluid; reduced force of ejaculation; frequency of urination

2000 elder health care should focus on primary prevention and health promotion. Still, many preventive health care needs of the elderly go unmet.

Older people grew up with a health care system that did not focus on preventive health activities. Studies have shown that older people go to the doctor primarily when something is wrong; have trouble with the idea of having tests done when they have no symptoms; and do not know when to request tests or what to expect from them (AARP, 1991, p. 15).

NCOA sponsors the Health Promotion Institute. This institute works to promote the ongoing development of preventive services that will enhance awareness among older Americans of the importance of health promotion activities. AARP sponsors the National Eldercare Institute on Health Promotion, which works to promote wellness among older Americans and to stimulate development of health promotion programs. Both organizations offer publications and materials on health education for seniors.

Health promotion activities can assist in changing or eliminating risk factors such as lack of exercise, cigarette smoking, excessive alcohol intake, high-cholesterol diets, and environmental exposures. Such activities can help to postpone or avoid chronic diseases and conditions. *Healthy People 2000* has set an objective to increase to at least 90% the proportion of people aged 65 and older who have the opportunity to participate in at least one organized health promotion program through a senior center, lifecare facility, or other community-based setting that serves older adults each year (USDHHS, 1991, p. 589). Health promotion activities such as regular physical examinations, exercise, safety, and good nutrition play a significant role in promoting healthy aging.

Physical Examinations

The report of the U.S. Public Health Service (1994), *Put Prevention Into Practice*, outlined a preventive care timeline for periodic health examination of adults extending to the

table 20-2 Physical Changes with Age—cont'd

Change	Implications
NUTRITION AND METABOLISM	
1. Vitamin and mineral deficiencies	1. Capillary fragility and bruising; anemia; malnutrition; bone demineralization; inflammation of mucous membranes
2. Altered digestive processes	2. Impaired taste, digestion, and absorption of food
3. Dentition: lost teeth, ill-fitting dentures	3. Impaired appetite; malnutrition; dehydration
4. Inadequate fluid intake	4. Dehydration; fluid and electrolyte imbalance
CARDIOVASCULAR SYSTEM	
1. Thickening and fibrosis of blood vessels	1. Atherosclerotic changes; increased risk for hypertension, heart ischemia, stroke, and myocardial infarction
2. Enlargement of left ventricle	2. Increased risk of congestive heart failure and impaired tissue perfusion; edema
3. Enlargement of right ventricle	3. Reduced oxygenation of blood, pulmonary hypertension
4. Impaired peripheral vascular circulation	4. Decreased tissue nourishment, edema
5. Diminished cardiac output	5. Decreased blood flow and tissue oxygenation
6. Calcification of cardiac valves	6. Heart murmurs and disorders
SKIN AND CUTANEOUS TISSUE	
1. Atrophy of sweat glands and sebaceous glands produce less sebum	1. Decreased perspiration; increased susceptibility to trauma, abrasions, bedsores; skin becomes drier; impaired heat dissipation
2. Deposits of melanin	2. "Age spots" occur
3. Thickening of finger and toenails	3. Splintering of nails; difficulty in cutting nails; increased risk of infection
4. Loss of subcutaneous fat and water in the epidermis	4. Wrinkling of skin; decreased turgor; slower wound healing
IMMUNE SYSTEM	
1. Decreased ability to make antibodies and mount an immune response	1. Increased risk of infection
SENSORY	
1. Lens of eye becomes more opaque and rigid; lens yellows	1. Decreased ability to focus on near objects (presbyopia); increased sensitivity to glare; increased difficulty with color discrimination; peripheral vision decreases
2. Size of pupil decreases	2. Need brighter light to see
3. Odor identification declines	3. Decreased appetite
4. Taste buds decrease in number	4. Decreased sense of taste and diminished appetite

Sexual Health History

- ❑ 1. Are you currently sexually active?
- ❑ 2. Are you currently active with more than one partner?
- ❑ 3. What kinds of protection do you and your partner use during sexual activity?
- ❑ 4. How has your illness and/or medications affected your sexual activity?
- ❑ 5. Do you have questions or concerns about your sexual activity?
- ❑ 6. Have you ever had a sexually transmitted disease, or knowingly been exposed to somebody with a sexually transmitted disease?
- ❑ 7. Have you ever had, or do you now have, discharge, rashes, or sores in the genital area?
- ❑ 8. Is there anything you would like to discuss concerning sexual issues?

From Letvak S, Schoder D: Sexually transmitted diseases in the elderly: what you need to know, *Geriatr Nurs* 17(4):159, 1996.
*Please put a check in the box next to any question you are unsure of how to answer, or which you would like to discuss further with your nurse or physician.

elderly. This timeline is presented in Appendix 17-1. Physical examinations can help to detect conditions early and prevent complications. For example, a sigmoidoscopy can detect polyps that 10 years later might have become cancer of the colon, and early detection of diabetes can help keep the disease and its related conditions under control. Physical examinations are a perfect time to discuss personal health habits regarding sleep, nutrition, exercise, alcohol, and smoking. They are also a time when the elder can share health concerns with the provider and work in partnership

Periodic health examination protocol

Age	20	30	40	50	60	70+
Physical exam and health risk assessment	Every 5 years		3 years	Every 2 years		Yearly
Blood pressure	Yearly					
Cholesterol	Every 5 years					
Breast and pelvic exam	Every 3 years		Yearly			
Pap smear	Yearly					
Mammography	Baseline at 35		2 years	Yearly		
Stool for blood			3 years	Yearly		
Proctosigmoidoscopy				Every 3 years (after 2 yearly negatives)		
Immunizations	Tetanus/diphtheria—every 10 years Influenza—yearly after age 65 Pneumovax—at age 65					

Figure 20-6 Periodic health examinations. *(From Annual checkups—who needs them,* Aging, *365:2, 1993.)*

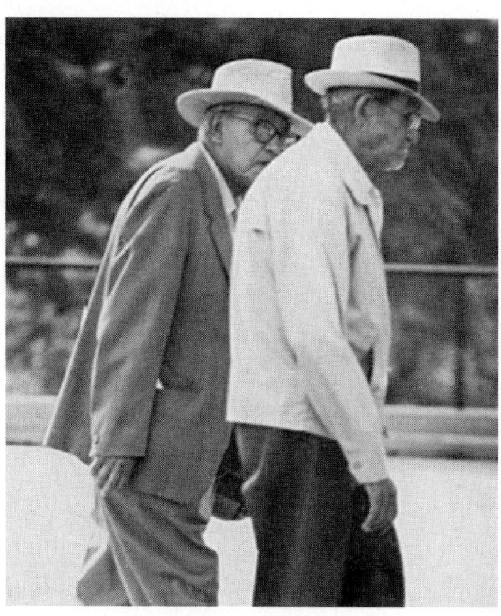

Figure 20-7 Nurses should stress the benefit of exercise to health. Exercising with a friend battles loneliness. *(Courtesy Ken Yamaguchi. In Castillo HM:* The nurse assistant in long-term care: a rehabilitative approach. *St. Louis, 1992, Mosby.)*

to develop a plan of care. A schedule of when periodic health examinations should be done is given in Figure 20-6.

Exercise

Regular exercise helps optimize physical and mental health throughout life. Physiological decline associated with aging may actually be the result of inactivity. Clinical evidence indicates that conditions such as osteoporosis, arterial and venous insufficiency, gastrointestinal stasis, and musculoskeletal stiffness are increased in inactive elders (Ham, Sloane, 1997, p. 105).

A survey by the National Center for Health Statistics showed that exercise can help prevent disease and extend and improve the quality of life; however, less than one fourth of older Americans exercise regularly (National Resource Center on Health Promotion and Aging [NRCHPA], 1991, p. 11). In research by O'Neill and Reid (1991) 87% of the elderly in the study perceived at least one major barrier that prevented their involvement in physical activity, such as an existing health problem or lack of knowledge about exercise resources and regimes (Figure 20-7).

Increased levels of physical activity are associated with reduced incidence of coronary heart disease, hypertension, obesity, stroke, osteoporosis, depression, and anxiety (Ham, Sloane, 1997, p. 105). Exercise has the potential to improve sleep, mobility, strength and balance, mood, and increase life span. *Healthy People 2000* has set objectives to increase the proportion of elderly people who engage regularly in light to moderate physical activity (USDHHS, 1995, p. 162).

According to Ham and Sloane (1997), "The right amount of exercise in old age is 'more exercise than yesterday.' For the sedentary older person the recommendation should be for slow reacquisition of regular, low-impact, unstressed but progressively increasing exercise" (p. 105). Research by Schaller (1996) indicated that Tai

Chi Chih was a safe and enjoyable form of exercise in older adults.

As with everyone else, older people with existing diseases and conditions should consult their primary care provider before beginning an exercise program. In general, swimming, walking, bicycling, and stationary cross-country skiing are all excellent exercises for the elderly (Ham, Sloane, 1997, p. 105). Many communities have YMCAs, YWCAs, and senior and fitness centers that offer senior exercise programs. Each person will want to assess what best meets his or her needs.

Safety

Accidents are one of the leading causes of death among the elderly. *Healthy People 2000* has numerous objectives that address the need to reduce in older adults accidental injuries from falls, motor vehicle accidents, and fires (USDHHS, 1995, p. 202). Factors that contribute to accidents are weakness, slowed reaction time, uncertain gait, changes in hearing and vision, and medications. Many accidents occur in the home and could be prevented if people followed simple safety rules and eliminated hazards in the home environment. Once an accident has occurred it is important to gather specific information on the location of the accident and environmental contributors to its occurrence.

Seventy percent of fall-related deaths occur in elders over age 75, and the mortality associated with falling increases logarithmically with age (Ham, Sloane, 1997, p. 312). Postural hypotension is frequently associated with falling in the elderly. Up to half of elderly patients hospitalized for a fall do not survive another year, and a fall is a potent marker of future morbidity (Ham, Sloane, p. 312). One in four community-dwelling elders experiences at least one episode of falling each year, and the incidence is greatly increased in nursing home residents (Sattin, 1992, p. 489). Fear of falls and their resultant injuries limits the activities of many older people.

Since most falls occur in or around the home, the home should be assessed for safety hazards and made as safe as possible. Stairs and bathrooms are the most dangerous locations for falls. Stairs should be adequately lighted, free of clutter, and equipped with handrails and nonskid surfaces. It may be helpful to outline the edge of each step with a luminescent or contrast tape or color and to paint top and bottom steps in colors that make them easily noticed. Bathrooms should have hand rails, nonslip adhesive surfaces in tubs and showers, and nonslip flooring.

Other safety precautions around the home include having enough light; having light switches within easy reach; using a light when getting up at night; using nonskid soles on shoes; eliminating throw rugs, casters on chairs, and extension cords; avoiding sedation; and placing distinct labels on medications and toxic substances. Smoking in bed should be eliminated. To avoid accidental scaldings and burns, lowering hot water heater temperatures and labeling hot and cold water faucets is helpful. Only safe home heating methods should be used to minimize the chance of smoke and fires. Carbon monoxide and smoke detectors should be a part of every elder's home.

Having a telephone or emergency responder system in the home is an important safety measure. The telephone and emergency numbers should be in a convenient, accessible location—often at the bedside. Telephone services such as "Friendly Caller" programs help give the elderly person contact with the outside world, reduce social isolation, and promote safety.

Crime and the elderly is another safety concern. Contrary to popular belief, the elderly have the lowest victimization rates of any age group in our society except for "personal larcency with contact" (i.e., purse snatching and pickpocketing) (Harris, 1990, p. 400). Common crimes against the elderly include purse snatchings, fraud, theft, vandalism, and harassment. Consumer fraud, confidence games, and medical quackery are major forms of crime against the elderly (Harris, p. 406). Research shows that the elderly rank fear of crime as a major concern (Harris, p. 401) and that this fear may add to their social isolation.

The nurse can be of assistance in making seniors aware of the health risks of accidents and in helping to prevent them. The nurse can also help older adults understand that safety is an area over which they have control, and that safety precautions can help to promote health and maintain quality of life. Older adults owe it to themselves to play it safe.

Nutrition

Nutrition is an important aspect of health across the life span. Researchers have estimated that 15% to 50% of those age 65 and older have poor nutrition or are malnourished (Greely, 1991). *Healthy People 2000* has set an objective to increase to at least 80% the receipt of home food services by people age 65 and older who have difficulty in preparing their own meals or are otherwise in need of home-delivered meals (USDHHS, 1991, p. 589).

A number of epidemiological studies have demonstrated that nutritional deficiencies are prevalent with older people and that older people are at a greater risk for malnutrition than other age groups (Lueckenotte, 1996, p. 206). Many older persons have at least one chronic condition that could improve with proper nutrition. Poor nutrition among older people occurs as a result of a number of problems such as illness, lack of proper hydration, oral health problems, poverty, medications, social isolation, and mobility limitations (Malnutrition, 1993, p. 4).

Nutrition plays an important part in maintaining health, independence, and quality of life for older Americans. Eating the proper foods can help older Americans to lower their risks of health problems such as high blood pressure, osteoporosis, diabetes, heart disease, and cancer (NRCHPA, 1991, p. 9). The aging process can actually be slowed through eating well (Greely, 1991).

The Nutrition Screening Initiative is a national program sponsored by the American Academy of Family Physicians, the American Dietetic Association, and NCOA. It is committed to the identification of nutritional problems in older persons, improved elder nutrition, and improved delivery of nutrition services to the elderly. The Initiative has developed a checklist that can be helpful to the nurse when initiating discussion about diet and nutrition (Figure 20-8).

Deficiencies in intake of protein, calcium, iron, and vitamins C and A are common among elderly persons. Foods such as cheeses, yogurt, and buttermilk may help to meet these deficiencies and are good sources of protein. Some suggestions for a longer, healthier life through good nutrition, along with select dietary recommendations for the elderly, are given in the Teaching Tips box.

Fluids are necessary to maintain kidney function, aid in the absorption of medications and high-fiber foods, decrease side effects of some medications, aid in expectoration, soften stools, and prevent dehydration. The aging process may reduce the thirst sensation, and some elders limit fluid intake to ease problems with urinary incontinence. Adequate water intake is an essential part of good nutrition.

In general, elders should eat a variety of foods; maintain a desirable weight; avoid fried and fatty foods; eat an adequate amount of fiber-rich foods; and avoid too much sugar and starch (Greely, 1991). If a person is not getting adequate nutrition from their daily diet then supplements should be taken.

GETTING SENIORS TO EAT WELL The community health nurse plays an important role in senior nutrition counseling, helping elders to realize that their physical, emotional, and economic status all play a part in good nutrition. Getting seniors to eat well and pay attention to nutrition is a complex challenge. Problems such as ill-fitting dentures, loss of teeth, and periodontal disease make chewing painful and can make it difficult to maintain good nutrition. Also, a decreased sense of smell directly affects the elderly person's ability to taste and enjoy food, and certain medications can depress appetite or taste sensations. Other factors, such as diminished efficiency of the digestive and excretory systems, reduced income, and loneliness and depression affect nutritional status.

Older people living alone are especially vulnerable to the problems of inadequate nutrition, often losing interest in meal planning and preparation. Eating with others helps to make mealtimes more enjoyable (Promoting, 1993, p. 9). The frail elderly may lack the dexterity and energy to feed themselves and thus pose a unique nutritional challenge.

The nurse should implement a nutritional assessment such as a 3-day diet recall to assist in evaluating a client's nutritional status and needs. Such a recall can lead to discussions of food preparation and preferences, buying habits, and eating problems, and can be an excellent teaching tool. Older persons have developed a lifetime of food practices, and the nurse needs to remember that nutritional habits are not easy to change. Also, cultural, ethnic and religious beliefs, as well as income, strongly influence nutritional practices (Figure 20-9).

Cutting food costs is difficult when food prices keep increasing and senior income remains relatively constant. The nurse can assist in low-cost food buying and preparation. Ingenuity in using dried legumes, beans, whole cereal grains, poultry, fish, dried fortified milk, and less expensive cuts of meat is often helpful. Although not always inexpensive, foods such as low-fat cheeses and yogurt are good sources of protein and keep well when refrigerated.

Many seniors are not aware of the meal programs in the community that can help to stretch their food budget, such as food stamps, Meals on Wheels, and meals at senior centers. Alternating meal preparation with someone else, and "Meal Clubs," where meal preparation responsibilities are shared, can help curb food costs, offer variety to meals, and provide companionship. Cooking in larger quantities and freezing foods may be a helpful idea. Many local restaurants offer senior discounts, and local churches frequently sponsor meals for seniors.

Serving foods in an attractive, pleasant manner often enhances appetite. Fixing foods with different textures and aromas and using flavor boosters such as commercially prepared flavor enhancers and spices can enhance appetite (Promoting, 1993, p. 9). Switching around from food to food during meals (after three bites) helps to prevent sensory adaptation in which the palate becomes less sensitive to taste and food becomes less tasty (Promoting, p. 9). Also, eating each food separately, rather than mixing them, helps increase the ability to taste the food. Good oral hygiene should be encouraged and helps promote appetite.

Physical barriers to proper nutrition need to be considered. Lack of transportation to cost-efficient grocery stores, restaurants, and food programs can pose a nutrition problem. Physical disabilities such as orthopedic problems and poor vision can inhibit the ability to shop. Shopping assistance may be available through local homemaker services, senior centers, or friends and family. Some grocery stores are now providing electric shopping carts that could be useful to the older shopper.

On a national level numerous resources on nutrition and the elderly exist, such as the U.S. Administration on Aging's National Eldercare Institute on Nutrition, which conducts research and provides information on nutrition for the elderly, American Dietetic Association Gerontological Nutritionist Practice Group, and National Meals on Wheels Foundation, which was created to promote public awareness and financially support senior meal programs. These organizations can assist the nurse in obtaining nutrition resources. Local nutritional services to the elderly are often coordinated through senior centers and area offices on aging. When the nutrition problems of the client are

Determine Your Nutritional Health

The warning signs of poor nutritional health are often overlooked. Use this checklist to find out if you or someone you know is at nutritional risk.

Read the statements below. Circle the number in the yes column for those that apply to you or someone you know. For each yes answer score the number in the box. Total your nutritional score.

	Yes
I have an illness or condition that made me change the kind and/or amount of food I eat.	2
I eat fewer than 2 meals per day.	3
I eat few fruits or vegetables, or milk products.	2
I have 3 or more drinks of beer, liquor, or wine almost every day.	2
I have tooth or mouth problems that make it hard for me to eat.	2
I don't always have enough money to buy the food I need.	4
I eat alone most of the time.	1
I take 3 or more different prescribed or over-the-counter drugs a day.	1
Without wanting to, I have lost or gained 10 pounds in the last 6 months.	2
I am not always physically able to shop, cook, and/or feed myself.	2
Total	

Total your nutritional score. If it's —

0-2 **Good!** Recheck your nutritional score in 6 months.

3-5 **You are at moderate nutritional risk.** See what can be done to improve your eating habits and lifestyle. Your office on aging, senior nutrition program, senior citizens center or health department can help. Recheck your nutritional score in 3 months.

6 or more **You are at high nutritional risk.** Bring this checklist the next time you see your doctor, dietitian or other qualified health or social service professional. Talk with them about any problems you may have. Ask for help to improve your nutritional health.

These materials developed and distributed by the Nutrition Screening Initiative, a project of:

American Academy of Family Physicians

The American Dietetic Association

National Council on the Aging, Inc.

Remember that warning signs suggest risk, but do not represent diagnosis of any condition.

Figure 20-8 Nutrition screening checklist. *(From Nutrition Screening Initiative:* Nutrition screening checklist, *Washington, D.C., 1992, a cooperative effort of the American Dietetic Association, the American Academy of Family Physicians, and the National Council on the Aging. Used with permission.)*

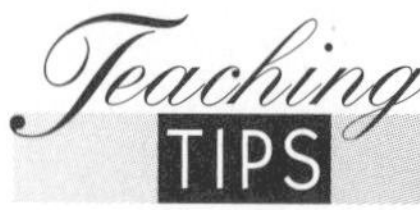

Nutrition for the Elderly

Suggestions for a Longer, Healthier Life through Good Nutrition

Establish good eating patterns now and stick to them. The quality of your diet becomes even more important as you age and is critical in your later years.

To strengthen your body's ability to combat infection and chronic disease, make sure you eat food containing immune-friendly nutrients such as vitamins E and B_6 and the mineral zinc.

To prevent your bones from becoming porous and brittle, choose food rich in vitamin D and calcium.

To ensure your digestive system stays healthy, active, and regular, include at least 20 grams of fiber in your diet every day.

To safeguard your vision and help delay later-life problems such as cataracts, increase your intake of vitamins C, E, and beta-carotene.

To reduce your risk of cardiovascular disease, limit fat, dietary cholesterol, and sodium and focus on sources high in vitamins B_6, B_{12}, and folate, as well as soluble fiber, calcium, and potassium.

To help keep your mind alert and your nervous system performing at its best, vitamins B_6, B_{12}, and folate should be in your diet.

To maintain your idea body weight and keep excess fat off, stay active and choose a diet low in fat, high in complex carbohydrates and dietary fiber.

To keep your appetite hearty and your muscles healthy, mix aerobic exercises (walking or swimming) with simple activities that strengthen muscle.

From Rosenburg IH: As you age: 10 keys to a longer, healthier, more vital life, *Worldview* 5(2):2-3, 1993.

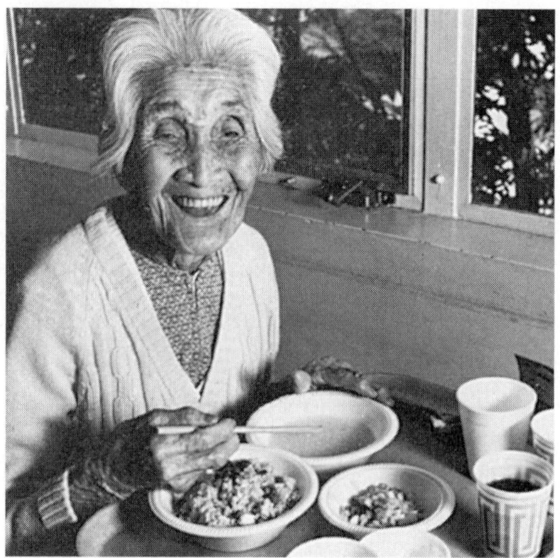

Figure **20-9** Chopsticks and Asian food make the meal enjoyable for this elderly Japanese lady. *(Courtesy Ken Yamaguchi. In Castillo HM:* The nurse assistant in long-term care: a rehabilitative approach, *St. Louis, 1992, Mosby.)*

beyond the scope of the nurse, a nutritionist or physician should be contacted. Many local health departments have nutritionists on the staff; nutritionists are also available through local hospitals and county extension services.

SELECTED HEALTH CONCERNS AMONG THE ELDERLY

Common causes of morbidity and mortality have already been mentioned. Discussion of some selected health concerns in relation to these conditions, such as medications, elder abuse and neglect, and depression follows.

Medications

Older people frequently have chronic disease conditions that require long-term and/or multiple-drug therapy. The elderly account for approximately 30% of all prescription drug use in the United States, more than 400 million prescriptions a year (NRCHPA, 1991, p. 5). By the year 2000 the elderly are expected to account for more than half of all prescription drug use (NRCHPA, p. 5). Additionally, it is estimated that older adults use 40% of all over-the-counter medication on a daily basis (Lueckenotte, 1996, p. 453). Taking all medications into consideration, elders take an average of seven medications daily (Duxbury, 1996, p. 762). Such polypharmacy puts the elder at increased risk of drug interactions and adverse drug reactions (Duxbury, 1996, p. 764; White, 1995, p. 545). Research has repeatedly cited overuse of medications in elders as a major health concern (Lueckenotte, 1996, p. 452).

It is estimated that at least 25% to 50% of elders in the community make errors in their medication regimens (Palmieri, 1991, p. 34), and many tend to self-medicate in terms of increasing or decreasing prescribed medication dosages. Research studies show that older people are frequently confused about their medicines and how to take them (NRCHPA, 1991, p. 5). About 25% of all hospital and nursing home admissions of older Americans result from taking prescriptions incorrectly (NRCHPA, p. 5).

Elders suffer side effects from medications 2 to 3 times more frequently than do younger patients (White, 1995, p. 545). Many drugs induce impairments in elders' mobility and can be a risk factor for falls and other injuries. The physiological changes that come with aging alter how older adults distribute, metabolize, and excrete drugs; make them susceptible to adverse drug effects; and can cause increased plasma levels of drugs (Palmieri, 1991, p. 33). Numerous medications can cause changes in behavior and mental status with elders (Medical Letter, Inc., 1993).

Healthy People 2000 has an age-related objective to increase to at least 75% the number of primary health care providers who routinely review with their patients age 65 and older all prescribed and over-the-counter medicines they are taking each time a new medication is prescribed (USDHHS, 1991, p. 590).

The nurse needs to carefully monitor the medications of elderly clients and explain their medication regimens. The community health nurse is in an excellent position to help clients avoid medication errors and comply with medication regimens. During home visits a medication history is essential. This can be initiated with questions such as, "Let's take yesterday, starting with when you woke in the morning. What was the first medicine you took? How much of the medicine do you take? How many times a day do you take the medication? What do you take the medicine for?" and repeating such questions for all medications involved. Checking a client's medication and assessing for side effects needs to be done on each visit. Appendix 20-1 provides a guide to use when doing a medication assessment with elderly persons. A medication assessment should be completed on a regular basis because factors that affect drug use can change dramatically in a very short time for the elder.

The nurse should be aware that Medicare does *not* pay for the cost of prescription drugs. Some older Americans do not take their prescribed medications properly because they cannot afford to buy them. Elders often omit medications or take less than the prescribed dosage to decrease cost.

Elder Abuse and Neglect

It has been estimated that between 5% and 10% of the elder population, more than 1,000,000 older Americans, are abused and neglected each year (U.S. House Select Committee on Aging, 1990). Mistreated elders are often frail, dependent, over age 70, and women. Typically family members, not strangers, are the perpetrators of this abuse (Ham, Sloane, 1997, p. 361). A major problem with elder abuse and neglect is the "invisibility" of the problem (Miller, 1995, p. 523). Research has suggested that most maltreatment is repeated and is seldom reported to authorities (Miller, p. 521).

Abuse may be *physical* (e.g., slapping, pushing, restraining), *psychological* (e.g., threats, intimidation), or *financial/material* (e.g., misuse or misappropriation of funds or property), or involve *violation of rights* (e.g., forced institutionalization). Without intervention it is unlikely that the abuse will go away, and it often tends to intensify over time (Lynch, 1997, p. 27).

Neglect can be passive, active, or self-neglect. It typically involves withholding necessities of life such as food, medications, and nourishment (Ham, Sloane, 1997, p. 361). *Passive neglect* is the unintentional failure to fulfill a caretaking obligation as a result of things such as ignorance or lack of ability. *Active neglect* is an intentional failure to fulfill a caretaking obligation. *Self-neglect* is a commonly reported form of neglect (National Aging Resource Center on Elder Abuse, 1992). Lack of knowledge regarding the elder's health needs can lead to neglect. Abandonment is a form of neglect and has been dubbed "granny dumping" by some (Hey, Carlson, 1991, p. 1). An example is elders being left at a hospital emergency room by caretakers who no longer want or can handle the responsibility of caregiving (Hey, Carlson, p. 1). Elder abuse is often not reported to appropriate protective agencies. As with other forms of family violence, when it is reported authorities may hesitate to become involved.

LEGISLATION Each state has elder abuse reporting and adult protective services legislation, but state laws vary greatly. Nurses are routinely identified under state protective service laws as mandatory reporters of suspected abuse or neglect. Each state will have a public agency, often the state department of human services, that is responsible for investigating cases of elder abuse.

SIGNS AND SYMPTOMS OF ABUSE AND NEGLECT Detecting elder abuse and neglect is not always easy. Signs and symptoms of elder abuse include bruises, lacerations, pressure sores, fractures; malnutrition; conflicting explanations about the elder's condition; a caregiver describing an elder as "clumsy" or "accident-prone"; sudden changes in the elder's physical or mental state; unusual fears exhibited by the elder; abnormal caregiver behavior; social isolation of the elder by a caregiver; and indifference or hostility displayed by the caregiver in response to questions. A recent, unexpected change in the financial status of the caregiver can be a sign of financial abuse.

A number of factors play a part in elder abuse, including crowded or inadequate family living conditions, marital problems in the caregiving family, insufficient income, increasing dependency needs of the elderly, pathological parent-child relationships (e.g., children who were mistreated by parents now mistreating parents), pathological caregivers, and functional impairment of caregivers (Harris, 1990, p. 409). Nursing research has also identified elder abuse risk factors that include functional disability, confusion, minority status, and poor social networks (Campbell, Harris, Lee, 1995).

DOCUMENTATION AND REPORTING According to Miller (1995, p. 541), in assessing cases of suspected abuse or neglect the health professional should document (1) background data (e.g., client's name, address, phone number, caregiver name, documentation of previous maltreatment); (2) signs of maltreatment or self-neglect (e.g., bruises, burns, broken bones); (3) severity of signs; (4) indicators of maltreatment intentionality (e.g., caregiver will not allow nurse to be alone with client); (5) symptoms of acute or chronic illness (e.g., incontinence); (6) functional incapacity (e.g., an inability to dress or toilet without assistance); (7) aggravating social conditions (e.g., client lives alone and is isolated); (8) source of information (e.g., agency referral); and (9) recommendations (e.g., opening the case for home health care services). A well-documented history of injury and illness is important. The nurse is usually mandated by state law to report suspected cases of elder abuse or neglect.

PREVENTION AND INTERVENTION Nursing research on elder abuse has resulted in the development of assessment tools for elder abuse, prevention strategies, and nursing interventions (Campbell, Harris, Lee, 1995). Prevention is the key to resolving the serious problem of elder abuse. Primary prevention activities include encouraging people to plan for future care needs while they are healthy and capable of making such decisions, providing adequate community resources to prevent caregiver burnout (e.g., respite care, financial aid, counseling), fostering personal self-esteem, and promoting positive attitudes about aging. Secondary prevention efforts focus on early casefinding and treatment (e.g., crisis intervention, Neighborhood Watches, and "buddy" systems). Tertiary prevention interventions involve family and caregiver rehabilitation activities in relation to counseling and care management, and in some cases the removal of the elderly person from the setting. However, community placement options for such elders are limited. Interventions can be complicated, and an abused elder may be loyal or fearful of the abuser, ashamed to acknowledge the abuse, or unaware of the services available to them (Lynch, 1997, p. 27). If the nurse suspects abuse she or he should try to interview the client privately, avoid asking leading questions, and keep questions simple and direct (Lynch, pp. 27-28).

Depression

Mental health is an important aspect of healthy aging. The United States has failed to ensure older persons' access to community mental health services, and many older persons have unmet mental health needs (USDHHS, 1991, p. 26). Depression is considered to be a significant problem for the elderly (Abrams, Beers, Berkow, 1995, p. 1216; USDHHS, 1991, p. 26). The prevalence of depression with elders tends to vary by setting, with major depression affecting 5% to 20% of elderly living in the community, 25% of hospitalized elderly, and as high as 40% of elderly nursing home residents (Ham, Sloane, 1997, p. 262).

Most of our knowledge about the etiology and treatment of depression has come from studies conducted on patients experiencing major depression under the care of psychiatrists and/or residing in hospital and nursing home settings (Baldwin, 1995; Caine, Lyness, King, 1993). Little research has been done on people under the care of their primary care provider and/or residing in community settings. Ham and Sloane (1997) state that "depression should be regarded as a communicable disease . . . if the depression has become persistent and unaddressed, the spouse or other family members may have become depressed themselves or begun to feel hopeless about the situation" (p. 262).

Signs and symptoms of depression in the elderly often do not follow the patterns seen in younger individuals. Some elderly become depressed for no obvious or clear reason (National Institute on Aging, 1992). Depression can result from things such as physical illness, medications, disability, financial problems, and loneliness. Signs and symptoms of depression and drugs that can cause symptoms of depression are given in the boxes on pages 621 and 622.

Results of a study by Kennedy, Kelman, and Thomas (1990) found that increasing disability and declining health were frequently responsible for depressive symptoms in late life and were more significant than social support, number of medical conditions, and life events in predicting depression. Others have reported that depression in older people is often related to experiencing a major loss such as retirement or death of a spouse or loved one (Staab, Hodges, 1996, p. 354). "An important component of depression among older adults may be a perceived lack of control over their lives or their current situation" (Staab, Hodges, p. 354).

The elderly frequently describe physical rather than emotional manifestations of illness, and as a result depression often goes undetected by families and health professionals (USDHHS, 1991, p. 26). Classic symptoms of depression in elders include feeling worthless, hopeless, helpless, irritable, and/or fearful; overwhelming sadness or grief; loss of interest in activities once enjoyed; sleeping and eating disturbances (including significant weight loss or gain); difficulty concentrating or thinking; recurring thoughts of death or suicide; and aches and pains that don't go away (Hogstel, 1994, pp. 209-210; Miller, 1995, p. 504). Some of the first symptoms noted are often decreased concentration, mobility, and zest for life, followed by signs of sleep and appetite disturbance, inattention to grooming and daily living tasks, and feelings of hopelessness and isolation (Huysman, 1996).

DEPRESSION: A TREATABLE CONDITION Depression is the most treatable of all mental illnesses (NIA, 1992). About 60% to 80% of people who are depressed can be treated successfully on an outpatient basis, and depression in older people typically responds to treatment (NIA). Many therapies are utilized to treat depression. Antidepressant drugs can improve mood, sleep, appetite, and concentration; however, it may take 6 to 12 weeks before there are real signs of progress (NIA).

Hospitalization may be effective in stabilizing depression among the elderly and provides an opportunity to monitor for suicidal tendencies (Huysman, 1996). Exercise and social interactions can be important interventions in affecting mood and relieving depression. Browning (1990) reported that a 20-minute session of low-impact aerobic exercise coupled with activities such as walking, cycling, swimming, and dancing can reduce stress. Some researchers recommend walking to alleviate depression (McAuliffe, 1994).

Unresolved depression can result in serious physical and psychological consequences. A fatal outcome of depression is suicide.

SUICIDE AND DEPRESSION Depression is one of the most common risk factors for suicide, and the suicide rate for depressed persons is at least eight times higher than that of the general population (U.S. Preventive Services Task Force, 1996, p. 541). *Healthy People 2000* addresses the need to reduce the incidence of suicide in the elderly (USDHHS, 1995, p. 194).

Suicide is a leading cause of death in older adults. Suicides among the elderly account for 25% of all suicides in the United States (Hogstel, 1994, p. 217). Men age 65+ have the highest rate of suicide in the United States (U.S. Preventive Services Task Force, 1996, p. 547).

A research study by Meehan, Saltzman, and Sattin (1991) demonstrated that the rate of elder suicide has increased in recent years. Important high-risk indicators for suicide include social isolation and loneliness; bereavement; low self-esteem; pain and illness; a sense of hopelessness; and previous suicide attempts. Few suicide prevention and intervention programs specifically target older persons, and few professionals are specifically trained in elder suicide prevention and counseling (AARP, 1989). AARP has published *Elder Suicide: A National Survey of Prevention and Intervention Programs* to increase understanding among the general public about this problem.

Health professionals "need to consider how current approaches to suicide prevention can better reflect the special circumstances of older persons" (Meehan, Saltzman, Sattin, 1991, p. 1200). About one half to two thirds of persons who commit suicide visit their primary care practitioners less than one month before the suicide, and 10% to 40% visit in the preceding week—giving practitioners a "window of opportunity" to assess, diagnose, and intervene (U.S. Preventive Services Task Force, 1996, p. 548). Another window of opportunity that is frequently overlooked is the "window" through which health care providers can look at "chronic suicide" activities evidenced by elders. Butler (1992) states that chronic suicide involves activities such as refusal to take medication, refusal to eat, and not following elementary safety procedures (such as walking out in traffic and falling down stairs). Such activities can result in death by "chronic suicide" (Butler).

Nurses and other health professionals need to take the suicidal thoughts of elders seriously. If older persons say they are going to kill themselves they usually mean it and are successful in carrying out the task (Butler, 1992). Nurses need to recognize the clinical symptoms and risk factors for depression, work to prevent depression, and facilitate early diagnosis and treatment (USDHHS, 1991, p. 26).

RURAL ELDERLY

Almost one out of four older Americans, 7.7 million people, lives in a rural setting, and the number continues to grow

Symptoms and Signs of Depression in Late Life

Symptoms

EMOTIONAL

Dejected mood or sadness
Decreased life satisfaction
Loss of interest
Impulse to cry
Irritability
Emptiness
Fearfulness and anxiety
Negative feelings toward self
Worry
Helplessness
Hopelessness
Sense of failure
Loneliness
Uselessness

COGNITIVE

Low self-esteem
Pessimism
Self-blame and criticism
Rumination about problems
Suicidal thoughts
Delusions:
- Of uselessness
- Of unforgivable behavior
- Nihilistic
- Somatic

Hallucinations:
- Auditory
- Visual
- Kinesthetic

Doubt of values and beliefs
Difficulty concentrating
Poor memory

PHYSICAL

Loss of appetite
Fatigability
Sleep disturbance:
- Initial insomnia
- Terminal insomnia
- Frequent awakenings

Constipation
Loss of libido
Pain
Restlessness

VOLITIONAL

Loss of motivation or "paralysis of will"
Suicidal impulses
Desire to withdraw socially

Observable Signs

APPEARANCE

Stooped posture
Sad face
Uncooperativeness
Social withdrawal
Hostility
Suspiciousness
Confusion and clouding of consciousness
Diurnal variations of mood
Drooling (in severe cases)
Unkempt appearance (in severe cases)
Occasional ulcerations of skin secondary to picking
Crying or whining
Occasional ulcerations of cornea secondary to decreased blinking
Weight loss
Bowel impaction

PSYCHOMOTOR RETARDATION

Slowed speech
Slowed movements
Gestures minimized
Shuffling slow gait
Mutism (in severe cases)
Cessation of mastication and swallowing (in severe cases)
Decreased or inhibited blinking (in severe cases)

PSYCHOMOTOR AGITATION

Continued motor activity
Wringing of hands
Picking at skin
Pacing
Restless sleep
Grasping others

BIZARRE OR INAPPROPRIATE BEHAVIOR

Suicidal gestures or attempts
Negativism, such as refusal to eat or drink and stiffness of the body
Outbursts of aggression
Falling backward

From Blazer DG: *Depression in late life*, ed 2, St. Louis, 1993, Mosby, p. 30.

Drugs That Can Cause Symptoms of Depression

ANTIHYPERTENSIVES
Reserpine
Methyldopa
Propranolol
Clonidine
Hydralazine
Guanethidine

ANALGESICS
Narcotic
Morphine
Codeine
Meperidine
Pentazocine
Propoxyphene
Nonnarcotic
Indomethacin

ANTIPARKINSONISM DRUGS
Levodopa

ANTIMICROBIALS
Sulfonamides
Isoniazid

CARDIOVASCULAR PREPARATIONS
Digitalis
Diuretics
Lidocaine

HYPOGLYCEMIC AGENTS

PSYCHOTROPIC AGENTS
Sedatives
Barbiturates
Benzodiazepines
Meprobamate
Antipsychotics
Chlorpromazine
Haloperidol
Thiothixene
Hypnotics
Chloral hydrate
Flurazepam

STEROIDS
Corticosteroids
Estrogens

OTHER
Cimetidine
Cancer chemotherapeutic agents
Alcohol

Source: Kane RL, Ouslander JG, Abrass IB, eds: *Essentials of clinical geriatrics*, New York, 1994, McGraw-Hill; Levenson AJ, Hall RCW, eds, *Neuropsychiatric manifestations of physical disorders in the elderly*, New York 1981, Raven Press. In Ham RJ, Sloane PD: *Primary care geriatrics: a case-based approach*, ed 3, St. Louis, 1997, Mosby, p. 264.

(Profile, 1993, p. 11). In many cases the elderly in these rural towns are the "oldest-old," those 85 and older. The health promotion needs of the rural elderly are extensive. The rural elderly have a greater incidence of chronic health problems than elderly living in metropolitan areas (Growing old, 1993, p. 19). Minority rural elders have poorer health than other rural elders (Growing old, p. 19).

The elderly in rural America are often isolated from access to health care services and have inadequate health care. Rural hospitals continue to close at an alarming rate. Many rural areas have a shortage of health care professionals. Studies have shown that rural areas have almost 44% fewer physicians than metropolitan areas (Where doctors, 1993, p. 13).

Numerous organizations are working to address the health care needs of the nation's rural elders. NCOA's National Center on Rural Aging (NCRA) works to increase service provision to the rural elderly. The National Resource Center for Rural Elderly (University of Missouri, Kansas City, Missouri) focuses on service provision, housing, and health care for the elderly and serves as an information clearinghouse. Elders who are members of AARP can obtain prescribed medications at a reduced cost by mail if there is no drugstore in their community. Community health nurses need to help link rural elders to such organizations and services and advocate for further services.

SIGNIFICANT LEGISLATION

Two extremely significant pieces of legislation for the elderly are the Social Security Act of 1935 and the Older Americans Act of 1965. The Social Security Act was discussed in Chapter 4, and the Older Americans Act is presented here.

Older Americans Act

Under President Lyndon B. Johnson, Congress passed the Older Americans Act (OAA) of 1965, which gave national attention to the needs of the elderly and authorized the Administration on Aging within the Department of Health and Human Services. It funded research and training in gerontology and facilitated development of regional, state, and local programs on aging. It proposed broad, comprehensive goals to improve the quality of life for older Americans. These goals are displayed in the following box.

Over the years the act has been amended to include the establishment of area agencies on aging, multipurpose senior centers (discussed later in this chapter), senior employment and volunteer programs, senior nutrition programs, health education and preventive health activities, senior transportation services, and in-home health care. The act is a major piece of legislation relating to services for older Americans. Appendix 20-2 presents some amendments to the act.

GOALS OF THE 1965 OLDER AMERICANS ACT

The Older Americans Act was designed to help elders achieve the following goals:

- An adequate retirement income
- The best possible physical and mental health available
- Suitable, affordable housing
- Necessary restorative services
- Employment without age discrimination
- Retirement in health, honor, and dignity
- Meaningful activity within the widest range of civic, cultural, and recreational opportunities
- Provision of efficient and coordinated community services
- Benefits from research knowledge that can sustain and improve health and quality of life
- Freedom, independence, and the free exercise of individual initiative in planning and managing their own lives

Social Security Act of 1935

The Social Security Act of 1935 mandates many programs that serve elderly people. The main provisions of the act that affect older Americans are the income support programs of Old Age, Survivors and Disability Insurance (OASDI) and Supplemental Security Income (SSI), and the health components of Medicare and Medicaid (see Chapter 4).

Other Legislation

Several other pieces of legislation have helped to improve the quality of life for the elderly. Examples of this legislation include the Age Discrimination in Employment Act of 1967, which prevented age discrimination in employment and protected workers from forced retirement; the Rehabilitation Act of 1973, which provided for rehabilitation services to Americans; the Research on Aging Act of 1974, which created the National Institute of Aging in the National Institutes of Health; and the Americans with Disabilities Act of 1990, which assured the rights of Americans with disabilities. These pieces of legislation have helped provide important services to older Americans.

SELECTED RESOURCES ON AGING

Many resources for older Americans are available in both the public and private sectors. Public-sector resources are supported by tax dollars and exist on federal, state, and local levels. Private-sector resources will vary greatly from community to community and are both voluntary (nonprofit) or proprietary (for-profit) in nature.

Government/Public Resources

Numerous agencies exist within federal, state, and local government to provide services to elders. The U.S. Department of Health and Human Services (USDHHS) and the Social Security Administration are major federal agencies involved in providing services to older people (see Chapter 5). Within the USDHHS agencies that provide extensive services to elders are the Administration on Aging and the National Institute on Aging.

ADMINISTRATION ON AGING The Administration on Aging is the principal agency charged with carrying out the provision of the Older Americans Act. The Administration publishes *Aging* magazine. Each year in May the Administration sponsors Older Americans Month. The Administration helps to fund and develop publications and documentaries on aging, including a Public Broadcasting System (PBS) documentary entitled *Our Nation's Health . . . Healthy Aging*.

NATIONAL INSTITUTE ON AGING The National Institute on Aging (1-800-222-2225) was established to conduct and support biomedical and behavioral research and training related to the aging process for the purpose of increasing knowledge about aging and the associated physical, psychological, and social factors resulting from advanced age. It has numerous free publications, including *A Resource Guide for Older Americans* and *Age Pages*.

SOCIAL SECURITY ADMINISTRATION The Social Security Administration (SSA) is a freestanding agency of the federal government discussed in Chapter 5. It administers the Social Security Act programs of Old Age, Survivors and Disability Insurance, "Social Security," and Supplemental Security Income (SSI) that are used extensively by senior citizens. Branches of Social Security Administration offices can be found in the local telephone directory under federal government listings.

ACTION This agency is an independent federal organization that administers volunteer programs. Its purpose is to mobilize Americans for voluntary service throughout the United States through programs that help meet basic human needs and support self-help efforts of low-income families and impoverished communities. ACTION offers Foster Grandparents, Retired Senior Volunteers Program (RSVP), and Senior Companions, and many older Americans are volunteers in these programs. Local Area Agencies on Aging often have information on ACTION programs.

OTHER FEDERAL AGENCIES Numerous other federal agencies provide assistance to the elderly. The Department of Agriculture offers many food and nutrition programs. The Department of Housing and Urban Development subsidizes low-cost public housing for the elderly. The Department of the Treasury offers assistance with income tax problems and filing taxes through the Internal Revenue Service. The Department of Labor enforces the Age Discrimination in Employment Act. The Department of the Interior issues Gold Age Passports (free) and Golden Eagle Passports (low-cost) for the federal park system to senior citizens. The Department of Transportation underwrites funding to assist in providing mass transportation that services the elderly. The Department of Defense offers programs for retired veterans, often through Veterans Administration hospitals. The U.S. Small Business Administration sponsors the SCORE program discussed earlier in this chapter.

STATE AND LOCAL AGENCIES ON AGING The Older Americans Act of 1965 provides funding to states to establish state and local agencies on aging. These agencies plan and coordinate programs for older people. Local agencies on aging can be located by calling the Federal Information Center or by checking the local telephone directories under county or city government listings.

SENIOR CENTERS The Older Americans Act of 1965 also provides funding for Senior Centers. These centers provide social, recreational, educational, and nutritional services for senior citizens. The first senior center was the William Hodson Senior Center established by the New York City Department of Welfare in 1943 (The first half-century, 1993, p. 2). Today more than 12,000 senior centers across the nation serve more than 7 million Americans (The first half-century, p. 2). The passage of the Older Americans Act of 1965 provided ongoing funding for such centers and designated them as the primary organizations for service delivery to the elderly in the community (The National Institute of Senior Centers, 1993, p. 10). In 1970 the National Institute of Senior Centers was formed (The National Institute of Senior Centers, p. 10). Today senior centers continue to provide valuable services for aging citizens; information about them is often found under local government listings in the phone book.

Private/Voluntary Resources

Private/voluntary resources are numerous and vary from community to community. On a national level two private, voluntary agencies that work actively for the elderly are the National Council on the Aging (NCOA) and the American Association for Retired Persons (AARP). These two groups, along with the activist Gray Panthers and other groups on aging, have lobbied for legislation, resources, and services for older persons.

NATIONAL COUNCIL ON THE AGING (NCOA) Established in 1950, the NCOA is a private, nonprofit organization that serves as a national resource for information and consultation and sponsors publications, special programs, advocacy activities, research, and training to meet older persons' needs and improve their lives. NCOA forms cooperative relationships with government and private agencies to educate the public and professionals about the aged and to provide services to the aged.

In 1987 NCOA and the Child Welfare League of America cofounded Generations United, a coalition of more than 100 national organizations dedicated to linking the needs and resources of generations. Generations United focuses on themes and programs that help to bring young and old together. NCOA also works closely with the Center for Understanding Aging (P.O. Box 246, Southington, Ct. 06489-0246) and Generations Together (University of Pittsburgh, 811 William Pitt Union, Pittsburgh, Pa. 15260) to promote aging education and intergenerational activities. Such affiliations have been successful in developing programs such as the Senior Center/Latchkey program that links seniors with young children home alone after school. NCOA is headquartered at 409 Third Street SW, Washington, D.C. 20024 (202-479-1200).

AMERICAN ASSOCIATION OF RETIRED PERSONS (AARP) The AARP was established in 1958 by Dr. Ethel Percy Andrus, founder of the National Retired Teachers Association. AARP today has over 30 million members across the United States in almost 4000 local chapters and is the largest nonprofit, nonpartisan membership organization in the world. The purposes of AARP are to enhance the quality of life for older persons; promote independence, dignity, and purpose for older persons; provide leadership in determining the role of older persons in society; and improve the image of aging. Membership in the group is limited to those age 50 years and older.

AARP publishes a bimonthly magazine, *Modern Maturity*, that offers retirement advice, travel ideas, and health tips, and also publishes the monthly *AARP News Bulletin*. It sponsors a tax assistance program to help older taxpayers, provides leadership in legislative issues, and is an advocate for the elderly.

Other community resources include senior centers, adult day care programs, home care agencies, family service agencies, geriatric counselors, health care professionals, churches, community service groups, and caregiver support groups. Increasingly, care management services are being developed in local communities to assist elders in maintaining their independence, and community health nurses are assuming major roles in carrying out these activities. The nurse needs to be aware of resources and services for the elderly in the community and be an advocate for service provision.

BARRIERS TO HEALTH CARE

Societal attitudes are barriers to all care, including health care. These attitudes often inhibit healthy aging, affecting resource availability and care given. Major barriers to health care for the elderly are access to health services and the cost of health services. A major access barrier is that of transportation. There is little public transportation in the United States, so the elderly person may have to rely on friends and family, taxis, Dial-a-Ride, and church or volunteer groups for transportation services. Seniors living in rural areas are especially affected by the problems of transportation and access to service. As a result of the Americans with Disabilities Act of 1990, buildings are now becoming more accessible for people who need to use wheelchairs, walkers, and other mobility appliances, but "accessibility" remains a problem.

Cost is another major barrier to health care. Many health care services are costly and may not be covered under private insurance, Medicare, or Medicaid. If services are too expensive the elderly may not use them. For example, Medicare does not pay for prescription drugs, and if an elderly person does not have these drugs paid for by private insurance or Medicaid he or she may not purchase them. The prices of food, medicine, doctors' visits, and gas continually rise, yet many older persons live on a fixed income and cannot afford the services they need.

THE NURSING ROLE

As early as 1925 an editorial in the *American Journal of Nursing* alerted nurses to the increasing need to prepare for care of the elderly (Editorial, 1925). The American Nurses Association (ANA), National League for Nursing (NLN), National Gerontological Nursing Association (NGNA), and the National Conference of Gerontological Nurse Practitioners (NCGNP) have helped to keep nurses aware of educational opportunities in gerontology and issues relevant to the health care of older people (Johnson, Connelly, 1990, p. iv).

The role of the nurse in working with the elderly client has been discussed throughout this chapter in reference to healthy aging, health promotion, and concerns of the elderly. Gerontological nursing involves assessing the health and functional status of elders; planning, providing, and coordinating appropriate nursing and health care services; and evaluating the effectiveness of care (ANA, 1995, p. 7). The nurse works to maximize the elder's functional ability in activities of daily living, strives to identify and build on elder strengths, and assists the client in maintaining independence (ANA, p. 7). The nurse may assume the role of advocate for the elderly client and help to link the client to community resources.

Graduates of nursing programs are entering practice where the majority of clients are over age 65 and many over 85 years old (Small, 1993, p. 27). Nurses need to be able to provide quality care to elderly clients by understanding the aging process; common problems of aging; functional abilities associated with aging; public policy and economics; health maintenance and promotion; long-term care needs; ethics and attitudes; and cultural variations and opportunities for professional development (Johnson, Connelly, 1990, p. 3).

The ANA established certification of gerontological nurses in 1973; as of January 1992 there were almost 10,000 certified gerontological nurses (LeSage, 1993, p. 19). The ANA's Council on Gerontological Nursing has been involved in many important gerontological nursing initiatives. NLN is committed to the improvement of education and practice in gerontological nursing and to the provision of quality long-term care (Waters, 1993, p. 23). Unfortunately, education in gerontology is frequently lacking in the educational programs of nurses and other health care professionals. No health profession has claimed service to the elderly as its unique task, leaving open a window of opportunity for nurses to step forward and assume primary responsibility for providing comprehensive health care to the elderly.

Standards of Practice

ANA's (1995) *Scope and Standards of Gerontological Nursing Practice* are presented in the box on the following page. These standards address the application of the nursing process to gerontological nursing, interdisciplinary collaboration, the integration of theory and research in practice, and professional performance.

Levels of Prevention

Getting older people to take part in health promotion activities can be a challenging but rewarding experience. The nurse can help the elderly client to see that "an ounce of prevention is worth a pound of cure." Community health nurses can assist people in taking responsibility for maintaining their health and promoting healthy aging.

When implementing health promotion and wellness activities for the elderly client, community health nurses emphasize primary prevention activities but use secondary and tertiary prevention activities as well (see Chapter 11). Such activities have the potential to facilitate wellness, reduce premature death and disability, maintain health and functional independence of older adults, and improve the overall quality of life (USDHHS, 1991, pp. 24, 587).

Primary prevention is integrally linked with health promotion and wellness. A goal of primary prevention activities is to help the elderly to maintain physical functioning and independence as long as possible (Alford, Futrell, 1992, p. 221; USDHHS, 1991, p. 587). Wellness programs for seniors are often located in local senior centers, churches, and fitness organizations.

Examples of *primary prevention interventions* that the community health nurse may implement include health education measures in relation to the normal changes of aging; need for preventive medical care (e.g. regular physical examinations, receiving immunizations for pneumonia and influenza); proper exercise, nutrition, and oral health; safety measures; and health assessment. These activities also include anticipatory guidance that can help prepare the individual and family for significant life changes such as retirement. Predisposition to conditions such as coronary artery disease can be altered with a preventive program of exercise, good nutrition, avoidance of smoking, and protection from stress.

Secondary prevention activities involve early diagnosis and treatment, including encouraging and facilitating regular medical and dental care and periodic screening for conditions (e.g., hypertension and diabetes); encouraging adherence to medical treatment regimens; carrying out self-monitoring activities such as breast and testicular self-examinations; and assessing for the warning signs of cancer. *Tertiary prevention* involves rehabilitative and restorative activities and includes physical, occupational, recreational, and speech therapy and adjusting to activities of daily living in relation to changing levels of functioning.

Scope and Standards of Gerontological Nursing Practice

STANDARDS OF CLINICAL GERONTOLOGICAL NURSING CARE

Standard I. Assessment

The gerontological nurse collects client health data.

Information obtained from the aging person, significant others, and the interdisciplinary team and nursing judgment based on knowledge of gerontological nursing are used to develop the comprehensive care plan. Interviewing, functional assessment, environmental assessment, physical assessment, and review of health records enhance the nurse's ability to make sound clinical judgments. Assessment is culturally and ethnically appropriate.

Standard II. Diagnosis

The gerontological nurse analyzes the assessment data in determining diagnosis.

The gerontological nurse evaluates health assessment data to identify the aging person's state of health and well-being, and treatment of and responses to illness, aging, and reduced activity. Each person responds to aging in a unique way. Nursing diagnoses form the basis for nursing interventions.

Standard III. Outcome Identification

The gerontological nurse identifies expected outcomes individualized to the client.

The ultimate goals of providing gerontological nursing care are to influence health outcomes and improve the aging person's health status. Outcomes often focus on maximizing the aging person's state of well-being, functional status, and quality of life.

Standard IV. Planning

The gerontological nurse develops a plan of care that prescribes interventions to attain expected outcomes.

A plan of care is used to structure and guide therapeutic interventions and achieve expected outcomes. It is developed in conjunction with the aging person and significant others.

Standard V. Implementation

The gerontological nurse implements the interventions identified in the care plan.

The gerontological nurse implements a care plan in collaboration with the aging person, significant others, and the interdisciplinary team. The gerontological nurse provides culturally competent direct and indirect care, using concepts of health promotion, illness prevention, health maintenance, rehabilitation, restoration, and palliation. The nurse educates and counsels the aging person and significant others involved in that person's care. In addition, the gerontological nurse supervises and evaluates both formal and informal caregivers to ensure that their care is supportive and ethical and demonstrates respect for the aging person's dignity. Gerontological nurses select interventions according to their level of practice.

Standard VI. Evaluation

The gerontological nurse evaluates the aging person's progress toward attainment of expected outcomes.

Nursing practice is a dynamic process. The gerontological nurse continually evaluates the aging person's responses to therapeutic interventions. Collection of new data, revision of the database, alteration of nursing diagnoses, and modification of the care plan are often required. The effectiveness of nursing care depends on ongoing evaluation.

STANDARDS OF PROFESSIONAL GERONTOLOGICAL NURSING PERFORMANCE

Standard I. Quality of Care

The gerontological nurse systematically evaluates the quality of care and effectiveness of nursing practice.

The dynamic nature of geriatric care and the growing body of gerontological nursing knowledge and research provide both the impetus and the means for gerontological nurses to improve the quality of client care.

Standard II. Performance Appraisal

The gerontological nurse evaluates his or her own nursing practice in relation to professional practice standards and relevant statutes and regulations.

The gerontological nurse is accountable to the public for providing competent clinical care and has an inherent responsibility to practice according to standards established by the profession and by regulatory bodies.

Standard III. Education

The gerontological nurse acquires and maintains current knowledge in nursing practice.

Scientific, cultural, societal, and political changes require a continuing commitment from the gerontological nurse to pursue knowledge, to enhance nursing expertise and advance the profession. Formal education, continuing education, certification, and experiential learning are some of the means for professional growth.

From American Nurses Association: *Scope and standards of gerontological nursing practice*, Washington, D.C., 1995, ANA.

Advanced Practice Nursing Roles

The advanced practice gerontological nurse holds a master's degree in nursing, preferably with a concentration in gerontological nursing (ANA, 1995, p. 9). Gerontological nurse practitioner and clinical nurse specialist programs are scattered throughout the nation, and nurses graduating from such programs fall under each state's nurse practice acts for their scope of practice. According to ANA, "Nurses prepared for advanced practice in gerontoloigcal nursing are experts in providing, directing, and delegating the care of aging persons, and they support other practitioners in a variety of settings" (p. 9).

Summary

Challenging and enriching opportunities exist for community health nurses in implementing health care for the elderly. Nurses need to be educated about aging and be familiar with the aging process. Nursing efforts need to focus on health promotion with the elderly and facilitation of wellness and healthy aging. Aging is a universal phenomena—everyone

Scope and Standards of Gerontological Nursing Practice—cont'd

Standard IV. Collegiality

The gerontological nurse contributes to the professional development of peers, colleagues, and others.

The gerontological nurse is responsible for sharing knowledge, research, and clinical information with colleagues and others through formal and informal teaching methods and collaborative educational programs.

Standard V. Ethics

The gerontological nurse's decisions and actions on behalf of clients are determined in an ethical manner.

The gerontological nurse is responsible for providing nursing services and health care that are responsive to the public's trust and client's rights. Co-workers and other formal and informal care providers must also be prepared to provide the care needed and desired by the aging person and to render services in an appropriate setting. Special ethical concerns in gerontological nursing care include informed consent; emergency interventions; nutrition and hydration of the terminally ill; pain management; need for self-determination by the aging person; treatment termination; quality-of-life issues; confidentiality; surrogate decision making; nontraditional treatment modalities; fair distribution of scarce resources; and economic decision making.

Standard VI. Collaboration

The gerontological nurse collaborates with the aging person, significant others, and health care providers in providing client care.

The complex nature of comprehensive care for aging persons and their significant others requires expertise from a number of different health care providers. Collaboration between consumers and providers is optimal for planning, implementing, and evaluating care. Meetings of the interdisciplinary team provide a forum to evaluate the effectiveness of the care plan and make necessary adjustments.

Standard VII. Research

The gerontological nurse uses research findings in practice.

Gerontological nurses are responsible for improving nursing practice and the future health care for aging persons by participating in research. At the basic level of practice, the gerontological nurse uses research findings to improve clinical care and identifies clinical problems for study.

Standard VIII. Resource Utilization

The gerontological nurse considers factors related to safety, effectiveness, and cost in planning and delivering client care.

The aging person is entitled to health care that is safe, effective, and affordable. Treatment decisions must maximize resources and maintain quality of care.

is aging. It is important to remember that the elderly person is a unique individual with unique health care needs. Our society's ageist attitudes often become self-fulfilling prophecies in old age and inhibit healthy aging. Nurses need to be aware of their own attitudes about aging and how these attitudes affect nursing care and caring.

Healthy People 2000 has addressed health needs of the elderly and established numerous national health objectives for this aggregate. Nurses frequently provide care to elderly clients and need to be aware of national health objectives, health concerns of the elderly, the physiological changes of aging, legislation that has an impact on the elderly, and community resources. Nurses are advocates for health care resources and services for the elderly and work to minimize barriers to care such as societal attitudes, inadequate resources and services, problems of accessibility, and transportation and limited income.

The expected growth of the population over 65 signals an expanding nursing role and opportunity to work with older people. Nurses need to be educated in gerontology. Nursing has the opportunity to be the leader in the delivery of health care services to the elderly. Planning and implementing policy for the elderly client is a significant challenge for community health nurses.

Critical *Thinking Exercise*

After reading this chapter you are aware of the *Healthy People 2000* national health objectives for older people and numerous needs, resources, and services in relation to the elderly client. What do you see as the greatest major health care concern for today's older Americans? What can nurses in your community do to help meet this health care need?

REFERENCES

Abrams WB, Beers, MH, Berkow MD: *The Merck manual of geriatrics*, Whitehouse Station, N.J., 1995, Merck Research Laboratories.

Alford DM, Futrell M: AAN working paper: wellness and health promotion of the elderly, *Nurs Outlook* 40(5):221-226, 1992.

American Association of Retired Persons (AARP): *Truth about aging: guidelines for accurate communications*, Washington, D.C., 1984, AARP.

American Association of Retired Persons (AARP): *Elder suicide: a national survey of prevention and intervention programs*, Washington, D.C., 1989, AARP.

American Association of Retired Persons (AARP): *Healthy older adults*, Washington, D.C., 1991, AARP.

American Association of Retired Persons (AARP): *A profile of older Americans 1995*, Washington, D.C., 1996, AARP.

American Nurses Association (ANA): *Scope and standards of gerontological nursing practice*, Washington, D.C., 1995, ANA.

Annual checkups—who needs them, *Aging* 365:2-3, 1993.

Baldwin RC: Antidepressants in geriatric depression: what difference have they made? *Int Psychogeriatrics* 7(Supplement):55-68, 1995.

Beckerman A, Northrop C: Hope, chronic illness and the elderly, *J Gerontol Nurs* 22(5):19-25, 1996.

Blazer DG: *Depression in late life*, ed 2, St. Louis, 1993, Mosby.

Bronte L: *The longevity factor: the new reality of long careers and how it can lead to richer lives*, New York, 1993, Harper Collins.

Browning MA: Depression. In Hogstel M, ed: *Geropsychiatric nursing*, St. Louis, 1990, Mosby.

Butler R: *Treatment of the aged*, Network for Continuing Medical Education, Continuing Medical Education Series, Video #629, 1992.

Caine ED, Lyness MM, King DA: Reconsidering depression in the elderly, *Am J Geriatric Psychiatry* 1:4-20, 1993.

Cameron M: *Views of aging: a teacher's guide*, Ann Arbor, 1967, Institute of Gerontology, University of Michigan–Wayne State University.

Campbell JC, Harris MJ, Lee RK: Violence research: an overview, *Scholar Inq Nurs Pract* 9(2):105-126, 1995.

Castillo HM: *The nurse assistant in long-term care: a rehabilitative approach*, St. Louis, 1992, Mosby.

Comfort A: *Say yes to old age: developing a positive attitude toward aging*, New York, 1990, Crown.

Duxbury AS: Geriatrics: unmasking "polypharmacy" problems and adverse drug effects, *Consultant* 4:762-764, 775-777, 1996.

Editorial, *Am J Nurs* 25(5):394, 1925.

Erikson EH: *The life cycle completed: a review*, New York, 1982, Norton.

Greely A: *Nutrition and the elderly*, Publication No. (FDA) 91-2243, Washington, D. C., 1991, U.S. Department of Health and Human Services.

Growing old in rural America: new approach needed in rural health care, *Aging* 365:18-25, 1993.

Ham RJ, Sloane PD: *Primary care geriatrics: a case-based approach*, ed 3, St. Louis, 1997, Mosby.

Harris DK: *Sociology of aging*, ed 2, New York, 1990, Harper & Row.

Hey RP, Carlson E: "Granny dumping": new pain for U.S. elders, *AARP Bull* 32(8):1, 16, 1991.

Hogstel MO: *Nursing care of the older adult*, ed 3, Albany, N.Y., 1994, Delmar.

Huysman AM: Depression in older people and its implications in health care, *Topics in Geriatric Rehab* 11(4):16-24, 1996.

Johnson BK: Older adults and sexuality: a multidimensional perspective, *J Gerontol Nurs* 22(2):6-15, 1996.

Johnson MA, Connelly JR: *Nursing and gerontology: status report*, Washington, D.C., 1990, Association for Gerontology in Higher Education.

Kane RL, Ouslander JG, Abrass IB, eds: *Essentials of clinical geriatrics*, New York, 1994, McGraw-Hill.

Kennedy GJ, Kelman HR, Thomas C: The emergence of depressive symptoms in late life: the importance of declining health and increasing disability, *J Community Health* 15:93-104, 1990.

Kraus LE, Stoddard S: *Chartbook on disability in the United States, an InfoUse Report*, Washington, D.C., March 1989, U.S. National Institute on Disability and Rehabilitation Research.

Kuhn ME: *Maggie Kuhn on aging*, Philadelphia, 1977, Westminister.

LeSage J: Initiatives in gerontological nursing education: the role of the American Nurses Association's Council on Gerontological Nursing. In Heine C, ed: *Determining the future of gerontological nursing education*, New York, 1993, National League for Nursing Press, pp. 17-22.

Letvak S, Schoder D: Sexually transmitted diseases in the elderly: what you need to know, *Geriatr Nurs* 17(4):156-160, 1996.

Levenson AJ, Hall RCW, eds: *Neuropsychiatric manifestations of physical disorders in the elderly*, New York, 1981, Raven Press.

Lueckenotte AG: *Gerontologic nursing*, St. Louis, 1996, Mosby.

Lynch SH: Elder abuse: what to look for, how to intervene, *AJN* 97:27-32, 1997.

Malnutrition: tackling a major problem, *Worldview* 5(2):4, 1993.

McAuliffe K: Out of the blues, *Walking*, March/April:42-44, 46-47, 1994.

McGuire SL, Gerber DE: Prevention starts early: aging education for children. In Edwards RB, Bittar EE: *Advances in bioethics: violence, neglect and the elderly*, Greenwich, Ct., 1996, JAI Press, pp. 189-202.

Medical Letter, Inc.: Drugs that cause psychiatric symptoms, *The Medical Letter on Drugs and Therapeutics* 35(901):65-70, 1993.

Meehan P, Saltzman L, Sattin R: Suicides among older United States residents: epidemiologic characteristics and trends, *Am J Public Health* 81(9):1198-1200, 1991.

Miller CA: *Nursing care of older adults: theory and practice*, ed 2, Philadelphia, 1995, Lippincott.

National Aging Resource Center on Elder Abuse: *Elder abuse: questions and answers (an information guide for professionals and concerned citizens)*, ed 2, Washington, D.C., 1992, The Center.

National Council on the Aging (NCOA): Public policy agenda 1993-1994, *Perspect Aging* 22(1):1-46, 1993.

National Institute on Aging (NIA): *Depression: a serious but treatable illness*, AgePage, Washington, D.C., 1992, NIA.

National Resource Center on Health Promotion and Aging (NRCHPA): *Medications and the elderly*, Washington, D.C., 1991, U.S. Government Printing Office.

Nutrition Screening Initiative: *Nutrition screening checklist*, A cooperative effort of the American Dietetic Association, the American Academy of Family Physicians, and the National Council on the Aging, Washington, D.C., 1992, Nutrition Screening Initiative.

O'Neill K, Reid G: Perceived barriers to physical activity by older adults, *Can J Public Health* 82(6):392-396, 1991.

Painter K: Better care and plain old luck are keys, *USA Today* April 7, 1993, pp. D1-2.

Palmieri DT: Clearing up the confusion: adverse effects of medications in the elderly, *J Gerontol Nurs* 17(10):32-35, 1991.

Promoting elderly appetites: a feast for the senses, *Worldview* 5(2):9, 1993.

Profile of the rural U.S., *Aging* 365:10-11, 1993.

Rosenburg IH: As you age: 10 keys to a longer, healthier, more vital life, *Worldview* 5(2):2-3, 1993.

Sattin RW: Falls among older persons: a public health perspective, *Annu Rev Public Health* 13:489-508, 1992.

Schaller KJ: Tai Chi Chih: an exercise option for older adults, *J Gerontological Nurs* 22(10):12-17, 1996.

Sheppard HL: Damaging stereotypes about aging are taking hold: how to counter them? *Perspect Aging* 19(1):4-8, 1990.

Skinner BF, Vaughn ME: *Enjoy old age: a program of self-management*, New York, 1983, Norton.

Small NR: National consensus conference on gerontologic nursing competencies. In Heine C, ed: *Determining the future of gerontological nursing education*, New York, 1993, National League for Nursing Press, pp. 27-31.

Staab AS, Hodges LC: *Essentials of gerontological nursing: adaptation to the aging process*, Philadelphia, 1996, Lippincott.

The first half-century of senior centers charts the way for decades to come, *Perspect Aging* 22(2):2-6, 1993.

The National Institute of Senior Centers and the senior center field: a chronology, *Perspect Aging* 22(2):10-11, 1993.

U.S. Bureau of the Census: *Sixty-five plus in America*, Washington, D.C., 1992, U.S. Government Printing Office.

U.S. Bureau of the Census: *Sixty-five plus in the United States*, Special Studies, P 23-190, Washington, D.C., 1996, U.S. Government Printing Office.

U.S. Department of Health and Human Services (USDHHS): *Healthy People 2000, full report, with commentary*, Washington, D.C., 1991, U.S. Government Printing Office.

U.S. Department of Health and Human Services (USDHHS), Public Health Service: National ambulatory medical care surgery: 1991 summary, *Vital and Health Statistics*, Series 13, No. 116, May 1994.

U.S. Department of Health and Human Services (USDHHS): *Income of the aged chartbook 1990*, Washington, D.C., 1992, U.S. Government Printing Office.

U.S. Department of Health and Human Services (USDHHS): *Healthy people 2000: midcourse review and revisions*, Washington, D.C., 1995, U.S. Government Printing Office.

U.S. House Select Committee on Aging: *Elder abuse: a decade of shame and inaction*, Washington, D. C., 1990, U.S. Government Printing Office.

U.S. Preventive Services Task Force: *Guide to clinical preventive services: report of the U.S. Preventive Services Task Force*, ed 2, Baltimore, 1996, Williams & Wilkins.

U.S. Public Health Service: *Put prevention into practice*, Waldorf, Md., 1994, American Nurses Publishing.

Upward trend, *AARP Bull* 37(11):12, 1996.

Waters V: National League for Nursing: initiatives in gerontological nursing education. In Heine C, ed: *Determining the future of gerontological nursing education*, New York, 1993, National League for Nursing Press, pp. 23-26.

Where doctors are few and far between, *Aging* 365:12-17, 1993.

White P: Pearls for practice: polypharmacy and the older adult, *J Am Ac Nurse Pract* 7(11):545-548, 1995.

Yoder MK: Starting a nurse-managed center for older adults: the needs assessment process, *Geriatr Nurs* 17(1):14-19, 1996.

SELECTED BIBLIOGRAPHY

Advice to elders: drink up for health, *Worldview* 5(2):5, 1993.

American Association for Retired Persons (AARP): *Growing together: an intergenerational sourcebook*, Washington, D.C., 1986, AARP.

Brower HT, Yurchuck ER: Teaching gerontological nursing in southern states, *Nurs Health Care* 14(4):198-205, 1993.

Conn VS: Self-management of over-the-counter medications by older adults, *Public Health Nurs* 9(1):29-36, 1992.

Hawranik P: Clinical possibility: preventing health problems after the age of 65, *J Gerontol Nurs* 17(11):20-25, 1991.

Hofland SL, Powers J: Sexual dysfunction in the menopausal woman: hormonal causes and management issues, *Geriatric Nurs* 17(4):161-165, 1996.

Hungelmann J, Kenkel-Rossi E, Klasser L, Stollenweek R: Focus on spiritual well-being: harmonious interconnectedness of mind-body-spirit—use of the JAREL spiritual well-being scale, *Geriatric Nurs* 17(6):262-265, 1996.

Kubler-Ross E: *On death and dying*, New York, 1969, Macmillan.

Marchi-Jones S, Murphy JF, Rosseau P: Caring for the caregivers, *J Gerontol Nurs* 22(8):7-13, 1996.

McGuire SL: Promoting positive attitudes toward aging among children, *J Sch Health* 56(8):322-324, 1986.

McGuire SL: Aging education in schools, *J Sch Health* 57(5):174-176, 1987.

McGuire SL: Promoting positive attitudes toward aging: literature for young children, *Childhood Education* 69(4):204-210, 1993.

McGuire SL: Promoting positive attitudes through aging education: a study with preschool children, *Gerontol Geriatrics Ed* 13(4):3-12, 1993.

Penn C, Lekan-Rutledge D, Joers AM et al: Assessment of urinary incontinence, *J Gerontol Nurs* 22(1):8-19, 1996.

Turner C, Quine S: Nurses' knowledge, assessment skills, experience, and confidence in toenail management of elderly people, *Geriatric Nurs* 17(6):273-277, 1996.

21

Clients with Long-Term Care Needs: Home Health, Hospice, and Other Services

Objectives

Upon completion of this chapter, the reader should be able to:

1. Describe the factors influencing the growing need for long-term care.
2. Discuss population groups at risk for needing long-term care services.
3. Identify the settings where long-term care services are provided.
4. Discuss the concept of home care and the range of home care services available in the community.
5. Describe how managed care affects the services provided by home care agencies.
6. Summarize governmental financing for long-term care.
7. Explain legislation influencing long-term care service delivery.
8. Discuss barriers to the provision of community-based long-term care service delivery.
9. Analyze the role of the community health nurse in long-term care.
10. Describe the difference between the services offered by hospice and traditional home care.
11. Discuss the role of an ethics committee in the home care setting.

Like good cheese
She sits idly waiting to be selected or needed
But the ugly mold of age
Repels life's amateurs
And turns them away
Ignorant of the quality inside

RUTH NAYLOR

This text stresses the importance of working with aggregates at risk in the community to prevent major community health problems. Of all the groups discussed, none is growing more rapidly or has more primary, secondary, and tertiary prevention needs than the population that requires long-term care: the elderly, the chronically ill, and the disabled across the life span. Members of these groups are often ignored by society because their qualities are not recognized.

Multiple institutional and community settings provide long-term care services for individuals across the life span. Although this chapter focuses on the role of the community health nurse in providing services at home for people who have long-term care needs, community health nurses must be aware of the role institutional settings play in long-term care because they provide extensive, formal long-term care services and consume a major portion of the long-term health care dollar.

In 1993 more than $100 billion was spent by individuals, families, and local, state, and federal governments on long-term care services. The need for these services and the expenditures required by clients to receive them are escalating rapidly. Families, the traditional providers of long-term care services, are less and less able to maintain this role as they cope with competing demands of jobs and family. Further, many people receiving these services, along with their families, are dissatisfied with them. The government at all levels, along with the private sector, is searching for better strategies to meet the needs of individuals and their families who need long-term care services (GAO, 1994c).

Since demand for long-term care is growing, the focus in this chapter is on examining the role of the community health nurse in this area of practice. Emphasis is placed on identifying current long-term care resources, gaps in the present system, and future needs of this rapidly growing population.

DEFINING LONG-TERM CARE

Long-term care services are those health, social, housing, transportation, and other supportive services needed by persons with physical, mental, or cognitive limitations, regardless of age or diagnosis, that are severe enough to compromise independent living (Harrington, Cassell, Estes et al, 1991). The need for long-term care is generally defined by a person's ability to independently carry out activities and routines of daily living. One of the more common ways to assess people's limitations is to measure their ability to perform self-care tasks, often called the activities of daily living (ADL). These include eating, bathing, dressing, getting to and using the bathroom, and getting in or out a bed and/or chair. Less severe limitations are often assessed through the ability of the person to perform household chores and social tasks, known as the instrumental activities of daily living (IADL). These tasks include activities such as shopping, doing light housework, keeping track of money, using the telephone, and preparing meals. Other activities such as the ability to attend school or behavioral problems are used for children or people with mental illness. In these instances self-care and household activities are not valid for assessing the need for long-term care services.

Site of Care

A distinction is often made between institutional long-term care and home- and community-based long-term care. The vast majority of people needing long-term care live at home or in small community residences. Twelve million people in this country report needing assistance with ADL; about 5.1 million of this group are so severely disabled that they need substantial assistance 24 hours a day. Of this severely disabled group 2.4 million live in institutions such as nursing homes; the remaining 2.7 million live at home or in community settings (GAO, 1994c). Table 21-1 depicts the fact that most people who need long-term care are not in institutional settings.

Age of Those Receiving Long-Term Care

The majority of people needing long-term care services (57%) are over the age of 65. However, a sizable proportion of this aggregate includes working-age adults and children. Figure 21-1 illustrates this fact. Estimating the long-term care needs of children is difficult because their age makes the usual assessments of ability to carry out ADL and IADL inappropriate. About 330,000 children live at home, unable to participate in major play or school activities as a result of problems such as epilepsy or cystic fibrosis. About 170,000 children are severely disabled with diseases such as cerebral palsy or mental retardation, and another 90,000 children live in institutions as a result of severe mental or physically handicapping conditions (GAO, 1994c).

table 21-1 Most People Needing Long-Term Care Are Not in Institutions

	Numbers in Thousands		
Age Group	In Institutions	At Home or in Community Settings	Total Population
Children	90	330	420
Working-age adults	710	4,380	5,090
Elderly	1,640	5,690	7,330
Total	**2,440**	**10,400**	**12,840**

Sources: Based on information from the U.S. Department of Health and Human Services, and the Institute for Health Policy Studies at the University of California, San Francisco. From GAO: *Long-term care: diverse, growing population includes millions of Americans of all ages*, Pub No. HEHS-95-26, Washington, D.C., November 1994c, U.S. Government Printing Office, p. 5.

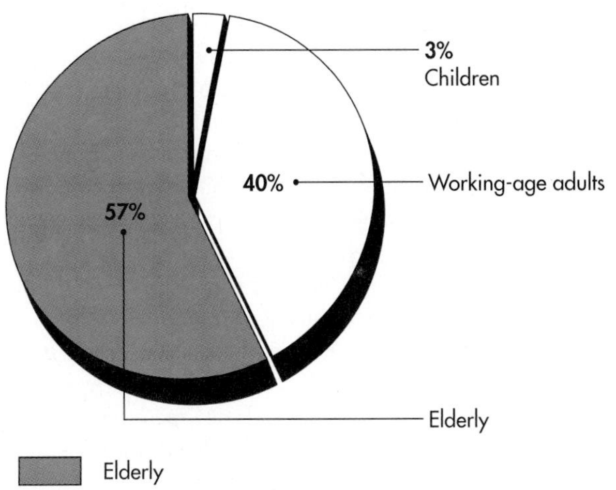

Note: Includes people needing long-term care in institutions or in the community. Children are those under age 18, working-age adults are those aged 18 to 64, and the elderly are those aged 65 and older.

Figure 21-1 Most people needing long-term care are elderly. (From GAO: Long-term care: diverse, growing population includes millions of Americans of all ages, *Pub No. HEHS-95-26, Washington, D.C., November 1994c, U.S. Government Printing Office, p. 6.)*

FACTORS INFLUENCING THE GROWTH OF LONG-TERM CARE SERVICES

Six factors in American society have influenced the need for increasing organized long term care services: epidemiological conditions, changes in informal support systems, sociodemographic factors, consumer preference, and increasingly sophisticated medical technology. Medicare had a powerful effect on these factors when it was created in 1965.

Epidemiological Conditions

Americans are living longer, the causes of death are changing, chronic illness is increasing, and the gap between male and female longevity is widening. It is crucial to the subject of long-term care to recognize that the rise in numbers and percentages of people in this country is among the very groups who need long-term care services the most. As medical technology and public health practice have advanced, an increasing number of vulnerable infants and disabled children and adults have been saved and life expectancy has risen dramatically, causing a significant expansion in the numbers of people 65 years of age and older. Persons in these population groups often have multiple chronic conditions and frequently require institutional or community-based long-term care services. Home health and other long-term care services are primarily delivered to the aging and the chronically ill.

A dramatic increase in the size of the elderly population is expected in the twenty-first century. Although not all elderly are at risk for needing long-term care services, they do have the greatest likelihood of needing this care. Projections for the number of elderly needing long-term care will reach 10 to 14 million by 2020, compared with 7 million today. The need for long-term care increases significantly after the age of 85 (the "oldest old"; see Chapter 20), and it is this aggregate of the elderly that is projected to grow the most rapidly (GAO, 1994c, p. 9).

People are living longer because they are dying of different diseases now than 80 years ago. Infectious diseases are no longer the leading cause of death as was the case in the early 1900s (see Chapter 1). Cancer, heart disease, and stroke are now the chief killers, and they are often degenerative and chronic. As previously mentioned, individuals affected by these conditions usually require long-term care services. It is clear that epidemiological factors and demographic changes will make significant demands upon the long-term care delivery system in the near future.

Informal Supports

Nine out of 10 persons who are disabled and who are not institutionalized receive unpaid care from family and friends. Almost 7 million Americans are unpaid caregivers to the elderly, with the majority of those caregivers being women. The average caregiver to the elderly in the United States is a married woman 45 years of age. Daughters outnumber sons three to one as caregivers of their elderly parents (Brakman, 1994, p. 26).

However, four consequences of industrialization—geographical mobility, rising incomes, urbanization, and careers for women—have all changed the ability of families to provide informal support. Although the mobility rate has been declining in the past several decades, a large number of people move from one residence to another, and many move significant distances. Of the 43 million persons who moved between March 1993 and March 1994, 7 million moved from one state to another (U.S. Bureau of the Census, 1996, p. 2).

Rising incomes allow people to live apart and to negate the dependence families have on one another. Small urban homes are not designed for intergenerational families. The average number of persons per household in 1995 was 2.62 people (Day, 1996). Industrialization has made it both possible and necessary for women to take on a career outside the home. During recent decades females have increasingly joined the paid labor force. This will make it more difficult for them to provide informal care for elderly relatives. It is anticipated that work obligations may conflict with caregiving responsibilities to a greater extent in the future than they do now.

Sociodemographic Factors

Three sociodemographic factors have increased the need for people to use formal long-term care services. These are the decline in the number of children a family chooses to have, the aging of the providers of care, and the increasing rates of divorce and remarriage. Simply summarized, there are fewer children to care for parents who are living longer lives. These children are also older when they are required to care for their parents. Further, divorce may change the bonds of affection and obligation, and children and stepchildren may face extremely difficult decisions about those for whom they should care. Aging persons themselves may be alone as the result of divorce or death.

Consumer Preference

People want to be treated and cared for at home rather than in institutional settings. Home has the advantage of providing security and familiarity, and it also reduces exposure to iatrogenically induced problems of hospitals and nursing homes. Costs can be less, and the client and family are able to be in charge of the client's care.

Medical Technology

What's new in home care? In the words of Judith P. Harris, Vice President of Patient Services for the Visiting Nurse Association of Greater Philadelphia, it is

> high technology. Just look at what is available in the home today that even a few years ago seemed an impossibility: some of the more progressive home care agencies offer services so patients can remain at home on ventilators. Home intravenous therapies now include total parenteral nutrition (TPN), hydration, antibiotics, pain management, chemotherapy, and drugs to treat AIDS-related infections. Specialty infusions include Lasix, Dopamine/Dobutamine, Desferoxamine and Neupogen. Patients may receive

> all types of gastrointestinal tube feedings. PICC lines (peripherally-inserted central catheters) can stay in place for a long time and reduce the number of times a patient needs to be stuck with a needle during the course of therapy. (Harris, 1992, p. 15)

The Creation of Medicare

Home care agencies of various types have been providing high-quality services for more than 100 years (see Chapter 1). However, the enactment of Medicare in 1965 greatly spurred the growth of this industry. Medicare made home care services, primarily skilled nursing and therapy of a curative or restorative nature, available to the elderly and, beginning in 1973, to certain disabled young Americans.

Between 1967 and 1980 the number of agencies certified to participate in Medicare doubled, from 1753 to 2924. From 1980 to 1985 they doubled again to about 5983. As of August 1995 the number of certified agencies grew to an all-time high of 8747 (National Association for Home Care, 1995).

Hospital-based and proprietary agencies have grown faster than other types of certified agencies; proprietary agencies make up about 40%, and hospital-based agencies about 25%, of all certified agencies. Table 21-2 depicts the growth in the number and kinds of Medicare-certified agencies from 1967 to 1995.

PROFILE OF THE LONG-TERM CARE POPULATION

The long-term care population includes people of all ages with a wide array of disabling conditions and assistance needs. Disability can result from mental disabilities such as traumatic brain injuries, mental retardation, or Alzheimer's dementia. Physical limitations can be the result of paraplegia, heart disease, asthma, and arthritis. Among both the

table 21-2 Number of Medicare-Certified Home Care Agencies, by Auspice, 1967-1995

	Freestanding Agencies						Facility-based Agencies			
Year	VNA	COMB	PUB	PROP	PNP	OTH	HOSP	REHAB	SNF	Total
1967	549	93	939	0	0	39	133	0	0	1753
1975	525	46	1228	47	0	109	273	9	5	2242
1980	515	63	1260	186	484	40	359	8	9	2924
1985	514	59	1205	1943	832	4	1277	20	129	5983
1986	510	62	1192	1915	826	4	1341	17	117	5984
1987	500	61	1172	1882	803	1	1382	14	108	5923
1988	496	55	1073	1846	766	1	1439	12	97	5785
1989	491	51	1011	1818	727	1	1465	10	102	5676
1990	474	47	985	1884	710	0	1486	8	101	5695
1991	476	41	941	1970	701	0	1537	9	105	5780
1992	530	52	1083	1962	637	28	1623	3	86	6004
1993	594	46	1196	2146	558	41	1809	1	106	6497
1994	586	45	1146	2892	597	48	2081	3	123	7521
1995	579	38	1161	3730	667	59	2357	3	153	8747

From National Association for Home Care (NAHC): *Basic statistics about home health care 1995*, Washington, D.C., 1995, NAHC, p. 2.
Source: HCFA, Office of Survey and Certification
VNA: Visiting Nurse Associations are freestanding, voluntary, nonprofit organizations governed by a board of directors and usually financed by tax-deductible contributions as well as by earnings.
COMB: Combination agencies are combined government and voluntary agencies. These agencies are sometimes included with counts for VNAs.
PUB: Public agencies are government agencies operated by a state, county, city, or other unit of local government having a major responsibility for preventing disease and for community health education.
PROP: Proprietary agencies are freestanding, for-profit home care agencies.
PNP: Private not-for-profit agencies are freestanding and privately developed, governed, and owned nonprofit home care agencies.
OTH: Other freestanding agencies are agencies that do not fit one of the categories for freestanding agencies listed above.
HOSP: Hospital-based agencies are operating units or departments of a hospital. Agencies that have working arrangements with a hospital, or perhaps are even owned by a hospital but operated as separate entities, are classified as freestanding agencies under one of the categories listed above.
REHAB: Refers to agencies based in rehabilitation facilities.
SNF: Refers to agencies based in skilled nursing facilities.

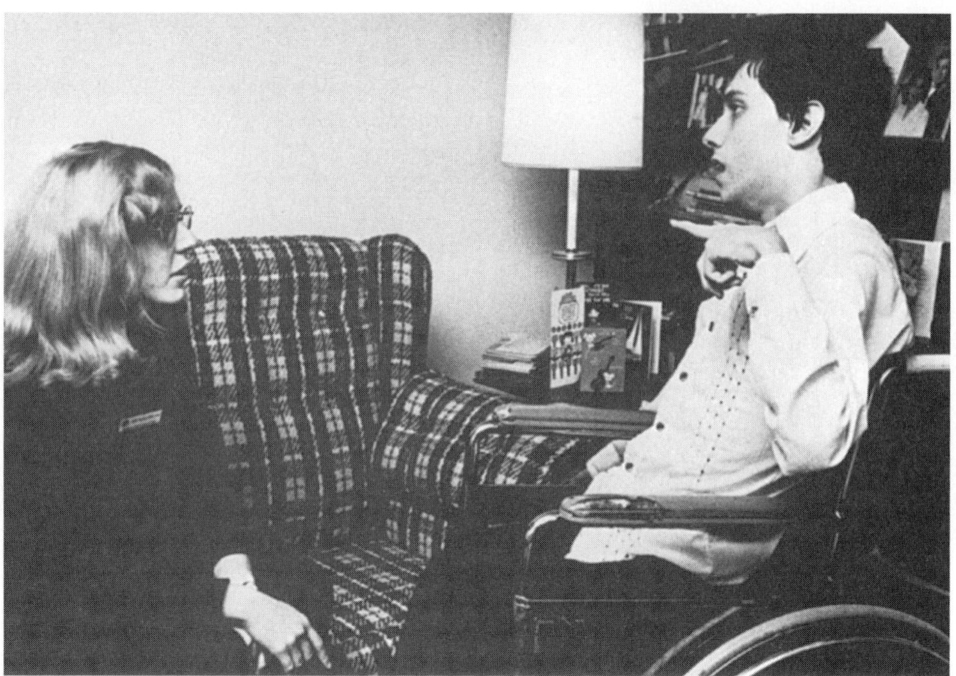

Figure 21-2 Young adults who are physically disabled frequently have extended health care needs that cannot be overlooked when plans for long-term care are developed. These young adults can become productive members of society when they have social and community supports that help them handle their disabling conditions. *(From Genesee Region Home Care Association, Rochester, N.Y.)*

elderly and nonelderly arthritis and heart disease are two of the most common reasons for long-term care services (GAO, 1994c, p. 12). Of the nonelderly, mental retardation is the third most common diagnosis underlying the need for service.

The range of services needed by clients and their families from the long-term care system varies greatly. Persons with mental disabilities often require supervision and protection as opposed to hands-on care. Not everyone with the same diagnosis needs the same level of care, and that level of care can change for the same person over time. Further, the needs of the elderly, working adults, and children vary over time because of the developmental life stage of each of these aggregates. Following is a profile of the aggregate of people using institutional and community-based long-term care services (GAO, 1994c, pp. 19-22):

Adults with ADL and IADL limitations: Persons age 18 to 64 and those 65 and over who need assistance with one or more ADL or IADL. An estimated 3.8 million persons need help with one or two ADL, and 1.3 million more need assistance with three of them.

Children with disabilities living at home: In August 1994 170,000 children under age 18 had limitations in at least one ADL (Figure 21-2).

Persons with severe mental disabilities: Approximately 1.4 million people have a level of cognitive impairment similar in severity to needing assistance with three or more ADLs. This includes persons of all ages with severe or profound mental retardation or another developmental disability, persons with severe mental illness, and persons with Alzheimer's disease or other mental illness.

Of the persons just described, 10.3 million live in the community. Of this group 3.1 million have severe disabilities, needing help with three or more ADLs, have severe cognitive or mental impairments, or have severe or profound mental retardation (Figure 21-3). Two thirds of them are elderly, two thirds live below the poverty line, and fewer than one in four has income at or above 300% of the poverty line ($22,000 for a single person in 1991)(AARP, 1995a, p. G6).

Cognitive Impairment

Causes of cognitive impairment in the elderly include dementia, delerium, toxic effects of medications, trauma, and psychiatric illness. Dementia is the most common cause and it implies a decline in cognitive function severe enough to interfere with social functioning. The estimated prevalence of dementia is 3% to 6% of community-based elderly persons, but the prevalence of dementia increases with age and is more common in institutional settings (Callahan, Hendrie, Tierney, 1995). The annual cost of caring for a client with Alzheimer's dementia (AD) is $47,000; total national costs in 1991 were $67 billion. The risk for AD increases with advancing age: the percentage of people who

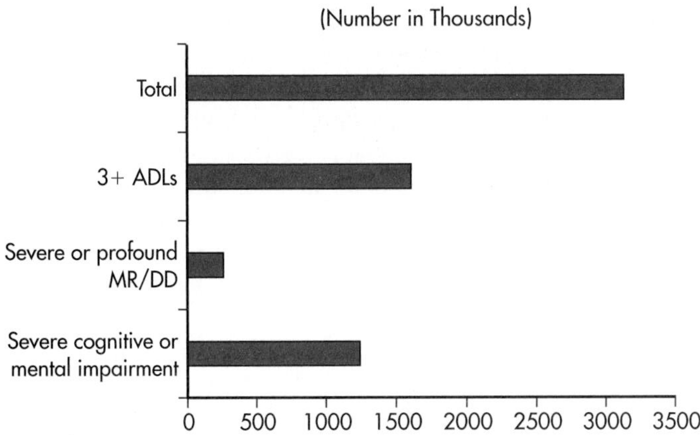

Figure 21-3 Persons in the community with severe disabilities by type of disability, 1993. *(From American Association of Retired Persons, Public Policy Institute:* Helping people with disabilities: the need for long-term care, *Washington, D.C., January 1995a, AARP, unpaginated.)*

suffer from AD or other dementias doubles with every decade of life (USDHHS, 1995).

Given the fact that people are increasingly living to a very old age, AD represents a major public health concern. Until a cure is found, providing and financing the long-term care needed by clients and their families presents a real challenge.

ALZHEIMER'S DEMENTIA Alzheimer's dementia is a degenerative brain disease that is marked by changes in behavior and personality and by an irreversible decline in intellectual abilities. In the person with AD the intricate process of communication between nerve cells in the brain breaks down. The destructive forces involved in AD ultimately cause nerve cell dysfunction, loss of connections between nerve cells, and death of some nerve cells in the brain. The death of neurons in key parts of the AD brain impairs thinking, memory, and judgment, and the deterioration advances in several stages that range from mild forgetfulness to severe dementia. The average duration of AD ranges from 4 to 8 years (USDHHS, 1995).

Two abnormal structures are found in the brain of the person with AD: amyloid plaques and neurofibrillary tangles. The plaques are outside and around neurons and contain dense deposits of an amyloid protein. The neurofibrillary tangles are twisted fibers inside neurons.

Risk factors for AD are under intense study. Aging itself does not result in AD; however, it is the most strongly associated risk factor for the disease. Family history is another important risk factor: a history of AD in a parent or sibling increases the odds of developing the disease by three to four times. Researchers believe that genetic factors may be involved in more than half the cases of the disease. Further, a severe head injury that leads to a loss of consciousness doubles the risk of developing AD. "These three factors—age, family history, and head injury—meet the accepted epidemiologic criteria for causal factors: they provide a plausible biological explanation, and their effects are strong and consistent" (USDHHS, 1995, p. 8).

Genetic research has found three gene alterations that are more common in AD patients than the general population: one, the ApoE4 gene on chromosome 19, has been linked to the most common form of AD, late-onset AD, which appears in older people. Researchers have also found genes on chromosomes 14 and 21 that are more common among people who develop AD in middle age. One gene on chromosome 21 has been associated with some early-onset familial AD; another gene on chromosome 14 has been associated with a larger portion of early-onset families who have members with AD.

Other risk factors being investigated include educational and occupational factors as well as the environment: aluminum and zinc have been postulated to be associated. However, there is no firm evidence at this point. Currently there is no way to prevent AD because its cause is unknown. No controllable risk factors are known, so there is no way to decrease the risk of getting the disease.

The onset of symptoms is usually noticed first by the affected person, family, friends, or peers at work rather than by health care professionals. The person usually hides early symptoms such as memory loss and decreased mental ability, possibly for years. Progression is insidious, with a diagnosis frequently made more than 4 years after the onset of symptoms. The average duration of Alzheimer's disease is 8 years, but duration is unpredictable: in some people it has remained as long as 25 years.

Most persons with AD are cared for at home for years before they are placed in a nursing home. Often this is a matter of choice. However, the fact that AD is a financial burden is a part of this decision. At this point no insurance policy offers home care benefits that cover the range of long-term services needed for a person with AD. Thus people at greatest risk cannot get coverage at all (Dittbrenner, 1994).

Alzheimer's disease causes mental anguish for the affected person and for the significant others. Caring for the individual places a constant burden on families and taxes their resources. Community health nurses play a major role in helping afflicted persons and their families to obtain appropriate care. A mental health model that focuses on adapting to the individual's behavior appears to benefit them more than a medical model focused on correcting a disability. A specific pattern of care is emerging that emphasizes medical evaluation and drug management, combined with mental health care in nursing homes and day care centers that coordinate their services with social and aging services.

Special care units (SCU) are programs designed specifically for persons with AD and other dementias. Programs vary widely from freestanding facilities that are specifically designed with highly trained staff members to wings of nursing homes that simply segregate persons with this diagnosis from others. The home care industry has also begun to develop special care programming. Today approximately 15,000 SCUs serving 50,000 persons have been developed. There is a lack of standardization about what constitutes an SCU versus a nonSCU: they vary in size, age of patients admitted, and whether there is segregation from other people. Accompanying this development has been a flurry of legislative and regulatory activity designed to ensure quality care in these settings (McConnell, 1994). The proliferation of special units means that for the first time in the United States staff members in nursing homes can develop methods of care specifically for their clients with AD. Better methods of care cannot be developed until there is formal research that describes, compares, and evaluates the methods being used. Continuing research will assist health professionals to answer these questions.

A variety of social and aging services are frequently available in the community to assist demented persons and their families to enhance the quality of their lives (see the box below). Community health nurses are often in a unique position to help families obtain needed services. The Alzheimer's Disease and Related Disorders Association (ADRDA) is a valuable resource for both health care professionals and clients. This association provides resource materials that help families establish an effective management program at home, offers group support services for families experiencing related stresses, and assists families in identifying community resources skilled in working with affected persons. Another valuable resource for clients, families, and health professionals is the Alzheimer's Disease Education and Referral Center, P.O. Box 8250, Silver Spring, Md. 20907-8250 (1-800-438-4380). However, many health care services do not address the needs of individuals with dementia. Persons especially likely to be unable to obtain adequate services are those without families, individuals from minority and ethnic groups, individuals experiencing disease onset in middle age, individuals residing in rural areas, veterans, and the poor (Dittbrenner, 1994; OTA, 1987, p. 45).

Support for informal caregivers is essential. The problems faced by families dealing with dementia are complex and very stressful and place them at high risk for experiencing financial difficulties in addition to health problems. "The primary needs of informal caregivers are respite care, information on the diseases and care methods, information about services, and a broadened range of services" (OTA, 1987, p. 63; Dittbrenner, 1994). The range of services for persons with dementia and their families is very limited in many communities.

There is no question that long-term care resources must be expanded. Statistical data show that the number of persons needing long-term services will increase dramatically in the next several decades. Defining at-risk aggregates in the community and subgroups within these aggregates who need these services, and pinpointing exactly at what intensity they need the services, will be the future challenge of health care providers.

Current research efforts are focusing on the gene on chormosome 14 that is responsible for one form of early-onset AD, as well as on how ApoE works as a risk factor for the disease. Other efforts are focusing on ways to enhance the use of imaging techniques such as magnetic resonance imaging, which assists researchers to identify initial changes in the hippocampus in AD, and positron emission computed tomography scans, which may eventually detect changes in brain metabolism that precede AD onset by as much as 20 years. Another crucial focus is on behavioral interventions for clients and training programs for caregivers (USDHHS, 1995). The country is making strides in dealing with this enormous public health problem.

FORMAL HOME CARE SERVICES

The founder of modern community health nursing, Lillian Wald, was introduced in the first chapter of this text. Wald and her contemporaries nursed the sick of all ages in their homes and also provided instructions to reduce illness and to promote health. The goals of these early home health care visits were to care for the sick, to teach the family how to care for the ill person, and above all to protect the public from the spread of disease (Buhler-Wilkerson, 1991, p. 7). Wald's work with the Metropolitan Life Insurance

CARE SERVICES FOR INDIVIDUALS WITH DEMENTIA

Adult day care	Homemaker services	Patient assessment	Respite care
Case management	Hospice services	Personal care	Skilled nursing
Chore services	Information and referral to services	Personal emergency response systems	Speech therapy
Congregate meals	Legal services	Physical therapy	Supervision
Dental services	Mental health services	Physician services	Telephone reassurance
Home delivered meals	Occupational therapy	Protective services	Transportation
Home health aide services	Paid companion/sitter	Recreational services	

From Office of Technology Assessment (OTA): *Losing a million minds: confronting the tragedy of Alzheimer's disease and other dementias*, Washington, D.C., 1987, U.S. Government Printing Office, p. 36.

Company to provide home health services was also described in Chapter 1. She was instrumental in developing a plan to extend nursing care to the Metropolitan's industrial policyholders during illness. The experiment was tremendously successful because the nurses, at a cost of five cents per policy, reduced the number of death benefits paid and also created the public image of a concerned humanitarian institution for the "Met." To provide this care across the country the organization used both existing visiting nurse associations and their own nurses. "For many visiting nurse associations, this new business partnership meant that without additional fund-raising, they could extend their services to more of the working class. Only three years later, Metropolitan Life Insurance Company was paying for one million nursing visits each year at a cost of roughly $500,000 per year. By 1916, the Metropolitan visiting nurse service was available to 90% of its 10.5 million policyholders living in 2,000 United States and Canadian cities" (Buhler-Wilkerson, p. 7-8) (Figure 21-4).

By the 1920s, 20 years later, care of ill people in their homes by nurses had declined. Infectious diseases such as smallpox and yellow fever were no longer the leading causes of death, and chronic diseases, much less dramatic in their impact, generated public concern. Further, patients of all classes began to seek hospital-based care since practitioners in this setting were better prepared than previously. Despite these changes, home care has been reaffirmed as an essential community service from a public health perspective throughout this century (Administration of Home Health Nursing, 1945; ANA, 1992; Bedside nursing care, 1945; Haupt, 1953; Olson, 1986; Stulginsky, 1993a).

Today home health care is the fastest growing industry in the United States. In fact, "it is poised to eclipse hospitals for the front-end care of many non-surgical patients in the years ahead" (Lumsdon, 1994, p. 45). Including certified and non-certified agencies total numbers of home care agencies grew from 11,765 in 1990 to 15,027 in 1994, and this growth shows little indication of slowing. The development of managed care plans, the downsizing of hospitals, and the emphasis on cost controls in health care are forcing dramatic changes for health professionals in home care. This chapter section discusses the impact of managed care on these services, the role of the nurse in this setting, reimbursement concerns, and the future of home health care. The philosophy of hospice care for the dying is also presented.

In 1992 the ANA refined the concept of home health nursing in its document *A Statement on the Scope of Home Health Nursing Practice*. This document defined home health nursing as a "synthesis of community health nursing and selected technical skills from other specialty nursing

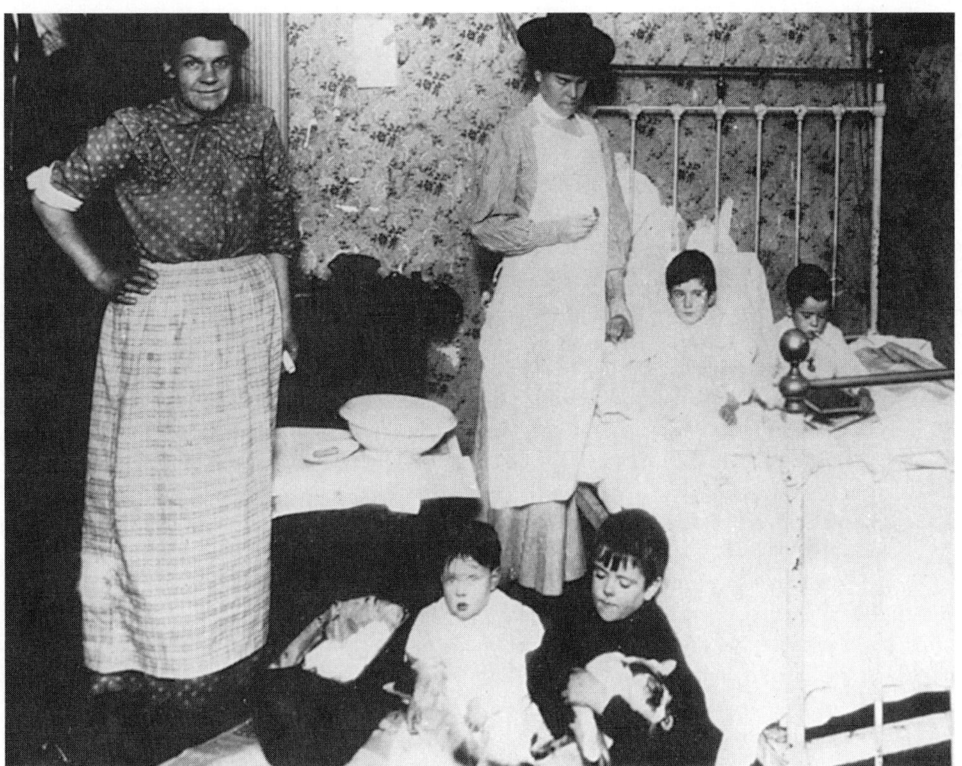

Figure 21-4 The increased emphasis being placed on home health care is not new. Home health care services have been provided by public health nurses in the United States since the late 1800s. Individuals across the life span benefit from these services. *(Courtesy the Metropolitan Life Insurance.)*

practices" (ANA, 1992, p. 5), such as medical-surgical nursing, gerontological nursing, and parent-child nursing. The health care deficits of the client determine the appropriate augmentation of other specialty skills with community health nursing practice. As discussed in Chapter 2, the home health nurse who practices within a community health nursing framework provides specialty focused skilled care beyond the individual and family. Nursing care from this perspective directs attention to aggregate needs, "with the predominate responsibility for care to the population as a whole" (ANA, p. 5). In line with this philosophy the home health nurse's role as a multidisciplinary care coordinator is important in facilitating the goal of care (ANA, p. 6). The Webster case situation in Chapter 2 illustrates the importance of the care coordinator role in facilitating the goal of care beyond the individual family.

Home care includes a broad range of homebased health and social services such as home management assistance, personal care, consumer education, and financial counseling services. Social home care services are covered under Title XX of the Social Security Act for clients who qualify for Title XX assistance (Title XX is discussed later in this chapter). These services are provided by diverse community agencies such as local departments of social service, family service organizations, and councils on agencies.

Home care visits at one time centered around visits to mothers and children, care of the chronically ill person, and an emphasis on health promotion. Today this specialty area of nursing is synonomous not only with acute care but also with intensive at-home care. Home health nurses are no longer exclusively generalists: advanced practice nurses are increasingly demanded by the medical community and used to address the complexity and acuity found in the home setting. The contemporary home health nurse is more likely than not "a generalist/specialist from an acute care setting where the emphasis is on individualized, holistic care and a curative short-term outcome" (Stulginsky, 1993a, p. 402).

Experienced home health nurses interviewed by Stulginsky (1993a) said that their practice was "meeting the acute and chronic care needs of patients and their families in the home environment. Inherent in this definition was an appreciation for the family's psychosocial resources, the neighborhood, and the presence or absence of community services." The patient was the controlling center of the provider's focus (Stulginsky, 1993a, p. 402).

Although both hospital-based nurses and home health nurses use acute care and high technology skills, the home visit requires nursing practice that is very different from the hospital setting. The competencies needed by nurses in home health were ascertained by interviews of expert nurses in home care (Stulginsky, 1993b). They are listed in the box below.

Multiple types of agencies (Table 21-3) provide home health care services. Both the government and private sectors of the health care delivery system are active in delivering home health services.

The Practical Wisdom of Expert Home Care Nurses

Build trust and rapport: Enter the home as a guest; sense "where people are"; do not enter the family's "space"; note the family's customs; negotiate visit times around family needs; honor time commitments

The first contact sets the tone: Since few people understand what home care is, the first visit is crucial to developing a lasting helpful relationship; define what nursing can and cannot do; work on mutually acceptable goals; speak slowly and allow processing; ascertain that families know where to call in emergencies

Assessing the home involves common sense and imagination: There is no baseline from home to home; listen, look, smell, look for patterns, space, touch, availability of supports; develop giant antennae

Setting limits to encourage self-care: Help people solve their own problems, help them look to the past to find their own strengths

Priorities remain fluid: Base priorities for visits on (1) potential threats to health, (2) degree of concern to the client, (3) ease of solution

Suspend one's own values: Accept things where they are and find common ground; communicate trust and respect in the family's ability to make good decisions

Teach survival to patients: Teach information that will keep the patient safe until the next visit; understand learner readiness; teaching while doing; enable and empower patients to do for themselves

Professional boundaries are rarely secure: With the familiarity of home visits, self-disclosure, accepting gifts and hospitality, and maintaining therapeutic distance are all boundaries one struggles with to find a place of comfort; rarely are those boundaries secure

Homes can be more distracting than clinical settings: There may be environmental (clutter, noise), behavioral (drug seeking, avoidance), or nurse initiated (fears of harm, reaction to lifestyle) distractions to providing care. Deal with them directly whenever possible

Nurses need to protect themselves: Threats to safety must be handled realistically; heed subtle and not-so-subtle messages from families

Making do is an essential skill: Equipment and supplies are not always available; adapting can be a challenge for both nurse and family

Time is the nurse's most precious resource: As a result of third-party reimbursement, paperwork is a home health nurse's biggest complaint; develop your own techniques for keeping this at a minimum

From Stulginsky MM: Nurses' home health experience. Part II: the unique demands of home visits, *Nurs Health Care* 14(9):476-485, 1993b.

The proliferation of home health care agencies provided an impetus for the development of *Standards of Home Health Nursing Practice* by the American Nurses Association in 1986. These standards guide agencies and nurses in providing care of the highest quality for home health care clients and are presented in the box on the next page.

Presented in the View from the Field are four case histories that represent the type of care offered by home health agencies. The case situations illustrate the direct service role, as well as the care coordinator role, of the home health care nurse. The Visiting Nurse Service of the Toledo District Nurse Association, the agency that published these case histories, has been caring for elderly and disabled persons for more than 83 years. Throughout these years this organization has provided millions of home visits to needy persons.

These case histories continue to reflect current practice and clearly illustrate that individuals across the life span need community-based home care services. They also reflect the increasing acuity of client care demands and the need for coordinated, multidisciplinary home health services. Most importantly, they show that skilled home-based nursing services can make a difference. They help families to strengthen their coping abilities, and they assist disabled persons to improve their functional capabilities and avoid unnecessary institutionalization.

MANAGED CARE AND HOME CARE

Increasing numbers of clients seen by home health nurses are part of managed care organizations. Nearly half of the population of the United States with private health insurance coverage was in some type of managed care arrangement in 1989 (Hadley, Langwell, 1991). Sixty-three percent of employees in the nation's largest corporations are now HMO members, up 41% from 2 years ago, and 28% of California's Medicare population is enrolled in a Medicare Risk HMO (Masso, 1995). "As of November 1995, fully half of the states were operating, waiting for approvals of, or developing statewide Medicaid managed care programs," (Children's Defense Fund, 1996, p. 21).

The significance of this activity for the profession is outstanding. Managed care companies will face strong incentives to lower costs, and the use of advanced practice nurses to replace physicians will expand (Buerhaus, 1994). Further, nursing interventions must be described and their cost and

table 21-3 Types of Home Health Care Agencies in the United States*

Type of Agency	Description of Agency
Official	A governmental or public agency, usually a local health department, which is supported by state and local taxes. Official agencies are mandated by law to provide certain specific services, such as communicable disease follow-up. They provide health promotion and disease prevention services as well as home health care.
Voluntary	A private, nonprofit agency whose operating funds come largely from individual contributions, fees-for-service, united community funds, contracts for service, grants, and other nonofficial sources of funding. Voluntary agencies are governed by a board of directors. These agencies are not required by law to provide specific types of services; they primarily, but not exclusively, provide home health care services. The visiting nurse associations traditionally have been the major voluntary organizations which provide home health care services in a local community.
Combination	A combined governmental (a local health department) and voluntary agency (a VNA), whose operating funds came from both official and nonofficial sources. This organizational structure was promoted for the purposes of preventing duplication of services, decreasing continuity of care difficulties and reducing the cost of delivering local health care services. A combination agency provides both health promotion/disease prevention and home health care services.
Private, nonprofit	A privately owned agency which is tax exempt because of its nonprofit status. Unlike voluntary agencies, these agencies are governed by the owner(s) of the organization. Their major source of revenue is fee-for-service. Private nonprofit agencies are usually established to provide home health care services only.
Proprietary	A private agency established to make a profit. These agencies are not eligible for tax exemption. They are governed by their owner(s), who are increasingly large corporations. Their major source of revenue is a fee for service. Like the private, nonprofit agencies, proprietary agencies are usually established to provide home health care services only.
Hospital-based	A home health care agency run and governed by a hospital. Sources of revenue and tax status vary depending on the type of hospital (governmental, voluntary, private, nonprofit, or proprietary) which has established the home health care agency. It is predicted that the numbers of hospital-based home health care agencies will increase dramatically in the next decade.

Modified from Health Care Financing Administration: *Medicare program: home health agencies—conditions of participation and reductions in recordkeeping requirements*, 42 CFR, Part 484, Sections 484.1 through 484.52, Washington, D.C., October, 1994b, U.S. Department of Health and Human Services; and Hirsh L, Klein M, Marlowe G: *Combining public health nursing agencies: a case study in Philadelphia*, New York, 1967, Department of PHN, NLN, p. 3.

*See Chapter 5 for further discussion of official and voluntary agencies.

Standards of Home Health Nursing Practice

STANDARD I. ORGANIZATION OF HOME HEALTH SERVICES

All home health services are planned, organized, and directed by a master's-prepared professional nurse with experience in community health and administration.

STANDARD II. THEORY

The nurse applies theoretical concepts as a basis for decisions in practice.

STANDARD III. DATA COLLECTION

The nurse continuously collects and records data that are comprehensive, accurate, and systematic.

STANDARD IV. DIAGNOSIS

The nurse uses health assessment data to determine nursing diagnoses.

STANDARD V. PLANNING

The nurse develops care plans that establish goals. The care plan is based on nursing diagnoses and incorporates therapeutic, preventive, and rehabilitative nursing actions.

STANDARD VI. INTERVENTION

The nurse, guided by the care plan, intervenes to provide comfort, to restore, improve, and promote health, to prevent complications and sequelae of illness, and to effect rehabilitation.

STANDARD VII. EVALUATION

The nurse continually evaluates the client's and family's responses to interventions in order to determine progress toward goal attainment and to revise the data base, nursing diagnoses, and plan of care.

STANDARD VIII. CONTINUITY OF CARE

The nurse is responsible for the client's appropriate and uninterrupted care along the health care continuum, and therefore uses discharge planning, case management, and coordination of community resources.

STANDARD IX. INTERDISCIPLINARY COLLABORATION

The nurse initiates and maintains a liaison relationship with all appropriate health care providers to assure that all efforts effectively complement one another.

STANDARD X. PROFESSIONAL DEVELOPMENT

The nurse assumes responsibility for professional development and contributes to the professional growth of others.

STANDARD XI. RESEARCH

The nurse participates in research activities that contribute to the profession's continuing development of knowledge of home health care.

STANDARD XII. ETHICS

The nurse uses the code for nurses established by the American Nurses Association as a guide for ethical decision making in practice.

From American Nurses Association (ANA): *Standards of home health nursing practice*, Kansas City, Mo., 1986, The Association, pp. 5-19.

effectiveness determined. These interventions then must be related to client satisfaction and other outcomes, and the public educated about this information. McCloskey and Bulechek's work with the Iowa Intervention Projection is a sound step in this direction (1996). Their research work has established 433 interventions, each having a label name, a definition, and a list of activities that a nurse does to carry out the intervention. The interventions are linked to the diagnoses of the North American Nursing Diagnosis Association (NANDA) (see Chapter 9). Future research with the intervention structure will enable nurses to begin to objectively identify the work that is done to nurse clients to health with the possibility of costing out care by intervention. Home health companies can begin to demonstrate objectively to insurers the cost of care by diagnosis and intervention.

Nurses in home care must understand that they are part of an industry, that the time spent and the outcomes achieved with clients and their families are carried out within the framework of the managed care setting: case managers authorize the kinds of services that the home care nurse can provide for clients, and those services need to lead to planned outcomes within a specific time frame. Nurses' approach to client care needs to change from a focus on "caring for the client" to a mindset that teaches the family/caregiver how to care for the client so that health care needs are met in the shortest possible time. Effective nurses have communication skills that appropriately convey the client needs to the case manager and other disciplines involved in the care. Nurses also need the skills to delegate to other levels of caregivers (see Chapter 23).

In managed care focus is on both outcomes achieved and quality of care given; clients have a major role in determining both what that quality is and what the outcomes will be. Nurses must be leaders and managers of their own caseloads to achieve the highest quality in the shortest amount of time (see Chapter 23). Nurses will use progressive technologies, will work with disciplines in collaborative efforts, and will provide primary and not specialty care (note the *Competencies Needed for Health Professionals* listed by the Pew Health Professions Commission and presented in Chapter 25).

As discussed in Chapter 23, successful nurses are comfortable with constant change. Home care organizations are changing care delivery systems and some of these include the following (Lumsdon, 1994):

A View from the Field VNS CARING IN TOLEDO, OHIO: FOUR CASE EXAMPLES

CASE EXAMPLE ONE

Sixteen-year-old boy run over by train, which inflicted massive trauma resulting in amputation of left hindquarter, amputation of arm, multiple pelvic fractures, fracture of transverse process, avulsion of urethra-prostate-testes and L-sileium exposing peritoneal sac, laceration L. ureter and L. iliac arteries, resulted in colostomy, supra-pubic cystotomy, hemipelvectomy, bilateral orchiectomy, skin grafts to hip sockets, etc.

After only five weeks in the hospital, client was allowed to go home (on Coordinated Home Care, saving over 30 hospital days) with a 24" × 24" graft in L pelvic area with open draining area. The VNS Home Care Coordinator managed this complex referral, coordinated arrangements for special dressing supplies and equipment and facilitated care throughout the period of need. The case nurse said, "The coordinator made it all come together and work." Clearly, the value of the coordinator having home care experience and familiarity with agency operations was evident.

Nursing visits were daily for two weeks, then reduced to three times a week as the family became more confident in care. Nursing activities included aseptic wound care, supervision of colostomy care, suprapubic catheter care, observation for complications with prompt intervention, instruction of family in all aspects of care and encouraging this adolescent to become independent in ADLs. To promote usual family activities, the nurse supported their decision to go on a weekend camping trip within the first two weeks and arranged to make visits at the local campsite.

Physical and occupational therapy services were provided for ADL's, gait training, transfers, strengthening and stump wrapping. Since this boy was left-dominant, he had to relearn all activities one-handed with the nondominant side. When a left arm prosthesis was secured, the OT (who herself has an upper extremity prosthesis) resumed visits to aid in learning its use.

A total of 129 home health visits were provided over a nine-month period to aid in his excellent recovery, and he has now returned to school.

Although several intervening hospitalizations were required for re-evaluations and surgical revisions, none were necessary for complications, e.g., infection.

This example of teamwork included various surgery specialists, numerous VNS staff, and, of course, the family.

CASE EXAMPLE TWO

A 70-year-old patient who had transhepatic biliary disease, probably cancer of head of pancreas, and a history of cancer of gallbladder was admitted to service after insertion of a transhepatic ring catheter which allows bile to drain from the common duct to the duodenum.

The patient and family were quite anxious re: involved procedures. The visiting nurse instructed the family in home care including such things as withdrawing of bile, irrigating ring catheter technique, dressing changes using

From Visiting Nurse Service (VNS) of Toledo: Eighty-three years of caring, *Caring* 3:61, 1984. Case examples were written by Janet Blaufuss, RN, former Executive Director of the Visiting Nurse Service of the Toledo District Nurse Association, Toledo, Ohio, 1984.

Continued

- High-risk maternity care; for example, pregnant women who develop gestational diabetes are cared for at home with a "packaged program."
- Neonatal care; for example, stabilized neonates who meet specific criteria are sent home in isolettes.
- Niche services in high-volume areas such as cardiology, oncology, respiratory ailments, and pregnancy are delivered in the home setting.

Outcomes in Nursing Care

The focus on quality assessment has moved from structure and process to the outcomes of care (Peters, Eigsti, 1991). Though all three are essential, in managed care the outcome of care is the bottom line. Shaughnessy's research (1996) has developed Medicare's OASIS: Standardized Outcome and Assessment Information Set for Home Health Care. OASIS is a data set with the following categories of items: demographics and client history, living arrangements, supportive assistance, body systems, ADL/IADL, medications, equipment management, and emergent care. The data are assessed on admission to a home health agency, at a point in time during care, and then upon discharge. OASIS is used for measuring outcomes defined as a change in health status between two or more time points; the instrument will likely be mandated by the Health Care Financing Administration to monitor outcomes of the care provided by Medicare-certified agencies. Because Medicare benefits typically account for about 60% to 85% of hospital-based home health agencies revenues (Lumsdon, 1994), OASIS has the potential for a national overview of the outcomes of care provided to adults in this country, and thus can provide HCFA with comparison data for all types of certified home health agencies.

ANALYSIS OF OTHER LONG-TERM CARE SETTINGS

Though the home is the site of care for the majority of people needing long-term care services, care in institutional settings, primarily nursing homes, constitutes about 85% of

A View from the Field VNS CARING IN TOLEDO, OHIO: FOUR CASE EXAMPLES—cont'd

aseptic technique, changing catheter plug, and teaching of signs of complications, in addition to monitoring hypertension status, nutrition/hydration, reactions to x-ray treatment, medications and pain control.

After verbal and demonstrative teaching, the family was able to provide the necessary care and patient was discharged in stabilized condition.

CASE EXAMPLE THREE

A 5-month-old infant who had been normal at birth developed pneumococcal meningitis with resulting hydrocephalus, severe neurologic deficits and seizure disorders. The mother, who was single and 16 years old, wanted to care for the child at home as long as possible so a referral was made to VNS.

At the time of hospital discharge, the child was totally unresponsive and had no purposeful movements, was on continuous gastric tube feedings with a Kangaroo pump, and required a suction machine and vaporizer. Nursing care consisted of providing and teaching re: dressing changes around the G-tube, tube irrigation, frequent repositioning, ROM, skin care and hygiene, relaxation and stimulation techniques, and use of Kangaroo pump. Additionally, the home care nurse assessed neurological and respiratory status and provided frequent intervention related to medication regimen, irritability, and seizure control. A home health aide assisted the mother with care, bathing and stimulation techniques. A total of 54 home health visits were provided over a five-month period.

The Maternal Child Health nurse supported this young mother in her difficult decision to place the child in an extended care unit for the developmentally disabled at one year of age (where she visits frequently and takes her home every other weekend) so she could return to school.

At the time of discharge from VNS, this young child could take water orally, respond to the mother and had some purposeful movement.

CASE EXAMPLE FOUR

A 76-year-old client had a long history of Crohn's disease and malabsorption syndrome, and after multiple admissions for weight loss, malnutrition and dehydration, a permanent subclavian line was inserted in early summer of 1981 for total parenteral nutrition. It became apparent that adequate nutrition could only be attained through TPN and she would need regular infusions of amino acids, electrolytes, minerals and, eventually, fatty acids through this subclavian line. VNS nurses worked closely with physicians, hospital nurses, nutritionists, pharmacists, social workers, and patient's family in planning for adequate predischarge teaching and adequate home support for this patient. Through a joint effort between VNS and the community hospital, the patient's elderly brother has been successfully managing her four-times-a-week home TPN infusion, and once-a-week lipid infusion. This patient has the original subclavian line in place (for over two years) and it has remained free of any signs and symptoms of infection for over two years. In addition to care for the subclavian line and TPN infusions, VNS has helped the brother learn to care for the patient's permanent colostomy and chronic abdominal fistula.

Patient's condition has deteriorated gradually over the last two years; she now has an indwelling foley catheter and is essentially bed bound, requiring the services of a home health aide. Patient appears to have suffered at least one CVA and has been hospitalized for erratic blood sugars, and abnormal blood values which reflects the necessary and frequent nursing intervention. Nutritionally she has remained stable, demonstrating a weight gain of sixteen pounds over two years (originally weight was 88 pounds and now is 104 pounds).

Through the joint efforts of VNS, the community hospital, and the family, this patient has been able to go home and remain at home, without serious nutritional compromise, over the last two years.

Medicaid expenditures for long-term care. In this country expenditures for nursing facilities are financed about equally by Medicaid and private out-of-pocket payments. In 1993 Medicaid provided $36.3 billion (48.3%) of the $75.2 billion spent on nursing facility care including care in intermediate care facilities for the mentally retarded. Private individuals paid $29.6 billion (39.4%) out of pocket. The remainder was covered by Medicare (7.6%), private insurance (0.1%), and other sources (GAO, 1994a).

Figure 21-5 depicts the Medicaid expenditures for long-term care services in 1993. Payments for institutional care far exceed the amount spent on noninstitutional care. Home health received 3.4%, personal care assistance in the home received 5.9%, and home and community based waiver services, programs designed to permit States flexibility in developing alternatives to institutional care, received 6.6%.

The importance of informal support networks in preventing institutionalization cannot be overestimated. As previously discussed, about 75% of the dependent elderly are cared for in their homes. Most families want to care for their disabled family members and keep them at home as long as possible. Often in doing so these families experience extreme financial costs and stress and place themselves at risk for experiencing health problems. Families usually opt for institutional care as a solution for dealing with their stress only after their personal resources for coping have become exhausted.

When visiting in the home environment community health nurses assess characteristics that place people at risk

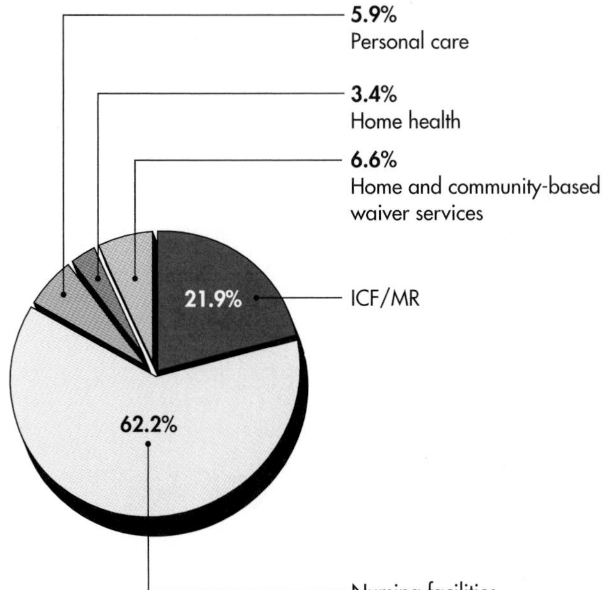

Note: Total spending was $42 billion.
Source: SysteMetrics.MEDSTAT, using preliminary data from HCFA-64.

Figure 21-5 Medicaid expenditures for long-term care services, 1993. *(From GAO:* Medicaid long term care: successful state efforts to expand home services while limiting costs, *Pub No. HEHS-94-167, Washington, D.C., August, 1994a, U.S. Government Printing Office, p. 21.)*

for requiring nursing home placement and should work with the client and family to explore other long-term care options. Adult day care programs, respite care, alternative family care homes, residential care facilities, and domiciliary care facilities are a few examples of such options.

Figure 21-6 shows the home and community-based services needed by the largest proportion of elderly persons needing assistance. Unfortunately few funds are available to assist clients with their greatest needs: personal care, housekeeping, meal preparation, and home chore service.

Community health nurses play a crucial role in assessing the level of care needed by clients who require long-term care services. Reducing inappropriate use of nursing home beds by people who are capable of living at home—a "gatekeeping mechanism"—can save costly and scarce health care resources and can better meet clients' physical and emotional needs.

Residential Options

A number of residential options other than nursing home care are open to people who either cannot or do not want to maintain an independent household and who have varying needs of help with ADL. They include board and care homes, also called rest homes, personal care homes, domiciliary homes, retirement homes, family care homes, and adult congregate living facilities, among others. They vary in price range from those who serve people on SSI (see Chapters 4 and 5) to those that advertise for the affluent. *Board and care homes* usually provide housekeeping and congregate meals and may include some oversight from staff members. Typically they do not provide a comprehensive range of services and do not claim to meet unscheduled needs. Every state has adopted a form of licensure for these facilities, but most states have unlicensed facilities (Kane, Wilson, 1993). *Continuing care retirement communities* usually have three levels of care; the level of care between independent living and a nursing home is a form of assisted living. These tend to be available only to aggregates who can afford the high fees. *Residential care in nursing homes,* usually on the same premises, has been available in many communities for some time. *Adult foster homes* generally serve the mentally and developmentally disabled adult rather than those with physical disabilities. *Congregate care* refers to complexes with separate apartments and some services such as housekeeping and meals. Personal care is usually not a part of congregate care. Finally, *home-sharing arrangements,* several individuals or families living together in a single family home, can work very well in some instances.

New models of assisted living are currently under development and study in the United States (Kane, Wilson, 1993). Interest is growing in community-based residential arrangements that offer personal care to persons who need assistance and that can respond to unscheduled (unexpected) needs for older persons. Developers in the private sector have built programs in response to consumer demand and funding mechanisms, and state regulation of them is currently under study. Separation of government funding for housing, housekeeping, and meal preparation from the funding for personal care and nursing services is a promising approach to the financing of assisted living. "If nurtured and encouraged in particular directions, we believe that the emerging phenomenon of assisted living could result in a widespread program offering a new paradigm for residential long-term care for disabled older people" (Kane, Wilson, p. 120). Such arrangements have the possibilities of retaining some independence for people and separating out the high-cost activities of personal care from the day-to-day costs of food and shelter.

GOVERNMENT LONG-TERM CARE FINANCING

The Health Care Financing Administration (HCFA) is the primary source of funding for long-term services. The major portion of public expenditures for long-term care services goes to institutional care, with the Medicaid program being the principal payor for this type of care. The Medicaid program pays for over half of all nursing home expenditures. It supports long-term institutional care in a variety of facilities, including skilled nursing facilities (SNFs), intermediate care facilities (ICFs), intermediate care facilities for the mentally retarded (ICFs/MR), and mental hospitals. The Medicare program pays for skilled and complementing skilled (home health aide services) home health care services, and care in skilled nursing facilities during acute phases of illness. This program does not support long-term care in nursing

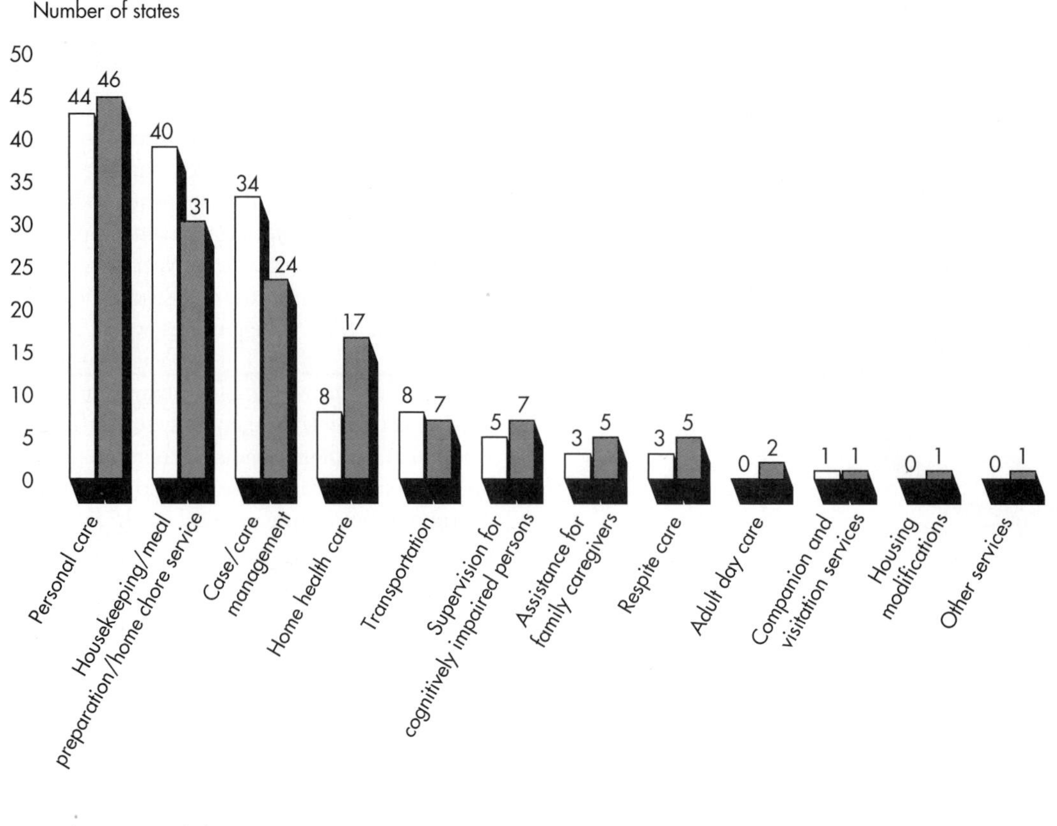

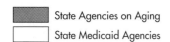

Figure 21-6 Home and community-based services needed by the largest proportion of elderly persons with severe disabilities. *(From GAO: Long-term care reform: states' views on key elements of well-designed programs for the elderly, Pub No. HEHS-94-227, Washington, D.C., September 1994b, U.S. Government Printing Office, p. 9.)*

homes and other facilities providing unskilled or custodial services.

Noninstitutional long-term care or home care is currently funded by four federal programs—Title XVIII (Medicare), Title XIX (Medicaid), Title XX (block grants to states for social services) of the Social Security Act, and Title III of the Older Americans Act. The basic characteristics of each of these programs are discussed in Chapter 4. The type of home care services financially supported by each program is next presented.

Medicare (Title XVIII)

The largest governmental expenditures for home health care services are made by Medicare. Both part A (hospital insurance) and Part B (supplemental medical insurance) of Medicare include provisions for home health care. Medicare reimburses a home health care agency for the following services if they are reasonable and necessary (HCFA, 1989b; HCFA, 1994):

- Part-time or *intermittent* skilled nursing services provided by or under the supervision of a registered nurse
- *Intermittent* physical, occupational, or speech therapy provided by or under the supervision of a qualified therapist
- *Intermittent* medical social services provided by or under the supervision of a qualified social worker
- *Intermittent* home health services provided by a home health aide who has completed a competency evaluation program and is supervised by a registered nurse who possesses a minimum of 2 years of nursing experience, at least 1 year of which must be in the provision of home health care, and who has a perfor-

mance review of 12 hours of inservice and training annually

- Medical supplies (other than drugs and medications) and the use of medical appliances
- Hospice services including short-term inpatient care, nursing care, therapy services, medical social services, home health aide services, physician services, and counseling.

Provisions of the Omnibus Budget Reconciliation Act of 1980 (Public Law 96-499) expanded the home health benefits offered by Medicare so that beneficiaries are permitted unlimited home health visits without the requirement for a prior hospital stay or payment of a deductible amount. To qualify for those benefits, Medicare beneficiaries must be *homebound;* the services must be prescribed and periodically reviewed by a physician (at least once every 62 days); and the client must need part-time or *intermittent, skilled* nursing care and/or therapy services (physical, occupational, or speech therapy). When home health aide services are needed, the registered nurse, or appropriate professional staff member if only therapy services are provided, must make supervisory visits (Table 21-5) to the client's residence on a regular basis (HCFA, 1994).

Landmark changes in the Medicare program have occurred as a result of a lawsuit brought against Medicare by the National Association for Home Care (NAHC) in the late 1980s. The suit contained two essential claims: (1) the challenge to the part-time or intermittent policy for length of care allowed clients, and (2) how "medical necessity" is interpreted to qualify a client for care. The successful conclusion to the lawsuit did not change Medicare regulations but did change HCFA's interpretation of them, so that more services could be provided. Several of these changes are noteworthy (Staggers' Lawsuit, 1988, pp. 1-3):

1. Clients are considered homebound if they attend adult day care centers, renal dialysis clinics, or outpatient radiation or chemotherapy facilities when the purpose is to receive medical care. Regarding adult day care patients, it is the agency's responsibility to demonstrate that attendance at the day center is for the purpose of receiving medical care.
2. A new skilled service is described—skilled nursing management and evaluation of a client care plan—that allows coverage for nurses who need to manage certain complex unskilled care cases.
3. Specific coverage standards are set out for venipuncture in stable and unstable patients. For example, a client receiving prothrombin whose blood test results indicate stability within the therapeutic range will qualify for a skilled nursing visit once a month to continue appropriate monitoring.
4. A client cannot be denied solely on the basis of having a chronic disease or terminal illness.
5. An order for "personal care" of a home health aide is allowed, with the boundaries of that personal care to be determined by the nurse following a care plan rather than by a physician.
6. Coverage of family counseling is specifically recognized as part of the function of a medical social services visit, in which family counseling is incidental to beneficiary counseling and designed to remove an impediment to the delivery of safe and effective care.

The skilled nursing management change generated a model for nurses to provide case management for persons at risk for rehospitalization. It is significant because for the first time Medicare eligibility rules do the following (Allen, 1994): (1) recognize and reimburse nurses as case managers in the home, (2) reimburse for prevention and health promotion in the home, and (3) acknowledge and reimburse chronic rather than exclusively acute care for its recipients.

The Medicare Home Health Agency Manual (HCFA, 1989a), known as HIM 11, was rewritten to address the changes noted in the Staggers' Lawsuit. It contains case examples clarifying coverage criteria and is useful on a daily basis for the staff nurse. Failure to comply with the conditions of participation results in an agency's loss of certification by Medicare and the ability to receive Medicare reimbursement.

With its statutory emphases on part-time acute and postacute treatment of illness, the Medicare program does not adequately address the long-term care needs of the aging population. The homebound and the part-time or intermittent skilled nursing criteria for eligibility make it impossible for many chronically ill or disabled aging persons to qualify for Medicare home health care benefits. To add to the problem of the emphasis on acute care, in 1994 noninstitutionalized Americans age 65 and over were projected to spend an average of $2519 out-of-pocket for health care (see Chapter 4 for definitions of out-of-pocket). Of this amount, 45% was spent on insurance premiums, 17% on physician services, 13% on home health care services, 10% on prescription drugs, 7% on hospital services, and the remaining 8% on vision and dental services and durable medical equipment (AARP, 1995b). Out-of-pocket expenses for older Americans rose 90%, on average, between 1987 and 1994, and the greatest increase on average was for home health services (defined as a relatively broad range of services provided in the home, including those delivered by paid health care providers and paid homemakers) (AARP). Figure 21-7 depicts in a striking manner the money spent by clients for home care services as compared to total health costs in 1994.

PROBLEMS WITH MEDICARE AND LEGISLATION ACTION

The Medicare Trust Fund will go bankrupt in 2001 if expenditures for home health care and hospital care continue to rise at present rates. Further, with the rapid growth in home care agencies there have been concerns about both the quality and appropriateness of some of the home care services provided (St. Pierre, Dittbrenner, 1995).

The first sections of this chapter discussed the factors that have influenced the needs for long-term care services in this

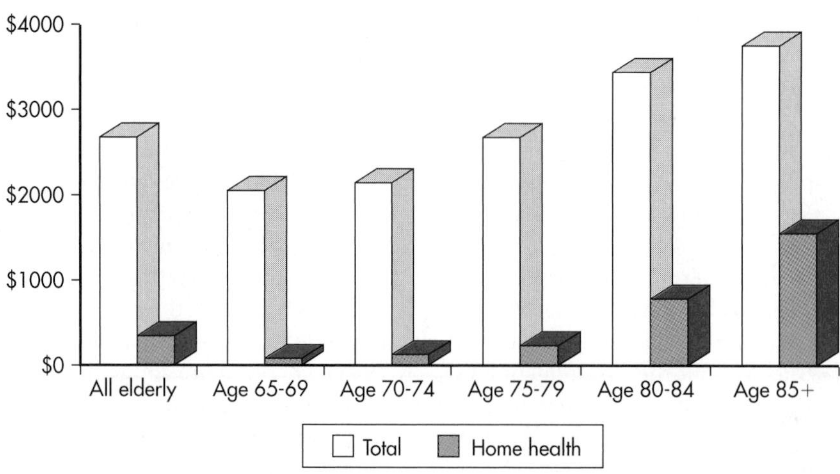

Figure 21-7 Average elderly out-of-pocket costs by age: home health care compared to total health costs, 1994. (*From AARP Public Policy Institute and The Urban Institute:* Coming up short: increasing out-of-pocket health spending by older Americans, *Washington, D.C., April 1995b, AARP, p. 7.)*

country. With the concomitant costs and needs associated with those services there have been almost yearly amendments to the Social Security Act to both restrict and expand home health care services. In 1993, for example, there was a reduction in payment to agencies providing hospice services, a repeal of the mandate requiring personal care services to be covered under states' Medicaid programs, an extension of social HMO demonstrations (discussed in the next section of this chapter), and an extension of monies for Alzheimer's dementia demonstration projects (NAHC, 1996). In 1994 much of the legislation for changes in home health care was part of Bill and Hillary Clinton's Health Security Bill, which was not passed into legislation. The Balanced Budget Act of 1995, which contained sweeping changes in both Medicare and Medicaid, was vetoed by President Clinton.

After the 1996 presidential campaign, many of the debates about Medicare and other health care costs had not reached resolution. However, current issues under discussion will affect the aggregate of persons needing long-term care services, as well as the providers of that care. The National Association for Home Care, 519 C Street N.E., Washington, D.C. 20002-5809 (202-547-7424) publishes an annual legislative blueprint that details the focus of their legislative efforts. Some that are current are listed in the box on the next page.

Medicaid (Title XIX)

The current Medicaid statute provides states with the authority to include a variety of home and community-based services in their Medicaid programs. Medicaid programs can cover case management, personal care services, day care, private duty nursing, and home health services. Unlike the requirements of the Medicare program, home health under Medicaid includes *skilled* and *unskilled* services. To qualify for home care benefits under Medicaid clients must meet income eligibility requirements, have the services ordered by a physician, and have the plan of care reviewed by a physician every 62 days. Clients do not need to be homebound to receive Medicaid benefits.

Since Medicaid is a state-administered program, the range of home care benefits offered varies from state to state. However, in order to be federally subsidized under Medicaid, a state must provide at least home health services. Personal care services are not mandated by the federal government. States also have the freedom to determine eligibility requirements and the amount of service they will reimburse under Medicaid. Some states extend home care benefits to the "medically needy," those persons who do not qualify for regular Medicaid benefits but who have inadequate financial resources to meet health care costs.

Section 2176 of the Omnibus Budget Reconciliation Act of 1981 (Public Law 97-35) expanded the range of long-term services that can be offered by the Medicaid program; this act established the Medicaid Waiver Authority to implement 2176 Waiver programs of home- and community-based care. "Under these programs, states can provide a comprehensive array of medical and social services including case management, homemaker and home health aides, personal care, adult day care, habilitation care and respite care to avoid more costly institutional care" (U.S. Senate, Committee on Finance, 1984, p. 78). These programs serve individuals in the community who would require the level of care provided in a skilled nursing facility or intermediate care facility if they did not receive 2176 Waiver services. The costs

National Association for Home Care Summary of 1996 Key Legislative Issues Around Medicare

1. *Preserve Medicare:* Medicare continues to be a target for significant reform due to spending reductions as Congress looks for ways to control growth in entitlements and achieve a balanced budget.
2. *Oppose coinsurance:* Congress should oppose any coinsurance proposal for home health services so that individuals who need medical care are not discouraged from using in-home services that could reduce the need for more costly institutional care.
3. *Oppose bundling:* The idea of bundling post-acute services into hospitals' diagnostic-related groups payments (including in the DRG reimbursement the care both in the hospital and homecare afterward) has been advanced in the past and may again receive attention as a "back door" approach to managed care. Bundling would cause major disruption to the health care industry, increase the federal regulatory burden, be anti-competitive, and erect a barrier (hospital approval) to access to services. For examples, hospitals could decide how much the home care agency would receive out of the DRG reimbursement sum and could even make the decision about the services the home care agency should provide for that money.
4. *Enact a prospective payment system for home care:* Congress should enact a prospective payment system for home care agencies that equitably and predictably pays for services while minimizing administrative burdens on providers. It should establish prospectively determined national payment rates for home health services that are indexed to keep pace with changes in the home care market.
5. *Oppose shifting Medicare coverage from Part A to Part B:* Proposals to shift Medicare home care payments from Part A to Part B would jeopardize home care by making it even more vulnerable to copayments and by eliminating its status as an entitlement program.
6. *Managed care:* There has been a growing shift to managed care for Medicare beneficiaries and Congress should explore ways to increase this enrollment as well as ensuring their choice to receive services under fee-for-service *or* managed care.

From National Association for Home Care (NAHC): *1996 Legislative Blueprint for action*, Washington, D.C., 1996, NAHC, pp. 8-9.

of the community-based waiver services cannot exceed the cost of institutional care.

As is the case with Medicare, home health services are only a small percentage of the total Medicaid expenditures. Of the $108 million spent nationally on Medicaid payments in 1994, more than 50% went to hospital and skilled nursing facility services. Home health care expenditures were about 6.5% of the total amount (NAHC, 1995, p. 3).

Medicaid costs for health care are rising rapidly, and legislators are looking for ways of increasing revenues and cutting costs. In 1980 about 9% of each state's cost went to fund Medicaid; in 1990 this amount was about 12.5%, and in 1994 20%. NAHC, in its 1996 Legislative Blueprint, is monitoring a number of issues under debate by legislators at every level of government that could affect the aggregate of low-income persons needing long-term care, as well as their providers. The box at right lists these issues. Concerned professionals will remain keenly aware of legislative debates and proposals.

Social Services Block Grants to States (Title XX)

The Title XX program was established by the 1975 Amendments to the Social Security Act. The Omnibus Budget Reconciliation Act of 1981 (Public Law 97-35) altered Title XX, reformulating it as a federally funded Social Services Block Grant. The Social Services Block Grant, like other block grants, provides the states freedom in determining the

National Association for Home Care 1996 Key Legislative Issues, Medicaid

Preserve Medicaid: Congress is considering dramatic change to Medicaid, one of them being a system of copayments for home visits to clients whose care is reimbursed by Medicaid. Since recipients of services are, by definition, very poor, many individuals would be forced to go without services.

Improve reimbursement to providers: Inadequate reimbursement for providers, home health care agencies, doctors, and therapists discourages them from participating in the Medicaid program and forces some to limit acceptance of the number of persons they can accept (in some states Medicaid home health reimbursement is as low as 60% of the reimbursement of Medicare accepted costs!).

Establish federal minimum standards of coverage for home health services under Medicaid: The general home health benefits are generally more limited in coverage and reimbursement than the Medicare home health benefits. In some states physical, occupational, and speech therapy are optional and frequently not available to Medicaid recipients in the home setting.

From National Association for Home Care (NAHC): *1996 legislative blueprint for action*, Washington, D.C., 1996, NAHC, pp. 8-9.

populations to be served and the types of services to be offered. The Social Services Block Grant program provides funding for a comprehensive array of social services directed toward the following goals:

- Achieving or maintaining economic self-support to prevent, reduce, or eliminate financial dependency
- Achieving or maintaining self-sufficiency, including reduction or prevention of dependency for daily care
- Preventing or remedying neglect, abuse, or exploitation of children and adults unable to protect their own interests, or preserving, rehabilitating, or reuniting families
- Preventing or reducing inappropriate institutional care by providing for community-based care, home-based care, or other forms of less intensive care
- Securing referral or admission for institutional care when other forms of care are not appropriate, or providing services to individuals in institutions

A broad range of home-based services can be provided by the states under Title XX, including homemaker, home health aide, home management, personal care, consumer education, and financial counseling services. As with Medicaid, the benefits offered under this program vary from state to state. In order to qualify for Title XX services, clients must meet income eligibility requirements.

For states to participate in the Title XX program they must establish a Comprehensive Annual Service Program plan that outlines the services they will provide to whom and by what methods. Federal spending under Title XX is capped, and funds are allocated among states on the basis of their populations. Social Services Block Grant funds aid states in meeting local needs not met by other social service agencies in the community. However, the limited funding for this program does not allow states to expand home care services significantly.

Title III Under the Older Americans Act of 1965

The Older Americans Act (OAA) of 1965 established the Administration on Aging in the Department of Health, Education, and Welfare and authorized a variety of health and social services projects for aging citizens (see Chapters 4 and 20). In 1978 amendments to the Older Americans Act consolidated several existing titles (Titles III, V, and VII) of the original act and revised and expanded Title III. Title III is now designed to encourage and help state and local agencies to concentrate resources on developing a comprehensive and coordinated system to serve elderly citizens age 60 and over.

Title III mandates a broad range of social services for the elderly, including but not limited to home health, home health aide, homemaker, and nutritional services. The only eligibility requirement for participation in the Title III program is that clients must be at least age 60. Unlike Medicare, clients do not need to be homebound and do not need skilled nursing care to qualify for home health benefits.

Title III is a state-administered program carried out under the direction of the Department of Health and Human Services. Federal expenditures under Title III are capped. In 1992 less than $200 million was spent by the OAA on community-based long-term care services, serving about 1.7 million people (AARP, 1994).

Other Programs Funding Home Health Care

Other programs that pay for home health care services include the following:

- *Private health insurance:* This is generally limited to physician-directed medical services, courses of therapy, and equipment. For the elderly, coverage under long-term care insurance is increasing.
- *Veterans Administration:* Veterans with a disability of 50% or more are eligible for home health care coverage. Services must be authorized by a physician and are provided through the VA network of providers.
- *CHAMPUS (Civilian Health and Medical Program of the Uniformed Services):* On a cost-shared basis this program covers skilled nursing care and other medical home care for dependents of active military personnel, retirees, and their dependents.
- *Social service organizations:* Organizations that operate with private charitable funding, such as the United Way, may offer a wide range of services, including most of the health and supportive home care services needed by clients. Depending on eligibility, agencies may require sliding scale payments, donations, or services without charge.
- *Private pay:* In spite of the many methods of reimbursing home care providers, when formal and informal health care services are considered, the majority of home care expenses are still paid for out-of-pocket (see definition in Chapter 4) because of the stringent limitations of coverage under both public and private financing programs.

BARRIERS TO ADEQUATE COMMUNITY-BASED LONG-TERM CARE

Various problems in the community and in the health care delivery system make it difficult for clients who have long-term care needs to avoid unnecessary institutionalization. These problems can be summarized under four categories: (1) lack of community resources, (2) acute-focused reimbursement mechanisms, (3) fragmentation and lack of coordination, and (4) family burnout.

Lack of Community Resources

A significant factor preventing many of the chronically disabled from obtaining adequate long-term care is the scarcity of formal alternatives to institutionalization. After it is ascertained by caregivers and families that an individual cannot live at home without support or health care, staying in the community depends upon social supports, adequate financial resources, and the availability of health and social services.

Many older people, especially those older than 75, have characteristics that place them at risk for being institutionalized. Unfortunately, the very dependent elderly often find it difficult to obtain needed services in the home.

The lack of adequate housing (and especially supportive congregate or domiciliary housing for people who live alone) for the frail elderly and disabled is a major barrier to community long-term care services. One problem with current housing arrangements is affordability: fuel prices, interest rates, and construction costs have all made housing costs difficult to manage on a limited income. Another problem is that households are becoming smaller; although rents are increasing, the number of people paying rent is decreasing as a result of increasing divorce rates and increasing numbers of aged and deinstitutionalized people living alone. In large cities single room occupancy (SRO) hotels, formerly a source of housing for many, are being converted into condominiums.

In some communities innovative housing programs sponsored by the Department of Housing and Urban Development have provided suitable alternatives to institutionalization. The National Housing Act, Section 202, provides a direct loan program based on the current securities marketed by the Treasury Department. The level of these interest rates makes housing projects attractive to builders; they are financially sound as well. Section 8 of the same act provides for direct subsidies to individuals who occupy Section 8 housing. The sponsors of such housing, usually nonprofit organizations, receive full market rent. However, the federal government pays a portion of the rent.

Acute-Focused Reimbursement Mechanisms

Another barrier to effective long-term care is inadequate financial coverage for needed long-term care services. The Medicare program was specifically designed to provide protection for acute-care needs. Once a client's condition becomes stable or once skilled services such as nursing, speech, or physical therapy are no longer needed, Medicare coverage for home health care ceases. Medicare specifically prohibits payment for custodial care. Care is considered custodial when it is for the purpose of meeting personal needs and could be provided by persons without professional skill or training; for example, help in walking, getting in and out of bed, bathing, eating, dressing, and taking medicine. These are precisely the functions needed by many clients with long-term care needs.

Other problems with Medicare home health benefits are that housekeeping and food services arrangements are not covered. One of the most serious problems is that services must be *intermittent* to be covered. For example, home health aides, in conjunction with other services and for a finite period of time, may work only a few hours a day, several days a week, and their hours may not exceed 32 per week. This type of care is often inadequate when a client needs help with activities of daily living on a constant basis.

Medicaid, the assistance program for the very poor, does cover long-term care, but clients must deplete their own resources to qualify as "medically needy" to receive these funds. However, for persons who meet the eligibility requirements, the Medicaid program more effectively meets the long-term care needs of clients than does Medicare. Services do not have to be skilled (a client may have custodial needs met) and the services may be delivered by a person who has received some training for personal care services.

Medicaid expenditures for home care remain small. Because Medicaid is a state-administered program, services vary considerably from state to state. In some states participation was limited in home and community-based services because these states viewed the services as (1) potentially costly and difficult to manage and (2) not permitting targeting of services to address the specific long-term care needs of the elderly (Justice, 1988). However, as states become more confident of their ability to manage home and community-based waiver programs, they apply for more and larger waivers (GAO, 1994).

Fragmentation and Lack of Coordination

It has consistently been documented that fragmentation and lack of coordination in the long-term care system make it extremely difficult for clients to obtain needed long-term care services. Consequently, a significant number of the noninstitutionalized population need but do not receive long-term care.

Existing formal long-term care services are provided by an array of state and local agencies that have differing eligibility requirements and finance mechanisms. Clients who have multifaceted needs frequently find it difficult, if not impossible, to identify the appropriate service provider. Many communities have no central organization or professional that assists the chronically impaired client in locating and coordinating needed long-term care services.

Obtaining needed long-term care services often places unnecessary hardships on the client. It is not unusual for clients to have to make separate trips to several agencies in order to arrange a comprehensive package of services. An aged client, for example, may have to apply separately for Medicaid, Meals-on-Wheels, transportation services, Title XX homemaker services, and home nursing services.

Fragmentation and lack of coordination have left many gaps in the long-term care delivery systems. Thus unnecessary institutionalization among high-risk groups continues, and the costs for long-term care services are rising dramatically. Efforts to develop comprehensive, coordinated systems for delivering community-based services must be expanded.

Family Burnout

An estimated 60% to 85% of all disabled or impaired people are helped by the family in a significant way. It has been demonstrated over the years that the family is the primary source of care for the frail elderly in the community. Some family members and friends provide this care out of a sense of responsibility, but most do so primarily because they care. Family caretakers play a pivotal role in helping chronically disabled family members to avoid institutionalization. Caring for impaired family members, however, can place a heavy and expensive burden on the family, especially when care is required for an extended period of time. Many chronically impaired persons have been placed in nursing homes because their families are unable to bear the emotional, physical, and financial strain of providing home care in the absence of support from community programs.

For long-term care programs to be effective, the needs of family caregivers, as well as dependent family members, must be addressed. As discussed previously, caregivers of the dependent disabled need respite care, information about services, a broad array of community- and home-based health and social services, and knowledge about health conditions and care methods.

METHODS FOR IMPROVING THE LONG-TERM CARE SYSTEM

With population estimates that project dramatic increases in the over-75 age group and with health care costs expanding, it is obvious that the present system is not meeting and will not in the future meet the need for long-term care services. A number of methods for improving the system have been suggested, including:

1. Expansion of noninstitutional forms of long-term care while developing disincentives to construction of more institutional capacity
2. Emphasis on appropriate discharge planning
3. Effective gatekeeping and initial placement of clients assessed as appropriate for institutionalization
4. Targeting home care services to the people who need them the most

Discharge planning is discussed in Chapter 10 and thus will not be expanded on here. It is important to remember, however, that chronically ill and disabled clients often need detailed discharge planning services.

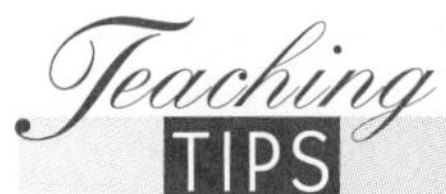

Establish a Caregiving Routine

1. Put Yourself in Control
   a. Plan a caregiving schedule that fits your own routine and activities.
   b. Plan your routine in partnership with: home care nurse, family members, and others.
   c. Use a calendar to write down the things you need to do. Include doctor appointments and ordering supplies.
   d. Get a spiral notebook and make a chart. Write down important information in the spaces, such as daily weights or blood sugars.
   e. Use your notebook for reminders you want to discuss with the physician or nurse. Take the notebook to the physician's office.
2. Ask for Help
   a. Think about how much help you need. You will often need more help in the beginning. It is helpful to have someone to call every day.
   b. It *is* okay to ask others for help. It is best to have someone to help you in case something unexpected happens.
3. Control Supplies and Medicines
   a. Start a list of all needed supplies.
   b. Keep supplies in a separate cabinet, closet, or room. Keep this place clean and organized.
   c. Sterility and cleanliness are the most important factors to help in avoiding infections.
4. Know What to Tell the Doctor or Nurse
   a. Record daily information as instructed by your nurse, such as blood sugars or urine output.
   b. Write any progress or changes in symptoms in your spiral notebook.
   c. Tell your physician or nurse about changes they have asked you to record. Examples are fever or weight changes.

Remember—everyone has good and bad days! Do not worry about one bad day. There are times when you may need professional support from a minister or counselor. Signs of depression include a loss of self-worth, frequent crying spells, loss of interest in family life, and difficulty concentrating or sleeping. Tell the physician or nurse about these signs if they occur. You *can* get help for depression.

Modified from Martin KS, Larson BJ, Gorski LA, Hayko DM, eds: *Mosby's home health client teaching guides: R_x for teaching*, St. Louis, 1997, Mosby, p. III-F-1-6.

Expansion of Noninstitutional Alternatives

A number of demonstration projects have been funded at the state and federal level to evaluate the appropriateness of expanding noninstitutional alternatives and decreasing capacity levels in institutional settings. In the state of New York, for example, the Nursing Home Without Walls program was initiated in 1978 to encourage noninstitutional alternatives as an appropriate cost-effective policy for long-term care of the elderly. Four components of the program included (1) intervention in the actual process of nursing home placement so that clients are exposed to home care before a nursing home placement decision is made, (2) cost containment with a limit set on the per capita cost of services, (3) case management of services so that social and medical services are integrated into the system, and (4) waivered services so that services not included in the Medicaid law, such as respiratory therapy and home improvement, can be offered to those needing them.

Another demonstration of the expansion of noninstitutional forms of long-term care is Enriched Housing. Enriched Housing serves that portion of the population who is able to live independently but needs some help with personal care, meal preparation, housekeeping, shopping, laundry, heavy cleaning, transportation, and 24-hour emergency coverage. The typical person entering this program does not have an informal support network to help him or her to live independently. The program differs from the Nursing Home Without Walls program in that the client must also need housing. In this program the person enters the housing secured by the program, usually a portion of a rent-subsidized building. Payment is generally through SSI (Figure 21-8).

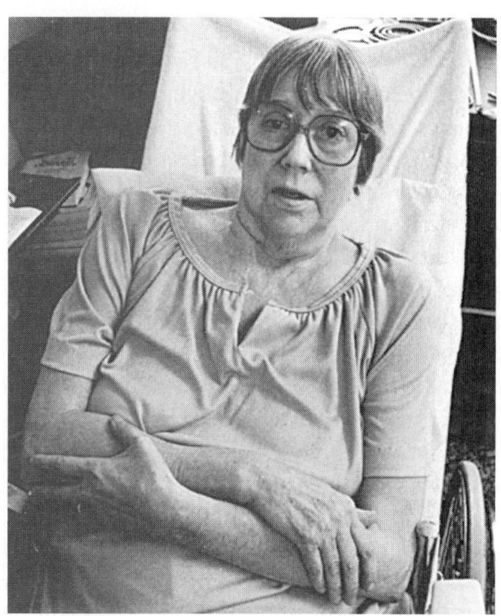

Figure 21-8 Jane Richards, who lost both legs to circulatory disease, lives at home rather than in a nursing home. *(Courtesy Anne Lennox/Times-Union.)*

Adult foster care is another mandated service in many states for people over 18 who are socially, mentally, or physically handicapped. Its purpose is to provide the opportunity for normal family and community life and help with problems. A foster home for adults is usually operated by individuals in their own homes and provides room, board, housekeeping, personal care, and supervision to four or fewer adults on a 24-hour basis. Those eligible for the program include people who receive TANF (Temporary Assistance to Needy Families) or SSI.

Economical shared or sheltered housing for the elderly and disabled deserves greater effort. Improved federal funding of long-term care services should accompany efforts to use volunteer efforts on behalf of this population. One mutual aid scheme, proposed in the 1980s (Sanger, 1983), and involving the exchange and banking of time in long-term care could be centered on congregate housing developments. These would ordinarily be built without adequate service supports. Residents could be admitted initially across a range of ages and disabilities. When able, they could be encouraged to help care for one another in a variety of ways. Those on waiting lists for apartments could be encouraged to help as well. In exchange, residents subsequently would receive aid from new and more able helpers. These exchanges are in existence today and can probably be increased in number and intensity by a mild effort to back them publicly. People who help others would be guaranteed help in return. If no one volunteered to provide that subsequent help, it would be financed publicly and delivered by paid workers. Time devoted to helping others would be backed hour for hour by the full faith and credit of the United States—probably the best form of currency since the silver certificate. In this way we could build faith in a currency of altruism. Adult day care centers are another noninstitutional alternative for people and families needing help. Day care centers provide assistance for adults who cannot be left alone during the day yet do not require 24-hour nursing care in an institution. A wide variety of services, including nutritious lunches; medical and social services; occupational, speech, and physical therapy; and health screening are often available to clients. Those who profit from this kind of service are persons with Alzheimer's disease, the physically impaired with diagnoses such as arthritis or stroke, the mentally impaired, and the socially impaired or isolated individual. Candidates are evaluated in their homes before enrollment, and the daily attendance fee is usually based on a sliding scale fee schedule.

Developing Effective Gatekeeping Mechanisms

Developing models, such as local area management organizations (LAMOs) and social–health maintenance organizations (S/HMOs), are another solution for dealing with the problems in the long-term care system. (Both are methods of financing and organizing health care for the elderly and are variations of the health maintenance organizations [HMOs] described in Chapters 4 and 5). Funding for LAMOs and S/HMOs comes from all public monies currently designated for short-term and long-term medical care, rehabilitation, and custodial services. The LAMO enrolls all people with functional deficits and provides the services necessary to help them at home, utilizing informal supports whenever possible. The S/HMO enrolls all elderly people, anticipating that low use of services by the relatively well elderly compensates for extensive use by the vulnerable severely ill. Both models function as gatekeepers into the long-term care system; case managers function as brokers for the services needed by the elderly population served, and they also certify the level of care needed.

HOSPICE CARE

Hospice is a humanistic approach to the care of the dying. One of the three main diagnoses of home care clients is cancer. This disease is a chronic one that requires services much more important than medical care. For the elderly, cancer often progresses slowly and thus leads to a longer period of home care than other diseases. Hospice presents a solution to many of the needs of this population group, as well as to clients across the lifespan who are dealing with the difficulties associated with cancer and other diseases.

The hospice concept is an approach to providing comprehensive care for terminally ill clients and their families: it is a way of dying rather than a place where dying people receive care. It focuses on helping people to die with dignity and on assisting families with the grieving process. It emphasizes relieving psychological and physical distress.

The hospice movement developed from the work of Cicely Saunders, a physician from England. She founded St. Christopher's Hospice in 1960, which became a model for similar programs in the United States. In the early 1970s the first American hospice was organized in New Haven, Connecticut.

The development of the hospice movement in the United States is relatively recent, beginning about 25 years ago. The authorization of the Medicare Hospice benefit under the Tax Equity and Fiscal Responsibility Act of 1982 spurred the growth of this industry. Many insurers and managed care companies use the Medicare standards for their own packages. The growing number of aging people, the tremendous growth in medical technology that extends life, the growing awareness and fear of cancer, and the involvement of educated consumers who desire a voice in treatment have all contributed to the growth of this movement in recent years. Further, cost containment has been another important issue since caring for the terminally ill in the cure-focused setting of a high-technology hospital is more expensive and less comfortable than the home setting. Since the inception of the movement the number of hospices has expanded significantly.

Hospice is a movement that emphasizes the following ideals (ANA, 1987):

- Help in dealing with emotional, spiritual, and medical problems
- Support for the entire family
- Keeping the patient in his or her home for as long as appropriate and making his or her remaining life as comfortable and as meaningful as possible
- Centrally coordinated home care, inpatient, acute, and respite care, and bereavement services
- Professional services from a health care team supplemented by volunteer services, as appropriate to individual circumstances
- Relief of pain and other symptoms

The 1990s have brought about a great change in the delivery of hospice care services. Where once care was primarily delivered in institutional settings, today care is almost exclusively outpatient or home-based. In the contemporary market-driven health care industry competition for patients is strong, and it is important for providers to know the difference between hospice and home care programs (Table 21-4). Further, with the advent of Medicare into the managed care industry, the differences between the goals of home care and hospice become even more pronounced. Hospice care deals with the intangibles of psychosocial and spiritual care interwoven with medical care. Home health care under managed care aims for observable outcomes within a specified time frame.

Under Medicare hospice is a comprehensive home care program that provides all the reasonable and necessary medical and support services for the management of a terminal illness. Medicare covers physician and nursing services, medical appliances and supplies, outpatient drugs for symptom management and pain relief, short-term respite care in an inpatient setting, home health aide and homemaker services, nutrition counseling, medical social services, physical and occupational therapy, and speech and language pathology services. Medicare clients receive hospice benefits when the physician certifies that they are terminally ill (defined as 6 months or fewer to live) and when the client chooses hospice care for terminal care rather than standard Medicare benefits. Care must also be provided by a Medicare-certified hospice. At the end of this chapter is the story of one family's experience with hospice; it depicts the focus on the family, comfort in dying, and the interdisciplinary nature of hospice care.

THE ROLE OF THE COMMUNITY HEALTH NURSE IN LONG-TERM CARE

Nurses are increasing their involvement with the growing at-risk long-term care population and are becoming leaders in caring for people who have long-term needs. In fact, long-term care is very likely to become a key growth area for professional nursing. Nurses already represent the largest number and percent of professional workers involved in long-term care; however, estimates suggest that there is a growing shortage of nurses in the areas of long-term care and gerontology.

Community health nurses should focus on seven areas to provide more adequate long-term care. These are prevention at all three levels among people across the life span, functional independence for clients rather than a cure, families' coping abilities, collaboration, evaluation of services, and responsible public policy making.

Use Levels of Prevention

Throughout this text the concepts of disease prevention and health promotion have been stressed. The importance of these concepts cannot be overemphasized, especially when one examines the problems encountered by long-term care population groups. To decrease the number of people

table 21-4 Comparison of the Medicare Home Health Benefit and Hospice Benefit

Service	Medicare Hospice Benefit*	Medicare Home Care Benefit†
Visiting nurse	Covered for skilled and supportive care	Covered for skilled care, if part time or intermittent
Physician	Private physician 80% covered under Part B; consulting hospice physician 100% covered	Not covered under home care, but 80% of approved charge covered under Part B
Social work and counseling services	Covered for patient and caregivers	Covered for patient
Pastoral counseling and chaplain services	Covered	Not covered
Home care aide	Covered, as specified in hospice plan of care	Covered, if part time or intermittent
Volunteers for patient and caregivers	Covered, as specified in hospice plan of care	Not included
Physical and occupational therapy, speech-language pathology	Covered, as specified in hospice plan of care	Covered, with some limitations on occupational therapy
Dietitian	Covered, as specified in hospice plan of care	Not covered for individual patients
Skilled continuous care/private-duty nursing during crisis periods	Covered	May be covered, where the need is finite and predictable
Inpatient care	Covered	Not covered under home care, but covered under hospital benefit
Respite care	Included	Not covered
Services to nursing facility residents	Included	Not covered
24-hour on-call services	Included	Not required, but frequently included
Bereavement counseling	Covered	Not included
Care management/coordination	100% covered, as specified in hospice plan of care	Included
Medications related to primary illness		Not covered
Durable medical equipment	Medical and personal care supplies covered	80% of approved amount covered
Supplies		Medical supplies covered

From Colburn K, Hively D: The hospice phenomenon in its second decade under medicare, *Caring* 12(11):8-9, 1995, p. 8.

*Medicare will pay for hospice care if all the following requirements are met: terminal illness is certified by a physician; patient elects hospice benefit; and hospice program is Medicare certified.

†There are additional services that can be provided in the home but are not included in the home care benefit. Medicare will pay for reasonable and necessary home visits if all the following requirements are met: patient needs skilled care; patient is homebound; care is authorized by a physician; and home care agency is Medicare certified.

needing long-term care, it is essential to concentrate our efforts on the primary prevention of chronic problems.

Since the prepathogenesis period of disease (see Chapter 11) begins early in life, primary prevention and health promotion interventions that address many problems encountered by chronically disabled persons and the aged must be introduced when working with young people. Health education programs that address such matters as lifestyle modification, stress management, retirement planning, and counseling services that help individuals to develop a risk profile, are examples of such interventions. Other examples are integrated throughout Chapters 15 to 20.

Community health nurses are uniquely able to apply the concepts of prevention as they work with clients who need long-term care. Primary, secondary, and tertiary preventive interventions are commonly implemented by nurses who provide home health care services. Examples of primary prevention interventions include accident prevention education and teaching about infection control. Helping a client with diabetes to learn how to self-administer insulin injections and to handle postsurgical wound care are examples of secondary prevention interventions.

Tertiary prevention, continuing care and rehabilitation, is frequently carried out with people who need long-term care. These people often need help with physical, occupational, and/or speech therapy to return to or maintain their optimal level of functioning. The challenge facing the community health nurse at the tertiary level of prevention is how to maintain an ongoing working relationship with clients so that the care plan can be adjusted in response to the client's and family's changing circumstances and conditions. Strategies that community health nurses can use to help clients manage chronic diseases include medical record coauthoring, self-monitoring, educational support groups, family involvement, and telephone or postcard contact with clients.

Help Families Cope

As discussed previously, nine out of 10 of the disabled elderly in the United States receive unpaid care from relatives and friends. The majority of caregivers are women. The current average caregiver to the elderly is 45 years old, female, and married. Among children who are primary caregivers, daughters outnumber sons three to one (Brakman, 1994).

However, community health nurses should not expect families and other informal supports to do the impossible—to provide care with no relief for long periods. Formal and informal caregivers share the responsibility for meeting the long-term care needs of clients. Often what the family caregiver wants from the formal caregivers, the nurse, and home health agency, is the following (Nottingham, 1995):

- Close involvement with a competent and caring professional who is part of an integrated health or social service delivery system
- Professionals who can relate easily and comfortably with families
- Cooperation, understanding, and support among formal and informal caregivers
- Families working with the professional who represents the formal service delivery system and both working jointly on what needs to be done
- Having their own knowledge and skills valued

Health care professionals have made the choice of careers that involve helping others cope with difficult situations. Informal caregivers have often not consciously made this choice, but both groups of caregivers need to take care of themselves. Health professionals should know the symptoms of burnout—emotional exhaustion that comes from excessive demands on one's energy, strength, or resources—and try to prevent those excessive demands from continuing for long periods without asking for help. The healthiest way to take care of another is to take care of yourself.

Health care policy changes under discussion would assist families with the problems of burnout (Brakman, 1994). First, since the vast majority of caregivers are women (wives, daughters, and daughters-in-law), society needs the message that the obligation of caregiving should be met by all adult children who have such responsibilities and not just daughters. This would have the effect of reshaping societal expectations about women as well as the discussion about the implications of obligations of gratitude for caregiving throughout the life cycle. Second, the state should support families who are caregivers of their adult members by providing financial subsidies for those who cannot afford to quit working. The Family and Medical Leave Act just

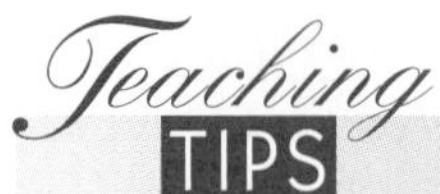

Caregiving: What Do I Need to Know?

1. Illness and treatment
   a. What do I need to know about the illness and the treatment?
   b. How does the treatment work?
   c. How much will this cost?
   d. Will my insurance pay for this?
2. Emergency care
   a. When should we call for help?
   b. Who should we call for help?
   c. Is fever an emergency?
3. Daily activities
   a. How will this illness and treatment affect everyday life?
   b. Can we still do "normal" things?
   c. Will we still be able to have sexual relations?
4. Treatments and procedures
   a. How do we keep the treatments sterile?
   b. What is the best way to sleep with tubing hooked up?
   c. How do we use the machine (for example, hook it up, keep it clean, and set the volume)?
5. Medicine and supplies
   a. How do we know if the medicine or treatment is not working?
   b. What do we do if the medicine does not seem to work?
   c. When should we order supplies?
   d. How can we cut costs on supplies and medicines?
6. Food and beverages
   a. What kinds of supplements are required?
   b. Should the diet for the rest of the family change?
7. Emotional reactions to illness
   a. What if the doctors do not seem to understand?
   b. How do we cope with loneliness, sadness, or depression?
   c. If our relationships with friends change, how do we handle the changes?
8. Home care services
   a. What type of help will home care provide?
   b. When do we call the home care nurse?
   c. Will insurance pay for home care?

From Martin KS, Larson BJ, Gorski LA, Hayko DM, eds: *Mosby's home health client teaching guides: R_x for teaching,* St. Louis, 1997, Mosby, p. III-F-1-6.

recently enacted does provide job protection for caregivers of children, spouses, and parents, but the leave is without pay for a limited time. Third, respite services must be widely available.

Respite services include a wide range of services intended to give temporary relief for families caring for members with disabilities. Recognition of this need has been very recent in the United States, and formal respite services are not widely available (Montgomery, 1995)

One of the 1996 key legislative issues of the National Association of Home care has been to promote respite care for family caregivers by including in-home respite care in the Medicare home health benefit. The recommendation from the National Association for Home Care included hours permitted under the benefit, criteria for eligibility, as well as the supervision and training of persons providing the respite care. NAHC also promoted respite care outside of the Medicare program (NAHC, 1996, p. 29).

An organization that exists solely for the purpose of assisting informal family caregivers is the National Family Caregivers Association, 9621 East Bexhill Drive, Kensington, Md., 20895-3104 (301-942-6430 or 1-800-896-3650). It is an invaluable resource for families and professionals.

Focus on Functional Independence

Clients with long-term care needs often have conditions that cannot be cured. The goal for their care is to help them maintain quality in their lives and continue to function at the highest possible level. With the cure orientation that pervades our health care system, this can be a difficult orientation for a community health nurse to develop and maintain. This orientation becomes easier to handle as one sees through practice that clients can live satisfying lives even when they have not been cured. Community health nurses play a significant role in assisting clients to achieve greater functional independence.

The National Eldercare Institute on Health Promotion can be a valuable resource for nurses who are assisting clients to achieve greater functional independence. The American Association of Retired Persons is the lead organization for the Institute; Meharry Medical College will focus efforts of the Institute on outreach to minority elders. The principal objectives and activities of this institute are presented in the box, above right.

National Eldercare Institute on Health Promotion

PRINCIPAL OBJECTIVES OF THE INSTITUTE INCLUDE:

- Serving as a knowledge base and program resource on health promotion, disease, and disability prevention for vulnerable older persons and their caregivers;
- Promoting the effective transfer, dissemination, and utilization of relevant information on health promotion to audiences across the continuum of care; and
- Providing training and technical assistance on health promotion and aging, focusing on agencies and organizations comprising the national, state, and community Eldercare coalitions.

ACTIVITIES OF THE INSTITUTE WILL INCLUDE:

- Linkages with other organizations and institutions through task forces, for example, with federal agencies and researchers;
- A library and database to respond to written and phone inquiries;
- Outreach to elders-at-risk through the development of program guides, publications, and audiovisual materials;
- Publication of the Institute newsletter, *Perspectives in Health Promotion and Aging;*
- Development of resource lists on health promotion topics for older adults;
- Training and technical assistance to professionals in the fields of health promotion and aging; and
- National conferences on health promotion and aging.

From National Eldercare Institute on Health Promotion: *Perspectives in health promotion and aging,* 7(1), Washington, D.C., 1992, AARP.

Collaboration

No one discipline can address the array of needs experienced by long-term care clients. The problems involved with long-term care demand that all members and levels of health care providers be involved. The community health nurse must be attuned to drawing on the health care team's sources whenever possible.

The community health nurse often functions as the coordinator of the health care team, an extremely important role that must not be neglected. The client can easily feel that care is fragmented if no one person has overall responsibility for complete care. Understanding the roles of each team member (Table 21-5) can facilitate planning and coordination. The role definitions presented in Table 21-5 should be regarded only as a starting point for developing effective team relationships. When entering any new service agency, spend time with each member of the team to determine how they function.

The central figures on any long-term health care team must be the client and his or her family. To achieve the highest level of functioning possible for the client, the client must be actively involved in establishing a plan of care appropriate to his or her needs. Engaging families in the therapeutic process is essential because often they have needs of their own that must be addressed. In addition, families are frequently participants in the rehabilitation process and provide continuing support for disabled family members after health care providers leave the home environment.

Evaluate Services

An integral part of working in any health care setting is evaluation. The evaluation process helps health care

table 21-5 Descriptions for Select Members of the Long-Term Health Care Team*

Discipline	Role Description
Community health nurse†	*An essential professional member of the health care team*—The professional nurse utilizes the nursing process to determine client needs, to establish a plan of care in conjunction with the client, to provide skilled nursing services, and to evaluate care delivered by the nursing team. Traditionally, the professional nurse has assumed a case management role on the health care team. As a care manager, the community health nurse focuses on determining the comprehensive needs of the client and the client's family, makes referrals to appropriate community resources as needed, and coordinates care among the multiple agencies providing services to a family.
Homemaker–health aide	*A paraprofessional who is trained to assist clients with personal care and light household tasks*—According to the Medicare conditions of participation for home health agencies, a home health aide's "duties include the performance of simple procedures as an extension of therapy services, personal care, ambulation and exercise, household services essential to health care at home, assistance with medications that are ordinarily self-administered, reporting changes in the patient's condition and needs, and completing appropriate records" (HCFA, 1989b, October). Home health aides providing only personal care must be supervised by professional nurses via supervisory visits to the client's home at least every *2 weeks* if skilled nursing or therapy service is also needed by the client. If the client needs only custodial care, home health aide supervisory visits must be made once every 62 days (HCFA, October 1994).
Nutritionist	*A professional team member who assists clients in meeting their basic nutritional needs*—The nutritionist assesses a client's nutritional status, helps the client to plan an adequate and appropriate dietary intake, suggests ways to plan economical nutritious meals, helps clients to learn about therapeutic diets, and teaches about food purchasing and preparation. These professionals are often used as resource persons by other members of the health care team.
Physician	*A professional team member who is either a doctor of medicine or osteopathy*—The Medicare conditions of participation for home health agencies specify that the physician must establish and authorize the client's plan of treatment in writing and must review this treatment plan at least once *every 62 days* to determine if care is appropriate and necessary (HCFA, October 1994). In addition to establishing a plan of treatment, the physician evaluates the client's medical status and provides medical care as needed. A physician also serves on a home health agency's professional advisory committee.
Social worker, medical	*A professional member of the home health care team who works with clients who are experiencing significant psychosocial, financial, or environmental difficulties*—Medical social workers apply the principles of social case work to help clients to enhance their emotional and social adjustment and to adapt to change. The primary purpose of their intervention is to reduce psychosocial, financial, and environmental barriers that are adversely affecting a client's health status or response to health care. Medical social workers provide direct counseling services, refer clients to community resources, assist clients in attaining needed social and health care services, and help plan for institutional community placements such as nursing home or extended-care facility placements. They also serve as resource persons for other members of the health care team who are dealing with difficult psychosocial, financial, or environmental problems.

Modified from Health Care Financing Administration (HCFA): *Medicare program: home health agencies—conditions of participation and reductions in recordkeeping requirements*, 42 CFR, Part 484, Sections 484.1 through 484.52, Washington, D.C., October 1989b, U.S. Department of Health and Human Services; and HCFA: *Medicare program: home health agencies—conditions of participation*, 42 CFR, Part 484, Section 484.1 through 484.52, Washington, D.C., October 1994, USDHHS.

*The central figures on any long-term health care team must be the client and his or her family.

†To be certified for Medicare and Medicaid funding, a home health agency must provide nursing services.

professionals to determine whether they are providing appropriate and quality services in an effective and efficient way. In this era of decreasing resources it is essential for community health professionals to monitor carefully how they use available resources. The needs of at-risk aggregates, such as those composing the long-term care population, can only be met if resources are allocated and used in a responsible manner.

Community health nurses at all levels must assume responsibility for evaluating the way in which nursing services are delivered. Although nursing administrators have the overall task of seeing that evaluation is done, staff-level professionals must be accountable for assessing their own practice. They must also supervise the care they have delegated to others, such as home health aides and homemakers. When community health nurses delegate or assign tasks to others, they are responsible for seeing that these tasks are performed in an acceptable way (see Chapter 23).

A variety of direct and indirect measures are currently used by community health nurses to evaluate the delivery of nursing services, such as direct observation of care, case management conferences, annual performance evaluations, and record reviews. The Standards of Home Health Nursing Practice (ANA, 1986) referred to earlier in this chapter

table 21-5 DESCRIPTIONS FOR SELECT MEMBERS OF THE LONG-TERM HEALTH CARE TEAM* — CONT'D

DISCIPLINE	ROLE DESCRIPTION
Therapists, occupational	*Professional members of the team who work with clients that have difficulty carrying out activities of daily living*—After determining the self-care activities most important to the client, the occupational therapist assesses the environment to identify safety hazards and barriers to self-care, recommends environmental modifications that would help the client to increase independence and to prevent accidents, and assists the client in learning techniques, such as the use of simple eating and dressing devices that promote effective and efficient client functioning. The occupational therapist focuses on helping the client to improve motor coordination and muscle strength so that the client can reach his or her maximum level of functioning.
Therapists, physical	*Professional members of the team who work with clients who have functional impairments related to neuromuscular problems*—After assessing the client's functional abilities, physical therapists help clients to preserve, restore, and improve neuromuscular functioning and to increase their self-care capabilities. Physical therapists carry out a broad range of activities to help clients reach their maximum level of functioning. Performing needed range-of-motion, strengthening, and coordination exercises; recommending the use of appropriate orthopedic and prosthetic devices; and teaching clients ambulation techniques and how to use assistive appliances are a few examples of the activities performed by physical therapists.
Therapists, speech-language	*Professional members of the team who work with clients who have communication problems*—After assessing the client's speech, language, and hearing abilities, speech therapists concentrate on helping clients to increase their functional communication skills. Based on client needs, the speech therapist may initiate exercises to increase functional speaking skills, teach esophageal speech, recommend the use of communication appliances such as intraoral devices or hearing aids, identify barriers in the environment which inhibit effective communication, and teach significant others in the environment how to communicate with the client.

should guide the development of an evaluation plan that includes criteria for measuring quality and methods for ensuring that care is consistent with professional standards (see Chapter 24). Requirements of reimbursement sources must also guide the development of evaluation measures. Community health nurses in home health agencies must, for example, fulfill the following evaluation requirements to receive Medicare reimbursement for health services provided by their agency (HCFA, 1989b; HCFA, 1994).

- Conduct an overall evaluation of the agency's total program at least once a year to examine to what extent the agency's program is *appropriate*, *adequate*, *effective*, and *efficient*
- Establish a professional *advisory* group that includes at least one physician, one registered nurse, one member who is neither an owner nor an employee of the agency, and appropriate representatives of other professional disciplines, such as social work, physical therapy, and speech therapy, who are providing service for the agency; the group must meet frequently to advise agency staff on professional issues and to participate in overall agency evaluation
- Review with the patient's physician the appropriateness of the plan of treatment as often as the severity of the patient's condition requires but at *least once every 62 days*.
- Have the registered nurse, or appropriate professional staff member if other services are provided, make a supervisory home health aide visit *at least every 2 weeks* if skilled nursing or therapy services are needed by the client or *once every 62 days* if only custodial care is needed
- Conduct a clinical record review on active and closed records *at least quarterly* to ensure that established policies are followed in providing services
- Employ only those home health aides who have completed a competency evaluation program

Two types of record reviews are conducted in the home health setting: quality care audit and utilization review. During the *quality care audit* process, health care providers focus on appraising the quality of care received by clients using predetermined standards of care, as evidenced by documentation in the client's record (see Chapter 24). During a *utilization review* the client's records are assessed for the purposes of evaluating the appropriateness of the client's admissions and discharges; the appropriate and adequate use of personnel; and over- and underutilization of services.

Staff-level community health nurses can play a very important role in all evaluation review procedures. Staff involvement in evaluation processes helps administrators to obtain a clearer picture about service delivery issues. As case managers, staff-level nurses are in a unique position to identify gaps in service and deficiencies of care.

Work Toward Responsible Public Policy

Thus far in this chapter, ample evidence has been presented to demonstrate that public policy for long-term care in this country is inadequate. Involvement in forming public policy can be at any one of a number of levels. These levels range from apathy and no participation to voting to holding public office. All levels require knowledge of the issues; community health nurses in long-term care possess this as an outcome of their experience.

Involvement in the political arena is both fun and professionally rewarding. Working with professional organizations such as the National Association for Home Care and the American Public Health Association is a good way to get started in the political arena. These organizations are making a concerted effort to analyze key health care issues and to promote strategies that may resolve some of the current health care delivery problems.

FACTORS INFLUENCING ETHICAL DECISION MAKING IN THE HOME

A number of factors make an impact on the ethical dilemmas and decisions that caregivers in the home environment encounter. Since home health care is the most rapidly growing segment of the health care industry, nurses will continue to be more frequently challenged by the ethical dilemmas confronting them. Burger, Erlen, and Tesone (1992) discuss the five factors that influence ethical decisions:

1. *Time*. Home nurses visit the family and client on an intermittent basis and thus have to assess quickly and determine what has value and meaning to those involved. They need to establish plans of care within the first few visits.
2. *Involvement*. Clients and caretakers are active partners in care and must assume responsibility for treatments when professionals are not present.
3. *Interdisciplinary communication*. The home setting presents limited opportunities for direct communication between professionals involved in the client's and family's care.
4. *Support system*. The accessibility, availability, and affordability of a caretaker affects options the client has. Without an appropriate caretaker there are few alternatives; financial constraints, time, and ability are other concerns.
5. Ethics committees are increasingly a part of the structure of home care agencies. Ethicists are part of these groups and can assist clients, their families, and professionals with situations where there is no "right" answer (ethical dilemmas). A frequently encountered example is the *conflict between health providers' desires to provide quality care that meets needs and the demands of third party payors;* for example, Medicare pays for skilled intermittent care, but all a client needs is an aide to watch him 24 hours a day for a short period of time to ensure his independence and safety.

Another dilemma centers around the implementation of the Patient Self-Determination Act of 1990. This legislation mandates that agencies that participate in Medicare and Medicaid provide information and education about advanced directives to clients so that they have the right to control their own health care decisions. With the medical technology that is available, advanced directives can help minimize people's fears of being kept on artificial life support after meaningful life for them has ceased. While there is little disagreement with the legislation, health providers may see conflicts between the decision a client makes and that made by his or her family; nurses may also question the cognitive ability of a client to make a decision.

Advanced directives are written documents by which competent persons can seek to influence their medical treatment in the event of serious illness and subsequent loss of consciousness. The "Living Will" is often referred to as a type of advanced directive, but it needs to be properly executed to be legally binding. The Durable Power of Attorney for Health Care is a more effective instrument as a proxy directive since a specific person is legally designated to make treatment decisions on behalf of another person. Nurses working in the home health care environment deal with the concept of advanced directives on a daily basis; it is one of the conditions of participation in the Medicare program and is part of the Joint Commission on Accreditation of Health Care Organizations (JCAHO) accreditation criteria.

The Rising Cost of the Elderly

By the year 2050 those over 65 in this country are expected to account for 20% of the population. With entitlements under the Social Security Act for those over 65, this aggregate receives 41% of their income from the government. Thirty-eight percent receive 80% or more of their income from the government, and only 35% receive their incomes from private pensions. Today spending for entitlements plus interest payments on the national debt amounts to 60% of the Federal budget. By the year 2013, if nothing is changed, these entitlements for the rising number of people over 65 will amount to 100% of the Federal budget (Thurow, 1996).

Discussion about these statistics clearly falls into the category of an ethical dilemma: how, in this country, do we combine justice and aging? There will continue to be discussions in this country about how to distribute the enormous resources available so that justice is served to all age groups.

Increasingly, state home health organizations are focusing on developing guidelines to facilitate ethical decision making in practice. The American Nurses Association also assists practitioners and administrators in dealing with ethical issues encountered in the clinical setting. The American Nurses Association can be reached by phone at 202-554-4444.

SUMMARY

Increasing numbers of people across the life span have long-term care needs that must be addressed by local communities throughout our nation. Elderly persons, who constitute the most rapidly growing population group in America, are particularly at risk for needing long-term care services. Although most elderly people experience good health, certain chronic, disabling illnesses do increase with aging.

The fastest-growing component of the United States health care delivery system is long-term care. Diverse and multiple social, health-related, and health care organizations deliver a variety of long-term care services to people in need. Despite the dramatic growth in the long-term care industry, many chronically disabled persons still do not receive the services they need. Developing strategies to eliminate barriers to adequate community-based, long-term care must receive greater attention by health care providers in this decade. There is no question that the aging of the American population will increase the need for long-term care services in the future.

Long-term care presents challenges and opportunities for the community health nurse. Developing solutions to overcome the deficiencies and to fill the gaps in the long-term care system will require major policy changes at all three levels of government. However, community health nurses at all levels of practice can be instrumental in effecting change in the health care delivery system. Innovative projects that more adequately address the needs of at-risk long-term care populations are beginning to emerge across the country.

CRITICAL *Thinking Exercise*

The story presented below recounts how three different families have coped with terminal illnesses using the hospice program (Fine, 1990). Think about how the goals of nursing care differ for these people as compared to a well-baby or school population. What interventions does the community health nurse in a hospice setting use as compared to those used in a well-baby clinic? How do you evaluate the importance of interdisciplinary functioning in the hospice setting? Would you consider having a career in hospice nursing? Discuss why you would or would not become a hospice nurse.

We thank Theresa M. Crist, MSNA, RN, Vice President Operations, American Nursing Care, Cincinnati, Ohio for her assistance with this chapter.

A View *from the* Field: THE HOME AS HOSPICE: THE TERMINALLY ILL CAN FIND HELP FOR THEMSELVES AND THEIR FAMILY

Once she accepted the truth, once her options were gone, Peg Johnson looked at the finite future—too short, too soon—and chose to face it at home. There, in her brave, new world, she took some small measure of control over what remained of her life in the ever-present shadow of death.

Johnson, dwarfed by the corduroy lounge chair in which she sat, spoke about her choice one recent afternoon. As she sat, pale and thin, feet elevated, the bulge of her belly prominent beneath a pale blue coverlet, she seemed at ease. Her spirit seemed strong.

"So far," she said. "I'm not saying that I'm going to be this way always. But I believe in God, and I think that helps."

Linda Trout helps, too. A nurse, she is the coordinator of the hospice program at Taylor Hospital in Ridley Park; Johnson has been a patient at the hospital on and off since she was diagnosed with colon cancer two years ago. Trout visits Johnson at her home in Prospect Park to treat, to advise, to talk, to listen.

In a sense, hospice is an old story made new.

"In the first part of the century, most people died at home," said Andrew Parker of the National Hospice Organization (NHO). "There was caring, there was comfort, there were people around. And then we moved into an era where most people die in a hospital . . . isolated and abandoned."

The recent hospice movement, begun in England in the 1960s, is a coordinated program of care—medical, psychological, social and spiritual—for the terminally ill and their families. Although hospice care sometimes is delivered in a separate facility, often it permits people to live, and die, in their own homes, cared for by their own families, surrounded by their own things. Since the first hospice opened in this country—in 1974, in Connecticut—the movement has expanded steadily to the present 1,700 hospices nationwide.

"Hospice makes two promises," Parker said. "You won't die alone, and you won't die in pain. And it delivers."

It was a terrible year, 1989.

In January, Helen Margaret Johnson, known as Peg—67 years old, mother of a grown son and daughter, widow for 13 years—underwent colostomy surgery. In April, she had heart surgery, a valve replacement. Chronic lymphocytic leukemia, diagnosed in 1982, remained a complication.

With all that, she carried on: "And I was doing pretty good, but they told me in the beginning that the cancer had spilled over to the pelvic area. I must have resigned myself, because nothing has been that difficult."

Her hospice care began on Oct. 3.

From Fine MJ: Home as hospice: the terminally ill can find help for themselves and their families, *The Philadelphia Inquirer*, Section I, January 28, 1990, p. 6.

Continued

A View from the Field THE HOME AS HOSPICE: THE TERMINALLY ILL CAN FIND HELP FOR THEMSELVES AND THEIR FAMILY—cont'd

Hospice generally means several things: that the patient has six months or less to live, that treatment is often palliative or centered on pain control, and that family members assume much of the care. It isn't for everyone, said Toni McClay, who runs Taylor's program: Some families simply cannot accept that a patient is beyond the point where recovery is possible.

That was not the case with Johnson. She has made her funeral arrangements, paid for her casket. Even so, she has not entirely given up: "I have friends of many faiths praying for me. Methodist. Presbyterian. Baptist. Episcopalian." A smile, wry and brief, crosses her lips. "It can't hurt."

On one visit, midafternoon on a Thursday, the affection between nurse and patient was evident. Trout bent to kiss Johnson's cheek, then sat down to talk with her and her daughter, Cathy Giarrusso, 44, who was visiting from Georgia. Two or three times a week, Trout, 37, makes house calls to Johnson, each visit lasting an hour or more. A social worker comes about twice a month, Johnson said, and the conversations "get some of the miseries off your mind." Taylor's three dozen hospice volunteers, who work with the staff of five nurses, make themselves available as needed.

Half an hour of breezy chitchat passed before Trout segued gracefully from social topics to medical ones.

"How's your appetite?" she asked gently.

"Not terrific," Johnson replied.

Persistent, painful sores in Johnson's mouth and throat had improved, but drinking citrus juices—once her favorite, now too acidic—still hurt. Trout recommended a "homemade mouthwash" of Epsom salts and peroxide.

Trout knelt at Johnson's side, took her blood pressure, dressed the site of a small skin cancer, inquired about her weight. (About 114, Johnson said, "but most of that is tumor.") Giarrusso reported her mother's temperature to be 99.3.

Johnson's forthrightness about her illness, her approaching death, had surprised Giarrusso. Such openness once was uncharacteristic of her mother, she said, but she is grateful for it—"It's easier to deal with someone who knows they're dying, rather than you know and they don't"—and thinks she knows its source.

Her mother, trying to protect her, had been evasive about her father's condition before his death in 1976. "So when I came here," Giarrusso recalled, "it was not quality time I had with him. He was in a coma and died three days after I got here."

This time, she and her mother have said what they wanted and needed to say to each other. During a visit in June, they even chose the casket together. Her brother, David—who lives in Philadelphia with his own family but stays with his mother one or two nights a week—found funeral-planning morbid and excluded himself from it.

According to Parker of the NHO, hospice care helps families get through the grieving process—partly by counseling and partly by their involvement in a family member's care.

"There's healing (of grief) going on when you're serving a loved one," Parker said. Most hospices also operate bereavement programs for the surviving family members, he said, because "loss is something that our culture doesn't deal with well."

Peg Johnson chose hospice care for the comfort of being at home, where she can set her own schedule for eating and sleeping, sitting up and lying down.

When her doctor suggested the hospice program, she was initially hesitant. "At the time, I thought it was a little soon," she said, "but it wasn't. You always think it's too soon."

Not every patient wants to know as much as Peg Johnson knows.

Anna Mills is one who doesn't.

Sunlight filters through the lace curtains of her living room and onto the hospital bed where she lies beneath a crocheted comforter. A large yellow cat named Mikey is asleep beside her.

Mills is chatty, smiling, uncomplaining and, at 85, dying of breast cancer. Since June, Linda Trout has been visiting the two-story brick twin that Mills shares with her daughter, Ann Bevan, and her niece, Anna Mae Happersett.

The house is homey and welcoming, overflowing with a lifetime's collection of dolls—"My babies," Mills calls them—baby dolls with china hands, fashion dolls in elaborate gowns, a Princess Di bought in the Bahamas.

Twice a week, Trout is greeted at the Ridley Park home like family. When Mills speaks of "my girls," the words encompass Ann and Anna Mae and Trout. As much as possible, Trout makes the visit appear to be a social call. When Mills admires the cameo brooch at Trout's throat, she and Trout discuss a shared love of antiques.

Trout is fond of the women, admiring of their closeness, respectful of Mills' choices.

"She is not aware of her diagnosis," Trout said, although the hospice worker suspects that Mills really knows the truth. "She has chosen not to recognize it," Trout said. "She thinks she's sick because she fell three years ago, and she thinks the pain she is having is from that."

A View from the Field — The Home as Hospice: The Terminally Ill Can Find Help for Themselves and Their Family—cont'd

Mills' evasion of the truth is explained by family history, Happersett said: "She's seen her husband go (from cancer). And she won't take needles . . . she's seen them give him needles constantly and torture him." Such avoidance can make home care a challenge—Mills will not enter the hospital, wear a catheter, accept injections—for both hospice workers and family members.

But denial is not uncommon, hospice workers agree. Most, however, say that their mission is to make patients and families as comfortable as possible, not to force them to confront unhappy truths.

"We respect people's right to be who they are, to have their own defenses," said Karen Neyer, 39, a hospice social worker at Lankenau Hospital on the Main Line. "We do not impose our standards on other people. We use the language they use. As we form a relationship, if there's a space to challenge, to open doors, we knock on them."

For Linda Trout, triumph meant finding a long-acting morphine pill that seems to be controlling the pain in Anna Mills' right leg, a result of her disease spreading to the bone.

In the kitchen, out of earshot, Trout calls Bevan at work to discuss the possibility of catheterizing Mills for bladder control, to spare her daughter and niece having to change absorbent bed pads numerous times a day.

"But, of course, if it causes her mental anguish, it's no good," Trout said into the telephone. "Whatever is best for her."

Bevan has agreed to discuss the matter with her mother, however, and Trout packs her carryall to depart. She bends to kiss Mills and straighten her yellow-flowered sheets. Mills beams.

"I love her," she said of Trout. "I love my girls."

Outside, in her car, Linda Trout reflects on the emotional nature of nursing patients who will all die.

"It's OK for me to cry," she said quietly. "And I do. It's a relationship for me that's gone. I get in my car and cry."

She began studying nursing only seven years ago and, then, only because her husband was diagnosed with leukemia. She wanted to learn how to care for him. At some point, however, it became her calling, her profession, and after his death, she found herself drawn to the terminally ill. This has remained true, even though she has since remarried.

"Disease has been here since the dinosaurs, and I can't change that," she said. "But if I can make it better . . . I don't think anyone should live in pain. Or die in pain."

She said that her work had changed her in subtle ways. "Probably, I live one day at a time now," she said. "And my friendships and family are more cherished."

For the Rev. Wesley K. Meixell, minister and widower, it is all over now, except for the memories—and the continuing support of the hospice program at Taylor Hospital.

His wife, Lorna, died on Oct. 22, 1988, after 35 years of marriage. The final seven months were a tumultuous time filled with fear and hope, pain and despair.

Lorna Meixell, an advertising artist at Franklin Mills, began suffering dizziness, weakness and loss of peripheral vision early in 1988. On March 23, she learned why: The diagnosis was glioblastoma, a rare and fatal brain tumor.

"The doctor told me no one survives that unless it's a miracle," Meixell recalled. He is pastor of Norwood United Methodist Church—and he put his faith in a miracle.

It was not to be. His wife's deterioration was gradual but steady. He remembered all the parishioners he had visited in hospitals over the years and their wishes to be at home. Right after Labor Day, his wife began receiving hospice care.

"She just felt better, being at home," he said. The hospice team was "very compassionate, very caring, all of them."

It began with a home-health aide, two hours a day, five days a week. By the end, a nurse was taking care of her eight hours a day. The Meixells' combined insurance paid for it all, 100 percent, he said. Most hospice care—65 to 70 percent—is covered by Medicare, the rest by private insurance or Medicaid; many hospice programs absorb the cost for uninsured patients.

"We do not turn anyone away," said Taylor's Toni McClay.

And after a patient's death, hospices do not abandon the survivors. Meixell still attends a monthly bereavement support group, most of whose members also lost spouses and understand the truth of Meixell's painfully learned knowledge: "Even if you're prepared for (death), it's still very hard to accept."

During his wife's illness, at the time of her death and afterward, the hospice team offered comfort and support, he said; "When she died, in those months—and even now—they said, 'If you're having trouble dealing with the loss, call us. Any time. Twenty-four hours a day.'"

REFERENCES

Administration of Home Health Nursing: Care of the sick by health departments, *Public Health Nurs* 37:339-342, 1945.

Allen SA: Medicare case management, *Home Healthc Nurse* 12(3):21-27, 1994.

American Association of Retired Persons (AARP), Center on Elderly People Living Alone, Staff, Public Policy Institute: *Home and community-based long-term care*, Fact Sheet 13R, Washington, D.C., 1994, AARP.

American Association of Retired Persons (AARP), Public Policy Institute: *Helping people with disabilities: the need for long term care*, Washington, D.C., January 1995a, AARP.

American Association of Retired Persons (AARP), Public Policy Institute and the Urban Institute: *Coming up short: increasing out-of-pocket health spending by older Americans*, Washington, D.C., April 1995b, AARP.

American Nurses Association (ANA): *Standards of home health nursing practice*, Kansas City, Mo., 1986, ANA.

American Nurses Association (ANA): *Standards and scope of hospice nursing practice*, Kansas City, Mo., 1987, ANA.

American Nurses Association (ANA): *A statement on the scope of home health nursing practice*, Kansas City, Mo., 1992, ANA.

Bedside nursing care by official agencies, *Public Health Nurs* 37:333-334, 1945.

Brakman SV: Adult daughter caregivers, *Hastings Cent Rep* 24(5):26-28, 1994.

Buerhaus P: Managed competition and critical issues facing nurses, *Nurs Health Care* 15(1):23-26, 1994.

Buhler-Wilkerson K: Home care the American way: an historical analysis, *Home Health Care Serv Q* 12(3):5-17, 1991.

Burger AM, Erlen JA, Tesone L: Factors influencing ethical decision-making in the home setting, *Home Healthc Nurse* 10(2):16-21, 1992.

Callahan CM, Hendrie HC, Tierney WM: Documentation and evaluation of cognitive impairment in elderly primary care patients, *Ann Intern Med* 122:422-429, 1995.

Children's Defense Fund: *The state of America's children yearbook 1996*, Washington, D.C., 1996, The Fund.

Colburn K, Hively D: The hospice phenomenon in its second decade under Medicare, *Caring* 12(11):8-9, 1995.

Day JC: Projections of the number of households and families in the United States: 1995 to 2010, U.S. Bureau of the Census, current population report, series P25-1129, Washington, D.C., 1996, U.S. Government Printing Office.

Dittbrenner H: Alzheimer's disease: the long goodbye, *Caring* 13(8):14-23, 1994.

Fine MJ: Home as hospice: the terminally ill can find help for themselves and their families, *The Philadelphia Inquirer*, Section 1, January 28, 1990, p. 6.

General Accounting Office (GAO): *Medicaid long-term care: successful state efforts to expand home services while limiting costs*, Pub No. HEHS-94-167, Washington, D.C., August, 1994a, U.S. Government Printing Office.

General Accounting Office (GAO): *Long-term care reform: states' views on key elements of well-designed programs for the elderly*, Pub No. HEHS-94-227, Washington, D.C., September 1994b, U.S. Government Printing Office.

General Accounting Office (GAO): *Long-term care: diverse, growing population includes millions of Americans of all ages*, Pub No. HEHS-95-26, Washington, D.C., November 1994c, U.S. Government Printing Office.

Hadley JP, Langwell K: Managed care in the United States: promises, evidence to date and future direction, *Health Policy* 19:91-118, 1991.

Harrington C, Cassell C, Estes C et al: Caring for the uninsured and underinsured: a national long-term care program for the United States, *JAMA* 266(1):3023-3029, December 4, 1991.

Harris JP: High tech is a boost to home health care, *Special Advertising Section: Health Care Career Forum, Philadelphia Inquirer*, September 16, 1992, p. 15.

Haupt AC: Forty years of teamwork in public health nursing, *Am J Nurs* 1:53, 1953.

Health Care Financing Administration (HCFA): *Medicare home health agency manual, HIM 11*, Washington, D.C., 1989a, USDHHS.

Health Care Financing Administration (HCFA): *Medicare program: home health agencies—conditions of participation and reductions in recordkeeping requirements*, 42 CFR, Part 484, Sections 484.1 through 484.52, Washington, D.C., October 1989b, USDHHS.

Health Care Financing Administration (HCFA): *Medicare program: home health agencies—conditions of participation*, 42CFR, Part 484, Sections 484.1 through 484.52, Washington, D.C., October 1994, USDHHS.

Health Care Financing Administration (HCFA): Medicare program: home health agencies—conditions of participation, 42CFR, Part 484, *Federal Register* 56:32967-32975, July 1991.

Hirsh L, Klein M, Marlowe G: *Combining public health nursing agencies: a case study in Philadelphia*, New York, 1967, Department of PHN, NLN.

Justice D: *State long-term care reform: development of community care systems in six states*, Washington, D.C., April 1988, National Governors Association.

Kane RA, Wilson KB: *Assisted living in the United States: a new paradigm for residential care for frail older persons*, Washington, D.C., 1993, AARP.

Lumsdon K: No place like home? *Hosp Health Netw*, October 5:45-52, 1994.

Martin KS, Larson BJ, Gorski LA, Hayko DM, eds: *Mosby's home health client teaching guides: R_x for teaching*, St. Louis, 1997, Mosby, p. III-F-1-6.

Masso AR: Managed care and alternate-site health care delivery, *J Case Manage* 1(1):45-51, 1995.

McCloskey JC, Bulechek GM (eds): *Nursing interventions classification (NIC)*, ed 2, St. Louis, 1996, Mosby.

McConnell S: Policy issues surrounding special care units, *Caring* 13(8):30-33, 1994.

Montgomery RJV: Examining respite care: promises and limitations. In Kane RA, Penrod JD, eds: *Family caregiving in an aging society: policy perspectives*, Thousand Oaks, Ca., 1995, Sage, pp. 29-45.

National Association for Home Care (NAHC): *Basic statistics about home health care, 1995*, Washington, D.C., 1995, NAHC.

National Association for Home Care (NAHC): *1996 legislative blueprint for action*, Washington, D.C., 1996, NAHC.

National Eldercare Institute on Health Promotion: *Perspectives in health promotion and aging* 7(1), Washington, D.C., 1992, AARP.

Naylor R: *Christian living*, March-April 1983, p. 21.

Nottingham JA: Navigating the seas of caregiving: allies and ideas for success, *Caring* 14(4):16-20, 1995.

Office of Technology Assessment (OTA): *Losing a million minds: confronting the tragedy of Alzheimer's disease and other dementias*, Washington, D.C., 1987, U.S. Government Printing Office.

Olson HH: Home health nursing, *Caring* 5(8):53-61, 1986.

Peters DA, Eigsti DG: Utilizing outcomes in home care, *Caring* 10:44-51, 1991.

Sanger AD: *Planning home care with the elderly—patient, family, and professional views of an alternative to institutionalization*, Cambridge, Ma., 1983, Ballinger.

Shaughnessy PW: *Using outcomes to build a continuous quality improvement program for home care*, 11th National Nursing Symposium on Home Health Care, University of Michigan School of Nursing, June 14, 1996.

Staggers' Lawsuit: *Part II, NAHC Report*, No. 275, Washington, D.C., August 12, 1988, NAHC, pp. 1-3.

Stulginsky MM: Nurses' home health experience. Part I: the practice setting, *Nurs Health Care* 14(8):402-407, 1993a.

Stulginsky MM: Nurses' home health experience. Part II: the unique demands of home visits, *Nurs Health Care* 14(9):476-485, 1993b.

St. Pierre M, Dittbrenner H: HCFA's home health initiative: the first comprehensive reassessment of the Medicare home health benefit, *Caring* 14(3):22-27, 1995.

Thurow LC: *The future of capitalism*, Boston, 1996, William Morrow.

U.S. Bureau of the Census: *Population profile of the United States: 1993*, current population reports, series P23-185, Washington, D.C., 1993, U.S. Government Printing Office.

U.S. Bureau of the Census: *How we're changing: demographic state of the nation: 1996*, series P23-191, Washington, D.C. 1996, U.S. Government Printing Office.

United States Department of Health and Human Services (USDHHS), Public Health Service: *Progress report on Alzheimer's disease 1995*, NIH Pub No. 95-3994, Washington, D.C., 1995, National Institute on Aging.

U.S. Senate, Committee on Finance: *Long-term health care: hearing before the subcommittee on health of the committee on finance*, United States Senate, ninety-eighth Congress, Washington, D.C., 1984, U.S. Government Printing Office.

Visiting Nurse Service of Toledo: Eighty-three years of caring, *Caring* 3:57-61, 1984.

SELECTED BIBLIOGRAPHY

Arras JD, Dubler NN: Bringing the hospital home: ethical and social implications of high-tech home care, Special Supplement, *Hastings Cent Rep* 24(5):S19-S28, 1994.

Bissonnette A, Hijjazi KH: Elderly homelessness: a community perspective, *Nurs Clin North Am* 29(3):409-416, 1994.

Cox DM, Sachs GA: Advance directives and the Patient Self-Determination Act, *Clin Geriatr Med* 10(3):431-443, 1994.

Davitt JK, Kaye LW: Supporting patient autonomy: decision making in home health care, *Soc Work* 41(1):42-50, 1996.

Dula A: The life and death of Miss Mildred: an elderly black woman, *Clin Geriatr Med* 10(3):419-430, 1994.

Esposito L: Home health case management, rural caregiving, *Home Healthc Nurse* 12(3):38-48, 1994.

Elias CJ, Inui TS: When a house is not a home: exploring the meaning of shelter among the chronically homeless older men, *Gerontologist* 33(3):396-402, 1993.

Erkel EA: The impact of case management in preventive services, *J Nurs Adm* 23(1):27-32, 1993.

Harris MD: Medicare update, reimbursement for pronouncement of death visits, *Home Healthc Nurse* 12(2):47-50, 1994.

Johnson EA: The public's future perspective on managed care, *Health Care Manage Rev* 20(2):45-47, 1995.

Klem CB: Attitudes of direct care staff in home healthcare toward advance directives, *Home Healthc Nurse* 12(3):55-59, 1994.

Mahowald MB: So many ways to think: an overview of approaches to ethical issues in geriatrics, *Clinical Ethics* 10(3):403-418, 1994.

Molloy SP: Defining case management, *Home Healthc Nurse* 12(3):51-54, 1994.

Mintz S: Family caregivers, *Caring* 14(4):7-9, 1995.

Reilly FE: An ecological approach to health risk: a case study of urban elderly homeless people, *Public Health Nurs* 11(5):305-314, 1994.

Remington Report: *Where to find information on the managed care market* 3(2):43-48, 1995.

Rotwein S, Boulmetis M, Boben PJ et al: Medicaid and state health care reform: process, programs, and policy options, *HealthC Financ Review* 16(3):105-140, 1995.

Spiller K: Shifting with the paradigm, a primer for embracing managed care, *The Remington Report* 3(2):18-20, 1995.

Winston MR: Dealing with depression and anger: reactions of family caregivers, *Caring* 13(8):52-59, 1995.

22

Aggregate-Focused Interventions and Settings

OBJECTIVES

Upon completion of this chapter, the reader should be able to:

1. Describe the differences between teaching, task, and supportive groups.
2. Understand how the community health nurse uses group process to target preventive health services for aggregates at risk.
3. Summarize the phases in the life of a group and leadership interventions that facilitate movement from one phase to the next.
4. Discuss how developments in society have contributed to the development of clinic and nursing center services.
5. Articulate how community health nurses establish and maintain clinic and nursing center services for aggregates at risk.
6. Describe the parish nursing and block nursing concept.

In every enterprise consider where you would come out.

PUBLIUS SYRUS

Just as a map provides alternative roads to a destination, various community health nursing roles and settings provide alternatives for addressing the health needs of clients in the community. Community health nurses have recognized throughout their history that multiple methods must be used to resolve the complex problems existing in society. They have worked collaboratively with professionals from other disciplines and community residents to reach underserved populations. National data concerning health disparities among Americans, health care access issues, and changing demographics (USDHHS, 1991, 1995) urgently propel community health nurses to continue to develop effective alternatives for intervening with diverse clients at risk. From both a cost containment and a quality perspective, it is important for community health nurses to consider aggregate-focused as well as individual- and family-focused interventions that take into account the client's unique environment. There is a growing recognition that health behavior is significantly influenced by environmental factors (Pederson, O'Neill, Rootman, 1994; Scherl, Noren, Osterweis, 1992). Health promotion interventions that focus only on changing individual behavior leave out important influences in the social cultural environment (Steckler, Allegrante, Altman et al, 1995). "To have enduring effects, interventions must have an impact on social norms and accepted ways of functioning that may be deleterious to health" (Clark, McLeroy, 1995, p. 277).

Although aggregate-focused nursing roles and interventions have been addressed in several chapters in this text, this chapter broadens discussion about the roles community health nurses assume and interventions they use when working with small groups and populations in the community. The emphasis is on examining how community health nurses use the group process to provide targeted preventive services and how they function in clinic, nursing center, parish, and neighborhood settings to address the needs of aggregates across the life span. Increasing evidence supports the fact that targeted, group-specific interventions and nontraditional as well as traditional approaches are needed to effectively work with the diverse populations in the community (Clark, McLeroy, 1995; Freudenberg, Eng, Flay et al, 1995; Marín, Burhansstipanov, Connell et al, 1995). The settings in which health care professionals function provide channels for reaching specific groups (Mullen, Evans, Forster et al, 1995).

INTERVENING WITH AGGREGATES THROUGH GROUP PROCESS

Community health nurses have long worked with groups of people to meet health care needs effectively. In this context *group* is defined as a gathering of people who are together for a specific reason. An example of the use of group work in community health nursing practice is a parent effectiveness training class. Parents in this situation come together to discuss ways to rear children effectively. A gathering of people at a bus stop does not meet the definition of a group.

Community-based agencies frequently use the group process as an aggregate-focused intervention strategy. Through group process, community health nurses are able to assist small client or community groups to learn new knowledge and skills, to support group members during stressful times, or to solve problems around issues important to the community, groups of individuals, and families. Community assessment and caseload analysis data help community health nurses identify needs common to aggregates within the community and the nurse's work area. For example, one community health nurse realized that she continually received numerous referrals from the intermediate school district to visit families with children who had developmental delays, and that many of these families were clustered close together. To help meet the needs of these families, the nurse formed a parent support group to serve the many primary and secondary preventive needs of this population.

A Brief Historical Perspective on Group Process

Kurt Lewin is generally considered to be the founder of modern group process. His research during World War II was aimed at increasing work production and changing food consumption patterns. Lewin found that group discussion and decision making helped people change their ideas much more effectively than lectures or even individual instruction (Lewin, 1947). Giving people information alone did not motivate them to change personal attitudes and behavior. Rather, discussion in groups helped persons become involved, conceptualize ideas, and take health action. Group participants learned something about their own behavior in group settings, and the information gained was relevant to their personal lives.

Another development in the group approach to health was *group psychotherapy*. It became a part of the treatment plan of psychologists and psychiatrists in the 1920s and 1930s, but it was not until the 1960s that group process and group psychotherapy came together (Loomis, 1979, p. 5). In the 1960s the *encounter group* movement proliferated, and the differences between sensitivity groups and psychotherapy groups blurred. It was realized that everyone, not just "sick" people, could benefit from group process.

"During the 1960s and 1970s, groups reached their zenith; then the group fever declined for a decade" (Corey, Corey, 1997, p. 5). In the 1990s, another surge of interest in the use of group work has emerged. Some see the group approach to care as a cost-effective way to address client needs in a managed care environment (MacKenzie, 1995; Sleek, 1995). Corey and Corey (1997) believe that groups are the treatment of choice, not a second-rate cost containment approach to helping people change. "Groups have immense power to move people in creative and more life-giving directions" (Corey, Corey, p. 5).

The terms *group process*, *group dynamics*, and *group interaction* all refer to the way groups work and provide methods to assess and observe group functioning. Groups are formed for a variety of psychological, social, and educational purposes such as losing weight, controlling drug usage and smoking, and giving support during divorce and death. Nurses are part of a group on the health team and in professional associations, parent-teacher organizations, League of Women Voters, and synagogues. Clearly group work is an integral part of life in the United States today.

Advantages and Disadvantages of the Group Process Approach

The definition of community health nursing states that promoting and preserving the health of populations is its goal (APHA, Public Health Nursing Section, 1996). Thus nurses are constantly viewing ways of helping people look critically at their own health behavior.

Telling people about healthy behavior is not enough—the nation's high infant mortality ranking among industrialized countries is verification of that statement. Telling parents ways to increase the likelihood of positive pregnancy outcomes has not been adequate to significantly reduce infant mortality in America. There must be a way of helping people value preventive health practices so that they will change their health behavior. Lewin's work, among that of many others, gives evidence that groups can help accomplish this. A major reason for using the group approach is that different kinds of people with similar concerns can work on these concerns together.

It must be emphasized that the group approach will not meet all clients' health needs. Some people will never feel secure enough to leave their own familiar surroundings, to find transportation, to have the needed energy and skill, or even to want to become part of a group. There are people who lack the social expertise, experience, and motivation required to become involved in a group. This behavior can be learned, but it requires patience and skill on the part of the nurse to teach it. An overwhelmed 17-year-old single mother with two children under 2 years of age who has exhibited poor bonding behaviors with her newborn probably needs an intense one-to-one relationship with a nurse before she can profit from a group discussion about parenting.

Situations that warrant a family-centered nursing approach are best handled in the home environment. Nurses gain valuable information about a family when they see individual family members interacting in their own surroundings. A database on the family system as discussed in Chapter 7 is very difficult to collect when the client is a member of a larger group.

Some people like to function in groups; others do not. These differences need to be respected because an individual's attitude and beliefs regarding the group experience will have an effect on group learning and outcomes. Successful group outcomes have been limited in situations where the group's culture (e.g., Hispanic) is not amenable to sharing problems with strangers or where the social conditions (e.g., lack of child care, long working hours, or dangerousness of neighborhood) make participation in groups less likely (Marín, Burhansstipanov, Connell et al, 1995, p. 353). Successful group outcomes have been achieved among some aggregates at risk (e.g., non-Hispanic whites) who are members of underserved groups (Clark, Janz, Dodge, Sharpe, 1992; Marín, Burhansstipanov, Connell et al, 1995).

When planned carefully, groups can have several advantages. Luft (1970, p. 30), in his classic writings on group process, identified that groups can be a source of strong interpersonal stimulation, can bring a wide variety of skills, information, or the cross-checking of facts to problem-solving discussions, and can promote commitment to shared goals. Others have found that the group process can foster hope (Piechowski, Ciha, 1988), can facilitate compliance with health promotion programs (Burlew, Jones, Emerson, 1991), and can increase intergenerational understanding (Myers, Poidevant, Dean, 1991). It can also help people alter ineffective patterns of functioning through observation of how other group members handle stressful situations; help group participants validate thoughts, feelings, and experiences; and facilitate the development of a social network (Corey, Corey, 1997).

It is important for community health nurses to understand the advantages and disadvantages of using the group process approach in meeting the needs of aggregates in the community. This understanding can assist nurses in identifying clients who may or may not be responsive to involvement in groups and outcomes that may or may not be achieved through the group process. When clients are not responsive to the group process, the nurse needs to seek other alternative interventions for meeting their needs.

Types of Groups in the Community Setting

According to Clark (1994), "nurses work primarily in three types of groups: task groups, teaching groups, and supportive or therapeutic groups" (p. 4). Types of "groups differ with respect to goals, techniques used, the role of the leader, training requirements, and the kind of people involved" (Corey, Corey, 1997, p. 9). Training requirements vary based on the type of strategies used by the group leader, the role of the leader, and the primary goal of the group. For example, a group leader guiding a teaching group needs a firm understanding of the principles of teaching and learning, and behavioral change theories. On the other hand, a leader conducting a support group needs strong counseling skills, and the leader working in a task group needs team-building, problem-solving, change-agent, and management skills. The task group leader may also need community organization and health planning skills if he or she is working in a group established to promote community capacity (Corey, Corey).

TASK GROUPS Task groups are usually developed to accomplish a specific task or goal and often within specified time limits. These groups "place a high priority on decision-making and problem-solving" (Clark, 1994, p. 4). Large, complex tasks often need more than one person, or a multidisciplinary team, to carry them out. The multidisciplinary team in the community health setting may include nurses, physicians, environmentalists, physical and occupational therapists, nutritionists, social workers, and other professional consultants meeting as a group to address the needs of aggregates in a community.

Within community health nursing practice numerous task groups are continuously formed to achieve specified goals and objectives. An example of a large-scale, aggregate-focused group effort designed to accomplish a specific task is the work groups established to develop the *Healthy People 2000* national health objectives. These work groups focused on developing goals for improving the health status among Americans and objectives for addressing the needs of aggregates at risk. The *Healthy People 2000* work groups had representation from an extensive list of national organizations from around the country. Another example of a large-scale task group established to address a major aggregate-focused health problem is the national Healthy Mothers, Healthy Babies Coalition. This coalition is a cooperative venture of national voluntary, health professional, and government organizations, and it has affiliated coalitions in the majority of the states. Its specific task or goal is to improve maternal and infant health through education (USDHHS, 1992).

Task groups exist at all levels of community health nursing practice. Nursing organizations have State Political Action Groups that address legislative concerns regarding the health of the people within given states. Community action groups, such as Mothers Against Drunk Driving (MADD), exist on national, state, and local levels and are becoming a powerful force in influencing the health care delivery system. These groups are involved in areas such as fundraising for innovative health planning activities, informing the public about major health problems, and influencing public policy through interactions with legislators and other public officials.

Clients within a group can also help each other accomplish tasks and reach desired goals. For example, one large senior citizen's center uses retired volunteer nurses, physicians, lay persons, and residents of the center to plan and implement a monthly health screening program. The retired workers and clients involved in this task group feel needed, and the clients screened feel they are helped "by people who understand them." Other examples of task groups involving clients and providers are community partnership groups, planning groups for local community agencies, and client care conference groups (Clark, 1994).

TEACHING GROUPS "The primary purpose of teaching groups is to impart information to the participants" (Clark, 1994, p. 6). Teaching implies that someone wants to learn, and as an outcome of the teaching there is an expected learning-behavior change. For group teaching to be effective it must be determined that the group learners have need for the information that is being taught. There are numerous teaching groups in the community setting. For example, groups assist clients in dealing with a new diagnosis of an illness such as diabetes, hypertension, multiple sclerosis, or asthma. Clients in these types of groups often must learn new methods of functioning and coping with changes in their lifestyle. Groups composed of clients with common problems often provide support in addition to helping participants increase their knowledge of a disease process and treatment options. Numerous topics can be dealt with in teaching groups such as parenting, childbirth, breast-feeding, weight loss, and care of a new colostomy.

Teaching groups should be carefully planned and related to the purpose of the group experience so that the desired outcome can be achieved. The community health nurse may focus on providing information unknown to group participants, such as when the nurse is working with a group of expectant parents who want to learn about labor and delivery processes. At other times the community health nurse focuses on the facilitator role, especially when group members are learning how to cope with changes in their lifestyle.

When establishing a teaching-learning group designed to promote behavior change, it is essential for the nurse to obtain baseline data about what is already known by the group, as well as the interests and needs of individual group members. This database can help the nurse select appropriate content, educational materials, and educational objectives and strategies (see Chapter 8).

Major functions of community health nurses include providing health education and facilitating problem solving through groups and one-on-one client education sessions. With the current emphasis on cost containment in the health care field, nurses use the group process, when appropriate, to reach the greatest number of clients while controlling costs. Community health nurses can make a significant contribution to the public's health through group work.

SUPPORTIVE OR THERAPEUTIC GROUPS The primary purpose of supportive or therapeutic groups is to help participants deal with emotions associated with normative and nonnormative stressors that could lead to crises (Clark, 1994, p. 7). Community health nurses work with clients across the life span who are experiencing such stressors. Most people are healthy, but during periods of rapid development and change, they may need help to manage stress and develop effective coping strategies. Examples of supportive groups are widow-to-widow programs, classes for lay caregivers, parenting groups for grandparents, and groups for parents who have disabled children. The thrust of supportive groups is to *prevent* future upsets by helping participants to learn ways to effectively express their emotions and methods of coping in potentially difficult situations (Clark, p. 7).

Because of the complex nature of many current health problems, community health nurses are increasingly initiating support groups for at-risk clients and/or their families. Support groups are established in a variety of settings including schools, clinics, industries, neighborhood centers, and other community facilities. They are developed for multiple purposes and have been used effectively with children, adults, and the elderly. For example, support groups have been used with the elderly to address death and dying, reality orientation for persons with dementia, remotivation for daily living, and reminiscence and life review (Burnside, 1994). Support or therapeutic groups can be an effective intervention for meeting the needs of aggregates experiencing stress. These types of groups can help individuals learn about different problem-solving techniques and expand their social network. This, in turn, can assist them in dealing more effectively with normative and nonnormative sressors.

Developing a Group

Before nurses think about using the group approach to meet health needs of aggregates at risk, they must become familiar with the policies of their employing agency. Some agencies will not permit nurses to form groups under their auspices. Others will actively support group efforts if they are compatible with agency philosophy and resources. The nurse must also know whether her or his workload can support the added responsibility of group work. This can be ascertained by discussion with the nurse manager. Chapter 23 deals more fully with this aspect of the nurse's role, that is, dealing with caseload management issues.

Since community health nurses work with populations within a county, a city, or a township, common needs that can be met by a group may be expressed by clients, staff nurses, or others (for example, school officials). If the client and the nurse are so inclined, almost any health need can be met by the group process except those for which clients need one-to-one relationships. The very young single mother referred to earlier is a client whose needs may not be met by the group process. Frequently it can be useful to combine group and individual intervention strategies. For example, one nurse had a family in her caseload that included a child with spina bifida and resultant paraplegia. The nurse visited the home to assess family functioning and the environment, as well as to help the mother with the child's daily routine. The nurse also referred the parents to a parent group at the intermediate

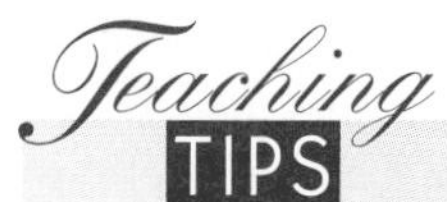

Individual and Group Teaching Methods

Cognitive

Discussion (One-on-One or Group)

May involve nurse and client or nurse with several clients
Promotes active participation and focuses on topics of interest to client
Allows peer support
Enhances application and analysis of new information

Lecture

Is a more formal method of instruction because it is controlled by teacher
Helps learner acquire new knowledge and gain comprehension

Question-and-Answer Session

Is designed specifically to address client's concerns
Assists client in applying knowledge

Role Play, Discovery

Allows client to actively apply knowledge in controlled situation
Promotes synthesis of information and problem solving

Independent Project (Computer-Assisted Instruction), Field Experience

Allows client to assume responsibility for completing learning activities at own pace
Promotes analysis, synthesis, and evaluation of new information and skills

Affective

Role Play

Allows expression of values, feelings, and attitudes

Discussion (Group)

Allows client to acquire support from others in group
Permits client to learn from other experiences
Promotes responding, valuing, and organization

Discussion (One-on-One)

Allows discussion of personal, sensitive topics of interest or concern

Psychomotor

Demonstration

Provides presentation of procedures or skills by nurse
Permits client to incorporate modeling of nurse's behavior
Allows nurse to control questioning during demonstration

Practice

Gives client opportunity to perform skills using equipment
Provides repetition

Return Demonstration

Permits client to perform skill as nurse observes
Is excellent source of feedback and reinforcement

Independent Projects, Games

Require teaching method that promotes adaptation and origination of psychomotor learning
Permit learner to use new skills

From Potter PA, Perry AG: *Basic nursing: theory and practice*, ed 3, St. Louis, 1995, Mosby, p. 242.

school, where they received support from families with similar problems.

Once a need common to a number of people has been established, decisions about group composition must be made. "In general, for a specific target population with given needs, a group composed entirely of members of that population (e.g., Parents Without Partners, clients who abuse drugs, or parents who have a disabled child) is more appropriate than a heterogeneous group" (Corey, Corey, 1997, p. 115). When potential group members are identified, the nurse should discuss with them the objectives that can be accomplished in a group setting. The important principle involved is that the nurse must have expected outcomes in mind for the group, the clients must have needs in mind, and the two should be congruent. This principle is also valid when the nurse is considering a referral to an already established group: the group experience must meet the needs of clients. A support group for new parents would probably not be helpful for a client with severe postpartum depression. However, this type of group could be very beneficial for couples who have a limited extended family network in the area and who enjoy interacting with other people.

To facilitate the implementation of the above principle, contracting is suggested when working with groups. A contract is a written statement of the mutual expectations of both client and nurse for each other. Chapter 9 discusses contracting with families. These same principles can be used when working with groups. Contracts provide a basis for evaluation of the progress that takes place. The key question to consider is whether you have met the expected outcomes you set out to achieve.

The setting plays a crucial role in groups. Several questions, such as those below, should be asked to determine whether a particular setting is appropriate.

- Is the group meeting in a place that is easily accessible, that can be reached by public transportation or personal cars easily?
- Is the meeting place near the population being served?
- Is the location of the meeting place safe after dark?
- Does the meeting room provide privacy and warmth?
- Do seating arrangements facilitate group interaction?
- Will the facility be consistently available?

Besides the setting, there are many other factors to consider when developing a group. The size of the group is a major consideration. The size of the group "depends on several factors: the age of the clients, the experience of the leader, the type of group, and the problems to be explored. For example, a group composed of elementary school children might be kept to three or four, whereas a group of adolescents might be made of six to eight people" (Corey, Corey, 1997, p. 116). Though there are no clear rules about group size, it is important to remember that group cohesiveness decreases as groups become larger (Clark, 1994). "Cohesiveness is the attraction of the group members for each other" (Clark, p. 49).

Another important variable to consider when developing a group is when the group should meet. If the group is composed of unemployed persons, daytime hours may be fine. Wage earners, on the other hand, who work during the day are likely to be free only in the evenings. The frequency and length of meetings and child care arrangements are other issues that need to be decided by the nurse and clients. If small children are to be brought along with clients, there needs to be a place with play equipment and a caretaker provided. None of these details have "right" and "wrong" answers, but it is essential that clients know them and help plan them.

Many nurses are hesitant to use the group approach to nursing care because they lack experience with this intervention strategy. Careful planning, staff development activities that facilitate the understanding of group dynamics, and guidance from professionals comfortable with this process will reduce fear.

The Life of a Group

It is important for nurses who lead groups to understand that a group goes through phases that include an orientation phase, a working phase, and a termination phase (Clark, 1994, pp. 126-127). During the orientation phase the group is introduced to its goals and purposes. Included in this phase are the time limitations, behavior expectations, and goal clarifications. The working phase encourages problem solving through intense discussion and sharing between members. The termination phase is not abrupt. This phase encourages expression of emotions, thoughts, feelings, and accomplishments associated with the group experience as well as related to separating from the group. This phase can provoke anxiety, and the leader must be prepared to help group members deal with the separation so that they do not leave feeling dejected (Clark, pp. 127-129).

The Community Health Nurse as Group Leader

Effective leadership is fundamental to a positive group experience. Group leaders perform three significant functions during early group sessions. First, they facilitate the development of a sense of cohesion and connectedness in the group. Cohesive groups are motivated to meet group goals as well as to satisfy group participants' needs. Secondly, group leaders provide sufficient structure for group interaction to maintain a secure group atmosphere that keeps anxiety at a tolerable level. And, lastly, group leaders identify group norms, or rules for behavior within the group (Clark, 1994, pp. 48-49, 123).

To succeed in implementing leadership responsibilities in a group, a nurse must have an awareness of how people interact with each other. Community health nurses must use basic interviewing and communication skills in all settings, and group work is no exception. Group participants generally want to share their feelings and thoughts, and this can be facilitated by asking open-ended questions, asking direct questions, and using other techniques such as reflection and role playing. Games and audiovisual aids are different methods that can be used to stimulate interaction between group members.

Table 22-1 is a summary of the interventions, and the goals for each intervention, that community health nurses use when they are group leaders. These leadership interventions can help the group move from the orientation to the working phase (Clark, 1994), and can promote positive group relationships. Having an awareness of group intervention strategies and why they are used helps group leaders to effectively guide the group process and develop criteria for evaluating group dynamics.

Abraham, Niles, Thiel et al, (1991) described (note summary below) how the group process can be used with elderly people and demonstrated how principles of group work and specific group interventions can be adapted for use with the depressed elderly, including those who have functional and cognitive impairments. They carried out educational group work in addition to group therapy and emphasized that even though education groups focus on learning and discussion instead of therapy, both are equally therapeutic.

It is unrealistic to expect that participants (in a group) will limit themselves to these (educational) topics and that no personal

table 22-1 A Summary of Leader Interventions

Type of Intervention	Goals of Intervention
Support	Provides supportive climate for expressing ideas and opinions, including unpopular unusual points of view. Facilitates members continuing with their ongoing behavior. Helps reinforce positive forms of behavior. Creates a climate in which silent members may feel secure enough to participate.
Confrontation	Aids in growth and development; helps unfreeze members from being stuck in one mode of functioning. Helps reduce some forms of disruptive behavior. Helps members deal more openly and directly with each other.
Advice and suggestions	Shares expertise, offers new perspectives. Helps focus group on its task and goals.
Summarizing	Helps keep group on its task by reviewing past actions and by setting agenda for future sessions. Brings to focus still unresolved issues. Organizes past in ways that help clarify; brings into focus themes and patterns of interaction.
Clarifying	Helps reduce distortion in communication. Facilitates focus on substantive issues rather than allowing members to be sidetracked into misunderstandings.
Probing and questioning	Helps expand a point that may have been left incomplete. Gets at more extensive and wider range of information. Invites members to explore their ideas in greater detail.
Repeating, paraphrasing, and highlighting	Helps members continue with their ongoing behavior, invites further exploration and examination of what is being said. Clarifies and helps focus on the specific, important, or key aspect of a communication. Sharpens members' understanding of what is being said or done.
Reflecting: Feelings	Orients members to the feelings that may lie behind what is being said or done. Helps members deal with issues they might otherwise avoid or miss.
Reflecting: Behavior	Gives members the opportunity to see how their behavior appears to others and to see and evaluate its consequences. Helps members to understand others' perceptions and responses to them.
Interpretation and analysis	Renders behavior meaningful by locating it in a larger context in which a causal explanation is provided. Helps members understand both the likely bases of their behavior and its meaning. Summarizes a pattern of behavior and provides a useful way of examining it and working to modify it through the insights gained.
Listening	Provides an attentive and responsive audience for those who participate. Models a helpful way for members to relate to one another; gives a feeling of sharing and mutual concern. Helps members sharpen their own ideas and thinking as they realize that indeed others are listening and concerned about what they are saying.

From Sampson E, Marthas M: *Group process for the health professions,* New York, 1981, Wiley, pp. 258-260.

issues will emerge. The key in education groups is how to handle such personal issues. This is done best by having the group leader use interpersonal (rather than therapeutic) skills, such as active and sensitive listening.

Education groups need as much structuring by the leader as therapy groups. Not only does this facilitate group activity, it also introduces a sense of safe group environment that is key to active participation. A sense of safety also encourages members to bring up topics of discussion that are personally relevant and important to them. In our groups, over the course of several meetings, topics became progressively more personal and pertinent to the concerns and fears that are so typical of long-term care residents. Whereas earlier subject material was safe and did not involve feelings and conflicts, this was not the case for later topics.

It is the succession of topics as well as their content that creates the group process. For instance, by having group members share their favorite poems, they were given a safe avenue for sharing what is important to them, what beauty means to them, as well as some feelings. In turn, this encouraged group interaction. Similarly, discussing Alzheimer's disease, expressing fears of developing the disease, and expressing concerns about residents with Alzheimer-type symptoms opened the way for personalizing specific concerns about growing old in later sessions. (Abraham, Niles, Thiel et al, 1991, p. 641)

Nurses who are interested in working with groups but who have never done so should ask for supervision and a preceptor to help them with the process. Effective communication with group members and agency personnel, careful scheduling, and attention to small details of organizing the group can help this to be a successful experience. Review of the literature is also helpful when community health nurses consider developing groups in the clinical setting. Corey and Corey (1997) and Clark (1994) have written readable, practical books for neophytes who are interested in creating a group and practicing group process skills.

THE EVOLUTION OF CLINIC AND NURSING CENTER SERVICES

Community health nurses have long worked in clinics. Beginning with the era of Lillian Wald, they have had to assume a considerable amount of responsibility, make independent judgments, and use skill in teaching clients. These competencies especially fitted them to work in the relatively independent clinic setting.

Early efforts at the beginning of the century to improve maternal-child health and to control communicable disease frequently resulted in the development of clinic services for underserved aggregates. For example, between 1900 and 1930 many milk dispensaries evolved into preventive health centers.

In her history of the origins of nursing centers, Glass (1989, p. 21) begins with the work of Lillian Wald and also describes the endeavors of Mary Breckinridge with the Frontier Nursing Service in Hyden, Kentucky (Figure 22-1); Margaret Sanger, the pioneer birth control activist in Europe and the United States; and a nurse settlement house in Orange, New Jersey. The three women named were pioneer feminists well-known to activists working for the health of women today. Wald's accomplishments with nursing clinics are detailed in Chapter 1. In 1923 Breckinridge used the principles of program planning, described in Chapter 14, to determine where nursing services were needed in rural, mountainous Kentucky. After surveying a three-county area covering 1000 square miles she concluded that a decentralized system of health care was essential. Based on her study, The Kentucky Committee for Mothers and Babies opened their first nursing center in Hyden, Kentucky, in September 1925. By 1930 there were six nursing centers, each serving a 5-mile radius, with the objectives of providing the following: skilled care for the sick of all ages and women in childbirth, the health education of the population, social services, and the advancement of economic independence (Glass).

Margaret Sanger (1870-1966) began her career as a visiting nurse in New York City. Her work with poor women and children stimulated her interest in birth control and women having control over their own bodies. Because the Comstock Act of 1873 declared birth control material obscene and prohibited the mailing of it, Sanger travelled to France to obtain information. She opened the first birth control clinic in America in 1916 in Brooklyn. She was shortly thereafter arrested and spent the first of her many sentences in jail. The establishment of today's Planned Parenthood Federation is to her credit, and her contributions to the health of women is inestimable.

These are dramatic, wonderful examples of the beginnings of nursing centers as we know them today. Additionally, large-scale demonstration projects were sponsored by the Metropolitan Life Insurance Company to combat tuberculosis and other communicable diseases, and included programs of mass screening and health assessment, as well as community education activities (Kalisch, Kalisch, 1986).

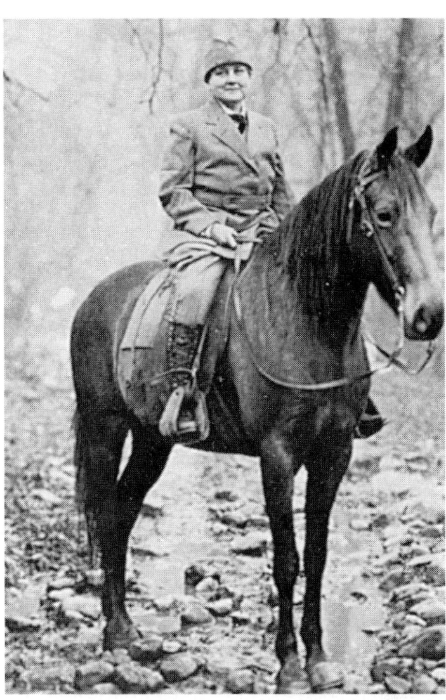

Figure 22-1 Mary Breckinridge founded the Frontier Nursing Service in Kentucky. Her nurses used horses to service families in the hills of Kentucky.

By the 1930s child health conferences and maternity conferences or clinics were well established. Books on public health nursing practice written at this time addressed the role of the nurse in the clinic and stressed the need for conferences to achieve a well-balanced child welfare program (Gardner, 1928; National Organization for Public Health Nursing, 1939).

Clinic services were developed in the beginning of the century because a significant number of families could not afford other types of care. They were also established to reach a large number of individuals very quickly during epidemics of communicable diseases. These services have been maintained over the century because early efforts dramatically demonstrated their effectiveness in improving maternal-child health and in combating communicable diseases.

The nurse practitioner movement of the 1960s and 1970s significantly altered the role of nurses in community-based clinics. This movement evolved to advance nursing practice in a variety of settings and to address the needs of disadvantaged aggregates across the life span. It was believed that well-trained nurses with expanded skills could help eradicate the problem of inaccessible and fragmented health care services, especially in underserved areas. Increasingly, local health departments and other community health clinics are using nurse practitioners to provide comprehensive services for at-risk aggregates (Lawler, Valand, 1988, pp. 187-188).

During the 1980s and the early 1990s there was tremendous growth in ambulatory care or clinic services, particularly because of the introduction of the prospective payment system for Medicare-sponsored hospital stays. As the length of hospital stays has decreased, patient acuity at discharge has increased. This has resulted in the need for increased continuing care after discharge and has shifted the responsibility for clients' care to their families and community-based providers. Further, to increase the efficiency of care, insurers have encouraged people to have preadmission testing done on an outpatient basis and have moved many surgeries such as lens implantation to an outpatient basis. As a result, the number of days being spent in community hospitals is decreasing significantly while the number of outpatient visits is rising dramatically. In fact, ambulatory care is one of the fastest growing specialties in nursing.

AGGREGATE-FOCUSED CLINIC SERVICES

Clinics, often called *ambulatory health services*, are centers that examine and treat ambulatory clients on an outpatient basis. They are frequently operated under the auspices of a larger institution such as a hospital, medical school, group practice, HMO, health department, church, or community organization. Defining their services is difficult because they vary from one institution to the next.

The clinic setting offers a wide range of preventive health services. Clinics may provide only primary intervention; this is usually the main focus in immunization clinics. Or clinics may provide screening, diagnosis, and treatment services, such as those provided by clinics treating sexually transmitted diseases, that identify the disease, administer appropriate treatments, and locate contacts of the infected client for screening.

Clinics may serve only a specific population. Well-baby clinics usually provide assessment services for children from birth to 5 years of age, and family planning clinics usually serve females of childbearing age. Other clinics may serve anyone who comes at any time with any problem, as do walk-in clinics of large teaching hospitals and neighborhood health care centers. Emergency rooms function as ambulatory clinics in many towns where there are no other resources.

The needs of aggregates at risk have also been addressed through the use of mobile clinics that target specific populations (McNeal, 1996). Communities are using these mobile units to provide a wide array of health care, including dental services, multiphasic screenings, immunizations, family planning and pregnancy testing, and acute and chronic disease treatment services. Mobile health care units help professionals to outreach in underserved areas and are often the only source of care for some aggregates at risk. Through the use of these units, many of the primary and secondary preventive needs of at-risk populations can be addressed.

Many official local health agencies provide multiphasic diagnostic and primary health care services through clinics on an ongoing basis. Frequently, these services are targeted to specific population groups. For example, the high rate of pregnancy and sexually transmitted diseases and other health problems among adolescents has created a need for population-specific interventions for this age group. Increasingly, services for teens are provided in settings, such as teen clinics and school-based clinics, that are easily accessible, safe and confidential (Blum, Beuhring, Wunderlich, Resnick, 1996; Ferretti, Verhey, Isham, 1996; Scott, 1996; Yawn, Yawn, 1997). The St. Paul Maternal and Child Health Program, one of the oldest school-based clinic projects, offers a wide range of services to students during school hours, such as immunizations, mental health counseling, prenatal care, family planning, and supportive group services (Maternal and Child Health Program, undated). Other significant health problems have also provided the stimulus for the development of clinic services by private and official community health agencies. Another example of this is how communities have responded to the needs of homeless populations by reaching out to them in a variety of nontraditional settings. In one inner-city community, a nurse's clinic was established in a soup kitchen as a walk-in clinic for the homeless. Clinic hours coincided with the times that the soup kitchen was open. In this situation nurses were able to provide health services in a familiar setting that met many of the physical and psychosocial needs of the homeless (Scholler-Jaquish, 1996).

As discussed previously, community health centers (CHCs) are also emerging across the country to assist medically underserved aggregates. These centers, federally supported under Section 330 of the Public Health Service Act, are located in every territory and state except Wyoming. They exist in both urban and rural settings and serve persons with special needs, such as coal miners with respiratory and pulmonary impairments, the elderly, people who are confined to their homes, and migrant and seasonal farmworkers. Most migrant health centers are operated together with CHCs. Data reveal that these centers have significantly influenced the health status of the population groups they are serving. Clients served by a CHC have a lower incidence of hospitalization than clients cared for in other health care settings. Studies have also shown a dramatic reduction in infant mortality in specific regions of the country after the establishment of a CHC: in the rural south, infant mortality decreased by 50%, and in Denver's CHC program it decreased by 25% (National Association of Community Health Centers, Inc., 1986).

The type of care provided through clinics may be episodic, in which only the immediate needs of the clients are handled, or comprehensive, providing all levels of preventive services: primary preventive, diagnostic, therapeutic, and rehabilitative services. Primary preventive and diagnostic services (e.g., screening for communicable diseases or health risks such as high blood cholesterol) are frequently the focus in clinics sponsored by official health agencies.

THE DEVELOPMENT OF NURSING CENTERS

"A nursing center is both a setting and a concept" (Riesch, 1992, p. 145). A number of terms are used to refer to nursing centers, including *nurse-managed care*, *community nursing center* or *organization*, or *nurse-run clinic*. These terms refer to organizations where nurses control practice and patient care and where education and research are paramount (Riesch, p. 145). Riesch reviewed the literature about nursing centers and defined them by three criteria: direct access by client/patient to the nurse, a nursing model of care, and holistic reimbursed services. Aydelotte and Gregory (1989) reported that, at the Second National Conference on Nursing Centers in 1984, the participants defined a nursing center as follows:

> Nurse-Managed Centers are organizations that provide direct access to professional nurses who offer holistic, client-centered health services for reimbursement. With the use of nursing models of health, professional nurses in NMC's diagnose and treat human responses to potential and actual health problems. Examples of professional nursing services include health education, health promotion, and health-related research. Services are targeted to underserved individuals and groups. An effective referral system and collaboration with other health care professionals are an integral part of NMC's. As models of professional nursing practice and research, NMC's are ideal sites for faculty and student practice. They are administered by a professional nurse. (Fehring, Schulte, Riesch, 1986, p. 63)

As indicated previously in this chapter, nursing centers were developed in the early 1900s by Lillian Wald, Mary Breckenride, and other pioneering public health nursing leaders. However, "the literature is devoid of reports of nursing center development until the 1960s" (Riesch, 1992, p. 147), when Lydia Hall established the Loeb Center in New York in 1963. The Center was described as being "close to public health nursing in an institutional setting" (Riesch, p. 147).

During the 1970s and 1980s nursing centers grew for several reasons: nursing faculty identified underserved populations and realized that these groups could serve as learning experiences for students. Further, monies from federal and state legislatures and private foundations and professional organizations assisted in the development of the concept (Riesch, 1992, p. 148). The Community Nursing Organizations Bill, signed into law in 1987, provided direct Medicare reimbursement to nurses and permitted the development of ten demonstration sites. "Nursing education has been the pacesetter in the development of nursing centers" (Courney, 1992, p. 1). The View from the Field at the end of the chapter showcases two academic nursing centers that demonstrate the variety of services delivered by nursing centers and gives some evidence of how students learn about models of care delivery that they can use in their own practice.

Nursing centers grew rapidly during the 1980s. An estimated 250 were in place across the country, serving 118,000 Americans, in 1990 (News, 1992, p. 70). About half were freestanding; others were affiliated with a hospital, a public health or home health agency, or a retirement community. Those not freestanding were usually housed in a school of nursing where students were assigned to the center for clinical experience (News, p. 70). Now there are approximately 500 nurse-managed centers in the United States (Ferretti, Verhey, Isham, 1996, p. 35).

Services Offered by Nursing Centers

Care offered by nursing centers may focus on health promotion and early casefinding services such as health education, health screening, and physical assessment or may span the entire range of primary care (Cole, Mackey, 1996; Ferretti, Verhey, Isham, 1996; Holman, 1990; Walker, 1994). The type of services provided and the conditions diagnosed and treated vary, based on the purpose of the nursing center and the characteristics of the population being served. Care in nursing centers is reimbursed in several ways, including out-of-pocket fees, Medicare or Medicaid, and private insurance. Reimbursement is also provided through other financing mechanisms such as private foundation support, managed care contracts, worker compensation funding, and federal research and demonstration grants (Ferretti, Verhey, Isham, 1996; Starck, Mackey, Adams, 1995).

ESTABLISHING AGGREGATE-FOCUSED CLINIC AND NURSING CENTER SERVICES

Community health nurses frequently assume a major role in planning, implementing, and evaluating services for aggregates with unmet needs. When establishing new health care services, the nurse uses the health planning process described in Chapter 14. Some specific factors to consider when setting up clinic services follow.

Determining the need for clinics and nursing centers is the first responsibility of a health care professional interested in developing such services. Factors to consider during this process are the health status, lifestyle patterns, and demographic characteristics of the population being studied; community resources available to the population under consideration; health care use patterns; and health care accessibility variables, such as location of resources and client referral processes. Chapter 13 describes how and where community health nurses obtain these data. When analyzing these data, it is important to examine trends over time and to identify strengths as well as limitations in the health care delivery system. The goal is to determine whether services are lacking or whether services are adequate but not used as a result of unique characteristics of the population being served or service delivery problems. For example, community health nurses have found that clients frequently do not use clinic services because their location makes them inaccessible or clients are unaware they exist. If a need is verified, careful planning should take place before starting a clinic.

Several organizational activities need to be accomplished to ensure effective and efficient service delivery. Establishing specific objectives helps the nurse determine what types of services to offer and what resources are needed to provide them. For example, the resources needed to staff a comprehensive child health conference would be significantly greater than those needed to staff an immunization clinic.

Prospective clients and collaborative agencies should be part of the planning team to help ensure that clients' needs can be met through the proposed clinic. When interagency collaboration is needed to achieve proposed goals, tasks and task characteristics must be clearly delineated according to scope, complexity, and uncertainty. "Task scope is the extent to which a multidisciplinary/multidimensional approach to the issue is required. Task complexity is reflected in the amount of time spent on a project and the duration of the project. Task uncertainty indicates the unpredictability of the outcome of the task" (Polivka, 1995, p. 111). Classifying tasks helps the staff of a clinic to determine what resources are needed to achieve desired outcomes.

Other organizational activities include determining the location for the clinic or center, securing necessary equipment and supplies, organizing facilities to ensure client privacy and effective and efficient service delivery, establishing procedures such as follow-up policies that promote quality care, obtaining adequate professional staff with the skills needed to manage client health needs, securing and training volunteers, and developing marketing strategies. All of these activities require careful thought and planning and include several components. For example, securing necessary equipment and supplies involves such things as identifying what is needed, determining where to purchase it, and establishing appropriate storage procedures for vaccines and other medications.

Determining a site requires special attention because location of a clinic or center influences the way it will be used. Some clients are affected more than others by the location, namely, the poor and the aged. Difficulty and expense of access are important, so a knowledge of the possible transportation alternatives is important. Accessibility also involves appointment delay time, waiting time, clinic or center hours, services offered, health care given, and client/professional relationships.

Evaluation procedures should be established during the organizational phase of planning. An overall evaluation of operations should occur at least once a year, but evaluation is an ongoing process that needs attention throughout the year. Procedures need to be established to evaluate overall operations and usage patterns. Questions for planners to consider when evaluating services are shared in a later section of this chapter and in Chapter 14.

The importance of adequate planning when establishing a clinic or nursing center cannot be overstressed. Neglecting significant details during the planning phase can result in poor use of services. For example, one health department decided to open a well-baby clinic because it was determined that a rural portion of a large county was underserved. The first decision made was to send a staff nurse to school for preparation as a pediatric nurse practitioner. However, steps of the planning process were not logically followed after preparing this staff nurse for new role responsibilities. Thus, even though there were no other facilities for well-child care in the area, the clinic closed because of lack of clients. It was isolated with no public transportation available, so clients could not use the service.

The Role of the Community Health Nurse in Clinics and Nursing Centers

The community health nurse can function in various ways to meet the health needs of aggregates. As previously discussed, the expanded role of the nurse has aided community health nurses in more adequately meeting the health care needs of people in clinics and nursing centers. As finances for health care delivery become an increasingly scarce commodity, health care agencies are shifting the emphasis from home visits to the use of clinics, nursing centers, and groups to meet the needs of people as aggregates. Often these agencies use an outreach approach to facilitate the identification of underserved clients who could benefit from clinic and nursing center services. Outreach activities include such things as working with community leaders to advertise services, meeting with community agencies (e.g., domestic violence centers and homeless shelters) that normally work with underserved populations to identify potential clients, and using lay workers to survey families in their neighborhood about unmet needs.

The client population being served in many clinics has become more complex and acute. Nurses no longer serve as schedulers and receptionists. Their roles have enlarged to include management of clients with both acute and long-term care needs, handling of complex treatments and procedures, client counseling, and health education. In addition, nurses are often the primary providers for many clients and their families. One study on elder client satisfaction with nursing services provided by a community-based nursing center found that access to services in the center "helped to increase the older adult's knowledge of healthy behaviors, prevented potential problems, and maintained or improved current level of health" (Scott, Moneyham, 1995, p. 186).

The range of activities implemented by a nurse in a clinic setting or nursing center will vary based on its objectives and the needs of clients. Common roles assumed by the nurse in most community health settings are discussed below.

MANAGER The role of manager was the main nursing function in clinics for many years. Nurses attended to the many details necessary for clinics to run smoothly: distributing client caseload, following up on clients with problems, bringing needed reports to physicians, preparing clients physically for examinations, performing procedures, supervising aides and practical nurses, and carrying out clerical work. Although all this is necessary, the nurse should perform *nursing* activities, that is, helping clients when they are unable to help themselves. The nurse should supervise other members of the health team as described in Chapter 23 so that they can carry out the functions that do not require the professional skills of a registered nurse. This means that the nurse will understand the different levels of functioning of team members and use them appropriately. Clerks and aides, as well as volunteers, can be valuable assets in the clinic. They can weigh and measure babies, file and pull records, label and carry specimens to the laboratory, act as receptionists, and take temperatures. Smooth flow of clients from waiting to examining rooms is important and can be facilitated by aides. As a manager, the community health nurse must understand that she or he is responsible for the care that these team members give. The nurse's supervision of team members is fundamental to the care given clients in the clinic setting.

GROUP LEADER AND TEACHER Many clinics and nursing centers have as one of their most important functions group sessions in which information is discussed that is designed to promote health. One example is an ostomy information clinic that disseminates information and helps clients cope with problems related to their ostomies. Another example is a prenatal education program in a nursing center in which the community health nurse meets with clients before appointments to share information about pregnancy, childbirth, child care, and role transition concerns. The concepts presented earlier in this chapter on developing and leading a group are applicable to the nurse's role in clinics as group leader and teacher.

PRACTITIONER The expanded role of the nurse has provided nurses with physical assessment and client management skills. Practitioners are able to identify the current health status of clients, including emotional and physical components, and to plan interventions that meet clients' needs. Practitioners carry out a variety of functions in both adult and child health clinics. Providing physical, mental, social, and emotional support, educating clients about their health conditions, and referring clients to needed community resources are examples of functions implemented by the practitioner. Practitioners often work with an interdisciplinary team and actively participate in client care conferences. They provide a continuum of nursing services, especially for clients who have chronic health conditions or preventive health needs.

EVALUATOR An integral part of working in these settings is evaluation. This process was discussed in depth in Chapter 14. Some specific questions to ask when evaluating services include the following: Are the objectives of the clinic or nursing center being met? If this is the immunization clinic in Smith County, for example, are children completely immunized at age 2 and upon school entrance? Are the numbers of clients being served increasing or decreasing? If the number of clients being served is changing, is it because the health service area population is changing or because clients feel that they are not being served adequately? The way clients feel about the care they receive determines whether they will use the health facility. Some method of client contact on a regular basis, either questionnaire or interview, is needed to provide data concerning this factor. Knowing who is served also means that a record system will be in operation so that number and kinds of visits can be tabulated easily. A good record system will also provide for continuity of care from one visit to the next and yet not be overly time-consuming.

COMMUNITY HEALTH NURSING IN NONTRADITIONAL PRACTICE SETTINGS

Increasingly, community health nurses are working with a team of health care providers in nontraditional settings to provide services for underserved populations. An important role for community health nurses on these teams is to promote the philosophy of community health practice: orientation to wellness rather than illness; family-centered versus individual-centered; continuous rather than episodic intervention; and population- and community-focused health planning. Regardless of where community health nurses function, these concepts should be central to their practice. As discussed in Chapter 2, it is *the nature of the practice*—not the setting—that distinguishes community health nursing from other specialty nursing areas. The concepts of community health nursing greatly enrich service delivery and nursing care in any setting.

Developing new ways of providing services for at-risk aggregates is essential in this era of cost containment. To handle the demands in the health care delivery system and the changing nature of current health problems, coordinated community-wide approaches targeted to specific populations must be emphasized. Community health nurses have unique skills and knowledge to address this challenge. The roles community health nurses have assumed in block nursing and parish nursing illustrate how these nurses have used their skills to work with communities in providing services for targeted aggregates at risk.

Block Nursing and Parish Nursing

Block nursing and parish nursing are two creative, alternative ways for addressing the needs of specific aggregates in the community. Both provide a nontraditional setting for practice and are based on a holistic philosophy that addresses health promotion as well as curative health services. These approaches to nursing practice assist clients in accessing health services and prevent institutionalization for many people in the community. Both settings provide opportunities for nurses to practice autonomous professional nursing and help to fill in the gaps of the traditional acute health care system (Armmer, Humbles, 1995; Jamieson, 1990).

Jamieson (1990) described *block nursing* as nursing on the block where the nurse lives, making services available based on need rather than reimbursement eligibility. Professional and volunteer community members, an informal network of family, friends, neighbors, church and civic groups, service groups such as Boy and Girl Scouts, and people who are part of the neighborhood provide many of the services needed. These include shopping, running errands, and providing respite care to relieve caregivers. Funding to pay for client assessments and direct care provided by aides/homemakers and nurses has come from sources such as grants, client fees, and demonstration projects. One block nurse program prevented hospitalization in 25% of its clients. Referrals for block nursing services frequently come by word of mouth from the neighborhood. Block nursing "is reminiscent of earlier eras when a nurse was involved with a total community and all its citizens" (Jamieson, p. 251).

Parish nursing meets many of the same needs as block nursing. However, churches and synagogues provide the system whereby the services are offered.

> Churches and synagogues have been promoting health and wholeness for centuries through the ministries of worship, music, sharing and caring. A new dimension is the addition of the nurse to the ministry team. For the past dozen years, nurses across the state and across the country have been using their nursing skills to demonstrate religious witness. Some are volunteers; some are paid; some just get mileage. Some train volunteers; others actually staff the program. Some minister to their congregations only; others reach out into their communities. *Parish nursing* takes many forms, depending on each congregation—its needs, visions, and resources (Parish nursing, 1993, p. 1).

The role of the parish nurse is relatively new. The first institutionally based parish nurse program emerged in 1984 and, as a result, more parish nurse programs are continuing to develop throughout the United States (Djupe, 1996). Currently, four types of parish nursing models exist, including (1) *hospital-sponsored*, where the nurse works for the institution; (2) *parish-based*, where the nurse is hired by the church; (3) *hospital-sponsored volunteer*, where nurses associated with specific institutions volunteer to provide resource information to the parishioners in their congregation; and (4) *congregation-based*, which is a volunteer model where the nurses from within a congregation volunteer to provide resources and services to the congregation (Armmer, Humbles, 1995, p. 66). Regardless of the model used, the parish nurse endeavors to provide holistic care by providing a variety of services through various roles. The most common roles of the parish nurse include *health educator*, *health counselor*, *resource* and *referral agent*, *volunteer coordinator*, and *facilitator* or *troubleshooter*, where the nurse helps bridge gaps between the parishioners and the health care system (Armmer, Humbles; Djupe, 1996; Dunkle, 1996).

Both block nursing and parish nursing are community-based and serve to meet needs that are not met by the traditional health care system. Both also build on the concept of nursing neighbors in one's community. Likely, not even the best national health care package will meet everyone's needs. Therefore, the idealism of these services should continue to be part of community health nursing. These non-traditional alternatives can serve as a guide for caring for others in unique and holistic ways.

Summary

Community health nurses carry out numerous roles and functions in a variety of settings to meet the health care needs and goals of aggregates at risk in the community. Some roles implemented by nurses in the community setting are manager, health educator, health counselor, resource and referral agent, group leader, practitioner, and health planner. This chapter addresses how nurses function in clinic, nursing center, parish, and neighborhood or block settings to address the needs of aggregates across the life span. It also addresses how nurses use the group process to provide targeted preventive services. The emphasis is on working cooperatively with clients in identifying appropriate ways to deliver community health nursing services.

Increasingly, with a focus on cost containment, health care agencies are using creative ways to meet the needs of aggregates in the community. It is important to remember that no one method will meet everyone's health needs and that nurses must assess clients before deciding which intervention will effectively and efficiently assist them. This kind of choice contributes to the challenge, excitement, and creativity of community health nursing. It brings nurses closer to clients in the community and provides a stimulus for developing innovative nontraditional practice. Nurses must become involved in planning for the future so that a viable role for nursing is maintained in the evolving health care system.

CRITICAL *Thinking Exercise*

The box on the next page contains descriptions of two academic nursing centers, demonstrating the variety of services offered by this segment of the health care delivery system. Think about the services that are offered and how they differ from the traditional clinic services that are part of many neighborhoods. Considering the characteristics of the community you are serving, identify populations at risk that could benefit from nursing center services. Additionally, identify potential locations for a nursing center and the type of services needed by at-risk groups in your community.

We would like to acknowledge Ella Mae Brooks, PhD, RN, for her help in developing this chapter.

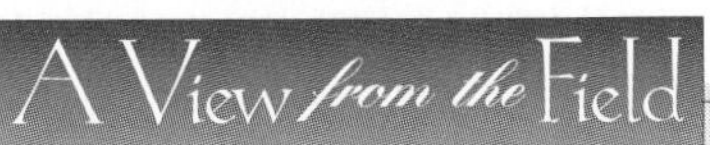
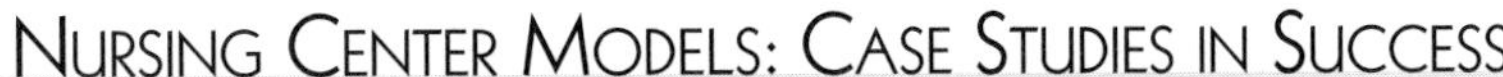

A View from the Field: Nursing Center Models: Case Studies in Success

SOUTHERN ILLINOIS UNIVERSITY AT EDWARDSVILLE COMMUNITY NURSING SERVICES

By Barbara C. Martin, EdD, RNC, Jacalyn Ryberg, MA, RNC, and Jacquelyn Clement, PhD, RN

The Southern Illinois University at Edwardsville (SIUE) Community Nursing Services provides an ideal setting for a community health experience. In this primarily black, inner city community, a clinical practicum for senior nursing students was developed with the local Head Start program in 1989.

Students were originally involved with case management for children with identified health problems. They worked with families to assure that the children had access to appropriate care. Working with families provided an excellent community health experience for nursing students and resulted in faster, more comprehensive resolution of health problems for Head Start children.

The program later expanded to include health screening services. The nursing students set up screening sites, collect blood samples, operate the screening test machines, identify health problems, and keep records.

As the students and faculty identify health problems, there is an increased opportunity to speak with the teachers, and on occasion parents. This dialogue facilitates information sharing and early intervention for the children.

In the summer of 1989, an elderly component was added to the practicum. In conjunction with the local housing authority, the students began to collect emergency data on a *Health Alert Form*. This form helps keep all pertinent data on the elderly residents of public housing in one accessible place.

The form is maintained in an opaque sleeve on the back of each apartment hall door. It is available to emergency teams, family members, and health care workers assuring continuity of care. Students visit the elderly in their homes, interview them, fill out the forms, and identify problems. In follow-up visits they do basic health education and medication teaching. They are also able to relate to problems of independent living that commonly occur upon hospital discharge.

Students appreciate the opportunity for practical application of the cultural concepts they learn in class as they are exposed to multigenerational families, elders in independent living settings, and accessing limited resources for those with limited financial assets.

As the nursing center grows, the educational experience opportunities for the students will expand. The potential benefits to clients, the community, the students, and the center are only limited by imagination.

UNIVERSITY OF TEXAS NURSING SERVICES—HOUSTON

By Glenda C. Walker, DSN, RN

In February 1991, The University of Texas School of Nursing at the Health Science Center in Houston (UTNS-H) opened an ambulatory nursing service center. The purposes of the UTNS-H were to provide educational and research opportunities for students and faculty.

At UTNS-H categories or clinical services include: high risk screening, health education, well child care, and home infusion therapy. Other services currently under development include: geriatric nursing care, women's health care, and psychiatric health care. When deviations from normal are found, patients are referred to either their private physician or the UT Family Practice clinic. When the patient needs follow-up monitoring and/or educational services, they are referred back to UTNS-H. This type of arrangement allows for cost-effective services delivered by the most appropriate provider with an emphasis on continuity of care.

UTNS-H also provides health education seminars on such topics as chronic disease, healthy lifestyles, stress management, and safety in the work place. In addition, ongoing health education classes are provided for patients who are referred to UTNS-H needing health education counseling, such as nutritional management of diabetes. UTNS-H encourages consumer/patient responsibility and accountability for the management of their health care.

Well child services provided by UTNS-H include: well baby exams (EPSDT), immunizations, TB skin tests, school physicals, and parenting classes. These services are provided at a variety of settings with an emphasis on easy access. For example, the UTNS-H pediatric nurse practitioner has provided EPSDT screenings at the City of Houston housing project apartments. In addition, a UTNS-H pediatric nurse practitioner provides well child services at a community-based health clinic five mornings a week. A collaborative agreement with UT Department of Pediatrics allows for supervision of the medical protocols, consultation regarding cases, and referrals to the department for those patients needing more extensive care.

UTNS-H provides home IV infusion services for patients who need continuing care within the home environment. A case management approach is utilized to meet the physical and emotional needs of the family and patients. It is believed that this approach will strengthen the coping resources of the family thereby minimizing costly rehospitalization.

As nursing embraces and lobbys for *Nursing's Agenda for Health Care Reform*, it is important for nursing centers to analyze how their activities correlate with that agenda. An initial analysis of UTNS-H activities and the agenda has proven successful for our current path.

From National League for Nursing, Council for Nursing Centers: *Connections*, New York, Winter 1992, NLN, p. 2.

REFERENCES

Abraham IL, Niles SA, Thiel BP et al: Therapeutic group work with depressed elderly, *Nurs Clin North Am* 26(3):635-650, 1991.

American Public Health Association (APHA), Public Health Nursing Section: *The definition and role of public health nursing: a statement of APHA public health nursing section*, Washington, D.C., 1996, APHA.

Armmer FA, Humbles P: Parish nursing: extending health care to urban African-Americans, *Nurs Health Care* 16(2):64-68, 1995.

Aydelotte MK, Gregory MS: Nursing practice: innovative models. In *Nursing centers: meeting the demand for quality health care*, Pub No. 21-2311, New York, 1989, NLN.

Blum RW, Beuhring T, Wunderlich M, Resnick M: Don't ask, they won't tell: the quality of adolescent health screening in five practice settings, *Am J Public Health* 86(12):1767-1772, 1996.

Burlew LD, Jones J, Emerson P: Exercise and the elderly: a group counseling approach, *J Specialists in Group Work* 16(3):152-158, 1991.

Burnside I: History and overview of group work. In Burnside I, Schmidt MG: *Coping with older adults: group process and techniques*, ed 3, Boston, 1994, Jones & Bartlett, pp. 24-37.

Clark CC: *The nurse as group leader*, ed 3, New York, 1994, Springer Publishing Co..

Clark NM, Janz NK, Dodge JA, Sharpe PA: Self-regulation of health behavior: the "Take PRIDE" program, *Health Educ Q* 19:341-354, 1992.

Clark NM, McLeroy KR: Creating capacity through health education; what we know and what we don't, *Health Educ Q* 22:273-289, 1995.

Cole FL, Mackey T: Utilization of an academic nursing center, *J Prof Nurs* 12:349-353, 1996.

Corey MS, Corey G: *Groups: process and practice*, Pacific Grove, Ca., 1997, Brooks/Cole Publishing.

Courney D: Information sharing is the key, *Connections, National League for Nursing's Council for Nursing Centers*, pp. 1-4, Winter 1992.

Djupe AM: Parish nursing. In Cohen EL: *Nurse case management in the 21st century*, St. Louis, 1996, Mosby, pp. 140-148.

Dunkle RM: Parish nurses help patients-body and soul, *RN* 59(5):55-57, 1996.

Fehring R, Schulte J, Riesch S: Toward a definition of nurse-managed centers, *J Community Health Nurs* 3:2, 59-67, 1986.

Ferretti CK, Verhey MP, Isham MM: Development of a nurse-managed, school-based health center, *Nurse Educ* 21:35-42, 1996.

Freudenberg N, Eng E, Flay B et al: Strengthening individual and community capacity to prevent disease and promote health: in search of relevant theories and principles, *Health Educ Q* 22(3): 290-306, 1995.

Gardner MS: *Public health nursing*, ed 2, New York, 1928, Macmillan.

Glass LK: The historic origins of nursing centers. In *Nursing centers: meeting the demand for quality health care*, Pub No. 21-2311, New York, 1989, NLN.

Holman E: Nursing centers—state of the art and future initiatives: services and marketing strategies. In *Perspectives in nursing 1989-1991*, Pub No. 41-2281, New York, 1990, NLN.

Jamieson MK: Block nursing: practicing autonomous professional nursing in the community, *Nurs Health Care* 11(5):250-253, May 1990.

Kalisch PA, Kalisch BJ: *The advance of American nursing*, ed 2, Boston, 1986, Little, Brown.

Lawler TG, Valand MC: Patterns of practice of nurse practitioners in an underserved rural region, *J Community Health Nurs* 5:187-194, 1988.

Lewin K: Group decision and social change. In Newcomb TM, Hartley EL, eds: *Readings in social psychology*, New York, 1947, Holt.

Loomis ME: *Group process for nurses*, St. Louis, 1979, Mosby.

Luft J: *Group process: an introduction to group dynamics*, ed 2, Palo Alto, Ca., 1970, Mayfield.

MacKenzie KR, ed: *Effective use of group therapy in managed care*, Washington, D.C., 1995, American Psychiatric Press.

Marín G, Burhansstipanov L, Connell CM et al: A research agenda for health education among underserved populations, *Health Educ Q* 22(3):346-363, 1995.

Maternal and Child Health Program: *St. Paul Adolescent Health Services Project*, St. Paul, Mn., undated, St. Paul-Ramsey Medical Center.

McNeal GJ: Mobile Health care for those at risk, *Nurs Health Care* 17(3):134-140, 1996.

Mullen PD, Evans D, Forster J et al: Settings as an important dimension in health education/promotion policy, programs, and research, *Health Educ Q* 22(3):330-347, 1995.

Myers JE, Poidevant JM, Dean LA: Groups for older persons and their caregivers: a review of the literature, *J Specialists in Group Work* 16(3):197-205, 1991.

National Association of Community Health Centers, Inc.: *Community health centers: a quality system for the changing health care market*, McLean, Va., 1986, National Clearinghouse for Primary Care Information.

National League for Nursing (NLN), Council for Nursing Centers: *Connections*, New York, Winter 1992, NLN.

National Organization for Public Health Nursing: *Manual of public health nursing*, ed 3, New York, 1939, Macmillan.

News, community nursing centers gaining ground as solution to health issues, *AJN* 92(7):70-71, 1992.

Parish nursing, *Penn Nurse* 48:1, July 1993, Pennsylvania State Nurses Association.

Pederson A, O'Neill M, Rootman I: *Health promotion in Canada: provincial, national, and international perspectives*, Toronto, 1994, Saunders.

Piechowski PA, Ciha TE, eds: *Project group work: an innovative approach to counseling in schools*, Des Moines, Ia., 1988, State of Iowa, Department of Education.

Polivka BJ: A conceptual model for community interagency collaboration, *Image J Nurs Sch* 27(2):110-115, 1995.

Potter PA, Perry AG: *Basic nursing: theory and practice*, ed 3, St. Louis, 1995, Mosby.

Riesch SK: Nursing centers. In Fitzpatrick JJ, Tauton RL, Jacox AK, ed: *Annu Rev Nurs Res*, vol 10, New York, 1992, Springer, pp. 145-162.

Sampson E, Marthas M: *Group process for the health professions*, New York, 1981, Wiley.

Scherl D, Noren J, Osterweis M, ed: *Promoting health and preventing disease*, Washington, D.C., 1992, Association of Academic Health Centers.

Scholler-Jaquish A: Walk-in health clinic for the homeless, *Nurs Health Care* 17(3):119-123, 1996.

Scott CB, Moneyham L: Perceptions of senior residents about a community-based nursing center, *Image J Nurs Sch* 27(3)181-186, 1995.

Scott MAK: Reducing the risks: adolescents and sexually transmitted diseases, *Nurse Pract Forum* 7(1):23-29, 1996.

Sleek S: Group therapy: tapping the power of teamwork, *The APA Monitor* 26(7):1, 38-39, 1995.

Starck PL, Mackey TA, Adams J: Nurse-managed clinics: a blueprint for success using the Covey framework, *J Prof Nurs* 11:71-77, 1995.

Steckler A, Allegrante JP, Altman D et al: Health education intervention strategies: recommendations for future research, *Health Educ Q* 22:307-328, 1995.

United States Department of Health and Human Services (USDHHS): *Healthy people 2000: national health promotion and disease prevention objectives, full report, with commentary*, Washington, D.C., 1991, U.S. Government Printing Office.

United States Department of Health and Human Services (USDHHS): *Healthy people 2000: consortium action*, Washington, D.C., 1992, U.S. Government Printing Office.

United States Department of Health and Human Services (USDHHS): *Healthy people 2000: midcourse review and 1995 revisions*, Washington, D.C., 1995, U.S. Government Printing Office.

Walker P: A comprehensive community nursing center model: maximizing practice income—a challenge to educators, *J Prof Nurs* 10:131-139, 1994.

Yawn BP, Yawn RA: Adolescent pregnancy: a preventable consequence? *The Prevention Researcher* 4(1):1-4, Winter, 1997.

SELECTED BIBLIOGRAPHY

Bremer A: Revitalizing the district model for the delivery of prevention-focused community health nursing services, *Fam Community Health* 10:1-10, 1987.

Bull CN, Bane SD: Growing old in rural America: new approach needed in rural health care, *Aging* 365:18-25, 1993.

Chafey K: Caring is not enough: ethical paradigms for community-based care, *Nurs Health Care* 17(1):10-15, 1996.

Corey G, Corey M: *I never knew I had a choice*, ed 6, Pacific Grove, Ca., 1997, Brooks/Cole.

Droege T: Congregations as communities of health and healing, *Interpretation* 49:117-129, 1995.

Hatch JW, Voorhorst S. The church as a resource for health promotion activities in the black community. In National Institutes of Health: *Health behavior research in minority populations: access, design, and implementation*, NIH Pub No. 92-2965, Washington, D.C., 1992, NIH.

Kinney CK, Mannetter R, Carpenter MA: Support groups. In Bulechek GM, McCloskey JC: *Nursing interventions: essential nursing treatment*, ed 2, Philadelphia, 1992, Saunders, pp. 326-339.

Malloch K, Laeger E: Nursing partnerships: education and practice, *Nurs Health Care* 18(1):32-35, 1997.

Matteson PS: Developing a clinical site at a day camp, *Nurse Educ* 20:34-37, 1995.

Merta RJ: Group work: multicultural perspectives: In Ponterotto J, Casus M, Suzuki A, Alexander CM, ed: *Handbook of multicultural counseling*, Newsbury Park, Ca., 1995, Sage, pp. 567-585.

Murphy B, ed: *Nursing centers: the time is now*, NLN Pub No. 41-2629, New York, 1995, National League for Nursing Press.

Ransdell LB: Church-based health promotion: an untapped resource for women 65 and older, *J Health Promotion* 9:333-336, 1995.

Redman B: *The practice of patient education*, ed 8, St. Louis, 1997, Mosby.

Selby ML, Riportella-Muller R, Sorenson JR, Walters CR: Improving EPSDT use: development and application of a practice-based model for public health nursing research, *Public Health Nurs* 6:174-181, 1989.

Smead R: *Skills and techniques for group work with children and adolescents*, Champaign, Il., 1995, Research Press.

Solari-Twadell PA: Parish nurse revitalizes church's community health role, *Nursing Matters* 6:13, 1995.

The Medicaid Access Study Group: access of Medicaid recipients to outpatient care, *N Engl J Med* 330(2)):1426-1430, 1994.

Thornton J: Developing a rural nursing clinic, *Nurse Educ* 7(2):24-29, 1983.

Wilson J: *How to work with self help groups: guidelines for professionals*, Aldershot, Hampshire, England, 1995, Ashgate Publishing Group.

Yu A, Gregg CH: Asians in groups: more than a matter of cultural awareness, *J Specialists Group Work* 18:86-93, 1993.

Zuvekas A: Community and migrant health centers: an overview, *J Ambulatory Care Manage* 13:13-21, 1990.

23

Utilizing Management Concepts in Community Health Nursing

Objectives

Upon completion of this chapter, the reader should be able to:

1. Explain how a staff-level community health nurse uses management skills in the practice setting.
2. Distinguish between the informal and formal structure of an organization.
3. Analyze how the structure of an organization influences the nurse's role in decision making.
4. Describe the five management functions used by community health nurses.
5. Discuss the elements involved in analyzing a caseload and a client care situation.
6. Differentiate between the terms *team nursing* and *primary nursing*.
7. Describe the implications of managed care for the community health nurse.
8. Describe factors to consider when scheduling community health nursing activities.
9. Explain factors that affect priority determination and intensity of community health nursing in caseload management.
10. Describe the use of delegation in community health nursing practice.
11. Identify selected ANA standards that can guide management practice in a community health nursing setting.
12. Explain how the principles of reengineering help health organizations to function effectively in contemporary society.
13. Describe the importance of the customer, change, and competition to health organizations.

> We are now entering an Age of Unreason, when the future, in so many areas, is there to be shaped, by us and for us—a time when the only prediction that will hold true is that no predictions will hold true; a time, therefore, for bold imaginings in private life as well as public, for thinking the unlikely and doing the unreasonable.
>
> CHARLES HANDY

The community is an exciting setting that provides challenging opportunities for community health nurses. An outstanding characteristic of community health nursing is the independence of its practitioners. In any one day, a community health nurse may decide what families to visit and in what order they will be visited. During that day the nurse may make a nursing diagnosis and carry out nursing interventions without nursing supervision, without a doctor's order, or without even talking to another nurse. That day, she or he may also receive new referrals and make decisions on their priority. Furthermore, the nurse may be carrying out nursing care indirectly through delegation to registered nurses, licensed practical nurses, or assistive personnel. When these health personnel are caring for clients under the nurse's supervision, the nurse is responsible for the act of delegation.

This independence and delegation in community health nursing practice must be accompanied by knowledge of management concepts. Knowledge of management concepts helps the community health nurse provide care, directly and indirectly, to families and aggregates and evaluate the quality of health services that the client receives. Available resources, such as finances and personnel, need to be managed so that maximum productivity, efficiency, and quality of care are achieved.

Managing the extensive amounts of data that community health nurses must collect and use is increasingly complex. Computerized management information systems are crucial for today's community health nurse manager: these systems are being used by agencies across the country to facilitate effective and efficient resource management. Staff nurses use these systems as well to schedule and document client care and to communicate with members of the health care team.

Whatever role a nurse assumes in the community setting, be it staff nurse, supervisor, or administrator, the nurse will participate in leadership and management functions to some degree. Community health nursing, like the management process, is a logical activity that helps clients, families, and aggregates make goal-directed changes. The nurse facilitates these changes through the work of others. Thus a conscious application of the management process to nursing care at any level can make the nurse more effective in arranging his or her own personal workload, as well as in functioning within a larger system.

This chapter briefly analyzes concepts of management and then examines how the community health nurse can use them. A limited discussion of the historical development of management thought is also shared. Knowledge of the evolution of management concepts provides the information an individual needs to formulate a personal philosophy of management.

THE HISTORICAL DEVELOPMENT OF MANAGEMENT CONCEPTS

Numerous leaders in the field of management contributed to its development. To list them all here would be an almost impossible task. When reviewing the development of management thought, however, one can see that modern concepts of management have evolved over time. Historically, emphasis was placed on analyzing the functions and processes of management tasks, without taking into consideration the needs of the worker (see Chapter 18). Later the trend was for managers to apply systems concepts (see Chapter 7) in the work environment to determine how to maintain employee satisfaction and to increase productivity and efficiency. Today the emphasis in on the people in organizations and the processes in which they participate to make responsive and competitive organizations that create valued services for their customers (clients).

Frederick Taylor is the founder of the scientific management movement. His belief was that planning tasks should be separate from performing them. In relation to this thought, he felt that managers should be responsible for planning and controlling tasks and that employees should assume responsibility for production. He conducted time-and-motion studies to determine the best way to accomplish tasks, to develop work standards, and to identify how to divide the work between managers and employees. Taylor's book, *The Principles of Scientific Management*, was published in 1911.

Henri Fayol expanded on Taylor's thoughts by identifying a composite of well-defined functions and tasks for managers. In 1916 he published his ideas about management, which included the notion that managers have five basic functions: planning, organizing, commanding, coordinating, and controlling. With some minor changes, these functions are still used by most authorities on management.

Significant criticism of management occurred during the first half of the twentieth century because managers emphasized task performance without looking at worker satisfaction. As a result of this criticism, modern management trends that focused on the importance of examining employee needs emerged. The classic Hawthorne experiment conducted by Elton Mayo clearly demonstrated to management the value of looking at employees as people.

The Hawthorne studies of the Western Electric Company during the 1920s and 1930s applied the principles of psychology, social psychology, and sociology to the understanding of organizational behavior. The researchers of this study began by investigating the relationship between physical conditions of work and employee productivity. However, they found that social variables were much more important to productivity. The outgrowth of the Hawthorne study was the concept of human relations, or the study of human behavior for the purposes of attaining higher production levels and personal satisfaction. The human relations concept has expanded into the behavioral science approach to management. A trend toward emphasizing employee satisfaction to increase production on the job is still visible. Employee motivation, the workplace as a social system, leadership within the organization, communication within the system, and personal and professional employee development are five major areas of concern to managers who use behavioral science methods and principles. Writings by Chris Argyris, Chester Barnard, Douglas McGregor, Kurt Lewin, Rensis Likert, Robert Tannenbaum, and others give a more in-depth perspective on the behavioral science movement.

The systems approach to management was another development among management concepts. With the systems approach, both the structure and the processes of an organization are analyzed. Emphasis is placed on examining how all the parts of an organization interact and interrelate to achieve the goals of the organization. Systems managers recognize that a change in one part of the organizational system affects all the other parts, just as practitioners using a systems approach recognize that a change (illness) in the family unit affects all other members of the family system (see Chapter 7).

Changing the manner in which systems are explored was described by Gleick (1987) in his book *Chaos*, which examined "the science of the global nature of systems" (p. 5). In contrast to Taylor's work and the work of others who followed Taylor in developing the science of management, Gleick examined systems holistically. Taylor and those who followed him used a reductionistic approach: complex phenomena could be understood by reducing them to their basic building blocks and looking at the mechanisms through which they interacted. For example, a health care agency would be analyzed department by department for its effectiveness under the science of reductionism. The sum of how each department functioned would result in the effectiveness of the organization. The science of chaos examines the system holistically and focuses on the dynamics of the overall system and the order that comes from the interactions of the parts of the whole. A basic tenet of the science of chaos was that the tiniest change in a system, be it the water dripping from a faucet or people working in an agency, causes profound changes in the system. "The simplest systems are now seen to create extraordinarily difficult problems of predictability" (Gleick, pp. 7-8). Further, though the conditions that bring about change and the change itself appear to be random, there is order in the chaos created in systems by miniscule changes (Gleick, pp. 7-8).

The importance of the science of chaos for managers, leaders, and all employees was discussed by Freedman (1992), who based his thoughts on the work of both Gleick (1987) and Senge (1990). Managers think that they know their organizations because they believe in the reductionistic theory of cause and effect. If the workers for whom they are responsible carry out their job descriptions, the objectives of the organization will be reached. However, the relationship between cause and effect is much more complicated than many people understand. People working in an organization, when asked what they do, describe the daily tasks that they do rather than the system in which they work. Frequently workers believe that they have little impact on this system. The science of chaos tells managers that their tiniest actions, along with the smallest thoughts and actions of employees, make a dramatic impact on the agency system. Senge (1990) reported that managers who master systems thinking have "learning organizations" (p. 37). Such organizations are highly decentralized, and decision making at the department level maintains order throughout to constantly adjust to change.

MANAGEMENT IN THE 1990s

The health care organizations of the past decades were well-suited to the growth that was occurring in this industry. The passage of Medicare and Medicaid in 1965, (see Chapters 4 and 5) and the development of private insurance plans, along with the increasing expectations of consumers for both quantity and quality in sickness care, brought about unprecedented growth in all sectors of the health care field. The standard pyramidal organizational structure (Figure 23-1) fit this high-growth environment because it could be easily enlarged. Nurses could be added at the bottom of the chart and management layers could be added above. It was also well-suited to control and planning. By breaking work into small units supervisors could ensure consistent and accurate performance. Budgets were easily approved and monitored, department by department, and planning was done in the same manner.

However, this kind of structure made delivery of a product—client care—increasingly complicated, and managing it became more difficult. The growing numbers of people in the middle of the chart—supervisors, and assistant directors, and administrators—added greatly to the cost of the direct care given to people. Further, distance increased between the persons who delivered client care—staff nurses—and the administrators of their agencies who planned and designed the care that was to be delivered. The all-too-common result became dissatisfied customers (clients), unhappy caregivers, and high costs.

Contemporary community health nurses are working in a challenging environment and confront daily the realization that the work world is a different place: old ways of doing things simply do not work any more. The economic crises facing all sectors of the global economy are not going to go away. "In today's environment, nothing is constant or predictable—not market growth, customer demand, product life cycles, the rate of technological change, or the nature of competition" (Hammer, Champy, 1993, p. 17).

The Three Cs: Customers, Competition, and Change

The successful community health nurse understands the three primary forces that, separately and in combination, are shaping health care organizations. These three forces, the three Cs, are Customers, Competition, and Change (Hammer, Champy, 1993, p. 16).

Customers, commonly called clients or patients in the health care industry, want to be treated as individuals. They want care that matches their unique needs and schedules. They are telling providers what they want and how they want it delivered. They are demanding, appropriately, quality service, and are defining what quality means for them. They are increasingly sophisticated and knowledgeable about the possibilities available to them.

Competition is the name of the game in the health care industry, driven by the costs of care. Health care expenditures in the United States increased from 9.2% of the gross national product (GNP) in 1980 to 12.1% of the GNP in 1990. In contrast, in Germany this same expenditure dropped from 8.4% in 1980 to 8.1% in 1990 (Schieber, Poullier, Greenwald, 1992). These costs have mandated a change in where care is delivered, resulting in the downsizing and/or closing of hospitals nationwide and the expansion of services delivered in the home setting. Since 1988 the home health care sector of the health care industry has had the largest relative employment increase of any industry (Dittbrenner, 1996, p. 11). In this kind of climate excellent agencies drive out those that are less than excellent because the lowest price, the highest quality, and the best service available from any of them quickly become the standard for all competitors. "Adequate is no longer good enough. If a company can't stand shoulder to shoulder with the world's best in a competitive category, it soon has no place to stand at all" (Hammer, Champy, 1993, p. 21).

The last C is *change*. Change today is pervasive, persistent, rapid, and normal. Though change may not be comfortable, it can be what we make it: an opportunity or a crisis. It can be a catalyst to make us think about what we are doing in different ways.

Reengineering

How does an agency meet the many needs of its customers in an era of unprecedented competition and change? One answer used by corporations all over the United States is a process called reengineering. *Reengineering* is defined as the "fundamental rethinking and radical redesign of business processes to achieve dramatic improvements in critical, contemporary measures of performance, such as cost, quality, service, and speed" (Hammer, Champy, 1993, p. 32).

Reengineering has five key concepts: process, teamwork, technology, leadership, and time (Boston Consulting Group, 1993, pp. 4-5). Each of these concepts will be discussed in the next section.

1. *Process*. Though the concept of quality processes has been discussed for many years in nursing and other businesses, with reengineering *complete* processes are designed end to end to service the customer (client). Rather than breaking work down into tasks and assigning them to different people, the emphasis is on the larger objective of what needs to be accomplished. For example, in one large home health agency the desired end result is quality care that assists clients in meeting their desired outcomes in the shortest time possible. Every nurse in the agency knows how to take client admission calls, make initial admission assessment visits, contact the insurance company to receive clearance to make visits, do all of the home visits needed to care for the client, and take care of all of the billing and paperwork. No longer do different individuals perform these separate tasks to admit new clients to care. The result is clients and families who are happier and a smoother process from beginning to end in the care of the client because only one person has been involved for the duration.
2. *Teamwork*. In reengineering teamwork is encouraged to find radical solutions to obstacles. Though teams have been a part of nursing for years, under reengineering teams are given permission and authority to make far-reaching suggestions and decisions and are given the power and authority to carry them out.
3. *Technology*. Communication and information technology provide new possibilities for creativity and reduce time and cost. Health care organizations have increasingly become full-fledged partners in using technology. In one large visiting nurse association each nurse is supplied with a laptop computer. Software designed for the company gives the nurse the ability to quickly individualize a nursing care plan for each client or family; documentation takes place at the client's bedside and then is transmitted via electronic mail to the agency's quality management center each evening from the nurse's home. Nurses need not visit the agency office each day because they receive messages quickly via electronic mail. Further, the agency office has almost immediate feedback about the clients being visited and the resources necessary to meet their needs.
4. *Leadership*. In reengineering managers become leaders—defined as persons who harness the learning and creative power of organizations. Their second priority is to generate results. Further, each person working in the organization is viewed as a leader and a manager: everyone has the responsibility to be visionary and to create possibilities, and each person also has the responsibility, power, and authority to get things done.
5. *Time*. Nurses must understand that "time is money" and that it is not possible to justify caring for clients without also thinking in terms of the time required to achieve what needs to be done. In some agencies the majority of home visits are reimbursed through managed care companies. These companies mandate the number of visits that nurses may make for given diagnoses. Successful nurses learn to accomplish quickly what needs to be accomplished within a time frame.

These are radically new ways of thinking for health care professionals, particularly nurses. However, it is crucial to understand that quality care for clients is provided in the context of a business organization. Quality care must be paid for; nurses, rightfully so, want appropriate reimbursement for their services. Community health nurses have to learn to "think the unlikely and do the unreasonable" (Handy, 1990, p. 5). Unwillingness to do so will make health care organizations increasingly uncompetitive in a world that is competitive.

THE ORGANIZATIONAL STRUCTURE OF HEALTH CARE DELIVERY

The number of health care delivery systems in which community health nurses may work is increasing. They work in diverse health and health-related organizations, each of which may have a differing organizational structure and way of delivering nursing services. Reflecting the intense change occurring in contemporary health care, organizational structures range from the pyramidal (Figure 23-1) to self-governance (Figure 23-2).

Nurses must know the organizational structure of their employing agencies so that they can determine how to use agency resources and to identify appropriate ways to effect change within the organization. Organizational structure encompasses the formal and informal patterns of behavior and relationships in an organization. This includes both formal and informal position allocations, as well as the chain of command and the channels of communication.

The Informal Organizational Structure

The informal organizational structure refers to the personal and social relationships of people who work together. Informal relationships have no formal power. However, they can have a major impact on the organization and its management. The way in which a manager is viewed by the staff does influence the manner and effectiveness of her or his management.

The Formal Organizational Structure

Formal organizational structure defines which people will do which tasks so that the objectives of the organization can be accomplished. It is the power structure of the organization. The rules, policies, procedures, control mechanisms, and financial arrangements of the organization are all part of the formal structure. The schematic organization is part of this formal structure and can be seen in an organizational chart.

ORGANIZATIONAL CHART An organizational chart diagrams the relationship among members of the organization and indicates the structure of authority, formal lines of communication, and levels of management and delegation. These all interrelate to accomplish the goals of the organization. Two types of organizational charts, pyramidal (Figure 23-1) and shared governance (Figure 23-2), are discussed in this section.

An organizational manual supplements an organizational chart by supplying information about the requirements of the various job positions represented on the chart. Organizational charts and manuals are useful tools that describe the formal relationships in a particular organization. Charts and manuals do not show the informal relationships that exist.

PYRAMIDAL. Figure 23-1 depicts a traditional, pyramidal organizational structure. There are two types of positions in this pattern: *staff* and *line*. The line structure is the basic framework for the organization. The staff nurse is in a direct line position and is accountable to the person directly above her or him on the organizational chart. The term *staff nurse* should not be confused with *staff personnel*. Staff personnel supplement the line personnel in an advisory capacity. Staff personnel are extensions of the administrator but usually have no authority to direct the actions of persons in line positions. Authority can, however, be delegated in several directions from both line and staff positions.

The line organization is characterized by a direct flow of authority from top to bottom. Each position has general authority over the one directly below it. Authority is inherent in line positions. For example, the assistant director of nursing has authority over the nursing supervisor, who in turn has authority over the staff nurse. Persons in staff positions, on the other hand, are delegated authority by top-level administrators (e.g., the nursing director) to carry out specific tasks and responsibilities. Authority is not inherent in staff positions.

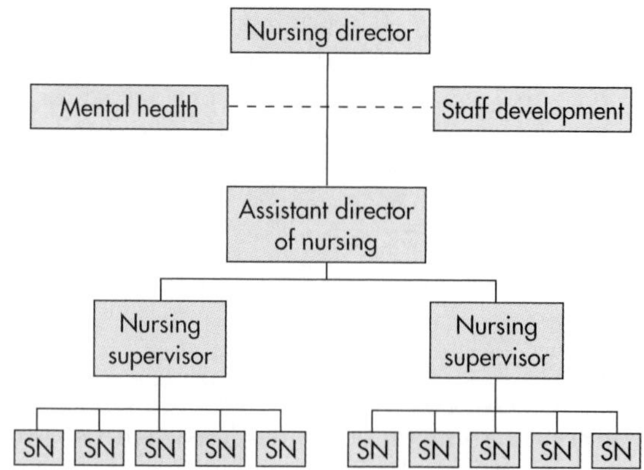

Figure 23-1 A pyramidal organizational chart showing staff and line positions.

SHARED GOVERNANCE. In recent years some health care organizations have implemented the concepts of reengineering. *Shared governance* alters organizational structures so that decision making is carried out by joint practice committees. Figure 23-2 depicts the shared governance model in use at the Henry Ford Hospital in Detroit. Although there is no single model of shared governance across health care organizations, all models in use empower staff nurses by giving them control over their nursing practice. Essential to empowering staff nurses is the transfer of power and accountability to the committees regarding the decisions to be made. In the Henry Ford Hospital model the Unit Governance Council is at the core of the structure. This council is composed of assistive personnel and nurses. The council's purpose is to govern issues related to practice, education, role, performance, and retention for the unit. The expected outcome is improved communication and decision making for the unit, as well as between the nursing councils, the department of nursing, and other hospital departments, committees, and task forces.

One important difference between the pyramidal organization and the shared governance organization is apparent from viewing each chart. In Figure 23-1 it is clear who is at the top. In Figure 23-2 there is no top; rather, there is a circle that facilitates equality in communication and decision making.

POWER RELATIONSHIPS. In any health care organizational structure a manager must have a basic understanding of organizational power relationships to manage effectively. Four types of power relationships evolve in any organization:

1. *Authority:* the power to direct the actions of others
2. *Responsibility:* the obligation to carry out or perform tasks in an acceptable way
3. *Accountability:* the obligation to answer for one's actions
4. *Delegation:* assigning and empowering one person to act for another with the responsibility for the act remaining with the person who assigned it

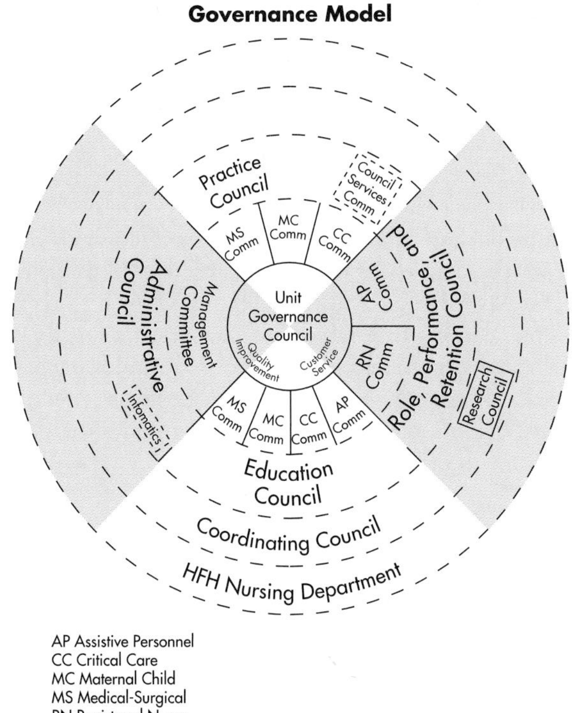

Figure 23-2 A shared governance organizational chart. *(From Department of Nursing, Henry Ford Hospital:* Images of nursing, *Detroit, Mi., Spring Edition 1995, The Department, p. 6. Reprinted with permission of the Henry Ford Health System. Authors are the Shared Governance Task Force.)*

Organizational structure and resulting power relationships in a health care agency assist personnel in all positions to carry out effectively the functions of management. Regardless of the type of structure, it would be impossible to manage if such a structure did not exist. Effective and efficient management can occur only when personnel understand what they are responsible for and to whom they are accountable. Ignoring the power relationships in an organization can create real difficulties. Illustrative of this are the actions taken by the community health nurse in the following scenario.

CASE *Scenario*

A community health nurse identified a need for a family planning program in two of the census tracts she served. Knowing that the county health department did not include these services, she independently arranged a group meeting in the clubhouse at a local park to discuss the need for these services with the people of the community. This was done without discussing the action with her supervisor.

Twenty community members attended the meeting. They quickly became emotionally involved in the issue and wanted immediate action taken by the health department to initiate such a service. The nurse became uncomfortable because she recognized that she did not have the power to make a definite commitment regarding the establishment of a new program. The community members became frustrated with the nurse's lack of action.

Had proper channels within the agency power structure been utilized, this situation would probably have been handled differently.

While examining this situation, the following questions quickly become obvious: Did the nurse have the authority to organize this meeting, and was she acting in a responsible and accountable manner? What were her objectives for the meeting, and did she clarify them for herself and the group?

When planning a meeting with a group such as the one above, it is crucial to seek the advice of individuals within the organization who have the authority to make decisions. When this is not done, it can result in stress and frustration for all parties involved. If the nurse had gone to her supervisor before the meeting, she would have been aware of the types of commitments she could make during the meeting. If, for instance, the health department did not have adequate resources to staff a family planning clinic, the group goal might have been to look at alternative ways to obtain funding for family planning services in the community, rather than discussing only how the health department might provide these services.

ORGANIZATIONAL POLICIES Another component of the formal organization structure that maximizes functioning is organizational policies. Policies define the limits of acceptable activities and provide structure and guidelines for employee decision making. They are generally developed to handle situations that occur consistently in daily practice. Policies that address how to handle referrals (see Chapter 10), when and how to conduct nursing audits (see Chapter 24), and benefits staff will have, such as travel allowances, are a few examples of policies commonly found in a community health agency. These types of policies provide direction for decision making.

When policies are absolute, with no flexibility, they are considered *rules*. Rules are usually established to ensure client and staff safety and quality of care. The following are examples of rules:

- "No home visits are to be made at night in census tract 3 without an escort."
- "No immunizations are to be given until an allergy history has been taken."
- "Every fifth record closed to service must be audited."

When nurses accept employment within a health setting, it is assumed that they accept responsibility for following, enforcing, and informing others about agency policies. This means that the conditions of employment should be clearly understood before the nurse accepts a position within an organization. Otherwise the nurse may end up in a situation where it is necessary to follow certain policies that are inconsistent with her or his philosophy of practice.

Nursing personnel at all levels may be involved in writing policies. Policy statements should include the following items:

1. Reason for establishing the policy (philosophy behind the policy)
2. Actual policy statement
3. Guidelines for implementing the policy
4. Lead persons or department interpreting the policy
5. Persons affected by the policy

If used effectively, policies can increase the efficiency and ease with which individuals carry out their functions within an organization. Difficulties with implementing a policy will occur, however, if employees do not understand the reason for the policy, if employee input is not obtained when the policy is being formulated, if the policy is not clearly written, or if policies become numerous and prevent necessary flexibility for nursing practice.

ANA STANDARDS

The American Nurses Association (ANA, 1991) has developed "Standards for Organized Nursing Services and Responsibilities of Nurse Administrators Across All Settings." The standards (see the box below) provide guidance to nurse administrators in addressing the rapid changes sweeping all settings where nursing care is delivered. Each of the nine standards has a rationale and criteria. Neophyte and experienced nurses can use the standards to make decisions about the most effective employment opportunities, and both experienced and inexperienced students and nurses need guidance in using them in the practice setting. Agencies that follow these standards or similar ones are likely to promote organizational and staff growth and provide direction for the delivery of quality nursing services as well.

The ANA has also addressed the need for lifelong professional learning by establishing standards for quality staff development programs (see the box on the following page). Nurses can use these standards to judge an employing agency's commitment to the care of clients and the professional growth of its staff.

DEFINING MANAGEMENT LANGUAGE

Management is the planning, organizing, directing, coordinating, and controlling of activities in a system so that the objectives of that system are met. For community health nurses, that system may be represented by any number of settings in which the nurse practices, such as a public health agency, an ambulatory care setting, a school, an industrial plant, or a home care organization.

ANA Standards for Organized Nursing Services and Responsibilities of Nurse Administrators Across ANA Settings

STANDARD I. PHILOSOPHY AND STRUCTURE

Organized nursing services have a philosophy and structure that ensure the delivery of effective nursing care.

STANDARD II. NURSE ADMINISTRATOR

Organized nursing services are administered by qualified and competent nurse administrators.

STANDARD III. FISCAL RESOURCE MANAGEMENT

The nurse executive determines and administers the fiscal resources of organized nursing services. The nurse executive has an interactive role in the determination of the organization's fiscal resource requirements and their acquisition, allocation, and utilization.

STANDARD IV. NURSING PROCESS

Within organized nursing services, the nursing process is used as the framework for providing nursing care to recipients.

STANDARD V. ENVIRONMENT FOR PRACTICE

An environment is created within organized nursing services that enhances nursing practice and facilitates the delivery of care by all nursing staff.

STANDARD VI. QUALITY ASSURANCE/IMPROVEMENT

Organized nursing services have a quality assurance/improvement program.

STANDARD VII. ETHICS

Organized nursing services have policies to guide ethical decision making based on the code for nurses.

STANDARD VIII. RESEARCH

Within organized nursing services, research in nursing, health, and nursing systems is facilitated; research findings are disseminated; and support is provided for integration of these findings into the delivery of nursing care and nursing administration.

STANDARD IX. CULTURAL, ECONOMIC, AND SOCIAL DIFFERENCES

Organized nursing services provide policies and practices that address equality and continuity of nursing services, and that recognize cultural, economic, and social differences among recipients served by the health care organization.

From American Nurses Association: *Standards for organized nursing services and responsibilities of nurse administrators across all settings*, Washington, D.C., 1991, ANA, pp. 3-10.

Administration is a term that is often mistakenly used interchangeably with *management*. The principles of management and administration are the same, but the scope of functioning for managers and administrators varies. For instance, both administrators and managers set goals, but the administrator sets goals for a department, whereas a staff nurse sets personal goals when managing her or his workload responsibilities.

Leadership is "shaping and sharing a vision which gives point to the work of others" (Handy, 1990, p. 134). In addition, leadership needs to be "endemic in organizations, the rule not the exception" (p. 133). For an organization to compete successfully to provide quality care, that vision must "reconceptualize the obvious, and connect the previously unconnected dream" (p. 133). At the same time that vision must make sense; it must be understandable to others. Leaders live the vision and believe in it completely. Finally, a leader realizes that unless others follow there is no leadership.

Successful employees at every level in an organization, be they staff nurses, secretaries, directors of departments, or assistive personnel, can and must be managers and leaders in the work that they do. An organization with employees who accept this responsibility has the capability to provide long-term quality care.

THE MANAGEMENT FUNCTIONS OF THE COMMUNITY HEALTH NURSE

The five management functions carried out by the community health nurse are planning, organizing, directing, coordinating, and controlling. These management functions help link the entire organizational system together and assist the nurse in effectively managing workload responsibilities. Managing is done on many levels by nurses, depending on their place in the organizational structure and their interests, skills, and educational backgrounds.

The director of nursing in an agency will probably spend more time managing at a level that affects all staff members than the staff nurse will. Staff nurses must, however, use management functions to deliver nursing services. Staff nurses can also influence how a director of nurses carries out management functions.

Management is a process that has both interpersonal and technical aspects and that uses human, physical, and

ANA Standards for Nursing Staff Development

STANDARD I. ORGANIZATION AND ADMINISTRATION

The Nursing Service Department and the nursing staff development unit philosophy, purpose, and goals address the staff development needs of nursing personnel. The organizational structure facilitates the provision of learning experiences for nursing service personnel.

STANDARD II. HUMAN RESOURCES

Qualified administrative, educational, and support personnel are provided to meet the learning and developmental needs of nursing service personnel.

STANDARD III. LEARNER

Nursing staff development educators assist nursing personnel in identifying their learning needs and planning learning activities to meet those needs.

STANDARD IV. PROGRAM PLANNING

The provider unit systematically plans and evaluates the overall nursing staff development program in response to health care needs, health care trends, nursing personnel's learning needs, and organizational needs and goals.

STANDARD V. EDUCATIONAL DESIGN

Educational offerings and learning experiences are designed through the use of educational processes and incorporate adult education and learning principles.

STANDARD VI. MATERIAL RESOURCES AND FACILITIES

Material resources and facilities are adequate to achieve the goals and implement the functions of the overall nursing staff development unit.

STANDARD VII. RECORDS AND REPORTS

The nursing staff development unit establishes and maintains a record keeping and report system.

STANDARD VIII. EVALUATION

Evaluation is an integral, ongoing, and systematic process which includes measuring its impact on the learner, patient, and organization.

STANDARD IX. CONSULTATION

Nursing staff development educators use the consultation process to facilitate and enhance achievement of individual departmental and organizational goals.

STANDARD X. CLIMATE

Nursing staff development educators foster a climate which promotes open communication, learning, and professional growth.

STANDARD XI. SYSTEMATIC INQUIRY

Nursing staff development educators encourage systematic inquiry and applications of the results into nursing practice.

From American Nurses Association: *Standards for nursing staff development*, Washington, D.C., 1990, ANA, pp. 7-13.

technological resources to achieve well-defined goals. The management process is cyclical; the functions overlap and do not always follow a sequential pattern.

Planning

Planning assists an organization in establishing a vision for the future. It means deciding in advance what must be done and what the organization wants to achieve. Without planning, no set goals will be accomplished.

Planning gives purpose and direction to the decision-making process. It is the management function most often neglected because of the emphasis placed on carrying out day-to-day activities, the attitude that planning takes too much time, and the tendency for individuals to resist change. Planning is an important activity because it helps the organization remain dynamic, identify standards, and determine what or who requires organization or direction. It increases the likelihood that activities will be orderly, predictable, and less costly. Most important, planning improves the quality and effectiveness of nursing care. Although planning does not guarantee the quality of outcomes, the evaluation aspects of this process help a manager identify strengths and needs within the organization.

Health care planning should include both the provider and the consumer. Emergencies may necessitate individual decision making and planning. In these situations it is important for the decision maker to explain to others involved in the process the circumstances and reasons for the emergency decision.

Planning uses past, present, and future information to project what services should be provided. Currently the impact of political, social, economic, and technical forces is directly influencing the types of services provided by community health agencies and the type of personnel needed to implement these services. For instance, in health departments that provide bedside care money allocated from taxes is increasingly scarce, and third-party payments for home health care are an increasingly larger part of the health department budget. This budget change comes about because of demographic changes in the population, as well as social and political policy about the appropriateness of tax money for tertiary health care. Some of the results of these changes include a greater emphasis on delivering home health care, greater use of ancillary personnel such as home health aides, and a greater focus on older people who need "hands-on" care rather than on clients who need health teaching and anticipatory guidance.

Careful planning is needed to successfully implement nursing services when the focus of these services has changed. Activities such as inservice education for staff, planning for increased time for the supervision of home health aides, and the added paperwork involved in carrying out a home health care program are a few examples of factors that should be considered when planning for increased home health services.

An example of a staff nurse putting the planning process into action would be when working with the nursing supervisor to establish a clinic for the homeless in the staff nurse's area. Together they would develop a written plan that might include the following:

1. Specific, measurable objectives related to establishment of the conference
2. Time schedule for achieving objectives
3. Process for carrying out the objectives, including necessary resources
4. Evaluation methods to measure the success of the plan in relation to completion of objectives
5. Timetable for periodic evaluation

A staff community health nurse also implements the planning function when structuring the workday and when carrying out caseload management activities. The data gathering, diagnosis, and goal-setting phases of the nursing process are used for activities such as those described above.

During planning many needs and goals may be identified, and priorities for them must be set. The following points should be considered when setting priorities.

ECONOMIC IMPACT Considering the results if something is or is not done is crucial. Although an immunization campaign against rubella may be costly, it is much less expensive socially and economically than paying for the care of children who have congenital deformities resulting from in utero rubella. The cost-benefit aspect must also be considered. In one community, for instance, the health department discontinued a screening clinic for the geriatric population because it was not cost effective. It cost the health department $40 per client to do the screening, and 90% of those screened had recently received the same screening from their private physicians and planned to do so again in the future. This was duplication of services at a high cost to the health department. Methods other than a screening clinic could be used to reach the 10% of the population not receiving the screening privately.

PRACTICALITY Is the program necessary? What is being done currently? Will enough people benefit from it to make it worthwhile? Are sufficient resources available, such as work force and money, to accomplish the stated goals? Is there enough organizational and community support to carry out the program? Does it meet the needs of the community? All of these are questions to be answered in relation to the practicality of the program.

FEASIBILITY Does the program fit the organization's policies and priorities? Are the resources available to carry out the program?

LEGAL REQUIREMENTS The organization must follow its legal mandates. The official health department, for example, has a legal mandate to control communicable disease. Home health agencies have regulations imposed by funding agencies; an example is Medicare, which mandates that home health aides have at least 12 hours of in service education on a yearly basis. Thus an agency using home health aides would need to carefully plan its staff development program so that this requirement was met.

URGENCY OF THE SITUATION An emergency situation is usually given top priority. In one urban community, for instance, a large Mexican restaurant used home-canned chili peppers that were improperly prepared. Many of the restaurant's patrons developed botulism. This produced an emergency health situation that required urgent action to pinpoint the source of the poisoning and all patrons affected by the botulism agent. The county health department launched an immediate epidemiological investigation to pinpoint the cause. Many other health department activities were stopped or modified so that this serious problem could be given top priority. Once priorities are established, a manager must organize activities so priority goals can be implemented.

Increasingly there are competing priorities and demands for the available resources in any one health care organization. Nurses need to be able to defend their request for new or enlarged programs. They also should be able to see the "larger picture" for the total organization and perhaps defer to another colleague or discipline when requests or priorities conflict.

Organizing

Organizing determines how a manager implements planning to achieve stated goals. The organizational structure, as previously discussed, facilitates decision making and assigning of tasks. Any organizational structure has three principal components: people, work, and relationships. The interrelationship of these three variables is analyzed during the organizing phase to determine the best way to organize activities. A manager's major concerns when organizing are fourfold:

1. *Analysis of the system*. Identifying strengths and needs of the present system to make it more effective and efficient in the future. Comparing present staff capabilities to the needs evidenced by clients being served is one example of how a system is analyzed.
2. *Analysis of functions*. Defining all the tasks that are involved in a particular job and determining the relationships between various jobs. A nurse and supervisor analyzing a staff nurse's responsibilities when she or he has a caseload of eight bedside care clients, 40 families needing health supervision, and work in six schools and two clinics weekly is an example of this principle.
3. *Assigning job responsibilities*. Grouping tasks to minimize duplication of effort and assigning responsibilities to individuals who have the knowledge and competence to carry out the job. Responsibility and authority limits should be clearly defined. Again, work with clients who need bedside care illustrates this principle. Assistive personnel should be assigned only basic physical care, and the community health nurse should assess and supervise the care given by the home health aide. If the health care organization has a union, labor agreements may dictate the extent to which managers can expand or contract a role. The agreement may also stipulate who can be selected for a particular position and can impose limitations on innovation and deployment of personnel to carry out assignments.
4. *Implementation*. Developing an atmosphere that allows for successful completion of the work to be done by identifying the structure of authority and support mechanisms in the system. Team meetings that provide support, case consultation, and identification of needs illustrate this concept.

Organizing requires a cooperative effort by a health care team working together to achieve the goals of the organization. This managerial function is familiar to community health nurses because they must organize the care of a family around the family's expressed needs and the resources of the health team working with them.

Directing

Effective programs and organizations include all levels of staff in the planning process so that information is disseminated by peers, at least in part, and "top-down" directing is minimized. The purpose of directing is to convey to workers what has occurred during the planning and organizing phases of management. The activities of directing include order giving, direction, leadership, motivating, and communicating.

Order giving involves helping an employee to identify what needs to be done in a way that fosters understanding and acceptance. A community health nurse who clearly and completely tells assistive personnel the details of the physical care needed by a client with a cerebrovascular accident and provides opportunity for the assistant to ask questions illustrates how effective order giving can be accomplished.

Direction refers to the effort made in an organization to ensure that all the work is done. Personal and professional guidance for people is basic to the concept of direction. In the community health setting, work activities are focused on the provision of services both to families and to the community. Thus the focus of direction should include guidance that helps staff to effectively intervene both with families and with the community. This helps staff to provide the services and the agency to achieve stated goals.

Employees are more likely to carry out directions if they assist in setting the goals and designing the interventions to reach them. When they are able to understand the justification for organizational goals and the strategies for meeting these goals, and when there is no doubt regarding what is expected of them, employees are able to carry out responsibilities without constant supervision. This, in turn, leaves more time for staff and supervisors to work on career development plans that focus on staff growth and challenging opportunities in the work setting. Most staff members desire these types of opportunities. However, supervision of home health paraprofessionals is frequently overlooked (Gilbert, 1992).

Motivating focuses on analyzing the needs of individual workers. Maslow's hierarchy of needs can provide a theoretical framework for examining worker needs. Maslow has developed a priority schema based on a continuum of needs beginning with those that are physiological and ending with self-actualization. He believes that a worker must satisfy lower-level needs (physiological) before the higher-level ones (self-actualization) become significant (Maslow, 1954). When working with other employees or when analyzing one's own behavior in the job setting, it may be found that work is not satisfying because lower-level needs are not being met. If this is the case, an effective manager attempts to build into the management system rewards that will help the employee to meet these basic human needs.

Communicating with workers is crucial. The manager must be able to convey what is to be done, how it is to be done, who is to do it, and why it is to be done and to provide feedback on the activity. This feedback should emphasize the strengths, as well as the weaknesses, inherent in the employee's activity.

Communication implies a two-way process. The manager uses skill to convey what needs to be done. Noticing staff members' responses, both verbal and nonverbal, is a critical part of the process. If the person does not hear what has been said, appropriate communication has not occurred. The interviewing skills that are a primary tool of community health nurses should be used in communicating with health care workers. These skills will help the manager to direct, coordinate, and control activities within the organization.

Coordinating

Coordination links people on the health care team together to function in such a way that objectives are achieved. A problem arises when health care workers look at objectives in different ways. One nurse may consider nursing in the school setting as a low priority. The supervisor may think it a high priority. Thus coordinating can mean managing conflict. Conflict can promote growth but it can also reduce productivity. Effective coordination reduces and prevents growth-restricting conflict.

Controlling

Controlling is the act of helping organizations achieve their goals by ensuring that employees perform their jobs effectively (carrying out the correct functions) and efficiently (quality and cost-effectiveness of the end product). In reengineered businesses, employees are trusted to use their own methods to achieve the purposes of the organization; therefore mistakes can and will be made. However, employees are urged to truly learn from their mistakes: mistakes are to be used as an opportunity for learning and not thought of as failures. Though not all mistakes can be forgiven (for example, those that affect client safety), most can be. Again, in reality, this is a different way of thinking for many people in the health professions, where "perfection" is the accepted norm.

A system called "performance management" assists managers in identifying the current learning requirements of individual employees, as well as ways to improve the employee's work performance (Benjamin, Penland, 1995). The system has five steps:

1. Agreeing about what competencies are needed by employees to carry out their role. Competencies need to be clear and written in explicit detail so that they are understandable to all parties. Use of a collaborative process between the formal manager and employee to develop the competencies is the expectation.
2. The competencies are next prioritized in order of importance according to the needs of the organization.
3. The employee and supervisor then rate the employee on the ability to perform each of the competencies. Each employee and supervisor must reach consensus on the ranking of the employee's performance.
4. The manager and employee develop goals for improving the employee's performance, and a performance improvement contract is written.
5. Both parties meet frequently on a formal and informal basis to examine the progress that is being made toward defined goals.

The performance management system reflects the management movement to actively involve staff members in decision making about strategies for delivery of quality services. The emphasis on competencies helps an organization to maintain a clear focus on staff, client, and organizational needs.

The staff nurse who delegates care to a home health aide can use the performance management system so that quality care is given consistently. The nurse and aide must be flexible in their expectations of each other; an aide who has an ill child at home may not work as well on that day as on another. If the nurse is concerned about a particular client care problem, such as the aide's lack of understanding about maintaining skin integrity, she or he can use conference time to discuss that problem but should not bring all other concerns to the conference. The nurse needs the supervisor's support when working with the home health aide so that the solutions to the nurse's concerns are enforceable and not opposed by the supervisor.

The controlling function can provide direction for growth and thus should be considered a positive function. It is important to examine *strengths* of workers, as well as areas of concern, when implementing the controlling function of management.

INFORMATION TECHNOLOGY IN COMMUNITY HEALTH NURSING

One of the five key elements of reengineering discussed at the beginning of this chapter is technology. Information technology opens new possibilities for delivering more quality services, as well as for decreasing time and cost. "What is new is that technology itself is not the driving force for change—the opportunity to create new value is" (Boston Consulting Group, 1993, p. 4). "A company that equates technology with automation cannot reengineer. A company that looks for problems first and then seeks technology solutions for them cannot reengineer" (Hammer, Champy, 1993, p. 83). Applying the power of modern information technology demands the ability to think deductively: to recognize a powerful solution and then seek the problems it might solve.

Currently computer applications are nationally marketed for the following areas (Kahn, 1996): generic business functions such as payroll and accounts payable; Health Care Financing Administration form preparation, electronic and hard billing, and accounts receivable; and clinical applications such as client assessments, physician orders, and chart notes. However, there is increasingly a broader use of technology. One of the best-known management information systems (MIS) for community and home health care is the one developed by the Visiting Nurse Association of Omaha, Nebraska. This system uses a classification scheme for client problems in community health nursing that adapts easily to a computerized system of record keeping (Martin, Scheet, 1992).

The computerized system developed by the Visiting Nurse Association of Greater Philadelphia is another example of how technology is being used in community health nursing practice. The agency received a foundation grant to develop a "fully integrated computer system that would increase the cost economics that voluntary, not-for-profit home health care providers require to survive in the extremely competitive home health care market" (Visiting Nurse Association of Greater Philadelphia, 1990-1992, p. 2). During the first 3 years of the grant the project developed and demonstrated a computerized voice messaging system for field and office staff to communicate with each other about client care and defined a comprehensive system for the development of care plans that could be computerized. During the final year the project developed a philosophy for satisfying the information needs of such an agency, produced a methodology for the identification of an agency's information management requirements, produced a methodology for the evaluation and selection of commercially available software, confirmed "open" architecture as the desired bridge between acquired software and internally developed systems, and developed several applications that track and control agency programs.

Milio (1996) has written a unique book, *The Engines of Empowerment: Using Information Technology to Create Healthy Communities and Challenge Public Policy*, that describes experiences of "ordinary people who are doing new things with computers to create healthier standards and styles of living. They are using these new tools to build social and economic renewal in their communities and to create *community*—the sense of shared responsibility that must accompany and complement viable communities" (p. 3). Milio's book is a masterful example of thinking deductively—of first finding solutions and then looking for problems.

When developing a computerized MIS, nurses must take into consideration nursing ethics. They must ensure that the rights of both client and staff are protected when information is computerized. Nurses must carefully monitor access to client and personnel data; limited access is permitted to these types of data when they are part of a computer information system.

The development of an MIS can create stress within an organization, especially when staff members have not previously worked with computers. When experiencing this stress, it helps to focus on what can be achieved long range through the use of an MIS. Initially it takes additional time out of one's schedule to become knowledgeable about the functioning of this type of system. However, a new system, if used effectively, can help an agency improve the delivery of client care services and can reduce indirect service time.

Outcomes in Community Health Nursing

Chapter 24 discusses how measuring quality in nursing care has moved from an emphasis on structure and process to a focus on outcomes of the care provided. Information technology can help nurses measure those outcomes.

The Outcome and Assessment Information Set (OASIS), discussed in Chapter 21, will provide agencies with the ability to measure outcomes of care delivered in the home setting, upon admission, at follow-up points, and at discharge for 12 different areas (see Chapter 21). Since the data set is designed to be tracked via computer, agencies will be able to make comparisons between reimbursers and other home health care agencies providing the same types of services. For example, does the number of visits authorized for a particular diagnosis make a difference in how quickly a client reaches the desired objective?

APPLYING MANAGEMENT CONCEPTS IN COMMUNITY HEALTH NURSING

In the community health nursing setting nurses have multiple responsibilities. They may have a large number of families in their caseload, as well as a number of other nursing services to be performed. In addition, community health nurses need to develop collaborative relationships with other disciplines to coordinate family care and to establish priorities for home visits and other activities, such as school and clinic services. Community health nurses must also learn how to effectively delegate tasks to other nursing personnel.

Organizing and scheduling community health nursing activities is not an easy task for an experienced practitioner; it is often overwhelming to a new staff member. These activities are easier to handle, however, if a new staff member applies management concepts while carrying out daily responsibilities.

Using Planning Functions of Management as a Staff Nurse

The nurse can more readily carry out responsibilities if the following planning activities of management are used.

SCHEDULING REGULAR CONFERENCES WITH THE NURSING SUPERVISOR Scheduling regular conferences with the nursing supervisor can assist the nurse in analyzing her or his caseload responsibilities and in establishing priorities for service (Figure 23-3). With the supervisor's help, the nurse should do both a case analysis of each family that is being seen and a caseload analysis of all the work that is being done. Since there is often rapid turnover of clients this discussion becomes crucial.

CASE ANALYSIS. The nurse should learn to "diagnose" each case by answering questions such as the following:

1. What are the health problems of this family as viewed by the family and the nurse?
2. What resources does the family have for meeting these problems?
3. What movement does the family wish to make?
4. What resources are there in the community for meeting these needs?
5. What nursing activities are needed to contribute to the solution of the problems and to bring family and community resources into proper relationship with family needs?
6. Are there some parts of the problems or needs that cannot be met at present with the resources available?
7. What has the family done to work toward solving the problem?
8. How effective have nursing interventions and family actions been in resolving current health problems?

Case analysis helps nurses look at their approach to families and alter it so that they can be more effective. A written summary, as well as supervisory conferences, facilitates case analyses. A written summary of work with a family, after a given number of visits in a specified time frame, helps nurses organize their care and their work. In some agencies this is part of the computerized MIS. The controlling function of management is in effect when case analysis is done as work with clients is being measured and corrections made.

CASELOAD ANALYSIS. Study of the caseload will also improve the planning ability of the nurse and will reveal gaps in service. A caseload analysis differs from a case analysis because it focuses more on examining the quantity of work the nurse is responsible for and the multiple activities assigned than on the needs of individual families. Caseload analysis is done to determine whether a nurse has sufficient time to implement all assigned responsibilities, to ascertain whether time is being used effectively and efficiently, and to identify whether the needs present in a caseload of families

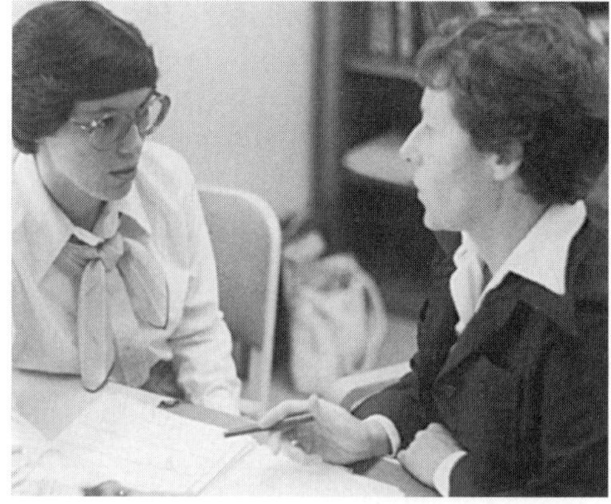

Figure 23-3 A staff nurse and supervisor in conference. Nurse/supervisor conferences are a common occurrence in community health nursing practice. Nurses find it helpful to discuss their caseloads and staff development issues on a regular basis.

reflect the needs of the population being served. Analysis of the caseload may be in relation to many aspects of service—the types and numbers of cases carried, the complexity of problems in the cases visited, the age groups served, the proportion of new referrals received, and the number of emergency or crisis situations, such as individuals with sputum testing positive for tuberculosis. In addition, it examines all the other activities a nurse engages in, such as school visits, clinic services, group work, committee meetings, coordination with other community agencies, and recording and planning time. When the caseload is studied, it is wise to graph or tabulate the findings so that they may be readily used and compared with caseloads in other areas or with the same area over time.

Simultaneous caseload study by several nurses may be encouraged occasionally to give a general picture of the services provided by the health agency and to allow for comparisons between nurses. When this was done in one health department, it was found that two of 15 census tracts had a disproportionate number of referrals. The result was that workload assignments were reallocated so that work was more evenly divided. The strength of such a procedure is its usefulness in helping the individual nurse to identify the uniqueness of cases in her or his own area and to examine whether there is adequate time to handle the demands of the workload. Freeman (1949, p. 358), in her classic writings on public health nursing supervision, emphasized that nurses should not try to develop an "average" in the caseloads they carry but should develop a caseload pattern that will provide optimum community service. This is a key principle to follow today because of the diverse health problems in society and the dramatic changes in the population structure of the United States. When making comparisons, nurses must keep in mind that caseloads should reflect community needs and population characteristics (see Chapter 13 for the method of determining these needs and characteristics). One nurse may have a higher geriatric clientele than another nurse because of the uniqueness of the census tract she or he serves. These data are a regular part of the MIS in some agencies.

USE A TICKLER SYSTEM A tickler system is a file wherein each family in the nurse's caseload has an identification card displaying data such as name, address, telephone number, and service classification. It assists in scheduling family visits and determining what families need service and when, as well as the type of service needed. When a nurse makes a home visit, the date of this visit and the month and day for the next visit are indicated on the card. The card is then placed under the appropriate month in an index file box. If a tickler system is used effectively, a new nurse can quickly identify priorities for home visiting by noting how frequently the previous nurse visited a family and when the nurse planned the next visit. When a staff nurse has a caseload of families, an organized method such as a tickler file for determining when to see whom is essential. This may be a part of the agency's MIS.

SET PRIORITIES This allows the nurse to put activities in order of importance or caseload priority. The following should be considered when establishing priorities:

NURSING KNOWLEDGE. The nurse has a strong theoretical background on which to base priorities for nursing service. This knowledge helps the nurse analyze the nursing service needs of families who have particular types of problems and direct interventions as well. The developmental framework discussed in Chapters 14 through 20 of this book, along with the nurse's knowledge of crisis theory, for instance, helps a nurse identify problems across the life span that present stress and, in some cases, crisis. For example, a single, pregnant adolescent may receive higher priority than a 25-year-old pregnant married woman. The first client is dealing with the developmental tasks of two age periods—the adolescent and the young adult—and thus is more likely to experience a crisis than the 25-year-old, who is dealing with developmental tasks of only one age period.

MANAGED CARE. By the year 2000 most health care at all levels—primary, secondary, and tertiary (preventive, acute, and rehabilitation services)—will be delivered through managed care companies. As described in Chapter 4, managed care provides a defined package of benefits to a specific population through a single "seamless" system. There are specific providers and specific services given for a defined length of time. This means that the number of visits provided to clients and the disciplines involved in care will be authorized by those companies. The nurse's priorities will be determined by the managed care company. Further, the nurse will have limited time to help the client and family achieve their desired outcomes. Nurses will need to be sure that their visits have been authorized so that the agency is reimbursed for services provided, and they will need communication skills to relay the needs of the client/family in a manner that elicits the needed services from the provider.

COMMUNITY NEEDS. Statistical data, input from consumers, and reports from other professionals can often alert the community health nurse to critical community problems or lack of health services in certain areas. For example, if the herd immunity for measles is 40% in a certain section of a county, the community health nurse needs to spend time planning for the provision of immunization service to the total population in this section. This may leave the nurse less time for home visiting. In the long run, however, an immunization campaign could reduce the time the nurse needs for home visits. It takes far more time to individually contact families who need to update their immunization status than to conduct a mass campaign that alerts the total community to the need for immunization protection.

AGENCY POLICIES AND PRIORITIES. A community health nurse is responsible for following agency policy. Some agency policies read: "Premature infants should be seen weekly for 6 weeks" or "All newborns in the community are to be visited once." If the nurse finds, after analyzing the caseload, that it is impossible to implement an agency policy, she or he should not ignore the policy, but rather should take concrete action to see that it is changed. Many agencies, for instance, have recently found that it is impossible to visit all newborns because of the multiple needs present in the community. Unfortunately, sometimes an old policy is not changed because staff do not take the initiative to have it changed. This can create frustration, especially if staff members are trying to implement an unrealistic policy.

Nursing services should also reflect agency priorities, which should coincide with communities' needs. If a community has a high geriatric population, a health department may place priority on delivering service such as home health care to the elderly. If an agency places a high priority on home health services, the staff nurse will have to schedule other health supervision visits (maternal-child health, school health, mental health) around home health services. If, on the other hand, community statistics reflect high infant and maternal mortality rates, maternal-child health cases at risk may receive top priority for follow-up. Priorities may vary from one census tract to another, depending on the needs evident in each census tract.

LEGAL MANDATES. Communicable disease follow-up by the official health department is mandated by law and as such must receive priority when caseload needs are analyzed. Communicable disease follow-up is also a high priority because of its potential threat to the community.

AGENCY RESOURCES.

1. *Staffing*. The availability of health personnel influences the type of services that can be provided. Where limited personnel and other resources exist, only clinic and crisis intervention services may be provided. If only limited resources are available, the community health nurse will have to examine carefully

what nursing services are essential and how the most people can be reached in the time available. Some agencies have increased clinic services and group work and decreased home visits because of personnel shortages. If changes such as these do not meet the needs of the population being served, careful documentation may help the agency obtain additional resources. Too often, however, nurses and other health professionals accept their current state and fail to document the need for increased resources.

2. *Funding*. Financing can affect the type and amount of staffing available within a health agency and also the type of services provided by a particular department. When nursing divisions in a health agency contract for special services, such as school health, family planning, and home health services, they often can expand their nursing staff, but usually there are conditions for the type of services that need to be provided, as well as a time frame designating when these services should be delivered. Health departments, for example, are sometimes paid for school health services by the board of education. Nurses in these instances may be required to visit the schools at least once a week from September through June.

FACTORS TO CONSIDER WHEN SCHEDULING COMMUNITY HEALTH NURSING ACTIVITIES The community health nurse has a work schedule that frequently changes. As previously discussed, guidelines help the nurse give priorities to work. Establishing priorities helps the nurse schedule activities more effectively. Several other factors need to be considered as the nurse schedules work. Ideally, at the beginning of each month the nurse will develop a calendar that identifies her or his scheduled activities for the month and allows the nurse to see how much time is available for other requests, such as new referrals. If new demands for service exceed the time available, the nurse will then have an organized calendar to share with the nursing supervisor that documents the excess demand and that helps rearrange priorities as necessary.

Nurses in a home health agency typically list all clients to be seen each day on a weekly calendar; they then inform the nurse manager of their plans for that day as priorities become apparent, such as referrals for new clients that must be seen immediately and early morning visits to check the effects of new medication orders. The nurse in this situation makes constant, urgent decisions about priorities, with flexibility as a guiding principle.

The community health nurse should consider the following parameters when scheduling community nursing activities for the coming month/week:

1. Schedule every case and activity requiring service during the month/week.
2. Schedule new visits around scheduled commitments.
3. Make daily visits at the same time each day, if possible.
4. Establish priorities for visits according to need and timing of visits, as illustrated by the following examples:
   A. Families with new babies: around feeding or bath time, to assess how these activities are handled by the family
   B. Crisis cases: as soon as possible
   C. IV medications: provide at specified times
   D. Infectious diseases: last in the day, if possible, to decrease potential for exposure to other families
5. Provide for follow-up of families with long-term and chronic diseases.
   A. Disabled or ill individuals
   B. Chronic problems
6. Set time aside for shared home visits, when care is delegated to:
   A. Home health aides/assistive personnel
   B. Licensed practical nurses
7. Plan time for:
   A. Office activities
      1. Planning visits for the week; planning activities for the next week
      2. Assignment of cases
      3. Supervisory conferences
         a. Ancillary personnel
         b. Supervisor
      4. Recording and reporting
      5. Follow-up
         a. Referrals
         b. Phone calls to agencies, physicians, families
      6. Team meetings
      7. Interdisciplinary conferences, e.g., hospice or case conference with protective service
   B. Clinic activities
      1. Setting up
      2. Time in clinic
      3. Follow-up and evaluation
   C. School activities
   D. Agency, committee, or community coalition activities

ORGANIZATIONAL STAFFING PATTERNS FOR COMMUNITY HEALTH NURSES Another area of concern to nurses who are managing the care of families and groups is the staffing pattern used in a health care organization. Some agencies use a system of primary nursing, whereas others use a team nursing system or a case management model. The method of staffing selected by an agency will determine how the nurse schedules and implements monthly and weekly activities.

PRIMARY NURSING. If this pattern of organization is used, the community health nurse is assigned a geographical area and is responsible for all open cases, new referrals, and schools in that district. The advantages of this method of assignment are several. First, the same nurse follows all clients over time, which results in better continuity of care. Second, this method allows for independent planning and decision making, which is often less time-consuming and, therefore, less expensive than group decisions. Last, one person serves a geographical area, which requires less travel time than if the same person would have to travel in several different geographical areas.

The greatest disadvantage for primary nursing is the lack of flexibility of work assignment. If an individual nurse becomes very busy with referrals or if the nurse becomes ill, coverage of the workload is difficult.

The primary nursing organizational pattern does not, or should not, eliminate peer and supervisory guidance with case analysis. Weekly team conferences (Figure 23-4) can be very important to the successful implementation of the primary nursing concept. The nurse can use weekly conferences to increase knowledge in specific areas, such as available community resources, or to analyze the needs of complex families, such as fragile families or families with limited resources who are dealing with complicated physical requirements.

TEAM NURSING. Other agencies use a team nursing method to deliver nursing services to clients in the community. This involves assigning a personnel team consisting of one or more community health nurses, RNs, LPNs, and HHAs/assistive personnel to serve a larger geographical area or larger caseload than that in a primary nursing assignment. Each member of the team covers the same geographical area. Team nursing offers the advantage of lending more flexibility to work assignments because there are several team members to share new referrals or care of clients. Perhaps its greatest advantage is that quality of service can improve as a result of the shared planning and problem solving that occurs in regularly planned team conferences. Disadvantages are that more time is needed for planning because of the number of people involved, and travel expenses are often increased.

If cases are divided between nurses who job-share or between part-time nurses, lack of continuity of care may result. This is a major complaint from clients who "see a different nurse every time" and their physicians. When cases are shared, the number of different personnel sharing cases should be minimized, and mechanisms to maintain effective and efficient communication should be established.

CASE MANAGEMENT. Case management aims, by case type, to achieve quality care at low cost. This is accomplished by standardizing resources with a very clear direction toward specific client interventions for like problems and with specific expected caregiver and system outcomes. Case managers promote collaboration among all disciplines to provide ongoing care from preadmission to postdischarge while involving the family in the process. Though this sounds like typical community health nursing, emphasis in case management models used by many community agencies is on *case types*. Illustrative of this concept is the case management focus on high-risk children at the Gloucester County Health Department in New Jersey. This health department uses the case management model to promote early identification, evaluation, diagnosis, and treatment of children with special needs and potentially disabling conditions. The case manager, a nurse who has a caseload of 300 families, is responsible for a team that counsels families, assesses the need for services, promotes and facilitates communication among the team providing services, and monitors the services received (ANA, 1988). With this model nursing personnel are used efficiently, expected client outcomes are well delineated, timely discharge is facilitated, material resources are used appropriately, and collaborative practice is promoted. (See Chapters 10 and 21 for discussion of case management from a generalized perspective.)

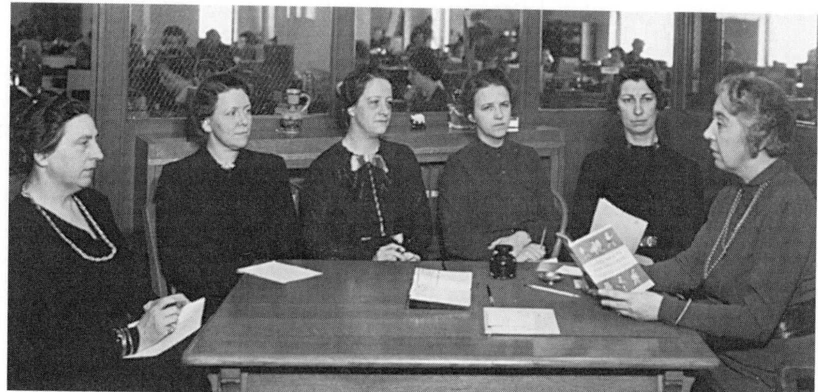

Figure 23-4 The value of team conferences to deal with client, staff, and agency issues has long been recognized in the field of community nursing. Depicted above is a staff conference being conducted by Alma Haupt (first right in picture), the Director of Metropolitan's first nursing service. This nursing service, founded in 1909, significantly influenced the development of management practices in public health nursing. Community health nurses at all levels find it essential to maintain supportive communication with their colleagues. This communication helps them to deal with workload demands, to maintain an objective perspective about practice issues, and to achieve cohesiveness among agency personnel. *(Courtesy Metropolitan Life Insurance Company.)*

The disadvantage is that this model is case-specific rather than general in scope.

Team nursing, primary nursing, and case management can work. Some advantages and disadvantages of each were shared so that nurses will recognize the importance of analyzing strengths and limitations of different organizational patterns. Examining both strengths and limitations helps nurses identify mechanisms that would minimize limitations when an agency selects a particular organizational pattern. It is possible to mix the patterns within an organization to fit the needs of various clients, nurse teams, and geographical areas.

Determining Priorities in Community Health Nursing Practice

When setting up a calendar for the month, the staff nurse may find that there is not enough time to carry out all the activities that she or he would like to be able to do. Community health nurses cannot meet all the health needs that are evidenced in the community setting. Money, time, and personnel are not limitless, and all three, in fact, are becoming scarcer commodities. As was indicated in Chapters 2, 11, and 13, responsibilities to aggregates in need are based on their vulnerability and their degree of risk. Thus one way of determining whom community health nurses will service is to set priorities for service. Several factors to consider when establishing priorities have already been discussed in the section that addresses how the community health nurse uses the planning function of management in the work setting. In addition to the variables mentioned in that section, such as funding, legal mandates, community needs, and agency priorities, determining priorities based on client needs is useful. In 1953 Ruth Rives wrote a classic work for public health nurses on the establishment of priorities according to client needs; it was updated in 1958. An update of Rives's article, which provides a basis for determining priorities for nursing services, is provided in Appendix 23-1. Many priorities defined by Rives are still entirely appropriate. Others have been added and some have been deleted.

USING VARIOUS LEVELS OF HEALTH PERSONNEL*

A variety of personnel are used in agencies to deliver community health nursing services. In nearly any community health setting, staff members are involved in offering nursing services who are prepared at various levels. In some agencies RNs (BSN-, AD-, and diploma-prepared), LPNs, and home health aides (HHAs)/assistive personnel are hired. In others only RNs and HHAs are available. In yet others, only BSN-prepared RNs are used. Knowledge of the educational preparation of these persons and the agency job descriptions are most helpful tools when nurses need to decide how to use personnel appropriately and determine what type of orientation and staff development is needed. Understanding a state's nurse practice act and the regulations regarding the practice of different levels of personnel is also essential.

HHAs/assistive personnel are often prepared through noncredit courses that provide 75 hours with at least 16 hours devoted to supervised practical training. Medicare regulations require that home health aides complete training and competency evaluation programs and have at least 12 hours of inservice training during each 12-month period. In the community setting HHAs can give personal care and assist with housekeeping, marketing, and preparation of meals. HHAs can give the kinds of personal care that can be taught easily to a family member if there is someone to teach.

The licensed practical nurse (LPN) is prepared to give physical care, to make observations about physical conditions, to carry out special rehabilitative measures after being instructed by the community health nurse, to continue the teaching of clients begun by the registered nurse, and to contribute to the nursing care plan of a client. There is a significant difference in the level of care given by LPNs and assistive personnel. The licensed practical nurse has knowledge and skill that helps in making limited patient assessments and contributing to the development of nursing interventions. HHAs have knowledge and skill to provide *unskilled* client care. Both the LPN and HHA, however, are prepared to function under the supervision of a registered nurse. They both make valuable contributions on the health care team.

The registered nurse (RN) prepared at the AD or diploma level has been prepared in institutions where there is a client-centered approach to care. The RN is usually highly skilled in the care of home health service clients who are ill and who need expert care and observations in the home. Because the RN often has developed expertise in technical procedures, she or he can teach these techniques to other staff and family members. The RN has skill and knowledge to assist in the development of the nursing care plan, especially with clients who have disease conditions. Because the RN's preparation has been primarily client-centered, she or he should receive orientation in relation to family-centered nursing practice, concepts related to analyzing the needs of populations, and principles relative to the coordination of care and prevention, if she or he is expected to implement all the services provided by community health nurses in a health department. This orientation is a necessity. It is unfair to expect the registered nurse, prepared at the AD or diploma level, to provide comprehensive community health nursing services. She or he has not been prepared to do so. If circumstances exist where only these RNs are available, an agency has the responsibility to

*We are indebted to Ruth Carey, former Vice President of Clinical Services, Michigan Home Health Care, Traverse City, Michigan, for the use of this material.

provide them with orientation and staff development opportunities that adequately prepare them to carry out the demands of the job.

The baccalaureate-prepared nurse has received education in community health with an emphasis on wellness and prevention and experience in the community health setting. She or he is expected to have a family-centered focus and to function in a comprehensive fashion. This entails identifying client strengths and needs and all variables that affect health and illness (physical, social, and emotional), facilitating identification of family health goals, and assisting families to reach their goals. The community health nurse initiates, plans, and evaluates care. In addition, she or he participates in planning for the health needs of the community and works in schools, clinics, and community groups, giving service and functioning as a planning participant to see that needed services are provided.

Another caregiver seen in the community setting is the Community/Public Health Advanced Practice Nurse (C/PHAPN), who is a clinical nurse specialist in community/public health. This nurse is prepared with a master's degree in nursing and the public health sciences and functions in clinical and administrative roles. The practice of this person is focused on a community and/or population and defines and implements the nursing aspects of the core public health functions of assessment, policy development, and assurance.

After orientation, which assists neophytes to the independence of the community as well as how to travel about safely and efficiently, nurses begin to develop familiarity with an organization's policies, procedures, and expectations. For the contemporary professional in the community setting, learning continues. The rapidly changing health care system and resulting complexities of care requirements make it important to have a sound staff development program in an organization.

Delegation as a Management Function in Community Health Nursing

To carry out the diverse responsibilities of the position, the community health nurse frequently assigns tasks to other health care personnel. When planning responsibilities for others, the community health nurse should:

1. Analyze the nature of the task to be delegated, considering the complexity and the time involved to complete it
2. Determine the capability of the individual staff member to handle the assigned responsibility, especially noting the staff member's educational and experience background and other workload responsibilities
3. Identify the willingness of the staff member to accept responsibility for the assigned activity
4. Determine how much time will be needed to supervise if tasks are delegated to others

Delegation is the process of designating tasks and bestowing on others the authority needed to accomplish these assigned tasks.

A synonym for delegation is *empowerment*. Thus when nurses assign a task for which they are responsible to another person, they are empowering that person to do that task. Carried out correctly, delegation requires instruction about what needs to be done, as well as attention to issues of employee motivation (McConnell, 1995). The key to appropriate delegation is to give the person assigned the task the equivalent authority and responsibility. Though delegation does not negate the personal responsibility that the nurse has for the care given, appropriate delegation does mean that the person being made responsible must be given sufficient authority to complete the task. And, as was discussed earlier, people need to be given the freedom to fail: mistakes need to be treated as a growth experience The nurse provides instruction, support, resources, explains the results expected, and gives overall direction; knowledgeable staff are empowered staff. For nurses educated and experienced in the primary care model, the use of assistive personnel is often a challenge for which they are not prepared. A change in mindset, from "doing it all myself" to trusting one's responsibilities for care to others requires not only the ability to judge what can be delegated but also the ability to empower that person to carry out the work and to trust them in the process.

Care given by assistive personnel or LPNs should never be increased so rapidly that it is impossible for the community health nurse to adequately supervise the care delegated to them. The community health nurse must have sufficient time available to apply the principles of the five management functions when carrying out the following supervisory activities with HHAs and LPNs:

1. Shared home visits with the LPN or HHA on the initial visit to a family (planning, organizing)
2. Development of nursing care plans on each family in the caseload, based on assessment data and input from the LPN or HHA (planning, organizing)
3. Regular conferences with the LPN or HHA to determine guidance and assistance needed in specific situations (directing, organizing, coordinating)
4. Periodic shared visits with the LPN or HHA for supervision and reevaluation of the status of the family (directing, coordinating, controlling)
5. Periodic review of family records to evaluate the status of the family and the level of nursing service (controlling)
6. Inservice education related to the needs of the staff and the families in the nurse's caseload (directing) when working with home health paraprofessionals; research shows that supervision is a critical component of assuring quality (Moore, 1990; Spiegel, 1987) and personnel retention (Donovan, 1989; Feldman, 1990).

INTERDISCIPLINARY COLLABORATION

One of the expectations for effective health professionals that is repeatedly identified in the literature is the need for interdisciplinary collaboration. It is also a focus of reengineering, discussed earlier in this chapter. The emerging health care system will require all health care professionals to "work effectively as a team member in organized settings that emphasize the integration of care" (Pew Health Professions Commission, 1995, p. 5). As integrated managed care systems become the dominant source of health care, nurses will be a part of teams and will relate to other social and academic organizations. Community health nurses have had a long history of collaboration with other disciplines, and we can continue to build on this strength. The box below lists some barriers to working in collaborative teams along with strategies for successful teams. Notice the themes that been repeated in this chapter: all levels of workers are managers and leaders; the emphasis on process; mistakes are made and learning must occur from mistakes; and trust is an important consideration.

Collaborative Interdisciplinary Teamwork

TYPES OF BARRIERS TO COLLABORATIVE TEAMWORK, WITH EXAMPLES

1. *Organizational barriers:* lack of knowledge and appreciation for the roles of other professionals; legal issues related to scope of practice and liability
2. *Barriers at a team level:* role and leadership ambiguity; team too large or too small; lack of a clearly stated purpose
3. *Barriers faced by individual team members:* multiple responsibilities and job titles; competition, naiveté; gender, race, and class issues

STRATEGIES FOR EFFECTIVE INTERDISCIPLINARY TEAMS

1. Agree on a unifying philosophy centered around the primary care of the patient and the community: define a vision of collaborative team care
2. Develop a commitment to the common goal of collaboration: simply believe in the power of the team
3. Learn about the contributions other disciplines bring to the team
4. Respect others' skills and knowledge: patients and their families and communities bring strengths to the interdisciplinary team
5. Establish positive attitudes about your own profession: when you are comfortable with yourself you will be able to value others
6. Develop trust between members
7. Be willing to share responsibility for patient care: trust others' abilities
8. Establish mechanisms for negotiation and re-negotiation of goals and roles over time: time and knowledge bring change to the team structure
9. Establish methods for resolving the conflicts that are inevitable among team members
10. Be willing to work continuously to overcome barriers: do not give up when the going gets rough

From Grant R: *Interdisciplinary collaborative teams in primary care: a model curriculum and resource guide,* San Francisco, Ca., January 1995, Pew Health Professions Commissions, unpaginated.

A DIVERSE WORKFORCE

By the year 2000 minorities will compose 29% of new entrants into the labor force, twice their current share. Black men will make up 7.7% of the labor force growth, black women will make up 12% of the labor force growth, and Hispanics will be 22% of that same aggregate. Immigrants will represent the largest share of the increase in the population and the workforce since the first World War, and two thirds of them or more are likely to join the labor force (Johnson, 1994, p. 81).

Effective leaders and managers will have the skills to work with people who do things differently than they do. They will understand that though all people are ethnocentric to some degree (thinking that their own ways of doing things are the "right ways"), the degree of ethnocentrism will lessen, and acceptance of people for who they are will become the norm.

Effective leaders and managers will make the effort to learn how others like to do things. For example, in Germany the common form of greeting is to shake hands, extended to women before men, and one is addressed formally (Mrs. and Mr.) even after years of working together. In Japan the group is the most important part of society and is emphasized for motivation in the workplace; in Korea, to accomplish something while causing unhappiness or discomfort for someone is to accomplish nothing at all. Leaders and managers acknowledge that diversity in a workplace can bring strength, that many ways of looking at a situation are ideal for solving problems. Culturally competent managers and leaders know that conflict is a natural part of working with people who do things differently. However, they have the skills to deal with that conflict and will help their colleagues to learn those skills. The box on the next page depicts seven skills that can be used by leaders and managers as they work with a culturally diverse workforce. Use of cross-cultural skills can result in people who are personally and professionally productive.

LIVING WITH CHANGE

Change was one of the three Cs discussed at the beginning of this chapter. Effective community health nurses will be comfortable with change because it is part of daily life. Thus lifelong professional and personal development will be their personal paradigm, the way they "see" the world.

Covey (1989), in his bestseller *The Seven Habits of Highly Effective People: Powerful Lessons in Personal Change*, described the characteristics of a person who believes in the concepts of reengineering. He emphasized the need to adapt to change and to see opportunities in the intense challenges of today's work world. He sees all persons as leaders and managers and emphasizes the need for teamwork. The box below presents his habits. He also has a page on the Internet (www.covey.com) and welcomes visitors. Nurses, neophytes, students, and those with experience are urged to make education, self-development, and self-renewal a part of life. Successful people are at peace with themselves and thus have the ability to work with others.

Seven Cross-Cultural Skills

1. *Show respect.* How can you demonstrate that you respect the people with whom you are working? Does your demonstration of respect mean the same thing to you that it does to the people with whom you are working?
2. *Tolerate uncertainty.* The ability to react to new, different, and unpredictable situations with little visible discomfort or irritation.
3. *Relate to people.* Are you concerned with the task side of the job rather than the people side? Do people feel a part of the work situation or do they feel used?
4. *Be nonjudgmental.* Do you withhold judgment and remain objective until you have enough information to understand another point of view?
5. *Personalize your observations.* Different people explain the world about them in different terms. Your knowledge and perceptions are valid only for you and not the rest of the world. What is right or true in one culture may not be right or true in another.
6. *Be empathetic.* Attempt to see things from another person's point of view.
7. *Be patient.* You may not be successful the first time and may not be able to get things done immediately, but be patient and persevere.

The Seven Habits of Highly Effective People

1. BE PROACTIVE.® The principles of personal vision
2. BEGIN WITH THE END IN MIND.® The principles of personal leadership
3. PUT FIRST THINGS FIRST.® The principles of personal management
4. THINK WIN-WIN.™ The principles of interpersonal leadership
5. SEEK FIRST TO UNDERSTAND, THEN TO BE UNDERSTOOD.™ The principles of empathetic communication
6. SYNERGIZE.® The principles of creative cooperation
7. SHARPEN THE SAW.® The principles of balanced self-renewal

From Covey SR: *The seven habits of highly effective people: powerful lessons in personal change*, New York, 1989, Simon & Schuster.

Summary

Community health nurses have multiple and diverse responsibilities in the practice setting, and they understand that they are both managers and leaders in carrying out responsibilities. They have found that by applying the principles of management they are more effective in dealing with the multiple and diverse demands in the work environment. Knowledge of the five functions of management is especially helpful. These functions are planning, organizing, directing, coordinating, and controlling. The use of a management information system supports these management functions by using data effectively and efficiently.

The development of management thought has changed over time. Reviewing the historical evolution of management helps nurses to understand why it is useful to implement the five functions of management in the work setting. Analysis of the evolution of management is also beneficial because it provides a basis for defining a personal philosophy of management and leadership.

The use of management concepts in the community health nursing setting is essential. Management principles help the community health nurse organize and schedule activities, establish priorities for nursing service, effectively and efficiently utilize time, and appropriately delegate responsibilities. All these tasks must be accomplished if the community health nurse is going to deliver quality care to clients in the community.

A changing health care climate and a diverse workforce contribute to a work setting that is stimulating and in flux. Principles of reengineering assist organizations with these changes in a productive manner.

Critical Thinking Exercise

Lieutenant General William G. Pagonis led 40,000 men and women who ran the theater logistics during the Persian Gulf War. Following are his remarks about leadership: "To lead successfully, a person must demonstrate two active, essential, and interrelated traits: expertise and empathy. In my experience, both of these traits can be deliberately and systematically cultivated; this personal development is the first important building block of leadership . . . The good news is that leaders are made, not born. I'm convinced that anyone who wants to work hard enough and develop these traits can lead" (1992, p. 118).

Describe the type of expertise you look for in a leader and share your perceptions of the concept *empathy* as it relates to leadership. Identify your strengths and needs in terms of these two leadership traits, expertise and empathy, and discuss how you would cultivate your leadership abilities.

We thank Paulette Worcester, RN, DNS, Assistant Professor, Miami University, Oxford, Ohio, for her assistance with this chapter.

REFERENCES

American Nurses Association (ANA): *Nursing case management*, Kansas City, Mo., 1988, ANA.

American Nurses Association (ANA): *Standards for nursing staff development*, Washington, D.C., 1990, ANA.

American Nurses Association (ANA): *Standards for organized nursing services and responsibilities of nurse administrators across all settings*, Washington, D.C., 1991, ANA.

Benjamin S, Penland T: How developmental supervision and performance management improve effectiveness, *Health Care Superv* 14(4):12-19, 1995.

Boston Consulting Group: *Reengineering and beyond*, Boston, 1993, The Group.

Covey SR: *The seven habits of highly effective people: powerful lessons in personal change*, New York, 1989, Simon & Schuster.

Department of Nursing, Henry Ford Hospital: *Images of nursing*, Detroit, Mi., Spring Edition 1995, The Department.

Dittbrenner H: Employment outlook: put on your sunglasses, *Caring* 15(5):10-12, 1996.

Donovan R: Worker stress and job satisfaction: a study of home care workers in New York City, *Home Health Care Serv Q* 16:97-114, 1989.

Feldman P: *Who cares for them? Workers in the home care industry*, New York, 1990, Greenwood.

Freedman DH: Is management a science? *Harvard Business Review* 70(6):26-38, 1992.

Freeman RB: *Techniques of supervision in public health nursing*, ed 2, Philadelphia, 1949, Saunders.

Gilbert N: Supervision of home health paraprofessionals: a quality of care issue, *Caring* 11:10-14, 1992.

Gleick J: *Chaos: making a new science*, New York, 1987, Viking.

Grant R: *Interdisciplinary collaborative teams in primary care: a model curriculum and resource guide*, San Francisco, Ca., January 1995, Pew Health Professions Commission.

Handy C: *The age of unreason*, Boston, 1990, Harvard University Press.

Hammer M, Champy J: *Reengineering the corporation: a manifesto for business revolution*, New York, 1993, Harper.

Johnson WB: Workforce 2000: executive summary. In Weaver G: *Culture, communication and conflict: readings in intercultural relations*, Needham Heights, Ma., 1994, Simon & Schuster, pp. 75-93.

Kahn E: A comprehensive computer system for the home health agency. In Schulmerich SC, Riordam TJ, Davis ST: *Home health care administration*, Boston, 1996, Delmar Publishers, pp. 87-108.

Martin KS, Scheet NJ: *The Omaha system: applications for community health nursing*, Philadelphia, 1992, Saunders.

Maslow AH: *Motivation and personality*, New York, 1954, Harper & Row.

McConnell CR: Delegation versus empowerment: what, how, and is there a difference? *Health Care Superv* 14(1):66-79, 1995.

Milio N: *The engines of empowerment: using information technology to create healthy communities and challenge public policy*, Chicago, 1996, Health Administration Press.

Moore F: What about the quality of care, *Caring* 9:16-26, 1990.

Pagonis WG: The work of the leader, *Harvard Business Review* 70(6):118-126, 1992.

Pew Health Professions Commission: *Critical challenges: revitalizing the health professions for the twenty-first century. The third report of the Pew Health Professions Commission*, San Francisco, Ca., November 1995, UCSF Center for the Health Professions.

Rives R: Priorities according to needs. In Stewart DM, Vincent PA, eds: *Public health nursing*, Dubuque, Ia., 1958, Brown.

Schieber G, Poullier JP, Greenwald LM: U.S. health expenditure performance: an international comparison and data update, *Health Care Financing Review* 13(4):14-15, 1992.

Senge PM: *The fifth discipline: the art and practice of the learning organization*, New York, 1990, Doubleday.

Spiegel A: *Home health care*, ed 2, Owing Mills, Md., 1987, National Health Publishing.

Visiting Nurse Association of Greater Philadelphia: *Software requirements, evaluation and selection for the voluntary home health agency*, Philadelphia, 1990-1992, The Association.

SELECTED BIBLIOGRAPHY

Beckhard R, Pritchard W: *Changing the essence: the art of creating and leading fundamental change in organizations*, San Francisco, 1992, Jossey-Bass.

Denton D: *Horizontal management: beyond total customer satisfaction*, New York, 1991, Lexington.

Everson-Bates S: First line managers in the expanded role: an ethnographic study, *J Nurs Adm* 22(3):32-37, 1992.

Glen P: *It's not my department: how America can return to excellence-giving and receiving quality service*, New York, 1992, Berkley.

Hall G, Rosental J, Wade J: How to make reengineering really work, *Harvard Business Review* 71(6):119-131, 1993.

Hammer M: Reengineering work: don't automate, *Harvard Business Review* 68(4):102-112, 1990.

Kerfoot K: Developing self-governed teams: the nurse manager's goal in shared governance, *Nurs Econ* 9(2):121-125, 1991.

Kerfoot K: From vertical to horizontal nursing management, *Nurs Econ* 11(1):49-51, 1993.

Kerfoot K, Uecker S: The techniques of developing self-managed teams: the nurse manager's role, *Nurs Econ* 10(1):70-71, 1992.

Kerfoot K, Green S: Redesign vs. fix-it-up: the case for reengineering, *Nursing Leadership and Manage* 1(4):1-4, 1993.

Kiernan MJ: *The eleven commandments of 21st century management*, Englewood Cliffs, N.J., 1996, Prentice Hall.

Manz C: *Mastering self-leadership: empowering yourself for personal excellence*, Englewood Cliffs, N.J., 1992, Prentice Hall.

Murphy R, Papazian-Boyce L: Seven barriers to work reengineering for patient-centered care, *Strategies for Health Care Excellence* 6(11):8-12, 1993.

Peters T: *Liberation management: necessary disorganization for the nanosecond nineties*, New York, 1992, Knopf.

Savage C: *Fifth generation management: integrating enterprises through human networking*, Maynard, Ma., 1990, Digital Press.

Wellins R, Byham W, Wilson J: *Empowered teams: creating self-directed work groups that improve quality, productivity, and participation*, San Francisco, 1991, Jossey Bass.

Wilson C: *Building new nursing organizations: visions and realities*, Gaithersburg, Md., 1992, Aspen.

24

Quality Processes in Community Health Nursing Practice

Objectives

Upon completion of this chapter, the reader should be able to:

1. Identify dimensions of quality in health care.
2. Discuss the concept of *total quality management* or *continuous quality improvement.*
3. Discuss the philosophical orientation of continuous quality improvement efforts.
4. Describe the components of a continuous quality improvement program.
5. Discuss the terms *structure, process,* and *outcome* as they relate to quality processes in community health nursing practice.
6. Discuss how standards and criteria guide measurement processes.
7. Discuss measurement issues in quality management.
8. Identify tools for collecting and displaying quality measurement data.

> One characteristic of a profession is the presence of a professional association that is cohesive, self-governing, and a source of professional self-discipline, standards, and ethics.
>
> JEROME P. LYSAUGHT, 1970, P. 41

"Self-review and self-regulation remain the hallmark of the healing professions" (Lohr, 1990, p. 11). Nurses share with all health care professionals the need to examine carefully the delivery of their services in light of changing societal demands. To validate itself as a profession and to maintain the right to govern practice, nursing must assume the responsibility for developing, implementing, and evaluating standards of excellence. The challenge for the late 1990s and beyond will be to use a multidisciplinary approach for continuous quality improvement while containing costs in a managed care environment.

EVOLUTION OF QUALITY PROCESSES IN NURSING

The professional's concern for quality improvement in health care delivery is not a recent phenomenon. Historical literature clearly identifies the fact that quality improvement has always been a primary focus in the health care industry (Lummis, 1996, p. 159). Throughout history professionals have worked to discover ways to decrease morbidity and premature mortality and to improve their practice. Evidence exists, dating back to the pre-Christian era, that supports the idea that public health surveillance and control measures have been instrumental in achieving desired outcomes related to the transmission of infectious diseases (Lummis). At that time these measures laid the foundation for developing effective quality improvement strategies.

Florence Nightingale established the foundation for quality in nursing practice during the latter half of the nineteenth century. She insisted that nurses needed formal education to carry out their role responsibilities, and she recognized the need for continuing education to remain current in practice (Reed, Zurakowski, 1996). Nightingale advocated for standards in practice that would guide all nurses in the delivery of quality professional interventions. Her focus on scientific inquiry, from both a practice and a research perspective, was aimed at improving quality in health care delivery. Her scientific investigations demonstrated that improvements in practice (e.g., increasing the size of the nursing staff) significantly reduced mortality during the Crimean War and led to Great Britain adopting the Audit Department Act of 1866. This act established procedures for evaluating quality on an ongoing basis (Lummis, 1996, p. 160).

During the early 1900s professional organizations campaigned for quality improvement in nursing practice. The initial objectives for the Nurses' Associated Alumnae of the United States and Canada, established in 1897 and known as the American Nurses Association (ANA) since 1911, focused on improving standardization in nurses' training. The

ANA advocated for licensure laws to protect the public from poorly trained nurses, and by 1912 thirty-three nurses associations had secured nurse practice acts (Christy, 1971).

Following ANA's focus, early public health nursing leaders pushed for standardization of public health/community health practice. The National Organization for Public Health Nursing (NOPHN), founded in 1912, grew out of a concern for the right of clients to receive care from qualified people. The NOPHN emphasized the importance of developing generally accepted standards for nursing care in the community (Gardner, 1975).

Professional nursing organizations have advocated for standards of excellence in practice throughout the twentieth century. The ANA has assumed a significant leadership role in setting standards for the profession and has diligently pursued as a major priority the development of a quality assurance program for nurses since 1966. All divisions of nursing practice under the ANA have developed and distributed standards of practice that are revised on a regular basis. The most recent ANA standards for community health nursing practice are delineated in the box below. These standards explicitly address the nurse's responsibility for ensuring quality in professional practice. To guide nurses in this endeavor, the ANA adopted a model for quality assurance in 1975. This model is discussed in a later section of this chapter.

Up until the 1960s major quality improvement efforts were primarily initiated by the health care professions. Societal influences during the 1960s, including concern for consumer protection, human rights, and health care as a right, changed this trend (Bull, 1996, p. 146). As the federal government became more actively involved in financially supporting health care for underserved populations under the Medicare and Medicaid programs, federal legislative action was taken to ensure accountability for quality care. The Professional Standard Review Organizations (PSROs), established by the 1972 amendments to the Social Security Act, were developed to ensure that federal monies spent for Medicaid, Medicare, and other federal health programs would be used effectively, efficiently, and economically. Peer Review Organizations (PROs) replaced PSROs by federal legislative action in 1982. Under the 1982 Tax Equity and Fiscal Responsibility Act (TEFRA) these structures were charged to review medical records for appropriateness, quality of care, and compliance with practice standards (Brecker, 1990; Bull, 1985).

Quality in health care service delivery became a national priority under the National Health Planning and Resources Development Act of 1974. This law mandated that health care professionals promote "equal access to quality health care at a reasonable cost" for all segments of the population (Papers on the National Health Guidelines, 1977, p. 1). It called for the development of national health planning goals and standards. As discussed throughout the text, national health goals were first published in 1979. The United States' *Healthy People* mandate continues to set

Standards of Community Health Nursing Practice

STANDARD I. THEORY

The nurse applies theoretical concepts as a basis for decisions in practice.

STANDARD II. DATA COLLECTION

The nurse systematically collects data that are comprehensive and accurate.

STANDARD III. DIAGNOSIS

The nurse analyzes data collected about the community, family, and individual to determine diagnosis.

STANDARD IV. PLANNING

At each level of prevention, the nurse develops plans that specify nursing actions unique to client needs.

STANDARD V. INTERVENTION

The nurse, guided by the plan, intervenes to promote, maintain, or restore health, to prevent illness, and to effect rehabilitation.

STANDARD VI. EVALUATION

The nurse evaluates responses of the community, family, and individual to interventions in order to determine progress toward goal achievement and to revise the data base, diagnoses, and plan.

STANDARD VII. QUALITY ASSURANCE AND PROFESSIONAL DEVELOPMENT

The nurse participates in peer review and other means of evaluation to assure quality of nursing practice. The nurse assumes responsibility for professional development and contributes to the professional growth of others.

STANDARD VIII. INTERDISCIPLINARY COLLABORATION

The nurse collaborates with other health care providers, professionals, and community representatives in assessing, planning, implementing, and evaluating programs for community health.

STANDARD IX. RESEARCH

The nurse contributes to theory and practice in community health nursing through research.

From American Nurses Association (ANA), Council of Community Health Nurses: *Standards of community health nursing practice*, Kansas City, Mo., 1986, ANA. Reprinted with permission of the American Nurses Association.

national goals and standards to improve quality of life among all at-risk aggregates. Model standards have been developed to assist local communities in achieving the goals specified in *Healthy People 2000* (APHA Model Standards, 1993).

Societal forces have significantly influenced the emphasis on quality since the 1980s. Health care providers are increasingly being challenged by legislative action, third-party payers, and consumers to assume accountability for the services delivered by members of their profession. Governmental officials, third-party payers, and influential consumer groups are all demanding that current professional practice keep up with societal changes and needs and that practice standards be maintained through quality review processes. A significant challenge that all health care professionals will need to address in the coming century is how to assess and continuously improve quality in a managed care environment.

QUALITY CHALLENGES IN A MANAGED CARE ENVIRONMENT

Health care providers will face several critical challenges during the twenty-first century as they strive to maintain quality in health care delivery. They will need to expand access to effective care, become more accountable to those who purchase and use health services, be able to use fewer resources more effectively, and be more reliant on outcomes data to guide appropriate practice. These challenges will need to be addressed within the context of a radically changing health care system that will serve an increasingly diverse population (Pew Health Professions Commission, 1995, pp. 4-6).

A major challenge for health care providers during the twenty-first century will be to maintain a focus on quality while containing costs in a managed care environment. Under a managed care system, health care providers have a powerful incentive to limit the use of health services: that is, financial gain. The more services providers perform for managed care clients, the less providers make (Managed care's conflicts of interest, 1995). "Clearly, there is a strong need for safeguards to ensure that cost savings are not achieved by denying needed services. If used, managed care plans should be designed carefully so that the pursuit of least costly care does not jeopardize quality of care or access to necessary services" (Managed care's conflicts of interest, p. 4).

A major concern of community health professionals is to ensure that all vulnerable populations have access to necessary health care services. Managed care programs try to pick the youngest and healthiest individuals and often exclude people because of preexisting conditions (Budetti, Feinson, 1993; Lawniczak, 1995). "There is increasing concern that managed care represents a potential threat to the health of vulnerable populations such as children and pregnant women, especially those who are poor" (Freund, Lewit, 1993, p. 94). In medically underserved areas, Medicaid managed care plans have frequently had to raise fees to providers to encourage them to participate in the plan, and often it is not possible to offer a reasonable choice of providers in poor neighborhoods (Freund, Lewit, p. 112). Additionally, in some areas egregious barriers to essential health care have been erected as a way to keep costs down and profits high (Children's Defense Fund, 1996).

Beery, Greenwald, and Nudelman (1996) propose that a national managed care public health network be established to develop strategies for improving the quality of health care services for economically disadvantaged groups. They believe that "managed care and public health have great potential for providing mutual assistance with significant benefit to society at large" (Beery, Greenwald, Nudelman, p. 306). Their proposed network would help advance the development of coalitions between managed care and public health and would encourage these coalitions to develop initiatives to safeguard the public good. Joining forces has the potential to advance quality in health care delivery for disadvantaged populations.

DEFINING QUALITY IN HEALTH CARE

As the emphasis on quality increases in the health care industry, numerous definitions of the term *quality in health care* are emerging in the literature. Most of these definitions imply a specified degree of excellence that is consistent with current professional standards and that results in positive client outcomes. A recent Institute of Medicine (IOM) study committee (Lohr, 1990), established to design a strategy for quality review and assurance in Medicare, examined over 100 definitions of quality of care. From knowledge gained from this process, the IOM study committee developed the following definition (Lohr):

> "Quality of care is the degree to which health services for individuals and populations increase the likelihood of desired health outcomes and are consistent with current professional knowledge." (p. 21)

Inherent in this definition are several key concepts. It implies that gradations or degrees of quality can be distinguished through measurement and that health care encompasses a broad set of services. It also implies that populations as well as individuals are proper targets for quality improvement efforts. Its goal orientation links the process of health care with outcomes and reflects the belief that the outcomes of care should have a net benefit or desired health results. Additionally, it highlights the constraints placed on professional performance by the current state of professional knowledge but underscores the importance of adhering to current professional standards (Lohr, p. 129). The IOM study committee believes that net benefit should "reflect considerations of patient satisfaction and well-being, broad health status or quality-of-life measures, and the processes of patient-provider interaction and decision making" (Lohr, p. 129).

A significant challenge confronting health care providers when examining quality of care is to identify dimensions of quality that can be measured and improved. The Joint Commission on Accreditation of Healthcare Organizations (JCAHO), a private accreditation organization dedicated to improving quality in client care, has identified nine dimensions of performance or quality that indicators may assess. These dimensions are identified and defined in the box at right. They examine whether an organization is *"doing the right thing"* (appropriateness, availability, and efficacy) and whether the organization is *"doing the right thing well"* (continuity, effectiveness, efficiency, respect and caring, safety, and timeliness) (JCAHO, 1993, p. 68). All of these dimensions of quality or performance can be defined, measured, and improved (JCAHO). For example, if an organization wanted to determine whether client care was coordinated (continuity) among health care providers, it could examine such things as how often appropriate follow-up care was offered to clients, whether an adequate referral network was available, and whether referrals were successfully implemented (Division of Programs for Special Populations, Bureau of Primary Health Care, 1996).

An in-depth analysis of the concept of quality in health care and quality measurement is beyond the scope of this book. Lohr (1990) and Schmele (1996) present a thoughtful discussion of both of these concepts. JCAHO (1993, 1994) devotes considerable attention to analyzing quality measurement.

DEFINITIONS OF THE DIMENSIONS OF PERFORMANCE

Appropriateness:
The degree to which the care/intervention provided is relevant to the patient's clinical needs, given the current state of knowledge

Availability:
The degree to which the appropriate care/intervention is available to meet the needs of the patient served

Continuity:
The degree to which the care/intervention for the patient is coordinated among practitioners, between organizations, and across time

Effectiveness:
The degree to which the care/intervention is provided in the correct manner, given the current state of knowledge, in order to achieve the desired/projected outcome(s) for the patient

Efficacy:
The degree to which the care/intervention used for the patient has been shown to accomplish the desired/projected outcome(s)

Efficiency:
The ratio of the outcomes (results of care/intervention) for a patient to the resources used to deliver the care

Respect and caring:
The degree to which a patient, or designee, is involved in his or her own care decisions, and that those providing the services do so with sensitivity and respect for his or her needs and expectations and individual differences

Safety:
The degree to which the risk of an intervention and the risk in the care environment are reduced for the patient and others, including the health care provider

Timeliness:
The degree to which the care/intervention is provided to the patient at the time it is most beneficial or necessary

From Joint Commission on Accreditation of Healthcare Organizations (JCAHO): *The measurement mandate: on the road to performance improvement in health care*, Oakbrook Terrace, Il., 1993, JCAHO, p. 69.

TOTAL QUALITY MANAGEMENT: THE EMPHASIS FOR THE 1990s AND BEYOND

The focus of quality efforts during the 1970s and early 1980s was on quality assurance. This process was viewed as a dynamic one through which health care professionals assumed accountability for the quality of care they provided. It was a commitment to excellence with an emphasis on ensuring that all health care professionals provided safe clinical care *equal to* or *better than* the standard of care designated appropriate for clients who had like characteristics.

During the 1980s the concept of quality assessment emerged. O'Leary (1991) believed that the term *quality assurance* was an "unfortunate semantic selection" because quality cannot be ensured but only improved. *Quality assessment* is currently being used synonymously with *quality assurance* by many health care professionals. "The activities now known as quality assurance . . . have evolved from their initial form (implicit peer-based discussions) through retrospective time-limited audits (in the 1970s) to their current form: ongoing monitoring, evaluation, and improvement, using well-chosen process and outcome indicators" (JCAHO, 1994, pp. 22-23). These activities focus on the clinical dimensions of client care and related governance, administrative, and support services that influence health outcomes (JCAHO).

As we advance toward the year 2000, the concept of total quality management (TQM), or continuous quality improvement (CQI), has come to the forefront and represents a significant philosophical shift in terms of the concept of quality. TQM moves away from the premise that problems are the result of errors by individual clinical professionals to the belief that the majority of problems arise from defects in the design of systems, products, and processes of production (Donabedian, 1993). In keeping with this idea, total quality management is viewed as a strategic mission shared by the entire organization (McLaughlin, Kaluzny, 1990). A major concept underlying JCAHO's *Agenda for Change*, launched in 1986 to stimulate greater attention to the quality of client care, is the belief that client outcomes are significantly influenced by all of the activities of a health care organization (JCAHO, 1990a, p. 4).

"Participative management is a predominant theme under TQM" (Smith, Discenza, Piland, 1993, p. 35). Leaders at all levels in the organization set the direction for TQM by promoting a shared vision, shared goals, and TQM values throughout the organization, empowering all employees to monitor their own work, evaluating and recognizing TQM progress, and acting as role models for TQM behavior (Melum, Sinioris, 1993, p. 60).

TQM puts responsibility for quality control in the province of frontline managers and employees through the use of quality circles and employee education and training in the methods of monitoring (Donabedian, 1993; McLaughlin, Kaluzny, 1990). *Quality circles* are small, structured problem-solving groups of employees from the same area who work on improving productivity, efficiency, and quality using a sound database (McLaughlin, Kaluzny; Mullins, Schmele, 1993).

Under TQM staff development, training, and educational activities have a different focus than the traditional models of human resource development. Emphasis is placed on helping employees deal with innovation and change. Training and educational activities are focused on reinforcing quality improvement processes rather than on imparting skills or knowledge to individuals (Smith, Discenza, Piland, 1993). These educational opportunities can assist staff in developing interdisciplinary teams that work toward achieving performance goals. An interdisciplinary approach to quality assessment and quality improvement is a major thrust in the continuous quality improvement model (Mold, Knapp, 1996).

In addition to creating a style of management that facilitates organization-wide involvement in quality improvement, TQM challenges the prevailing concept of *customer*. It demands that change be based on the needs of the customer, not the values of the providers (McLaughlin, Kaluzny, 1990). "A customer is anyone who receives and benefits from the product of someone else's labor" (Melum, Sinioris, 1993, p. 60), including *internal* consumers of one's labor. Within this context the recipient of clinical services—the client—is not the only focus when implementing quality improvement activities. Attention is placed on meeting the needs of all customers, such as personnel from other divisions within an organization, physicians and nurses in private practice, referral agencies, and third-party payers. In line with this philosophy, *evaluation of customer satisfaction* is seen as a significant component of the quality assessment process.

AN INTEGRATED QUALITY MANAGEMENT PROGRAM

"Total quality management (TQM) is a management system designed to create customer-focused, high performing organizations by involving all employees in process improvement efforts" (Gaucher, Kratochwill, 1993, p. 10). It is a synergistic approach between all components in an organization that promotes high quality health care. It requires an integrated program (Figure 24-1) that includes but is not limited to the following components (Koch, Fairly, 1993, p. 4):

- Quality assessment and improvement
- Infection control
- Utilization management
- Risk management/safety

An integrated quality management program is a broad and encompassing endeavor that addresses organization-wide performance improvement according to specified standards (Katz, Green, 1997). As previously mentioned, the performance improvement framework examines *what is done* and *how well it is done* (JCAHO, 1994). JCAHO believes

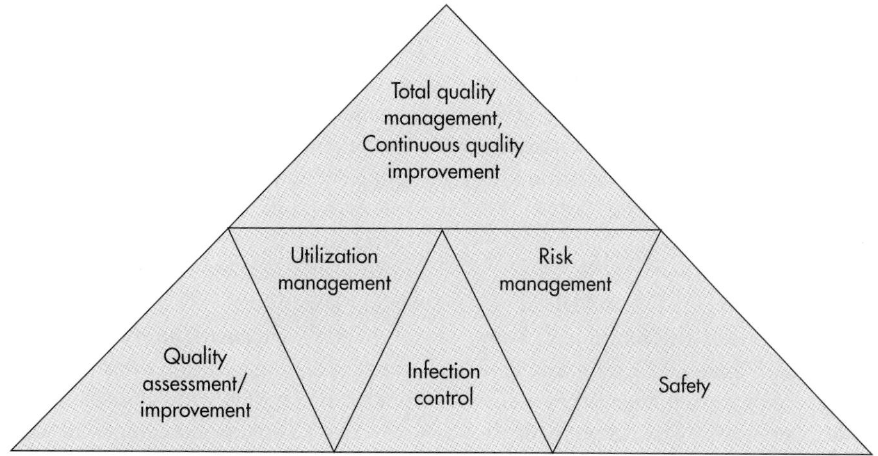

Figure 24-1 **Integrated quality management.** *(From Koch MW, Fairly TM:* Integrated quality management: the key to improving nursing care quality, *St. Louis, 1993, Mosby, p. 5.)*

that an organization's level of performance is reflected in client outcomes, in the cost (or efficiency) of its services, and in clients' and others' satisfaction (p. 11).

A well-established, integrated TQM program helps agencies monitor strengths and problems over time, review organizational processes and services, protect the consumer from adverse outcomes, and guard the agency from loss. It also assists agencies in maximizing resource management and educating the consumer and agency staff about reasonable and acceptable health care services at affordable prices (Koch, Fairly, 1993, pp. 5-6). An organization that cultivates an environment facilitating the achievement of these goals will maintain a competitive edge in the coming decade.

QUALITY ASSURANCE/ASSESSMENT AND IMPROVEMENT

"Quality assessment and improvement (QA/QI) is the systematic monitoring process that identifies opportunities for improvement in patient (client) care delivery, designs ways to improve the service, and continues to evaluate follow-up actions to make certain that improvement occurs" (Koch, Fairly, 1993, p. 17). Quality assurance/assessment and improvement is a complex process designed to evaluate the structure, process, and outcome aspects of health care delivery, with an emphasis on implementing measures to improve care when deficiencies are identified (Donabedian, 1988). All aspects of community health nursing practice, including services to individuals, families, aggregates, and the community as a whole, are monitored through a quality assessment and improvement process.

Desirable attributes of a quality assurance program are displayed in the box, above right. A successful quality assurance (QA) program provides practitioners with timely information for addressing a full range of quality care issues including overuse and underuse of services, the relevancy of interventions to clients' clinical needs, the caring and respect dimensions of performance, and system forces that influence health care delivery. A successful QA program is designed to foster active client and provider participation and focuses on improving client outcomes. In a QA program emphasis is on evaluating client outcomes against standards consistent with current professional knowledge, taking action to improve unacceptable practice, and continuously improving performance (Lohr, 1990).

Desirable Attributes of a Quality Assurance Program

- Addresses overuse, underuse, and poor technical and interpersonal quality
- Intrudes minimally into the patient-provider relationship
- Is acceptable to professionals and providers
- Fosters improvement throughout the health care organization and system
- Deals with outlier practice and performance
- Uses both positive and negative incentives for change and improvement in performance.
- Provides practitioners and providers with timely information to improve performance
- Has face validity for the public and for professionals (i.e., is understandable and relevant to patient and clinical decision making)
- Is scientifically rigorous
- Positive impact on patient outcomes can be demonstrated or inferred
- Can address both individual and population-based outcomes
- Documents improvement in quality and progress toward excellence
- Is easily implemented and administered
- Is affordable and is cost-effective
- Includes patients and the public

From Lohr KN, ed: *Medicare: a strategy for quality assurance*, vol 1, Washington, D.C., 1990, National Academy Press, p. 49.

THE ANA QUALITY ASSURANCE MODEL

In the mid-1970s the ANA adopted a QA model, developed by Dr. Norma Lang, to depict the multiple components of evaluating client care (Figure 24-2). This model illustrates that QA is a dynamic process, influenced by values and guided by standards of practice. "One strength of the model is that it suggests ongoing evaluation. The arrows around the circle indicate that the process is continuous, with subsequent evaluations incorporating previous findings as well as changes in values" (Bull, 1996, p. 149). Bull believes that this model "has stood the test of time and remains viable today" (p. 149).

There has been significant debate in the literature about the strengths and shortcomings of the QA model and the value of the industrial model of quality (TQM/CQI). Tilbury (1992, p. 12) suggests that the ANA generic model of QA can be applied to CQI with the addition of activities to monitor the new, higher level of quality achieved after action has been taken. She contends that the "differences in how the model is applied lie more in how the quality assessment and improvement processes are implemented than in the particular steps undertaken" (Tilbury, p. 12). For example, concurrent and terminal monitoring of performance, involving staff at *all* levels in the organization, is the norm under the CQI system. Under the traditional QA structure retrospective chart reviews by QA personnel were emphasized (Tilbury).

JCAHO supports the integration of QA and CQI concepts. This organization's framework for improving performance incorporates the strengths of QA while broadening its scope to reflect the complexity of external and internal environmental influences on the quality of health care. During its accreditation process JCAHO examines how well health care organizations understand and align their

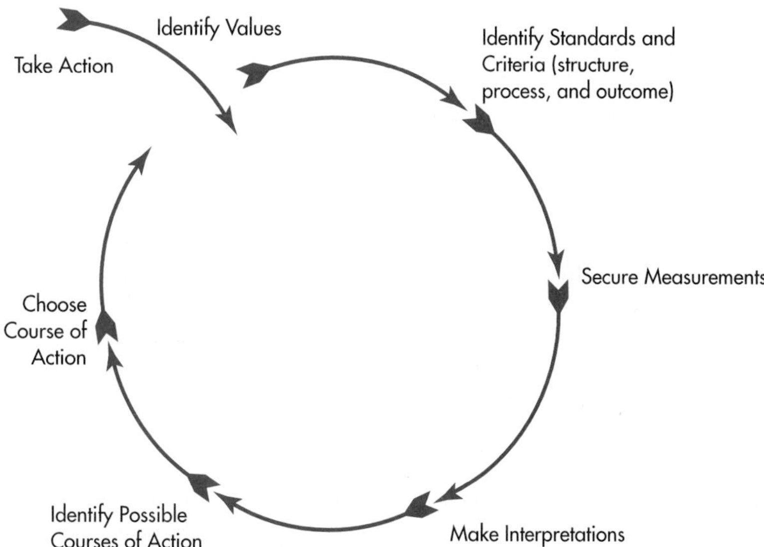

Figure 24-2 A quality assurance model. *(Modified from American Nurses Association:* A plan for implementation of the standards of nursing practice, *Kansas City, Mo., 1975, ANA, p. 15.)*

mission with identified community needs and how well they carry out cross-disciplinary, multidepartmental functions essential to client care (JCAHO, 1994, pp. 7-8).

Donabedian (1996), a world-renowned authority on health care QA, provided a thought-provoking analysis of the similarities and differences between the health care model of quality (QA) and the industrial model of quality (TQM/CQI). He concluded that despite differences in vocabulary, "the industrial model has many affinities to ours [health care model]: in its emphasis on service to the consumer; in its recognition of the worthiness, dignity, devotion, and skill of all workers; in its refusal to blame individuals for inherent deficiencies of systems and processes; in its reliance on education rather than punishment; in its reliance on leadership rather than dictation; and in its emphasis on internal self-amelioration rather than external regulation" (Donabedian, pp. 102-103). Donabedian believes that both health care professionals and industrial personnel have learned from each other. However, he cautions health care professionals not to deflect attention from clinical effectiveness to the efficiency of supportive activities as they embrace the concepts of CQI. The reader is encouraged to review in depth Donabedian's analysis of QA models.

KEY COMPONENTS OF QUALITY ASSURANCE/ASSESSMENT

Regardless of the terminology used, all quality assurance/assessment (QA) programs have several key elements. Organizations with well-established QA programs have articulated their values about quality health care and have linked these values with their mission, vision, and philosophy statements. Additionally, these organizations have developed performance standards and have established ongoing evaluation processes that are designed to assess and continuously improve quality outcomes.

Mission, Philosophy, and Values

Fundamental to sound QA efforts are well-defined statements that describe an organization's mission, philosophy, vision for responding to anticipated changes in the environment, and quality of care values. These statements provide direction for all organizational activities and a blueprint for action (Katz, Green, 1997).

An organization's *mission* statement identifies the overall business of the organization (Katz, Green, 1997). In other words, it describes the purpose of the organization by delineating the nature of services to be provided, the recipients of services, and the expected level of excellence to be achieved. For example, some organizations work toward being premier centers of excellence that provide a full range of acute and community-based services to all clients within the community served. Other organizations propose to provide quality, competent home care to all clients in the community who need skilled home health services. Or they may propose to provide high-quality health promotion and disease prevention services to all vulnerable populations within the community. Mission statements in the community health setting usually reflect the value that the community is the unit of service and focus organizational efforts on designing and delivering preventive health care services for vulnerable populations.

An organization's *philosophy* statement builds upon its mission statement. It describes beliefs about how things should be done to successfully carry out the business of the organization. A philosophy is "a written statement of an organization's beliefs about customer service, staff practice, and governance" (Katz, Green, 1997, p. 305). The box below presents an example of a philosophy statement that addresses these three domains. A well-written philosophy statement reflects professional as well as managerial values.

Beliefs and values influence how we think, how we act, and how we evaluate events and actions. In terms of QA and improvement, they affect commitment to the concept of quality and how quality is defined. Identifying values in relation to quality is difficult because many forces influence the delivery of health care services. Available resources, consumer needs and wants, and professional philosophies all determine the scope of practice in the community. For example, it is unrealistic to assume that an organization can plan clinical services without taking into consideration the restrictions of limited resources. Organizations must develop realistic mission and philosophy statements consistent with the resources available or potentially available to them. Being "all things to all people" is an impossible goal that can lead to frustration and quality performance problems.

Standards and Criteria Guide Quality Measurement

Organizational mission and philosophy statements reflect the values and beliefs of an agency and guide the activities of all personnel. They do not provide measurable elements by which a practitioner can judge the quality of care given by health care providers. Standards and criteria must be developed so that the measurement of quality is possible. *Standards* are "broad statements of agreed-upon quality for a given element of care" (Schmele, 1996, p. 591). "Standards define a set of rules, actions or outcomes. Rules constitute the structure of the service, actions are the process of how the service is carried out, and outcomes define the results of the service" (Katz, Green, 1997, p. 9). For example, in the ANA community health nursing standards, one identical outcome is "to promote, maintain, or restore health, to prevent illness, and to effect rehabilitation" (Standard V).

Criteria are used to measure the achievement of a standard. Criteria are measurable statements that address the *intent* of a standard and reflect the level of accomplishment of that standard (Schmele, 1996, p. 589). An objective, measurable criterion showing the degree to which a standard has been met is labeled an *indicator* (Schmele, p. 590).

Philosophy Written in Three Domains

Excellence in Service

We believe . . .

- That each of our patients, regardless of circumstances, possesses intrinsic value from God and should be treated with dignity and respect.
- That each encounter with patients and families should portray compassion and concern.
- That each patient should receive quality care that is cost-effective, competitive, and based on the latest technology.
- That patient confidentiality and privacy should be preserved.
- That meeting the needs of patients and other customers should always be our number one priority.

Excellence in Practice

We believe . . .

- That the primary duty of health care professionals is to restore and maintain the health of patients in a spirit of compassion and concern.
- That the scientific process is an integral part of practice as health care professionals.
- That collaboration within the health care team is essential to meet the holistic needs of patients, which include physical, psychosocial, and spiritual aspects of care.
- That we should aggressively promote patient and family education to allow each individual the opportunity to prevent illness and/or achieve optimal health.
- That we are accountable to patients, patients' families, and to each other for our professional practice.
- That monitoring and evaluating health care services is our responsibility and is necessary to continuously improve care.
- That we should pursue professional growth and development through education, participation in professional organizations, and support of research.

Excellence in Leadership

We believe . . .

- That we should provide a progressive environment, utilizing current technology, guided by responsible stewardship to promote the highest quality patient care and employee satisfaction.
- That we should encourage and support collaborative decision making by those who are closest to the situation, even at the risk of failure.
- That compassion should be characterized in our day-to-day personal interactions as well as being a motivating factor in management decisions.
- That we should be sensitive to individual needs and give support, praise, and recognition to encourage professional and personal development.
- That we should possess an energy level and personal style that empowers and inspires enthusiasm in others.
- That we should consider suggestions and criticisms as challenges for improvement and innovation.
- That justice should be applied equitably in all employment practices and personnel policies.

From Katz JM, Green E: *Managing quality: a guide to system-wide performance management in health care*, ed 2, St. Louis, 1997, Mosby, p. 93.

Community health agencies would examine such things as immunization rates, the incidence and prevalence of disease, and quality of life and level of functioning indicators to determine how well their staff were performing in relation to the ANA standard discussed above (Standard V). A specific outcome or performance indicator might be "improve the immunization rates for 2-year-olds served by the agency's well-child clinics from 72% to at least 90% by 1998." This performance indicator is directed toward decreasing vaccine-preventable diseases and is consistent with national standards *(Healthy People 2000)*. If it is not achieved, undesirable outcomes (e.g., an increase in vaccine-preventable diseases) may result.

Structure-Process-Outcome Measurement Approach

Donabedian's (1966) structure-process and outcome conceptual framework has guided quality measurement efforts for several decades and is widely used today (Katz, Green, 1997; Lohr, 1990; Schmele, Donabedian, 1996). This framework proposes that an effective quality management system evaluates quality from three perspectives: structure, process, and outcome. It provides a framework for examining both system-level and client-level outcomes against specified standards. It is based on the belief that *"good structure increases the likelihood of good process, and good process increases the likelihood of good outcome"* (Schmele, Donabedian, p. 378).

Structural standards assist organizations in appraising the environment in which health care is provided (Donabedian, 1969). The structure of an organization "comprises the relatively stable characteristics of the providers of care, the tools and resources they have at their disposal, and the physical and organizational settings where they work" (Schmele, Donabedian, 1996, p. 378). Structural criteria essentially measure an agency's capability to provide quality health care. Structural measures examine such variables as resource availability, the qualifications of staff, staff-client ratios, and adherence to legal standards. Licensure, certification, accreditation, and model professional standards provide guidelines for agencies by which to evaluate their structural characteristics. One such standard requires that agencies have adequate resources to achieve their stated outcomes. Criteria used to measure this standard include variables like staff qualifications, level of funding, and space and equipment needs.

Process standards describe how care should be delivered (Donabedian, 1969). Process criteria focus on measuring activities carried out by health care providers to assist clients in achieving desired health outcomes. They are designed to evaluate how the *clinical process* is used in the delivery of health services to clients. Process standards and criteria determine whether clinical interventions were appropriate to the needs of the family or a specified at-risk aggregate. For example, the working group on homeless health outcomes (Division of Programs for Special Populations, Bureau of Primary Health Care, 1996) believes that the Health Care for the Homeless (HCH) Program plays a critical role in *reengaging* homeless people in the health and social service systems and that this dimension of service needs to be evaluated during quality assessment efforts. Specifically, a QA team would examine whether the HCH program provides access for homeless people to a wide range of comprehensive services (standard). A process indicator (criterion) to measure this standard might be "homeless clients received care for acute illness within 24 hours." Another might be "outreach activities facilitate client access to domestic violence services."

Outcome standards focus attention on the end results of care (Donabedian, 1969). Clinical outcome measures examine change in a client's current or future health status that can be attributed to antecedent health care (Schmele, Donabedian, 1996, p. 378). An example of an aggregate-focused outcome standard is "reduce infant mortality by the year 2000." An outcome indicator (criterion) established to measure this standard might read "reduce the infant mortality rate to no more than 7 per 1000 live births-baseline: 10.1 per 1,000 live births in 1987" (USDHHS, 1991, p. 368). "The outcome of care can be compared to the picture on a puzzle box: it is what the consumer and provider see as a result of the structure (the pieces) and process (fitting the pieces together)" (Peters, Eigsti, 1991, p. 45).

Outcome measures are being used to monitor the process of care (success, failure, or complication of an intervention), the client's health status (short-term or long-term functional level of the client), and organizational outcomes including the cost of quality care (Finnigan, Abel, Dobler et al, 1993; JCAHO, 1993; Peters, Eigsti, 1991). Selected reasons for focusing attention on outcomes of health care delivery are displayed in the box on the next page. Accreditation bodies, funders of services, and consumers are increasingly demanding that health care organizations measure the quality of their outcomes. "There is agreement within the health care field, among purchasers and users of health care services, that external evaluation should be more focused on actual performance (outcomes) and less on the capability (structure and process) to perform" (Marrelli, 1994, p. 2).

Priorities for Quality Measurement

General consensus is that quality monitoring efforts that are all-inclusive can seldom be achieved, are costly, and tend to cause frustration and anxiety among staff. Quality monitoring efforts need to be focused on measuring the *critical desired outcomes* that the health care provider can influence and on the *key organizational functions and related processes* that have the greatest impact on client outcomes. Examples of desired outcomes that health care providers can influence are improved health status, improved level of functioning, and improved quality of life. A key function that can significantly influence these client outcomes is the care,

Selected Reasons for Measuring Outcomes of Care

- To demonstrate improvements in clients' health status, level of functioning, and quality of life.
- To know what works and what does not, and to be able to make appropriate interventions more effective.
- To build support for specific interventions that are effective with specific vulnerable populations.
- To assist with and assess internal quality improvement efforts.
- To demonstrate positive impact on public health and social issues.
- To assess cost-effectiveness.
- To assist in resource allocation.
- To exchange successful strategies.
- To increase client satisfaction.

Modified from Division of Programs for Special Populations, Bureau of Primary Health Care: *The working group on homeless health outcomes: meeting proceedings*, Rockville, Md., June 1996, The Division, pp. 3-4.

treatment, and service function, which encompasses the care or service planning process (JCAHO, 1996, p. 147). "A function is a goal-directed, interrelated series of processes . . . A process is a goal-directed, interrelated series of actions, events, mechanisms, or steps" (JCAHO, 1993, p. 253, 263). For example, the care or service planning process is an interdisciplinary process that encompasses the same steps as the nursing process. Other examples of key processes that significantly affect client outcomes are the hiring processes of an organization that are designed to recruit qualified providers and an organization's infection control and safety surveillance processes.

Four criteria are commonly used to determine which processes to review during quality monitoring efforts. "The predetermined criteria against which to measure and/or prioritize processes include deciding which are high-volume, high-risk, problem-prone, and high-cost" (Katz, Green, 1997, p. 78). These criteria are defined as follows (JCAHO, 1990b, p. 29; Katz, Green, 1997, pp. 78-80):

1. *High-volume* processes are those that occur frequently or involve a large number of clients, employees, or organizational systems (e.g., care planning for high-risk mothers and infants).
2. *High-risk* processes include those in which harm or lack of significant benefit may occur if the activity is either performed or not performed (e.g., giving a wrong medication or not giving a medication).
3. *Problem-prone* processes are those that have tended in the past to produce problems for staff or clients (e.g., wound infections after surgery or falls among elderly clients in a cluttered home environment).
4. *High-cost processes* are those that result in large expenditures for the organization or that can significantly deplete client or organizational resources immediately or over time (e.g., processes not covered by insurance or daily travel by the client to an ambulatory care center).

After the prioritizing process, structure, process, and outcome standards flow from the key organizational functions and related processes and indicators measure whether these standards have been achieved (Hoesing, Kirk, 1990, p. 12). *Indicators are not direct measures of quality.* Rather, markers can be used to assess organizational performance and to identify potential performance issues that need further evaluation (JCAHO, 1990b). For example, a community health agency that places priority on addressing the needs of high-risk pregnant women may use "the number of mothers served by the agency who received prenatal during the first trimester" as an indicator of performance. This indicator employs the rationale that pregnant women who receive prenatal care during their first trimester are more likely to have positive pregnancy outcomes than women who do not, and that if this rate is significantly lower than the norm opportunities for improving client service delivery exists.

Thresholds for Evaluation

Indicators focus an organization's attention on important processes and outcomes to monitor during quality improvement efforts. *Thresholds* help an organization *evaluate* data and determine when an intensive evaluation is needed to identify why a variance from the norm is occurring. When outcome, process, and structure indicators are developed, thresholds for evaluation and a time frame for goal achievement are also established.

A "threshold for evaluation is a level or point at which the results of data collection in monitoring and evaluation trigger intensive evaluation of a particular important aspect of care to determine whether an actual problem or opportunity for improvement exists" (JCAHO, 1990a, p. 141). In other words, a threshold is the percentage of time the indicator should be met within a given time period (Anderson, Singleton, 1992). Thresholds for evaluation can range from 100% of the time to 0% of the time. However, JCAHO (1990a) believes that since thresholds of evaluation are designed to take into account the multiple factors that affect health care delivery—such as socioeconomic and educational status of clients and caregivers, severity of a client's illness, and professional experience of staff—it is not effective or productive to set all thresholds for evaluation at 100%. For example, taking into consideration the varying characteristics of family caregivers, it is not realistic to expect that instruction to caregivers on appropriate infant feeding practices be completed by the first home visit 100% of the time.

"The setting of threshold parameters for clinical indicators is guided by past performance of the organization, experts in the field, or empirical findings reported in the literature" (Wagner, 1996, p. 414). For example, based on experience, the Baltimore County Public Health Nursing division set thresholds for assessment, family evaluation,

Questions Asked to Guide the Data Collection Process

- What are the goals for collecting the data?
- Who should collect the data?
- In which domain should the data be collected?
- For what purpose should the data be collected?
- What are the data sources?
- How much data should be collected?
- What tools should be used?
- What bias exists?

From Katz JM, Green E: *Managing quality: a guide to system-wide performance management in health care*, ed 2, St. Louis, 1997, Mosby, p. 163.

Goals for Data Collection

- Set up a system to ensure accuracy of information on which to base future decisions.
- Avoid all punitive measures associated with the results of collected data.
- Pinpoint the exact areas of the organization that contain the performance improvement opportunities.
- Establish the degree to which improvement has occurred after the implementation of an improvement action plan.
- Collect data at regular intervals on all critical processes to demonstrate sustained improvement.
- Collect both subjective and objective data.

From Katz JM, Green E: *Managing quality: a guide to system-wide performance management in health care*, ed 2, St. Louis, 1997, Mosby, p. 163.

and planning at 90%; for follow-up at 85%; and for client outcomes at 75% (Zlotnick, 1992, p. 134). Although quality management efforts are aimed at improving threshold parameters, these parameters must be realistic based on available resources and the characteristics of the clients being served. It is, for example, difficult for community health nurses to achieve desired outcomes 100% of the time when they are working with vulnerable families who are experiencing multiple physical and psychosocial problems.

Benchmarking

Organizations that strive toward excellence in health care service delivery use the benchmarking process to identify appropriate standards and indicators for quality monitoring and thresholds for evaluation. "*Benchmarking* means to study someone else's processes in order to learn how to improve one's own. *Internal benchmarking* occurs within an organization. *External benchmarking* occurs between organizations that produce the same product or provide the same service" (JCAHO, 1993, p. 28). Organizations use the benchmarking process to identify what is possible and how others have achieved higher levels of performance (Czarnecki, 1996; McKeon, 1996).

To successfully benchmark, organizations need to identify what to benchmark, develop an internal database for comparing performance, establish partnerships with other organizations or units within their organization that are willing to benchmark, and collect and evaluate *comparative* measures of performance (Czarnecki, 1996; Wagner, 1996). Benchmarking requires a commitment to excellence and continuous performance improvement as well as resources for carrying out benchmarking activities. Benchmarking can assist organizations in establishing realistic standards of excellence and in remaining competitive in the health care environment. Health care organizations are being challenged by consumers and purchasers of health care services to document how their outcomes compare with health care industry outcomes.

Secure and Use Performance Measures

TQM is a factual problem-solving process designed to monitor and evaluate organizational performance. After key functions, processes, standards, and indicators are specified, tools and methods for measuring performance must be selected. The quality improvement team answers several questions before securing methods for measuring organizational performance. These questions are displayed in the box, above left. "Both process and outcome must drive all data collection" (Katz, Green, 1997, p. 163). Usually multiple goals are established for the data collection process (see the box above). An organization that has a sound management information system (Figure 24-3) is more likely to accomplish multiple data collection goals than organizations that rely on traditional data recording procedures. Saba and McCormick (1996) have compiled an excellent overview of the development of computer applications in community health as well as a description of the major types of community health computer systems.

A performance management team usually collects data from multiple sources (e.g., users and purchasers of health care services, staff, managers, and organizational records) and uses multiple methods to collect these data. Some of the methods used for collecting performance data are record audits, utilization review procedures, interviews, customer surveys, observation of clients and their environment, focus groups, and staff self-reviews. The goals established for data collection drive the selection of data collection methods. Data collection efforts should be very specific and pertinent to the standard and indicators being measured (Hoesing, Kirk, 1990). For example, if the goal is to evaluate the care planning process and the standard specifies that this process should be individualized to address each client's problems and needs, the record audit tool used to measure this standard should have criteria measures to evaluate whether care has been individualized for each client. One such measure

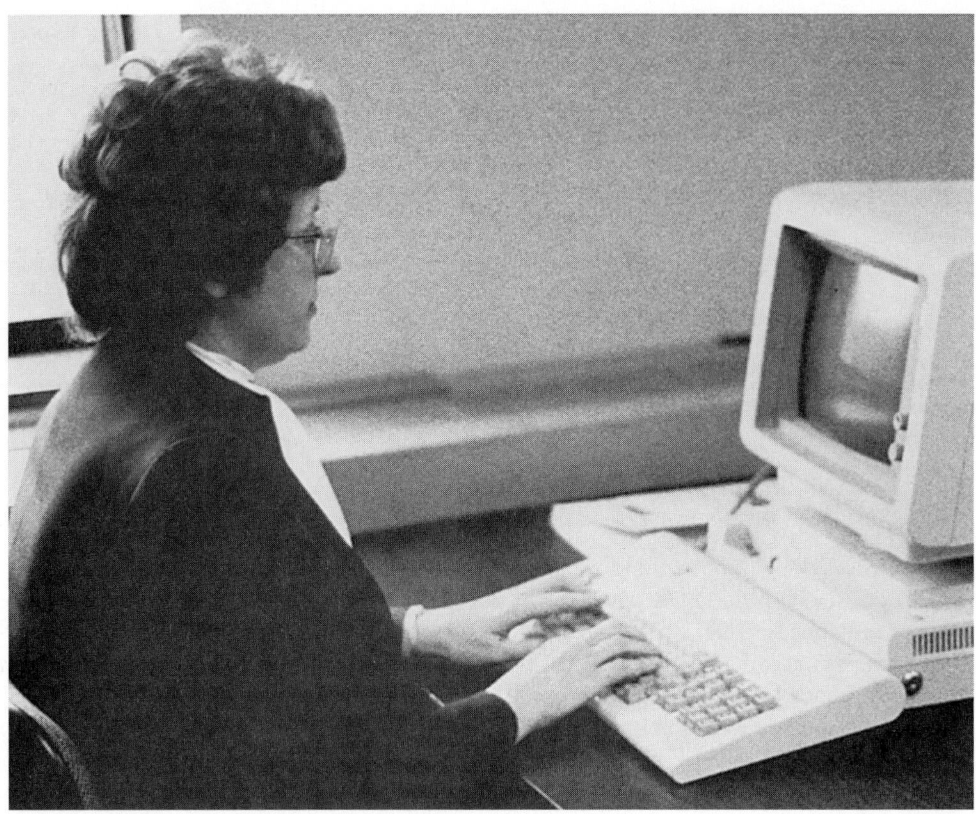

Figure 24-3 Community health nurses are using computers to facilitate recording of quality assessment and improvement efforts and other documentation processes. Computerized information systems help health care providers effectively and efficiently document client data and clinical services and obtain easy access to planning data. This, in turn, provides managers with information needed to support current or projected staffing patterns and relevant clinical programs. *(Courtesy Henry Parks, photographer.)*

might be "the health care provider has documented the problems and needs of the client." Another might be "the health care provider has documented that the client has received information about his or her medical condition."

Record Audit

A commonly used method for collecting performance data in community health is the record audit. Both concurrent and retrospective record auditing are carried out in community health agencies. Organizations subscribing to TQM or CQI emphasize concurrent review to learn about the process of care and services rather than the performance of individuals (Anderson, Singleton, 1992, p. 69; Peters, 1992). In other words, emphasis is placed on learning how the system is currently performing, with a focus on identifying how it can be improved. The concept underlying this emphasis is that there is always room for improvement, and if punitive measures are avoided improvement is more likely to occur (Peters).

A record audit encompasses a systematic review of a specified number of service records in a given period for the purpose of evaluating the care planning process and client outcomes. Katz and Green (1997) have established guidelines for determining sample size for record audit reviews and other measurement procedures (Table 24-1). As would be expected, the purpose of the review influences the sample size. A *routine review* is done to track trends over time. A *query review* occurs when data demonstrate that threshold parameters have not been achieved and the reasons for this can not be explained. An *intensive review* is conducted when negative client outcomes have been identified. A *sentinel event review* is done when a serious event (e.g., a medication error that compromises a client's quality of life) occurs (Katz, Green, p. 165).

Record audits are structured to ensure consistency of interpretation by all reviewers. This structure is obtained through the use of an audit tool that has a set of care standards, indicator measurements for each care standard, and a quality rating scale. Indicators are predetermined, measurable characteristics of a variable (care standard) that are used to evaluate clinical performance from both a process and an outcome perspective. One process indicator used to determine how well nurses complete assessments might read, "community health nurses collect and record data in relation to a client's family history." An outcome indicator used to assess continuity of care could

table 24-1 KATZ-GREEN GUIDELINES FOR DATA COLLECTION

TYPE OF STUDY	SAMPLE SIZE
Routine review	5% or 30 (whichever is greater)
Query review	10% or 60 (whichever is greater)
Intensive review	15% or 90 (whichever is greater)
Sentinel event	100% (every event)

From Katz JM, Green E: *Managing quality: a guide to system-wide performance management in health care*, ed 2, St. Louis, 1997, Mosby, p. 165.

be "all clients will be visited within 24 hours of referral to agency."

Each agency should have its own set of standards and indicators for its quality improvement program. These standards should address requirements of regulatory bodies. An agency functioning under a TQM philosophy empowers staff to select appropriate performance indicators, based on a review of the professional literature.

As previously mentioned, record audits are not used to evaluate individual staff performance but rather system performance that facilitates or inhibits the delivery of effective and efficient clinical services. With this philosophy, staff are encouraged to identify opportunities for improvement in clinical practice and to actively participate in matters affecting delivery of client care (Mills, 1992). This is not meant to imply that staff do not appraise their own performance. All staff are responsible for CQI, including examining ways to improve their own performance.

Staff Performance Appraisals

One of the most exciting aspects of a CQI program is the opportunity for staff to expand their competencies and to grow in a supportive environment. Organizations guided by the CQI model of QA/QI encourage staff and managers to work together in the development of performance management and career advancement plans. These plans are designed to increase job satisfaction as well as job performance and assist human resource departments in implementing competency-based orientation and staff development programs (Benjamin, Penland, 1995).

Ongoing appraisal of one's professional performance is absolutely critical in today's rapidly changing health care environment. This appraisal can provide a safeguard for quality client care, promote professional development, and facilitate the identification of professional strengths and opportunities for professional improvement. Staff performance appraisal processes also aid organizations in identifying system barriers that impede the effective and efficient delivery of clinical services.

The performance appraisal process is based on specified standards of performance and specific indicators (criteria) for measuring these standards. "Performance standards are derived from job analysis, job descriptions, job evaluation, and other documents detailing the qualitative and quantitative aspects of jobs. They are established by authority, which may be the agency in which they are used or a professional association such as the American Nurses Association" (e.g., community health nursing standards identified earlier in this chapter) (Swansburg, 1996, p. 630).

Managers and staff focus on identifying the critical components of service delivery when developing performance standards and personnel specifications. Standards established to appraise the performance of professional health care workers focus attention on how well the professional uses the care planning process. For example, the job description (Table 24-2) for a community health nurse would carefully address the role of nurse in using the nursing process to provide competent, quality care. Job descriptions are structure standards that outline "the requisite knowledge, skills, attitudes, responsibilities, and scope of authority of a specific position within an organization for the organization to function at maximum performance" (Katz, Green, 1997, p. 95).

A variety of tools and methods are used to appraise staff performance against specified standards. Some examples of these methods are peer, manager, and self-ratings, direct observation of staff in the clinical setting, and performance interview appraisals (Swansburg, 1996). Nurses who actively participate in the development of tools and methods for measuring staff performance will be more satisfied with the results. Take the initiative to become involved. It will be a learning experience that will have long-lasting effects on the delivery of your nursing care.

Client Reporting Measures

"Today, more than ever, the voice of the patient (client) is crucial for the continuous improvement of health care processes and clinical outcomes. As the medical care system shifts services to ambulatory and home care settings, patients' (clients') active participation in treatment and their compliance with instructions become even greater determining factors in successful clinical outcomes" (Barkley, Furse, 1996, p. 427). Most health care organizations use some type of client reporting measure to seek input from clients about their level of satisfaction with the health care delivery process and its outcomes and to rate the quality of care they received (Lohr, 1990). Organizations accrediated by JCAHO must document that they have sought client input and have used this input to improve organizational performance as needed.

Organizations are using a variety of methods to obtain input from clients about their perceptions of the quality of care they received and their level of satisfaction with this care. Examples of these methods are telephone or face-to-face interviews, client satisfaction and quality rating surveys, focus groups, and client representation on advisory boards.

table 24-2 Milwaukee Visiting Nurse Association's Job and Personnel Specifications for a Public Health Nurse II

Section A—job description and specifications

Job Summary: Under supervision, has responsibility for case management of patients and families with a wide variety of complex health and social problems, including multiproblem families. Is expected to be able to function independently in most situations. Identifies need for consultation or supervisory help. May be assigned additional responsibilities which require leadership ability.

Duties and Responsibilities	Basic Requirements
1. Functions independently in case management of complex situations, using supervision appropriately.	Interviewing skills. Physical assessment skills.
2. Admits patients and family members and gives service utilizing the nursing process.	Knowledge of health problems and illnesses.
a. Assessment—collects physiological, psychosocial, and financial data. Can identify the need for further data and pursues sources of data independently.	Knowledge of normal growth and development. Ability to make nursing judgments based on scientific nursing principles.
b. Assesses family members' health status and coping ability. Able to evaluate the family as a unit.	Knowledge of data sources within the community.
c. Identifies covert and overt nursing health and social problems of patients and families based on data collection.	Knowledge of family dynamics. Ability to see and interpret relationships in data and to arrive at a nursing care plan.
d. Implements nursing care plan as outlined. Adapts nursing procedures to the home setting.	Ability to identify objective parameters for evaluation of nursing care plan.
e. Evaluates results of care plan in terms of expected outcomes and takes appropriate action.	
3. Recognizes and interprets behavior patterns as influenced by basic physical and emotional needs, cultural and socioeconomic differences. Sensitive and accepting of these needs and differences and adapts plan of care accordingly.	Knowledge of cultural and socioeconomic factors. Knowledge of behavioral principles. Knowledge of self. Sensitivity and ability to listen. Knowledge of dependent and independent nursing functions.
4. Contacts physician to report alterations in patient's health status, to secure and share information, or to obtain medical orders.	Ability to collaborate with other disciplines regarding health care.
5. Independently identifies need for consultation and initiates referral.	Knowledge of consultants available and their role in the agency.
6. Independently refers patients and families to other VNA or community services.	
7. Communicates with other disciplines and services inter-agency and intra-agency to promote continuity and coordination of services.	Knowledge of community resources. Knowledge of agency procedures. Ability to write clear, concise, informative reports.
8. Teaches patients and families nursing procedures and good health practices. Interprets to patient and family the implications of the diagnosis—includes the patient and family in goal setting and plan of care according to their ability.	Knows teaching/learning principles. Ability to adapt to patient and family level of understanding and ability.

Reproduced by permission of the Milwaukee Visiting Nurse Association, Milwaukee, Wis. undated.

Client reporting measures can provide information about a variety of clinical care concerns and outcomes and client satisfaction issues. A major challenge for a quality management team is to identify the type of client data needed to assess system-level and client-level outcomes. Client reporting measures that are sensitive to *specific* aspects of care (e.g., interpersonal dimensions of care, continuity of care and access issues, and specified outcomes of care) and to *change over time* are valuable measures for documenting improvement and excellence (Lohr, 1990). Client reporting measures must be valid and reliable and address differing client characteristics. Bushy (1995) firmly believes that ethnocultural factors can no longer be ignored when seeking client input. These factors significantly influence if services are acceptable and appropriate for target populations.

The increasing diversity of the American population challenges health care providers to examine carefully their continuous quality monitoring efforts to determine whether they address quality improvement from a cultural perspective. Chapters 7 and 9 identify cultural parameters to consider when developing performance standards and measurements that evaluate the achievement of these standards. The *Healthy People 2000* national health objectives (USDHHS, 1991) assist health care providers in

table 24-2 Milwaukee Visiting Nurse Association's Job and Personnel Specifications for a Public Health Nurse II—cont'd

Duties and Responsibilities	Basic Requirements
9. Plans for the use of ancillary agency personnel and supervises their performance.	Knowledge of the legal functions of the RN, LPN, H-HHA. Knowledge of the legal functions of the RN, LPN, H-HHA in the agency.
10. Organizes and manages caseload efficiently.	Good organizational skills.
a. Plans travel routes for optimum economy and efficiency.	Knowledge of area and travel routes.
b. Establishes priorities within own caseload.	Ability to use maps.
c. Plans frequency of visits.	
d. Completes necessary records and reports as required within set time limits.	
11. May be assigned additional responsibilities. (Committees, research, etc.)	
PROFESSIONAL CONDUCT:	
1. Accepts agency philosophy, purpose, and objectives.	Knowledge of philosophy, purpose, and objectives.
2. Follows agency policies and procedures.	Knowledge of policies and procedures.
3. Demonstrates good inter-personal relationships.	Recognizes how behavior affects others.
4. Uses proper resources to deal with stress.	
PROFESSIONAL GROWTH:	
1. Participates in performance evaluation.	Motivated towards self-improvement.
2. Takes responsibility for own professional growth.	
Section B—personnel specifications	
1. Wisconsin professional nurse registration.	
2. Graduate of baccalaureate program accredited by the National League of Nursing and American Public Health Association.	
3. Two years current experience in community health nursing.	

targeting appropriate performance outcomes for populations belonging to different ethnic groups.

Analyze Data/Make Interpretations

Data from all clinical assessment procedures should be examined to make interpretations about clinical performance. One tool alone, such as the record audit, cannot provide a sufficient database to determine performance strengths or opportunities for improvement. Additionally, data from multiple sources are often needed to identify the real reasons for inadequate care.

The purpose of QA activities is to identify discrepancies, or *variance*, between established standards and criteria and actual clinical practice. Evaluation assessments should be specific enough to identify both strengths and areas needing improvement in the current level of clinical care. In general, most agencies have found that both exist. If either is found lacking when analyzing evaluation data, the measurement tools and the process for using these tools should be reevaluated. The tools may be too general and broad to discriminate between safe and unsafe care. On the other hand, the tools may be appropriate, but staff may need additional orientation to use them effectively. It is not uncommon to find providers assuming that certain care was given, even if it was not documented in the family service record. This may be an inappropriate assumption that covers up deficiencies in client care.

To identify variance between standards and actual practice, measurement data must be organized and grouped so that a composite picture is clearly presented. Summary reports should be developed so that the combined results of multiple efforts can be examined and patterns of care identified. Interpretations about overall agency performance must be based on *patterns* occurring over time, rather than on selected record reviews at a given time. Figure 24-4 is a sample of a summary report that displays the results of multiple records audits. This summary report helps agency staff quickly identify strengths and opportunities for improvement. It also allows for comparisons from one audit review to another, because change is depicted numerically.

There are several ways to display and summarize data such as the use of tables, histograms, graphs, and charts (see Chapter 13). Presented in the box on page 717 is a brief discussion of some common tools used to help understand the underlying causes of assessments results. A case study analysis using the "fishbone" cause-and-effect diagram is presented later in this chapter.

Monthly Summary Report

Nursing audit report ______________________
(Month) (Day) (Year)

____
/s/ Chairperson, Nursing Audit Committee

Number of family folders reviewed [ ]

	Outstanding	Satisfactory	Incomplete	Unsatisfactory
Overall evaluation by number of family folders				

Category name	Outstanding	Satisfactory	Incomplete	Unsatisfactory	Total
I. Observation of situation					
II. Evaluate total situation and draw up plans for nursing plans					
III. Implementation of nursing plans					
IV. Coordination of other services–intra- and interagency					
V. Recording format					

Function	Outstanding	Satisfactory	Incomplete	Unsatisfactory
I.	49-64	33-48	17-32	0-16
II.	49-64	33-48	17-32	0-16
III.	28-36	19-27	10-18	0-9
IV.	15-20	10-14	5-9	0-4
V.	12-14	8-11	4-7	0-3

Record score range

149-198 = Outstanding
100-148 = Satisfactory
51-99 = Incomplete
0-50 = Unsatisfactory

Summary of comments:

Figure 24-4 Oakland County Division of Health, Public Health Nurse Family Record Audit: Monthly Summary Report. *(Reproduced by permission of the Nursing Division, Oakland County Division of Health, Pontiac, Mi.)*

Identify, Choose, and Implement Action Strategies

Once strengths and opportunities for improvements have been delineated, alternative strategies for improvement should be identified. Additionally, health care providers should receive positive feedback about their strengths. Positive feedback provides an incentive for maintaining excellence in performance and for active participation in performance improvement efforts.

To identify action strategies for improvement, health care providers must first analyze why variance between established standards and actual performance is occurring. For example, perhaps record documentation demonstrates very little follow-up and evaluation of provider interventions. This may be occurring for a variety of reasons, including lack of knowledge, inadequate caseload management skills, insufficient time allocated for documentation, and poor staff morale. Discourse among providers to find the reasons for performance concerns should occur before action strategies are identified. Otherwise selected strategies may be inappropriate. If the documentation problem noted above, for example, was a result of unrealistic time allocations for recording, an action strategy designed to improve staff's understanding of follow-up and evaluation processes would be inappropriate for improving the identified documentation problem.

Data Display Tools

FLOW CHARTS

A flow chart graphically represents the sequence of events or steps that are required in a particular process or to produce a specific output.

CAUSE-AND-EFFECT DIAGRAM

The cause-and-effect diagram looks like a fishbone with the effect being the desired outcome and the causes represented by the "spines." The causes are usually divided into four categories: materials, methods, manpower, and machines. This tool is referred to as a fishbone diagram or Ishikawa, named after a leading QI authority in Japan.

RUN CHART

The run chart displays events or observations over time.

PARETO CHART

The pareto chart displays data in a ranking order comparing factors used to determine priorities, a way to sort out the "vital few" from the "trivial many."

HISTOGRAM

The histogram displays a graphic summary of how frequently something occurs.

CONTROL CHART

The control chart distinguishes common cause and special cause variation. It appears as a run chart with statistically determined upper and lower limits above and below the average.

SCATTER DIAGRAM

The scatter diagram demonstrates the relationship between two variables.

From Koch MW, Fairly TM: *Integrated quality management: the key to improving nursing care quality*, St. Louis, 1993, Mosby, p. 65.

Before staff choose an appropriate action strategy for improvement, they should discuss the advantages and disadvantages of each suggested strategy, taking into consideration organizational resources. Refer again to the situation in which record audits reflect inadequate follow-up and evaluation of provider interventions. If the reason identified for this situation is lack of knowledge of evaluation processes, action strategies might include conducting a total staff continuing education program that focuses on evaluation, holding weekly individual supervisory and staff conferences to discuss evaluation issues, or self-study by individual staff members. If only a few staff are having difficulty with evaluation, a staff development program for all personnel might be very costly to the organization.

Once staff choose an appropriate action strategy, it is important to develop a plan for implementing this strategy. Planning for action increases the likelihood that action will occur and increases the probability that activities will be orderly and predictable. Although the entire staff should be involved in developing action strategies, it is important to identify who or what is expected to change (Koch, Fairly, 1993, p. 65). Without such a plan it is difficult to coordinate change activities and to monitor their progress.

Taking action to improve performance is one of the most significant components of a QA/QI program. It demonstrates that health care providers do assume accountability for the care provided to clients served by the organization.

Action strategies and related changes must be carefully documented and evaluated to determine whether improvement has occurred. Other actions may be needed if the selected one does not result in the desired change. The quality assessment and monitoring cycle should continue even when expected performance is achieved. Ongoing monitoring is an important aspect of a total quality management program.

Monitor Quality Improvement Actions

Ongoing monitoring is essential to maintain quality performance over time. Emphasis should be placed on continuous improvement rather than on simply solving identified problems (Anderson, Singleton, 1992). A sound QA program sets in place strategies to identify whether improvement is sustained or whether new or additional improvement actions are needed. Such a program also maintains a focus on the future and continuously examines the need for new performance measurements or for actions and educational programs that will help staff members to gain the skills needed to handle job requirements and QA activities.

"Continuous improvement is like a chain reaction. Improvement in one area contributes to improvement in another area" (Smith, Discenza, Piland, 1993, p. 44). For example, poor performance is costly to an organization from both a direct and indirect perspective. Poor quality control can directly increase financial outlays for malpractice insurance and can cause costly insurance billing errors, excessive overtime, and the ordering of unnecessary clinical procedures. Indirectly poor performance can lead to such things as dissatisfied or lost clients, a bad reputation in the community, lack of client care follow-up, and upset or frustrated staff (Milakovich, 1991). Improving performance can help reduce both visible (direct) and hidden (indirect) costs for an organization.

Continuous quality monitoring helps an organization identify variance between established standards and actual performance and maintain the gains achieved through improvement actions. The CQI process encourages staff to actively participate in identifying potential and actual opportunities for improvement and to examine how environmental factors make an impact on service delivery. Environmental factors such as the evolutionary nature of the treatment of disease and changing technology, demographic characteristics of the population, and socioeconomic conditions in society continuously influence the health care delivery process (Cesta, 1993). This in turn requires a continuous focus on how the system can improve to address these changes.

INTEGRATED QUALITY MANAGEMENT PROCESSES

Escalating health care costs and complex changes in health care delivery have resulted in increased concern over cost containment and legal issues affecting community-based health care agencies. This has led to an emphasis on utilization review, risk and safety management, and infection control activities.

Utilization review, or *management*, is a process designed to evaluate "the appropriateness of client admissions and discharges; the appropriate and adequate use of personnel; and over- and under-utilization of services" (NLN, 1985, p. 48). This process focuses on the delivery of services in a cost-effective and efficient manner and uses a client record review to identify whether the amount and type of services provided were appropriate to the needs of the clients and appropriate for the agency to provide. Client classification systems and intensity rating instruments assist agencies in predicting the kind and amount of service needed by client groups with specific characteristics. Although client classification systems and rating instruments have been more widely used in acute care settings, several community-oriented ones are available (Ballard, McNamara, 1983; Churness, Kleffel, Onodera, Jacobson, 1988; Daubert, 1979; Hardy, 1984; Harris, Santoferraro, Silva, 1985; Hays, 1992; Hays, Kroeger, Tachenko-Achord, Peters, 1995; Martin, Scheet, 1992; Sienkiewicz, 1984).

Risk and safety management is a process designed to identify, evaluate, address, and prevent potential and actual risks that increase the chances of legal liability (Tehan, Colegrove, 1987). Tehan and Colegrove (p. 71) believe that home care agencies face significant risk in relation to the delivery of client care services, assessment of caregiver competency, and employee health and safety. Nonprofit and public community agencies face similar risks (Knapp, 1989). Community-based agencies must currently improve performance with increasingly limited resources while delivering unprecedented complex client services and containing costs. This position has exposed agencies to increased risks and safety issues and has provided a stimulus for agencies to expand their risk and safety management programs. A risk and safety management program focuses on such matters as the monitoring of staff selection, orientation, and on-going educational processes; the development of policies to ensure client and employee safety; the evaluation of unsafe client and employee incidents; and the development of educational materials to enhance caregiver/client competency.

Infection control is a process focused on disease prevention, intervention, and recognition (Koch, Fairly, 1993). The concepts and principles of epidemiology discussed in Chapter 11 form a foundation for an effective infection control program. The epidemiological process and the infection control process encompass the same steps (Friedman, Chenoweth, 1996). Control actions are generally directed toward breaking the chain of transmission for infection. Examples of infection control activities are reporting and monitoring infection rates; maintaining an infection control surveillance system; orienting or providing inservice for staff about infection control issues; establishing infection control policies and procedures, including policies regarding the disposal of infectious wastes and universal precautions; and instructing clients on infection control techniques (Koch, Fairly, 1993). Community health nurses have numerous opportunities for exposure to infectious diseases. It is imperative that infection control policies and procedures be followed in all community-based settings.

Although utilization review, risk and safety management, infection control, and QA programs have distinctive and separate foci, they are interrelated and have a significant impact on each other. For example, selected aspects of utilization review focus on the provision of optimal or quality care. Underutilization of clinical services such as limited referral to other community agencies and too few home visits can adversely influence client outcomes. Underutilization of resources can impede client progress.

An ultimate goal of each component of CQI is improved or positive outcomes (Figure 24-5). To accomplish this goal, all CQI efforts should be integrated and coordinated to achieve a balance among the goals of the four programs. If this coordination is lacking, an agency may

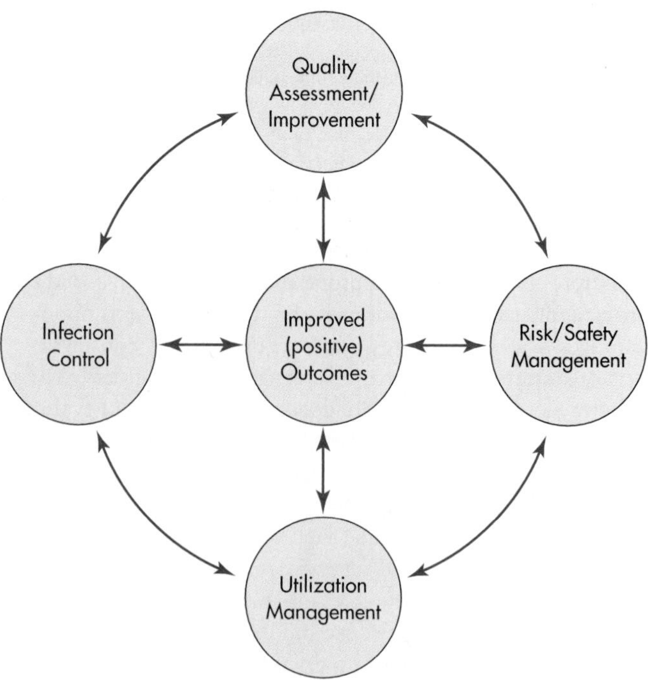

Figure 24-5 Integrated quality management model: improved (positive) outcomes. *(From Koch MW, Fairly TM: Integrated quality management: the key to improving nursing care quality, St. Louis, 1993, Mosby, p. 124.)*

neglect aspects of each of these components (Harris, 1988, p. 400). Integrated quality management is the key to improving performance, including client outcomes (Koch, Fairly, 1993).

A case scenario can best illustrate how CQI efforts are integrated and coordinated to address the important processes in an organization. The following case scenario represents a typical home care client (Koch, Fairly, 1993, pp. 235-236).

CASE *Scenario*

Mr. N. is a 55-year-old white male who retired early from a lucrative law practice because of a debilitating stroke (Figure 24-6). He has a history of hypertension and workaholic behavior. He has been in a rehabilitation center and has now returned home for continued support.

He is overweight and has been unable to care for himself since the cardiovascular accident. He has several children in town, including a son who is a nurse at a local hospital. His wife employs an attendant from 10 PM to 6 AM each day to care for Mr. N. She also has a housekeeper who is available for light assistance to Mr. N. during the day. There is good family support. Mr. N.'s private insurance covers intermittent visits by a home care nurse each week.

Figure 24-6 demonstrates the proactive CQI planning process for this case, utilizing the fishbone cause-and-effect diagram described earlier in this chapter. According to Koch and Fairly (1993), this process "analyzes the possible root causes to produce a positive patient care outcome in each case" (p. 234). The possible root causes of positive outcomes for Mr. N. were defined in terms of issues related to infection control, risk/safety management, utilization management, and QA/QI. Under the QA/QI component the authors identified a need to examine the important aspects of Mr. N's care using three priority indicators defined earlier in this chapter: high-volume (HV), high-risk (HR), and problem-prone (PP). Though Mr. N had excellent supports and was doing well, the fishbone diagram demonstrated potential risk factors. Koch and Fairly's book is an excellent resource for expanding knowledge of these concepts, as well as the concept of TQM.

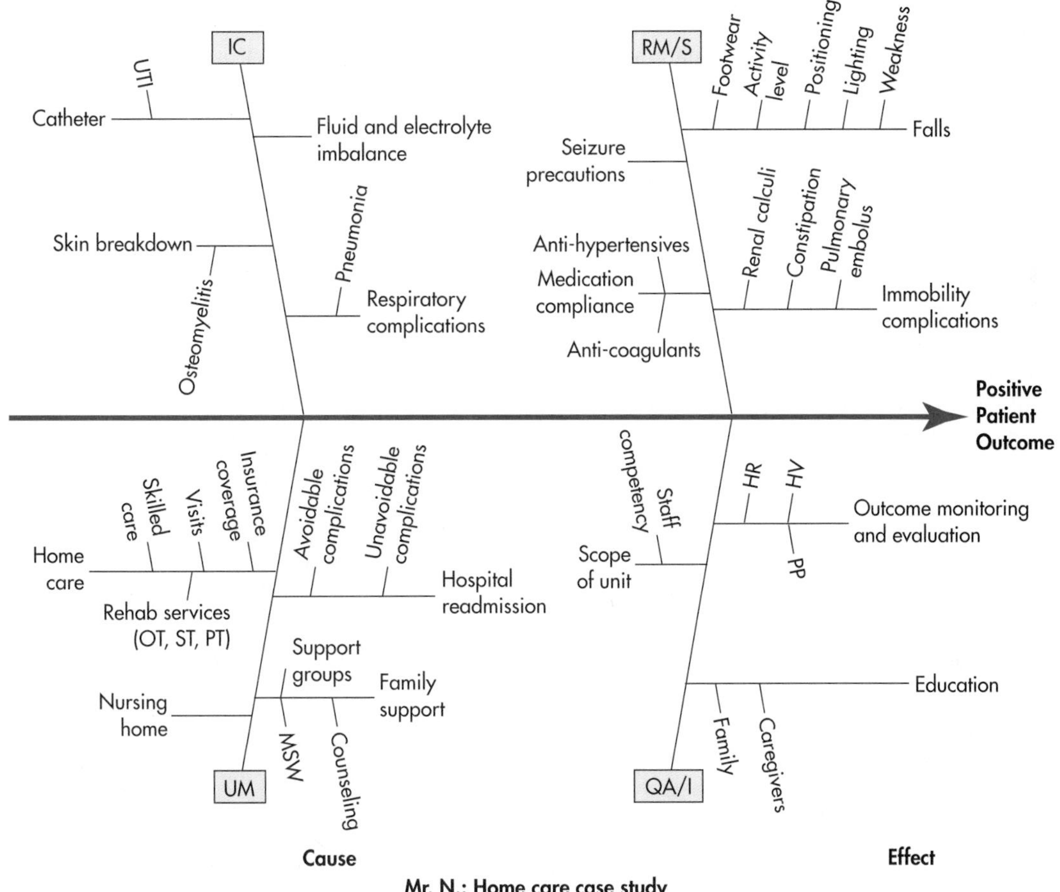

Figure 24-6 Integrated quality management "fishbone" diagrams: home care case study. *IC,* infection control; *UM,* utilization management; *RM/S,* risk management/safety; *QA/I,* quality assessment/improvement; *HV,* high-volume; *HR,* high-risk; *PP,* problem-prone. (*Redrawn from Koch MW, Fairly TM:* Integrated quality management: the key to improving nursing care quality, *St. Louis, 1993, Mosby, p. 238.*)

PARTNERS IN QUALITY IMPROVEMENT

Individual health care providers, professional organizations, service agencies, and clients all share responsibility for maintaining and improving quality standards for clinical practice. Input from the client is essential for determining values important to recipients of care. Client feedback is also crucial for the identification of improvements needed in practice on an ongoing basis. It is important that clients affect all components of a CQI program, because client needs form a foundation from which client services emerge. Organizations that remain viable in the marketplace are ones that are customer-focused in all aspects of health care delivery.

Implementing a TQM program is an exciting, challenging endeavor that promotes a client-focused system, team-building, and interdisciplinary functioning. All members of the health care team work with the client to improve health care service delivery. Through collaborative efforts all members of the health care team can help an organization maintain a competitive edge in the health care market. Such a challenge is worth working towards.

SUMMARY

As we advance toward the year 2000, emphasis on quality in health care delivery is increasing. Nurses share with all health care professionals the need to examine carefully the delivery of their services in light of changing societal demands. An exciting approach to quality appraisal and monitoring, *total quality management* or *continuous quality improvement*, has emerged. This concept is client-oriented with a focus on achieving excellence by identifying opportunities for performance improvement. It promotes team-building and interdisciplinary functioning.

Total quality management is a dynamic process that examines how significant organizational and clinical processes facilitate or inhibit quality performance. Quality assessment, utilization review, risk and safety management, and infection control activities are systematically implemented with a focus on improving client and system outcomes. An integrated and coordinated approach is essential to achieve a balance among all quality management components. Quality management is a factual problem-solving process that uses a variety of methods for assessing and improving quality. Crucial to the successful implementation of a total quality management program is an organizational philosophy that promotes a commitment to quality improvement, a participative management leadership style, and a shared vision that places the client in the forefront.

CRITICAL *Thinking Exercise*

Using data from a client situation in which you have been involved, identify issues related to infection control, risk/safety management, utilization management, and quality assessment and improvement that needed to be addressed (see Figure 24-6).

Taking into consideration the environmental conditions existing when you were caring for the identified client/family, discuss strategies that would improve service delivery performance.

REFERENCES

American Nurses Association (ANA): *A plan for implementation of the standards of nursing practice*, Kansas City, Mo., 1975, ANA.

American Nurses Association (ANA), Council of Community Health Nurses: *Standards of community health nursing practice*, Kansas City, Mo., 1986, ANA.

APHA: *Model Standards: The guide to implementing model standards: eleven steps toward a healthy community*, Washington, D.C., 1993, American Public Health Association.

Anderson P, Singleton EK: From QA to QI in a home health agency. In Dieneman J: *CQI: continuous quality improvement in nursing*, Washington, D.C., 1992, American Nurses Publishing, pp. 63-73.

Ballard S, McNamara R: Quantifying nursing needs in home health care, *Nurs Res* 32(4):236-241, 1983.

Barkley WM, Furse DH: Changing priorities for improvement: the impact of low response rates in patient satisfaction, *J Qual Improvement* 22(6):427-433, 1996.

Beery WL, Greenwald HP, Nudelman PM: Managed care and public health: building a partnership, *Public Health Nurs* 13:305-310, 1996.

Benjamin S, Penland T: How developmental supervision and performance management improve effectiveness, *Health Care Superv* 14(2):19-28, 1995.

Brecker C: The government's role in health care. In Kouner A, ed: *Health care delivery in the United States*, New York, 1990, Springer, pp. 297-328.

Budetti P, Feinson C: Ensuring adequate health care benefits for children and adolescents, *The Future of Children* 3(2):37-59, 1993.

Bull M: Quality assurance: its origins, transformation, and prospects. In Meisenheimer C, ed: *Quality assurance: a complete guide to effective programs*, Rockville, Md., 1985, Aspens, pp. 8-12.

Bull MJ: Past and present perspectives on quality of care in the United States. In Schmele JA: *Quality management in nursing and health care*, Albany, N.Y., 1996, Delmar, pp. 141-157.

Bushy A: Ethnocultural sensitivity and measurement of consumer satisfaction, *J Nurs Care Qual* 9(2):16-25, 1995.

Cesta TG: The link between continuous quality improvement and case management, *JONA* 23:55-61, 1993.

Children's Defense Fund: *The state of America's children, yearbook 1996*, Washington, D.C., 1996, The Fund.

Christy TE: The first 50 years, *Am J Nurs* 71:1778-1784, 1971.

Churness UH, Kleffel D, Onodera ML, Jacobson J: Reliability and validity testing of a home health patient classification system, *Public Health Nurs* 5:135-139, 1988.

Czarnecki MT: Benchmarking: a data-oriented look at improving health care performance, *J Nurs Care Qual* 10(3):1-6, 1996.

Daubert EA: Patient classification system and outcome criteria, *Nurs Outlook* 27:450-454, 1979.

Division of Programs for Special Populations, Bureau of Primary Health Care: *The working group on homeless health outcomes: meeting proceedings*, Rockville, Md., June 1996, The Division.

Donabedian A: Evaluating the quality of medical care, *Milbank Q* 44:166-206, 1966.

Donabedian A: Some issues in evaluating the quality of nursing care, *Am J Public Health* 59:1833-1836, 1969.

Donabedian A: The quality of care: how can it be assessed? *JAMA* 260:1743-1748, 1988.

Donabedian A: *Models of quality assurance*, materials prepared for the Eighth National Nursing Symposium on Home Health Care, The University of Michigan School of Nursing, Ann Arbor, Mi., June 1993.

Donabedian A: Models of quality assurance. In Schmele JA: *Quality management in nursing and health care*, Albany, N.Y., 1996, Delmar, pp. 88-103.

Finnigan SA, Abel M, Dobler T et al: Automated patient acuity: linking nursing systems and quality measurement with patient outcomes, *JONA* 23:62-71, 1993.

Freund DA, Lewit EM: Managed care for children and pregnant women: promises and pitfalls, *The Future of Children* 3(2):92-122, 1993.

Friedman C, Chenoweth C: Infection control. In Schmele JA: *Quality management in nursing and health care*, Albany, N.Y., 1996, Delmar, pp. 507-519.

Gardner MS: Typewritten remiscences, Feb. 5, 1948, NOPHN Archive Microfilm #25. In Fitzpatrick ML, ed: *The National Organization for Public Health Nursing 1912-1952: development of a practice field*, New York, 1975, National League for Nursing, p. 17.

Gaucher E, Kratochwill EW: The leader's role in implementing total quality management, *Quality Manage Health Care* 1:10-18, 1993.

Hardy JA: A patient classification system for home health patients, *Caring* 3(9):26-27, 1984.

Harris MD: *Home health administration*, Owings Mills, Md., 1988, National Health Publishing.

Harris MD, Santoferraro C, Silva S: A patient classification system in home health care, *Nurs Economics* 3:276-282, 1985.

Hays BJ: Nursing care requirements and resources consumption in home health care, *Nurs Res* 41(3):138-143, 1992.

Hays BJ, Kroeger RA, Tachenko-Achord SA, Peters DA: Determining intensity of need of high-risk maternal and infant clients, *J Nurs Care Qual* 9(2):67-75, 1995.

Hoesing H, Kirk R: Common sense quality management, *JONA* 20(10):10-15, 1990.

Joint Commission on Accreditation of Healthcare Organizations (JCAHO): *Quality assurance in home care and hospice organizations*, Oakbrook Terrace, Il., 1990a, JCAHO.

Joint Commission on Accreditation of Healthcare Organizations (JCAHO): *Primer on indicator development and application: measuring quality in health care*, Oakbrook Terrace, Il., 1990b, JCAHO.

Joint Commission on Accreditation of Healthcare Organizations (JCAHO): *Transitions: from QA to CQI—using CQI approaches to monitor, evaluate, and improve quality*, Oakbrook Terrace, Il., 1991, JCAHO.

Joint Commission on Accreditation of Healthcare Organizations (JCAHO): *The measurement mandate: on the road to performance improvement in health care*, Oakbrook Terrace, Il., 1993, JCAHO.

Joint Commission on Accreditation of Healthcare Organizations (JCAHO): *Framework for improving performance: from principles to practice*, Oakbrook Terrace, Il., 1994, JCAHO.

Joint Commission on Accreditation of Healthcare Organizations (JCAHO): CAMHC: *1997-98 comprehensive accreditation manual for home care*, Oakbrook Terrace, Il., 1996, JCAHO.

Katz JM, Green E: *Managing quality: a guide to system-wide performance management in health care*, ed 2, St. Louis, 1997, Mosby.

Knapp MB: Legal concerns affecting nonprofit community agencies that serve the elderly, *Quality Rev Bull* 15(3):86-91, 1989.

Koch MW, Fairly TM: *Integrated quality management: the key to improving nursing care quality*, St. Louis, 1993, Mosby.

Lawniczak J: Can managed care save Medicare? *Caring* 15:24-29, 1995.

Lohr KN, ed: *Medicare: a strategy for quality assurance*, vol 1, Washington, D.C., 1990, National Academy Press.

Lummis M: The quality improvement movement: an epidemiologist's viewpoint. In Schmele JA: *Quality management in nursing and health care*, Albany, N.Y., 1996, Delmar, pp. 158-173.

Lysaught JP: *An abstract for action*, New York, 1970, McGraw-Hill.

Managed care's conflicts of interest, *Caring* 14:4, 1995.

Marrelli TM: The relationship between quality and accreditation, *T.M. Marrelli's Home Care Nurse News* 1(1):1-2, 1994.

Martin KS, Scheet NJ: *The Omaha System: a pocket guide for community health nursing*, Philadelphia, 1992, Saunders.

McKeon T: Benchmarks and performance indicators: two tools for evaluating organizational results and continuous quality improvement efforts, *J Nurs Care Qual* 10(3):12-17, 1996.

McLaughlin CP, Kaluzny AD: Total quality management in health: making it work, *Health Care Manage Rev* 15:7-14, 1990.

Melum MM, Sinioris ME: Total quality management in health care: taking stock, *Quality Manage Health Care* 1(4):59-63, 1993.

Milakovich ME: Creating a total quality health care environment, *Health Care Manage Rev* 16:9-20, 1991.

Mills MEC: Some implications of CQI for nursing administration. In Dienemann J: *CQI: continuous quality improvement in nursing*, Washington, D.C., 1992, American Nurses Publishing, pp. 31-43.

Mold JW, Knapp KR: Interdisciplinary teamwork. In Schmele JA: *Quality management in nursing and health care*, Albany, N.Y., 1996, Delmar, pp. 125-140.

Mullins D, Schmele JA: Reconsideration of the quality circle process as a contemporary management strategy, *Health Care Superv* 12:14-22, 1993.

National League for Nursing (NLN), Council of Home Health Agencies and Community Health Services: *Administrator's handbook for the structure, operation and expansion of home health agencies*, New York, 1985, NLN.

O'Leary DS: CQI—a step beyond QA, *Quality Review Bull* 17(1):4-5, 1991.

Papers on the National Health Guidelines: *Baselines for setting health goals and standards*, DHEW Pub No. HRA 77-640, Washington, D.C., 1977, Health Resources Administration.

Peters DA, Eigsti D: Utilizing outcomes in home care, *Caring* 10:44-51, 1991.

Peters DA: A new look for quality in home care, *JONA* 22:11-26, 1992.

Pew Health Professions Commission: *Critical challenges: revitalizing the health professions for the twenty-first century*, San Francisco, 1995, UCSF Center for the Health Professions.

Reed PG, Zurakowski TL: Nightingale: foundations of nursing. In Fitzpatrick JJ, Whall AL: *Conceptual models of nursing: analysis and application*, ed 3, Stamford, Ct., 1996, Appleton & Lange, pp. 27-54.

Saba VK, McCormick KA: *Essentials of computers for nurses*, ed 2, New York, 1996, McGraw-Hill.

Schmele JA, Donabedian A: The application of a model to measure the quality of nursing care in home health. In Schmele JA: *Quality management in nursing and health care*, Albany, N.Y., 1996, Delmar, pp. 375-394.

Schmele JA: *Quality management in nursing and health care*, Albany, N.Y., 1996, Delmar.

Sienkiewicz JI: Patient classification in community health nursing, *Nurs Outlook* 32:319-321, 1984.

Smith HL, Discenza R, Piland NF: Reflections on total quality management and health care supervisors, *Health Care Superv* 12:32-45, 1993.

Swansburg RC: *Management and leadership for nurse managers*, ed 2, Boston, 1996, Jones & Bartlett.

Tehan J, Colegrove SL: Risk management and home health care: the time is now. In Fisher K, Gardner K, eds: *Quality and home health care: redefining the tradition*, Chicago, 1987, JCAHO.

Tilbury MS: From QA to CQI: a retrospective review. In Dienemann J, ed: *CQI: continuous quality improvement in nursing*, Washington, D.C., 1992, American Nurses Publishing, pp. 3-14.

U.S. Department of Health and Human Services (USDHHS): *Healthy people 2000: national health promotion and disease prevention objectives, full report, with commentary*, Washington, D.C., 1991, U.S. Government Printing Office.

Wagner PS: Guide to identifying, collecting, and managing data. In Schmele J: *Quality management in nursing and health care*, Albany, N.Y., 1996, Delmar, pp. 408-458.

Zlotnick C: A public health quality assurance system, *Public Health Nurs* 9(2):133-137, 1992.

SELECTED BIBLIOGRAPHY

Agency for Health Care Policy and Research: *Report to Congress: progress of research on outcomes of health care services and procedures*, Rockville, Md., 1991, The Agency.

Al-Assaf AF, Schmele JA, eds: *The textbook of total quality in healthcare*, Delray Beach, Fl., 1993, St. Lucie Press.

Berwick DM, Godfrey AB, Roessner J: *Caring health care: new strategies for quality improvement*, San Francisco, 1990, Jossey-Bass.

Bryant JM, Field MR, Schaedler P: Risk management. In Schmele JA: *Quality management in nursing and health care*, Albany, N.Y., 1996, Delmar, pp. 520-538.

Camp RC, Tweet AG: Benchmarking applied to health care, *J Qual Improvement* 20:229-238, 1994.

Carlin E, Carlson R, Nordin J: Using continuous quality improvement tools to improve pediatric immunization rates, *J Qual Improvement* 22(4):277-288, 1996.

Carter JH, Meridy H: Making a performance improvement plan work, *J Qual Improvement* 22(2):104-113, 1996.

Ceglarek JE, Rife JK: Developing a public health nursing audit, *J Nurs Adm* 10:37-43, 1977.

Davis ER: *Total quality management for homecare*, Gaithersburg, Md., 1994, Aspen.

Field MJ: *Setting priorities for clinical practice guidelines*, Washington, D.C., 1995, National Academy Press.

Flynn BC, Ray DW: Current perspectives in quality assurance and community health nursing, *J Community Health Nurs* 4:187-197, 1987.

Friedman MM: Designing an infection control program to meet JCAHO standards, *Caring* 15(7):18-25, 1996.

Harrington C: Quality, access, and costs: public policy and home health care, *Nurs Outlook* 36:164-166, 1988.

Harris MD, Dugan M: Evaluating the quality of home care services using patient outcome data, *Home Healthc Nurse* 14:463-468, 1996.

Hodges LC, Icenhour MC, Tate S: Measuring quality. In McCloskey J, Grace HK, eds: *Current issues in nursing*, ed 4, St. Louis, 1994, Mosby.

Lang NM, Clinton JF: Assessment of quality of nursing care. In Werley HH, Fitzpatrick JJ, eds: *Annual review of nursing research*, vol 2, New York, 1984, Springer.

McLaughlin C, Kaluzny A: *Continuous quality improvement in health care: theory, implementation, and applications*, Gaithersburg, Md., 1994, Aspen.

Rantz M: Quality measurement in nursing: Where are we now? *J Nurs Care Qual* 9(2):1-7, 1995.

Rice R, Jordan J: Implementing an infection control program for the community-based healthcare facility, *JONA* 22:18-22, 1992.

Seago ML, Conn CD: Outcome-based quality improvement demonstration, *Caring* 15(6):67, 1996.

25

Challenges for the Future

Objectives

Upon completion of this chapter, the reader should be able to:

1. Analyze societal trends that will influence community health nursing practice in the twenty-first century.
2. Articulate competencies for nursing practice in the coming century.
3. Discuss evolving ethical issues in community health nursing practice.
4. Identify the importance of nursing research in promoting the health of the nation.
5. Explain how political involvement can shape the health care delivery system.
6. Discuss the concept of health care for all.

We are made wise not by the recollections of our past but by the responsibilities for our future.

GEORGE BERNARD SHAW

Diversity and change will be the driving forces for the profession in the coming millennium, and these will be fueled by other trends that will continue to blossom well into the twenty-first century. The profession is at a fork in the road where it must respond to the first major restructuring of the U.S. health care system and the enormous implication this has for nursing (Scott, 1993). Concurrently, the profession is faced with unprecedented societal changes that are significantly influencing client need and client-provider relationships. Clearly the environment is calling for innovation in service delivery and a reformulation of health care provider roles.

SOCIETAL TRENDS

Many new things are occurring in the world today. Among these are altered demographics, increasing globalization, a knowledge explosion, technological innovation, and increasing consumer involvement (Brownson, Kreuter, 1997; Parks, 1997). "To be competitive in a rapidly changing environment will require an unprecedented understanding of changing health care markets, the need for developing new global competencies and capabilities, and a shift from tangible assets to an appreciation of the value of knowledge and technology" (Parks, p. 1).

Demographics

Changing demographics will have a profound effect on community health nursing service delivery in the coming century. Significant shifts in the age structure of the population, increasing diversity among Americans, and changing family patterns will influence both client need and service delivery strategies.

There is no debate about the graying of American society. Between 1900 and 1994 the elderly population increased 11-fold, compared with only a 3-fold increase for the younger population (U.S. Bureau of the Census, 1996). "Growth in the elderly population in the United States has outpaced the non-elderly since 1900, and is projected to continue through the middle of the next century: by 2040 . . . one in every five Americans will be 65 years or older" (Institute for Health and Aging, 1996). The continuing aging of our society will shift the emphasis of service delivery from acute to chronic care. This shift will require the development of "new and effective interventions for promoting healthy lifestyles among the elderly to improve quality of life and reduce the complications due to disabling conditions" (Brownson, Kreuter, 1997, p. 57).

There is also no debate about the growing ethnic diversity among the young as well as the old in America. Changes in immigration laws since the mid-1960s and differential fertility rates and age distribution patterns among minority groups have dramatically altered the ethnic mix in the United States (Day, 1993). It is projected that this trend will continue throughout the coming century. By the year 2050 the non-Hispanic white share of the U.S. population is projected to steadily fall from 76% in 1990 to 53% in 2050. The fastest-growing ethnic group (with the highest rate of increase) will be the Asian and Pacific Islander population, while the ethnic group adding the largest number of people to the population will be the Hispanic-origin population (Day). The practitioner of the future will need substantive transcultural knowledge to achieve favorable health outcomes (Leininger, 1997). There will be an increased need for health care providers to understand the most relevant health risks among differing ethnic populations and to develop culturally relevant interventions to address these risks (Marín, Burhansstipanov, Connell et al, 1995). Segments of ethnic minority populations continue to rely heavily on nontraditional healing alternatives. The continuing challenge for the twenty-first century will be to bridge the cultural gap between traditional and nontraditional medicine.

Continuing shifts in family patterns and the growing income inequality among American families will also present service delivery challenges in the coming century. With an increasing number of women entering the workforce, child and elder care arrangements are becoming more complex. This could provide the opportunity for community health nurses to develop specialized clinical niches, such as day care centers for ill children who cannot attend school or case management services for elderly clients who want to live independently in their own homes.

Although many dual-income families may be increasingly able to purchase needed health care services, the growing income inequality between the rich and poor is likely to continue in the coming century. This, coupled with the fact that many places of employment are no longer providing health care benefits, will make it difficult for vulnerable populations to access essential health care services. The community health nurse will continue to play a pivotal role in linking persons to essential personal health services in the twenty-first century.

Increasing Globalization

The globalization movement has brought both challenges and opportunities for the health care provider worldwide. "As free trade increasingly becomes a reality, free exchange of ideas and information between [professional] communities is increasingly becoming a reality" (Parks, Bajus, 1994, p. 783). This allows care providers to move more quickly in solving worldwide health problems. It permits strategic brokering, that is, connecting people who can solve problems with those who can identify them (Reich, 1991). This promotes collective action for community health.

Preventing the spread of disease, preserving the environment, and reducing poverty will be major worldwide challenges in the future. As we move toward a global society, the link between poverty, health disparities, and environmental degradation has become increasingly apparent (Hudson-Rodd, 1994). It also has become readily apparent that immigration, international travel, and free trade among nations fuel the spread of new and re-emerging infectious diseases (CDC, 1994). In the past 20 years at least 30 new infectious diseases have been identified internationally, and this number is projected to increase in the future (Seymour, 1997). The renewed interest in strengthening the international public health surveillance system will continue in the coming century.

An Explosion of Knowledge and Information Technology

In a world where knowledge doubles every 5 years (Society for Healthcare Planning and Marketing, 1995), it is imperative for health care professions to develop strategies for lifelong learning to prevent knowledge obsolescence. Additionally, "to remain a vital part of a complex, managed, information driven system, health professionals must be able to manage and use the large volumes of scientific, technological, and patient information in a way that helps them deliver effective clinical care in the context of community and system needs" (Pew Health Professions Commission, 1995, p. 6). Fortunately, the proliferation of information technologies will continue to provide exciting opportunities for self-renewal as well as for developing new approaches to health care delivery (Brownson, Kreuter, 1997). Interactive multimedia systems will help people "to learn anything, anytime, anywhere" (Halal, Liebowitz, 1994, p. 21).

Milio (1995), a nursing leader in the field of community health, is challenging public health professionals to move beyond informatics and create an electronic community infrastructure that provides worldwide linkages between international, national, and local governmental and community organizations. She proposes that such a structure would allow health care professionals to provide information and referral services to local residents and clients, promote awareness and understanding of major health problems among community citizens and policymakers, and support worldwide cooperative efforts focused on the early identification of health concerns and solutions to address these concerns. Community health professionals will increasingly develop health-related partnerships to pursue powerful goals aimed at developing healthy, healing communities.

Technological Innovation

In addition to information technology, numerous technological advances, such as virtual reality, robotics, and telemedicine/telenursing will continue to expand and significantly influence community health nursing service delivery in the future. For example, home telemedicine systems are currently allowing nurses in some settings to make a "video visit" to a client's home. It is projected that these systems will become common in many local communities and will have the potential to improve and expand care to vulnerable populations. Additionally, they have the potential to reduce costs in a managed care environment (Mahmud, Lenz, 1995).

Of all the technologies affecting the health care system in the future, the greatest impact will come from telematics (Bezold, 1987, p. 78). The field of telematics includes diagnostic software, record keeping, and the communication of knowledge about health care and individual client observations to almost anywhere in the world. Telematics also has the capability of developing a client profile that includes biochemical definitions of illness, health, and wellness for that person. Medical recordkeeping will continue to become more sophisticated, and systems will be able to monitor the outcomes of different modalities of care.

Telematics will allow consumers to be involved both in their own health care and in monitoring the outcomes produced by various providers. Therapies, including drugs, that are deemed to be successful or unsuccessful will be quickly apparent to the public. However, the use of telematics is not risk free. Questions of privacy, accuracy, and liability will become paramount for ethics committees in health care organizations, as well as for consumers who are currently demanding to become more involved in their own care.

Increasing Consumer Involvement

The twenty-first century will prove itself as the *golden era* of the consumer. Currently, sophisticated consumers are demanding more say in health care decision making and are being encouraged by health care providers to actively participate on the health care team. As information technology becomes more prevalent in the home and other settings such as public libraries, churches, and community centers, observers will witness a geometrical acceleration of this trend. Consumers will be able to readily access information needed to effectively solve problems about personal health issues as well as community health concerns. Governmental officials are already using electronic town hall meetings to seek citizen input about issues critical to the health of the nation. Electronic town hall meetings are the wave of the future (Snider, 1994), and they will greatly facilitate politicians' efforts to assess health needs. This in turn will help policymakers to make more knowledgeable judgments about critical health policy issues.

Community health professionals have actively promoted the position that the consumer should be the central focus in the new health care delivery system. "Public health, in a reformed health care system, will forge partnerships between communities and all levels of government. Communities and public health agencies—together—will keep the public healthy" (APHA, 1993, unnumbered forward). Community partnerships are advancing community development efforts as well as community action for health. Provider organizations are working with communities as partners to solve health concerns and to create environments that prevent health problems. These endeavors will grow in the future (Brownson, Kreuter, 1997).

As educated consumers become increasingly focused on health promotion and risk-reduction activities to improve their quality of life, community health nurses will assume a pivotal role in helping clients to promote health and prevent disease. Community health nurses are uniquely positioned to address preventive health care concerns and to facilitate self-care among a variety of client groups. Future advances in information technology will strengthen nurses' ability to help clients readily access essential health information and develop creative approaches to health education. The challenge for all health care providers will be to effectively and efficiently use technology to benefit diverse client groups, including the "haves" and the "have nots."

COMPETENCIES FOR NURSING PRACTICE IN THE TWENTY-FIRST CENTURY

In response to changing societal trends, the health care delivery system has undergone dramatic change, and this change will be even more encompassing in the twenty-first century. The health care practitioner in the future will be functioning in a highly integrated, managed care environment focused on delivering cost-effective, high-quality, community-based services. As the health care environment continues to change, community health nurses will be trailblazers in developing models for interdisciplinary care in a variety of community settings (Ferretti, Verhey, Isham, 1996). It is envisioned that schools, neighborhood clinics, work sites, and other community settings will become practice sites for providing holistic family- and population-focused care. The concept of neighborhood nursing is reemerging. "Neighborhood nursing is grounded in the public health nursing mission of promoting healthy communities by collaborating with consumers where they live, work, and go to school" (Reinhard, Christopher, Mason et al, 1996, p. 223).

Health care practitioners of tomorrow will need a number of skills to remain competitive in the evolving health care environment. The general consensus is that practitioners of the future need strong critical thinking skills to assist them with problem identification and problem solving (Bennison, 1996; Ibrahim, House, Levine, 1995; Misener, Alexander, Blaha et al, 1997; Reich, 1991). Having these skills helps the practitioner anticipate and plan for the future. It is also generally believed that health professionals will need effective communication skills; cultural skills; political competencies; business, management, and leadership skills; and lifelong learning skills. From a community health nursing perspective, the practitioner will need a strong knowledge base from nursing, social, and public health sciences (APHA, 1996).

The Pew Health Professions Commission (O'Neil, 1993; Pew Health Professions Commission, 1995; Shugars, O'Neil, Bader, 1991) argues that health care practitioners of tomorrow must have new attitudes as well as expanded skills to meet society's evolving health care needs. The specific competencies recommended by this Commission are identified in the box on the next page. These competencies highlight the need for health care professionals to shift their focus from acute, disease-oriented health care delivery to an "increased reliance on primary care, disease prevention and cost containment" (Pew Health Professions Commission, 1995, p. 1). They also reflect a need to remain committed

Competencies Needed by Practitioners for 2005

PRACTITIONERS FOR 2005 SHOULD:

- Care for the Community's Health
- Expand Access to Effective Care
- Provide Contemporary Clinical Care
- Emphasize Primary Care
- Participate in Coordinated Care
- Ensure Cost-Effective and Appropriate Care
- Practice Prevention
- Involve Patients and Families in the Decision-Making Process
- Promote Healthy Lifestyles
- Assess and Use Technology Appropriately
- Improve the Health Care System
- Manage Information
- Understand the Role of the Physical Environment
- Provide Counseling on Ethical Issues
- Accommodate Expanded Accountability
- Participate in a Racially and Culturally Diverse Society
- Continue to Learn

From Shugars DA, O'Neil EH, Bader JD, eds: *Healthy America: practitioners for 2005, an agenda for action for U.S. health professional schools*, Durham, N.C., 1991, The Pew Health Professions Commission, p. x.

to the ethical tenets of the profession while appreciating the value of knowledge and technology.

ETHICS IN COMMUNITY HEALTH NURSING PRACTICE

Rapid changes in the health care delivery system have made life more complex and have provoked dilemmas never before faced by consumers or health care providers. It is becoming increasingly difficult for professionals in many situations to discern what should or should not be done. Chapter 10 presents a scenario demonstrating some of the questions raised by the participants in sophisticated health care of a child; should a child have to live his or her life in a hospital? Is such a life of enough quality to make it meaningful? Is the terrible expense for the care of one such child possible, and what will happen when increasing numbers of children need the same care? How justly are the rest of the children in the family being treated when one family member consumes so much time?

The ability to preserve lives that once could not be saved, advances in information technology, and governmental cutbacks in health care spending have made it increasingly difficult for community health nurses to examine the concept of human rights and choices. Community health nurses must now make decisions about how to protect client rights on the information superhighway, whose rights prevail, and which client they should serve when resources are not sufficient for meeting the needs of *all* client groups. They must also examine how their choices about the delivery of health care services have affected various consumers and consumer groups. It is anticipated that these issues will intensify in the future and that new ethical issues will emerge (Kidder, 1995). A recent survey conducted by The Electronic Privacy Information Center (Kalish, 1997), for example, reflects an urgent need to establish procedures for protecting the privacy of computer users. The Federal Trade Commission is currently conducting hearings to determine whether the computer industry can police itself or whether government regulation is needed to protect personal computer users. Gaining an understanding of ethics can help nurses better deal with these complex and often confusing practice issues.

Ethics is the study of choices made by individuals and groups in their relationships with one another. The development of a code of ethics is basic to a profession because it provides a means for that profession to regulate its practice. It also helps its members make choices relative to clinical practice concerns.

> A code indicates a profession's acceptance of the responsibility and trust with which it has been invested by society. Upon entering the profession of nursing, each person inherits a measure of the responsibility and trust that has accrued to nursing over the years and the corresponding obligation to adhere to the profession's code of conduct and relationships for ethical practice. (ANA, 1985)

The American Nurses Association adopted its code of ethics in 1950 and revises it periodically. The most recent revision was published in 1985. Professional codes of ethics are statements encompassing rules that apply to persons in professional roles and that are *voluntarily* adopted by the group themselves (Beauchamp, Childress, 1994). Many national organizations involved in promoting quality health and health related services have developed a code of ethics for their membership. These codes are designed to preserve the basic rights of clients in an honest and ethical manner.

Implicit in codes of ethics are several fundamental principles. The general consensus is that health care professions have a responsibility to respect a client's right of self-determination in decision making *(autonomy)*, to do good *(beneficience)*, to avoid harm *(nonmaleficience)*, and to act fairly *(justice)* when allocating health care resources (Beauchamp, Childress, 1994). Hayne, Moore, and Osborne (1990) argue that nursing ethics is at a turning point and that the profession needs to understand the ethic of caring as well as the ethic of justice. The care-based approach to ethical inquiry focuses on the nurse-client relationship and the moral obligation of the professional to protect and promote the well-being of clients in a compassionate and empathic manner (Lowdermilk, Perry, Bobak, 1997). The value of caring in the nurse-client relationship is central to this approach. In the coming century increased emphasis will be placed on developing a theory of nursing ethics that delineates the uniqueness of ethics in the nurse-client relationship.

In a perfect world everyone's rights and choices are respected. However, in the real world some people are more respected than others (lawyers receive more respect than sanitation workers), and some people are often not respected at all (the poor and the disabled). Human choices are affected by one's attitude and environment. For example, some nurses believe that selective abortion should be the right of all women. Others believe, because of cultural influences or personal or religious beliefs, that abortion is categorically wrong. Changes in our society are making choices such as these much more difficult and are presenting ethical dilemmas for professionals in all health care settings.

In the community setting ethical dilemmas include multiple-option situations such as how to deal with conflicting needs of clients and caregivers, when to hospitalize a terminally ill client, resolving conflicts between what is ordered and what is needed, allowing "death with dignity," maintaining agency standards of productivity while competently meeting increasingly complex care needs of clients, giving pain medication even if early death might be an unavoidable consequence of pain control, and providing service based on payer regulations (Lund, 1989; Michigan Home Health Association, 1990; Pignatello, Moulton, Eng, 1988). In the coming century community-based health care practitioners will increasingly need to address ethical challenges such as the rightness of shifting health care costs to informal care providers, the appropriate role of the family in medical decision making, and the fair distribution of the care burden in a family setting (Fleck, 1997).

What to do *when* (not if) an ethical crisis occurs is the key question the health care practitioner will be asking in the future (Clemen-Stone, 1997). Currently community health professionals are experiencing unprecedented demands and client care complexities on a daily basis. With the revolutionary changes occurring in the health care delivery system, there is no question that these demands and complexities will increase in the future and that most professionals will experience an ethical dilemma during their career.

"Practitioners of the future must be able to frame their work in ethically sensitive ways and provide education and counseling for patients, families, and communities in situations where ethical issues arise" (Pew Health Professions Commission, 1995, p. 6). Community health organizations are increasingly establishing ethics committees to help practitioners carry out this responsibility (Abel, 1990; D'Olimpio, 1995; Skipper, 1992). Ethics committees play a key role in promoting an understanding of ethical practice through education, consultation, and the development of standards for ethical practice. "Regardless of the setting, the primary purpose of ethics committees is to provide a structural format for individuals within an organization to increase their awareness of ethics and its application to clinical practice" (Haddad, 1992, pp. 8, 10). Ethics committees play a vital role in helping practitioners to resolve ethical dilemmas. This role will become more paramount in the coming century.

Dubler (1993) writes compellingly on the need to bring clients' preferences and rights, family concerns, legal rules, and ethical principles into harmony in the coming decade. As health care delivery shifts from the institution to the community, this will be a critical challenge for community health nurses. Health care reform efforts focused on cost containment will also present a critical need to monitor carefully clinical service delivery from an ethical perspective. There is a significant potential for unethical practice when a professional is influenced by a cost containment arrangement. Acts of omission could be particularly problematic in these types of arrangements.

"The most pressing issues facing health care reform and change are fundamental concerns having to do with how social resources are spent, how decisions are made, how individuals take responsibility for their health and what role society plays in ensuring against risk" (Pew Health Professions Commission, 1995, p. 6). All of these issues have a potential for creating ethical conflicts. Recent debates about health care rationing have already caused significant ethical distress among health care providers, the lay public, and policy makers. Challenges such as these will intensify in the future and will require all the involved participants to make a morally and emotionally responsible judgment (Yankelovich, 1992).

The critical ethical concern for community health nurses in the future will be to ensure that cost-effective, quality health care is available to people in need. To achieve this goal, practitioners of the future must analyze social and health care situations from an ethical perspective that addresses community as well as individual needs. Practitioners will also need to shape health policy through research and political action. Health care reform will not evolve from interventions focused on individuals. Strong, collective community action for health, supported by sound research and health policy, is needed to resolve the nation's current health crises.

NURSING RESEARCH

Better health through nursing research was the theme of the 1996 International Nurses' Day (Holzemer, Tierney, 1996). The focus on this day was to highlight the fact that nursing care can make significant, cost-effective contributions that improve the quality of people's lives. This will be the continuing challenge for practitioners in the coming century. To remain competitive in the evolving health care system, professionals will need to demonstrate that they can provide high-quality, cost-effective care that is measurable (Hadley, 1996). Demonstrating the outcomes of health promotion interventions will be particularly challenging for nurses in the future.

The nursing profession has actively promoted the position that nurses must engage in research to enhance the health of the nation. "The National Institute of Nursing Research (1995) supports research on the biological and

Mandates for the National Institute of Nursing Research

- Reduce the burden of illness and disability by understanding and easing the effects of acute and chronic illness;
- Improve health-related quality of life by preventing or delaying the onset of disease or slowing its progression;
- Establish better approaches to promoting health and preventing disease; and
- Improve clinical environments by testing interventions that influence patient health outcomes and reduce costs and demand for care.

From National Institute of Nursing Research (NINR): *Mission statement*, Bethesda, Md., 1995, NINR.

behavioral aspects of critical health problems that confront the Nation (see the box above). Particular emphasis is placed on subsets of the population who have special health problems and needs, such as older people, women, minorities, and residents of rural areas" (p. 1). Nursing research priorities resulting from the second conference on research priorities in nursing practice are displayed in the following box. An example of a current National Institute of Nursing Research (NINR) initiative is the research funded by NINR to examine safe recovery after shortened hospitalization. This research is demonstrating "that a model consisting of a carefully planned hospital early discharge program with follow-up care in the home by nurse specialists can result in improved recovery of patients at substantially reduced health care costs" (NINR, 1996, p. 8).

Community health nursing, by definition, deals with vulnerable populations that have special health problems and needs. Thus nurses in this practice area are uniquely positioned to identify significant, researchable questions related to NINR's research priorities. Nurses at all levels of practice are needed to identify relevant research issues and to document outcomes of nursing practice.

Priorities Resulting from Second Conference on Research Priorities in Nursing Practice National Center for Nursing Research

1—COMMUNITY-BASED NURSING MODELS (1995)

Develop and test community-based nursing models designed to promote access to, utilization of, and quality of health services by rural and other underserved populations.

2—HEALTH-PROMOTING BEHAVIOR AND HIV/AIDS (1996)

Assess the effectiveness of bio-behavioral nursing interventions to foster health-promoting behaviors of individuals of different cultural backgrounds—especially women—who are at high risk for HIV/AIDS, incorporating bio-behavioral markers.

3—COGNITIVE IMPAIRMENT (1997)

Develop and test bio-behavioral and environmental approaches to remediating cognitive impairment.

4—LIVING WITH CHRONIC ILLNESS (1998)

Test interventions to strengthen individuals' personal resources in dealing with their chronic illness.

5—BIO-BEHAVIORAL FACTORS RELATED TO IMMUNOCOMPETENCE (1999)

Identify bio-behavioral factors and test interventions to promote immunocompetence.

From National Center for Nursing Research: *Priorities resulting from second conference on research priorities in nursing practice*, Bethesda, Md., February 1993, The Center.

POLITICAL INVOLVEMENT

The most powerful approach that nurses can take to shape the future is the political approach. It is vital that nurses understand, actively participate in, and provide leadership in politics and the political process. Nurses make up the largest group of health care providers in the country, and numbers alone give them a powerful majority. Today's nurses are becoming more politically active, visible, and powerful and are providing leadership in health care delivery. Practitioners in the future will need to expand their political involvement to ensure that people in need have consumer-accessible care.

Politics can be defined as the art of influencing the actions of others for the purposes of promoting specified goals and protecting one's interests (Kalisch, Kalisch, 1981). Political action usually involves activities directed toward influencing the behavior of governmental officials and other individuals in powerful positions. Politics and nursing are inseparable and, in fact, politics *is* an integral part of nursing. The relationship between federal legislation and health care (costs, programs, education, and services) cannot be denied. The federal government is heavily involved in health care and has a great influence on it through legislation and funding. The political arena is where health care decisions are made, decisions that will bear on health care for all of us.

"The nursing profession has a long history of political activism that has been heightened in recent years through the politics of health care reform" (Cohen, Mason, Kouner et al, 1996, p. 259). Nursing's political involvement in health action has evolved through several stages (Table 25-1) and reflects a movement from a reactive stance to a proactive stance. It has progressed from the "buy in," or stage of awareness where the profession recognized the importance of political activism, to the stage of political sophistication where nursing has gone beyond self-interest and is proactively campaigning on behalf of the public. The challenge for the future will be to "lead the way" in health care policy. At this stage, "nurses become the initiators of crucial health policy ideas and innovations as instigators,

table 25-1 THE PROGRESS OF NURSING THROUGH FOUR STAGES OF POLITICAL DEVELOPMENT

	STAGE 1 (BUY-IN)	STAGE 2 (SELF-INTEREST)	STAGE 3 (POLITICAL SOPHISTICATION)	STAGE 4 (LEADING THE WAY)
Nature of action	Reactive, with a focus on nursing issues	Reactive to nursing issues (e.g., funding for nursing education) and broader issues (e.g., long-term care and immunizations)	Proactive on nursing and other health issues (e.g., Nursing's Agenda for Health Care Reform)	Proactive on leadership and agenda-setting for a broad range of health and social policy issues
Language	Learning political language	Using nurse jargon (e.g., caring, nursing diagnosis)	Using parlance and rhetoric common to health policy deliberations	Introducing terms that reorder the debate
Coalition building	Political awareness; occasional participation in coalitions	Coalition forming among nursing organizations	Coalition forming among nursing groups; active and significant participation in broader health care groups (e.g., Clinton task force on health care reform)	Initiating coalitions beyond nursing for broad health policy concerns
Nurses as policy shapers	Isolated cases of nurses being appointed to policy positions, primarily because of individual accomplishments	Professional associations get nurses into nursing-related positions	Professional organizations get nurses appointed to health-related policy positions (e.g., nurse position on ProPAC)	Many nurses sought to fill nursing and health policy positions because of value of nursing expertise and knowledge

From Cohen SS, Mason DJ, Kouner C et al: Stages of nursing's political development: where we've been and where we ought to go, *Nurs Outlook* 44:259-266, 1996, p. 260.

leaders, or formulators of health policy" (Cohen, Mason, Kouner et al, p. 263).

There are several different ways to achieve one's goals in the legislative arena (deVries, Vanderbilt, 1992). Nurses are actively involved in writing letters, sending telegrams, making phone calls, arranging meetings with officials and legislators, making political contributions, and attending political meetings. They are also involved in political campaign efforts aimed at helping a candidate get elected, in taking an active role in the political aspects of professional organizations, in lobbying, and in running for political office (Cohen, Mason, Kouner et al, 1996).

Individual and collective political action by nurses has significantly strengthened the political power of nursing. "By 1996, 71 nurses held elected positions in state legislatures, and many more were members of legislative staffs in Congress or state governments" (Cohen, Mason, Kouner et al, 1996, p. 262). In recent years nurses have also been appointed to high-level positions in federal agencies (Figure 25-1) and on federal panels.

Additionally, nurses now sit on local and state boards of health; in policy positions for local, state, national, and international governments and organizations; and in the executive offices of many corporations. Meyer (1992) has developed three case studies that demonstrate how nurses use the skills of the profession and the political process to produce change for themselves, nursing, and their patients. They are worth reviewing because they show how the political process is real and usable for all nurses.

HEALTH CARE FOR ALL: A MAJOR CHALLENGE FOR THE FUTURE

The American Public Health Association (APHA) has openly and aggressively championed the right to health care for all in the United States. This is a significant goal, but one that will take much time and effort to achieve. In 1963 President Lyndon Johnson shared with the American public that "Yesterday is not ours to recover but tomorrow is ours to win or lose." The battle to win in the twenty-first century is the health care system's ability to extend access to health care services and ultimately to improve the quality of life among Americans. We must move ahead to a better health care delivery system. We must focus on the future rather than lament about the past, and we must learn from our mistakes. Although data suggest that significant difficulties in our health care system presently prevent the nation from providing comprehensive health care, these obstacles can be overcome. The United States has had a long list of accomplishments in health care delivery and has a strong potential for achieving major public health accomplishments.

The twenty-first century will bring many health care challenges. "Health for all" in a managed care environment will be the major one. This will involve *taking action* to address emerging threats to the health of the public while

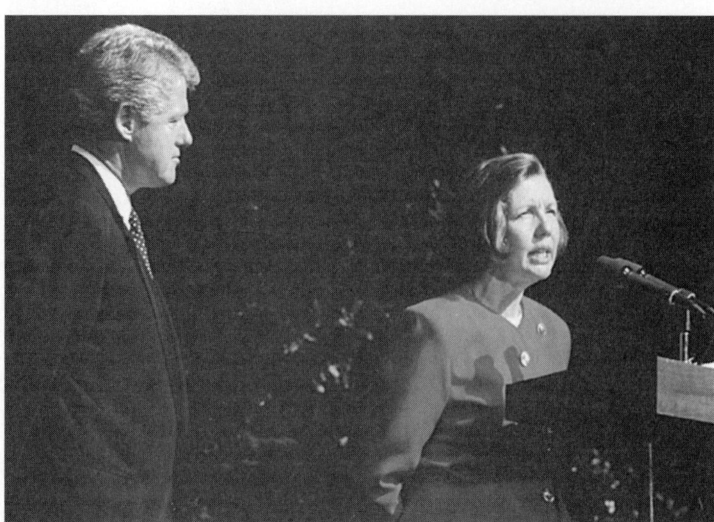

Figure 25-1 Kristine M. Gebbie accepted her appointment as AIDS Policy Coordinator while President Clinton looked on in 1993. While she is no longer in this position, it was significant to have a nurse appointed to a prominent federal-level health policy position.

containing continuing long-existing threats and health care costs. These threats include *immediate crises*, such as the AIDS epidemic and inadequate health care for disadvantaged aggregates; *enduring problems*, such as injuries, chronic illness, and infant mortality; and *impending crises* such as long-term care needs of populations across the life span and control of toxic wastes (Institute of Medicine, 1988, p. 1).

The "health for all" challenge emphasizes access to health care that will enable all people to lead productive and satisfying lives. It involves addressing the inequities in society and within the health care system that prevent people from achieving health, and it focuses on the shared responsibility of people for their own health. This battle requires implementing strategies that promote broad-based planning for health and development rather than for health services only. It demands a strong emphasis on political action, policy formulation, multidisciplinary practice, sound managerial functioning, and constituency building (Institute of Medicine, 1988; Maglacas, 1988). Constituency building is a "must." Current and future threats to our nation's public health will require collective action if they are to be resolved.

In 1993 100 years of public health/community health nursing was celebrated. This is a splendid opportunity to reflect on the rich heritage that Florence Nightingale, Lillian Wald, and many others provided for us. The health problems of today are much like the ones these women faced: communicable diseases, high infant mortality, and poverty. Wald and Nightingale viewed these problems as political ones, and emphasized that the public's health had to improve to change these problems. That fact is as true today as it was 100 years ago. Let us take on the mantle of developing a scientific basis for the nursing care of aggregates. Let us also use the stories of our sisters of the past to guide us in our future while recognizing that since our circumstances are new we must develop innovative population-focused interventions.

Summary

Community health professionals face many challenges. They are being asked to assume responsibility for care of unprecedented complexity and to plan services for multiple, diverse population groups. They must make some difficult decisions about the best means of allocating scarce resources, which often presents ethical dilemmas not easily solved. Competition has increased the number of selected types of community-based services, especially reimbursable home health care, but has not necessarily strengthened services for those most in need.

Sophisticated technology, spiraling health care costs, demographic changes, and increasing consumer involvement in health care decision making are dramatically influencing future directions in the health care delivery system. There is an increasing reliance on primary care, disease prevention, self-care, and cost containment. These trends present both challenges and opportunities for health care providers and consumers alike. To shape the future, health professionals must be risk takers. They must handle ethical dilemmas and engage in research activities to document the need for and the effectiveness of preventive health services, and they must be politically *active*. They must also develop new global competencies and capabilities and become technologically literate.

Let us as community health nurses think about the future so that we have the very best one possible! Let us follow Lillian Wald's ways and lead the way. Lillian Wald demonstrated the value of creating new practice roles and innovative service delivery strategies. That is our challenge for the twenty-first century.

CRITICAL *Thinking Exercise*

The accompanying A View from the Field is a news release about a nurse who was "the first nurse ever appointed director of a county health district in Texas . . ." (Mikulencak, 1993). The title of the article is "Public health stands as a proven model for future delivery systems." Do you believe this is feasible? Can community health nurses make a significant impact on the health care systems of this country? Justify your answers.

A View *from the* Field — PUBLIC HEALTH STANDS AS A PROVEN MODEL FOR FUTURE DELIVERY SYSTEMS

When Karen Wilson became the first nurse ever appointed director of a county health district in Texas, a headline in an area newspaper read "Nursing the Public Health."

The headline captures the essence of what many nurses feel is part of the solution to America's health care crisis—the utilization of public health nurses in existing public health structures.

"Public health nurses are experts at immunization, prenatal care, well child care, screening programs, outreach into the community, education—all that is critical in a health care reform package," said Wilson, MPH, MN, RN, who now directs a staff of 43 at the Williamson County and Cities Health District in Georgetown, Texas. "The emphasis must be reshifted to preventive care and early identification of problems, and that's been the business of public health for decades."

Mike Nilsson, RN, a public health nurse from Clearwater, Fla., firmly believes that the Administration's task force on health care reform must take into account a proven model of delivery.

"We don't need a new model. We know what works. We may fine tune it. We may upgrade it. We may computerize it. But the basis is there," he said. "I want Hillary's task force to come out and say that prevention is needed from the very beginning, and in order to make that work we're going to put 'x' amount of dollars, whether it's millions or billions or whatever, into rebuilding the public health system in this country."

Wilson believes that public health nurses should have a greater voice in health care reform discussions because of their expertise. She says that not only does the public health structure emphasize wellness and prevention, but it addresses issues of access and how to provide care to underserved populations. Ensuring access is a key tenet of *Nursing's Agenda for Health Care Reform* and continues to be one of the greatest challenges facing the President's Task Force on National Health Care Reform.

"Public health nurses just laugh when they hear that the new buzzwords are case management and care coordination because that's what public health nurses have done since day one. It's helping clients get into the health programs they need," Wilson said.

In Wilson's district, a case management team of nurses, social workers, nutrition staff and clerical staff meet often to solve problems jointly. Wilson notes that the "the more people who can form that safety net, the less likely that someone will fall through the cracks in the system."

Yet, often the groups who need health care the most will not seek it out in the present medical model of delivery, said Nilsson. "Before it was vogue, we were out in the minority communities, the communities with inadequate transportation, in the schools. We went into the homes to speak to teenagers and young women about prenatal and postnatal care or well-baby services. We discussed the whole spectrum of care."

Nilsson said, however, he has witnessed a "deterioration" of the public health system in his state and elsewhere due to a number of factors such as inadequate funding. "If the legislators and decision-makers don't value or understand prevention—if they don't see the value of public health nurses—they eliminate them." He said that legislators may not understand the "whole theory behind upfront prevention dollars—that it may take five years and cost in the short-term, but it will save you from spending thousands of dollars on the other end to take care of crack babies or a child who develops a chronic problem because of a measles outbreak."

Wilson said that current systems make it difficult for some populations to receive all the services they need—where clients must apply for Medicare and Medicaid in one office, health screenings in another office, and housing subsidies in still another location. She advocates a system where clients can "come in and tell their story one time to determine eligibility for a multiplicity of programs at once." A strength of public health nurses, she adds, is that they recognize the "needs of the whole person" and that some health care needs must wait until a family deals with more urgent social or survival needs.

Nilsson said that he hopes the administration recognizes the untapped resources of public health because "the potential is so great and we've got so much to offer."

"Our country has a lot of strong programs and a lot of experts" already available to address issues related to reform, Wilson added. "This doesn't have to be reinvented."

From Mikulencak M: Public health stands as a proven model for future delivery systems, *Am Nurse* 25(6):18, 1993.

REFERENCES

Abel PE: Ethics committees in home health agencies, *Public Health Nurs* 7:256-259, 1990.

American Nurses Association (ANA): *Code for nurses with interpretive statements*, ANA, Pub Code No. G-58, Kansas City, Mo., 1985, ANA.

American Public Health Association (APHA): *Public health in a reformed health care system: a vision for the future*, Washington, D.C., 1993, APHA.

American Public Health Association (APHA): Public Health Nursing Section: *The definition and role of public health nursing*, Washington, D.C., 1996, APHA.

Beauchamp T, Childress J: *Principles of biomedical ethics*, ed 4, New York, 1994, Oxford University Press.

Bennison K: Recommendations for the preferred future of nursing, *J Nurs Adm* 26:5-6, 1996.

Bezold C: Health trends and scenarios: implications for the health care professions. In Meyers JA, Lewin ME, eds: *Charting the future of health care: policy, politics, and public health*, Washington, D.C., 1987, American Enterprise Institute for Public Policy Research.

Brownson RC, Kreuter MW: Future trends affecting public health: challenges and opportunities, *J Public Health Management Practice* 3(2):49-60, 1997.

Centers for Disease Control and Prevention (CDC): *Addressing emerging infectious disease threats: a prevention strategy for the United States*, Atlanta, 1994, CDC.

Clemen-Stone S: What to do when (not if) an ethical crisis occurs, *Michigan Home Health Association News* 6:1-2, 1997.

Cohen SS, Mason DJ, Kouner C et al: Stages of nursing's political development: where we've been and where we ought to go, *Nurs Outlook* 44:259-266, 1996.

Day JC: *Population projections of the United States, by age, sex, race, and Hispanic origin: 1993 to 2050*, U.S. Bureau of the Census, current population reports, P25-1104, Washington, D.C., 1993, U.S. Government Printing Office.

deVries CM, Vanderbilt MC: *The grass roots lobbying handbook*, Washington, D.C., 1992, ANA.

D'Olimpio JT: The hospice ethics committee, *Caring* 14:31-34, 1995.

Dubler NN: Commentary: balancing life and death—proceed with caution, *Am J Public Health* 83(1):23-25, 1993.

Ferretti CK, Verhey MP, Isham MM: Development of a nurse-managed, school-based health center, *Nurs Educator* 21(5):35-42, 1996.

Fleck LM: Just caring: ethical issues in high-tech home care, *Michigan Home Health Association News* 6(2):1, 3, 7-10, 12, 1997.

Haddad AM: Developing an organizational ethos, *Caring* 11:4, 7-8, 10-11, 1992.

Hadley EH: Nursing in the political and economic marketplace: challenges for the 21st century, *Nurs Outlook* 44:6-10, 1996.

Halal WE, Liebowitz J: Telelearning: the multimedia revolution in education, *The Futurist* 28(6):21-26, 1994.

Hayne Y, Moore S, Osborne M: Nursing ethics: a turning point, *Nurs Forum* 25:10-12, 30, 1990.

Holzemer W, Tierney A: How nursing research makes a difference, *Int Nurs Rev* 43:49-52, 1996.

Hudson-Rodd N: Public health: people participating in the creation of healthy places, *Public Health Nurs* 11(2):119-126, 1994.

Ibrahim MA, House RM, Levine RH: Educating the public health workforce for the 21st century, *Fam Community Health* 18:17-25, 1995.

Institute for Health and Aging, University of California, San Francisco: *Chronic care in America: a 21st century challenge*, Princeton, N.J., 1996, Robert Wood Johnson Foundation.

Institute of Medicine: *The future of public health*, Washington, D.C., 1988, National Academy Press.

Kalisch BJ, Kalisch P: *Politics of nursing*, Philadelphia, 1981, Lippincott.

Kalisch P, Kalisch BJ: *The advance of American nursing*, ed 3, Boston, 1995, Little, Brown.

Kalish DE: Cyberspies often haunt web sites, survey says, *Ann Arbor News*, June 9, 1997, pp. A-1, A-12.

Kidder RM: Tough choices: why it's getting harder to be ethical, *The Futurist* 29(5):29-32, 1995.

Leininger M: Future directions in transcultural nursing in the 21st century, *Int Nurs Rev* 44:19-23, 1997.

Lowdermilk DL, Perry SE, Bobak IM: *Maternity and women's health care*, ed 6, St. Louis, 1997, Mosby.

Lund M: Nursing home dilemmas, *Geriatr Nurs* 10:298-300, 1989.

Maglacas AM: Health for all: nursing's role, *Nurs Outlook* 36:66-71, 1988.

Mahmud K, Lenz J: Personal telemedicine system: a new tool in the delivery of home care, *The Remington Report* 3(2):30-34, 1995.

Marín G, Burhansstipanov L, Connell CM et al: A research agenda for health education among underserved populations, *Health Educ Q* 22:346-363, 1995.

Meyer C: Nursing on the political front, *Am J Nurs* 92(10):56-64, 1992.

Michigan Home Health Association, Ethics Committee: *Ethical dilemmas experienced by professionals in home health care*, unpublished research project, East Lansing, Mi., 1990, The Association.

Mikulencak M: Public health stands as a proven model for future delivery systems, *Am Nurse* 25(6):18, 1993.

Milio N: Beyond informatics: an electronic community infrastructure for public health, *J Public Health Management Practice* 1(4):84-94, 1995.

Misener TR, Alexander JW, Blaha AJ et al: National delphi study to determine competencies for nursing leadership in public health, *Image J Nurs Sch* 29:47-51, 1997.

National Center for Nursing Research: *Priorities resulting from second conference on research priorities in nursing practice*, Bethesda, Md., February 1993, The Center.

National Institute of Nursing Research (NINR): *Mission statement*, Bethesda, Md., 1995, NINR.

National Institute of Nursing Research (NINR): *Planned initiative for 1997 and beyond*, Bethesda, Md., 1996, NINR.

O'Neil EH: *Health professions education for the future: schools in service to the nation*, San Francisco, 1993, The Pew Health Professions Commission.

Parks S: The future in dietetics. In Winterfeldt E, Ebro L, Bogle M: *The profession of dietetics: present practices, future trends*, Gaithersburg, Md., 1997, Aspen.

Parks S, Bajus B: Challenging the future—an evolving global perspective for the profession, *JADA* 94:782-784, 1994.

Parks S, Storey R, Bajus B: *Challenging the future: shaping food and nutrition choices for a healthier America*, Chicago, 1994, ADA.

Pew Health Professions Commission: *Critical challengers: revitalizing the health professions for the 21st century*, San Francisco, 1995, UCSF Center for the Health Professions.

Pignatello CH, Moulton P, Eng MA: Ethical concerns of home health administration: the day-to-day issues. In Harris MD, ed: *Home health administration*, Owings Mills, Md., 1988, National Health.

Reich RB: *The work of nations: preparing ourselves for 21st century capitalism*, New York, 1991, Alfred A. Knopf.

Reinhard SC, Christopher MA, Mason DJ et al: Promoting healthy communities through neighborhood nursing, *Nurs Outlook* 44:223-228, 1996.

Scott K: ANA: making health care reform work for all nurses, *Am Nurse* 25:1, 3, June 1993.

Seymour J: Old diseases, new danger, *Nurs Times* 93:22-24, 1997.

Shugars DA, O'Neil EH, Bader JD, eds: *Healthy America: practitioners for 2005, an agenda for action for U.S. health professional schools,* Durham, N.C., 1991, The Pew Health Professions Commission.

Skipper M: Launching an agency ethics committee, *Caring* 11:12-15, 1992.

Snider JH: Democracy on-line: tomorrow's election to electorate, *The Futurist* 28(5):15-19, 1994.

Society for Healthcare Planning and Marketing: *Environmental assessment, 1995-1996: renaissance for health care,* Chicago, 1995, American Hospital Association.

U.S. Bureau of the Census: 65 + *in the United States,* current population reports, Special Studies, P23-190, Washington, D.C., 1996, U.S. Government Printing Office.

Yankelovich D: How public opinion really works, *Fortune,* October 5, 1992, pp. 9-13.

SELECTED BIBLIOGRAPHY

Abrenheim JC, Moreno J, Zuckerman C: *Ethics in clinical practice,* Boston, 1994, Little, Brown.

Arras JD, Dubler NN: Bringing the hospital home, ethical and social implications of high-tech home care, *Hastings Cent Rep* 24(5): suppl, 519-528, 1994.

Campinha-Bacote J: The quest for cultural competence in nursing care, *Nurs Forum* 30(4):19-24, 1995.

Clarke HF, Beddome G, Whyte NB: Public health nurses' vision of their future reflects changing paradigms, *Image J Nurs Sch* 25(4): 305-309, 1993.

Collopy B, Dubler N, Zuckerman C: The ethics of home care, autonomy and accommodation, *Hastings Cent Rep* 20(2):Suppl, 1-16, 1990.

Fischer C: Information challenges of the integrated health care delivery system, *Remington Report* 5(2):24-25, 27, 1997.

Fletcher JC, Engelhard CL: Ethical issues in managed care, a report of the University of Virginia study group on managed care, *VMQ* 122(3):162-167, 1995.

Fry S: Dilemma in community health ethics, *Nurs Outlook* 31:176-179, 1983.

Fry S: Toward a theory of nursing ethics, *Adv Nurs Sci* 11(4):9-22, 1989.

Gordon RL, Baker EL, Roper WL, Omenn GS: Prevention and the reforming U.S. health care system: changing roles and responsibilities for public health, *Annu Rev Public Health* 17:489-509, 1996.

Hornblower M: Great expectations: Slackers? Hardly. The so-called Generation X turns out to be future go-getters who are just doing it—but their way, *Time* June 9, 1997, pp. 58-60.

Institute of Medicine: *2020 vision, health in the 21st century,* Washington, D.C., 1996, National Academy Press.

Kiernan MJ: *The eleven commandments of 21st century management,* Englewood Cliffs, N.J., 1996, Prentice Hall.

Livingston D, Oettinger E, Kenny D: *The Ethics Committee Handbook,* Seattle, 1996, Care Source.

Mahowald MB: So many ways to think, an overview of approaches to ethical issues in geriatrics, *Clin Geriatr Med* 10(3):403-418, 1994.

Milne TL: Toward a population focus: the transition of a local health department, *J Public Health Management Practice* 3(1):42-50, 1997.

Pearson TA, Spencer M, Jenkins P: Who will provide preventive services? The changing relationship between medical care systems and public health agencies in health care reform, *J Public Health Management Practice* 1(1):16-27, 1995.

Salmon ME: Public health policy: creating a healthy future for the American public, *Fam Community Health* 18(1):1-11, 1995.

The Commonwealth Fund: *Health care reform: what is at stake for women?* New York, 1994, The Fund.

Uphold CR, Graham MV: Schools as centers for collaborative services for families: a vision for change, *Nurs Outlook* 41:204-211, 1993.

Wetle T: A taxonomy of ethical issues in case management of the frail older person, *J Case Management* 1(3):71-75, 1992.

Williams CA: Beyond the Institute of Medicine report: a critical analysis and public health forecast, *Fam Community Health* 18(1): 12-23, 1995.

Appendix 1-1

Selected Significant CHN/PHN Leaders

Leader	Contributions
Clarissa (Clara) Barton (1821-1912)	The first woman to take to the battlefield as a volunteer nurse and relief worker during the Civil War; founder of the American Red Cross
Mary Beard (1876-1946)	One of the founders of the National Organization for Public Health Nursing; an advocate of preventive health services and a worker for the Rockefeller Foundation
Mary Breckinridge (1877-1965)	Founder of the Frontier Nursing Service, public pioneer in nurse-midwifery and in bringing modern nursing to rural America
Charity Collins (1882-*)	The first black public health school nurse in the country
Lavinia Lloyd Dock (1858-1956)	Helped develop the American Nurses Association; prolific author and educator; historian; advocate of social reform and women's rights
Ruth Freeman (1906-1982)	Nurse, educator, and author, using an interdisciplinary outlook that related academic work to the real world; prolific writer; worked to persuade personnel in public health to view nurses as team members
Mary Sewall Gardner (1871-1961)	Author of the first public health nursing text; founder of the National Organization for Public Health Nursing
Pearl McIver (1893-1976)	The first nurse on the staff of the U.S. Public Health Service, which she expanded into a modern and extensive agency to serve the needs of the U.S. public
Mary Adelaide Nutting (1858-1948)	First professor of nursing in an American university, occupying the first endowed chair in nursing; a reformer of nursing education
Margaret Sanger (1879-1966)	Pioneer in the birth control movement, launching the American Birth Control League, which became the Planned Parenthood Federation of America
Ada Mayo Stewart (1870-1945)	First occupational health nurse in the United States
Lina Rogers Struthers (1870-1946)	First school nurse in the United States, chosen by Lillian Wald while a nurse at the Henry Street Settlement House
Lillian Wald (1867-1940)	Leader of the public health nursing movement in the United States; developed the Henry Street Settlement House in New York and improved the lot of immigrants on the Lower East Side; established playgrounds for children who had none; placed the first nurse in a public school setting; developed innovative financing for nursing services; helped to found the National Child Labor Committee; formed the New York State Bureau of Industries and Immigrations and the Joint Board of Sanitary Control to enforce basic sanitary rules; helped develop the forerunner of the ACLU; prolific writer and teacher

Modified from Kaufman M, Hawkins WJ, Higgins LP, Friedman AH, eds: *Dictionary of American nursing biography*, Westport, Ct., 1988, Greenwood Press; and Kalisch P, Kalisch BJ: *The advance of American nursing*, ed 3, Boston, 1995, Little, Brown.
*Dates unknown.

Appendix 6-1

Federal Agencies Involved in Environmental Health: United States

DEPARTMENT OF AGRICULTURE
- U.S. Forest Service
- Soil conservation

DEPARTMENT OF COMMERCE
- Ocean research and monitoring

DEPARTMENT OF DEFENSE
- Pollution control in defense facilities

DEPARTMENT OF ENERGY
- Energy policy
- Nuclear energy

DEPARTMENT OF HEALTH AND HUMAN SERVICES
- National Institute of Environmental Health Services (publishes *Environmental Health Perspective*)
- *Healthy People* documents
- National Institute of Occupational Safety and Health
- Agency for Toxic Substances and Disease Registry
- Food and Drug Administration
- National Center for Environmental Health

DEPARTMENT OF HOUSING AND URBAN DEVELOPMENT
- Public housing
- Urban parks
- Urban planning

DEPARTMENT OF THE INTERIOR
- U.S. Fish and Wildlife Service
- National Wildlife Refuge System
- Public lands
- National parks

DEPARTMENT OF JUSTICE
- Environmental litigation

DEPARTMENT OF LABOR
- Occupational Safety and Health Administration

DEPARTMENT OF STATE
- International environmental health policy

DEPARTMENT OF TRANSPORTATION
- Monitors airplane noise
- Monitors oil pollution

COUNCIL ON ENVIRONMENTAL QUALITY
- Coordinates and monitors environmental policy

ENVIRONMENTAL PROTECTION AGENCY
- Primary agency in charge of protecting and enhancing the U.S. natural environment
- Enforces U.S. environmental health legislation
- Implements environmental research

FEDERAL EMERGENCY MANAGEMENT AGENCY
- Develops federal emergency response guidelines
- Works in cooperation with the American Red Cross

NUCLEAR REGULATORY COMMISSION
- Licensing and regulation of nuclear energy and power

TENNESSEE VALLEY AUTHORITY
- Electric power

NATIONAL LIBRARY OF MEDICINE
- Toxicology Data Network (TOXNET). A continuously available computerized system that includes:
  Hazardous Substance Data Bank
  Toxic Chemical Release Inventory
  Registry of Toxic Effects of Chemical Substances
  Chemical Carcinogenesis Research Information System
  Developmental and Reproductive Toxicology
  Environmental Teratology Information
  Environmental Mutagen Information

Modified from Sexton K, Perlin SA: The federal environmental health workforce in the United States, *Am J Public Health* 80(8):913-920, 1990; Office of the Federal Register: *U.S. Government Manual 1995-96*, Washington, D.C., 1995, U.S. Government Printing Office.

Appendix 7-1

Bloch's Ethnic/Cultural Assessment Guide

Categories	Guideline Questions/Instructions	Data Collected
CULTURAL		
Ethnic origin	Does the patient identify with a particular ethnic group (e.g., Puerto Rican, African)?	
Race	What is the patient's racial background (e.g., Black, Filipino, American Indian)?	
Place of birth	Where was the patient born?	
Relocations	Where has he or she lived (country, city)? During what years did patient live there and for how long? Has he or she moved recently?	
Habits, customs, values, and beliefs	Describe habits, customs, values, and beliefs patient holds or practices that affect his or her attitude toward birth, life, death, health and illness, time orientation, and health care system and health care providers. What is degree of belief and adherence by patient to his or her overall cultural system?	
Behaviors valued by culture	How does patient value privacy, courtesy, respect for elders, behaviors related to family roles and sex roles, and work ethics?	
Cultural sanctions and restrictions	*Sanctions*—What is accepted behavior by patient's cultural group regarding expression of emotions and feelings, religious expressions, and response to illness and death? *Restrictions*—Does patient have any restrictions related to sexual matters, exposure of body parts, certain types of surgery (e.g., hysterectomy), discussion of dead relatives, and discussion of fears related to the unknown?	
Language and communication processes:	What are some overall cultural characteristics of patient's language and communication process?	
Language(s) and/or dialect(s) spoken	Which language(s) and/or dialect(s) does patient speak most frequently? Where? At home or at work?	
Language barriers	Which language does patient predominantly use in thinking? Does patient need bilingual interpreter in nurse-patient interactions? Is patient non–English-speaking or limited English-speaking? Is patient able to read and/or write in English?	
Communication process	What are rules (linguistics) and modes (style) of communication process (e.g., "honorific" concept of showing "respect or deference" to others using words only common to specific ethnic/cultural group)? Is there need for variation in technique of communicating and interviewing to accommodate patient's cultural background (e.g., tempo of conversation, eye/body contact, topic restrictions, norms of confidentiality, and style of explanation)? Are there any conflicts in verbal and nonverbal interactions between patient and nurse? How does patient's nonverbal communication process compare with other ethnic/cultural groups, and how does it affect patient's response to nursing and medical care? Are there any variations between patient's interethnic and interracial communication process or intracultural and intraracial communication process (e.g., ethnic minority patient and White middle-class nurse, ethnic minority patient and ethnic minority nurse; beliefs, attitudes, values, role variations, stereotyping [perceptions and prejudice])?	
Healing beliefs and practices		
Cultural healing system	What cultural healing system does the patient predominantly adhere to (e.g., Asian healing system, Raza/Latina Curanderismo)? What religious healing system does the patient predominantly adhere to (e.g., Seventh Day Adventist, West African voodoo, Fundamentalist sect, Pentacostal)?	

Modified from Bloch B: Bloch's assessment guide for ethnic/cultural variations. In Orque MS, Bloch B, Monrroy LSA, eds: *Ethnic nursing care: a multicultural approach*, St Louis, 1983, Mosby, pp. 63-69.

Bloch's Ethnic/Cultural Assessment Guide (cont'd)

Categories	Guideline Questions/Instructions	Data Collected
Cultural health beliefs	Is illness explained by the germ theory or cause-effect relationship, presence of evil spirits, imbalance between "hot" and "cold" (yang and yin in Chinese culture), or disequilibrium between nature and man? Is good health related to success, ability to work or fulfill roles, reward from God, or balance with nature?	
Cultural health practices	What types of cultural healing practices does person from ethnic/cultural group adhere to? Does he or she use healing remedies to cure *natural* illnesses caused by the external environment [e.g., massage to cure *empacho* (a ball of food clinging to stomach wall), wearing of talismans or charms for protection against illness]?	
Cultural healers	Does patient rely on cultural healers [e.g., medicine men for American Indian, Curandero for Raza/Latina, Chinese herbalist, hougan (voodoo priest), spiritualist, or minister for Black American]?	
Nutritional variables or factors	What nutritional variables or factors are influenced by the patient's ethnic/cultural background?	
Characteristics of food preparation and consumption	What types of food preferences and restrictions, meaning of foods, style of food preparation and consumption, frequency of eating, time of eating, and eating utensils are culturally determined for patient? Are there any religious influences on food preparation and consumption?	
Influences from external environment	What modifications if any did the ethnic group that the patient identifies with have to make in its food practices in White dominant American society? Are there any adaptations of food customs and beliefs from rural setting to urban setting?	
Patient education needs	What are some implications of diet planning and teaching to patient who adheres to cultural practices concerning foods?	
SOCIOLOGICAL		
Economic status	Who is principal wage earner in patient's family? What is total annual income (approximately) of family? What impact does economic status have on lifestyle, place of residence, living conditions, and ability to obtain health services?	
Educational status	What is highest educational level obtained? Does patient's educational background influence his or her ability to understand how to seek health services, literature on health care, patient teaching experiences, and any written material patient is exposed to in health care setting (e.g., admission forms, patient care forms, teaching literature, and lab test forms)? Does patient's educational background cause him to feel inferior or superior to health care personnel in health care setting?	
Social network	What is patient's social network (kinship, peer, and cultural healing networks)? How do they influence health or illness status of patient?	
Family as supportive group	Does patient's family feel need for continuous presence in patient's clinical setting (is this an ethnic/cultural characteristic)? How is family valued during illness or death? How does family participate in patient's nursing care process (e.g., giving baths, feeding, using touch as support [cultural meaning], supportive presence)? How does ethnic/cultural family structure influence patient response to health or illness (e.g., roles, beliefs, strengths, weaknesses, and social class)? Are there any key family roles characteristic of a specific ethnic/cultural group (e.g., grandmother in Black and some American Indian families), and can these key persons be a resource for health personnel? What role does family play in health promotion or cause of illness (e.g., would family be intermediary group in patient interactions with health personnel and making decisions regarding his care)?	

Continued

Bloch's Ethnic/Cultural Assessment Guide (cont'd)

CATEGORIES	GUIDELINE QUESTIONS/INSTRUCTIONS	DATA COLLECTED
Supportive institutions in ethnic/cultural community	What influence do ethnic/cultural institutions have on patient receiving health services (e.g., institutions such as Organization of Migrant Workers, NAACP, Black Political Caucus, churches, schools, Urban League, community clinics)?	
Institutional racism	How does institutional racism in health facilities influence patient's response to receiving health care?	
PSYCHOLOGICAL		
Self-concept (identity)	Does patient show strong racial/cultural identity? How does this compare to that of other racial/cultural groups or to members of dominant society? What factors in patient's development helped to shape his or her self-concept (e.g., family, peers, society labels, external environment, institutions, racism)? How does patient deal with stereotypical behavior from health professionals? What is impact of racism on patient from distinct ethnic/cultural group (e.g., social anxiety, noncompliance to health care process in clinical settings, avoidance of utilizing or participating in health care institutions)? Does ethnic/cultural background have impact on how patient relates to body image change resulting from illness or surgery (e.g., importance to appearance and roles in cultural group)? Any adherence or identification with ethnic/cultural "group" identity? (e.g., solidarity, "we" concept)?	
Mental and behavioral processes and characteristics of ethnic/cultural group	How does patient relate to his external environment in clinical setting (e.g., fears, stress, and adaptive mechanisms characteristic of a specific ethnic/cultural group)? Any variations based on the life span? What is patient's ability to relate to persons outside of his ethnic/cultural group (health personnel)? Is he withdrawn, verbally or nonverbally expressive, negative or positive, feeling mentally or physically inferior or superior? How does patient deal with feelings of loss of dignity and respect in clinical setting?	
Religious influences on psychological effects of health/illness	Does patient's religion have a strong impact on how he relates to health/illness influences or outcomes (e.g., death/chronic illness, cause and effect of illness, or adherence to nursing/medical practices)? Do religious beliefs, sacred practices, and talismans play a role in treatment of disease? What is role of significant religious persons during health/illness (e.g., Black ministers, Catholic priests, Buddhist monks, Islamic imams)?	
Psychological/cultural response to stress and discomfort of illness	Based on ethnic/cultural background, does patient exhibit any variations in psychological response to pain or physical disability of disease processes?	
BIOLOGICAL/ PHYSIOLOGICAL (Consideration of *norms* for different ethnic/cultural groups)		
Racial-anatomical characteristics	Does patient have any distinct racial characteristics (e.g., skin color, hair texture and color, color of mucous membranes)? Does patient have any variations in anatomical characteristics (e.g., body structure [height and weight] more prevalent for ethnic/cultural group, skeletal formation [pelvic shape, especially for obstetrical evaluation], facial shape and structure [nose, eye shape, facial contour], upper and lower extremities)?	

Bloch's Ethnic/Cultural Assessment Guide (cont'd)

CATEGORIES	GUIDELINE QUESTIONS/INSTRUCTIONS	DATA COLLECTED
Racial-anatomical characteristics—cont'd	How do patient's racial and anatomical characteristics affect his or her self-concept and the way others relate to him or her? Does variation in racial-anatomical characteristics affect physical evaluations and physical care, skin assessment based on color, and variations in hair care and hygienic practices?	
Growth and development patterns	Are there any distinct growth and development characteristics that vary with patient's ethnic/cultural background (e.g., bone density, fat folds, motor ability)? What factors are important for nutritional assessment, neurological and motor assessment, assessment of bone deterioration in disease process or injury, evaluation of newborns, evaluation of intellectual status, or capacity in relationship to motor/sensory development in children? How do these differ in ethnic/cultural groups?	
Variations in body systems	Are there any variations in body systems for patient from distinct ethnic/cultural group (e.g., gastrointestinal disturbance with lactose intolerance in Blacks, nutritional intake of cultural foods causing adverse effects on gastrointestinal tract and fluid and electrolyte system, and variations in chemical and hematological systems [certain blood types prevalent in particular ethnic/cultural groups])?	
Skin and hair physiology, mucous membranes	How does skin color variation influence assessment of skin color changes (e.g., jaundice, cyanosis, ecchymosis, erythema, and its relationship to disease processes)? What are methods of assessing skin color changes (comparing variations and similarities between different ethnic groups)? Are there conditions of hypopigmentation and hyperpigmentation (e.g., vitiligo, mongolian spots, albinism, discoloration caused by trauma)? Why would these be more striking in some ethnic groups? Are there any skin conditions more prevalent in a distinct ethnic group (e.g., keloids in Blacks)? Is there any correlation between oral and skin pigmentation and their variations among distinct racial groups when doing assessment of oral cavity (e.g, leukoedema is normal occurrence in Blacks)? What are variations in hair texture and color among racially different groups? Ask patient about preferred hair care methods or any racial/cultural restrictions (e.g., not washing "hot-combed" hair while in clinical setting, not cutting very long hair of Raza/Latina patients). Are there any variations in skin care methods (e.g., using Vaseline on Black skin)?	
Diseases more prevalent among ethnic/cultural group	Are there any specific diseases or conditions that are more prevalent for a specific ethnic/cultural group (e.g., hypertension, sickle cell anemia, G6-PD, lactose intolerance)? Does patient have any socioenvironmental diseases common among ethnic/cultural groups [e.g., lead paint poisoning, poor nutrition, overcrowding (prone to tuberculosis), alcoholism resulting from psychological despair and alienation from dominant society, rat bites, poor sanitation]?	
Diseases ethnic/cultural group has increased resistance to	Are there any diseases that patient has increased resistance to because of racial/cultural background (e.g., skin cancer in Blacks)?	

Appendix 7-2

Family Assessment Guide

Family name ______________________ Family ID no. ______________
Source of referral ______________________
Reason for referral ______________________
Occupational status ______________________
Health insurance ______________________
Medical emergency plan ______________________
Preventive health care ______________________
Community agencies involved with family ______________________
Family composition: Map family constellation; include health problems of individual members.

Date			Rating		
1st	2nd	Assessment Parameters	1st	2nd	Significant Data
		1. *Structural characteristics* a. Family composition b. Financial resources c. Educational experiences d. Allocation of family and personal roles e. Division of labor f. Distribution of power and authority g. Cultural influences • Health beliefs and attitudes • Family goals • Norms for social behavior • Spiritual beliefs • Beliefs about folk diseases and medicine h. Activities of daily living • Dietary habits • Child-rearing practices • Housekeeping • Sleeping arrangements • Laundry facilities • Transportation • Child care arrangements i. Family health status/practices • Health history • Health status of family members (relevant diagnoses and treatment regimens) • Knowledge of health problems • Health risk factors (e.g., dietary, substance abuse, or current stressors) • Prevention practices (primary, secondary, and tertiary) • Care arrangements for ill family members			

Note: Code for recording assessment data—use a different color ink for the first and second assessment or rating (generally it takes several home visits to complete a family assessment). Rating scale: 1 = strength; 2 = problem; 3 = anticipatory guidance warranted; 4 = problem—family does not wish to change this area of functioning at this time; 5 = not applicable. Family functioning should be rated every 4 months to assist in evaluating family progress and nursing intervention strategies.

Family Assessment Guide (cont'd)

Date			Rating		
1st	2nd	Assessment Parameters	1st	2nd	Significant Data
		1. *Structural characteristics—cont'd* i. Family health status/practices—cont'd • Source of preventive and curative health care • Barriers to health care 2. *Process characteristics* a. Atmosphere of home b. Communication patterns c. Decision-making processes • How decisions are made • How decisions are implemented d. Conflict negotiation e. Achievement of developmental tasks f. Adaptation to change g. Autonomy of individual family members 3. *Relationships with external systems* a. How family boundaries are established b. Use of information from environment c. Contact with extended families d. Interactions with friends and neighbors e. Attitudes about community systems • Health • Welfare • Educational • Others (describe) f. Use of the referral process • Ability to seek assistance • Level of independence 4. *Environmental characteristics* a. Neighborhood • Accessibility of facilities to meet basic needs • Availability of recreational, educational, religious, and other resources • Safety (physical and psychosocial) b. Housing • Suitability in relation to family needs • Condition of structural components • Suitability of home furnishings • Sanitation (water source, sewage and garbage disposal, and housekeeping practices) • Accident hazards • Barriers to family mobility			

Professionals and volunteers working with family (identify person and agency) ______________________

Summary of family strengths (based on categories rated No. 1) ______________________

Description of family priorities and assistance desired ______________________

Specific factors to consider when developing and implementing a family care plan ______________________

Assessor ______________________ Date __________

Assessor ______________________ Date __________

Assessor ______________________ Date __________

Appendix 8-1

Life Change Events

Events	LCU Values	Events	LCU Values
FAMILY			
Death of spouse	100	Changing to a new school	20
Divorce	73	Change in residence	20
Marital separation	65	Major change in recreation	19
Death of a close family member	63	Major change in church activities	19
Marriage	50	Major change in sleeping habits	16
Marital reconciliation	45	Major change in eating habits	15
Major change in health of family	44	Vacation	13
Pregnancy	40	Christmas	12
Addition of new family member	39	Minor violations of the law	11
Major change in arguments with wife	35		
Son or daughter leaving home	29	**WORK**	
In-law troubles	29	Being fired from work	47
Wife starting or ending work	26	Retirement from work	45
Major change in family get-togethers	15	Major business adjustment	39
		Changing to different line of work	36
PERSONAL		Major change in work responsibilities	29
Detention in jail	63	Trouble with boss	23
Major pesonal injury or illness	53	Major change in working conditions	20
Sexual difficulties	39		
Death of a close friend	37	**FINANCIAL**	
Outstanding personal achievement	28	Major change in financial state	38
Start or end of formal schooling	26	Mortgage or loan over $10,000	31
Major change in living conditions	25	Mortgage foreclosure	30
Major revision of personal habits	24	Mortage or loan less than $10,000	17

From Rahe RH: Subjects' recent life changes and their near-future illness reports, *Ann Clin Res* 4:250-265, 1972. This study report was supported by the Bureau of Medicine and Surgery, Department of the Navy, under Research Work Unit MF51.524.002-5011-DD5G (Report No. 72-31). Opinions expressed are those of the author and are not to be construed as necessarily reflecting the official view or endorsement of the Department of the Navy.

Appendix 8-2

Youth Adaptation Rating Scale

- Graduation (.57)
- Pet dies (.55)
- Fights with parents (.67)
- Getting pressure about having sex (.63)
- Caught cheating or lying repeatedly (.73)
- Getting a major illness/injury/car accident (.81)
- Becoming religious or giving up religion (.63)
- Referral to the principal's office (.47)
- Getting acne/warts (.45)
- Trouble getting a date when it was not a problem before (.61)
- Problems developed with teachers/employers (.59)
- Making career decisions (college, majors training, etc.) (.64)
- Starting to go to weekend parties/rock concerts (.35)
- First day of school (.37)
- Going on first date/starting to date (.53)
- Death of a parent/guardian (.95)
- Not getting promoted to next grade (.76)
- Getting caught using drugs (.86)
- Getting attacked/raped/beat up (.84)
- Getting a ticket or other minor problems with law (.58)
- Parents getting a divorce/separation (.83)
- Getting expelled/suspended (.71)
- Fad pressure (.43)
- Breaking up with boy/girlfriend (.57)
- Getting minor illness (cold, flu, etc.) (.30)
- Arguments with peers/brothers/sisters (.46)
- Starting to perform (speeches, presentations, musical or drama performances) (.60)
- Getting a bad report card (.59)
- Getting fired from a job (.63)
- Going into debt (.72)
- Being stereotyped/discriminated/having bad rumors spread about you (.70)
- Death of a close family member (.94)
- Death of a boy/girlfriend/close friend (.94)
- Getting V.D. (.86)
- Getting someone pregnant/getting pregnant (.92)
- Taking finals/SAT test (.61)
- Moving to a different town/school/making new friends (.67)
- Getting a car (.35)
- Trying to get a job/job interview (.49)
- Getting an award, office, etc. (.36)
- Making a team (drill, athletic, debate) (.44)
- Getting married (.73)
- Getting beat up by parents (.86)
- Taking the driver license test (.55)
- Getting a new addition to the family (.45)
- Going to the dentist or doctor (.37)
- Going to jail/reform school (.88)
- Starting to use drugs (.82)
- Getting braces (.45)
- Going on a diet (.41)
- Losing or gaining weight (.49)
- Changing exercise habits (.21)
- Pressure to take drugs (.71)
- Moving out of the house (.56)
- Falling in love (.66)
- Getting a bad haircut (.57)
- Getting glasses (.49)
- Family member moving out (.47)

From Beall S, Schmidt G: Development of a youth adaptation rating scale, *J Sch Health* 54(5):197-200, 1984.
Note: The number after each item is the ratio value or degree of severity. This ratio value was determined by dividing the total value for each item by the highest possible score. Events with a high ratio value produce greater stress and require a greater degree of adaptation than do events with a lower ratio value.

Antepartum Nursing Assessment Guide

Client's name ______________________

EDC ______ GRAV ______ PARA ______ ABORT ______ DATE MED. CARE STARTED ____________

M.D. ______ HOSP. ______ SIGNIFICANT MEDICAL HISTORY OF PREGNANCIES ______________

____

Mother's opinion of previous pregnancy, delivery, and newborn (NB) ______________________________

____

Current Pregnancy	Yes	No	First Assessment, Comments Trimester 1 2 3 Date ____	Yes	No	Second Assessment, Comments Trimester 1 2 3 Date ____
MEDICAL SUPERVISION						
Medical appointments made						
Plans to keep						
Dental appointments made						
Plans to keep						
Dental care completed						
Ct understanding of doctor's orders is:						
SIGNS AND SYMPTOMS						
Nausea						
Vomiting						
Heartburn						
Spotting						
Bleeding						
Edema						
Leg cramps						
Varicosities						
Backache						
Dyspnea						
Constipation						
Hemorrhoids						
Dysuria						

Printed with permission and modified from the Nursing Division, King County Health Department, 1000 Public Safety Building, Seattle, Washington.

Antepartum Nursing Assessment Guide (cont'd)

			First Assessment, Comments			Second Assessment, Comments
Current Pregnancy	Yes	No	Trimester 1 2 3 Date _____	Yes	No	Trimester 1 2 3 Date _____
SIGNS AND SYMPTOMS—cont'd						
Urinary frequency						
Fetal movements						
Braxton Hicks						
Other						
PERSONAL MANAGEMENT						
Weight Gain						
Normal						
Diet—type ______________ Breakfast Lunch Dinner Snacks Dislikes Fluid intake pattern Comments						
Sleep—No. of hours						
Health Habits						
Physical activity						
Substance use (specify)						
Safety practices						
Preventive care						
Clothing						
Supportive						

Continued

Antepartum Nursing Assessment Guide (cont'd)

Client's name ______________________

EMOTIONAL (COMPLETE WITH CLIENT'S FEELINGS TOWARDS)

Current Pregnancy	First Assessment, Comments Trimester 1 2 3 Date _____	Second Assessment, Comments Trimester 1 2 3 Date _____
PERSONAL MANAGEMENT—cont'd		
Pregnancy		
Motherhood		
Changes in self-image		
Mood swings		
Pregnancy and parenthood affecting personal family goals		
Husband-wife social and sexual relationships		
Stresses created by emotional and physical changes of this pregnancy		
Anxiety re: labor and delivery		
Social and financial family stability re: future plans for NB		
Past and present personality difficulties		
Fetus		
Father's awareness of, interest and attitude		

Antepartum Nursing Assessment Guide (cont'd)

Client's name ____________

	First Assessment, Comments			Second Assessment, Comments		
	Yes	No	Trimester 1 2 3 Date ____	Yes	No	Trimester 1 2 3 Date ____
PLANS FOR DELIVERY						
Made plans for hospitalization						
Make arrangements for care of family at home						
Knows what to expect of hospital routine						
Knows signs of labor						
Knows what to expect during labor and delivery						
Knows what to expect PP						
PLANS FOR NEWBORN						
Plans to breast feed						
Plans to bottle feed						
Adequate layette and equipment						
Plans to have help PP						
Knows what to expect of NB						
FAMILY PLANNING						
Knows methods of birth control						
Wants information on family planning						

What kind of help does family want from CHN?

____

____

____

What kind of help does family want from CHN?

____

____

____

Postpartum Nursing Assessment Guide

Client's name ______________

GRAV _______ PARA _______ M.D. ______________

HOSPITAL _______ SIGNIFICANT MEDICAL HISTORY OF PREGNANCIES ______________

Check items which best describe client or complete with notation.

	First Assessment Date _____		Second Assessment Date _____	
Postpartum Exam	**Yes**	**No**	**Yes**	**No**
Temp _______				
BREASTS				
Physical appearance:				
Normal				
Engorgement				
Soreness				
Soft				
Cracked				
Redness				
Caked				
Inverted				
Lactation:				
Leaking				
Filling				
Nursing				
Not nursing				
"Dry up" pills				
ABDOMEN				
Fundus (firmness, position)				
C-section (incision)				
RECTOVAGINAL				
Laceration				
Episiotomy:				
None				
Clean				

Printed with permission and modified from the Nursing Division, King County Health Department, 1000 Public Safety Building, Seattle, Washington.

Postpartum Nursing Assessment Guide (cont'd)

	First Assessment Date _____		Second Assessment Date _____	
Postpartum Exam	**Yes**	**No**	**Yes**	**No**
RECTOVAGINAL—cont'd				
Episiotomy—cont'd				
Healing				
Painful				
Hemorrhoids				
Other				
LOCHIA				
Rubra				
Serosa				
Alba				
Clots				
No. pads per day				
VOIDING				
No difficulty				
Anuria				
Dysuria				
Frequency				
Burning				
BOWELS				
Constipated				
No difficulty				
Other				

First assessment date __________ *Second assessment date* __________

Personal Health Practices (Describe what the client is doing about the following.)

A. Care
   Bathing ____________________
   Peri-care ____________________
   Breast care ____________________

B. Rest ____________________
   Sleep ____________________
   Recreation ____________________
   Exercise and activity ____________________

Continued

Postpartum Nursing Assessment Guide (cont'd)

C. Foundation garment ______

D. Diet—Type ______

Breakfast ______

Lunch ______

Dinner ______

Snacks ______

Dislikes ______

Fluid intake ______

Comments ______

E. Sexual relations ______

PSYCHOSOCIAL (Describe mother's feeling or reaction to the following.)

Pregnancy ______

Labor ______

Delivery ______

Newborn ______

Motherhood ______

Family's reaction to labor, delivery, NB ______

Other ______

MEDICAL SUPERVISION	YES	NO	YES	NO
Medical appointments made				
Plan to keep				
Dental care up to date				

Client's understanding of doctor's orders is ______

FAMILY PLANNING

Future family plans (method, problems) ______

What kind of help does family want from CHN? ______

Appendix 9-3

NANDA Nursing Diagnoses Grouped by Gordon's Functional Health Patterns*

HEALTH-PERCEPTION—HEALTH-MANAGEMENT PATTERN

Health-Seeking Behaviors (Specify)
Altered Health Maintenance (Specify)
Ineffective Management of Therapeutic Regimen (Specify Area)
Risk for Ineffective Management of Therapeutic Regimen (Specify Area)
Effective Management of Therapeutic Regimen
Ineffective Family Management of Therapeutic Regimen
Ineffective Community Management of Therapeutic Regimen
Health-Management Deficit (Specify Area)
Risk for Health-Management Deficit (Specify Area)
Noncompliance (Specify Area)
Risk for Noncompliance (Specify Area)
Risk for Infection (Specify Type/Area)
Risk for Injury (Trauma)
Risk for Perioperative Poisitioning Injury
Risk for Poisoning
Risk for Suffocation
Altered Protection (Specify)
Energy Field Disturbance

NUTRITIONAL-METABOLIC PATTERN

Altered Nutrition: More than Body Requirements or Exogenous Obesity
Altered Nutrition: Risk for More than Body Requirements or Risk for Obesity
Altered Nutrition: Less than Body Requirements or Nutritional Deficit (Specify Type)
Ineffective Breastfeeding
Interrupted Breastfeeding
Effective Breastfeeding
Ineffective Infant Feeding Pattern
Impaired Swallowing (Uncompensated)
Risk for Aspiration
Altered Oral Mucous Membrane (Specify Alteration)
Fluid Volume Deficit
Risk for Fluid Volume Deficit
Fluid Volume Excess
Risk for Impaired Skin Integrity or Risk for Skin Breakdown
Impaired Skin Integrity
Pressure Ulcer (Specify Stage)
Impaired Tissue Integrity (Specify Type)
Risk for Altered Body Temperature
Ineffective Thermoregulation
Hyperthermia
Hypothermia

ELIMINATION PATTERN

Colonic Constipation
Perceived Constipation
Intermittent Constipation Pattern
Diarrhea
Bowel Incontinence
Altered Urinary Elimination Pattern
Functional Incontinence
Reflex Incontinence
Stress Incontinence
Urge Incontinence
Total Incontinence
Urinary Retention

ACTIVITY-EXERCISE PATTERN

Activity Intolerance (Specify Level)
Risk for Activity Intolerance
Fatigue
Impaired Physical Mobility (Specify Level)
Impaired Bed Mobility
Transfer Deficit
Impaired Locomotion
Impaired Ambulation
Risk for Disuse Syndrome
Risk for Joint Contractures

From Gordon M: *Manual of nursing diagnosis*, 1997-1998, St. Louis, 1997, Mosby, pp. xviii–xx.
*Boldface type indicates diagnoses currently accepted by the North American Nursing Diagnosis Association (NANDA). Others are either diagnoses received by NANDA for development or not accepted by NANDA but found to be useful in clinical practice.

Continued

NANDA Nursing Diagnoses Grouped by Gordon's Functional Health Patterns (cont'd)

ACTIVITY-EXERCISE PATTERN—cont'd

Total Self-Care Deficit (Specify Level)
Self-Bathing—Hygiene Deficit (Specify Level)
Self-Dressing—Grooming Deficit (Specify Level)
Self-Feeding Deficit (Specify Level)
Self-Toileting Deficit (Specify Level)
Altered Growth and Development: Self-Care Skills (Specify Level)
Diversional Activity Deficit
Impaired Home Maintenance Management (Mild, Moderate, Severe, Potential, Chronic)
Dysfunctional Ventilatory Weaning Response (DVWR)
Inability to Sustain Spontaneous Ventilation
Ineffective Airway Clearance
Ineffective Breathing Pattern
Impaired Gas Exchange
Decreased Cardiac Output
Altered Tissue Perfusion (Specify)
Dysreflexia
Disorganized Infant Behavior
Risk for Disorganized Infant Behavior
Potential for Enhanced Organized Infant Behavior
Risk for Peripheral Neurovascular Dysfunction
Altered Growth and Development

SLEEP-REST PATTERN

Sleep-Pattern Disturbance
Delayed Sleep Onset
Sleep Pattern Reversal
Sleep Deprivation

COGNITIVE-PERCEPTUAL PATTERN

Pain (Specify Type and Location)
Chronic Pain (Specify Type and Location)
Pain Self-Management Deficit (Acute, Chronic)
Uncompensated Sensory Loss (Specify Type/Degree)
Sensory Overload (Sensory-Perceptual Alteration)
Unilateral Neglect
Sensory Deprivation (Sensory-Perceptual Alterations)
Knowledge Deficit (Specify Area)
Altered Thought Processes (Specify)
Attention-Concentration Deficit
Acute Confusion
Chronic Confusion
Impaired Environmental Interpretation Syndrome
Uncompensated Memory Loss
Impaired Memory
Risk for Cognitive Impairment
Decisional Conflict (Specify)
Decreased Intracranial Adaptive Capacity

SELF-PERCEPTION—SELF-CONCEPT PATTERN

Fear (Specify Focus)
Anxiety
Mild Anxiety
Moderate Anxiety
Severe Anxiety (Panic)
Anticipatory Anxiety (Mild, Moderate, Severe)
Reactive Situational Depression (Specify Situation)
Risk for Loneliness
Hopelessness
Powerlessness (Severe, Moderate, Low)
Low Self-Esteem
Chronic Low Self-Esteem
Situational Low Self-Esteem
Body Image Disturbance
Risk for Self-Mutilation
Personal Identity Disturbance

NANDA Nursing Diagnoses Grouped by Gordon's Functional Health Patterns (cont'd)

ROLE-RELATIONSHIP PATTERN

Anticipatory Grieving
Dysfunctional Grieving
Altered Role Performance (Specify)
Unresolved Independence-Dependence Conflict
Social Isolation or Social Rejection
Social Isolation
Impaired Social Interaction
Altered Growth and Development: Social Skills (Specify)
Relocation Stress Syndrome
Altered Family Processes (Specify)
Altered Family Process: Alcoholism
Altered Parenting (Specify Alteration)
Risk for Altered Parenting (Specify Alteration)
Parental Role Conflict
Weak Parent-Infant Attachment
Risk for Altered Parent-Infant/Child Attachment
Parent-Infant Separation
Caregiver Role Strain
Risk for Caregiver Role Strain
Support System Deficit
Impaired Verbal Communication
Altered Growth and Development: Communication Skills (Specify Type)
Risk for Violence

SEXUALITY-REPRODUCTIVE PATTERN

Altered Sexuality Patterns
Sexual Dysfunction
Rape Trauma Syndrome
Rape Trauma Syndrome: Compound Reaction
Rape Trauma Syndrome: Silent Reaction

COPING—STRESS-TOLERANCE PATTERN

Ineffective Coping (Individual)
Avoidance Coping
Defensive Coping
Ineffective Denial or Denial
Impaired Adjustment
Post-Trauma Response
Family Coping: Potential for Growth
Compromised Family Coping
Disabling Family Coping
Ineffective Community Coping
Potential for Enhanced Community Coping

VALUE-BELIEF PATTERN

Spiritual Distress (Distress of Human Spirit)
Potential for Enhanced Spiritual Well-Being

Appendix 9-4

Sample Clinical Path

CLINICAL PATH DIABETES MELLITUS (DM), adult, juvenile, ketoacidosis, PVD ICD-9 Code(s) 250.9, 250.91, 250.11, 250.70

Patient Name ______ Pt. ID No. ______ SOC Date ______ Discharge Date ______

Date Noted	Expected Outcomes	Achieved Y	Achieved N	Achieved Date	Variance Codes	Date Noted	Nursing/Functional Diagnoses	Date Closed
	1. Stable endocrine status by visit no. _____ as noted by blood glucose in range of ______ to ______.						Cardiac output, decreased Outcome(s) no. _____:	
	2. Patient/caregiver demonstrates compliance with treatment regimen, to include dietary and exercise requirements, as well as general health issues by visit no. _____.						Coping, ineffective family/patient Outcome(s) no. _____:	
	3. Patient/caregiver demonstrates understanding and compliance with blood glucose testing, insulin administration, and medication regimens as evidenced by return demonstration by visit no. _____.						Denial, ineffective Outcome(s) no. _____: Knowledge deficit: medication and therapeutic regimen Outcome(s) no. _____:	
	4. Patient/caregiver demonstrates understanding of home safety, general emergency measures related to disease condition, infection control, and proper disposal of contaminated wastes by visit no. _____.						Management of therapeutic and medication regimen, ineffective Outcome(s) no. _____: Nutrition, altered: high risk for body requirements Outcome(s) no. _____:	

Date Noted	Expected Outcomes	Achieved Y	Achieved N	Achieved Date	Variance Codes	Date Noted	Nursing/Functional Diagnoses	Date Closed
	5. Other:						Tissue perfusion, altered: peripheral, renal Outcome(s) no. ____:	
	6. Other:						Noncompliance (specify) Outcome(s) no. ____:	
	7. Other:						Other: Outcome(s) no. ____:	
							Other: Outcome(s) no. ____:	

From Marrelli TM, Hilliard LS: *Home care and clinical paths: effective care planning across the continuum*, St. Louis, 1996, Mosby, pp. 105-106.

Continued

Sample Clinical Path (cont'd)

Assessments/Instructions/Interventions	VS No._		VS No._		VS No._		VS No._		VS No._		VS No._		VS No._		VS No._		VS No._		VS No._	
Explain patient rights and responsibilities.																				
Assess for home safety management.																				
Assess vital signs.																				
Assess endocrine status.																				
Assess hydration and nutrition status.																				
Assess weight.																				
Assess coping skills of patient/family/caregiver.																				
Assess patient/caregiver's strengths/weaknesses related to therapeutic regimen.																				
Assess patient/caregiver's willingness and ability to provide home therapeutic regimen.																				
Assess patient/caregiver's understanding of disease process and compliance with therapeutic regimen.																				
Refer to: Dietitian for nutritional needs and safe allowances.																				
Instruct on home safety.																				
Instruct on medication regimen and compliance issues.																				
Instruct patient/caregiver on signs of hypoglycemia and hyperglycemia and emergency measures related to those conditions.																				
Instruct patient/caregiver on blood glucose testing.																				

ASSESSMENETS/INSTRUCTIONS/INTERVENTIONS	VS No._	VS No._	VS No._	VS No._	VS No._	VS No._	VS No._	VS No._	VS No._	VS No._
Instruct patient/caregiver on self/caregiver administration of insulin.										
Instruct patient/caregiver on home maintenance program (including exercise and correct nutritional allowances). ______ on visit no. ___										
Venipuncture for ordered laboratory tests.										
Other:										
Other:										
Other:										
MEDICAL SUPPLIES/HOME MEDICAL EQUIPMENT NEEDS 1. Glucometer 2. Insulin syringes/insulin 3. Other ______										

Variance codes

1. Patient related
2. Situation related
3. Systems related

Team member signature ______ Initials ___

Team member signature ______ Initials ___

Team member signature ______ Initials ___

Case manager name ______

______

Patient signature (involved in care planning)

Appendix 10-1

Discharge Questionnaire

The staff on (unit name) wants to make your return to the community as easy for you as possible. The nurse who is primarily responsible for helping you plan your discharge is ________. He or she will help you and your family reach any resources you may need for your health care at home. There are many agencies, including home care, which assist people in the community with health care problems.

Please complete the following questions with your family as soon as you feel able. Your discharge nurse will be in contact with you within a few days of your admission.

DATA #1

When you get home

1. With whom will you live? ____________________
2. Will they be able to help with your care if needed? ____________________
3. Will you have difficulty getting around your home—stairs, small bathroom, low bed, safety problems, to the telephone, to shower, or bathtub? ____________________
4. Will you have any problems in getting any of the following—transportation, food, medicine, heat, place to stay, child care, pet care, water supply? ____________________
5. Will you need any of these to function at home—wheelchair, brace, cane, walker, crutches, special equipment? ____________________
6. How much of the following will you be able to do? (Please mark appropriate column.)

	INDEPENDENT	WITH FAMILY	UNABLE TO
Turning in bed			
Bathing			
Dressing			
Eating			
Sitting			
Standing			
Transfers to tub			
Transfers to toilet			
Walking			

DATA #2

1. Have you had a problem with any of these areas recently?
   a. Eyes/ears
   b. Mouth/throat/teeth
   c. Skin
   d. Lungs/breathing
   e. Breasts
   f. Heart/blood vessels
   g. Stomach/bowel
   h. Bladder/kidneys/urine
   i. Genitals
   j. Mental status
   k. Nerves/muscles
2. Will you have difficulty getting to your physician, nurse, or therapist often enough to have these checked? ____________________

DATA #3

Please mark any of the following areas that you would like to know more about:

1. Your disease/illness/accident
   a. What caused it
   b. What can be done to prevent a repeat
   c. How to recognize a repeat
   d. How it will affect you later

Please mark any of the following areas that you would like to know more about:

2. Your medication
   a. What it does
   b. How much to take
   c. When to take it
   d. What side effects to be aware of

From Stone M: Discharge planning guide, *Am J Nurs* 79:1445-1447, 1979.

Discharge Questionnaire (cont'd)

DATA #3—cont'd

3. Your treatments, procedures, or exercises
   a. What they do for you
   b. How to do them
   c. How often to do them
   d. What difficulties to be aware of
4. Supplies or equipment you'll use at home
   a. What it does
   b. When to use it
   c. How to get more or to get repairs
5. Your nutrition
   a. How it affects you
   b. Special diets—how much to eat, when to eat, what to avoid
   c. How much and what to drink
6. Preventive health practices
   a. How to examine your breasts
   b. Pap smears
   c. Birth control
   d. Effect of cigarettes
   e. Effect of alcohol and drugs
   f. Dental health
   g. Seat belt
   h. Immunizations (yourself or children)
   i. Exercise
7. Other ______________________________

DATA #4

1. Which of these agencies are you involved with?
   a. VNA/Home Health
   b. Senior Citizens
   c. Vocational Rehabilitation
   d. Social Welfare
   e. Planned Parenthood
   f. Mental Health Agency
   g. Diet Club
   h. Alcoholics Anonymous
   i. Cancer Society
   j. Ostomy Club
   k. Meals-on-Wheels
   l. Diabetes Association
   m. Dialysis Association
   n. MS Society
   o. MD Society
   p. Association for the Blind
   q. Other ____________
2. Please mark any of the areas that you would especially like to discuss with your discharge nurse.
   a. Finances, jobs
   b. Drugs, alcohol
   c. Caring for children or elderly relatives
   d. Emotional or nerve problem
   e. Sexuality
   f. Family or marital relationships
   g. Grieving
   h. School or work
   i. Problem, retirement
   j. Spiritual needs
   k. Legal problems
   l. Other ____________

STOP HERE. YOUR DISCHARGE NURSE WILL HELP YOU COMPLETE THE FORM. Ask to see him or her if you haven't met yet, especially if you think you might go home soon.

Assessments (To be done by RN and patient)

1. Will there be a need for help with physical care at home?
2. Will there be a need for a nurse or therapist at home to assess physical status, disease process, or exercise and therapy?
3. Will the patient or family need more health education about any of the areas above (Data #3), either during hospitalization or at home?
4. Will the patient or family need more information or assistance with any of the psychosocial areas listed in Data #4?

Plan (To be done by patient and nurse together)

Consider the four assessments above. If there are *no* yes responses, proceed to section B and complete. If there are any yes responses, you *must* select either part 1 or part 2 of section A before completing section B.

A. 1. No referral necessary, but must have further education before discharge regarding ______________
   2. Refer to: (see above list of agencies) ______________

B. 1. Equipment or supplies to leave with patient ______________
   2. Transfer plan ______________
   3. Medical follow-up ______________
   4. Surgical follow-up ______________

Enteric Infections Case History

All Other Persons in Household

	Name	Age	Relation	History of Recent Illness	Laboratory Data
1.					
2.					
3.					
4.					
5.					
6.					
7.					
8.					
9.					
10.					

Visitors to Household During Past Month

	Name	Age	Relation	Address	Laboratory Data
1.					
2.					
3.					
4.					
5.					
6.					

Case Laboratory Data

Specimens							
Blood	Feces	Urine	Bile	Date	Positive	Negative	Laboratory

Informant ____________________

Investigation by ____________________

Health Dept. ____________________

Please use ink in making out histories

Date ____________________

From Michigan Department of Public Health, Division of Epidemiology: *Enteric infections case history,* Lansing, Mi., undated, MDPH.

Enteric Infections Case History (cont'd)

ENTERIC INFECTIONS ____________________ CASE HISTORY
(Insert type)

DIVISION OF EPIDEMIOLOGY
Michigan Department of Public Health

No. ________

Name ____________________ Birth date __________ Birthplace __________

Address ____________________

Occupational address ____________________

Physician ____________________ Address ____________________

Health officer ____________________ Address ____________________

CLINICAL HISTORY: Date of onset ____________________ Diarrhea ____________________

Vomiting _______ Temp. _______ Weight loss _______ Other symptoms ____________________

____________________ Duration of symptoms ____________________

Present condition ____________________

Previous pertinent history, if any ____________________

Source of water: ___ Well ___ Municipal ___ Other (specify) ____________________

Source of milk: ___ Pasteurized (name dairy) ____________________

___ Unpasteurized (source) ____________________

Source of food: ___ Restaurant (name) ____________________

___ Private home, other than given ____________________

___ Other (specify) ____________________

Sewage disposal ___ Privy ___ Septic tank ___ Municipal

____

Additional epidemiological data pertaining to this case:

Appendix 11-2

Notifiable Infectious Diseases, Noninfectious Conditions, and Health Risk Behavior: United States*

INFECTIOUS

Acquired immunodeficiency syndrome
Anthrax
Botulism**
Brucellosis
Chancroid**
Chlamydia trachomatis, genital infection
Cholera
Coccidioidomycosis**
Congenital rubella syndrome
Congenital syphilis
Cryptosporidiosis
Diphtheria
Encephalitis, California
Encephalitis, eastern equine
Encephalitis, St. Louis
Encephalitis, western equine
Escherichia coli 0157:H7
Gonorrhea
Haemophilus influenzae, invasive disease
Hansen disease (Leprosy)
Hantavirus pulmonary syndrome
Hemolytic uremic syndrome, post-diarrheal**
Hepatitis A
Hepatitis B
Hepatitis C/non-A, non-B
HIV infection, pediatric
Legionellosis
Lyme disease
Malaria
Measles
Meningococcal disease
Mumps
Pertussis
Plague
Poliomyelitis, paralytic
Psittacosis
Rabies, animal
Rabies, human
Rocky Mountain spotted fever
Rubella
Salmonellosis**
Shigellosis**
Streptococcal disease, invasive, group A**
Streptococcus pneumoniae, drug-resistant**
Streptococcal toxic-shock syndrome
Syphilis
Tetanus
Toxic-shock syndrome
Trichinosis
Tuberculosis
Typhoid fever
Yellow fever**

NONINFECTIOUS CONDITIONS

Elevated blood lead levels
Silicosis
Pesticide poisoning/injuries

HEALTH RISK BEHAVIOR

Prevalence of cigarette smoking

From Centers for Disease Control and Prevention (CDC): Infectious diseases designated as notifiable at the national level*—United States, 1996, *MMWR* 25(3):42, 1996; CDC: Notifiable disease surveillance and notifiable disease statistics—United States, June 1946 and June 1996, *MMWR* 25(45):531, 537, 1996.
*Although varicella is not a nationally notifiable disease, the Council of State and Territorial Epidemiologists recommends reporting of cases of this disease to CDC.
**Not currently published in the weekly tables.

Common Communicable Diseases

Disease	Etiological Agent	Primary Reservoir	Incubation Period	Mode of Transmission	Period of Communicability	Symptoms	Treatment
Hepatitis A (infectious)	Virus	Humans	15-50 days (30 days average)	Person-to-person by fecal-oral route	Maximum infectivity during the incubation period and continuing for a few days after onset of jaundice; no carrier state	Abrupt and "flu-like" with loss of appetite, nausea and vomiting, abdominal discomfort, jaundice, dark brown urine, light brown stool (may be asymptomatic)	No specific treatment (bedrest, increased fluids, no alcoholic beverages, no fried or fatty foods)
Hepatitis B (serum)	Virus	Humans	2 weeks-9 months (60-90 day average)	Percutaneous or permucosal exposure to infected body fluids (blood, saliva, semen, and vaginal fluids)	Weeks before onset of symptoms and infective for entire clinical course; carrier state can exist	Onset is gradual with symptoms similar to those of hepatitis A	Same as hepatitis A
Rubella (German measles)	Virus	Humans	14-21 days	Usually person-to-person (direct contact or droplet spread)	At least 4 days before rash and at least 4 days after onset of rash; very contagious	Mild febrile illness with a macular rash (adults may experience more serious illness); rash on scalp, body, and limbs; usually lasts 1-3 days	No specific treatment (bedrest, increase fluids)
Measles	Virus	Humans	7-21 days (10 days average)	Usually person-to-person (direct contact or droplet spread)	At least 4 days before rash and at least 4 days after onset of rash; very contagious	Resembles a bad cold with eyes and nose running, red blotchy rash beginning usually on face (often behind ears) and then becoming generalized, cough, Koplik spots, more severe symptoms than in rubella; lasts about 4 days	No specific treatment (bedrest increase fluids, place in darkened room if eyes hurt)

Data from Vaughan G: *Mummy, I don't feel well*, London, 1970, Causton & Sons, Ltd.; Tennessee Department of Health and Environment: *Protect them from harm*, Murfreesboro, Tn., 1983, Lancer; Benenson AS: *Control of communicable diseases manual*, ed 16, Washington, D.C., 1995, American Public Health Association.

Continued

Common Communicable Diseases (cont'd)

Disease	Etiological Agent	Primary Reservoir	Incubation Period	Mode of Transmission	Period of Communicability	Symptoms	Treatment
Mumps	Virus	Humans	14-26 days (18 days average)	Person-to-person (direct contact with saliva or droplet spread)	At least 6 days before parotitis and up to 9 days after; very infective about 2 days before symptoms	Pain and swelling in one or both parotid glands, fever, pain on opening and shutting mouth (may need to use a straw to drink)	No specific treatment (bedrest, increase fluids)
Chickenpox	Virus	Humans	12-21 days (14 days average)	Person-to-person (direct contact; droplet or airborne spread)	2 days before vesicles and 6 days after vesicles appear; very contagious	Sudden onset; maculopapular rash that becomes vesicular and leaves a crusty scalp; generalized rash, itchy	No specific treatment (topical applications for itching, bedrest, encourage fluids, dress in loose clothing and caution person not to become overheated)
Pink eye	Multiple agents	Humans	24-72 hours	Person-to-person by direct contact, also through contaminated clothing, fomites	Entire course of disease, until redness and discharge have disappeared	Lacrimation, eye irritation, and redness of lids; photophobia and mucopurulent discharge	Treatment dependent on causative agent
Ringworm	Fungi	Humans	4-14 days (variable)	Direct skin-to-skin or indirect contact from items such as chairs, barber clippers	As long as lesions are present	Scalp: scaly patches of temporary baldness, crusty lesions, hair may become brittle Body: flat, spreading ring-shaped lesions that are red on the periphery and vesticular or pustular in center Feet: "athlete's foot" characterized by scaling or cracking of the skin between the toes, itching	Topical fungicide: oral medication as prescribed

Scabies	Mite (*Sarcoptes scabiei)*	Humans	2-6 weeks for initial infestation; 1-4 days for reinfection	Direct skin-to-skin contact; transfer may occur from clothing	As long as condition is present—until mites and eggs are destroyed by treatment	Papular or vesicular; may evidence "burrows" on skin like grayish-white threads; lesions prominent around webs of fingers, wrists, elbows, belt line; intense itching	Kwell lotion
Pediculosis	Louse	Humans	2 weeks (8-10 days average)	Direct person-to-person or indirect contact with infected personal belongings	As long as eggs or lice are alive	Scalp: itching; swollen lymph nodes; can often see nits or lice in hair Pubic: itching; swollen glands	Kwell lotion or shampoo
Giardiasis	*Giardia lamblia,* a flagellate protozoan	Humans	5-25 days or longer (7-10 days average)	Ingestion of cysts in fecally contaminated water or food; person-to-person by hand-to-mouth transfer of cysts from feces	Entire period of infection	Chronic diarrhea, steatorrhea, abdominal cramps, bloating, frequent loose and pale greasy stools, fatigue, weight loss	Atabrine is drug of choice; metronidazole (Flagyl) is also effective; furazolidone pediatric suspension for young children and infants; enteric precautions should be used
Salmonellosis	Numerous serotypes of salmonella (bacterial); *S. typhimurium* is the most common	Humans and domestic and wild animals, including poultry, swine, cattle, rodents, and pets (e.g., dogs, cats, turtles, chickens)	6-72 hours (12-36 hours average)	Ingestion of organisms in food contaminated by feces; person-to-person by fecal-oral route	Entire period of infection, sometimes over 1 year; antibiotics can prolong this period	Acute enterocolitis, with sudden onset of headache, abdominal pain, diarrhea, nausea, and sometimes vomiting; dehydration; fever nearly always present; anorexia and loose bowels persist for days	Rehydration and electrolyte replacement with oral glucose-electrolyte solution; antibiotics (ampicillin or amoxicillin) for infants under 2 months, the elderly, and the debilitated, or patients with prolonged symptoms (antibiotics may prolong carrier state)

Continued

Common Communicable Diseases (cont'd)

Disease	Etiological Agent	Primary Reservoir	Incubation Period	Mode of Transmission	Period of Communicability	Symptoms	Treatment
Shigellosis	Shigella (Group A, *S. dysenteriae;* Group B, *S. flexneri;* Group C, *S. boydii;* Group D, *S. sonnei*); bacterial	Humans	1-7 days (1-3 days average)	Person-to-person by fecal-oral route	During acute infection and until infectious agent is no longer present (usually within 4 weeks)	Diarrhea accompanied by fever, nausea, and sometimes toxemia, vomiting, cramps, and tenesmus; blood, mucus, pus in stool	Fluid and electrolyte replacement; antimotility agents contraindicated; antibiotic therapy (e.g., ampicillin, tetracyclines), based on antibiogram of isolated strain, for patients with severe symptoms
Tuberculosis	*Mycobacterium tuberculosis* and *M. africanum* primarily from humans, and *M. bovis* primarily from cattle	Humans	From infection to demonstrable primary lesion 4-12 weeks; risk after infection may persist for a lifetime as a latent infection	Person-to-person (airborne droplet); ingestion of unpasteurized milk or dairy products	As long as sputum is positive for tubercular bacilli; children with primary tuberculosis are generally not infectious	Imperceptible onset of cough that progressively worsens and is associated with production of mucopurulent sputum Hemoptysis, chills, myalgia, sweating, anorexia, weight loss, or low-grade fever that persists over weeks to months may occur	Drug therapy with a combination of antimicrobial drugs (e.g., isoniazid, rifampin, and pyrazinamide) Rest/maintain adequate fluid and caloric intake
Impetigo	Bacteria (often *streptococci* or *staphylococci*)	Humans	Variable, but commonly 4-10 days	Person-to-person contact with lesions or secretions and mildly infectious through fomites	As long as purulent lesions continue	Draining, crusty skin lesions that may resemble ringworm or dry scales; often accompanied by fever, malaise, headache and loss of appetite	Antibiotics such as penicillin and erythromycin and antibiotic creams and lotions

Appendix 12-1

Commonly Acquired Sexually Transmitted Diseases

Disease	Usual Symptoms	Diagnosis	Possible Complications	Treatment	Special Considerations
GONORRHEA* (clap, dose, drip)					
Cause: *Neisseria gonorrhoeae* bacterium	Appear in 2-10 days or up to 30 days *Women:* 80% have no symptoms; may have puslike vaginal discharge; lower abdominal pain; painful urination *Men:* Thick, milky discharge from penis and/or painful urination; 10%-20% have no symptoms *Men and women:* Sore throat, pain and mucus when defecating; often no anal symptoms	*Women:* Culture from vagina, cervix, throat and/or rectum *Men:* Smear or culture from penis, rectum, and/or throat	*Women:* Pelvic inflammatory disease (10%-20% of cases) (see PID on the next page) *Men:* Narrowing of urethra; sterility; swelling of testicles *Men and women:* Arthritis, blood infections, dermatitis, meningitis, and endocarditis *Newborns:* Eye, nose, lung, and/or rectal infections	Ceftriazone plus doxycycline or tetracycline or spectinomycin Ceftriazone	3-10 days after treatment and again in 4-6 weeks a culture test should be done (to show cure)

Data from Venereal Disease Action Coalition: *Sexually transmitted diseases: a community information and resource guide*, Detroit, 1983, United Community Services of Metropolitan Detroit, pp. 9-11; Centers for Disease Control: 1989 sexually transmitted diseases treatment guidelines, *MMWR* 38(No. S-8):4-40, 1989; Centers for Disease Control and Prevention: 1993 sexually transmitted diseases treatment guidelines, *MMWR* 42(No. RR-14):3-59, 1993.

Symbols indicate that a particular STD may also be contracted in the following ways:

*Infants: while in birth canal of an infected mother.

†Increased risk through use of the intrauterine device (IUD) as a method of contraception.

‡Fluid from chancre coming in contact with cuts in the skin; infants: while in infected mother's womb.

§Sharing wet towels with an infected person.

‖Change in pH balance of vagina from pregnancy, diabetes, birth control pills, antibiotics, stress, douching.

¶Puncture of skin with contaminated needle; using toothbrush, razor, etc., of an infected person.

#May be spread by fingers from one hairy area to another; or by sharing linen or clothing of an infected person.

**Close physical contact (sexual or nonsexual).

Continued

Commonly Acquired Sexually Transmitted Diseases (cont'd)

Disease	Usual Symptoms	Diagnosis	Possible Complications	Treatment	Special Considerations
NONGONOCOCCAL URETHRITIS/CERVICITIS* (NGU, NGC)					
Common cause: *Chlamydia trachomatis* Other causes: *Ureaplasma urealtyticum; Trichomonas vaginalis; Candida albicans* and *herpes simplex virus*	Appear in 1-3 weeks *Women* (NGC): Usually have no symptoms; may have frequent uncomfortable urination; vaginal discharge *Men* (NGU): Mild to moderate discomfort on urination; thin, clear, or white morning discharge from penis	*Women:* No highly definitive diagnostic tool is currently available for chlamydial infection; culture (to rule out gonorrhea) and a vaginal smear (to rule out trichomonas and yeast) *Men:* Culture (to rule out gonorrhea) and a smear	*Women:* Pelvic inflammatory disease (see PID below), cervical dysplasia (currently under study), ectopic pregnancy, and infertility *Men:* Prostatitis, epididymitis *Newborns:* Eye infections, pneumonia	Doxycycline or azithromycin (erythromycin for pregnant women)	
PELVIC INFLAMMATORY DISEASE (PID)[†]					
Affects only women Usual causes: *Neisseria gonorrhoeae; Chlamydia trachomatis;* enteric bacteria	Onset of symptoms varies; abnormal vaginal discharge; severe pain and tenderness in lower abdominal/pelvic area; painful intercourse and/or menstruation; irregular bleeding; chills and fever; nausea, vomiting	History, culture, and examination to rule out other problems (ectopic pregnancy, appendicitis, etc.); pelvic ultrasound; laparoscopy	Sterility; chronic abdominal pain; chronic infection (of the fallopian tubes, uterus and/or ovaries); ectopic pregnancy, death	*Inpatient:* Cefoxitin IV in combination with doxycycline or clindamycin and gentamicin IV *Ambulatory:* Cefoxitin IM in combination with ceftiaxone and doxycycline or tetracycline; bedrest and no sex for at least 2 weeks	Usually the result of untreated gonorrhea or chlamydial infection Scarring of fallopian tubes may increase risk of future ectopic pregnancies IUD, if present, should be removed and replaced by another form of birth control Careful medical follow-up is essential
HUMAN PAPILLOMA VIRUS INFECTION/CONDYLOMATA ACUMINATA (HPV, genital/venereal warts)					
Cause: Human papilloma virus	Appear in 1-6 months; firm, flesh-colored or grayish-white warts on vulva, anus, lower vagina, penis, scrotum, mouth, throat; lesions on cervix usually not visible to the naked eye; itching	Clinical examination and Pap smear of colposcopy for lesions on cervix	Blockage of vaginal, rectal, or throat openings; cervical dysplasia; cancer (currently under study)	Cryotherapy with liquid nitrogen or cryoprobe; podophyllin benzoin (contraindicated in pregnancy) or trichloroacetic acid; electrocautery	Warts and invisible lesions are highly contagious; both will continue to multiply until completely removed

HERPES, GENITAL OR ORAL (cold sores; fever blisters on mouth)					
Causes: herpes simplex virus I (HSV I; oral); herpes simplex virus II (HSV II; genital)	May occur immediately or as late as 1 year after contact or not at all; some people exhibit few or no symptoms Itching, tingling sensation followed by painful blister-like lesions that appear in clusters at the site of infection (i.e., lips, nose, inner and outer vaginal lips, clitoris, rectum, thighs, buttocks); blisters dry up and disappear generally leaving no scar tissue HSV II symptoms in women may include increased vaginal discharge, painful intercourse and urination; painless lesions on cervix may go undected *Primary episodes:* HSV II—some experience fever, body aches, flulike symptoms, swollen lymph nodes near infected areas *Recurrent episodes:* HSV I and HSV II—generally lessen in frequency and severity over time	Culture from sore, clinical examination or Tzanck smear Definitive diagnosis only possible when lesions are present	*Oral:* Autoinoculation to skin or eyes *Genital:* Possible increased risk of cervical cancer; disturbance of bladder or bowel functioning (neuralgia); meningitis (nonfatal) *Newborns:* Blindness, brain damage, and/or death to baby passing through birth canal of mother with active lesions	No known cure at present The following may be helpful in reducing symptoms and/or recurrences: oral acyclovir; stress reduction techniques (yoga, meditation, etc.); keeping sores dry/clean; healthy diet and exercise; inpatient therapy in severe cases: acyclovir IV	HSV I can be found genitally and HSV II can be found orally due to oral-genital sex or autoinoculation Recurrent attacks are unpredictable but often appear at times of high stress, when fatigued, after vigorous intercourse, around menstruation, at times of other illnesses, etc. Research is inconclusive regarding whether herpes is occasionally contagious when there are no active lesions Many experience difficult, but not insurmountable, adjustments in self-image and sexual behavior *Women:* Should have Pap smears twice yearly and if pregnant, inform their health care provider (of their herpes); cesarean delivery is indicated if mother has active lesions at the time of delivery; *cervical lesions may go undetected because they are not painful*

Continued

Commonly Acquired Sexually Transmitted Diseases (cont'd)

Disease	Usual Symptoms	Diagnosis	Possible Complications	Treatment	Special Considerations
SYPHILIS[#] (syph, lues, pox, bad blood)					
Cause: *Treponema pallidum* (spirochete bacterium)	First stage—(appears in 10-90 days, average 3 weeks): painless sores (chancres) where bacteria entered body (genitals, rectum, lips, breasts, etc.) Second stage—(1 week to 6 months after stage 1): rash; flulike symptoms; mouth sores; genital/anal sores (condylomata lata); inflamed eyes; patchy balding Latent stage—(10-20 years after stage 2): None Final stage—See possible complications	Blood test; clinical examination	*Adult:* Blindness, deafness (usually reversible); brain damage; paralysis, heart disease, death *Newborns:* Damage to skin, bones, eyes, teeth, and/or liver; death	Penicillin (tetracycline or doxycycline for penicillin-allergic patients; doxycycline used in nonpregnant patients only)	Many women will not notice chancre because it is painless and may be deep inside vagina Complications can be prevented if treated at 1st or 2nd stage Return for blood test 1 month after treatment and once every 3 months for 1 year
VULVOVAGINITIS					
Causes: *Trichomonas vaginalis* (protozoa)[§]; *Candida albicans* (fungus)[‖]; *Gardnerella/Haemophilus vaginalis* (bacteria)	A. *Trichomoniasis* (Trich, TV, A, B, C Vaginitis) appear in 1-6 weeks *Women:* Thin, foamy yellow-green or gray vaginal discharge with foul odor; burning, redness, itching and/or frequent urination	*Women:* Vaginal smear; microscopic identification; urinalysis; culture (to rule out gonorrhea); clinical examination *Men:* Hard to diagnose	A. None	A. Metronidazole (Flagyl)	A. All partners should be treated even if they have no symptoms Cautions about Flagyl: very high doses have been shown to cause cancer in laboratory animals Should not be taken by pregnant or breast-feeding women

VULVOVAGINITIS—cont'd					
	Men: Usually no symptoms. May have slight, clear morning discharge from penis; itching after urination				Alcohol should be avoided when taking Flagyl because it may cause severe headaches and nausea
	B. Candida infections (yeast, monilia); onset of symptoms varies *Women:* Thick, white, cottage cheese–like, foul-smelling discharge that adheres to the vaginal walls; intense itching and irritation of genitals *Men:* usually no symptoms; dermatitis on penis		B. *Newborns:* Mouth and throat infections	B. Miconazole nitrate, clotrimazole, butaconazole, or teraconazole intravaginally	A, B, and C. Recurrent infections are common and can be prevented: tub bathing during menstruation, loose clothing and cotton panties; also avoid use of bubble bath, deodorant tampons, scented soaps, vaginal sprays, and douches (because these may irritate the vagina and/or change the pH balance)
	C. *Gardnerella infections;* onset of symptoms varies *Women:* Thin, foul-smelling, yellow-gray discharage; may have some vaginal burning		C. None	C. Metronidazole (Flagyl) or clindamycin (effective in 50%-60% of cases)	
HEPATITIS B Cause: hepatitis B virus	Appear in 1-6 months, but often no clear symptoms	Blood tests; clinical examination	Chronic hepatitis; chronic acute hepatitis; cirrhosis; liver cancer; death	Bed rest; lots of fluids; a light, healthy diet and no alcohol; no specific drug therapy	Often confused with flu or a bad cold and thus not treated early Recovery usually 2-3 months

Continued

Commonly Acquired Sexually Transmitted Diseases (cont'd)

Disease	Usual Symptoms	Diagnosis	Possible Complications	Treatment	Special Considerations
HEPATITIS B—cont'd	General flulike symptoms; liver deterioration marked by darkened urine, lightened stool, yellowed eyes and skin, skin eruptions, enlarged and tender liver				Will not recur once cured Hepatitis B vaccine will provide immunity
PEDICULOSIS PUBIS# (crabs, cooties, lice) Cause: *Phthirus pubis* (crab louse)	Appear in 4-5 weeks Intense itching in hairy areas (usually begins in pubic hair)	Clinical examination; self-examination may reveal blood spots on underwear, eggs or nits	None	Lindane (Kwell) cream, lotion, or shampoo (not recommended for pregnant or breast-feeding women); pyrethrins and piperonyl butoxide applications	Common soap will not kill crabs All clothes and linen must be washed in hot water or dry-cleaned or removed from human contact for 1-2 weeks
SCABIES** (the itch) Cause: *Sarcoptes scabiei* (parasite mite)	Appear in 4-6 weeks Severe itching and raised reddish tracts; may appear anywhere on body and are caused by the mite burrowing under the skin	Clinical examination; microscopic observation	Secondary bacterial infection (from scratching)	Lindane (Kwell) cream, lotion, or shampoo (not recommended for pregnant or breast-feeding women) or crotamiton (Eurox) cream or lotion	Common soap will not kill the mites Alll clothing and linen must be washed in hot water or dry-cleaned or removed from human contact for 1-2 weeks

Appendix 13-1

Community Assessment Guide

Community ____________________ Date ____________________

CHECK (✓) APPROPRIATE COLUMN*	STRENGTH	POTENTIAL NEED	PROBLEM	DESCRIPTION/COMMENTS
I. *People* A. Vital and demographic statistics 1. Population density				
2. Population composition a. Sex ratio				
b. Age distribution				
c. Race distribution				
d. Ethnic origin				
3. Population characteristics a. Mobility				
b. Socioeconomic status				
c. Level of unemployment				
d. Educational level				
e. Marriage rate				
f. Divorce rate				
g. Dependency ratio				
h. Fertility rate				
i. Head of household				
4. Mortality characteristics a. Crude death rate				
b. Infant mortality rate				
c. Maternal mortality rate				
d. Age-specific death rate				
e. Leading causes of death				
5. Morbidity characteristics a. Incidence rate (specific diseases)				
b. Prevalence rate (specific diseases)				
B. History of community (e.g., founding, cultural groups)				
C. Values, attitudes, and norms				

*Place check in only one column—strength, potential need, or problem.

Note: The material presented in Chapters 3, 4, 5, 11, 13, and 14 and the cultural assessment tool in Chapter 7 are especially helpful to the nurse when using this assessment tool. The nurse initially collects available data and then adds to this assessment on an ongoing basis.

Continued

Community Assessment Guide (cont'd)

CHECK (✓) APPROPRIATE COLUMN	STRENGTH	POTENTIAL NEED	PROBLEM	DESCRIPTION/COMMENTS
D. Individual and family living practices 1. Types of families				
2. Number of children per family				
3. Leisure activities				
II. *Environmental* A. Physical 1. Natural resources				
2. Geography, climate, terrain				
3. Roads/transportation				
4. Boundaries				
5. Housing (types available by percent, condition, percent rented, percent owned)				
6. Other major structures				
B. Biological and chemical 1. Water supply				
2. Air (color, odor, particulates)				
3. Food supply (sources, preparation)				
4. Pollutants, toxic substances, animal reservoirs or vectors				
5. Flora and fauna				
6. Is this a predominantly urban, suburban, or rural community? (How is land used?)				
III. *Systems* A. Health 1. Preventive health care practices and facilities (list)				
2. Treatment health care facilities (e.g., acute care, medical, and surgical hospitals) (list)				
3. Rehabilitation health care facilities (e.g., alcoholism) (list)				
4. Long-term health care facilities (e.g., nursing homes) (list)				

Community Assessment Guide (cont'd)

CHECK (✓) APPROPRIATE COLUMN	STRENGTH	POTENTIAL NEED	PROBLEM	DESCRIPTION/COMMENTS
A. Health—cont'd 5. Respite care services for special population groups (list)				
6. Hospice care services (list)				
7. Catastrophic health care facilities and services (list)				
8. Special health services for population groups (what and how provided) a. Preschool				
b. School age				
c. Adult or young adult				
d. Occupational health				
e. Adults and children with disabling conditions				
9. Voluntary health care resources				
10. Sanitation services				
11. Health work force (population ratios)				
12. Health education activities				
13. Methods of health care financing (approximate percent) a. Private pay				
b. Health insurance				
c. HMO				
d. Medicaid/Medicare				
e. Worker's Compensation				
f. Uninsured				
g. Underinsured				
14. Prevalent diseases and conditions (list)				
15. Linkages with other systems				
16. Health care resource overall availability				
17. Health care resource overall use				

Continued

Community Assessment Guide (cont'd)

Check (✓) Appropriate Column	Strength	Potential Need	Problem	Description/Comments
B. Welfare 1. Official (public) welfare resources a. General (list; e.g., Department of Social Services)				
b. Safety and protection (list; e.g., fire department)				
2. Voluntary welfare resources (list)				
3. Transportation resources (public and private)				
4. Facilities to meet needs (e.g., shopping areas, public housing)				
5. Special services for population groups (list)				
6. Resource accessibility				
7. Resource use				
C. Education 1. Public educational facilities (list)				
2. Private educational facilities (list)				
3. Libraries (list)				
4. Educational services for special populations a. Pregnant teens				
b. Adults				
c. Developmentally disabled children and adults				
d. Other				
5. Resource accessibility				
6. Resource use				
D. Economic 1. Major industry and business (list)				
2. Banks, savings and loans, credit unions (list)				
3. Major occupations (list)				
4. General socioeconomic status of population				

Community Assessment Guide (cont'd)

CHECK (✓) APPROPRIATE COLUMN	STRENGTH	POTENTIAL NEED	PROBLEM	DESCRIPTION/COMMENTS
D. Economic—cont'd 5. Median income				
6. Percentage of population below poverty level				
7. Percentage of population who are retired				
E. Government and leadership 1. Elected official leadership (list with title)				
2. Nonofficial leadership (list with title affiliations)				
3. City offices (location, hours, services)				
4. Accessibility to constituents				
5. Support of community resources				
F. Recreation 1. Public facilities (list)				
2. Private facilities (list)				
3. Recreational activities frequently used (list)				
4. Leisure activities frequently used (list)				
5. Coordination with educational recreation facilities and programs				
6. Programs for special population groups a. Elderly				
b. People who are disabled				
c. Others				
7. Resource accessibility				
8. Resource use				
G. Religion 1. Facilities by denomination (list)				
2. Religious leaders (list)				
3. Community programs and services				

Continued

Community Assessment Guide (cont'd)

CHECK (✓) APPROPRIATE COLUMN	STRENGTH	POTENTIAL NEED	PROBLEM	DESCRIPTION/COMMENTS
G. Religion—cont'd 4. Resource accessibility				
5. Resource use				
IV. *Community dynamics* (describe) A. Communication (diagram and describe) 1. Vertical (community to larger society)				
2. Horizontal (community to itself)				
3. Specific resources (e.g., television, radio, newspapers)				
V. *Major sources of community data* A. Government (list, e.g., local health department, city planning office)				
B. Private (list, e.g., chamber of commerce; key informants)				

QUESTIONS FOR THE COMMUNITY HEALTH NURSE

1. In general, are resources readily available and accessible?
2. What does the community see as its major strengths and needs?
3. How self-sufficient is the community in meeting its perceived needs?
4. What does the community health nurse see as the community's major strengths and needs?
5. How does the community's health status indicators compare to state and national indicators?
6. Are there established health coalitions to address community needs?
7. Health care
   a. How does the community view and use the health care system? (Specify cultural barriers.)
   b. What does the community see as its health care needs?
   c. What are the goals and major activities of the health system?
   d. How self-sufficient is the community in meeting its health needs?

Community Assessment Guide (cont'd)

COMMUNITY HEALTH CARE GOALS AND ACTIVITIES TO IMPLEMENT THEM

DATE	GOALS	ACTIVITIES TO IMPLEMENT

Assessor ____________________ Date __________
Assessor ____________________ Date __________
Assessor ____________________ Date __________

Appendix 13-2

Ongoing National Health Data Collection Systems and Health Surveys

System/Survey	Purpose	Lead Agency
DATA COLLECTION SYSTEMS		
National Vital Statistics System	Collect and publish data on births, deaths, marriages, and divorces in the United States	National Center for Health Statistics
National Notifiable Diseases Surveillance System	Provide weekly provisional information on the occurrence of notifiable diseases	Epidemiology Office of CDC
AIDS surveillance	Epidemiologic surveillance of AIDS	National Center for Infectious Diseases
Abortion surveillance	Epidemiologic surveillance of abortions	National Center for Chronic Disease Prevention and Health Promotion
National Traumatic Occupational Fatalities Surveillance System	Monitor occupational fatalities	National Institute for Occupational Safety and Health
Estimates of National Health Expenditures	Compile annually estimates of health expenditures by type of expenditure and source of funding	Office of the Actuary, Health Care Financing Administration
Surveillance, Epidemiology, and End Results Program	Provide data on all residents diagnosed with cancer during the year and current follow-up information on all previously diagnosed patients	Eleven population-based registries throughout the nation and Puerto Rico under contract of the National Cancer Institute
Behavioral Risk Factor Surveillance System	Monitor key health risk behaviors (e.g., alcohol use, smoking behaviors, and AIDS attitude and knowledge awareness) in the U.S. population	State health departments in cooperation with CDC
HEALTH SURVEYS		
National Survey of Family Growth	Provide national data on the demographic and social factors associated with childbearing, adoption, and maternal and child health	National Center for Health Statistics
National Health Interview Survey	Identify annually changes in illnesses, injuries, impairments, chronic conditions, and utilization of health resources	National Center for Health Statistics

From National Center for Health Statistics: *Health, United States, 1994*, Hyattsville, Md., 1995, U.S. Government Printing Office, pp. 259-277; Rafferty AP, McGee HB, Skarupski KA: *Results from Michigan's Behavioral Risk Factor Survey*, Lansing, Mi., 1995, Michigan Department of Public Health, pp. v-vi.

Ongoing National Health Data Collection Systems and Health Surveys (cont'd)

System/Survey	Purpose	Lead Agency
HEALTH SURVEYS—cont'd		
National Health and Nutrition Examination Survey	Estimate through health interviews and examination the national prevalence and reasons for secular trends of select diseases and risk factors and contribute to an epidemiologic understanding of these diseases (e.g., cardiovascular, respiratory, arthritis, hearing, and diabetes)	National Center for Health Statistics
National Home and Hospice Care Survey	Provide annual information about the demographic and health characteristics of home health and hospice patients and characteristics of agencies serving these patients	National Center for Health Statistics
National Household Surveys on Drug Abuse	Monitor trends in use of marijuana, cigarettes, alcohol, and cocaine among persons 12 years of age and older	Substance Abuse and Mental Health Services Administration
Monitoring the Future Study	Epidemiological annual survey of drug use and related attitudes among college and high school seniors and 8th- and 10th-graders	University of Michigan's Institute for Social Research under contract of the National Institute of Drug Abuse
Annual Survey of Occupational Injuries and Illnesses	Collect annual statistics on occupational injuries and illnesses	Bureau of Labor Statistics of Department of Labor

Appendix 15-1

Child Preventive Care Timeline

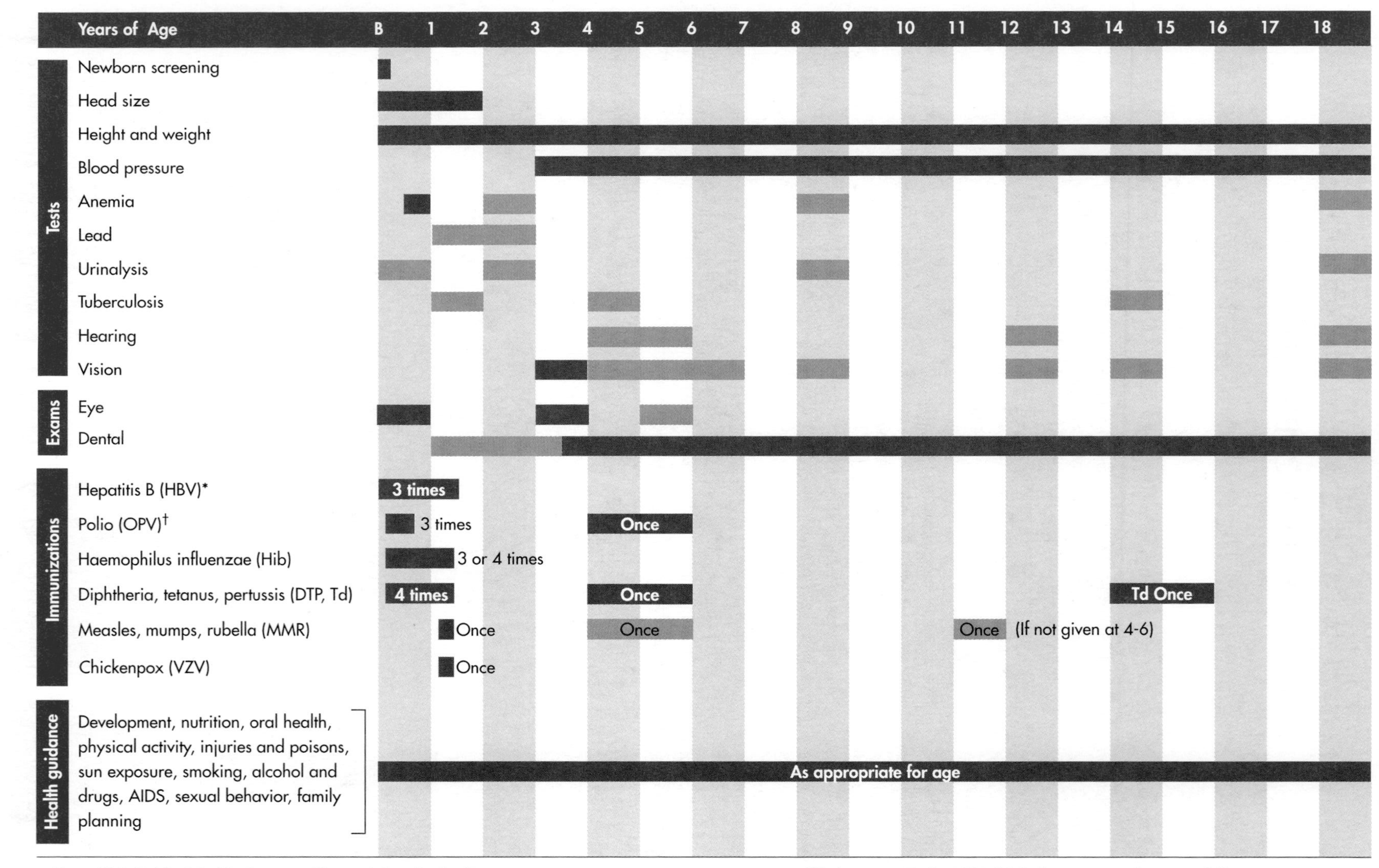

From U.S. Public Health Service: *Clinician's handbook of preventive services: put prevention into practice*, Washington, D.C., 1994, U.S. Government Printing Office, p. xviii.

Key: Recommended by all major authorities. Recommended by some major authorities.

Please note: Children with special risk factors may need more frequent and additional types of preventive care.

Some examples: RISK FACTORS		PREVENTIVE SERVICE(S) NEEDED	
Exposure to TB.	Sexually active.	TB test	AIDS test, hepatitis immunization
	High risk sexual behavior.	Pap test (females): syphilis, gonorrhea, chlamydia tests	AIDS, TB tests, hepatitis immunization
	Drug abuse.		

*See Figure 15-13 for the latest recommended childhood immunization schedule. Immunization schedules are changed on an ongoing basis.

†Two poliovirus vaccines are currently licensed in the U.S.: inactivated poliovirus vaccine (IPV) and oral poliovirus vaccine (OPV). The Advisory Committee on Immunization Practice (ACIP) routinely recommends IPV at 2 and 4 mos; OPV at 12-18 mos and 4-6 yr. IPV is the only poliovirus vaccine recommended for immunocompromised persons and their household contacts.

Appendix 15-2

Guide to Contraindications and Precautions to Vaccinations*

TRUE CONTRAINDICATIONS AND PRECAUTIONS	NOT TRUE (VACCINES MAY BE ADMINISTERED)
GENERAL FOR ALL VACCINES (DTP/DTaP, OPV, IPV, MMR, Hib, HBV)	
CONTRAINDICATIONS	
Anaphylactic reaction to a vaccine contraindicates further doses of that vaccine	Mild to moderate local reaction (soreness, redness, swelling) following a dose of an injectable antigen
Anaphylactic reaction to a vaccine constituent contraindicates the use of vaccines containing that substance	Mild acute illness with or without low-grade fever
Moderate or severe illnesses with or without a fever	Current antimicrobial therapy
	Convalescent phase of illnesses
	Prematurity (same dosage and indications as for normal, full-term infants)
	Recent exposure to an infectious disease
	History of penicillin or other nonspecific allergies or family history of such allergies

From Centers for Disease Control and Prevention (CDC): Standards for pediatric immunization practice, MMWR 42(No RR-5):12-13, 1993.

Continued

DTP = Diphtheria-tetanus toxoid and pertussis vaccine
DTaP = Diphtheria and tetanus toxoids and acellular pertussis vaccine
OPV = Oral poliovirus vaccine
IPV = Inactivated poliovirus vaccine
MMR = Measles-mumps-rubella vaccine
Hib = *Haemophilus influenzae* type b vaccine
HBV = Hepatitis B vaccine

*This information is based on the recommendations of the Advisory Committee on Immunization Practices (ACIP) and those of the Committee on Infectious Diseases (Red Book Committee) of the American Academy of Pediatrics (AAP) as of October 1992. Sometimes these recommendations vary from those contained in the manufacturer's package inserts. For more detailed information, providers should consult the published recommendations of the ACIP, AAP, American Association of Family Practice Physicians, and the manufacturer's package inserts.

†The events or conditions listed as precautions, although not contraindications, should be carefully reviewed. The benefits and risks of administering a specific vaccine to an individual under the circumstances should be considered. If the risks are believed to outweigh the benefits, the vaccination should be withheld; if the benefits are believed to outweigh the risks (for example, during an outbreak or foreign travel), the vaccination should be administered. Whether and when to administer DTP to children with proven or suspected underlying neurologic disorders should be decided on an individual basis. It is prudent on theoretical grounds to avoid vaccinating pregnant women. However, if immediate protection against poliomyelitis is needed, OPV, not IPV, is recommended.

‡For children with a personal or family (siblings or parents) history of convulsions, acetaminophen should be considered before DTP is administered and thereafter every 4 hours for 24 hours.

§There is a theoretical risk that the administration of multiple live-virus vaccines (OPV and MMR) within 30 days of one another if not administered on the same day will result in a suboptimal immune response. There are no data to substantiate this lack of response.

‖Persons with a history of anaphylactic reactions following egg ingestion should be vaccinated only with extreme caution. Protocols that have been developed for vaccinating such persons should be consulted (*J Pediatr* 1983, 102:196-9; *J Pediatr* 1988; 113:504–6).

¶Measles vaccination may temporarily suppress tuberculin reactivity. If testing cannot be done the day of MMR vaccination, the test should be postponed for 4-6 weeks.

Guide to Contraindications and Precautions to Vaccinations (cont'd)

True Contraindications and Precautions	Not True (Vaccines May Be Administered)
DTP/DTaP	
CONTRAINDICATIONS Encephalopathy within 7 days of administration of previous dose of DTP **PRECAUTIONS**[†] Fever of ≥40.5°C (105°F) within 48 hrs after vaccination with a prior dose of DTP Collapse or shocklike state (hypotonic-hyporesponsive episode) within 48 hrs of receiving a prior dose of DTP Seizures within 3 days of receiving a prior dose of DTP[‡] Persistent, inconsolable crying lasting ≥3 hrs within 48 hrs of receiving a prior dose of DTP	Temperature of <40.5°C (105°F) following a previous dose of DTP Family history of convulsions[§] Family history of sudden infant death syndrome Family history of an adverse event following DTP administration
OPV[§]	
CONTRAINDICATIONS Infection with HIV or a household contact with HIV Known altered immunodeficiency (hematologic and solid tumors; congenital immunodeficiency; and long-term immunosuppressive therapy) Immunodeficient household contact **PRECAUTION**[†] Pregnancy	Breast-feeding Current antimicrobial therapy Diarrhea
IPV	
CONTRAINDICATION Anaphylactic reaction to neomycin or streptomycin **PRECAUTION**[†] Pregnancy	
MMR[§]	
CONTRAINDICATIONS Anaphylactic reactions to egg ingestion and to neomycin[‖] Pregnancy Known altered immunodeficiency (hematologic and solid tumors; congenital immunodeficiency; and long-term immunosuppressive therapy) **PRECAUTION**[†] Recent (within 3 months) immune globulin administration	Tuberculosis or positive skin test Simultaneous TB skin testing[¶] Breast-feeding Pregnancy of mother of recipient Immunodeficient family member or household contact Infection with HIV Nonanaphylactic reactions to eggs or neomycin
Hib	
None identified	
HBV	
None identified	Pregnancy

Appendix 15-3

Accident Prevention at Various Age Levels

Typical Accidents	Normal Behavior Characteristics	Precautions
FIRST YEAR		
Falls Inhalation of foreign objects Poisoning Burns Drowning	After several months of age can squirm and roll, and later creeps and pulls self erect Places anything and everything in mouth Helpless in water	Do not leave alone on tables, etc., from where falls can occur Keep crib sides up Keep small objects and harmful substances out of reach Use infant car seat Have syrup of ipecac at home
SECOND YEAR		
Falls Drowning Motor vehicles Ingestion of poisonous substances Burns	Able to roam about in erect posture Goes up and down stairs Has great curiosity Puts almost everything in mouth Helpless in water	Keep screens in windows Place gate at top of stairs Cover unused electrical outlets; keep electric cords out of easy reach Keep in enclosed space when outdoors; when not in company of an adult Keep medicines, househood poisons, and small sharp objects out of sight Keep handles of pots and pans on stove out of reach and containers of hot food from edge of table Protect from water in tub and in pools Use safety belts and car seats
2-4 YEARS		
Falls Drowning Motor vehicles Ingestion of poisonous substances Burns	Able to open doors Runs and climbs Can ride tricycle Investigates closets and drawers Plays with mechanical gadgets Can throw ball and other objects	Keep doors locked when there is danger of falls Place screen or guards in windows Teach about watching for automobiles in driveways and in streets Keep firearms locked up Keep knives, electrical equipment out of reach Teach about risks of throwing sharp objects and about danger of following balls into street Use safety belts and car seats
5-9 YEARS		
Motor vehicles Bicycle accidents Drowning Burns Firearms	Daring and adventurous Control over large muscles more advanced than control over small muscles Has increasing interest in group play; loyalty to group makes child willing to follow suggestions of leaders	Use seat belts Teach techniques and traffic rules for cycling Encourage skills in swimming Keep firearms locked up except when you can supervise their use

Modified from Vaughn VC, McKay RJ, Behrman RE, eds, and Nelson WE, senior ed: *Textbook of pediatrics*, ed 11, Philadelphia, 1979, Saunders, p. 264. Modified from Shaffer TC: *Pediatr Clin North Am* 1:426-427, May 1954.

Appendix 16-1

Clinical Manifestations of Potential Child Maltreatment

PHYSICAL NEGLECT

Suggestive Physical Findings

Failure to thrive

Signs of malnutrition, such as thin extremities, abdominal distention, lack of subcutaneous fat

Poor personal hygiene, especially of teeth

Unclean and/or inappropriate dress

Evidence of poor health care, such as nonimmunized status, untreated infections, frequent colds

Frequent injuries from lack of supervision

Suggestive Behaviors

Dull and inactive; excessively passive or sleepy

Self-stimulatory behaviors, such as finger-sucking or rocking

Begging or stealing food
Absenteeism from school
Drug or alcohol addiction
Vandalism or shoplifting
} in older child

EMOTIONAL ABUSE AND NEGLECT

Suggestive Physical Findings

Failure to thrive

Feeding disorders, such as rumination

Enuresis

Sleep disorders

Suggestive Behaviors

Self-stimulatory behaviors, such as biting, rocking, sucking

During infancy, lack of social smile and stranger anxiety

Withdrawal

Unusual fearfulness

Antisocial behavior, such as destructiveness, stealing, cruelty

Extremes of behavior, such as overcompliant and passive or aggressive and demanding

Lags in emotional and intellectual development, especially language

Suicide attempts

PHYSICAL ABUSE

Suggestive Physical Findings

Bruises and welts
- On face, lips, mouth, back, buttocks, thighs, or areas of torso
- Regular patterns descriptive of object used, such as belt buckle, hand, wire hanger, chain, wooden spoon, squeeze or pinch marks
- May be present in various stages of healing

Burns
- On soles of feet, palms of hands, back, or buttocks
- Patterns descriptive of object used, such as round cigar or cigarette burns, "glovelike" sharply demarcated areas from immersion in scalding water, rope burns on wrists or ankles from being bound, burns in the shape of an iron, radiator, or electric stove burner
- Absence of "splash" marks and presence of symmetric burns
- Stun gun injury—lesions circular, fairly uniform (up to 0.5 cm), and paired about 5 cm apart (Frechette and Rimsza, 1992).

Fractures and dislocations
- Skull, nose, or facial structures
- Injury may denote type of abuse, such as spiral fracture or dislocation from twisting of an extremity or whiplash from shaking the child
- Multiple new or old fractures in various stages of healing

Lacerations and abrasions
- On backs of arms, legs, torso, face, or external genitalia
- Unusual symptoms, such as abdominal swelling, pain, and vomiting from punching
- Descriptive marks such as from human bites or pulling the hair out

Chemical
- Unexplained repeated poisoning, especially drug overdose
- Unexplained sudden illness, such as hypoglycemia from insulin administration

From Wong DL: *Whaley and Wong's nursing care of infants and children*, ed 5, St. Louis, 1995, Mosby, p. 704. Source: Frechette A, Rimsza ME: Stun gun injury: a new presentation of the battered child syndrome, *Pediatrics* 89(5):898-901, 1992.

Clinical Manifestations of Potential Child Maltreatment (cont'd)

PHYSICAL ABUSE—cont'd

Suggestive Behaviors

Wary of physical contact with adults
Apparent fear of parents or going home
Lying very still while surveying environment
Inappropriate reaction to injury, such as failure to cry from pain
Lack of reaction to frightening events
Apprehensive when hearing other children cry
Indiscriminate friendliness and displays of affection
Superficial relationships
Acting-out behavior, such as aggression, to seek attention
Withdrawal behavior

SEXUAL ABUSE

Suggestive Physical Findings

Bruises, bleeding, lacerations or irritation of external genitalia, anus, mouth, or throat
Torn, stained, or bloody underclothing
Pain on urination or pain, swelling, and itching of genital area
Penile discharge
Sexually transmitted disease, nonspecific vaginitis, or venereal warts
Difficulty in walking or sitting
Unusal odor in the genital area
Recurrent urinary tract infections
Presence of sperm
Pregnancy in young adolescent

Suggestive Behaviors

Sudden emergence of sexually related problems, including excessive or public masturbation, age-inappropriate sexual play, promiscuity, or overtly seductive behavior
Withdrawn, excessive daydreaming
Preoccupied with fantasies, especially in play
Poor relationships with peers
Sudden changes, such as anxiety, loss or gain of weight, clinging behavior
In incestuous relationships, excessive anger at mother for not protecting daughter
Regressive behavior, such as bed-wetting or thumb-sucking
Sudden onset of phobias or fears, particularly fears of the dark, men, strangers, or particular settings or situations (e.g., undue fear of leaving the house or staying at the daycare center or the babysitter's house)
Running away from home
Substance abuse, particularly of alcohol or mood-elevating drugs
Profound and rapid personality changes, especially extreme depression, hostility, and aggression (often accompanied by social withdrawal)
Rapidly declining school performance
Suicidal attempts or ideation

Appendix 16-2

Middle Childhood Developmental Chart*

Health professionals should assess the achievements of the child and provide guidance to the family on anticipated tasks. The effects are demonstrated by health supervision outcomes.

Achievements During Middle Childhood	Tasks for the Child	Health Supervision Outcomes
Responsibility for good health habits	Maintain good eating habits	Sense of personal competence
Ability to play in groups	Practice good dental hygiene	Sense of self-efficacy and mastery
One or more close friendships	Participate in athletic or exercise programs	Active role in health supervision and promotion
Identification with peer groups	Maintain appropriate weight	Optimal nutrition
Competence as member of family, community, and other groups	Wear bicycle helmet, seat belt, and contact sports mouth guard	Satisfactory growth and development
Ability to express feelings	Avoid alcohol, tobacco, and other drugs	Good health habits
Belief in capacity for success	Resist peer pressure to engage in risk-taking behaviors	Injury prevention
Understanding of right and wrong	Control impulses	Personal safety
Awareness of safety rules	Resolve conflict and manage anger constructively	Social competence
Ability to read, write, and communicate increasingly complex and creative thoughts	Assume responsibility for belongings, chores, and good health habits	Promotion of developmental potential
Responsibility for homework	Play with and relate well to siblings and peers	Prevention of behavioral problems
School achievement	Communicate well with parents, teachers, and other adults	Promotion of family strengths
	Be industrious in school	Enhancement of parental effectiveness
		Success in school

From Green M, ed: *Bright futures: guidelines for health supervision of infants, children, and adolescents*, Arlington, Va., 1994, National Center for Education in Maternal and Child Health, p. 148.
*Middle childhood: 5-11 years

Appendix 16-3

Adolescence Developmental Chart*

Health professionals should assess the achievements of the adolescent and provide guidance to the family on anticipated tasks. The effects are demonstrated by health supervision outcomes.

Developmental Achievements	Tasks for the Adolescent	Health Supervision Outcomes
Responsibility for good health habits	Maintain good eating habits and dental hygiene	Self-efficacy and mastery
Somatic and sexual growth and development	Exercise regularly and maintain appropriate weight	Independence
Social and conflict resolution skills	Use seat belt and helmet	Active role in health supervision and promotion
Good peer relationships with the same and opposite sex	Avoid alcohol, tobacco, and other drugs	Optimal nutrition
Capacity for intimacy	Practice abstinence or safer sex	Satisfactory growth and development
Responsible sexual behavior and a sexual identity	Engage in safe and age-appropriate experimentation	Good health habits
Coping skills and strategies	Manage negative peer pressure	Reduction of high-risk behavior
Appropriate level of autonomy	Learn conflict resolution skills	Injury prevention
Personal value system	Protect self from physical, emotional, and sexual abuse	Promotion of developmental potential
Progression from concrete to formal operational thinking	Develop self-confidence, self-esteem, and own identity	Prevention of behavioral problems
Academic and career goals	Develop ability to interact with peers, siblings, and adults	Sense of responsibility and morality
Educational or vocational competence	Continue process of separating from family	Promotion of family strengths
	Develop sense of responsibility for others	Enhancement of parental effectiveness
	Be responsible for school performance	Educational/vocational success
	Development good oral and written language skills	

From Green M, ed: *Bright futures: guidelines for health supervision of infants, children, and adolescents*, Arlington, Va., 1994, National Center for Education in Maternal and Child Health, p. 20.

*Adolescence: 11-21 years

Appendix 17-1

Adult Preventive Care Timeline

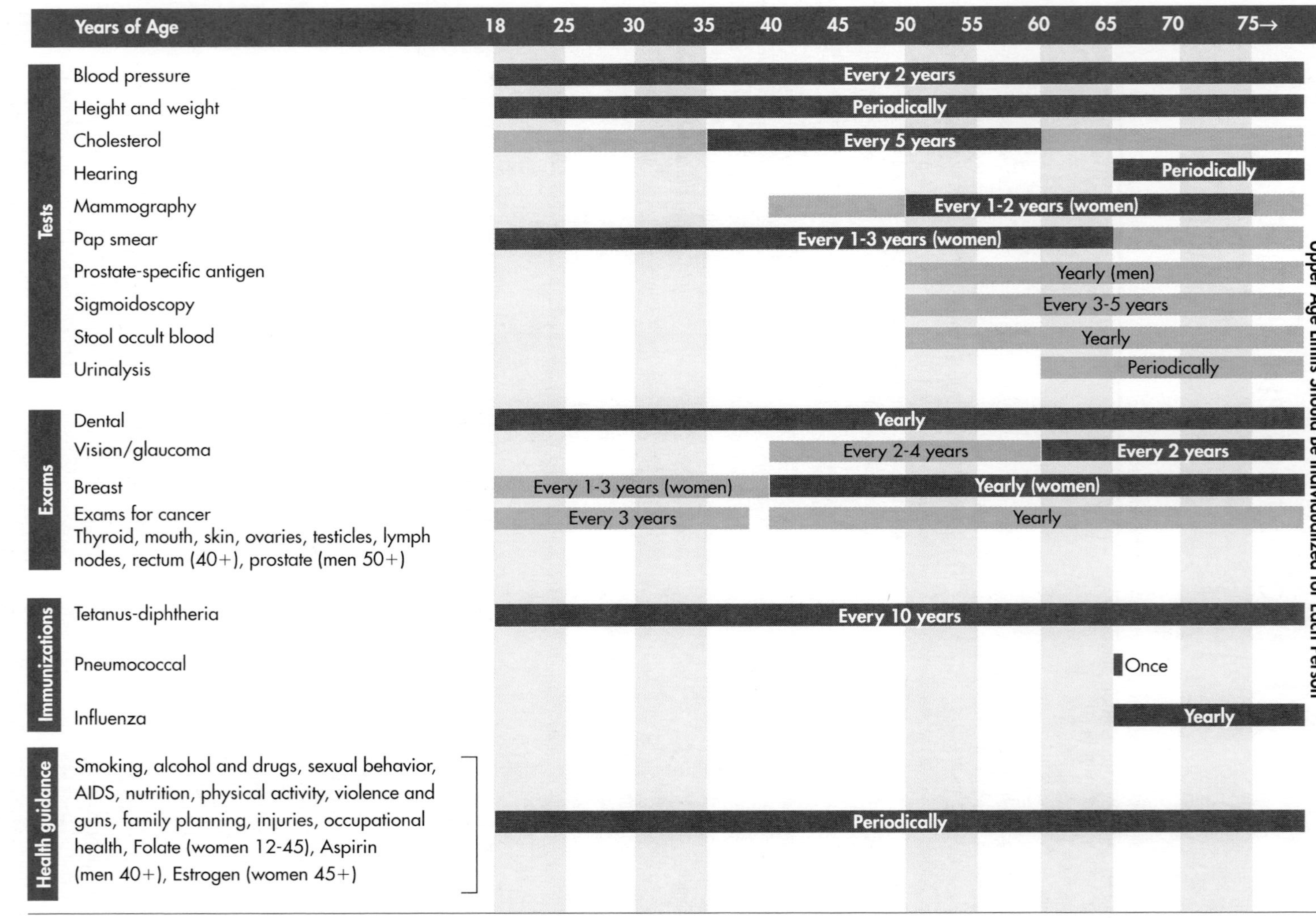

Years of Age
18
25
30
35
40
45
50
55
60
65
70
75→
Tests
Blood pressure
Every 2 years
Height and weight
Periodically
Cholesterol
Every 5 years
Hearing
Periodically
Mammography
Every 1-2 years (women)
Pap smear
Every 1-3 years (women)
Prostate-specific antigen
Yearly (men)
Sigmoidoscopy
Every 3-5 years
Stool occult blood
Yearly
Urinalysis
Periodically
Exams
Dental
Yearly
Vision/glaucoma
Every 2-4 years
Every 2 years
Breast
Every 1-3 years (women)
Yearly (women)
Exams for cancer
Thyroid, mouth, skin, ovaries, testicles, lymph nodes, rectum (40+), prostate (men 50+)
Every 3 years
Yearly
Immunizations
Tetanus-diphtheria
Every 10 years
Pneumococcal
Once
Influenza
Yearly
Health guidance
Smoking, alcohol and drugs, sexual behavior, AIDS, nutrition, physical activity, violence and guns, family planning, injuries, occupational health, Folate (women 12-45), Aspirin (men 40+), Estrogen (women 45+)
Periodically
Upper Age Limits Should Be Individualized for Each Person
Key:
Recommended by all major authorities.
Recommended by some major authorities.

From U.S. Public Health Service: *Clinician's handbook of preventive services: put prevention into practice*, Washington, D.C., 1994, U.S. Government Printing Office, p. xix.

Appendix 18-1

Assessment Guide for Nursing in Industry

1. Community in which industry is located	1. Just as industry affects the community, so the community affects industry.
a. Description of the community	a. Use three or four key descriptive words.
1. Size in area and population	1. How far do the employees travel to work and are the workers neighbors?
2. Climate, altitude, rainfall	2. Are there times or seasons that are more hazardous than others?
3. Pollution (noise, radiation, etc.)	3. Can the workers' dermatitis or hearing loss be attributed to the community or is it work related?
4. Housing	4. Is there adequate, safe housing in the area? Must the worker spend too great a percentage of his or her salary on housing?
5. Transportation	5. Is there safe, adequate transportation to work as well as to a hospital or school?
6. Schools	6. Do children have to be bused to school or attend overcrowded classes?
7. Sanitation	7. Are roaches and rats common to the area?
8. Protection: fire, police, etc.	8. Are the workers and the industry protected?
9. Trends	9. Is the area becoming more urban? Residential? Rundown? Deserted?
b. Population	b. How alike or different is the population of the industry from that of the community?
1. Age distribution	1. Are the families of child-rearing age or of retirement age?
2. Sex distribution	2. Are there more men or more women?
3. Ethnic and religious composition	3. Are there certain customs or languages that are predominant in the community?
4. Socioeconomic characteristics	4. What is the level of education of the community? What is the mean community income?
c. Health information	c. Is it an ill or well community?
1. Vital statistics	1. What is the infant mortality rate, birth rate, average life expectancy? Usually the local health department has this information.
2. *Disease incidence and prevalence*	2. *What are the leading causes of morbidity and mortality?*
3. *Health facilities available*	3. *What physical facilities and professional services are available?*
4. Community resources	4. Are there day-care centers, drug rehabilitation facilities, Alcoholics Anonymous groups, etc.?
2. The company	2. The official name and address of the company.
a. Historical development	a. Get a perspective on how, why, and by whom the company was founded and compare it with the present situation.
b. Organizational chart	b. What is the formal order of the system and to whom will the nurse be responsible?
c. *Policies*	c. *If there is a policy manual, try to obtain a copy. Are the workers aware of the manual?*
1. Length of the work week	1. How many days a week does the industry operate?
2. Length of work time	2. Are there several shifts? Breaks? Is there paid vacation?

From Serafini P: Nursing assessment in industry, *Am J Public Health* 66(8):755-760, 1976. (Author's name is now P. Serafini Blanco.)

Continued

Assessment Guide for Nursing in Industry (cont'd)

2. The company—cont'd	
c. *Policies*—cont'd	
3. *Sick leave*	3. Is there a clear policy, and do the workers know it?
4. *Safety and fire provisions*	4. Is management aware of situations or substances in the plant which represent danger? Are there organized fire drills? *The Federal Register* is the source of information for federal standards and serves as a helpful guide.
d. Support services (benefits)	d. What is the attitude of management concerning worker benefits?
1. Insurance programs	1. *Is there a system for health insurance and life insurance, and is it compulsory?* Does the company pay all or part? *Who fills out the necessary forms?*
2. Retirement program	2. Are the benefits realistic?
3. Educational support	3. Can the worker further his or her education? Will the company help financially?
4. Safety committee	4. The programmed Red Cross First Aid course is excellent. For information consult your Red Cross. *If there is no committee, do certain people routinely handle emergencies?*
5. Recreation committee	5. Do the workers have any communication with or interest in each other outside the work setting?
e. Relations between worker and management	e. This is difficult information to get, but it is important to know how each perceives the other.
f. Projection for the future	f. If the company is growing, workers may see themselves as having a secure future; if not, they may be worried about their job security. How will plant expansion affect the need for nursing services?
3. The plant	3. Draw a small map to scale, labeling the areas. When an accident occurs, place a pin in the exact location on your map. Different-color pinheads can be used for keeping statistics.
a. General physical setting	a. What is the gross appearance?
1. The construction	1. What is the size and general condition of buildings and grounds?
2. Parking facilities and public transportation stops	2. How far does the worker have to walk to get inside?
3. Entrances and exits	3. How many people must use them? How accessible are they?
4. Physical environment	4. Comment on heating, air conditioning, lighting glare, drafts, etc.
5. Communication facilities	5. Are there bulletin boards, newsletters?
6. Housekeeping	6. Is the physical setting maintained adequately?
7. Interior decoration	7. Are the surroundings conducive to work? Are they pleasing?
b. The work areas	b. Get permission to examine them. Use *The Federal Register* as a guide.
1. Space	1. Are workers isolated or crowded?
2. Heights: workplace and supply areas	2. *Falls and falling objects are dangerous and costly to industry.*
3. Stimulation	3. Is the worker too bored to pay attention?
4. Safety signs and markings	4. Is danger well marked?
5. Standing and sitting facilities	5. Are chairs safe and comfortable? Are there platforms to stand on, especially for wet processes?

Assessment Guide for Nursing in Industry (cont'd)

3. The plant—cont'd	
b. The work areas—cont'd	
6. Safety equipment	6. Do the workers make use of hard hats, safety glasses, face masks, radiation badges, etc.? Do they know the safety devices the OSHA regulations require?
c. Nonwork areas	c. Where are they located? Is there easy access?
1. Lockers	1. If the work is dirty, workers should be able to change clothes. Are they taking toxic substances home?
2. Hand-washing facilities	2. If facilities and supplies are available, do workers know how and when to wash their hands?
3. Rest rooms	3. How accessible are they and what condition are they in?
4. Drinking water	4. Can a worker leave the job long enough to get a drink of water when he or she wants to?
5. Recreation and rest facilities	5. Can a worker who is not feeling well lie down? Do workers feel free to use the facilities?
6. Telephones	6. Can a worker receive or make a call? Does a working mother have to stay home because she can't be reached at work?
7. Ashtrays	7. Are people allowed to smoke in designated areas? Is it safe?
4. The working population	4. Include worker and management, but separate data for comparison.
a. General characteristics	a. Be as accurate as possible, but estimate when necessary.
1. *Total number of employees*	1. Usually, if an industry has 500 or more employees, full-time nursing services are necessary.
2. General appearances	2. Heights, weights, cleanliness, etc.
3. *Age and sex distribution*	3. Certain screening programs are specific for young adults whereas others are more for the elderly. Some programs are more for women; others are more for men. Is there any difference between the day and evening shift? Are the problems of the minority sex unattended?
4. Race distribution	4. Does one race predominate? How does this compare with the general community?
5. Socioeconomic distribution	5. Great differences in worker salaries can sometimes cause problems.
6. Religious distribution	6. Does one religion predominate? Are religious holidays observed?
7. Ethnic distribution	7. Is there a language barrier?
8. Marital status	8. Widowed, single, divorced people often have different needs.
9. *Educational backgrounds*	9. *Can all teaching be done at approximately the same level?*
10. Life-styles practiced	10. Are certain life-styles frowned upon?
b. Type of employment offered	b. What percentage of the work force is blue-collar and what percentage is white-collar?
1. Background necessary	1. What educational level is required? Skilled vs. unskilled?
2. Work demands on physical condition	2. Strength needed: sedentary vs. active.
3. Work status	3. Part-time vs. full-time; overtime?

Continued

Assessment Guide for Nursing in Industry (cont'd)

4. The working population—cont'd	
c. Absenteeism	c. Is there a record kept? By whom? Why?
1. *Causes*	1. *What are the five most common reasons for absence?*
2. Length	2. Absenteeism is costly to the employer. There is some difference between one 10-day absence and ten 1-day absences by the same person.
d. Physically disabled	d. Does the company have a policy about hiring the disabled?
1. Number employed	1. Where do they work? What do they do?
2. *Extent of disabilities*	2. Are they specially trained? Are they in a special program? Do they use prosthetic devices?
e. Personnel on medication	e. Know what medication and where the employee works.
f. Personnel with chronic illness	f. At what stage of illness is the employee? Where does the employee work? Will he or she be able to continue at this job?
5. The industrial process	5. What does the company produce and how?
a. Equipment used	a. Portable vs. fixed; light vs. heavy.
1. General description of placement	1. Mark each piece of large equipment on the scale map.
2. Type of equipment	2. Fans, blowers, fast moving, wet or dry.
b. Nature of the operation	b. Get a brief description of each state of the process so that you can compare the needs and abilities of the workers with the needs of the job.
1. *Raw materials used*	1. *What are they and how dangerous are they? Are they properly stored?* Check *The Federal Register* for guidelines on storage.
2. Nature of the final product	2. Can the workers take pride in the final product or do they make parts?
3. Description of the jobs	3. Who does what? Where? Label the map.
4. Waste products produced	4. What is the system for waste disposal? Are the pollution control devices in place and functioning?
c. *Exposure to toxic substances*	c. *Describe the toxins to which the worker is exposed and the extent of exposure.* Include physical and emotional hazards. Remember that chronic effects of industrial exposure are subtle; a person often gets used to having mild symptoms and won't report them. *The Federal Register* contains specifications for exposure to toxins and some states issue state standards.
d. Faculties required throughout the industrial process	d. The need for speed, hearing, color vision, etc., can help determine the types of screening programs necessary.

Assessment Guide for Nursing in Industry (cont'd)

6. The health program	6. Outline what is actually in existence as well as what employees perceive to be in existence.
a. Existing polices	a. Are there informal, unwritten policies?
1. Objectives of the program	1. Are they clear?
2. *Preemployment physicals*	2. Are they required? Are they paid for by the company? Is the information used to deselect?
3. First-aid facilities	3. What is available? What is not available?
4. *Standard orders*	4. Is there a company physician who is responsible for first aid or emergency policy? If so, work closely with him or her in planning nursing services.
5. *Job descriptions for health personnel*	5. If there are no guidelines to be followed, write some.
b. Existing facilities and resources	b. Sometimes an industry that denies having a health program has more of a system than it realizes.
1. Trained personnel	1. *Who responds in an emergency?*
2. Space	2. Where is the sick worker taken? Where is the emergency equipment kept?
3. *Supplies*	3. *Make a list and describe the condition* of each item.
4. *Records and reports*	4. What exists? The Occupational Safety and Health Act requires that employers keep three types of records: a log of occupational injuries and illnesses, a supplemental record of certain illnesses or injuries, and an annual summary (forms 100, 101, and 102 are provided under the act). Good records provide data for good planning.
c. *Services rendered in the past year*	c. Describe as specifically as possible.
1. Care needed	1. Chronic or acute? Why?
2. Screening done	2. Where? By whom? Why?
3. Referrals made	3. By whom? To whom? Why?
4. Counseling done	4. Often informal counseling goes unnoticed.
5. Health education	5. What individual or group education was offered by the company?
d. *Accidents in the past year*	d. Including those occurring after work hours, as some of these accidents may be directly or indirectly work related.
e. *Reasons employees sought health care*	e. List the five major reasons.

Appendix 19-1

Legislation and Voluntary Efforts for the Disabled: United States

1798 U.S. Congress establishes a marine hospital to provide for disabled seamen (England had established such a facility in 1588).

1902 Goodwill Industries is originated by a minister, Dr. Edgar Helms, to provide employment opportunities for people who are disabled.

1918 Federal Board of Vocational Rehabilitation established to provide vocational rehabilitation services to the disabled veterans of World War I.

Massachusetts becomes the first state to establish public provisions to aid in the vocational rehabilitation of disabled citizens.

1920 The first Vocational Rehabilitation Act (Public Law 565) is passed. Services under the act were primarily for physically disabled military personnel. This act was administered by the Vocational Rehabilitation Administration.

1935 Social Security Act is passed, resulting in increased federal appropriations to states for vocational rehabilitation with direct relief provided for the disabled. Amendments to this act have provided for SSI, Disability Insurance, Medicare, and Medicaid.

1943 Amendments to the Vocational Rehabilitation Act of 1920 broaden vocational rehabilitation services to include facilitating a disabled person to engage in competitive employment and include such services as diagnosis, medical and surgical treatment, prescriptions, hospitalization, books, tools, and occupational equipment.

Baruch Committee on Physical Medicine is established by the son of Dr. Simon Baruch, a confederate army surgeon and pioneer in the field of physical medicine. The committee supports research and scholarship in physical medicine.

1944 The Public Health Act of 1944 (Public Law 78-410) provides for professional education, training, and research on many disabling conditions.

1945 Joseph Bulova School of Watchmaking establishes a training program in watchmaking for people who are disabled. Forerunner of many companies offering employment and training opportunities to the disabled.

1946 National Mental Health Act (Public Law 79-487) authorizes extensive federal support for mental health research, diagnosis, prevention, and treatment, establishing the National Institute of Mental Health and state grant-in-aid programs for mental health under the U.S. Public Health Service.

1947 The Department of Rehabilitation and Physical Medicine is started at New York University College of Medicine at Bellevue Hospital under the direction of Dr. Howard Rusk. The first comprehensive program in rehabilitation at Bellevue was made possible by a grant from the Baruch committee. This department served as a model for the development of rehabilitation centers all over the world.

1953 Establishment of the Department of Health, Education, and Welfare with the Office of Vocational Rehabilitation as a part.

1954 Federal provisions made to support training and education programs for professional rehabilitation personnel in the form of scholarships, stipends, research, and construction grants.

1956 Amendments to the Social Security Act give benefits to workers and their families during periods of extended disability.

The Mental Health Study Act (Public Law 84-812) authorizes grants to facilitate a program of research into resources and methods of care for the mentally ill. The act authorized grants for participation in a national study and reevaluation of the human and economic problems of mental illness.

1963 Mental Retardation Facilities and Community Mental Health Centers Construction Act of 1963 (Public Law 88-164) provides assistance in combating mental retardation through grants for construction of research centers and facilities for people who are mentally retarded. It provides assistance in improving mental health services through construction of community mental health centers.

1965 Amendments to the Vocational Rehabilitation Act of 1920 provide for increased flexibility in financing and administrating state rehabilitation programs and for assisting in the expansion and improvement of rehabilitation services financed by a state-federal payment sharing plan. The word *handicapped* was

Note: Laws that have had, or have the potential for having, major impact on the person who is disabled are indicated by an asterisk.

Legislation and Voluntary Efforts for the Disabled: United States (cont'd)

1965 (cont'd)
substituted for *physical disability*. The Federal Board of Vocational Education is established.

Medicaid and Medicare are established by federal law. Both programs provide essential health and health-related services for individuals who are disabled (see Chapter 4).

The Mental Retardation Facilities and Community Mental Health Centers Construction Act Amendments of 1965 (Public Law 89-105) authorize assistance in meeting the initial cost of professional and technical personnel for comprehensive community mental health centers.

1968 Architectural Barriers Act (Public Law 90-480) is passed. The act mandated that almost any public building constructed or leased by federal funds must be accessible to the physically disabled, and that all construction after 1968 using federal funds ensure building accessibility to disabled persons with no exceptions allowed. The act affected many educational settings and was enforced by the Architectural Barriers Compliance Board. However, the mandates of this law were ignored, and in 1978 Congress created a compliance board to enforce the law (Goldman, 1984).

1971 Developmental Disabilities Act* (Public Law 91-517) is passed. The act states that each state would receive federal funds to establish and maintain services that are required by developmentally disabled children and adults. These services include diagnosis, evaluation, treatment, personal care, special living arrangements, training, education, sheltered employment, recreation, counseling, protective and sociolegal services, information services, transportation services, and follow-up services.

Urban Mass Transportation Act (Public Law 91-453) is passed. The act states that special efforts would be made in federally funded mass transportation to include usage by persons who are disabled.

1973 Rehabilitation Act of 1973* (Public Law 91-453) is a landmark piece of legislation that replaced the 1920 act. It authorizes vocational rehabilitation services: emphasizes services to those with severe disabilities, expands the federal role in service and training programs, defines services necessary for rehabilitative programs, establishes the National Architectural and Transportation Barriers Board, and begins affirmative action programs to facilitate employment of the disabled. This act is the basis for rehabilitation services and programs.

Social Security Act of 1935 amendments eliminate previous categories of Aid to the Blind, Aid to the Aged (Old Age Assistance), and Aid to the Disabled under which direct financial assistance was given to people who were disabled. Supplemental Security Income is established as of January 1, 1974, under which the aged, blind, and disabled could qualify.

1974 Rehabilitation Act Amendments of 1974 (Public Law 93-576) authorizes the White House Conference on the Disabled.

Numerous transportation legislation including the following:

1. Amtrak Improvement Act (Public Law 93-140) stated that the Amtrak corporation must ensure that the disabled would not be denied transportation because of the disability. Provisions did not apply to commuter and short-haul service.
2. Federal Aid Highway Act (Public Law 93-87) stated that funding could not be approved for any state or federal highway not granting reasonable access for the movement of the physically disabled across curbs.
3. National Mass Transportation Act (Public Law 93-503) stated that mass transit funds could not be approved unless the rates charged persons who are disabled were reduced rates from regular fare.
4. Federal Bus Act (Public Law 93-37) stated that all federally funded projects to improve bus transportation must include plans to facilitate usage by people who are disabled.

1975 Developmental Disabilities Assistance and Bill of Rights Act* (Public Law 94-103) creates a system of advocacy on the state level to pursue legal and other actions necessary to eliminate the problems facing citizens with mental retardation, epilepsy, autism, and cerebral palsy and also expands the national effort to protect the rights of the developmentally disabled.

Education for All Handicapped Children Act (Public Law 94-142) passes. Enabled by September 1, 1980, a free, appropriate public education to all persons aged 3 to 21 years

Continued

Legislation and Voluntary Efforts for the Disabled: United States (cont'd)

1975 (cont'd)
old regardless of disabling condition involved. Recently the federal government has tried to deregulate the act, but proposed changes created such a furor among the disabled, their families, and advocates that the changes were withdrawn.

1977 Reorganization of the Department of Health, Education, and Welfare with creation of the Office of Human Development. The Administration for Handicapped Individuals (AHI) is under the Office of Human Development and oversees (1) Rehabilitation Services Administration, (2) President's Committee on Mental Retardation, (3) Architectural and Transportation Barriers Compliance Board, (4) White House Conference on Handicapped Individuals, (5) Developmental Disabilities Office, and (6) Office of Handicapped Individuals.

Federal Aviation Act of 1958 amends (Public Law 95-163) to provide special rates (reduced) on a space-available basis to persons with severe visual or hearing impairments and other physically or mentally disabled people as defined by the Civil Aeronautics Board, as well as any attendant required by such persons.

1978 Rehabilitation Act Amendments establish the Council on the Handicapped to function as a steering committee to make recommendations to the President concerning the needs of disabled individuals and establish the National Center for Rehabilitation Research.

1980 Mental Health Systems Act* (Public Law 96-398) gives the states more authority to plan community mental health centers, to increase the quality of mental health services, and to reach more people. Includes advocacy provisions and a Bill of Rights of Mental Health.

Civil Rights of Institutionalized Persons Act* (Public Law 96-247) authorizes actions for redress in cases involving deprivations of rights of institutionalized persons that were secured or protected by the Constitution of the United States. The act states that when an action has been commenced in any court of the United States seeking relief from conditions that deprive persons residing in such institutions of any rights, privileges, or immunities secured or protected by the Constitution or laws of the United States that causes them to suffer grievous harm, the Attorney General of the United States may intervene.

1982 Telecommunications for the Disabled Act (Public Law 97-140) amends the Communication Act of 1934 to provide that persons with impaired hearing are insured reasonable access to telephone service by requiring that all coin-operated telephones, telephones frequently used by hearing-impaired persons, and emergency telephones provide an internal means of coupling with hearing aids. Retrofitting could be required on coin-operated and emergency telephones.

The Surface Transportation Assistance Act (Public Law 97-424) encourages removal of architectural barriers.

1984 Rehabilitation Amendments (Public Law 98-221) modifies the definition of severely disabled and places the age limit for disability benefits at 16 years. Made the National Council on the Handicapped an agency independent from the Department of Education.

Developmental Disabilities Assistance and Bill of Rights Act (Public Law 98-527) formally establishes a Bill of Rights for the developmentally disabled.

1986 Protection and Advocacy for Mentally Ill Individuals Act of 1986* (Public Law 99-319) establishes protection and advo-

Legislation and Voluntary Efforts for the Disabled: United States (cont'd)

1986 (cont'd)

cacy services for individuals who are mentally ill. Restated the Bill of Rights for mental health patients. Promotes the establishment of family support groups for the families of people with Alzheimer's disease.

Education of the Deaf Act (Public Law 99-371) consolidates several free-standing statutes relating to federally supported educational institutions for the deaf into one effective piece of legislation.

Rehabilitation Amendments (Public Law 99--506) emphasize the rehabilitation needs of disabled Native Americans, provide funding for disability technology, and expand the influence of the National Council on the Handicapped.

Employment Opportunities for Disabled Americans Act (Public Law 99-643) amends the Social Security Act to improve employment opportunities for disabled Americans.

Air Carrier Access Act of 1986 greatly improves access to air transportation for people who are disabled.

1988 Numerous pieces of technology-related legislation including:

1. Hearing Aid Compatibility Act of 1988 (Public Law 100-394) requires telephones manufactured or imported into the United States after August 16, 1989 be hearing aid–compatible.
2. Technology-Related Assistance for Individuals with Disabilities Act of 1988 (Public Law 100-407) establishes a competitive grant program to enable participating states to develop and implement programs to promote technology-related assistance to individuals with disabilities.
3. Telecommunications Accessibility Act (Public Law 100-542) ensures that the federal telecommunication system is fully accessible to hearing-impaired persons who use telecommunications.

Protection and Advocacy for Mentally Ill Individuals Amendments Act of 1988 (Public Law 100-509) amends the 1986 act to reauthorize the act and to establish a governing authority for protection and advocacy in each state.

1990 The Americans with Disabilities Act* (Public Law 101-336) was passed. A landmark piece of legislation designed to provide a clear and comprehensive mandate to end discrimination against individuals with disabilities. It addresses such issues as housing, employment, public transportation, and communication services.

The 1975 Education for All Handicapped Children Act (Public Law 94-142) was renamed the Individuals with Disabilities Education Act (IDEA), (Public Law 101-476). Consistent with the Americans with Disabilities Act, Public Law 101-476 changed terminology (handicapped to disability) to reflect a more positive focus on individuals who have functional limitations.

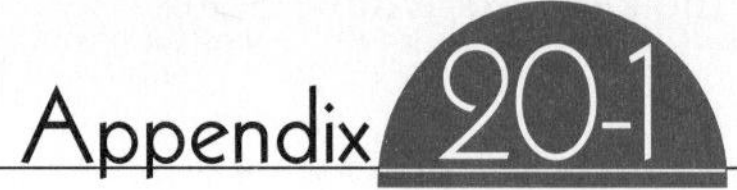

Seniors Substance Abuse Project

ASSESSMENT FORM

Name ______________________________ ID# __________

Occupation ______________________________

Language in the home ______________________________

Current living arrangements ______________________________

____

Number of children ______________________________

Significant others ______________________________

____

RELEASE OF INFORMATION

I, ____________________, agree to participate in a Seniors Substance Abuse Project conducted by the Kent County Health Department. I authorize Donna Spruit, R.N., from the Kent County Health Department to release information regarding my medication and health status to ______________________________

______________________________ (doctor or agency).

I also authorize ____________________ (doctor or agency) to give information regarding my medication and health status to Donna Spruit, R.N.

Recipients of substance abuse services have rights protected by State and Federal Law and promulgated rules. For information, contact Seniors Project Supervisor, Kent County Health Dept., 700 Fuller, N.E., GR, MI., 49503, 616-336-3040, or the Office of Substance Abuse Services, Recipient Rights Coordinator, P.O. Box 30035, 3500 North Logan, Lansing, MI 48909.

Client's signature ______________________________

Date ______________________________

Witness ______________________________

Relationship to Client ______________________________

Interviewer's name ______________________________ Date __________

Site of interview ______________________________

Seniors Substance Abuse Project (cont'd)

Seniors Project Questionnaire

ID# ______________

Date ______________

KNOWLEDGE OF MEDICATIONS

List each medication (including over-the-counter and home remedies) the client is taking in the left-hand column. In the center column, write down what the client says is the reason [for] taking this drug. Include how much and how often he [or she] claims to take each in the right column. Use the client's words if possible. It is important that the *client's perceptions* be recorded, not the interviewer's.

Name of Drug	*Reason for Taking*	*Amount and Frequency (with Meals/without Meals)*

Continued

Seniors Substance Abuse Project (cont'd)

SENIOR SUBSTANCE ABUSE QUESTIONNAIRE MEDICATION USE/MISUSE

Risk Factor Analysis *Date:* ________________ *ID#* ________________

Evaluate the status of risk factor and circle the number on the left which best describes the client's risk. 0 for not-at-all to 5 for very much a problem. On the right of each risk factor write in any comments which may help clarify the specific situation, e.g., "diet implications"—*special weight reduction 1500 cal. diet, lo Na lo chol.*; "side effects"—*C/O dry mouth, excessive tiredness;* "sensory deprivation"—*poor vision, cataracts both eyes.*

0 1 2 3 4 5 Cost ________________
0 1 2 3 4 5 Confusion ________________
0 1 2 3 4 5 Diet implications ________________
0 1 2 3 4 5 Difficulty opening safety closures ________________
0 1 2 3 4 5 Depression ________________
0 1 2 3 4 5 Drug intolerance ________________
0 1 2 3 4 5 Forgets to take medication ________________
0 1 2 3 4 5 Fear of taking medication ________________
0 1 2 3 4 5 Inappropriate storage:
____ temperature, humidity ________________
____ removal from original container ________________
____ medication stored at bedside ________________
0 1 2 3 4 5 Language barrier ________________
0 1 2 3 4 5 Lack of knowledge regarding meds ________________
0 1 2 3 4 5 Living alone ________________
0 1 2 3 4 5 Multiple prescriptions ________________
0 1 2 3 4 5 Multiple pharmacies ________________
0 1 2 3 4 5 Multiple physicians ________________
0 1 2 3 4 5 Physician hopping ________________
0 1 2 3 4 5 Outdated medications ________________
0 1 2 3 4 5 Over-the-counter use ________________
0 1 2 3 4 5 Reading disability ________________
0 1 2 3 4 5 Sensory deprivation ________________
0 1 2 3 4 5 Side effects ________________
0 1 2 3 4 5 Stopping medication ________________
0 1 2 3 4 5 Stretching medication ________________
0 1 2 3 4 5 Sharing medication ________________
0 1 2 3 4 5 Not following prescribed regimen ________________
0 1 2 3 4 5 Transportation difficulty ________________
0 1 2 3 4 5 Use of household remedies (e.g., baking soda) ________________
0 1 2 3 4 5 Mood-altering drugs ________________
0 1 2 3 4 5 Use of alcohol ________________
0 1 2 3 4 5 Other (list):
0 1 2 3 4 5 ________________
0 1 2 3 4 5 ________________
0 1 2 3 4 5 ________________
0 1 2 3 4 5 ________________

Total Risk Factor Score ________

Interviewer's Signature ________________

Seniors Substance Abuse Project (cont'd)

SENIORS SUBSTANCE ABUSE QUESTIONNAIRE GUIDE
RISK FACTOR ANALYSIS

Review each risk factor with client and determine applicability. Rate the risk factor from 0 (not applicable, no risk) to 5 (high risk), and circle the appropriate number. This analysis requires your professional judgment and is based upon your assessment of the client and his personal situation.

Cost

Clients may consider some of their medications to be very costly. If their income level is low and/or fixed, they may not be able to afford these medications. Determine their priority for expenses—medications may not be high priority, and therefore, the risk of omission is increased.

Confusion

Rate this according to how well oriented the client seems to be. Does he relate appropriately to time and place, etc.?

Diet Implications

Is the client on a special diet such as low sodium, low cholesterol, weight reduction, diabetic? Some medications contain sodium, i.e., Mylanta, Maalox. Some medications are to be taken on an empty stomach, while others are to be taken with meals. Milk is to be avoided with certain drugs. It is important to determine whether the client adheres to these recommendations.

Difficulty Opening Safety Closures

Patients with arthritis may have increased difficulty opening safety caps. They may omit a dose just because of the hassle or worse yet, they may transfer drugs to an unmarked container. (See inappropriate storage.) Determine how likely this risk is. Client may be unaware that easy-open caps are available from the pharmacy.

Depression

Is the client now depressed or does he have a history of depression? Because of the many losses suffered by the elderly, some degree of depression is fairly common. Depression may influence adherence to a medical regimen. Likewise, depression may be a side effect of some drugs.

Drug Intolerance or Allergy

History of intolerance or allergy would have implications for current drug use. It would be important that this information be readily available in case of emergency. Rate this risk according to the severity and likelihood of recurrence.

Forgets to Take Medication

Does the client state that he/she sometimes forgets to take medication? Determine how likely this is. This risk may go hand-in-hand with confusion, or it may stand alone. Not all persons who forget to take medication are confused. They may be overwhelmed by the number of medications they are to take or they may be distracted by other activities. Listen for key phrases like, "Don't know if I remembered." Client may be threatened or embarrassed to admit forgetfulness. Good, non-threatening interviewing will be helpful here.

Fear of Taking Medication

Some clients are reluctant to take drugs, even those that are prescribed. Determine if the client has any such reluctance. Some clients may be very open and verbal about this fear. Rate this risk according to how likely it is that the client would not take needed medication.

Inappropriate Storage

TEMPERATURE, HUMIDITY Medications are subject to deterioration in certain temperature extremes and high humidity. Storage in the bathroom is undesirable. Storage in the refrigerator is required for certain drugs and contraindicated for others. Check labels or check with pharmacist if necessary.

REMOVAL FROM ORIGINAL CONTAINERS Many clients are tempted to put all pills together in one container, especially when they travel. This is a very unsafe practice. All medications should remain in the original containers until needed. It is considered safe to place medications in special dispensers. These are best when divided by time of day they are to be taken. This helps the problem of forgetfulness. However, a list of what each drug is should be available nearby for emergency information, especially if traveling.

MEDICATION STORED AT BEDSIDE Although this may seem like a very convenient storage site, it runs the risk of error if the client should happen to take medications when not fully awake. Also, too easy access may make over-using certain medications more likely, such as pain medication or mood-altering drugs. Having to go to the storage site allows a more purposeful effort and hopefully a more accurate dosage.

LANGUAGE BARRIER Labels and directions written in a language not understood by a client could lead to misuse. Also, if the client does not understand verbal instructions given by the doctor or pharmacist, there is increased potential for misuse.

Continued

Seniors Substance Abuse Project (cont'd)

LACK OF KNOWLEDGE REGARDING MEDICATIONS See first part of Questionnaire, "Knowledge of Medications." How well does the client understand what the medications he/she is taking are for, how to take them, how much to take, and how often?

LIVING ALONE This may or may not be a risk factor, depending on how well the client has adapted to living alone. Living alone can be a problem if there is no support system to encourage the client to take good care of himself/herself. Motivation to comply with a medical regimen will be affected in some cases.

Multiple Prescriptions

The more medications the clients are taking, the more likely they are to have a problem with adverse drug interactions, side effects, inclusion about dosage and schedule, etc.

Multiple Pharmacies

Going to more than one pharmacy to have prescriptions filled is undesirable. The pharmacist may be unaware of other drugs being taken by the client and he/she will be hampered in his/her ability to do a drug profile and advise the client on possible incompatibility of certain drugs.

Multiple Physicians

Since the elderly tend to have a number of chronic illnesses, they frequently find themselves being treated by a number of specialists, e.g., internist, rheumatologist, cardiac specialist, gastroenterologist. This is sometimes unavoidable, and it is important that each physician be aware of what drugs the other has prescribed. The client has responsibility for conveying that information.

Physician Hopping

This is different from "multiple physicians." Here clients go from one doctor to another within a short span of time because they are not satisfied with their care. This can be a dangerous and fruitless practice and frequently results in multiple prescriptions for similar drugs, e.g., mood-altering drugs, antibiotics, pain medication. The client rarely informs the new doctor of his recent previous visits to other doctors. There are clients who have gotten three prescriptions for the same drug from three different doctors and ended up taking all three, and therefore, three times the desired dosage.

Outdated Medication

All drugs should be discarded once they are outdated. *Saving drugs* is a potentially dangerous practice because they can change in composition and may be harmful if used. Also their presence in the medicine chest could result in someone accidentally taking the old drug instead of the desired one. The risk factor can be most accurately evaluated by a home visit where the medicine chest can be viewed or by asking the client to bring all drugs to the next visit.

Over-the-Counter Use

Clients who regularly use over-the-counter drugs run the risk of drug interactions, especially if they are taking other prescription medication. Sometimes clients do not count over-the-counter drugs as "real" drugs. They do not realize that these drugs also have side effects and contraindications. The more over-the-counter drugs used by the client and the greater the frequency, the higher the risk rating they would receive from this risk factor.

Reading Disability (Comprehension)

This is not to be confused with the "language barrier" problem. What is considered here are perceptual difficulties that could be the result of a stroke (aphasia) or possibly a life-long condition. If a client is unable to read and understand the information on the label, it would signal a risk of misuse.

Sensory Deprivation

Visual, auditory, or other sensory-related problems that may influence the client's ability to follow directions or correctly self-administer medications, e.g., reduced vision or blindness, loss of feeling in fingertips, deafness.

Side Effects

Undesirable effects caused by the drug may influence a client to avoid taking a needed drug, e.g., disagreeable taste, dry mouth, dizziness, nausea, drowsiness, lingering bad taste in mouth, impotence.

Stopping Medication

When the client stops taking a prescribed drug before the desired therapeutic results are obtained, this is a medication misuse. This risk factor could occur as a result of unpleasant side effects, cost, emotional reasons, denial of illness, symptoms reduction (blood pressure medication, antibiotics), embarrassment.

Seniors Substance Abuse Project (cont'd)

Stretching Medication

The client tries to make the medication last longer by skipping doses or taking less than the prescribed dose. This is usually done for financial reasons or because the client desires to minimize the amount of drugs he/she is taking.

Sharing Medication

Usually a misplaced friendship gesture. The friend tells the client that this drug worked for him, "why doesn't he/she take one." A very dangerous practice.

Not Following Prescribed Regimen

This may or may not be a *deliberate* act on the part of the client. It could be the result of "confusion," "forgetfulness," or "stretching medication." Adjusting dosage schedules ad lib can be potentially hazardous depending upon the drug and its intended action.

Transportation Difficulty

This may not be a problem unless it results in not getting a prescripton filled or related effect such as not making a follow-up visit to the doctor, which might be a necessary component in monitoring a drug's effectiveness.

Use of Household Remedies

The use of such items as baking soda for upset stomach could be a problem if the client were on a low sodium diet and/or hypertensive, since baking soda is high in sodium.

The household remedy would need to be evaluated as to the contents, amount taken, and frequency.

Mood-Altering Drugs

This category of drug runs a risk of its own because of the nature of the drug and the condition it is intended to alleviate. These drugs may be habit forming. A depressed client may overdose himself.

Use of Alcohol

Some drugs interact or are increased by the use of alcohol. It would be important to determine how much and how often the client utilized alcohol. A history of alcohol abuse would be significant.

Asking the following questions developed by John A. Ewing, Director for the Center for Alcohol Studies at the University of North Carolina may be helpful:

1. Have you felt the need to cut down your drinking?
2. Have you ever felt annoyed by criticism of your drinking?
3. Have you had guilty feelings about drinking?
4. Do you ever take a morning eye-opener?

If two or three questions receive a positive response, the likelihood that the person is an alcoholic is high.

Add up the total risk factor score and place in the designated space. By looking over the form, you can determine which risk factors you can help eliminate or reduce through intervention. Write up a plan with the client. After six to eight weeks, readminister the tool and determine if the total risk factor score has been lowered.

Reproduced by permission of and modified from the Nursing Division, Kent County Health Department, Grand Rapids, MI; Wanda Bierman, RN, MS, Family Health Services Supervisor and Donna Spruit, RN, Geriatric Services, Principal Developers.

Appendix 20-2

The Older Americans Act of 1965: Significant Amendments and Changes

1967 *Older Americans Act; Amendments of 1967 (Public Law 90-42)*—Authorized studies to look at the availability and adequacy of training resources in gerontology and to evaluate present and future trends and needs for such personnel and programs. Resulted in increased funding and training in the field of gerontology. Placed new emphasis on providing services to seniors.

1969 *Older Americans Act; Amendments of 1969 (Public Law 91-69)*—Mandated increased state planning for act programs through state agencies on aging. Increased the emphasis on coordination with local programs and program evaluation. Authorized grants to states and communities for model projects on services to the elderly. Established the National Older Americans Volunteer Program (NOAVP). NOAVP's main purpose was to help retired persons avail themselves of opportunities for voluntary service in their communities and helped to subsidize this through provision of transportation, meals, and other necessary services needed for them to participate. Major components of NOAVP were: (1) *Retired Senior Volunteer Program (RSVP)* and (2) *Foster Grandparents.*

1972 *Older Americans Act; Amendments of 1972 (Public Law 92-258)*—Amended the act to provide grants to states for the establishment, maintenance, operation, and expansion of low-cost meal projects, nutrition training, and education, as well as opportunity for social contacts for the elderly. Established the Nutrition Program for the Elderly and brought the nutrition of the elderly into the national limelight. From this legislation sprang many senior nutrition services.

1973 *Older Americans Act; Comprehensive Amendments of 1973 (Public Law 93-29)*—Established the Federal Council on Aging and the National Information and Resources Clearinghouse for the Aging. Required that a sole state agency administer the provisions of the act in conjunction with local agencies on aging. Established Multipurpose Senior Centers and Older Readers Services. These multipurpose centers combined social, recreational, health, and nutrition aspects for seniors into one accessible program. These centers also placed a new and increasing emphasis on the social needs of seniors and attempted to decrease social isolation for seniors through a community-based program.

1974 *Older Americans Act; Amendments of 1974 (Public Law 93-351)*—Provided for increased funding for transportation for the elderly, especially transportation services that facilitated the elderly in using the nutrition programs and multipurpose centers already designated under the act. The transportation needs of the elderly living in rural areas were explored. This same year a separate presidential proclamation declared May to be Older Americans Month, and this tradition has been carried on by a presidential proclamation each year since.

1975 *Older Americans Act; Amendments of 1975 (Public Law 94-135)*—Established social services programs especially for seniors. A significant part of these amendments involved two separate acts: *Age Discrimination Act of 1975* and *Older Americans Community Service Employment Act of 1975.* Both of these acts carry the same public law number as the amendments and are incorporated into the amendments. The Age Discrimination Act prohibited discrimination on the basis of age, largely in relation to employment. The Community Service Employment Act section of the amendments provided for community service employment for seniors where they were eligible to receive a wage. Most employment programs under the act, before this time, had involved voluntary employment for seniors. These amendments also attempted to attract more qualified people into the field of gerontology through increased funding for training.

1978 *Comprehensive Older Americans Act; Amendments of 1978 (Public Law 95-478)*—The Amendments of 1978 were extensive and provided for improved and increased programs for older Americans. These amendments called for a great reduction in the paperwork necessary to run the program; increased planning, coordination, evaluation, and administration efforts; and facilitated the quality of programs. They also established the Advisory Council on Aging; provided for area agencies on aging to contract for legal services and to carry out demonstration projects on the legal services necessary for older Americans; provided for exploring alternative work modes for older Americans such as the Senior Environmental Protection Corps with the Environmental Protection Agency (EPA); provided for grants to Indian tribes for older American services to tribes members; set up a White House Conference on Aging for 1981 (there had previously been such

The Older Americans Act of 1965: Significant Amendments and Changes (cont'd)

1978 (cont'd)
conferences in 1961 and 1971); provided for a study of racial and ethnic discrimination in programs for older Americans; and outlined the programs of (1) *Congregate Nutrition Services* and (2) *Home Delivered Nutrition Services for the Elderly*. In addition, these amendments mandated development and implementation of national labor policy for the field of aging; discussed the concept of "preretirement" education and planning services; authorized special projects on long-term care and alternatives to institutionalization such as adult day care, supervised living in public or non-profit housing, family respite, preventive health services, home health and homemaker services, home maintenance programs, and geriatric health maintenance organizations; and authorized demonstration projects for community model programs to improve and expand social services, and nutrition services, and to promote the well-being of older Americans. High priority for placement of these demonstration projects was given to rural areas and rural agencies on aging.

1981 *Older Americans Act; Amendments of 1981 (Public Law 97-115)*—Emphasized the provision of nutritional programs in congregate settings and facilitated access to such programs. These amendments also encouraged the formation of university-affiliated and other multidisciplinary centers on aging as well as long-term care projects, and brought migrant and seasonal farm workers and organizations more in line with the provisions of the act.

1984 *Older Americans Act; Amendments of 1984 (Public Law 98-459)*—Often referred to as the Older Americans Personal Health Education and Training Act. Provided for a comprehensive array of community-based, long-term care services to appropriately sustain older people in their communities and homes. Authorized the designing of a uniform, standardized *program of health education and training* for older Americans with direct involvement of graduate educational institutions of public health in the design of such a program and direct involvement of graduate education institutions of public health, medical sciences, psychology, pharmacology, nursing, social work, health education, nutrition, and gerontology in the implementation of such a program. Planned for such education and training programs to be carried out in multipurpose senior centers as already provided for under the act.

1986 *Older Americans Act; Amendments of 1986 (Public Law 99-269)*—Amended the Older Americans Act to increase the federal contribution to senior nutrition programs covered under the act to about 57 cents per meal. Mandated that the Secretary of Agriculture and the Secretary of Health and Human Services jointly disseminate to state agencies, area agencies on aging, and providers of nutrition services covered under the act information concerning the existence of *all* federal commodity processing programs in which they would be eligible to participate, and the procedures necessary to participate in such programs.

1987 *Older Americans Act; Amendments of 1987 (Public Law 100-175)*—Often referred to as the Health Care Services in the Home Act of 1987. Established grants to states for *in-home health care services* for the frail elderly, for periodic *preventive health* services to be provided at senior centers or appropriate alternative sites, and to implement programs with respect to the prevention of abuse, neglect, and exploitation of the elderly. Authorized a 1991 White House Conference on Aging, and reauthorized the Act through fiscal year 1991. Required a direct reporting relationship between the Commissioner on Aging and the Secretary of Health and Human Services; added an outreach program on Supplemental Security Income, food stamps, and Medicaid benefits; increased funds for administration of area agencies on aging and community service employment projects; added a Demonstration Project Authority in areas of health education and promotion, volunteerism, and consumer protection from home care services; and added a program for grants to assist older Hawaiian natives.

1992 *Older Americans Act; Amendments of 1992 (Public Law 102-375)*—A four-year reauthorization of the Older Americans Act that established a study committee to look at the quality of home care services for older adults; established funding for in-school intergenerational activities where older adults could serve as tutors, teacher aides, living historians, speakers, playground supervisors, lunchroom assistants, and other roles; directed more services to minorities and rural elderly; placed increased emphasis on health promotion for the elderly; increased funding for senior nutrition programs and added supportive services for family caregivers of the frail elderly; and authorized a White House Conference on Aging before December 31, 1994.

Priorities in Community Health Nursing

PURPOSES

1. To identify target population groups requiring community health nursing service
2. To identify realistic spacing of nurse service contacts according to identified target population group
3. To use levels of prevention and health promotion in planning nursing service to a community

CODE

- *Classification I: intensive visiting* is defined as visits spaced daily to 3 times a week
- *Classification II: periodic visiting* is defined as visits spaced every 1 to 2 weeks
- *Classification III: widely spaced visiting* is defined as visits spaced every 2 to 3 months

	I. Intensive Visiting	II. Periodic Visiting	III. Widely Spaced Visiting
COMMUNICABLE DISEASE			
A. Tuberculosis (by law a priority)	To families who 1. Have young adults and unexamined contacts living in crowded home conditions with a client who has positive sputum 2. Have a recently diagnosed client with positive sputum 3. Have a diagnosed client with positive suptum, who is recalcitrant 4. Have a recently diagnosed client without positive sputum 5. Have a client who is immunosuppressed (AIDS, chronic illness, receiving chemotherapy)	To families who 1. Have the client with positive sputum hospitalized; have no young adults in the family; have good living standards but have some unexamined contacts 2. Need preparation for the hospital admission of the client 3. Need preparation for the discharge of the client	To families who 1. Have an arrested client returned to good home conditions 2. Have had all contacts examined and the client hospitalized under adequate medical supervision 3. Are under adequate medical supervision, with the source of infection located
B. Acute reportable dangerous communicable diseases	To families who 1. Have been contacts to reportable dangerous communicable disease 2. Have a diagnosed client needing home care 3. Have food handlers as a case/contact to *Salmonella*	To families who 1. Are unimmunized 2. Have a client under medical care but complications develop 3. Need follow-up for defects after recovery from acute stage	To families who 1. Are known to have immunization against communicable disease 2. Are receiving adequate medical care 3. Have a typhoid carrier in the home
C. Sexually transmissible diseases	To clients who 1. Need treatments and education on the prevention and spread of disease	To clients who 1. Need follow-up clinical examinations (for example, spinal taps)	

Modified from Rives R: Priorities according to needs, *Nurs Outlook* 6:404-408, 1958. Updated for the 3rd edition, by F. Armignacco, Director of Patient Services and Community Nursing, Monroe Co. Department of Health, Rochester, NY; updated for the 4th edition by L. Randar, RN, MPH, Director, Division of Nursing, Philadelphia Department of Health, Philadelphia, Penn. Updated for this edition by Joyce Kachelries, RN, BSN, Clinical Nursing Supervisor, Family Home Care, Hamilton, Ohio.

Priorities in Community Health Nursing (cont'd)

	I. Intensive Visiting	II. Periodic Visiting	III. Widely Spaced Visiting
C. Sexually transmissible diseases—cont'd	2. Have known contacts they will name 3. Need examination, advice on treatment, and education on how to arrest and prevent the transfer of infection 4. Need posttreatment observation 5. Need to be convinced of the necessity of the treatment ordered by the doctor 6. Need to be taught how to prevent further manifestations of the disease 7. Have babies born of mothers with active STD 8. To families who need instruction and assistance to care for a person with AIDS		
HOME CARE OF THE SICK			
A. Cardiovascular disease	To clients who 1. Have cardiac failure or have had an acute cardiac episode from any cause 2. Have a chronic cardiac disability requiring active treatment: medical, nursing, dietetic 3. Have had a CVA and require active treatment: medical, nursing, occupational, and physical therapy 4. Have cardiac surgery	To clients who 1. Have a congenital heart disease: nonoperable, postoperative 2. Have a murmur of undetermined origin with a history of rheumatic fever 3. Have congenital heart disease (to be followed until a thorough medical evaluation is completed) 4. Have diagnosed, untreated, uncontrolled hypertension	To clients who 1. Have a history of rheumatic fever, but no clinical heart disease 2. Are under medical care, stabilized for cardiovascular diagnoses
B. Diabetes	To clients who 1. Are newly diagnosed, not stabilized by diet or insulin 2. Cannot take own insulin (blind, aged, low mentality, and so forth) 3. Have difficulty understanding diet or administering their own insulin 4. Have uncontrolled diabetes	To clients who 1. Are newly diagnosed, administering own insulin but still needing supervision 2. Are suspected of having diabetes	To clients who 1. Are under medical care, stabilized as to diet or insulin, or both

Continued

Priorities in Community Health Nursing (cont'd)

	I. Intensive Visiting	II. Periodic Visiting	III. Widely Spaced Visiting
B. Diabetes—cont'd	5. Have diabetes with gangrene 6. Have diabetes complicated by an infection To caregivers who 1. Will be the persons maintaining the regimen of medications, diet, foot care, and daily assessments		
C. Kidney disease	To clients who 1. Are on dialysis 2. Have co-morbidities such as wound care 3. Need help with medications and diet and understanding disease	To clients who 1. Understand medications and diet but are not stabilized 2. Have other medical problems	To clients who 1. Are under medical care and are stabilized
D. Cancer	To clients who 1. Are discharged from a hospital and need active nursing care, instruction for themselves, and interpretation of their physical and emotional needs to the family 2. Have symptoms suspicious of cancer; need medical supervision, completion of all tests and examinations, and, if required, treatment on the earliest possible date 3. Are diagnosed but who, without consulting the physicians, have interrupted their treatment or discontinued having medical checkups 4. Are under observation for malignancy but delinquent from regular medical supervision (the urgency of a patient's problem can be determined only by the attending physician) 5. Have hospice/terminal care needs 6. Need complex, high-technology interventions such as TPN intravenous feedings, dobutamine IV, or pain control	To clients who 1. Have precancerous lesions and are delinquent for periodic checkups (cervical erosions, leukoplakias, keratoses, mastitis, and others) 2. Have cancer apparently treated successfully but are not reporting for medical reexamination (cancer of the skin with no apparent recurrence) 3. Have advanced disease and need care (some of these clients may need to be in intensive visiting classification) 4. Have families that have been taught to carry out medical orders but need support in continuing medical supervision	To clients about whom 1. Information is needed for statistical purposes (cured, deceased, or other)

Priorities in Community Health Nursing (cont'd)

	I. Intensive Visiting	II. Periodic Visiting	III. Widely Spaced Visiting
E. Other noncommunicable diseases, acute or chronic	To clients who 1. Are acutely ill and need nursing care 2. Are helpless or bedridden and need nursing service 3. Are senile and do not receive adequate home care 4. Are acutely ill or helpless but have families who can be taught how to give the necessary care 5. Are receiving terminal care	To clients who 1. Are acutely ill or helpless but whose families can provide care under nursing supervision 2. Need encouragement to continue medical care 3. Need emotional support to carry out health instructions	To clients who 1. Are under adequate medical supervision and are given good home care (by the family, a registered nurse, or a practical nurse)
HEALTH TEACHING AND SUPERVISION			
A. Maternity-antepartum	To women who 1. Are primiparas 2. Are under 17 or over 40 years of age 3. Are single parents 4. Are of low socioeconomic status 5. Are hypertensive 6. Have poor nutrition 7. Are not under medical care 8. Have had six or more pregnancies 9. Have had conditions associated with pregnancy resulting in infant deaths 10. Have had complications in past pregnancies or have signs of complications in the present pregnancy, including psychosomatic disturbances 11. Have a chronic disease, such as tuberculosis, diabetes, syphilis, anemia, nephritis, cardiac disease, or rheumatic fever 12. Have previously had premature deliveries 13. Are HIV-positive and/or drug abusers	To women who 1. Have adequate medical supervision for apparently normal pregnancies 2. Are in good physical and mental condition 3. Are able to follow advice 4. Have questions and desire help	(No antepartum clients in this category)

Continued

Priorities in Community Health Nursing (cont'd)

	I. Intensive Visiting	II. Periodic Visiting	III. Widely Spaced Visiting
B. Maternity-postpartum	To women who 1. Have nursing problems or breast complications, such as engorgement or abscess 2. Are not receiving adequate medical supervision or competent nursing care 3. Had complications or accidents of labor: stillbirths, abortions, or other difficulties resulting in a mishap to the mother or baby 4. Delivered prematurely 5. Had multiple births 6. Delivered a baby with a congenital defect 7. Had a baby that died during the first month of life 8. Evidence of poor maternal-infant bonding 9. Have no or few support systems 10. Are economically stressed (low socioeconomic status)	To women who 1. Had problems but are making normal progress 7 days after delivery 2. Have adequate medical supervision 3. Are coping but need guidance and support related to care of the baby, the family's adjustment, and socioeconomic variables	To women who 1. Are receiving good care and supervision 2. Are stabilizing in parenting skills and family adjustment
C. Infancy (higher priority is given to infants, regardless of whether they are firstborn, when they live in low economic districts where the mortality rate is highest)	To infants who 1. Are premature 2. Are newborn, especially if firstborn 3. Have difficulty in breastfeeding 4. Have consistently lost weight 5. Are being weaned 6. Have inadequate medical care 7. Have a reportable dangerous communicable disease 8. Have a physical disability resulting from a birth injury or a congenital defect—"high tech" babies such as those on respirators and who have been hospitalized at length 9. Need immunization 10. Are from substandard, poorly managed homes, or homes where there are problems of inadequate parenting 11. Are considered difficult babies by parents	To infants who 1. Are past the first month and are gaining weight slowly 2. Are not being fed properly 3. Have questionable physical and emotional delays	To infants who 1. Are receiving adequate medical supervision 2. Are receiving good home care

Priorities in Community Health Nursing (cont'd)

	I. Intensive Visiting	II. Periodic Visiting	III. Widely Spaced Visiting
C. Infancy—cont'd	12. Are born to drug abusers 13. Are born to mothers who are HIV-positive 14. Fail to thrive 15. Are low birth weight		
D. Preschool period	To children who 1. Have a reportable dangerous communicable disease 2. Have a physical defect 3. Need immunization 4. Need dental care 5. Have nutritional deficiencies 6. Are inconsistently disciplined 7. Are from homes where there is inadequate parenting 8. Are reported for suspected child abuse and neglect	To children who 1. Are insecure 2. Have lost weight 3. Lack medical supervision 4. Have poor health habits 5. Deviate from normal physical and emotional behavior	To children who 1. Have adequate medical supervision 2. Have good home care
E. School health	To children who 1. Have acute health problems a. Communicable diseases: immunization reactions or complications developing from acute communicable diseases b. Skin conditions: scabies, impetigo, ringworm, pediculosis c. Other: pregnancy, unexpected loss or gain of weight, abuse, neglect, diabetes, epilepsy 2. Have had an accident in school requiring hospitalization 3. Need immediate attention for defects discovered on physical examination: vision, hearing, cardiac, kidney, scoliosis, or other serious defects 4. Need follow-up of incidents indicating intense or serious emotional disturbance 5. Need follow-up as a contact of a diagnosed dangerous communicable disease 6. Have growth and other developmental delays	To children who 1. Need follow-up of allergies: hives, eczema, asthma 2. Have inadequate medical care 3. Have not had diagnosed defects corrected within a reasonable period of time 4. Are on medication for more than 3 weeks' duration during the school year 5. Need to be observed in relation to their growth pattern (those with structural scoliosis, those wearing braces, and so forth) 6. Need follow-up of minor defects: poor eating and health habits, poor dental and personal hygiene, foot and posture problems	To children who 1. Have a chronic health condition that is stabilized and under medical care 2. Have a congenital defect that does not require remedial work at the time

Continued

Priorities in Community Health Nursing (cont'd)

	I. Intensive Visiting	II. Periodic Visiting	III. Widely Spaced Visiting
F. Adult health	To clients who 1. Are in normative or nonnormative crisis 2. Are disorganized as a family and at risk for abuse and neglect of self, children, or spouse 3. Are homeless, in need of health and welfare services, but have not yet established contact with community resources 4. Have suspected dangerous communicable or chronic disease symptoms 5. Have no medical supervision for diagnosed physical, emotional, psychosocial problems 6. Are needing help adapting to chronic illness: heart disease, arthritis, multiple sclerosis, depression, etc.	To clients who 1. Are in crisis but have support systems 2. Recognize their disorganization and are working on ordering their lives 3. Are recently established in a home environment and are working with community resources 4. Have diagnosed disease and are receiving medical treatment; need help with referral to resources 5. Are needing help dealing with developmental tasks of parenting: sexuality and death education tasks of their children	To clients who 1. Have needed nursing care, are currently coping well, but are at risk for physical, emotional, and psychosocial problems
G. Health of aging people	To clients who 1. Have no medical supervision 2. Have symptoms of a dangerous communicable, nutritional, or chronic disease 3. Have a diagnosed disease and need help following the treatment plan 4. Have no support systems 5. Have evidence of normative or nonnormative maturational crisis especially in relation to: loss of income, loss of spouse, loss of friends 6. Have evidence of intentional or unintentional alcohol or drug abuse 7. Are unable to maintain an environmentally safe housing situation	To clients who 1. Have a diagnosed medical problem 2. Have a complex treatment regimen and are following it 3. Are able to live independently but need referral sources and support	To clients who 1. Are under medical supervision 2. Have readily available support systems

Index

G

I